CLINICAL LABORATORY SCIENCE: Strategies for Practice

with 76 Contributors

Associate Editors

Janet Duben-Von Laufen
MS, CLS, MT (ASCP)

Karen Karni
PhD, CLS

Marie Pezzlo
MA, MT (ASCP), SM (AAM)

Glenda D. Price
PhD, CLS

Virginia Sullivan Randolph
MA, CLS, MT (ASCP)

Sharon L. Zablotney
PhD, CLS

Medical Consultant

Dianne F. Johnson
MD, MT (ASCP)

J. B. Lippincott Company
PHILADELPHIA
London Mexico City New York St. Louis São Paulo Sydney

CLINICAL LABORATORY SCIENCE: Strategies For Practice

EDITED BY

Brenta G. Davis, *EdD, CLS, MT (ASCP)*
UNIVERSITY OF TENNESSEE, MEMPHIS
MEMPHIS, TENNESSEE

Michael L. Bishop, *MS, CLS, MT (ASCP)*
DUKE UNIVERSITY MEDICAL CENTER
DURHAM, NORTH CAROLINA

Diana Mass, *MA, CLS, MT (ASCP)*
ARIZONA STATE UNIVERSITY
TEMPE, ARIZONA

Acquisitions Editor: Lisa A. Biello
Sponsoring Editor: Richard Winters
Manuscript Editor: Lorraine D. Smith
Copy Editor: Mary Norris
Indexer: Ellen Murray
Interior Design: Rita Naughton
Cover Design: Donald Giordano
Production Manager: Kathleen P. Dunn
Design/Production Coordinator: Paul Fry
Compositor: Circle Graphics
Printer/Binder: R. R. Donnelley & Sons Company

6 5 4 3 2 1

Library of Congress Cataloging in Publication Data
Clinical laboratory science : strategies for practice / edited by Brenta G. Davis,
Michael L. Bishop, Diana Mass ; associate editors,
Janet Duben-Von Laufen . . . [et al.] ; 76 contributors.
p. cm.
Includes bibliographies and index.
ISBN 0-397-50860-3
1. Diagnosis, Laboratory. I. Davis, Brenta G. II. Bishop, Michael L.
III. Mass, Diana.
[DNLM: 1. Diagnosis, Laboratory. 2. Technology, Medical. QY 4 C6415]
RB37.C593 1989
616.07′5—dc19
DNLM/DLC
for Library of Congress 88-9050
CIP

The authors and publisher have exerted every effort to ensure that drug selection and dosage set forth in this text are in accord with current recommendations and practice at the time of publication. However, in view of ongoing research, changes in government regulations, and the constant flow of information relating to drug therapy and drug reactions, the reader is urged to check the package insert for each drug for any change in indications and dosage and for added warnings and precautions. This is particularly important when the recommended agent is a new or infrequently employed drug.

To my family and friends for their support, but especially for their unfailing good cheer.

Brenta G. Davis

To Sheila and Christopher for their patience, understanding, and support throughout this effort . . . and to my parents for preparing me for the challenges.

Michael L. Bishop

To my mother and father, Ella and Joseph Rotman, for their guidance, to my husband, Monty, for his encouragement, and to my daughter, Jacquelyn, for enriching our lives.

Diana Mass

Contributors

Associate Editors

JANET DUBEN–VON LAUFEN, MS, CLS, MT (ASCP)
Assistant Professor
Senior Education Coordinator
Program in Medical Technology/Cytogenetics
School of Allied Health Sciences
The University of Texas Health Science Center
Houston, Texas

KAREN KARNI, PhD, CLS
Director, Division of Medical Technology
Department of Laboratory Medicine and Pathology
University Hospital and Clinic
Minneapolis, Minnesota

MARIE PEZZLO, MA, MT (ASCP) SM (AAM)
Senior Supervisor
Medical Microbiology Division
University of California
Irvine Medical Center
Orange, California

GLENDA D. PRICE, PhD, CLS
Dean, School of Allied Health Professions
University of Connecticut
Storrs, Connecticut

VIRGINIA SULLIVAN RANDOLPH, MA, CLS, MT (ASCP)
Division Director, Associate Professor
Clinical Laboratory Sciences
School of Health Related Professions
University of Alabama at Birmingham
Birmingham, Alabama

SHARON L. ZABLOTNEY, PhD, CLS
Associate Dean
College of Natural Sciences
Professor of Medical Technology, Microbiology, and Pathology
Michigan State University
East Lansing, Michigan

Chapter Contributors

Joan E. Aldrich, MS
Assistant Professor
The University of Texas Southwestern Medical Center
Dallas, Texas

Holly Alexander, PhD
Clinical Microbiologist
Wesley Medical Center
Wichita, Kansas

Brian D. Andresen, PhD
Senior Scientist
Lawrence Livermore National Laboratory
Livermore, California

Benjamin J. Andrusaitis, MS, MT (ASCP)
Assistant Professor of Medical Technology
Fitchburg State College
Fitchburg, Massachusetts

Judith T. Barr, ScD
Associate Dean
College of Pharmacy and Allied Health Professions
Associate Professor
Medical Laboratory Science Program
Northeastern University
Boston, Massachusetts

Kathleen Becan–McBride, EdD, CLS, MT(ASCP)
Program Director and Professor
Program in Medical Technology/Cytogenetics
Professor, Division of Interdisciplinary Studies
School of Allied Health Sciences
Associate Professor, Department of Pathology and Laboratory Sciences
Associate Professor, Graduate School of Biomedical Sciences
The University of Texas Health Science Center
Texas Medical Center
Houston, Texas

Michael L. Bishop, MS, CLS, MT(ASCP)
Department of Hospital Laboratories
Duke University Medical Center
Durham, North Carolina

Michael Boroch, MBA, RRT
President, Health Network Associates
Houston, Texas

Peggy L. Bottjen, MS, MT(ASCP)
Assistant Supervisor
Clinical Laboratory
University of Nebraska Medical Center
Omaha, Nebraska

Linda H. Brooks, MS, MT(ASCP)
Director, Infection Control and Environmental Safety
American Hospital Association
Chicago, Illinois

Scot C. Buessow, PhD
Immunology Division
SmithKline Bio-science Laboratories
Van Nuys, California

JoLynne Campbell, DPH, MSPH
Assistant Professor of Medical Technology
College of Health Related Professions
Wichita State University
Wichita, Kansas

Louis B. Caruana, PhD, CLS, MT(ASCP)
Associate Professor
Department of Allied Health Sciences
Southwest Texas State University
San Marcos, Texas

V. Michelle Chenault, MA, CLS, MT(ASCP)
Assistant Professor and Field Coordinator
Winston-Salem State University
Winston-Salem, North Carolina

R. Lyle Christensen, PhD
Assistant Professor of Medical Technology and Pathology
Michigan State University
East Lansing, Michigan

Patricia Collins, MS, MT(ASCP) SM
Associate Professor of Medical Technology
University of Kentucky
Lexington, Kentucky

Suzanne W. Conner, MA, CLS/ClDir
Education Coordinator/Staff Development
Children's Hospital Medical Center
Akron, Ohio

Kozy M. Corsaut, MS, MT(ASCP)
Education Coordinator
Program of Medical Laboratory Technology
Allied Health Sciences
Stark Technical College
Canton, Ohio

Julia R. Crowley, EdD
Professor of Medical Technology
School of Allied Health Sciences
School of Graduate Studies
Medical College of Georgia
Augusta, Georgia

Brenta G. Davis, EdD, CLS, MT(ASCP)
Professor
Department of Clinical Laboratory Sciences
University of Tennessee, Memphis
Memphis, Tennessee

Catherine Conley Downs, MA, CLS, MT(ASCP)
Faculty Associate
Clinical Laboratory Sciences Program
Department of Botany/Microbiology
College of Liberal Arts and Sciences
Arizona State University
Tempe, Arizona

Madeline G. Ducate, MS, MPH, MT(ASCP)SM
Clinical Assistant Professor
School of Associated Health Professions
University of Medicine and Dentistry of New Jersey
Scientific Associate
G.H. Besselaar Associates
Princeton, New Jersey

Sharon S. Ehrmeyer, PhD
Associate Professor
School of Allied Health Professions
University of Wisconsin at Madison
Madison, Wisconsin

Paul G. Engelkirk, PhD, CLSpM, MT(ASCP)
Associate Professor
Program in Medical Technology/Cytogenetics
School of Allied Health Sciences
The University of Texas Health Science Center at Houston
Houston, Texas

Douglas W. Estry, PhD, MT(ASCP)
Assistant Professor of Medical Technology and Pathology
Michigan State University
East Lansing, Michigan

Kevin D. Fallon, PhD
Assistant Professor of Anesthesiology
The University of Texas Medical School at Houston
Houston, Texas

Deborah T. Firestone, MA, MT(ASCP), SBB
Clinical Assistant Professor of Medical Technology
School of Allied Health Professions
State University of New York
Stony Brook, New York

H. Elise Galloway, MS, CLS
Higher Education Administration
University of South Carolina
Mount Pleasant, South Carolina

Mary J. R. Gilchrist, PhD
Director, Clinical Microbiology
Assistant Professor of Pediatrics
Children's Hospital Medical Center
Cincinnati, Ohio

Linda Gorman, MS, CLS
Associate Professor
College of Allied Health Professions
University of Kentucky
Lexington, Kentucky

H. Jesse Guiles, CLS, MT(ASCP)SC
Assistant Professor of Clinical Laboratory Sciences
School of Health Related Professions
University of Medicine and Dentistry of New Jersey
Newark, New Jersey

Bethany W. Hurtuk, PhD, CLS, MT(ASCP)
Clinical Assistant Professor of Chemistry
Cleveland State University
Cleveland, Ohio

James Jackson, PhD, CLS, MT(ASCP)
Associate Professor and Chairman
Medical Technology Department
Wichita State University
Wichita, Kansas

Sharon Jackson, EdM, MT(ASCP)
Assistant Professor of Medical Technology
University of Florida
Gainesville, Florida

Dianne F. Johnson, MD, MT(ASCP)
Pathology Laboratories of Arkansas
Little Rock, Arkansas

Cynthia Karr, PhD, MT(ASCP)
Associate Professor
Medical Technology Educational Department
College of Health Related Professions
Medical University of South Carolina
Charleston, South Carolina

Consuelo M. Kazen, MS, MT(ASCP)SC
Department of Biochemistry
The University of Texas Health Science Center at San Antonio
San Antonio, Texas

Janice M. Klaassen, MS, CLS, MT(ASCP)SM
Laboratory Manager
Southwest Medical Associates
Las Vegas, Nevada

Robin Gaynor Krefetz, EdM, CLS, MT(ASCP)
Associate Professor and Director, Medical Laboratory Technology Program
Community College of Philadelphia
Philadelphia, Pennsylvania

Hal S. Larsen, PhD, CLS, MT(ASCP)
Chairman, Department of Medical Technology
Texas Technical University Health Sciences Center
Lubbock, Texas

Craig Lehman, MS, CC(NRCC)
Vice-Chairman and Associate Professor
Department of Medical Technology
School of Allied Health Professions
State University of New York
Health Sciences Center
Stony Brook, New York

Bernhard Ludvigsen, PhD
Associate Professor
Medical Technology Program
College of Allied Health Professions
University of South Alabama
Mobile, Alabama

Peggy Luebbert, MS, MT(ASCP)SC
Instructor in Medical Technology
University of Nebraska Medical Center
Omaha, Nebraska
Memorial Hospital of Dodge County
Fremont, Nebraska

Shirley MacManigal, PhD, CLS, MT(ASCP)
Dean, School of Allied Health
Texas Technical University Health Sciences Center
Lubbock, Texas

Diana Mass, MA, CLS, MT(ASCP)
Faculty Associate and Director
Clinical Laboratory Sciences Program
Department of Botany/Microbiology
College of Liberal Arts and Sciences
Arizona State University
Tempe, Arizona

Mary Ann McLane, MS, CLS
Assistant Professor of Clinical Laboratory Sciences
College of Allied Health Professions
Temple University
Philadelphia, Pennsylvania

Barbara Smith Michael, MS, CLS, MT(ASCP)
Education Resources Coordinator and Instructor
Program in Medical Technology/Cytogenetics
School of Allied Health Sciences
The University of Texas Health Science Center
Houston, Texas

Herb Miller, PhD, MT(ASCP)
Associate Professor of Medical Technology
Rush University
Rush–Presbyterian–St. Luke's Medical Center
Chicago, Illinois

Sharon M. Miller, PhC, CLS, MT(ASCP)
Associate Professor and Director
Medical Technology Program
School of Allied Health Professions
Northern Illinois University
De Kalb, Illinois

Barbara J. Minard, MT(ASCP)SH, SI
Adjunct Faculty, Medical Technology Department
Wichita State University
Technical Coordinator of Immunohematology
HCA/Wesley Medical Center
Wichita, Kansas

Maria Luisa J. Morsi, MS, RD
Assistant Professor
Department of Nursing
College of Allied Health Professions
Temple University
Philadelphia, Pennsylvania

Jon O. Nilsestuen, PhD, RRT
Associate Professor
Program Director
Respiratory Therapy Program
The University of Texas School of Allied Health Sciences
Houston, Texas

Jane Sidney Oliver, MA
Director of Professional Affairs
American Society for Medical Technology
Washington, D.C.

Martha Savage Payne, MPA, CLS, MT(ASCP)
Assistant Professor of Clinical Laboratory Sciences
University of Tennessee, Memphis
Memphis, Tennessee

Laura Martin Rahlfs, MBA, CLS, MT(ASCP)SH
Houston, Texas

Lucy J. Randles, MA, CLS/ClDir
Director, Cooperative Medical Technology Program of Akron
Children's Hospital Medical Center
Akron, Ohio

Lauren A. Roberts, MS, CLS, MT(ASCP)
Faculty Associate
Clinical Laboratory Sciences Program
Department of Botany/Microbiology
College of Liberal Arts and Sciences
Arizona State University
Tempe, Arizona

Larry Schoeff, MS
Associate Professor of Medical Laboratory Sciences
College of Associated Health Professions
University of Illinois at Chicago
Chicago, Illinois

Michael Sealfon, PhD, MT(ASCP)
Adjunct Clinical Instructor
Cleveland State University
Laboratory Manager
Mt. Sinai Medical Center
Cleveland, Ohio

Mary Lee Seibert, EdD
Dean, College of Allied Health Professions
Temple University
Philadelphia, Pennsylvania

Robert M. Shoemaker, EdD, CLS, MT(ASCP)
Laboratory Supervisor
Temple University Hospital
Senior Medical Technologist
Roxborough Memorial Hospital
Philadelphia, Pennsylvania

Linda A. Smith, MS, MT(ASCP)BB
Associate Professor, Medical Technology Program
The University of Texas Health Sciences Center at San Antonio
San Antonio, Texas

Thomas Spillman, PhD, DABCC
Assistant Professor of Clinical Pathology
The University of Texas Medical School at Houston
Associate Director of Clinical Chemistry
Hermann Hospital
Houston, Texas

Michael W. Sullivan, MS, MT(ASCP)
Instructor in Medical Technology
University of Alabama at Birmingham
Birmingham, Alabama

Cheryl Swinehart, MS, CLS
Assistant Professor
Division of Medical Technology
University of Minnesota
Minneapolis, Minnesota

Jacqueline Swoyer, BA, MT(ASCP)
Administrative Technologist
Department of Anatomical and Clinical Pathology
St. Paul–Ramsey Medical Center
St. Paul, Minnesota

Kerry A. Upton, MT(ASCP)
Section Supervisor
Toxicology/Special Chemistry Laboratory
University Hospital
University of Alabama at Birmingham
Birmingham, Alabama

Alexander Von Laufen, BA
Neuropsychological Examiner
Baylor Institute for Rehabilitation
Dallas, Texas

Patricia Walsh, PhD
Professor and Director of Graduate Studies
Medical Technology Department
University of Health Sciences
The Chicago Medical School
North Chicago, Illinois

Alan H. B. Wu, PhD
Assistant Professor of Pathology and Laboratory Medicine
The University of Texas Medical School at Houston
Director of Clinical Chemistry
Hermann Hospital
Houston, Texas

Foreword

Clinical laboratory science applies scientific laboratory methods to diagnostic and therapeutic problems of clinical medicine. The goal of the clinical laboratory scientist should be to enhance the diagnostic accuracy of the physician as well as to monitor a patient's response to therapy.

In years past, the role of the clinical physician was relatively straightforward in regard to laboratory testing. The physician would order a test and the laboratory would dutifully perform the study, regardless of whether or not it seemed appropriate. The laboratory functioned more or less as a cafeteria, providing any item in any quantity to the physician-customer. The advent of cost-containment programs has changed this picture significantly in the last few years. Quite apart from cost containment, however, laboratory scientists have become increasingly concerned with the strategies of testing as well as the interpretation of test results. The concepts of sensitivity, specificity, predictive value, and efficiency of tests are now widely understood and applied.

With the blossoming of clinical laboratories in the last decade, the physician has been and will continue to be faced with a continually expanding menu of tests and studies from which he must order wisely and interpret the forthcoming results correctly. The increasing complexity of clinical laboratory science forces the physician to run the risk of being incompletely informed. Many physicians will seek out the necessary information and interpretive guidelines to make optimal and cost-effective use of laboratory studies without additional aid. However, when a relationship of support and trust develops between the clinician and the laboratory scientist, there is an important and useful bidirectional transfer of information and the potential for more effective and efficient use of the physician's time and skills. The understanding of important clinical information by the clinical laboratory scientist allows for a better understanding of the patient's and physician's needs regarding laboratory tests. Moreover, if the laboratory scientist understands the clinical problem, appropriate screening and definitive testing procedures can be suggested that will more efficiently result in the correct diagnosis.

A good example of synergistic interaction between the clinical laboratory scientist and the physician occurs in the coagulation laboratory. The laboratory scientists in this area of the laboratory have a great deal of knowledge about these specific and sophisticated tests. Coupling clinical information with insightful test selection can expedite the interpretation of the results and the timely and appropriate treatment of the patient.

The clinical laboratory scientist's interest in the use and interpretation of tests has been present for many years. Initially it may have been stimulated by observing the patient's clinical condition during collection of blood samples or the charting of laboratory results. Both activities provided opportunities to review the clinical course and to understand the use of laboratory results in diagnosis and treatment. The trend of the clinical laboratory scientist to move toward a more direct involvement in the interpretation of laboratory tests has continued. Educational sessions at professional meetings and case presentations or articles in various journals are increasingly devoted to this subject. In many situations, physicians ask the clinical laboratory scientist about the interpretation of a particular test result. This may be a query about the reference or normal range or a possible diagnostic interpretation of the study; the laboratory scientist is expected to provide an appropriate and informed response in these situations.

There is, therefore, a need for clinical laboratory scientists to know more than just the *how* of tests, but also the *why,* and thus the need for a focus on a variety of major disease groups for which laboratory testing is an integral part of the diagnostic process. The authors of this text have done a remarkable job of focusing on the interpretive aspects of testing, but without trying to displace the physician's or clinical pathologist's role in the process. The discussions on the interpretation of laboratory data must be seen as an *addition* to the primary function of the laboratory scientist, that is, the flawless performance of testing done on a scientific basis, rather than as a *substitution* for this most important function. The added information should make laboratory work significantly more interesting and challenging for clinical laboratory scientists as well as useful to clinicians.

It is important to note that with this added dimension to the role of the clinical laboratory scientist comes an additional responsibility to the patient, who at times will ask the clinical laboratory scientist why a test had been ordered and the meaning of its result. Appropriate professional ethics should govern the response to the patient in these cases; yet the laboratory scientist cannot remain mute to these questions and must be prepared to respond.

We believe that readers will find the pages of this text filled with interesting and useful information as well as insights that will make their chosen profession even more rewarding in the years to come and their contribution to health care even more valuable.

John A. Koepke, MD
Department of Hospital Laboratories
Duke University Medical Center
Durham, North Carolina

Kenneth A. Schneider, MD
Director, Hospital Laboratories
Department of Pathology
Duke University Medical Center
Durham, North Carolina

Preface

HOW TO USE THIS BOOK AND PROSPER!

The clinical laboratory is changing and clinical laboratory scientists are changing with it. Even before the advent of prospective payment, technological advances were creating new and different roles for us. Because of these changes, the skills that are valued now in the clinical laboratory are quite different from those that were necessary for success in the past. Quality has been, and will always be, the *sine qua non* of the clinical laboratory, but an important new dimension has been added to considerations of quality: that of ***proper utilization*** of the laboratory for efficient and effective diagnosis and treatment of the patient.

This book is based on the premise that the demands on the clinical laboratory have become so complex that merely reporting raw data without insight and understanding of the physician's needs can be counterproductive for the patient. Today it is no longer sufficient for laboratory results to be accurate and precise. They must also be useful in the sense that they do not confuse the issue for the physician or add unnecessarily to costs because the results contribute nothing toward a diagnosis. Laboratory skills today often have less to do with performing a test than with determining whether the test should be done at all; with ensuring that follow-up testing is appropriate; and with assisting the clinician in asking the right laboratory question rather than using a "shotgun" approach to diagnostic testing. More is no longer better.

If we are to meet these needs and participate fully in this expanded view of clinical laboratory practice, we must understand clearly the bases on which clinical questions are formulated and acted upon by clinicians. We must know how to use our scientific and technical expertise to assist the clinician in choosing the right tests for a given patient and thus reach an accurate, timely, and cost-effective diagnosis. In doing this, we are in a unique position to integrate data from all of the laboratory disciplines in a relevant way. It is in this context—as we help the clinician to choose and interpret wisely from the great variety of tests available—that laboratory data become the *means,* not the end, of clinical laboratory science practice.

"Clinical Laboratory Science: Strategies for Practice" approaches the profession from this standpoint. We have assumed that our readers are familiar with normal physiology, and have addressed laboratory test methodology and related technical considerations elsewhere . This book does *not* address the "how to" of methodology; there are many excellent texts that do so. Instead, it addresses the "why" and the "when" of laboratory testing by means of a disease-oriented organization and content based on the perspective of the user of laboratory findings.

Thus the book begins with an Introduction that describes why clinicians choose laboratory tests and the process by which test results are used to evaluate differential diagnoses, derived from the patient's presenting symptoms, history, and physical findings, so that a final diagnosis evolves from laboratory data. The disease-oriented sequence of sections dealing with organ systems is generally ordered by acuity; for example, disorders of the heart or lungs can have an immediate and grave outcome for the patient who is not treated properly or promptly. The individual chapters, in turn, are organized to facilitate the clinical laboratory scientist's understanding of the circumstances under which one particular test or method might be valuable and another less so. Accordingly, there is great emphasis on the characteristics of laboratory analyses and the pathophysiology of various disease processes that result in significant, abnormal laboratory findings. At the same time, the clinical manifestations that also derive from the pathophysiologic process are discussed so that the laboratory scientist can interact meaningfully with clinicians making test choices in a given clinical situation. Similarly, brief discussions of treatment are provided, particularly treatment as it affects specific laboratory findings, so that the assistance and contribution of the clinical laboratory scientist can continue beyond the initial diagnosis.

The reader who finds these concepts of clinical laboratory science practice to be innovative or unusual would do well to read the Foreword of this text, as well as the Introduction and the chapter on the development of consultation skills. These initial sections, together with this Preface, are designed to provide a foundation and rationale for the remainder of the text. Except for a few chapters in which a different organization seemed more logical, the reader will find discussions of etiology and pathophysiology leading to a description of clinical manifestations, which in turn lead to discussion of effective and efficient laboratory approaches to the clinical questions involved. In many cases, algorithms to aid in test choices and interpretation are provided. The concluding sections of most chapters include a brief discussion of treatment and one or more case studies that illustrate the topics addressed therein. Lists of all the algorithms and case studies can be found in the Index.

Several conventions are followed throughout the text. The term *clinical laboratory scientist* as used is equivalent to a term that is, perhaps, more familiar: *medical technologist.* When discussing clinical laboratory test results, conventional units are followed by Système Internationale (SI) units in parentheses unless otherwise indicated. Peripheral blood cell counts are reported in thousands per cubic millimeter. Finally, although gender neutrality has been achieved in the greater portion of the text, the conventional usage of the pronoun *he,* to indicate both men and women, is followed in rare instances. To do otherwise in these cases would risk muddling perfectly good prose, and we chose not to do so.

Although this text is designed primarily for clinical laboratory science practitioners and students, it is hoped that other health-care professionals who have an interest in better utilization of the clinical laboratory might also find it helpful. The clinical laboratory is a powerful tool in quality patient care if it is properly used, and to that end this book has been written.

Brenta G. Davis
Michael L. Bishop
Diana Mass

Contents

Introduction

CLINICAL LABORATORY UTILIZATION: The Role of the Clinical Laboratory Scientist

Judith T. Barr

This introduction describes the "new age" laboratory that is developing as a result of profound economic and technological changes in health-care delivery, requiring clinical laboratory scientists to undertake challenging new roles in clinical laboratory science practice. Among these roles will be increased interaction and collaboration with attending physicians and others to enhance the medical efficacy and cost effectiveness of their patient care efforts. If clinical laboratory scientists are to fulfill their essential new roles involving expertise in laboratory utilization, they must understand *how* and *why* clinicians use the laboratory so that useful and effective interactions between these professionals can take place. The discussions below explore these issues in some detail and should be helpful to clinical laboratory scientists in successfully meeting the challenges that the new laboratory environment presents.

THE CHANGING LABORATORY

More than 4 billion clinical laboratory tests were performed in the United States in 1982 at an estimated cost of $20 billion.[1] Most were performed by clinical laboratory scientists using their technical skill and knowledge of test methodologies, instrumentation, and quality control. Unfortunately many of those tests probably did not benefit from the clinical laboratory scientist's knowledge of pathophysiology, appropriate test utilization, and test data synthesis and interpretation. That has not been the traditional role of the laboratory, and until recently there was little opportunity to change this tradition.

Now, however, a new role for the laboratory and the clinical laboratory scientist is evolving due not only to changes in the health-care system but to changes in technology as well. This new direction will challenge laboratory scientists to apply their knowledge and accept new responsibilities—responsibilities that require them to extend beyond the *process* of producing a test result and to interface with clinicians in a collaborative effort to improve both the laboratory's *input* and its *output.*

For most clinical laboratory scientists, this is a new view of their role and responsibility: To maximize the value of a laboratory test and the clinical laboratory scientist's contribution to patient care, the three primary phases of laboratory utilization must be considered. First, the input—is the test appropriate for the clinical condition and is the specimen and its time of collection correct? Next, the process—within clinically relevant guidelines is the test result accurate and precise, and is the process responsive to the turnaround time needs of clinicians? And third, the output—are the results being properly interpreted and integrated into proper patient care or is data overload confusing or misleading physicians? Study of all three phases is critical. An accurate and precise laboratory result is of no value if the test was not clinically indicated, the laboratory's precision was *beyond* that needed for clinical judgments, or the result was misinterpreted. It must be realized that such tests are of little value because they unnecessarily consume limited health-care resources and lead potentially to patient harm.

Central to the current changes in the delivery of clinical laboratory services is the adoption of an increased role for the clinical laboratory scientist, assisting the clinician in the appropriate utilization of laboratory services. To implement this new role, we must understand why clinicians order laboratory tests, the cognitive process involved in ordering, why there is such variation in test ordering patterns, and how the clinical laboratory scientist can assist in the effective and efficient use of the clinical laboratory. We must also understand the traditional laboratory, which is changing, and the "new age" laboratory, which is emerging as a result of those changes.

The Traditional Laboratory

The traditional role of the clinical laboratory has been to perform tests—to specialize in the *process* of producing names and numbers. Specimens are received, requested analyses performed, and results released. As depicted in the traditional laboratory model (illustrated on the opposite page), little laboratory input or communications occur prior to the test being received or after the result is released. Within this model, the major emphasis is on the quality of the test performance and the internal organization and production features of the laboratory. Here, neither clinical appropriateness of test requests nor interpretation of test results are considered major concerns of the clinical laboratory.

Adopting quality control and automation principles from industry, traditional laboratories have produced large quantities of high quality data at low unit cost. During the previous era of retrospective payment mechanisms, large laboratory volume generated needed revenues to support other, defi-

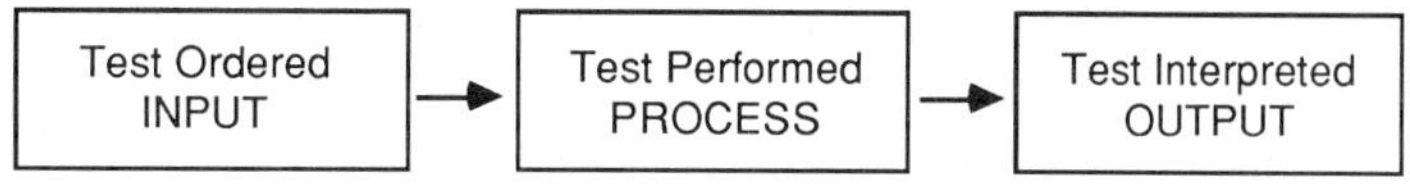

The traditional laboratory model.

cit-producing, hospital operations. In that period, the number of laboratory tests rose at an annual rate of 10%, but generally the increased testing was not associated with improved patient outcome.[2]

This situation led one laboratory observer to comment that "a significant proportion of the clinical laboratory tests ordered in the United States are not really needed for effective diagnosis and treatment," and that "the most important factor underlying the overuse of laboratory tests is physician behavior."[3]

Recently, incentives have changed under prospective payment systems, such as Diagnosis Related Groups (DRGs). No longer is the laboratory viewed as a revenue-generating profit center; it is now a consumer of limited hospital resources, a cost center. In response to these new economic forces, the traditional laboratory has focused on reducing costs by increasing the internal efficiency of producing test results. More structured cost-accounting methods have been introduced, work flow patterns analyzed, staffing and scheduling improved, and better volume discounts and leasing agreements negotiated. Discrete analyzers and other methodologies, using smaller reagent volumes, have yielded additional savings. From a cost-containment standpoint, however, there is a much greater payoff in attempting to reduce the numbers of unneeded tests ordered than in attempting to reduce the unit cost or charge per test.[3]

Moreover such efficiencies, although necessary, have not enabled clinical laboratory scientists to better integrate the process of laboratory testing into the total care of the patient nor have these efficiencies enabled the traditional laboratory to better control the use of services. To respond to the pressures of prospective payment systems and to increase the clinical relevance of their services, clinical laboratory scientists now must expand their views of the role and function of the clinical laboratory. Rather than focusing only on its internal *efficiency,* the laboratory must also examine its *effectiveness.* This involves not only the internal process of producing results (process), but also outreach efforts to increase appropriate laboratory utilization (input) and assist physicians by providing additional information to accompany numerical results (output). Laboratories must now assume some responsibility for the input and output components of their services. To achieve these goals, a new model of the clinical laboratory must be defined, that of the "new age" laboratory.

The "New Age" Laboratory

The "new age" laboratory broadens the mission of the traditional laboratory. In this model, clinical laboratory scientists expand beyond their traditional role as generators of test data to integrate themselves into all phases of the production of laboratory information and to influence the utilization of the department's resources and services. As depicted in the illustration on page XXXIV, laboratory scientists in the "new age" laboratory will interact and collaborate with clinicians to improve the clinical appropriateness of test requests (input), to improve the clinical relevance of the laboratory's offerings and procedures (process), and to assist the clinician in the proper interpretation of laboratory information (output).

To improve laboratory utilization, clinical laboratory scientists in the "new age" laboratory must influence the test-ordering behavior and data interpretation of clinicians. To develop strategies to affect clinician behavior, laboratory scientists must examine why tests are ordered, the influences and cognitive steps in the laboratory utilization process, and how variation in test utilization patterns

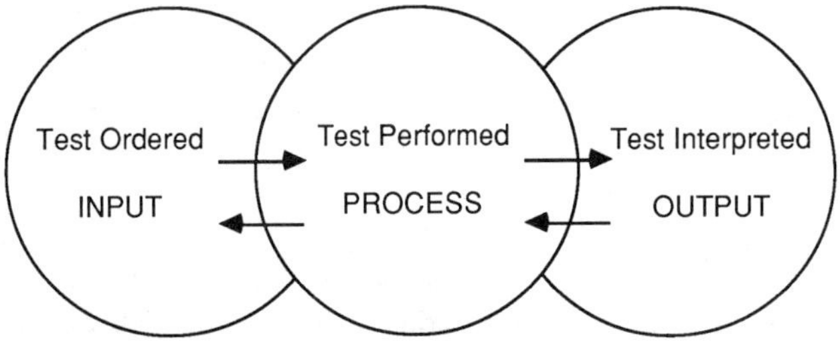

The "new age" laboratory.

can be reduced. Then, in collaboration with clinicians, laboratory-based strategies, targeted to areas of weakness in the test-ordering process, can be developed to improve appropriate utilization and reduce unnecessary testing.

LABORATORY UTILIZATION

Why Clinicians Order Tests

When physicians at a major medical center were asked why they had ordered one or more of the 11 most frequently requested tests or panels, they indicated that 37% of their requests were for diagnostic purposes, 33% for monitoring, and 32% for screening. Only 1% of the tests were said to be ordered for medicolegal protection, 1% were for repeated testing because a previous result was not available, and none were for presentation to senior staff.[4]

In addition to diagnosis, screening, and monitoring of disease, laboratory tests are also recognized to be useful in the determination of the severity of disease, the determination of the appropriate management of patients, the monitoring of therapy, and the prediction of response to treatment.[5]

Others have identified "the need to be complete" as a major impetus for test ordering. This compulsion to rule out or document every possibility, no matter how remote, creates much unnecessary testing.[6–10] Medical school faculty and hospital attending staff reinforce this mentality by criticizing the omission of one laboratory test rather than rewarding restraint and thoughtful use of diagnostic tests.[7]

Lastly, physicians also use laboratory tests as a form of communication with patients, colleagues, and potential referral specialists.[11–15] Laboratory tests can be used to show the patient and other physicians that something is being done, and can be used to reassure and please patients. Patients expect tests to be ordered, and physicians can both please the patient and signal the end of an office visit by ordering a test.

Given these reasons, what is the sequence of thoughts and events in the laboratory utilization process that leads the clinician from the clinical assessment of a patient, through the test order and its performance, to the integration of the results into patient care? One model of the laboratory utilization process is developed below.

A Utilization Model

A model of laboratory utilization must capture the interrelationship between the primary variables associated with laboratory test ordering and the sequential cognitive, organizational/environmental, and action processes leading from a clinical assessment, through the selection and ordering of a test, to the laboratory's performance of the test, and ultimately to the clinician's integration of the result into patient care. Institutional, laboratory, and medical staff characteristics and policies are known to affect the utilization pattern within a hospital. Also important are the characteristics of individual clinicians and the type and severity of each patient's illness.

Set in the context of public health, insurance, and institutional policies, the illustration opposite

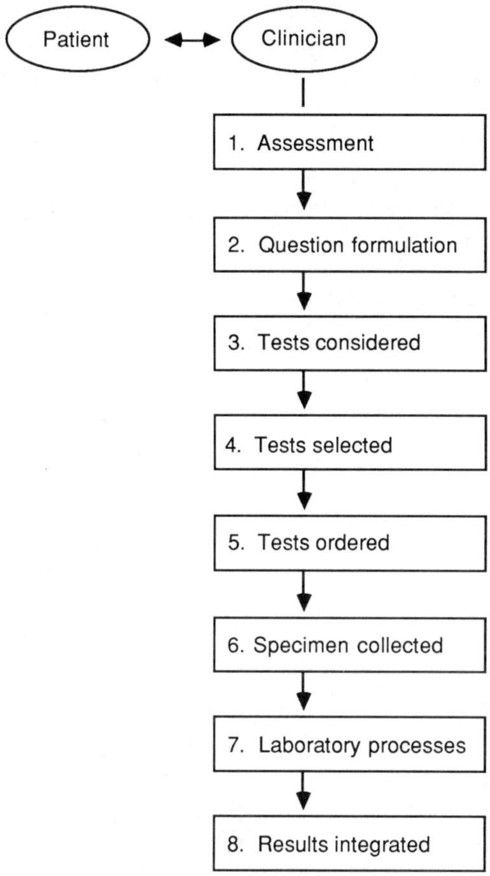

Steps in the laboratory utilization process.

expands the earlier input–process–output model by graphically displaying an eight-step sequence of clinicians' thoughts and actions in the laboratory utilization process. Although many feedback loops exist between various steps in the process, a simplified sequential model is presented. This model carefully dissects and analyzes the input phase, while the process and output phases, each represented by only a single, consolidated step, would be further elaborated in other models.

STEPS IN THE PROCESS

Starting with the clinician's assessment of the patient's clinical condition, the laboratory utilization process proceeds in eight steps to the application and integration of the test result into patient care. In Step 1, the clinician assesses the patient's status. Based on the condition of the patient, the clinician, in Step 2, formulates clinical questions that must be answered to guide further management of this patient. In Step 3, a variety of tests are considered that might be used to answer the questions raised in the earlier step. Step 4 involves the mental selection of a specific test or tests from the universe of those considered; in Step 5, that cognitive selection is converted into an action resulting in the placement of an order for the selected tests. In Step 6 a specimen is collected, and in Step 7, the laboratory accepts the specimen and conducts the analysis. Step 8 involves the integration of the results with the patient's condition. Steps 1 through 6 are part of the input phase; Step 7 is the process; and Step 8 is the output phase.

The entire test ordering model is set within the context of "environmental" policies external to the specific patient and clinician, but that influence the use or nonuse of laboratory tests. For example, public health policies may require or suggest that a particular test be ordered for a specific clinical condition, independent of the particular patient's condition or clinician's ordering practices. Several other examples of these "environmental" factors are an institution's standard operating procedures for admission and preoperative testing, an insurance company's denial of coverage if certain tests are used inappropriately, or establishment of clinical management protocols.

CONDITIONS AFFECTING EACH STEP IN LABORATORY UTILIZATION

Each step in the laboratory utilization model is affected by conditions or characteristics that influence the clinician's thoughts and actions. These factors can range from the severity of a patient's condition to the characteristics of the clinician's educational preparation and view of uncertainty and risk, or to the characteristics of the hospital and its clinical staff. Several of these important conditions and characteristics are incorporated into an amplified picture of the laboratory utilization process, illustrated here.

The first step in the process is the clinician's assessment of the patient's condition. This involves the interaction of the factors that are dependent upon the patient's clinical condition (*e.g.*, type of illness, severity of illness, patient's wishes) and the clinician's observational abilities and competence in physical assessment and in separating abnormal from normal signs. If the clinical sign is recognized, the first step has been completed successfully. However, if the symptom is overlooked, it is unlikely that a clinically indicated test will be performed.[16]

Following the clinician's assessment of the patient, the clinician next converts the observations into questions concerning diagnostic possibilities or changes in clinical status.[17, 18] All clinicians go through this question-posing step; whether or not they consciously analyze this step is largely de-

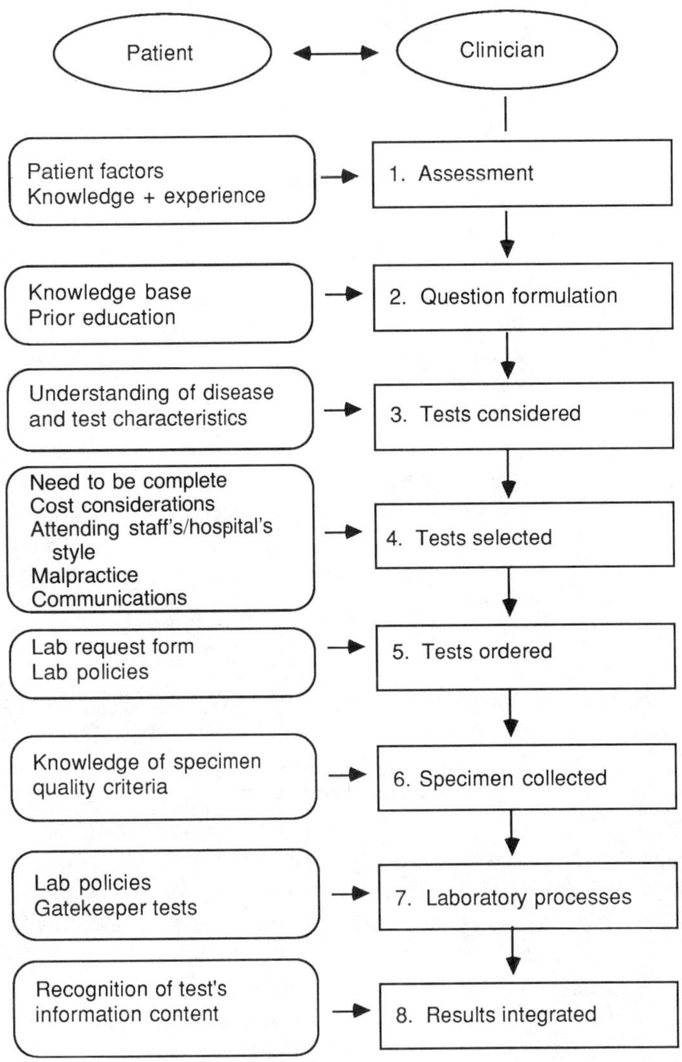

Conditions affecting the laboratory utilization process.

pendent on their educational preparation. The more focused the questions, the more likely that targeted, rather than "shotgun," test ordering will occur. The quality of the framing and focusing of the questions is dependent upon individual clinician characteristics as well as prior education.[19, 20]

Given a clinical presentation and the resultant framed question(s), the clinician considers the array of tests that can be ordered to answer the question. What tests are considered in this third step is dependent upon such factors as the clinician's ability to link the pathophysiology of the clinical condition with possible tests to answer the question,[19] experience with patients with similar clinical findings,[21] and understanding of the information content of each test and its ability to separate diseased from nondiseased populations.[17] An additional factor is the laboratory's packaging and pricing of the tests as profiles/panels or discrete analytes. If a panel is offered, it is more likely that a panel, rather than individual tests, will be considered.[22]

Given the universe of considered tests, the clinician now must select the specific test(s). Many factors influence this fourth step: the trade-off between the "need to be complete" versus the need to contain costs,[10] the degree of uncertainty the clinician can tolerate (the more uncertain the clinician, the more tests are ordered to reduce that uncertainty),[21, 23] malpractice issues (tests used to document that everything, no matter how remote, was considered),[9] and the need to use the test to communicate to other clinicians or the patient.[15] Other factors influencing selection of tests include the style and expectation of attending staff and chief of service (the ordering pattern of those in power is emulated by others),[24–28] the type of medical speciality,[29–31] the teaching status of a hospital or floor,[32–36] and the payment mechanism for the laboratory charges.[2, 4, 26, 27, 37–39]

At this step, for each test considered, the clinician should ask whether any result of that specific test would change the course of action. Generally, if the answer is no, the test should not be selected.

In the fifth step, the test selected by the clinician is converted into a test order. This step can be influenced, and hence limited, by institutional policies and laboratory order forms.[40] For example, the clinician may decide that a daily standing order for electrolyte testing is appropriate, but the institution may have a policy against standing orders. Or the clinician may select a single test, but may be induced to order more when the laboratory request slip offers that test as part of a panel. Or the institution may impose barriers to ordering that are designed to discourage the conversion of the mental selection of a test of little value into an action of placing an order for that test.

The sixth step involves the collection of the specimen for the ordered test. In this step, it is vital that proper sampling time criteria are followed (*e.g.*, glucose monitoring, therapeutic drug monitoring, cardiac isoenzymes) and that specimen quality is assured (*e.g.*, prevention of oxygen exposure to anaerobic cultures, hemolysis in venipuncture process). Whether proper specimen collection occurs is dependent primarily upon the knowledge base of those collecting the specimen and the ability of the laboratory to evaluate specimen quality and block those samples judged to be unacceptable.

In the seventh step, the laboratory accepts the specimen and conducts the analysis. Whether the test received by the laboratory is actually performed is dependent upon the screening or "gatekeeper" policies of the laboratory and institution. As described above, the laboratory may receive a specimen, but whether a test is performed is affected by the laboratory's ability to evaluate specimen quality.

Another laboratory policy in this step can actually block the performance of a test order, even though the specimen quality was acceptable. This policy is based on certain "reasonableness" or gatekeeper criteria. Examples of this form of laboratory policy include a limit on the frequency of repeat urine cultures, the omission of the white blood cell (WBC) differential when the WBC count is normal, and the policy to omit performing a lactate dehydrogenase (LD) isoenzyme order when the LD level is normal.

In the eighth step, the test result is released to

the clinician who integrates it with the clinical condition. The quality of this step is dependent upon the timely (and possibly consultative) response of the laboratory, the prepared mind of the clinician to recognize the information content of a result and his ability to properly apply it to the patient's condition.[41, 42] To assist clinicians with this step, annotated computer reports have been designed to suggest diagnostic possibilities.[43, 44] For results indicating that further testing is necessary, laboratories are developing protocols that automatically trigger a follow-up sequence of testing.[45–50] This assures that the initial abnormal result is not overlooked and that the appropriate definitive tests are performed.

This model explicitly identifies the "clinician," rather than the physician, during the laboratory utilization process. Recognizing that patient assessment and test ordering are now performed, officially and unofficially, by a variety of practitioners (nurse practitioners, physician assistants, dentists, nurse midwives, clinical pharmacists, and nurses), the model suggests that strategies to improve laboratory utilization must be addressed to more than the physician population, and that different practitioner populations may require alternative types of interventions to improve the process.

Variation in Utilization

Given this overview of the numerous factors influencing the steps in the laboratory utilization process, it is not surprising that there is a large variation among clinicians in their use of laboratory services.[26, 28, 51–53] Variations as large as seventeenfold have been documented among physicians treating the same patient population.[28] Different clinicians will treat the same patient differently,[53] and the same clinician will treat different patients differently.[15] Overall, although a singular model of laboratory utilization has been described in this section, there is great variation in just how a clinician approaches a case and progresses through each step in the model.

A number of factors can explain this variation—type and severity of illness, clinicians' educational preparation and personal characteristics, clinician–patient relationship, social and economic considerations, institutional and regional norms, and colleague expectations. Underlying them all, however, is a lack of standardization, or even consensus, in many of the steps in the laboratory utilization process.

Algorithms, which reduce variation by developing a logical sequence of tests for a given situation, are important interventions that should be combined with other strategies in a comprehensive program to improve the utilization process. Many algorithms can be found throughout the chapters in this text that will assist laboratory scientists in fulfilling their consultative role. Although algorithms can give direction, clinicians who wish "to be complete" or who are unable to cope with a degree of uncertainty are likely to order more than the algorithm-indicated tests. The discussion that follows will examine additional methods to improve the laboratory utilization process.

METHODS TO IMPROVE LABORATORY UTILIZATION

Although many attempts have been made to modify the test-ordering behavior of physicians, few have met with sustained success. Educational programs to improve test selection, cost awareness, and decision-making ability have been introduced into medical school curricula and sponsored by hospitals for their residents and attending staff. Other strategies have included rationing of laboratory tests, incentives to reduce utilization, and relative rank feedback programs.

The strategies that have met with most success, however, achieved their effectiveness by changing policies and procedures, and hence, by establishing new clinical and administrative guidelines by which tests were ordered. Rather than relying on persuasive educational programs to modify laboratory utilization, these new strategies directly intervened in the test-ordering process by redefining previous "routine" procedures (*e.g.*, eliminating microscopic examination for both "routine" urinalysis and complete blood counts), by identifying "gatekeeper" tests (*e.g.*, requiring abnormal creatine kinase (CK) level before CK isoenzymes are performed), and by creating "barriers" between steps (*e.g.*, requiring additional forms or other types of justification for test selection).

Still, numerous medical educators have argued that the answer to inappropriate laboratory utilization lies not in these latter types of restricted access to testing, but rather by changing the ordering behavior of physicians by systematic instruction in clinical decision making,[54, 55] appropriate use of clinical testing,[19] and the development of sequentially logical testing patterns based on priorities of cost effectiveness.[56] Therefore, to determine which strategy, or combination of strategies, would be most effective and efficient to improve laboratory utilization within an institution, the clinical laboratory scientist should be familiar with the variety of both nonlaboratory as well as laboratory-based interventions.

Educational Programs in Medical Schools and Hospitals

Laboratory utilization educational programs in medical schools are designed primarily to influence Steps 2–4—the question formulation, test consideration, and test selection steps (see the schematic on page XL). At this time students are first guided in converting a clinical assessment into a set of questions, linking those questions to a group of tests, and then selecting the best test in the group to answer the question.

Educational programs in hospitals include such varied interventions as simple passive distribution of information through lectures, newsletters, and booklets covering clinical appropriateness of certain tests or ordering strategies; feedback to physicians of patient-specific cost information and/or individual physician's ordering intensity relative to others in a group; and clinical appropriateness chart reviews with the house staff conducted by the attending staff. In this context passive and active audits and other forms of feedback are considered informational inputs and, as such, are part of the educational process. This type of intervention is aimed primarily at improving Step 4—the selection of the specific test based on its ability to answer a clinical question.

The results of studies that have examined the effect on physician test-ordering behavior by educational efforts are quite mixed. These studies, primarily conducted in a retrospective reimbursement environment and targeted at Step 4 in the laboratory utilization process—the test selection step—suggest the following: (1) "single dose" educational programs have limited effect; (2) feedback to the requesting clinician about laboratory charges per hospital stay is relatively inexpensive and appears to have some effect; (3) interactive chart audits focused on clinical appropriateness are costly but are successful, and (4) the attending physician's attitude is a major contributing factor to the success of any intervention[19, 28, 41, 57–67]

Rationing

Another strategy, rationing, limits the type or number of tests that the clinicians are permitted to order. This intervention is also aimed at restricting the test selection step—Step 4.

This strategy was implemented in one hospital where it had been found that only 5% of the hematology and chemistry tests ordered during hospitalizations were used in the diagnosis and treatment of the patient. It was also found that unnecessary follow-up tests were ordered without a change in the patient's condition, profiles were ordered when only one or two values were of interest, and tests were repeated at too frequent intervals.

Based on these findings, it was suggested that if tests were rationed, physicians would be more selective and reduce superfluous or redundant tests. Thus, a study was initiated where each house officer was restricted to a total of eight

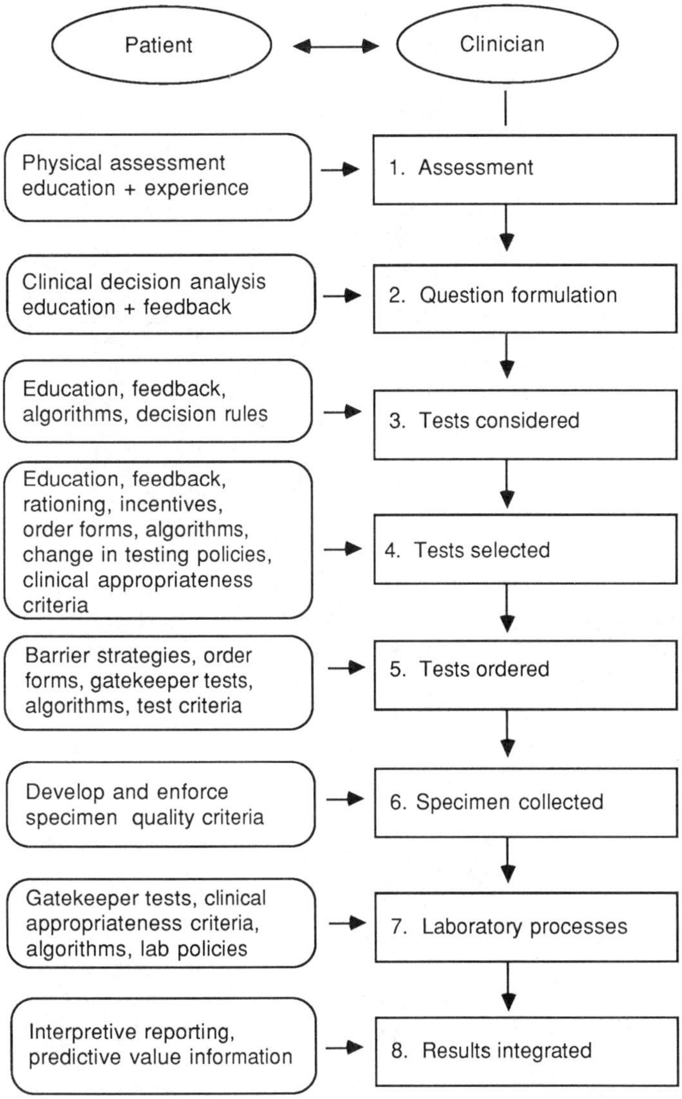

Strategies to modify the laboratory utilization process.

chemistry and hematology tests per patient per day. As a result of this intervention, the number of laboratory tests per patient was reduced by 25% without eliminating essential information, and the number of significant tests increased from 5% to 23%.[68]

Incentives

Two major forms of incentives are available to modify physicians' utilization; *positive* incentives rewarding appropriate ordering patterns, and *negative* incentives penalizing overutilization and incorrect utilization. These strategies also are designed to limit the test selection step—Step 4.

In one study where a small, positive financial incentive was offerred to a group of medical residents to decrease testing in the latter period of their first postgraduate year, it was found that either a program of positive incentives had no effect, or the size and nature of the incentive offered in this study was insufficient to induce a change in behavior.[61]

Under retrospective reimbursement and fee for service payment systems, both the hospital and physician had an incentive to overutilize the laboratory. Now, with a major component of the hospital reimbursement tied to prospective payment mechanisms and with a growing segment of the population covered by health maintenance organizations and other forms of prepaid group practices, laboratory tests ordered for completeness or strictly educational purposes no longer generate revenue. Now they are a financial liability to the institutions.

For the laboratory community, this financial *disincentive* will provide the stimulus to examine critically the services that it offers and to cooperate with administrators, third-party payers, and clinicians to promote a more rational and cost-effective use of clinical laboratory services. For physicians, the consequences will be increased financial accountability. One commentary recommended making physicians financially liable for tests they order that are judged to be unnecessary.[69]

Administrative Changes

Rather than relying on the individual clinician to voluntarily modify test-ordering behavior, physician organizations, third-party payers, and hospital and laboratory administrators are reassessing what laboratory services and standard operating procedures can be modified or eliminated. Based on these and independent investigators' evaluations, five administrative or system changes that have been recommended will be described: (1) Modify or eliminate uniform and preoperative testing (Steps 4 and 5); see schematic on page XL; (2) Eliminate standing orders (Steps 2–5), (3) Modify test request forms and the process by which tests are ordered (Steps 5 and 6); (4) Develop clinical appropriateness criteria for selected tests (Steps 4–6); and (5) Structure algorithms to guide diagnostic testing (Steps 3–5).

ROUTINE TESTING

Evidence is mounting that routine admission and preoperative testing are unnecessary and expensive.[70–76] One study calculated that admission testing added 5% to the total cost of hospital care and was not associated with any evidence of benefit to the patient.[73] Routine preoperative testing also did not contribute to patient outcome; some recommended that it be eliminated for asymptomatic and clinically normal patients who are undergoing elective minor surgery,[73] while others question whether any unindicated, routine preoperative testing should be performed at all.[75–76]

STANDING ORDERS

The elimination of standing orders is another method used to increase appropriate laboratory utilization. The logic behind this administrative change is that physicians should formulate a diagnostic or monitoring strategy each day and not rely on repetitive daily orders. With more thought given to the value of each test, the logic continues, the physician should order only the needed and appropriate tests while eliminating the unnecessary ones. While appearing to be a logical test reduction action,[77] few studies have evaluated its effectiveness and in these, results are mixed.

TEST REQUEST FORMS

Unlike many other strategies, modifications involving the design and use of test request forms can be under the control of the laboratory. At least two types of modifications are possible: redesign of test presentation on the ordering form, and use of request form as a type of "barrier" intervention.

In the first case, it has been suggested that the organization of laboratory request forms encourages unfocused ordering and should be improved.[40, 78] In response to this problem, Wong[79] created a problem-oriented form to be used for thyroid testing. The old form with four boxes to indicate if T_3 uptake, T_4, T_3, and/or TSH were ordered was replaced with a form offering a thyroid function screen, hyperthyroid panel, hypothyroid panel, or "other" thyroid test. This problem-oriented test form eliminated the problematic test selection phase by having the clinician select the *clinical problem* directly rather than the individual laboratory tests. As a result, T_3 requests declined 38% and thyrotropin by 68%. In commenting on this study, Lundberg[78] suggested that "the simplest, easiest, and cheapest, and probably most effective way to guide physicians to use a laboratory correctly is by designing test request forms properly."

Other modifications of test request forms have included the alphabetical, rather than organ-clustered, listing of tests; the replacement of a chemistry panel or profile with the individual listing of its constituent tests; and the elimination of highly specialized, and overutilized, tests from the routine test request slips. These types of forms are used to stimulate the ordering of a specific test to answer a specific question, rather than the unfocused ordering induced by poorly designed forms.

Another use of the test request form is to make the process of ordering a test more difficult. This blocks the conversion of a test selected in Step 4 to a test ordered in Step 5. By increasing the "price" the clinician must "pay" to have the test performed, it is suggested that only those tests that are highly valued will be advanced through the barrier. Several of these "barrier" interventions include: writing the order in a laboratory order book rather than simply checking off the test on the form; requesting approval to order restricted tests,[80] and justifying the test order by indicating a clinical condition on an additional test form.[81, 82] The effect of the first two has not been determined; several evaluations of the latter method offer important lessons for laboratory-based interventions.

The use of an additional or supplemental form has been reported to be successful in achieving test reductions of 25%–44%.[81–82] The decrease in testing also was associated with an improvement in the clinical appropriateness of the tests that rose from only 50% of the tests being clinically indicated prior to the supplemental form to an appropriateness level of 80% after the form was introduced.[82]

This type of intervention is one of the first that permits the laboratory to control directly one of the input variables into the laboratory. Hard copy forms are only the first examples. In institutions with computer-assisted test ordering, interactive programs can be developed that require clinicians to justify test selection. This will not only enable the laboratory to further manage, but also to provide assistance during, the test-ordering process.

CLINICAL APPROPRIATENESS CRITERIA

Laboratories are beginning to implement guidelines that place restrictions on the performance of selected tests. For example, the clinical utility of the once common complete blood count with differential and routine urinalysis with microscopic examination is under scrutiny. Both types of microscopic examinations are labor intensive, but contribute little additional clinical information when the white cell count is normal,[83–86] or the chemical screening of the urine is negative.[87, 88] Therefore, laboratories are limiting these follow-up tests to specimens with out-of-range cell counts or positive chemical screens. It is interesting to note that a Canadian hospital removed the differential white count from its requisition slips as early as 1973.[80]

The development of criteria to judge the clinical appropriateness of test requests should be a collaborative effort between clinicians and laboratory scientists and is likely to improve all aspects of laboratory utilization.

ALGORITHMS

Algorithms, or protocols, have been developed to guide clinicians in the sequence and selection of diagnostic tests. Previously published algorithms have emphasized diagnostic accuracy (hematuria[45, 46] and hypercalcemia[47, 48]) and cost effectiveness. Others have focused on a reduction in unnecessary test requests.[49, 50, 89, 90]

It is to be expected that efficiencies achieved by algorithms will make their use attractive in a prospective payment period. This text is an important contribution to improved testing and cost reduction in this regard because it includes a number of these tools. Not only can this information be used to assist clinicians in their test ordering, but it can also be used to develop triggered algorithms. When a primary result is abnormal, these algorithms could automatically initiate a properly structured sequence of clinically informative testing (triggered automatic test sequence—TATS).[40] This would improve the appropriateness of testing by preventing batch or untargeted ordering, and decrease the diagnostic time involved in the regular physician-initiated sequential testing.

Finally, within the laboratory, multistage protocols have been implemented to structure the laboratory processing of requests. In these algorithms, certain screening or primary tests must be abnormal before further diagnostic study is performed. The less expensive primary tests serve as "gatekeepers" to the more expensive follow-up tests. For example, an algorithm was developed to differentiate between pleural effusions that were transudates or exudates. Only those specimens meeting the exudate criteria would then have additional testing.[91] Similar staged strategies have been developed for immunoelectrophoretic analyses[92] and thyroid testing.[93]

THE ROLE OF THE CLINICAL LABORATORY SCIENTIST

In extending the role of the clinical laboratory scientist to assist clinicians in the proper utilization of the laboratory, much attention will be centered on the use of clinical appropriateness criteria and algorithms to ensure the most effective and efficient selection of tests, as well as their useful interpretation.

In order to function at this consultative level of collaboration with other professionals, clinical laboratory scientists must acquire both the content relevant to a disease oriented, clinical approach to laboratory testing *and* the interactive skills necessary to establish themselves as the appropriate providers of this important service. Clinical laboratory scientists have for some time acquired the necessary content, although they must now view it from a somewhat different perspective—through the eyes of the consumer of laboratory services. The development of the consultative skills necessary to become recognized as a useful resource in issues concerning laboratory utilization is a newer component of the laboratory scientist's body of knowledge. Patience and persistence in providing the unique expertise that integrates the right clinical question with the proper scientific/technical means to answer the question will benefit the patient, the physician, and the profession of clinical laboratory science.

REFERENCES

1. American Hospital Association: MediTrends: The Hospital Research and Educational Trust. Chicago, American Hospital Association, 1986
2. Conn RB: Clinical laboratories, profit center, production, industry or patient-care resource? N Engl J Med 298: 422–427, 1978
3. Sheinbach J: The clinical laboratories: Problems of cost containment as a challenge. In Benson ES, Rubin M (eds): Logic and Economics of Clinical Laboratory Use, pp 33–38. New York, Elsevier North-Holland Biomedical Press, 1978
4. Wertman BG, Sostrin SV, Pavlova Z, Lundberg GD: Why do physicians order laboratory tests? JAMA 243:2080–2082, 1980
5. Young DS: The role of the laboratory in clinical decision making. In Connolly DP, Benson ES, Burke MD, Fenderson D (eds): Clinical Decisions

and Laboratory Use, pp 69–79. Minneapolis, University of Minnesota Press, 1982

6. Krieg AF, Gambino R, Galen RS: Why are clinical laboratory tests performed? When are they valid? JAMA 233:76–78, 1975
7. Landau RL: Professors of medicine, stand up! Arch Intern Med 143:212–213, 1983
8. Hardison JE: To be complete. N Engl J Med 300:193–194, 1979
9. Feinstein AR: The "chagrin factor" and qualitative decision analysis. Arch Intern Med 145:1257–1259, 1985
10. Reuben DB: Learning diagnostic restraint. N Engl J Med 310:591–593, 1984
11. Epstein AM, Hartley RM, Charlton JR, Harris CM et al: A comparison of ambulatory test ordering for hypertensive patients in the United States and England. JAMA 252:1723–1726, 1984
12. Sox HC, Marguiles I, Sox CH: Psychologically mediated effects of diagnostic tests. Ann Intern Med 95:680–685, 1981
13. Woo B, Woo B, Cook EF, Weisberg M et al: Screening procedures in the asymptomatic adult: Comparison of physicians' recommendations, patients' desires, published guidelines, and actual practice. JAMA 254:1480–1484, 1985
14. Mills KA, Reilly PM: Laboratory and radiological investigations in general practice. II: Expectation and outcome: Brit Med J 287:1111–1113, 1983
15. Holmes MM, Rovner DR, Elstein AS, Holzman GB et al: Factors affecting laboratory utilization in clinical practice. Med Decis Making 2:471–482, 1982
16. Connelly DP, Johnson PE: The medical problem solving process. Hum Pathol 11:412–419, 1980
17. Weinstein MT, Fineberg HV: Clinical decision analysis. Philadelphia, WB Saunders, 1980
18. Johnson PE: Cognitive models of problem solvers. In Connolly DP, Benson ES, Burke MD, Fenderson D (eds): Clinical Decisions and Laboratory Use. Minneapolis, University of Minnesota Press, 1982
19. Burke MD, Connelly DP: Systematic instruction in laboratory medicine. Hum Pathol 12:134–144, 1981
20. Epstein AM, Begg CB, McNeil BJ: The effects of physicians' training and personality on test ordering for ambulatory patients. Am J Public Health 74:1271–1273, 1984
21. Tversky A, Kahneman D: Judgment under uncertainty: Heuristics and biases. Science 185:1124–1131, 1974
22. Golden W: Financial unbundling reduces outpatient laboratory use. Arch Intern Med 147:1045–1048, 1987
23. Greenland P, Mushlin AI, Griner PF: Discrepancies between knowledge and use of diagnostic studies in asymptomatic patients. J Med Educ 54:863–869, 1979
24. Eisenberg J: Sociologic influences on decision-making by clinicians. Ann Intern Med 90:957–964, 1979
25. Epstein AM, Begg CB, McNeil BJ: The effects of group size on test ordering for hypertensive patients. N Engl J Med 309:464–468, 1983
26. Freeborn DK, Baer D, Greenlick MR, Bailey JW: Determinations of medical care utilization: Physicians' use of laboratory services. Am J Public Health 62:846–853, 1972
27. Pineault R: The effect of prepaid group practice on physicians' utilization behavior. Med Care 14:121–136, 1976
28. Schroeder SA, Kenders K, Cooper JK, Piemme TE: Use of laboratory tests and pharmaceuticals: Variation among physicians and effect of cost audit on subsequent use. JAMA 225:969–973, 1973
29. Noren J, Frazier T, Altman I, DeLozier J: Ambulatory medical care: A comparison of internists and family–general practitioners. N Engl J Med 302:11–16, 1980
30. Everett GD, Chang P, deBlois CS, Holets TD: A comparative study of laboratory utilization behavior of "on-service" and "off-service" housestaff physicians. Med Care 21:1187–1191, 1983
31. Garg ML, Mulligan JL, McNamara MJ, Skipper JK et al: Teaching students the relationship between quality and cost of medical care. J Med Educ 50:1085–1091, 1975
32. Jones KR: The influence of the attending physician on indirect graduate medical education costs. J Med Educ 59:789–798, 1984
33. Busby DD, Leming JC, Olson MI: Unidentified educational costs in a university teaching hospital: An initial study. J Med Educ 47:243–253, 1972
34. Schroeder SA, O'Leary DS: Differences in laboratory use and length of stay between university and community hospitals. J Med Educ 52:418–420, 1977
35. Williams BT, Dixon RA: Biochemical testing for acute medical emergencies in four district general hospitals. Brit Med J 1:1313–1315, 1979

36. Martz EW, Ptakowski R: Educational costs to hospitalized patients. J Med Educ 53:383–386, 1978
37. Epstein AM, Krock SJ, McNeil BJ: Office laboratory tests: Perceptions of profitability. Med Care 22:160–166, 1984
38. Schroeder SA, Stowstack JA: Financial incentives to perform medical procedures and laboratory tests. Med Care 16:289–298, 1978
39. Rice TH: The impact of changing Medicare reimbursement rates on physician-induced demand. Med Care 21:803–815, 1983
40. Barr JT: Improved laboratory utilization and information production: the administrator's new role. J Med Tech 3:511–521, 1986
41. Ward PCJ, Harris IB, Burke MD, Horwitz C: Systematic instruction in interpretive aspects of laboratory medicine. J Med Educ 51:648–656, 1976
42. Ward PC, Harris LB, Horwitz CA, Burke MD: Systematic instruction in interpretive aspects of laboratory medicine. J Med Educ 1:618–621, 1976
43. Hobbie RK, Reece RL: Interpretative reporting by computer. Hum Pathol 12:127–134, 1981
44. Young DS: Interpretation of clinical chemical data with the aid of automatic data processing. Clin Chem 22:1555–1559, 1986
45. Brewer ED, Benson GS: Hematuria: Algorithms for diagnosis. 1. Hematuria in the child. JAMA 246:877–880, 1981
46. Benson GS, Brewer ED: Hematuria: Algorithms for diagnosis. 2. Hematuria in the adult and hematuria secondary to trauma. JAMA 246:993–995, 1981
47. Wong ET, Freier EF: The differential diagnosis of hypercalcemia. An algorithm for more effective use of laboratory tests. JAMA 247:75–80, 1982
48. Lum G, Deshotels SJ: The clinical usefulness of an algorithm for the interpretation of biochemical profiles with hypercalcemia. Am J Clin Pathol 78:479–484, 1982
49. Orient JM, Kettel LJ, Sox HC, Sox CH et al: The effect of algorithms on the cost and quality of patient care. Med Care 21:157–167, 1983
50. Wachtel T, Moulton AW, Pezzullo J, Hamolsky M: Inpatient management protocols to reduce health care costs. Med Decis Making 6:101–109, 1986
51. Fineberg HV, Funkhouser AR, Marks H: Variation in medical practice: A review of the literature. In Egdahl R, Walsh DC (eds): Industry and Health Care Vol 1: Health Cost Management and Medical Practice Patterns, pp 143–168. Cambridge, Ballinger, 1985
52. Schroeder SA, Schliftman A, Piemme TE: Variation among physicians in use of laboratory tests: Relation to quality of care. Med Care 12: 709–713, 1974
53. Hlatky MA, Lee KL, Botvinick EH, Brundage BH: Diagnostic test use in different practice settings. Arch Intern Med 143:1886–1889, 1983
54. Connelly C, Steele B: Laboratory utilization: Problems and solutions. Arch Pathol Lab Med 104:59–62, 1980
55. Kassirer JP, Pauker SG: Should diagnostic testing be regulated? N Engl J Med 299:947–949, 1978
56. Kassebaum DG: Teaching laboratory test use. J Med Educ 60:420–421, 1985
57. Garland MJ: Integrating cost awareness with ethics in the undergraduate medical curriculum. J Med Educ 60:44–52, 1985
58. Freeman RA: Cost containment. J Med Educ 51:157–158, 1976
59. Spiegel CT, Knapp BA, Newman MA, Birnbaum PS et al: Modification of decision-making behavior of third-year medical students. J Med Educ 57:769–777, 1982

59a. Garg ML, Gliebe WA, Kleinberg WM: Student peer review of diagnostic tests at the Medical College of Ohio. J Med Educ 54:852–855, 1979

60. Williams SV, Eisenberg JM, Kitz DS, Carroll JG et al: Teaching cost-effective diagnostic test use to medical students. Med Care 22:535–542, 1984
61. Rhyne RL, Gehlbach SH: Effects of an educational feedback strategy on physician utilization of thyroid function panels. J Fam Pract 8:1003–1007, 1979
62. Karas S: Cost containment in emergency medicine. JAMA 243:1356–1359, 1980
63. Martin AR, Wolf MA, Thibodeau LA, Dzau V et al: A trial of two strategies to modify the test-ordering behavior of medical residents. N Engl J Med 300:1330–1336, 1980
64. Eisenberg JM: An educational program to modify laboratory use by house staff. J Med Educ 52:578–581, 1979
65. Schroeder SA, Myers LP, McPhee SJ, Shawstack JA et al: The failure of physician education as a cost containment strategy. JAMA 252:225–230, 1984
66. Wones RG: Failure of low cost audits with feedback to reduce laboratory test utilization. Med Care 25:78–82, 1987
67. Everett GD, deBlois CS, Chang P, Holets T: Effect

of cost education, cost audits and faculty chart review on the use of laboratory services. Arch Intern Med 143: 942–944, 1983.

68. Dixon RH, Laszlo J: Utilization of clinical chemistry services by medical house staff: An analysis. Arch Intern Med 134:1064–1067, 1974
69. Eisenberg JM, Rosoff AJ: Physician responsibility for the cost of unnecessary medical services. N Engl J Med 299:76–80, 1978
70. Korvin CC, Pearce RH, Stanley J: Admissions screening: Clinical benefits. Ann Intern Med 83:197–203, 1975
71. Hampton JR, Harrison MJG, Mitchell JRA, Prichard JS et al: Relative contributions of history-taking, physical examination, and laboratory investigations to diagnosis and management of medical outpatients. Brit Med J 2:486–489, 1975
72. Sandler G: Costs of unnecessary tests. Brit Med J 2:21–24, 1979
73. Durbridge TC, Edwards F, Edwards RG, Atkinson M: Evaluation of benefits of screening tests done immediately on admission to hospital. Clin Chem 22:968–971, 1976
74. Delahunt B, Turnbull PRG: How cost effective are routine preoperative investigations? NZ Med J 92:431–432, 1980
75. Kaplan EB, Sheiner LB, Boeckmann AJ, Reizen MF et al: The usefulness of preoperative laboratory screening. JAMA 253:3576–3581, 1985
76. Lundberg GD: Is there a need for routine preoperative laboratory tests? JAMA 253:3589, 1985
77. Sussman E, Goodwin P, Rosen H: Administrative change and diagnostic test use: The effect of eliminating standing orders. Med Care 22:569–572, 1984
78. Lundberg GD: Laboratory request forms (menus) that guide and teach. JAMA 249:3075, 1983
79. Wong ET, McCarron MM, Shaw ST: Ordering of laboratory tests in a teaching hospital: Can it be improved? JAMA 249:3078–3080, 1983
80. Gray G, Marton R: Utilization of a hematology laboratory in a teaching hospital. Am J Clin Pathol 59:877–882, 1973
81. Novich M, Gillis L, Tauber AI: The laboratory test justified: An effective means to reduce routine laboratory testing. Am J Clin Pathol 84:756–759, 1985
82. Barr JT: Design and analysis of interventions to modify utilization of therapeutic drug monitoring: Doctoral dissertation. Cambridge, Massachusetts: Harvard University, 1987
83. Rich EC, Crowson TW, Connelly DP: Effectiveness of differential leukocyte count in case finding in the ambulatory care setting. JAMA 249:633–636, 1983
84. Rock WA, Grogan JE: Demand versus need versus physician prerogatives in the use of the WBC differential. JAMA 249:613–616, 1983
85. Shapiro MF, Hatch RL, Greenfield S: Cost containment and labor-intensive tests: The case of the leukocyte differential count. JAMA 252:231–234, 1984
86. Wesson SK, Mercado T, Austin M, Schumacher HR: Differential counts and overuse of the laboratory. Lancet 1:552, 1980
87. Shaw ST, Poon SY, Wong ET: "Routine urinalysis": Is the dipstick enough? JAMA 253:1596–1600, 1985
88. Valenstein P: New roles for the urine dipstick. Medical Laboratory Observer 18(2):63–66, 1986
89. Young DW: An aid to reducing unnecessary investigations. Br Med J 281:1610–1611, 1980
90. Taylor TR, Shields S, Black R: Study of cost-conscious computer-assisted diagnosis in thyroid disease. Lancet 2:79–83, 1972
91. Peterman TA, Speicher CE: Evaluating pleural effusions: A two-stage laboratory approach. JAMA 252:1051–1053, 1984
92. Rao KMK, Bordine SL, Keren DF: Decision making by pathologists: A strategy for curtailing the number of inappropriate tests. Arch Pathol Lab Med 106:55–56, 1982
93. Hardwick DF, Morrison JI, Tydeman J, Cassidy PA et al: Structuring complexity of testing: A process oriented approach to limiting unnecessary laboratory use. Am J Med Tech 48:605–608, 1982

Part I

CONSULTATION SKILLS

Glenda D. Price, Associate Editor

Chapter 1

Consulting As a Professional Role for the Clinical Laboratory Scientist

Mary Lee Seibert / Glenda Price

Historically physicians, with good reason, have guarded their right to be the sole determiner of patient care. Today, however, as health care becomes increasingly complex, no one person can keep abreast of all information and developments that might benefit any given patient. Similarly, rapid advances in clinical laboratory technology have made it nearly impossible for physicians and other health-care providers to stay abreast of available tests and their implications for diagnosis and treatment. The clinical laboratory scientist is a natural link between the clinical laboratory and other providers or patients on matters of test selection, specimen collection, interpretation of test results in light of specimen quality and sources of interference, and patient education. Laboratory professionals are expected to provide information, solve problems, analyze situations, and implement decisions related to laboratory testing.

Participating in the process of ordering tests and interpreting and correlating test results requires a new cooperative relationship between physicians and the clinical laboratory scientist. Physicians must be willing to share this responsibility and accept advice; laboratory scientists must be able to acknowledge appropriate boundaries. Each professional must recognize the other's expertise and complement each other's abilities to best benefit the patient. This is, in fact, the essence of the consulting relationship. Separating the activities that are the practice of medicine, and therefore the exclusive right of the physician, from those that are not is the challenge.

The laboratory scientist is qualified to provide assistance and guidance to physicians and other health-care professionals as they establish or use clinical laboratories in private practice settings. The broad-based education of clinical laboratory scientists in all aspects of laboratory practice prepares them to act as evaluators and problem solvers for health-care professionals whose expertise is in other areas of patient care. In this way, consultation has emerged as an important role for the clinical laboratory scientist.

CONSULTANT ROLES

A consultant is a person with recognized expertise in a given discipline who is asked by a client to apply that expertise to a given situation. Consultants are found in virtually every segment of industry, education, government, and health care. They may be employed by the organization they consult for, or they may be brought into the organization for a specific purpose. Clients may be physicians, other health-care providers, patients, organizations, or agencies. Many clients are unsure about their need for help and reluctant to ask for assistance even with their most important problems. When clients do ask for help, consultants must be particularly sensitive and respond skillfully to clients' implied as well as stated needs.

The Internal Consultant

An internal consultant is employed by the organization for which he consults. An example of this arrangement is the clinical laboratory scientist employed by a teaching hospital who attends patient rounds in order to consult with physicians on selecting laboratory tests. The internal consultant role is one that usually does not require the establishment of a formal consultant-client relationship each time service is provided, but all other responsibilities described below apply. When clinical laboratory scientists who are internal consultants earn the respect of their colleagues in the organization, they often become essential participants on the health-care team.

The consultant within the hospital environment can function in a variety of ways to improve patient care and enhance the efficiency of the facility. One important activity that should be increased is the clinical laboratory scientist's involvement in interpreting and integrating laboratory data in the management of the patient's condition. Too often the role of the laboratory has been perceived to begin with receipt of a specimen and end with reporting of a result.

Laboratory professionals should be involved in ordering tests. What test will provide the most information? What type of specimen should be obtained? Under what conditions should the specimen be collected? When and how often? Involvement in discussions with physicians about the patient's situation could avoid delays and inadequate or inappropriate samples, reduce the patient's trauma due to unnecessary venipunctures, and improve the cost effectiveness of patient care.

The laboratory's responsibility does not end when an accurate test value is obtained. The clinical laboratory scientist must ensure that the physician, nurse, therapist, pharmacist, or other health-care provider understands the *meaning* of the results. The care these persons give depends on such understanding. Whether the test results are inconclusive or appropriate, subsequent steps are indicated; the laboratory scientist should discuss these steps with the physician or follow up with institutionally sanctioned protocols.

Management within the institution is another vital consultant role. In addition to the usual staffing, budgeting, purchasing, and communications areas, the laboratory consultant can provide important input in collective bargaining, Equal Employment Opportunities Commission (EEOC) guidelines, and legal requirements. The laboratory practitioner may become the institution's expert in any one of a number of management arenas and provide expert advice to other units of the hospital. Opportunities exist, and there is a need for such individuals.

Another aspect of management includes institutional information systems. The selection, purchase, and use of a computer system and decisions concerning access to information, input to the data base, and direct lines of communication should include the clinical laboratory scientist. Factors such as system flexibility for management and educational purposes will affect that system's cost effectiveness.

Providing in-service education is another frequently overlooked consultative role. Health care is constantly undergoing rapid change, and all practitioners must maintain their competence by attending in-service education for laboratory personnel and providing programs for other health-care professionals as well. Instruction on new tests, new equipment, modified procedures, cautions, and complications is needed. The laboratory consultant should serve this role and meet this need.

Patients are increasingly involved in their own health care and becoming interested in all aspects of health. Information required to foster health-promoting behavior or enable the patient to provide self-care can and should be communicated by the clinical laboratory scientist. Patient education on the meaning of laboratory tests, *why* they are performed, and, in some instances, *how* they are performed is the laboratory scientist's responsibility. More frequent patient–clinical laboratory scientist interaction is necessary to generate trust.

The laboratory professional is qualified to serve as a consultant to risk management, infection control, patient relations, respiratory care, and nuclear medicine. Assuming this consultative role, however, means leaving the laboratory and becoming involved in general institutional affairs. It means volunteering for additional responsibility. See page 6 for an example of a position description for an internal consultant.

The External Consultant

An external consultant has a private consulting business or at least does not work in the client's organization. External consultants are hired to perform a specific function agreed on in advance. Generally, when the consultation has been completed, the consultant has no further ties to the client or the client's organization. The expectations of both client and consultant are detailed in an initial letter of agreement or contract. The relationship usually terminates when the consultant delivers the final report and recommendations.

The clinical laboratory scientist who becomes an external consultant has, in effect, started a business. Just as in any other business venture, the consultant must recognize legal limits of liability and function competently within those limits. The possibility of incorporation should be investigated. Some amount of venture capital will be needed to purchase liability (malpractice) insurance, business cards, office supplies and equipment, and a telephone answering machine or service. The clinical laboratory scientist starting a consulting business might find it helpful to take advantage of some of the many books and workshops available to assist individuals who wish to start a small business.

In short, consultation outside of the hospital is a

Sample Position Description: Internal Consultant

Position title: Laboratory Information Officer
Qualifications: Bachelor's degree in clinical laboratory science, certification plus appropriate advanced degree (e.g., M.S., M.B.A.; M.S. in related scientific discipline; Ph. D)
Good communications and interpersonal skills
Five years of experience in clinical laboratory science

General Responsibilities

The individual fulfilling this role will be responsible for providing information concerning the laboratory's services to physicians, nurses, therapists, other health-care providers, and patients. This information may include ordering specific tests, interpreting test results, correlating test data from various sections of the laboratory, preparing patients for testing, performing appropriate follow-up procedures, and describing expected results following therapy. Information will also be technical, such as the time needed to perform specific tests and the nature of the specimens required. The position also carries responsibility for follow-up of problems associated with venipuncture and other specimen collection techniques.

Specific Duties

1. Daily patient rounds to respond to questions raised during phlebotomy
2. Participation in grand rounds
3. Responding to telephone inquiries about laboratory services
4. Monitoring ordering patterns for efficiency and cost effectiveness
5. Working with human resources department to provide educational programs for patients and other health care professionals
6. Working with risk management department to identify, prevent, or solve problems related to the laboratory
7. Communicating with the originating site when inappropriate specimens are received in the laboratory
8. Providing information to laboratory personnel on changes in practice, trends, and new methods
9. Other communication as necessary to ensure maximal efficient use of the laboratory service

growing opportunity for laboratory practitioners. Many institutions, organizations, industrial firms, and insurance companies require the information that can be provided by a laboratory scientist. The establishment of small independent laboratories and physician office laboratories is increasing. Experts are needed to assist in the development of these facilities. Laboratory owners need advice on the following:

1. Test menu
2. Equipment
3. Cost/fees
4. Staffing

5. Hours of operation
6. Legal requirements
7. Quality control
8. Methodology
9. Space requirements/physical layout

Individuals with knowledge and experience in these areas can perform an invaluable service. Perhaps the fastest growing segment of the laboratory marketplace is over-the-counter testing. It is predicted that as many tests will be performed by clients in their own homes by 1990 as are performed within laboratory facilities. Individuals interested in monitoring their own health through self-testing need advice on which tests to purchase, how to perform the procedure, how to interpret the results, and when to seek further assistance from their physician. Working with the pharmacist, the clinical laboratory scientist can provide this consultation.

Consultants to industry on laboratory equipment and supplies, services to laboratories by industry, and new research avenues are needed. Experienced laboratory practitioners are in the best position to offer such consultation. Consultants to community groups on the development of health-promotion and disease-prevention programs are frequently sought. Laboratory practitioners must step forward to fulfill this need. Consultants to the media for health-related programming and articles are valued contributors to these activities. Again, the expertise of the laboratory professional could be useful.

Numerous opportunities exist for clinical laboratory scientists to serve as consultants. The only limitations are those that they place on themselves.

CONSULTANT RESPONSIBILITIES

The wide variety of potential consultant roles for the clinical laboratory scientist makes it difficult to state a set of responsibilities that apply to all situations. A consultant must be an expert, a planner, an analyzer, an independent thinker, a problem solver, and, above all, a master of interpersonal relations. The consultant's "stock in trade" is the ability to analyze problems quickly and thoroughly and propose potential solutions to clients in such a way that the solutions appear to emerge naturally as the interaction proceeds. It is not unusual for the problem identified by the client to be overshadowed by a more significant and complex one. Thus, the consultant must explore and identify all facets of the problem thoroughly before attempting to suggest a solution. Solving the wrong problem or recommending a solution to the right problem that will not be implemented is not helpful to any client. Much of the value of a consultant lies in the expertise to identify and define accurately the real problems and needs of clients and to resolve these needs. General consulting functions are discussed below; however, any given consultation dictates the function indicated. Informal, internal consultation with attending physicians about the ordering of laboratory tests obviously does not require the same level of activity as formal, external consulting.

Providing Information

The most common function of a consultant is to provide information to clients. Information is often all a client wants. Consultants should always determine what relevant information is already available on a problem before attempting to collect more data or even provide more information from their own background and experience. The consultant must understand exactly why certain information is important to the client and how the client wishes to use that information.

Consultants must clearly identify their clients' needs. This exploration may result in the asking of questions that appear impertinent or irrelevant by both consultants and clients, but they are often necessary to elicit information to meet underlying needs and triangulate data for actual problem identification.

Providing information to clients may require surveys, cost studies, feasibility studies, or just using one's expertise and background in the field to provide up-to-date information. Sometimes, however, the information the client really needs to address differs from the information the consultant is asked to provide. For example, an owner of a physician office laboratory asked a consultant to solve a technical problem that was resulting in incorrect laboratory findings. Upon investigation, the consultant found that the problem was a lack of proper personnel training, not technical difficulties with the equipment or reagents.

At the beginning of a consultation, a client may ask a seemingly simple question and expect to receive a simple answer within a short time. Simple questions can often have complex answers. A thorough investigation is required to determine the scope of the problem. Keep clients apprised of complexities and any delays encountered during the consultation process so that they can determine how far they are willing to go to pursue the answer to the question. At times, the answer may not be worth the client's time, effort, and money required to find it.

Often clients need only to make better use of available data to answer questions and solve problems. A consultant who wishes to develop an ongoing relationship with a client will find that helping a client to use available information to solve problems quickly and inexpensively can establish a high level of confidence and trust in the consultant's abilities.

Consultants must remember that they function at the client's pleasure, although not as his subordinate. Health-care professionals who are consultants often have difficulty stopping work on a problem before an acceptable solution is reached. Although that characteristic is laudable, it is not always appropriate in a consultation. Information gathered and shared may never be used by the client, no matter how accurate and appropriate it may be for solving the problem. The client may determine that the consultation is over just as the consultant was on the verge of acquiring the requested information. The consultant may regard the client as applying the information inappropriately. The consultant has no control over these client actions and no responsibility for their results. Consultants are responsible for keeping accurate and complete records of their activities and presenting a written report of results and recommendations.

Identifying and Solving Problems

Clients will sometimes approach consultants with a problem they want solved. For example, a group of physicians wishing to set up a laboratory in their private practice may engage a laboratory scientist as a consultant to determine what tests would be cost effective for them to do in-house, what space and equipment they will need, and what staff will be necessary to perform the testing. Or, a laboratory manager may ask a consultant how to restructure the laboratory to adapt to changes in technology, or the best way to decrease staff levels in response to a hospital administration's demand to cut costs.

Seeking solutions to such problems is certainly an appropriate function for a consultant laboratory scientist; however, it is the consultant's responsibility to determine the overall extent of the problem before attempting to solve it. Relevant questions to ask may include the following:

- What attempts have been made to solve the problem? With what results?
- Does the client have a solution in mind that has not been tried?
- Are any related aspects of the client's business not going well?
- Who besides the client must accept the solution to the problem for it to be implemented?
- Does the client have any predetermined limitations such as space use or amount of money available?
- Do solutions exist that you know will not be implemented?

At the beginning of the consultation process it is wise to work with the problem *as it has been defined by the client.* At the same time, the consultant should look for underlying issues that might shed light on related factors or subjects that may be uncomfortable for the client to discuss openly. For example, the need for a group practice to set up its own laboratory may be a desire of one or two of the physicians in the group who want to "keep up with the Jones'," while the others are satisfied with the service they have been receiving from another laboratory. In this case, any solution recommended by the consultant that addresses the original question of setting up a laboratory will meet opposition from some of the physicians in the practice. A feasibility study of the costs and benefits of developing an in-house clinical laboratory might be a more appropriate activity for initially addressing the problem. Depending on the results of the feasibility study and their acceptance, the consultation may continue or end. This reshaping can emerge gracefully if the consultant is sensitive to underlying issues and skillful in communicating with the client.

The most valuable consultant is one who can determine the exact nature of a client's problem while being sensitive to the client's comfort. The process of having an "outsider" come into the organization to diagnose the nature of a problem can often create stress between the consultant and the client, even though the client has requested the consultation. Including the client in the exploration of the complexities of the problem is helpful, since a client who is actively involved in the process is more likely to discuss personal involvement with issues bearing on the problem and accept suggestions.

Making Recommendations

A formal consultation usually concludes with a written report summarizing the situation and recommending action. The consultant may also be asked to present an oral report. Written and oral reports should be accurate and concise representations of the information gathered and the analysis of the problem. Any recommendations should include alternative plans for action with an explanation of each alternative in terms of projected outcomes, costs, and benefits. In situations where a consultation consists of only a short discussion with a client and the providing of information without research, the consultant should follow up with a written report to the client. Written reports protect the consultant from potential misuse of the recommendations and provides the client with a written record for business and tax purposes. Even when consultations are provided informally and no charge is made for the service, good business practice dictates that a written report be prepared for the client.

If the consultant's recommendations are to be viewed as credible and have much chance of being implemented, the recommendations must be stated in such a way to demonstrate an in-depth knowledge of the problem and a sensitivity to the client's environment and constraints. All recommendations must be tailored to the client's specific ability to carry them out. A consistent, logical sequence of steps to solve a problem in one environment may not work in another. There will be situations where strong and unpopular recommendations must be made to ensure quality performance and improved patient care. Consultants should not skirt around the issue when these situations arise, or they will jeopardize any credibility that has been established with the client. However, if the client has been actively involved in the consulting process, the resulting recommendations are more likely to be implemented. Clients should not receive a surprise at the final report, particularly if it is a surprise they are not going to like.

Assisting with Implementation

Occasionally a consultant is asked to assist a client in implementing the recommended changes. Participation in the implementation of change represents a *modification* of the relationship between the client and the consultant. There is considerable debate about the appropriateness of this management role for a consultant. If there is already a manager in the organization, the potential for real conflict exists.

The extent of collaboration between client and consultant during consultation may set the tone for the continuation of the engagement into the implementation phase. If there was not a collaborative relationship during the consultation, then the client may only want to use the consultant's findings to implement unpopular decisions. On the other hand, if active collaboration was part of the consultation, then continuation into the implementation phase may be a natural progression for the consultant. The consultant knows better than anyone else how the recommendations were meant to be implemented and may bring new ways of problem solving and innovation into the work setting.

Preparation for Consulting

The preliminary preparation of a clinical laboratory scientist for a consulting role begins with entry-level professional education. It is at that time that theoretical concepts and their practical application in the field of clinical laboratory science come together to form the foundation for consulting expertise. The seasoning and new knowledge gained during several years of varied and increasingly responsible professional practice and the acquisition of advanced education in related aspects of practice round out the preparation for the substantive aspects of consulting. This preparation and its resultant professional expertise is only the first step to being a successful consultant. It is certainly an essential step, but expertise alone will not ensure success.

The consulting role requires that clinical laboratory scientists be able to sell their expertise. This entails marketing expertise, which, in turn, requires excellence in communications. The consultant must be able to gain the client's trust. In an ongoing relationship clients learn to trust consultants by relying on their past records of success with other clients. At the beginning, the consultant must convey self-confidence without appearing arrogant.

Dress and demeanor must be businesslike. Although physical appearance does not necessarily represent character and qualifications, we do know that appearance most assuredly makes up a substantial component of first impressions. There are many books available on appropriate dress for success in the business world, and anyone considering a consultant role would do well to read one. Adaptations may be appropriate for particular settings, but the pattern of dress should always be equivalent to that of the client.

Perhaps the most important preparation a consultant can have is in the area of communication. The ability to communicate effectively can compensate for shortcomings in the extent of a consultant's expertise. A client will often prefer to engage a consultant who is able to work quietly within the organization while solving a problem than one who solves the problem while destroying employee morale and upsetting the organization through inappropriate remarks.

Preparation in the area of communications can be direct, such as taking courses and participating in workshops, or it can be indirect, such as observing good communications and emulating those patterns in one's own behavior. It is helpful to obtain analysis and feedback from others. Identifying a friend or colleague to act as a sounding board or even as a mentor may be quite valuable.

Communication skills that are particularly important to consultants include listening, questioning, and conveying potentially disturbing information in ways that result in positive action. A consultant must demonstrate a style of communication that inspires confidence and promotes cooperation.

The successful consultant is one who is recommended for further consultations by satisfied clients. Word-of-mouth is not a replacement for marketing consultant services, but results do speak louder than promises. Building a satisfied clientele takes nurturing and follow through.

CONSULTING WITHIN ETHICAL AND LEGAL BOUNDARIES

One of the major dangers inherent in the consultative process is the possibility of going beyond one's abilities or the limit of one's legal and ethical boundaries. Care must be taken to ensure that no harm is caused through advice provided by a consultant. At the same time, the consultant should not be limited by tradition and past practice or constrained by fear.

The scope of practice for many health-care professionals is embodied within legal practice acts by state governments. In the absence of such acts for laboratory personnel in most states, the practitioner must rely on a code of ethics and the generally acknowledged scope of practice. The body of knowledge that has been delineated for the profession also represents an acceptable basis for establishing professional boundaries. Establishing the boundaries of one's expertise without infringing on the professional rights and responsibilities of others is perhaps one of the most difficult tasks of the consultant. In this arena there is no substitute for experience.

Several moral/ethical problems that face the individual wishing to be a consultant are described below. Appropriate answers to the questions raised must be found within consultants' knowledge and expertise as well as their individual value systems.

Confidentiality

The confidential nature of patient information is not new to the laboratory scientist; however, there are additional dimensions to this problem for the consultant. When participating in decisions concerning the ordering of tests and the preparation of patients for testing, how much information is acceptable to release concerning another patient to illustrate a situation? Is it ethical to share knowledge gained in one consultative role in another? Is personal information gained about employees during the data-gathering phase of a consultation confidential or can or should it be shared with the employer?

Client-Consultant Relationship

It is clear that the success of a consultation depends on pleasing the client; however, consultants must determine how far they wish to go in assisting the client in meeting their objective. Does the consultant have a moral obligation to withdraw from a relationship if it becomes clear that the client is using the process purely for personal gain? How does the consultant avoid the problem of providing a report that simply mimics the client's wishes rather than providing an in-depth analysis of the problem? Is the consultant obliged to provide information to others in the client's organization if there is reason to believe that they require such information but are unlikely to obtain it from the client?

Compliance With Rules and Regulations

The entire health-care delivery system, including laboratories, is heavily regulated by both voluntary and governmental rules. Many times these rules place extra burdens on a facility for personnel, process, and physical requirements. Avoiding or circumventing the regulations may be the intent of clients as they employ a consultant. Experience gained through years of practice or superior knowledge of the rules may provide the consultant with information that although technically within the law, will allow the client to diminish the impact of the regulation. Is it ethical to participate in this process?

Inside Information

A laboratory scientist with an active consulting practice may at some time provide consultation for organizations or institutions that are competitors. So as not to violate a confidence, care must be taken to avoid using inside information to the new client's competitive advantage. In developing a marketing plan for laboratory services for one client, how does the consultant avoid the use of inside information concerning the weaknesses of a competitor who had been a former client?

These are by no means all the ethical questions that may arise in the course of consultation activities; however, they illustrate the variety of issues that must be carefully and thoughtfully considered by the consultant. No amount of scientific and technical expertise will make up for casual ethics or lack of knowledge about the legal parameters relevant to the laboratory.

BIBLIOGRAPHY

Dutton R: Procedures for designing an occupational therapy consultation contract. AJOT 40:160–166, 1986

Ellis JA, Helbig S: The Health Care Consultant as a Change Agent. Chicago, American Medical Record Association, 1981

Helbig S, Ellis JA: A Selected and Annotated Bibliography for Consultants in the Health Care Field, Chicago, American Medical Record Association, 1980

Siver EW: The 10 commandments for choosing and using consultants. Risk Management June, pp 64–74, 1983

Turner A: Consulting is more than giving advice. Howard Business Review, September/October, pp 120–129, 1982

Zielke EA: Full-time consulting: The business of starting a business. J Am Med Rec Assoc, October pp 32–39, 1982

Part II

CARDIOVASCULAR DISORDERS

Karen Karni, Associate Editor

Diseases of the heart and blood vessels, cardiovascular diseases (CVD), account for almost half of all deaths in the United States. Most are related to one type of arteriosclerosis—atherosclerosis. The most frequent cause of CVD death is heart attack (55%), followed by stroke (16%), hypertensive disease (3%), and rheumatic fever and rheumatic heart disease (1%). It is thought that 63 million Americans have one or more forms of CVD, with 58 million having high blood pressure. According to the American

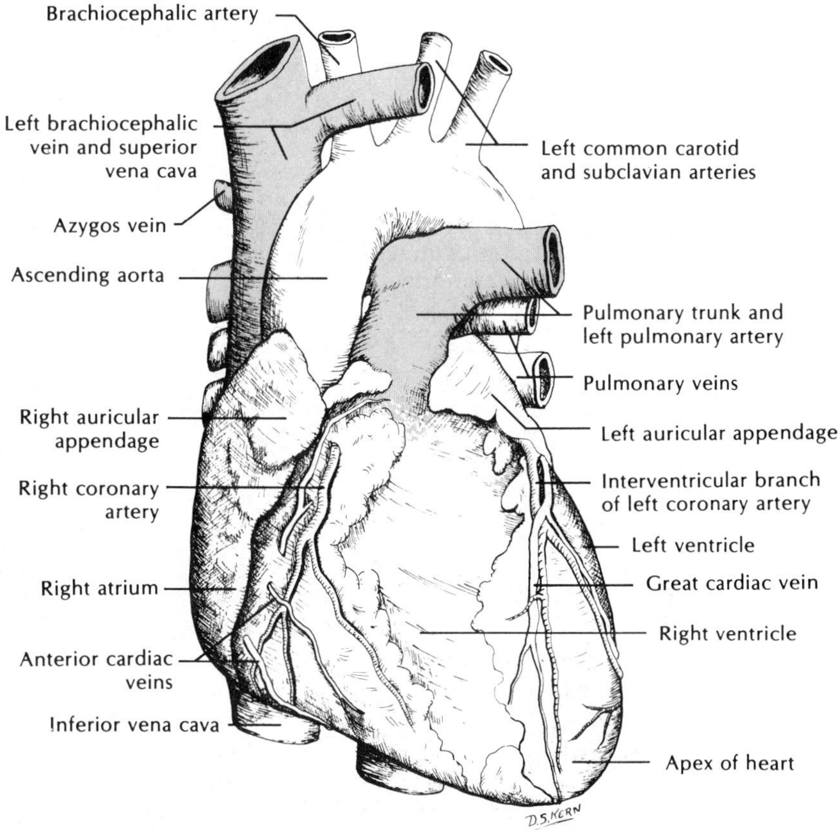

Anterior aspect of the heart. (Christensen JB, Telford IR: Synopsis of Gross Anatomy With Clinical Correlations, 5th ed, p 123. Philadelphia, JB Lippincott, 1988)

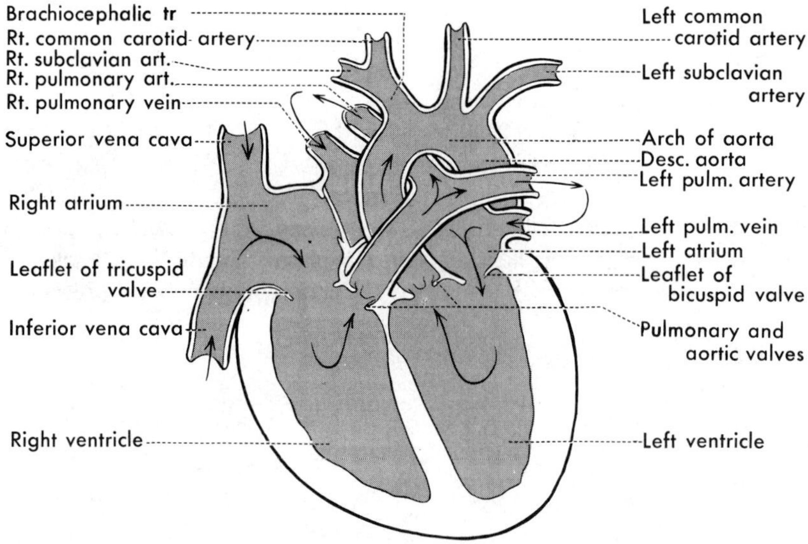

Diagram of the heart and the great vessels connected to it. Arrows indicate the directions of blood flow. (Hollinshead WH, Rosse C: Textbook of Anatomy, 4th ed. p 78. Philadelphia, JB Lippincott, 1985)

Heart Association, the cost of CVD in 1987 was estimated at $85.2 billion, including hospital and physician costs, nursing services, medications, and lost productivity.

Disruption of cardiac function is one of the more serious medical emergencies and requires prompt, effective action by health-care professionals. This section includes those cardiovascular disorders in which the clinical laboratory plays a vital role at some point in the course of the disease. The various features of the heart discussed in this section are diagrammed in the illustrations on page 15 and above. It should be recalled that the heart is contained within the *pericardium,* a layered sac containing a small amount of serous fluid that permits the heart to move freely within the sac.

BIBLIOGRAPHY

American Heart Association: 1987 Heart Facts. Dallas, The American Heart Association, 1987

Department of Health and Human Services: Vital and Health Statistics, Series 10, No. 160. National Centers for Health Statistics, U.S. Public Health Service, 1985

Chapter 2

Myocardial Infarction

Bethany W. Hurtuk

ETIOLOGY AND PATHOPHYSIOLOGY

In the majority of cases an acute myocardial infarction (AMI) is the result of reduced blood supply to some area of myocardial tissue, caused by atherosclerosis. In addition, some sudden event such as coronary thrombosis may unfavorably alter the already precarious balance between myocardial oxygen demand and need in the atherosclerotic patient. Alternatively, the myocardial supply of oxygen in a patient with insignificant atherosclerosis may be suddenly reduced by a superimposed occlusive thrombosis or vasospasm. Whatever the sequence of events, as the blood flow decreases, the myocardium becomes ischemic and eventually necrotic.

At the cellular level biochemical changes occur when blood flow to the myocardium decreases. Aerobic glucose metabolism is replaced by the Embden-Meyerhoff pathway. Pyruvate, the end product of the anaerobic glucose metabolism, is reduced to lactate, which begins to accumulate. To provide the energy needed, myocardial uptake of glucose increases, resulting in increased glycogenolysis, which leads to more pyruvate that is converted to lactic acid. The result is intracellular acidosis, which decreases glycolysis. Also, free fatty acids cannot be oxidized and, instead, tend to accumulate in the cells.[1]

Loss of the energy necessary to maintain ionic equilibrium of the myocardial cell membrane results in ionic changes within the cell that cause loss of cellular integrity. Sodium accumulates, and potassium is lost. With the increased sodium comes an influx of chloride, and the cell begins to swell.[1]

Hence, as ischemia progresses, anatomical changes are observable at the cellular level. The mitochondria swell, the myofibrils become stretched, and in the sarcolemma there are areas of separation. The cell membrane is damaged.[1] Ultimately, the infarction occurs, the myocardial cells are no longer intact, and cellular contents appear in the general circulation.

CLINICAL MANIFESTATIONS

A patient who experiences AMI may have a history of angina or central chest pain or pressure that begins during a period of exertion and subsides when the activity is stopped. The pain usually lasts a few minutes. As narrowing of the arteries becomes more severe, the pain may occur at rest. Eventually blood supply ceases, resulting in myocardial infarction.

A deep heavy pain in the center of the chest is the most frequent complaint of individuals suffering from AMI. The pain commonly begins when the patient is resting, but if it begins during activity, stopping the activity does not relieve the pain. Anxiety, sweating, nausea, vomiting, and weakness usually accompany the pain, and pallor may also occur in conjunction with coolness of the extremities. In an attempt to relieve the pain, the patient may squirm and stretch in bed. In 15% to 20% of cases pain is absent; however, the patient may experience confusion, loss of consciousness, arrhythmia, a sensation of profound weakness, or a drop in arterial blood pressure. In elderly individuals a sudden onset of breathlessness, often progressing to pulmonary edema, is common.[2]

LABORATORY ANALYSES AND DIAGNOSIS

Even though physical examination may provide enough evidence to diagnose a myocardial infarction, other confirmatory tests may be helpful, particularly the electrocardiogram (ECG), blood tests for evidence of tissue necrosis, and elevations in some serum enzyme levels. An ECG characteristic of AMI would show pathologic Q waves and ST-segment and T-wave changes. However, such an ECG may not be present in patients with AMI and should therefore not be used alone for diagnosis.[2]

Tissue necrosis in AMI is evident with the presence of polymorphonuclear leukocytosis. This reaction appears a few hours after the onset of pain and lasts for 3 to 7 days. The leukocyte level often reaches $12.0-15.0 \times 10^3/mm^3$, with higher levels being associated with larger infarcts. The erythrocyte sedimentation rate also rises but more slowly than the leukocyte count and may stay elevated for 1 to 2 weeks.[2]

Enzymes that are present in high concentrations in cardiac cells and that are released into the general circulation with cellular necrosis are the primary laboratory analytes used to identify AMI. Following AMI, each enzyme that appears in the serum in increased amounts does so for a certain time period, depending on the size of the enzyme and its half-life in the blood stream. Smaller enzymes enter the general circulation sooner than larger enzymes as the integrity of the cellular membrane deteriorates. The pattern of serum enzyme elevation aids in both diagnosis and monitoring of the infarction (Fig. 2-1). The serum enzyme levels roughly depend on the extent of cellular damage.[2, 3] Once the damage has occurred, the rise and eventual decrease in enzyme levels are helpful in monitoring patient recovery and ensuring that another infarction has not occurred. Successful treatment aids recovery and prevents further infarction but does not quicken return of enzyme levels to normal. The specific enzymes that may elevate and at which time intervals they may elevate are outlined in the following discussion.

Creatine Kinase

Creatine kinase (CK) is the first enzyme to show a serum elevation following AMI, with elevation onset 4 to 8 hours after infarction, a peak 12 to 24 hours following infarction, and a duration of 3 to 4

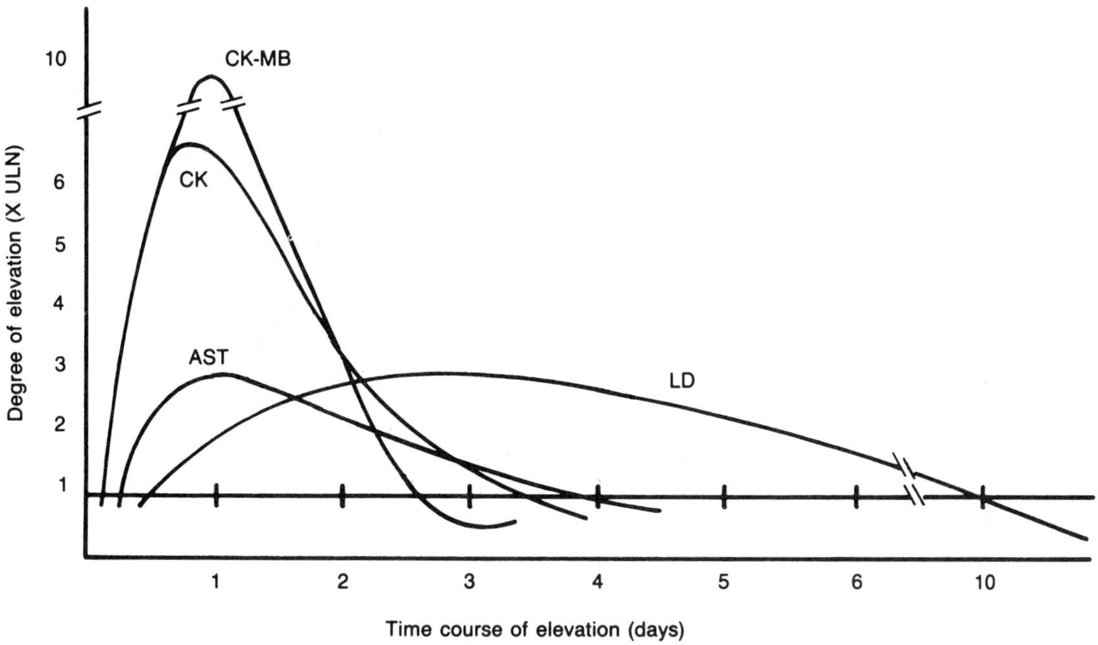

Figure 2-1 **Time activity curves of CK, CK-MB, and LD following acute myocardial infarction. CK (more specifically CK-MB) increases initially, followed by AST and LD. (From Bishop ML, Duben-Von Laufen JL, Fody EP [eds]: Clinical Chemistry, p 233. Philadelphia, JB Lippincott, 1985)**

days (see Fig. 2-1). The enzyme may be elevated from five to ten times normal. An elevation of more than eight times normal is usually related to a serious infarct with a risk of mortality.

Since CK is present in body tissues other than the heart, several other abnormalities may result in elevations of total CK; therefore, measurement of total CK is not as sensitive an indicator of AMI as is the isoenzyme of CK, CK-MB. The isoenzyme is found mostly in the heart and is responsible for most of the increase in the total CK in AMI (see Fig. 2-1). A CK-MB increase of at least 6%, together with other enzyme increases, is a reliable indication that AMI has occurred. It is believed that the grams of infarcted tissue can be estimated by analyzing the CK-MB time curve.[2] CK-MB is especially useful in differentiating AMI from a pulmonary embolism, which causes symptoms similar to those of AMI. CK-MB is usually normal following a pulmonary embolism.[3]

There are other instances in which CK-MB is elevated, but the patient has not suffered AMI. Angina pectoris and coronary insufficiency result in elevated CK-MB, as do coronary bypass surgery and electrical cardioversion.[2, 3]

Aspartate Aminotransferase

The second enzyme to show a serum elevation following AMI is aspartate aminotransferase (AST), which begins to elevate 8 to 12 hours and peaks at 24 hours following the infarction (see Fig. 2-1). AST is usually elevated 2 to 3 times the reference range when peaked and remains elevated for about 5 days. An AST level more than five times the reference range increases the risk of mortality.

AST levels should not be used to aid in the diagnosis of myocardial infarction without the other enzyme levels discussed in this chapter, because several pathological conditions also result in AST elevations. These include (1) right ventricular failure with hepatic congestion, (2) cardiac operations, (3) acute pancreatitis, (4) pregnancy-induced hypertension (toxemia of pregnancy), (5) infarction of intestine, kidney, or spleen, (6) burns or crush injuries, (7) hypothyroidism, (8) primary muscle disease, (9) hemolytic crisis, (10) extensive central nervous system damage, and (11) administration of opiates, salicylates, or warfarin-type anticoagulants.[2]

Lactate Dehydrogenase

Following AMI, lactate dehydrogenase (LD) is the last enzyme to show serum elevation. LD also remains elevated longer than either CK or AST (see Fig. 2-1). The elevation begins 12 to 24 hours after the infarction, peaks at 72 hours at 2 to 3 times the reference range, and remains elevated for about 10 days. Hence LD measurements are useful for detecting an infarction that occurred more than 4 days before enzyme analysis, after CK and AST levels have already returned to normal. However, since LD is present in several different parts of the body, an increase in total LD is not indicative of AMI.

To aid in the diagnosis of AMI, LD isoenzyme analysis may be performed. After AMI the LD-1 isoenzyme increases, often to a level higher than that of LD-2 (LD-2 is usually higher than LD-1), a situation commonly called a "flipped" LD pattern. LD-1 may be elevated with no increase in the total LD and is said to have a sensitivity of more than 95% as an indicator of AMI.[2] Especially in conjunction with increased CK-MB levels (discussed above), the "flipped" LD is indicative of AMI. The LD pattern may also be "flipped" in cases of renal cortex infarct, megaloblastic anemia, and intravascular hemolysis, but the CK-MB is not elevated in these instances.

Since each enzyme that elevates does so within its own characteristic time frame, it is recommended that laboratory analyses for diagnosis of AMI be performed as a "cardiac profile." Blood samples should be collected initially and then at specific intervals, usually every 12 hours for the next 48-hour period, and the enzymes that may increase in AMI should be quantitated on each sample. The enzyme analyses that may be performed without delay will depend on the services available in the laboratory. For example, isoenzyme tests are often not available at night. Total AST, CK, and LD levels are usually considered adequate for making immediate decisions regarding patient care. However, the CK-MB level and later the LD-1 level and LD-1/LD-2 provide more sensitive information to confirm or rule out the diagnosis of AMI.

OTHER RELATED LABORATORY FINDINGS

Even though the enzymes discussed in this chapter are the primary laboratory analyses that aid the physician in diagnosing AMI, several other laboratory findings are affected as well. Myoglobin, a protein found in muscles, is elevated early and briefly following myocardial infarction. Hence, myoglobin levels are helpful for early detection of AMI. However, because there are significant amounts of myoglobin in skeletal muscle, the specificity of the analyte is low, so CK or CK-MB levels are preferred instead of myoglobin levels.[4]

Arterial blood gases may also appear abnormal following AMI. Hypoxemia, a deficiency of oxygen, is the condition usually found and is caused by poor aeration of the lung bases. Hence, oxygen therapy is provided to minimize myocardial damage at the location of the infarct, and arterial blood gases are frequently analyzed to verify adequate oxygenation.[5]

Certain serum lipoprotein levels may be altered by AMI. Specifically, there is an immediate 10% to 60% decrease in low-density lipoprotein levels and a gradual increase in very-low-density lipoprotein levels over a 10-to 30-day period following the infarction.[5]

TREATMENT

When AMI is suspected, prompt and effective treatment is necessary to minimize the mass of infarcted tissue and prevent death due to arrhythmia. Hence, treatment may be initiated on the basis of clinical manifestations before other test results are obtained. One important goal of treatment is to save the infarcted area by maintaining a balance between supply and demand of oxygen to the myocardium. Appropriate therapy includes relief of pain, rest, sedation, and a quiet atmosphere to lower the heart rate and thus reduce oxygen consumption. Additionally, oxygen is usually given to raise the arterial Po_2. Morphine to relieve the pain and chlordiazepoxide or diazepam for sedation are commonly prescribed. When arrhythmias are present, additional medication such as procainamide, lidocaine, or quinidine is prescribed. In the presence of heart failure a digitalis glycoside, usually digoxin, is given. For infarcts caused by an occlusive thrombus near an atherosclerotic plaque in a coronary artery, a thrombolytic agent such as streptokinase is indicated. Other medications may also be given, depending on the patient's specific condition.[2, 4]

CASE STUDY

A 58-year-old, heavy-set man had been shoveling snow in his driveway. A neighbor noticed the man lying on the ground as though he had fainted or fallen and hit his head. The neighbor called for help and began cardiopulmonary resuscitation. The patient was taken to the hospital and admitted.

Questions

1. What is one of the most common disorders that the patient might have suffered besides a blow on the head?
2. What laboratory test might be done initially to help diagnose the patient's condition?
3. What should the physician do if the laboratory test referred to in question #2 is normal?

Discussion

1. The patient may have suffered a myocardial infarction. Shoveling snow is one of the most strenuous tasks someone who is susceptible to a myocardial infarction may undertake. A middle-aged overweight man may have a tendency for atherosclerosis.
2. A CK isoenzyme analysis would be very helpful. Evidence of a cerebral accident might show as an increase in CK-BB, while evidence of a myocardial infarction might show as an increase in CK-MB.
3. A "cardiac profile" should be ordered a few hours after the patient has arrived at the hospital and again 24 hours later. From the repeated testing the physician may observe the typical increases and decreases in enzymes following a myocardial infarction.

REFERENCES

1. Braunwald E (ed): Heart Disease: A Textbook of Cardiovascular Medicine. Philadelphia, WB Saunders, 1980
2. Petersdorf RG, Adams AD, Braunwald E et al (eds): Harrison's Principles of Internal Medicine, 10th ed. New York City, McGraw-Hill, 1983
3. Bishop ML, Duben-Von Laufen JL, Fody EP (eds): Clinical Chemistry Principles, Procedures, Correlations. Philadelphia, JB Lippincott, 1985
4. Kaplan LA, Pesce AJ: Clinical Chemistry Theory, Analysis, and Correlation. St. Louis, CV Mosby, 1984
5. Henry JB: Clinical Diagnosis and Management by Laboratory Methods. Philadelphia, WB Saunders, 1984

Chapter 3

Infectious Processes

V. Michelle Chenault

The infectious processes of the cardiovascular system include pericarditis, myocarditis, endocarditis, and rheumatic heart disease. These conditions are often caused by the same organisms, and it may be difficult to differentiate one disorder from another. To further complicate diagnosis and treatment, disorders may occur concomitantly or sequentially (*e.g.*, rheumatic heart disease and bacterial endocarditis).

ETIOLOGY AND PATHOPHYSIOLOGY

Pericarditis

The pericardium is a serous membrane composed of a single inner layer of mesothelial cells and a fibrous outer layer. These two layers, visceral and parietal, respectively, surround the heart and have a number of functions, including holding the heart in its fixed anatomical position and minimizing friction between the heart and surrounding tissues.[1]

Pericarditis is the term applied to any alteration of the pericardium, whether inflammatory or infectious. Pericarditis can result from therapeutic agents, uremia, connective tissue diseases, malignant diseases, or autoimmune diseases as well as from infection. Several other causes exist and the acute and chronic syndromes have some degree of overlap.

Acute pericarditis lasts a few weeks and may be due to a number of causes listed on page 24. The disorder may be associated with accumulation of a pericardial effusion.

Chronic pericarditis lasts for 6 months or more, and certain chronic infections such as tuberculosis and chronic renal insufficiency are possible causes. Effusive, fibrous adhesive, chylous, or calcific pericarditis disorders are more prone to be manifested in a chronic form.

Infections may spread to the pericardium through the blood stream, a contiguous infection, a penetrating trauma, infective endocarditis, rupture of a hepatic abscess through the diaphragm, or an esophagopericardial fistula.

Most pericardial infections, including viral infections and, most commonly, tuberculous infections, are followed by constrictive pericarditis. Constrictive pericarditis may also follow idiopathic pericarditis, connective tissue disease, trauma (including surgery), neoplastic diseases, and radiation therapy.

Constrictive pericarditis results when the healing of an acute fibrinous or serofibrinous pericarditis is followed by the destruction of the pericardial cavity. The heart is encased in a tissue that forms a firm scar and contracts, interfering with the filling of the ventricles during diastole. Immunosuppressive therapy, cardiovascular surgery, and hemodialysis have also been associated with bacterial pericarditis.

Although bacterial pericarditis is uncommon in very young children, it appears to be more common in children than adults. The prognosis is poor and the mortality is high, especially in infants less than 1 year of age.

In adult patients, the most common organisms found are *Staphylococcus aureus* followed by various streptococci. In pediatric patients, in addition to *S. aureus, Hemophilus influenzae* and meningococci are the most frequent etiologic agents. In infants and children under the age of 4 years, pneumococcal pericarditis is encountered as part of a generalized infection. With gram-negative organisms, multiple microbial infections are often seen.

Bacterial pericarditis is almost always purulent. The fluid accumulates rapidly in the sac and may cause obstruction to the inflow of blood to the ventricles (cardiac tamponade). The viral causes of pericarditis include Coxsackie A or B virus, influenza, mumps, chickenpox, herpes simplex, and others (see the display on page 24). By far the most common agents are the Coxsackie virus, especially group B. When the viral causative agent cannot be detected, a diagnosis of acute idiopathic or nonspecific pericarditis is often made. Except for firm identification of the virus, no features or clinical manifestations distinguish viral from bacterial etiology.

Viral pericarditis occurs most frequently in

Etiology of Pericarditis*

1. Idiopathic (nonspecific)
2. Connective tissue diseases and arthritis: rheumatic fever, scleroderma, rheumatoid arthritis, Takayasu's arteritis, polyarteritis nodosa, Wegener's granulomatosis, systemic lupus erythematosus
3. Uremia; also in association with hemodialysis
4. Acute bacterial infection: pneumococcus, staphylococcus, influenza bacillus, infective endocarditis, tularemia, meningococcemia, gonococcal septicemia
5. Trauma, including thoracic surgical procedures, diagnostic procedures, transvenous cardiac pacemaker insertion, nonpenetrating chest trauma
6. Tuberculosis
7. Fungus infections: *Candida,* histoplasmosis, blastomycosis, coccidioidomycosis, sporotrichosis
8. Radiation
9. Neoplastic disease
10. Drugs: e.g., hydralazine, psicofuranine, procainamide, isonicotinic acid hydrazide, anticoagulant therapy, penicillin, phenylbutazone, diphenylhydantoin, methysergide
11. Dissecting aortic aneurysm
12. Chylopericardium
13. Viral disease: e.g., Coxsackie A virus, Coxsackie B virus, infectious mononucleosis, adenovirus, echovirus, mumps virus
14. Protozoal infections: amebiasis, toxoplasmosis
15. Miscellaneous infections: actinomycosis, Reiter's syndrome, echinococcal disease, agents of the psittacosis-lymphopathia venereum group, mycoplasma, Behcet's syndrome, Whipple's disease, *Nocardia*
16. Miscellaneous: sarcoidosis, myxedema, amyloid disease, multiple myeloma, acute pancreatitis, esophageal-pericardial fistula, hypereosinophilic syndrome
17. Delayed postmyocardial-postpericardial-injury syndromes:
    (a) Postmyocardial infarction (Dressler's syndrome)
    (b) Postcardiotomy (postthoracotomy syndrome or postpericardiotomy syndrome)
    (c) Postcardiac trauma syndromes (penetrating and nonpenetrating trauma)
    (d) Postinfectious syndromes with viral infections; histoplasmosis; meningococcemia, gonococcemia

*Recurrent pericarditis is said to occur in 7% of patients with active chronic hepatitis. The cause of this disease is unknown. (Data from reference number[6])

young adults. It is often associated with pneumonitis and pleural effusions and runs its course in a few days to 2 weeks. Recurrences occur in about one-fourth of patients, but this tendency decreases within 2 years after the initial episode.

Fungal pericarditis is found in patients who have been extensively treated with immunosuppressive drugs or with prolonged courses of potent antibiotics. Pericarditis may also be caused by *Actinomyces israelii* and *Nocardia asteroides.* The anaerobic *A. israelii* thrives in necrotic tissue. The organism may be spread from the esophagus and mediastinum, a necrotic pulmonary focus, or an infected lesion in the mouth. It is almost invariably fatal. *Nocardia* may be a pathogen or an opportunistic organism. Patients may develop a constrictive pericarditis, or they may die of cerebral complications.

No mycobacteria other than *Mycobacterium tuberculosis* have been reported to cause pericarditis. Although the incidence of tuberculous pericarditis has declined in the last decade, it remains an important cause of pericarditis. The disorder usually accompanies tuberculosis elsewhere in the body, most commonly the lungs and predominantly affects males. Those with impaired immunologic defenses are also at great risk. Tuberculous pericarditis may also appear in patients with diabetes mellitus, abnormal plasma proteins, and chronic renal disease who are undergoing hemodialysis.

Pericarditis may also result from infection with *Entamoeba histolytica* when a hepatic abscess ruptures through the diaphragm into the pericardium. The pericardial fluid resembles "anchovy paste material,"[2] and the trophozoite of *E. histolytica* may be isolated from the fluid.

Myocarditis

The myocardium is the middle layer of the chambers of the heart and its thick contractile wall. Myocarditis is the focal or diffuse inflammatory process caused by infectious agents, chemical poisons, or hypersensitive states such as rheumatic fever.

Infectious myocarditis may be caused by any of the bacteria, viruses, fungal agents, rickettsia, protozoa, and metazoa. The most common infectious agents in the United States are viruses and include Group B Coxsackie, echovirus, influenza, polio, mumps, measles, and varicella viruses. Bacteria such as *Corynebacterium diphtheriae* and *Streptococcus pneumoniae* have also been implicated. Chagas' disease is a major cause of myocarditis in South America; however, the causative agent, *Trypanosoma cruzi,* is rare in the United States. Myocarditis caused by the Group B Coxsackie virus is most frequently associated with acute pericarditis, especially in infants.

Fungal myocarditis seen in patients receiving steroid, radiation, or immunosuppressive therapy or chemotherapy or those patients with lymphoma. The most common cause is *Candida.* Infections with *Candida* may be limited to the lining of the heart or be systemic with vascular involvement.

Toxoplasmosis, Chagas' disease, Trypanosomiasis, and malaria have in common parasitic agents that cause myocarditis (see Chapter 58).

Endocarditis

The chambers of the heart are lined by a thin, serous endothelial layer known as the *endocardium.* Endocarditis is an intravascular infection of the lining membrane of the heart, and valvular endocarditis is the term used to describe inflammation of only the membrane covering the valves. Inflammation of the general lining of the chambers of the heart is called *mural endocarditis.* The terms acute, subacute, and chronic (bacterial) endocarditis are no longer used because of confusion in the definitions and a lack of differences in the clinical presentation and bacteriology. In this chapter, the term *infectious endocarditis (IE)* will be used to describe infections of the heart valves and endocardium from bacterial, viral, fungal, and rickettsial agents.

Normally, the endothelial surface is resistant to microbial infection; however a nonbacterial thrombotic vegetation (NBTV) can be produced in the circulatory system in cases of endothelial damage or by hypercoagulability. It is found most often on the left side of the heart and the low-pressure side of the valves.[3] This distribution is similar to that found in infective endocarditis and rheumatic valvular lesions. Most of the endocardial intravascular infections are the result of microbial dissemination and proliferation within this platelet-fibrin vegetation.

The infection may be caused by normally indigenous organisms or highly pathogenic organisms. The course of the illness may be acute or chronic and is fatal unless treated. The source of infection is often unknown. However, alcoholics, drug addicts, and patients undergoing hemodialysis are especially susceptible. Also, patients who have undergone prosthetic valve surgery or open heart surgery and those with congenital heart defects have a particular predisposition to the incidence of IE. The mean age of the patients is 55 years with the advent of antibiotics. In the preantibiotic era, the mean age was 39 years. The disease is more common in men.

All valves (mitral, aortic, tricuspid, and pulmonary) may be involved, and valves damaged by arteriosclerosis, syphilis, and rheumatic fever are particularly susceptible. Organisms can enter the blood stream from the mouth, gastrointestinal tract, genitourinary tract, and cardiorenal system and from miscellaneous minor or severe infections.[4] The most common causative organisms of IE are staphylococci and streptococci.

Bacterial agents for IE are numerous and dependent on population and geography. In addition to streptococci and staphylococci other causative agents include *S. pneumoniae, Candida, Pseudomonas aeruginosa, Serratia marcescens,* and gram-negative bacilli such as *Hemophilus, Brucella, Bordetella, Francisella, Pasteurella,* and others such as *Aspergillus,* and *N. gonorrhea.* The association of these organisms with particular conditions is summarized in Table 3-1. IE is usually caused by only one organism; however, multiple microbial infections can occur in parenteral drug addicts or in patients who have undergone prosthetic valve surgery. Bacterial IE may recur within 4 weeks after treatment has been halted, but a new infectious agent may be the problem if infectious carditis occurs 6 weeks after treatment has stopped.

Table 3-1 ***Etiologic Associations of Endocarditis with Pathological Conditions***

Condition	Associated Bacterial Agent
Alcoholism	Pneumococcus
Septic thrombophlebitis Infected intravenous catheters Total parenteral nutrition Arteriovenous shunts Infection (cutaneous, bone, lung)	*Staphylococcus*
Bacteremia of streptococcal skin or puerperal infection	Group A streptococcus
Intravenous drug users or surgery (sutures or protheses)	Staphylococci, coliform bacilli, *Candida*
Males with prostatism or females with genitourinary tract infections	*Streptococcus fecalis* (enterococcus)
Dental manipulation or extraction	Viridans streptococci
Osteomyelitis	
Septic arthritis	

The causative agents of viral endocarditis include Coxsackie B and echovirus. Although they have produced endocardial lesions in humans, there is no evidence that vegetation, like that produced in bacterial endocarditis, is produced.

The infectious process of fungal endocarditis is usually fatal unless surgery for valve replacement is used with antifungal therapy. The most common fungal agent is *Candida albicans,* but other common agents include *Aspergillus* and *Histoplasma.*

The infections are opportunistic and may accompany diabetes mellitus, lymphoma, and leukemia and appear in patients taking antibiotics, cytotoxic drugs, and steroids. Drug addicts and patients who have had open heart surgery or previously diseased valves are also susceptible. The majority of the patients with fungal endocarditis have a large amount of vegetation causing valve dysfunction.

Rheumatic Heart Disease

Rheumatic valvular heart disease (RVHD) was one of the principal causes of death and disability in children and adolescents in the United States 30 years ago. Now its severity has lessened due to the use of antibiotics and better diagnostic techniques; however, in patients more than 40 and the elderly, it is a common cause of heart disease. The condition causes scarring and deformity of the heart valves.

The underlying cause is rheumatic fever, a severe inflammatory disease that occurs as the result of a group A hemolytic streptococcal infection.

All the layers of the heart (pericardium, myocardium, endocardium) may be involved in RVHD, and the term rheumatic pancarditis is used to describe this general involvement. Although group A streptococcal infections have long been associated with RVHD, the mechanism by which the crippling disorder affects heart tissue has not been totally elucidated. It is known, however, that throat infections initiate the process, that *Streptococcus* produces tissue-damaging exotoxins, and that immunologic phenomena are in some way involved. For example, human leukocyte antigens (HLA) have been shown to be involved in the pathogenesis of RVHD.

The course and clinical syndromes of RVHD vary, although carditis is the major manifestation. The consequences of chronic RVHD are aortic insufficiency, aortic stenosis, mitral insufficiency, or, most common in adults, mitral stenosis.

Rheumatic endocarditis most commonly involves the mitral valve. The endocardium thickens, and inflammatory cells and mucoid material accumulate; this leads to mitral or aortic regurgitation. This disorder progresses to the most severe form of permanent cardiac damage.

Rheumatic pericarditis produces effusion without constriction. In rheumatic myocarditis, the myocardium is thickened and small foci of necrosis (Aschoff bodies) can be seen in the tissue. These are only seen in rheumatic fever[5] and may be found in the tissue of patients years after the last attack. The disorder is difficult to distinguish from other causes of myocarditis and may actually be a pancarditis.

CLINICAL MANIFESTATIONS

Pericarditis

Fever, upper respiratory manifestations, and anorexia are the most common symptoms noted on admission. The diagnosis of infectious pericarditis should be considered in any patient with septicemia, an immunosuppressed state, or a recent cardiac operation with the symptoms described. Development of a pericardial friction rub, or ECG or radiologic changes of the pericardium also indicate this condition. Chest pain is absent in the majority of cases. The clinical features are summarized below.

Features of Bacterial Pericarditis

- Fever
- Chills
- Night sweats
- Dyspnea
- Cough
- Chest pain
- Tachycardia
- Pericardial rub
- Decreased blood pressure
- Pulsus paradoxus
- Elevated cardiovascular pressure
- Hepatomegaly

Adapted from reference number[6]

The seven major features of pericarditis are (1) pain over the precordium; (2) pericardial friction rub; (3) cardiac tamponade; (4) signs simulating right heart failure; (5) radiologic changes; (6) ECG changes; and (7) fever.[6] The most common symptoms are chest pain and a pericardial friction rub.[7] The pain associated with pericarditis can be dull or sharp and is aggravated by deep breathing, thoracic motion, coughing, or turning in bed.

Myocarditis

The signs or cardiovascular manifestations of viral myocarditis, the most common form of the disease, will not help the physician diagnose the specific causative virus. The initial symptoms in infants are nonspecific: lethargy, fever, and difficulty in feeding. Later symptoms include tachycardia, cyanosis, arrhythmias, cardiac enlargement, and heart failure. Adults experience chest pain, fatigue, palpitation, and dyspnea.

Endocarditis

Infectious endocarditis is a common cause of "fever of undetermined origin." Infectious endocarditis should be suspected in all patients with a fever, heart murmur, and anemia. In addition to fever, patients experience weakness, fatigue, weight loss, splenomegaly, cardiac murmurs, anemia, mucocutaneous petechiae, and emboli. The latter are pieces of fibrin that have separated from the site of infection and may involve the brain, spleen, kidney, gastrointestinal tract, heart, or extremities. Infectious aneurysms may be caused by emboli in the major arteries, and ruptures are fatal. Coronary emboli may cause myocardial infarctions. Although a myocardial infarction due to coronary emboli is clinically unusual, it is seen in 50% of the autopsies of patients who die of bacterial endocarditis. Cerebral emboli cause death in 50% to 80% of patients. The most common fatal complication is congestive heart failure due to valvular dysfunction.

Older patients and patients with extremely virulent causative agents develop neurological complications. This has been shown to be significant in about one-third of the patients who have infectious endocarditis, and a higher mortality rate is associated with this development.

Rheumatic Heart Disease

A heart murmur of the mitral or aortic valves may be the first sign of acute rheumatic carditis. Other signs are tachycardia, increased heart size, pericardial friction rub or effusion, and signs of congestive heart failure. Irregular movements of the facial muscles or limbs (Sydenham's chorea) may be one of the first signs prompting the physician to suspect carditis from RVHD. Some patients complain of joint pain (arthralgia).

LABORATORY ANALYSES AND DIAGNOSIS

Pericarditis

Diagnosis is confirmed by aspiration, examination, and culture of the pericardial fluid.

The following clinical laboratory findings are most useful. The white blood cell count is elevated but seldom exceeds $20.0 \times 10^3/mm^3$ and may be normal. The differential white blood cell count may show a modest increase of polymorphonuclear leukocytes. The erythrocyte sedimentation rate (ESR) is increased. The myocardial serum enzymes are usually normal. Blood cultures or cultures of the pericardial fluid may reveal the cause of pericarditis and should include methods to recover mycobacteria, fungi, and viruses. The pericardial fluid is usually clear but may be blood tinged. There is an increased number of white blood cells in the fluid, mostly lymphocytes. Chest x-ray films may detect evidence of tuberculosis or fungal disease. Lymph node enlargement, particularly in endemic areas, has been associated with a histoplasmosis infection of the pericardium. Complement fixation tests are used for *H. capsulatum.* These tests and the serological tests for viral disease are determined at 2- and 3-week intervals. Antinuclear antibody studies are useful to differentiate connective tissue disease causes of pericarditis from infectious causes.

Myocarditis

Although viral myocarditis is the most common form it is not always easy to identify the agent. Because the virus must be isolated early in the illness, the specimens commonly used are throat washings, feces, blood, pericardial fluid, or myocardial biopsy. A current infection can be indicated by a fourfold increase in virus neutralizing antibody, complement fixation, or hemagglutination inhibition titers. A recent infection can be evidenced by a rising antibody titer to a specific virus. The stage of the infection can be assessed using the immunoglobulin class. IgM antibody appears first and peaks in two to three weeks. IgG appears later and is the main antibody after the first month of the disease. Immunofluorescence can be used to identify the antigen in body fluid or tissue. Electron microscopy is used to identify the virus in tissue. Other laboratory tests used, such as white blood cell count, myocardial enzymes, and ESR, although increased, are nonspecific.

Endocarditis

Because the endocardium is not accessible to direct examination, the blood culture is the most valuable tool in diagnosis of infectious endocarditis. Blood cultures should be drawn in pairs (aerobic and anaerobic) every few hours for at least eight hours when the temperature is rising and before therapy. Negative blood cultures have been reported to occur in 10% to 33% of all patients. The possible causes of negative blood cultures are variable. The following display outlines an approach for those patients with a negative blood culture.

Diagnostic Approach to the Patient with Culture-Negative Endocarditis

General

1. History: epidemiology (attention to animal exposure, travel history, immune status)
2. Physical examination: particular attention to optic fundus for chorioretinitis.
3. Culture techniques: aerobic, anaerobic, hypertonic bottles; optimal blood to medium ratio; hold 4 to 6 weeks; close inspection of culture bottles; blind subculture at least once each week; +/− add penicillinase if patient has taken beta-lactam antibiotics before cultures.
4. Consider culturing other sites: bone marrow, +/− petechiae.
5. Examine peripheral smear for intraleukocytic microorganisms.
6. Acute and convalescent serologic testing for: *Chlamydia psittaci, Brucella,* including *B. canis,* Q fever, *Aspergillus* sp., *Histoplasma capsulatum, Candida albicans,* teichoic acid antibodies.
7. Consider nonbacterial causes: check antinuclear antibodies, anti-DNA antibodies, LE prep, rheumatoid factor, anti-streptolysin O, skin or muscle biopsy (Remember that some of these will be abnormal in patients with infective endocarditis.)

Special Circumstances

1. Recoverable embolus: culture for pyogenic bacteria, fungi, mycobacteria, stain sections with Gram's stain, and special stains for fungi, acid-fast microorganisms.
2. Valvular material from surgery or autopsy: culture and stain as above.
3. Patient has xenograft valve: consider *Mycobacterium chelonei.*

Freedman AL (ed): Treatment of Infective Endocarditis, p. 158. New York, Grune & Stratton, 1981

The hematological findings include an elevated ESR, leukocytosis with neutrophilia, normocytic, normochromic anemia, thrombocytopenia, and activation and coagulation abnormalities. Reticulocytosis is demonstrated with effective antibiotic therapy. Serological tests are particularly helpful in negative-blood-culture patients. The serum immunoglobulins are elevated initially but return to normal during convalescence. There are elevated levels of circulating immune complexes that can be demonstrated with a positive rheumatoid factor (RF) test. Intravenous drug abusers with IE frequently have a positive RF test, and they often have values higher than the general population even if they do not have IE. After effective antibiotic therapy, the RF titers return to normal in two to three weeks. The anti–gamma globulin latex fixation test and the test for cryoglobulins are also positive in patients with IE.

Rheumatic Heart Disease

A combination of tests should be used to diagnose RVHD because there is not one definitive procedure. Patients have an elevated ESR, a positive C-reactive protein test, leukocytosis, increases in serum complement, alpha$_2$ globulin, gamma globulin, and mucoproteins. Evidence of a streptococcal infection may be demonstrated by a positive throat culture or antibody determinations. Elevated serial antistreptolysin O (ASO) titers are reliable indicators of rheumatic fever. The ASO test should be repeated at two week intervals. The Streptozyme test is a hemagglutination procedure and a sensitive screen for streptococcal infections; however, it is only qualitative.

TREATMENT

Pericarditis

Treatment of the underlying disorder after the causative infectious agent is determined usually resolves the pericarditis. Appropriate antibiotics and surgical drainage should be used if the pericarditis is due to bacterial or mycotic infections. Anticoagulants should not be administered in most cases of pericarditis because they may precipitate bleeding into the pericardial space.[8] Corticosteroids diminish the inflammation and are therefore used to control pain, fever, and effusion. Analgesics may also be used for pain.

Myocarditis

Septic myocarditis should be treated using the appropriate antibiotics for the causative agent. Patients with viral myocarditis should be treated with bedrest, observation of complications, and adrenal steroid therapy. Short-acting digitalis, controlled salt intake, and diuretics are needed to manage congestive heart failure. The viral disease is most often self-limited, although one of the most common reasons for a heart transplant in young adults is viral myocarditis. This mode of therapy has been successful in those with severe disease resulting in irreversible heart failure.

Endocarditis

Treatment must be instituted as soon as the causative agent is determined. The best prognosis can be ensured when treatment is begun early in the illness, when the effective antimicrobial agent is selected, and when treatment is continued over a long period. Effective antibiotic treatment should be determined using the MIC (minimal inhibitory concentration) and the MBC (minimal bactericidal concentration) techniques for sensitivity testing. The disk sensitivity methods are not adequate for infectious endocarditis. Tests of serum bactericidal activity (SBA, Schlicter Test), although not generally available, may be useful in determining the effectiveness of the antibiotic treatment. The disappearance of microscopic hematuria can also help judge the effectiveness of treatment. Surgery for valve replacement may be required in addition to antibiotic therapy.

Infective endocarditis is a severe, life-threatening illness which is fatal in 50% of patients. The

Committee of Rheumatic Fever and Bacterial Endocarditis of the American Heart Association (AHA) has developed recommendations for prevention of infective endocarditis in conjunction with the Council on Dental Therapeutics of the American Dental Association. These recommendations are based on the known prevalence of particular causative agents and the efficacy of various antibiotics in preventing infectious endocarditis in patients at high risk. The display below summarizes the procedures and conditions that require prophylaxis for endocarditis.

Rheumatic Heart Disease

The mortality and morbidity of this disease can be reduced with early diagnosis, careful monitoring, and prevention of recurring episodes. With the advent of antibiotics, few patients die of initial attacks.

All patients diagnosed with rheumatic fever should be given antibiotics as soon as possible even if throat cultures are negative. They should be observed closely for heart murmurs, cardiomegaly, and signs of cardiac failure. Bedrest is recommended for patients who have abnormal heart sounds. The length of the confinement and the amount of ambulation permitted are individual and depend on the specific symptoms. Analgesics and adrenal corticosteroids should be administered in combinations dependent on the patient's symptoms and to prevent relapses of rheumatic activity. These medications do not help the chorea. Sedatives and tranquilizers should be used to help control the involuntary movements and the emotional side-effects. Prophylaxis with penicillin against group A streptococci may be required for up to 5 years.[9]

If rheumatic carditis does not respond to treatment and the mitral valve is hopelessly damaged, mitral valve replacement should be considered; however, the disease is usually self-limiting and subsides in 8 to 12 weeks.

CASE STUDY

A 37-year-old man was admitted to the hospital because of intermittent fever, malaise, hematuria,

Procedures and Conditions that Require Endocarditis Prophylaxis

- All dental procedures (including routine professional cleaning) likely to cause gingival bleeding
- Tonsillectomy
- Adenoidectomy
- Bronchoscopy, especially with a rigid bronchoscope
- Surgical procedures involving the respiratory mucosa
- Surgery or instrumentation of the genitourinary tract, especially urethral or prostatic manipulations
- Urethral catheterization, whether the urine is infected or not
- Surgery and instrumentation of the lower gastrointestinal tract and gall bladder
- Obstetrical infections, including septic abortion or peripartum infection
- Surgery on any infected or contaminated tissues, including incision and drainage of abscesses

Bisno AL: Treatment of Infective Endocarditis, p. 294. New York, Grune & Stratton, 1981

and arthralgia. He reported that he had been experiencing flulike symptoms for about 2 weeks. He had no previous history of heart disease, but his mother told him he had rheumatic fever at six years of age. During lunch 1 week before the symptoms began, he broke a tooth that was later extracted. On physical examination a diastolic murmur was audible.

The following test results were obtained on admission:

Hgb = 10.9gm/dL (1.69 mmol/L)
Hct = 33%
WBC = $18.0 \times 10^3/mm^3$
ESR = elevated
C-reactive protein positive
Blood culture positive for viridans streptococci
Other laboratory tests essentially normal

Questions

1. What is this patient's disorder?
2. What is the best treatment for this disorder?
3. What other tests or procedures could help assess the severity of the damage to the cardiac tissue?
4. What is the prognosis?
5. Should prophylactic antibiotics be used with this patient?

Discussion

1. The disorder is infectious endocarditis resulting from viridans streptococci within platelet fibrin vegetation from childhood rheumatic fever.
2. A regimen of penicillin for four weeks and concomitant streptomycin for the first two weeks has been shown to be very effective in preventing relapses.
3. An echocardiogram would demonstrate vegetation larger than 2 mm and lesions of the valves. Surgical intervention should be used to remove infected tissue, correct defects, or restore valvular function.
4. Untreated, the prognosis is poor. Mortality can be reduced by early diagnosis, appropriate antibiotic therapy, and prevention of recurring infections.
5. Antimicrobial prophylaxis should be used in this patient for any future surgery on any infected or contaminated tissue, surgery of the genitourinary tract, respiratory mucosa, or gastrointestinal tract, and all dental procedures.

REFERENCES

1. Braunwald E: Pericardial disease. In Isselbacher KJ (ed): Harrison's Principles of Internal Medicine, 9th ed., p 1149. New York City, McGraw-Hill, 1980
2. Shabetai R: The Pericardium, p 385. New York, Grune & Stratton, 1981
3. Pelletier LL, Petersdorf RG: Infective endocarditis. In Isselbacher KJ (ed): Harrison's Principles of Internal Medicine, 9th ed., p 1112. New York City, McGraw-Hill, 1980
4. Freedman LR: Infective Endocarditis and Other Intravascular Infections, pp 31–32. New York, Plenum Publishing, 1982
5. Stollerman GH: Rheumatic fever. In Isselbacher KJ (ed): Harrison's Principles of Internal Medicine, 9th ed., p 1091. New York City, McGraw-Hill, 1980
6. Fowler NO: Infectious pericarditis. In Fowler NO (ed): The Pericardium in Health and Disease, p 157. New York, Futura Publishing, 1985
7. Shabetai R: The Pericardium, p 351. New York, Grune & Stratton, 1981
8. Shabetai R: Diseases of the pericardium. In Chung EK (ed): Quick Reference to Cardiovascular Diseases, p 242. Philadelphia, JB Lippincott, 1982
9. Stollerman GH: Rheumatic fever. In Isselbacher KJ (ed): Harrison's Principles of Internal Medicine, 9th ed., p 1095. New York City, McGraw-Hill, 1980

BIBLIOGRAPHY

Berkow R, Talbott JH (eds): The Merck Manual, 13th ed. Rahway, NJ, Merck, Sharp and Dohme Research Laboratories, 1977

Olsen EGJ: The Pathology of the Heart, 2d ed. Baltimore, University Park Press, 1980

Isselbacher KJ (ed): Harrison's Principles of Internal Medicine, 9th ed. New York City, McGraw-Hill, 1980

Chung EK: Quick Reference to Cardiovascular Diseases, 2d ed. Philadelphia, JB Lippincott, 1983

Robinson JA, O'Connell JB (eds): Myocarditis: Precursor of Cardiopathy. Lexington, MA, The Collamore Press, 1983

Lundberg GD (ed): Using the Clinical Laboratory in Medical Decision Making. Chicago, American Society of Clinical Pathologists, 1983

Freedman LR: Infective Endocarditis and Other Intravascular Infections. New York, Plenum Publishing, 1982

Bisno AL (ed): Treatment of Infective Endocarditis. New York, Grune & Stratton, 1981

Lab Manage 23:23–26, 1985

Selzer A: Principles and Practice of Clinical Cardiology, 2d ed. Philadelphia, WB Saunders, 1983

Stapleton JF: Essentials of Clinical Cardiology. Philadelphia, FA Davis, 1983

Cohn PF: Clinical Cardiovascular Physiology. Philadelphia, WB Saunders, 1985

Guyton AC: Textbook of Medical Physiology. Philadelphia, WB Saunders, 1981

Chapter 4

Hypertensive Disorders

Brian D. Andresen

Attempts to measure blood pressure began early in the 18th century, but it was not until 1896 that an Italian physician, Riva-Rocci, developed and made measurements with a prototype sphygmomanometer, incorporating the first pressure cuff, ascending mercury (Hg) column, and pressure scale.

Today, blood pressure is routinely measured and is generally the first indicator of hypertension. Nevertheless, statistics indicate that only half of all Americans who suffer from hypertension are ever aware of their illness, and only 50% of those who are diagnosed receive adequate treatment.

ETIOLOGY AND PATHOPHYSIOLOGY

Hypertensive disorders are characterized by systolic and diastolic blood pressures exceeding 140/90 mm Hg. A blood pressure that consistently exceeds a diastolic value of 90 mm Hg is observed in approximately 15% to 25% of the U.S. adult population. For reasons that are not entirely clear, the reported incidence of hypertension in black persons is more than twice that in whites.

Repeated measurements of blood pressure over 200/140 mm Hg are very serious. Untreated, this "malignant" form of hypertension can quickly lead to death. "Benign" forms of hypertension typically reveal no apparent symptoms until the advanced stages. Unaware of the disorder, the patient is at risk of heart, eye, kidney, and brain injury, and of early death as a result of long-term physiological damage. Subtle arteriosclerotic changes are also present in the benign hypertensive patient, which can lead to a severely compromised blood flow in the extremities and brain. High blood pressure forces the heart to pump harder than normal because of increased vascular resistance. Over time, the overworked heart may fail.

Hypertension is most common in adults over the age of 65 years. Approximately 35% to 50% of the elderly have blood pressures over 160/90 mm Hg. Many of these persons suffer from congestive heart failure, heart disease, ventricular hypertrophy, and vascular complications. In addition, strokes and other cardiovascular complications can be precipitated by sustained high blood pressure. Thus the identification and management of hypertension is most important.

Children have significantly lower blood pressures than those of adults. Blood pressure gradually increases with age through puberty. Only 1% to 2% of children under age 14 years have pressures over 140/90 mm Hg. It has been suggested that children with slightly elevated blood pressures have an increased risk of developing hypertension as adults. The parents of hypertensive offspring often have elevated blood pressures as well, which suggests that a hereditary component is involved.

Hypertensive patients can be classified using two different approaches.[1, 2] One method is by *the degree of hypertension,* which is important prognostically. The second method is to classify the hypertensive patient according to *the underlying etiology.* The latter approach is most important for selecting the appropriate therapy.

Degree of Hypertension

Patients can be categorized according to the degree of their hypertension. Hypertension that is immediately life-threatening is termed *malignant.* Hypertension that is not immediately life-threatening is termed *benign,* although long-term benign hypertension can also be life-threatening eventually. It may persist for decades, leading to physiological complications and a shorter life span than the average, age-matched, nonhypertensive patient.

Malignant hypertensive patients have a very poor prognosis. If untreated, 60% die in six months and 80% die within one year.[3] Untreated, malignant hypertension leads to inflammation and necrosis of the arterioles. The arteriopathy can be visualized on physical examination by changes in the ocular fundus, which reveals hemorrhages, exudates, and papilledema. Papilledema under these circumstances usually results from ischemia of the optic nerve as a consequence of a damaged vasa nervorum and does not imply increased pressure of the cerebrospinal fluid. Similar vascular lesions can be found in the kidneys, where the severity of the disease is reflected by proteinuria, hematuria, red blood cell casts, and progressive renal failure.

Primary Hypertension

Although hypertension can be caused by a number of conditions, more than 90% of patients have "primary," "idiopathic," or "essential" hypertension, in which the etiology is unknown.[4] There is typically no common profile for patients with primary hypertension, and it is believed that a mosaic of interacting factors causes the disease. Generally, all hypertension is considered primary until discovery of a distinct etiology that may respond to a specific therapy.

The mosaic of factors leading to primary hypertension includes age, race, posture, salt intake, emotional state, hormonal balance, and medication, all of which can interact to influence blood pressure. An initial consideration in primary hypertension is a defect in the transport of sodium in the renal tubules. In theory, the renal retention of sodium would lead to expanded intravascular volume and increased vascular resistance and signal the release of angiotensin. As a result, cardiac output would be elevated and blood pressure would increase. The increase in pressure and fluid exchange should promote sodium excretion; this may not be the case, however, if a faulty autoregulatory mechanism prevents adequate tissue perfusion.

Ingestion of sodium appears to be very important in the etiology of primary hypertension.[5] Various studies have shown that populations consuming relatively small amounts of sodium (less than 60 to 80 mEq/day [60–80 mmol/day]) have little hypertension and minimal or no increase in blood pressure with age.

It has also been suggested that most sodium-associated hypertension is caused by an imbalance in the interaction of sodium and the blood pressure regulatory mechanisms, which include sympathetic function, angiotensin, vasopressin, and vascular reactivity. Various abnormalities in sodium and calcium transport in the red blood cell and leukocyte membranes of patients with primary hypertension have also been reported. These findings lead to further speculation that membrane defects in vascular smooth muscles may be involved in the pathogenesis of high blood pressure.

Primary hypertension can be further subdivided into two groups based on abnormalities in either the *hemodynamic* or the *renin-angiotensin system.*[6] Hemodynamic abnormalities are most often associated with *labile hypertension.* This subclassification of primary hypertension is generally applied when cardiac output increases yet vascular resistance remains unchanged or is considered "inappropriate" to match cardiac output. If the sympathetic nervous system function is altered in an essential hypertensive patient by increased visual or emotional stress, extremes of heat or cold, or heavy or mild forms of exercise, an exaggerated response can be evoked among heart rate, cardiac output, renal renin release, and blood pressure. In the labile hypertensive patient the imbalance in hemodynamics is accentuated and may evolve into fixed or established hypertension. Unfortunately, the mechanisms involved in labile hypertension are not yet well enough understood to enable the development of an adequate drug regimen or other treatment.

The status and possible role of the renin-angiotensin system in patients with primary hypertension has been thoroughly investigated, and studies point to a variety of causative factors. Renin is a proteolytic enzyme that catalyzes the conversion of a tetradecapeptide substrate to angiotensin-I, which is later converted by a variety of tissues to angiotensin-II (Fig. 4-1). False substrates, diminished receptor sites, and poor conversion due to a variety of biochemical factors may lead to altered levels of angiotensin-II and essential hypertension. In comparisons with normotensive control patients, almost 70% of patients with essential hypertension have normal plasma renin activity (PRA) levels, 20% to 25% have abnormally low PRA levels, and 5% to 10% have high PRA levels[1] (see also Chap. 18).

Recent research points to inappropriate levels of newly identified renal vasodilator substances in the primary hypertensive patient.[7] For example, researchers have reported that reduced levels of renal kallikrein, the enzyme that catalyzes the formation of the vasodilator bradykinin, are observed in the urine of the hypertensive patient.

Prostaglandins, particularly of the E series, can also cause renal vasodilation, natriuresis, and renin release. However, the role of prostaglandins in hypertension is not well understood.

Secondary Hypertension

HYPERTENSIVE EMERGENCIES

Secondary hypertension is identified with a specific disease state responsible for the elevated blood pressure.[3] Only 5% to 10% of cases of hypertension in the United States are secondary. Although this form of hypertension is much less prevalent

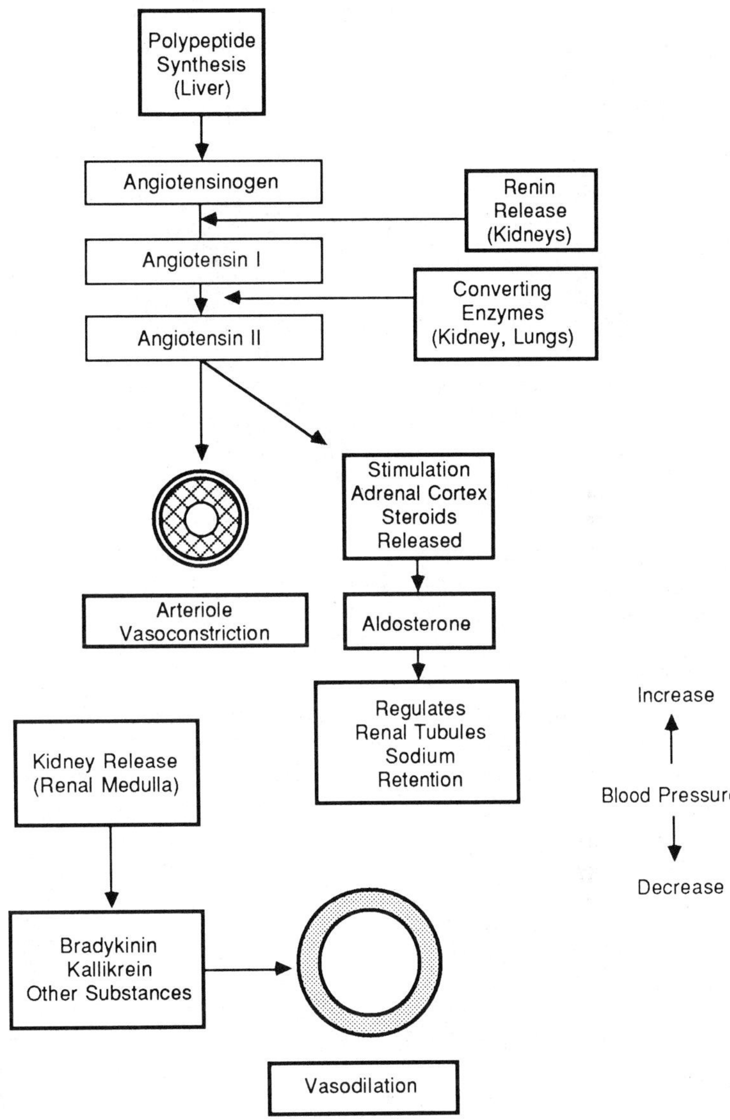

Figure 4-1 **Renin-angiotensin system.**

than primary hypertension, it is important to identify the etiology of secondary hypertension because the underlying problem, even when relatively serious, may often be cured if identified.[8] The patient with secondary hypertension can be further classified as either a candidate for diagnostic procedures or a person in hypertensive crisis. The former state is not considered life-threatening, and there is time for thorough laboratory studies. The latter state, however, requires immediate emergency care to prevent irreversible or lethal complications of the disease.[1, 9] A display on page 38 lists situations mandating immediate emergency treatment for hypertensive crisis.

Hypertensive Emergencies

1. Malignant hypertension
   (a) Rapid funduscopic changes with necrotizing arteriolitis
   (b) Hypertensive encephalopathy
2. Hypertension associated with:
   (a) Acute left ventricular failure
   (b) Coronary insufficiency
   (c) Aortic dissection or a leaking aneurysm
   (d) Intracranial hemorrhage
   (e) Postoperative bleeding

CLINICALLY DEMONSTRABLE HYPERTENSION
Although they are eventually life-threatening, other forms of secondary hypertension are more subtle in their initial stages. If left untreated, however, these disease states may also develop to a crisis level. The following display lists several disorders clearly responsible for secondary hypertension that can typically be associated with certain target tissues.[4]

Disorders Responsible for Secondary Hypertension

1. Renal (parenchymal and vascular)
2. Adrenal (cortical and medullary)
3. Neurogenic
4. Parathyroid or thyroid (Hyperthyroid and myxedema)
5. Coarctation of aorta (thoracic and abdominal)
6. Toxemia of pregnancy (preeclampsia and eclampsia)
7. Drug-induced (therapeutic and abusive)
8. Increased left ventricle stroke volume
9. Decreased aortic distensibility (arteriosclerosis and coarctation)

Renal (See also Part 4)

Parenchymal Hypertension Mild and severe diseases of the vascular and parenchymal tissues of the kidney are associated with hypertension.[6, 10, 11] Several important disease states associated with parenchymal deterioration are highlighted below.

Hypertension is observed in both acute and chronic glomerulonephritis. In the acute disease, volume overload is usually the most prominent feature. In the chronic disease, the hypertension usually is not severe unless associated with high levels of urea, creatinine, and other nonprotein nitrogen substances in the serum.

Pyelonephritis may also induce hypertension by causing renal failure or by interfering with intrarenal circulation. The severity of the hypertension does not parallel the severity of the renal disease, and renin concentrations may remain normal.[12]

The type of hypertension that commonly develops in patients with diabetic nephropathy is related to impaired renal function often generated from intercapillary glomerulosclerosis or from chronic pyelonephritis. Plasma renin activity measurements in diabetics are often low due to volume

Parenchymal Disease States
Glomerulonephritis
Chronic pyelonephritis
Diabetic nephropathy
Interstitial nephritis
Polycystic kidney
Connective tissue disease
Hydronephrosis
Hypernephroma
Juxtaglomerular (JG) cell tumor
Wilms's tumor
Solitary renal cyst
Perinephritis
Renal hematoma
Fibrous constriction (Ask-Upmark kidney)

expansion, sympathetic neuropathy, or a combination.

Hypertension associated with polycystic kidney disease has not been correlated to renin concentration. In contrast, renal compression caused by hematomas, perinephritis, and renal scars or obstructions may cause renin-dependent hypertension.[11]

Severe hypertension is often associated with connective tissue disorders such as scleroderma and systemic lupus erythematosus. The resultant hypertension may in turn accelerate the development of renal insufficiency, which further accelerates the underlying disease state.

Abnormal parenchymal growths, such as renal cell carcinomas and cysts or other large intrarenal masses occasionally cause hypertension, presumably by interfering with renal circulation with subsequent stimulation of renin release.[12] Hyperreninemia is also observed with many other types of renal tumors or compression lesions that cause hypertension.[13] Juxtaglomerular (JG) cell tumors and hemangiopericytomas of the kidney may produce severe hypertension with hyperreninemia, secondary hyperaldosteronism, and marked hypokalemia. These tumors, which are more common in the young, tend to be small and may be missed radiologically unless selective renal angiography is performed. Wilms's tumor and some rare forms of extrarenal malignancies also may produce reninlike material and cause severe hypertension.

Renal Vascular Disease The display above (right) lists various disease states associated with renal vascular diseases.[11, 13, 14] All are associated with abnormalities of the blood flow and perfusion of the kidney. One or both kidneys may be involved.

Hypertension is secondary to these renovascular diseases in only 1% to 2% of patients.[15, 16] Although almost half of secondary hypertensive patients have some type of renovascular lesion, only a few of these lesions actually cause the hypertension. Generally, atherosclerosis is more common in men and involves the proximal portion of the renal artery. Fibrous dysplasia, either from infection or congenital abnormalities, is more often diagnosed in women and affects the middle and distal portions of the renal vessels. Fibromuscular hyperplasia may also involve arteries elsewhere in the body, leading to ischemia of other organs and additional blood pressure elevations.

Renal Vascular Diseases

Atherosclerotic, thrombotic, or embolic obstructions
Fibromuscular hyperplasia
Aneurysm or dissecting aneurysm
Inflammation (infection)
Hypoplasia

Adrenal Hypertension (See also Chap. 37)

Abnormalities of the adrenals can be classified broadly as mineralocorticoid excess syndromes.[6, 7, 8] Steroids that are important in hypertension are seen in Figure 4-2. Steroid production abnormalities can be grouped into aldosterone-producing adenoma, adrenocortical hyperplasia, Cushing's syndrome, and metabolic errors for steroid hydroxylation (hydroxylase deficiencies). Hypertension is secondary to primary hyperaldosteronism in approximately 1% of hypertensive patients. Of these, approximately 75% have an isolated primary, aldosterone-producing adenoma. The remaining 25% are termed *idiopathic* and typically possess hyperplastic, nodular masses on one or both adrenal glands. Patients with primary hyperaldosteronism have spontaneous hypokalemia, an inability to concentrate urine, tetany, glucose intolerance, and overall depressed muscle strength. Abnormally low plasma renin activity (PLA) values are another important feature of hyperaldosteronism. In fact, the triad of *hypertension, hypokalemia,* and *low plasma renin levels* is highly suggestive of mineralocorticoid excess.

Cushing's syndrome is the abnormal overproduction of cortisol or related corticosteroids,

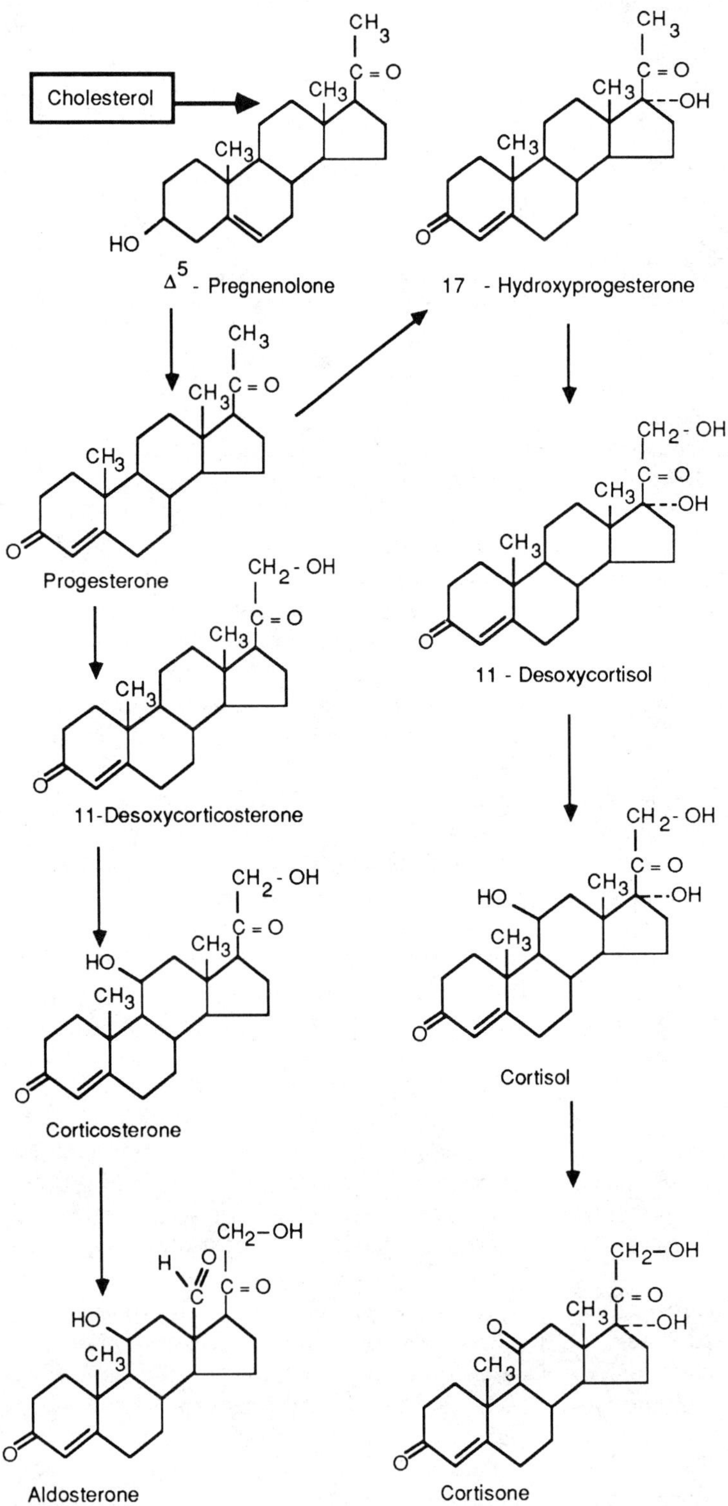

Figure 4-2 Biosynthesis of corticosteroids.

resulting in a constellation of clinical signs and symptoms.[17] One of these is hypertension. However, the hypertension in most patients with Cushing's syndrome is not directly related to mineralocorticoid excess and is of unknown etiology. In addition, there is a group of patients with essential hypertension who have some similarities to patients with mineralocorticoid excess but have normal aldosterone secretions.

Genetic defects involving enzymatic reactions that hydroxylate at the 17, 11, 18, or 19 carbon position of cortisol have also been identified as contributing to hypertension (see Fig. 4-2). Most of these enzyme deficiencies result in excess production of desoxycorticosterone (DOC). Hydroxylation at carbon 18 or 19 generates 18-hydroxy-DOC and 19-hydroxy-DOC, both of which are associated with hypertension.

Pheochromocytoma is usually derived from the adrenal medulla and is a rare chromaffin tissue tumor that causes excess secretion of catecholamines, resulting in hypertension.[18] Catecholamines are biosynthesized from phenylalanine (Fig. 4-3) and are very important in a variety of regulatory processes. Interest in pheochromocytoma arises because the tumor can cause a dramatic and potentially lethal elevation of blood pressure. The tumors are found in only 0.1% to 0.3% of the hypertensive population and originate in the adrenal medulla in approximately 90% of these patients. In the remaining 10%, the catecholamine-generating tumors originate from the Zuckerkandl's organs, paraganglionic cells of the sympathetic nervous system, bladder, aorta, or carotid.

Pheochromocytoma is easily diagnosed[8] and surgically correctable. Most signs and symptoms can be related directly to an overproduction of catecholamines secreted by the tumor. However, patients can be misdiagnosed as having disorders such as thyrotoxicosis, severe anxiety, diabetes mellitus, or hyperventilation. Onset at an early age is often characteristic of pheochromocytoma. There is also a familial association, and family members should be screened to identify asymptomatic individuals. Familial pheochromocytoma may be associated with other neural crest tissue tumors. These include tumors of the pituitary and pancreas and medullary carcinoma of the thyroid and parathyroid gland. Other associated disorders are cerebellar hemangioblastoma and retinal angioma. Approximately 10% of pheochromocytoma patients have malignant diseases that metastasize. When the metastatic lesions are slow-growing, death usually results from hypertension rather than from the malignancy.

Neurogenic Hypertension

Many types of neurological conditions may cause hypertension. These can include intracranial lesions, tumors, hematomas, subdural hygromas, carotid sinus denervation, familial dysautonomia, and spinal cord transection. In addition, various peripheral neuropathies, including those seen with infectious polyneuritis, tabes dorsalis, porphyria, and lead poisoning, may cause hypertension.[19]

Thyroid and Parathyroid Diseases (See also Chaps. 35 and 36)

Myxedematous patients tend to have hypertension that, when correctly diagnosed, can be corrected by the administration of thyroid hormone.[20] Approximately one-third of patients with hyperparathyroidism have hypertension,[2] which can often be attributed to renal parenchymal damage due to nephrolithiasis (stones) and nephrocalcinosis (salt deposits). The observed hypertension usually disappears when the hypercalcemia is corrected. Elevated angiotensin levels, which are also common with hyperthyroidism, may play a role in the hypertension.

Coarctation of the Aorta

Hypertension is often associated with a congenital defect leading to a constriction in the aorta.[1, 21] The constriction is usually located distal to the insertion of the ductus arteriosus and near the subclavian artery, but can be in any portion of the aorta. It occurs most frequently in males and is associated with Turner's syndrome and other cardiac abnor-

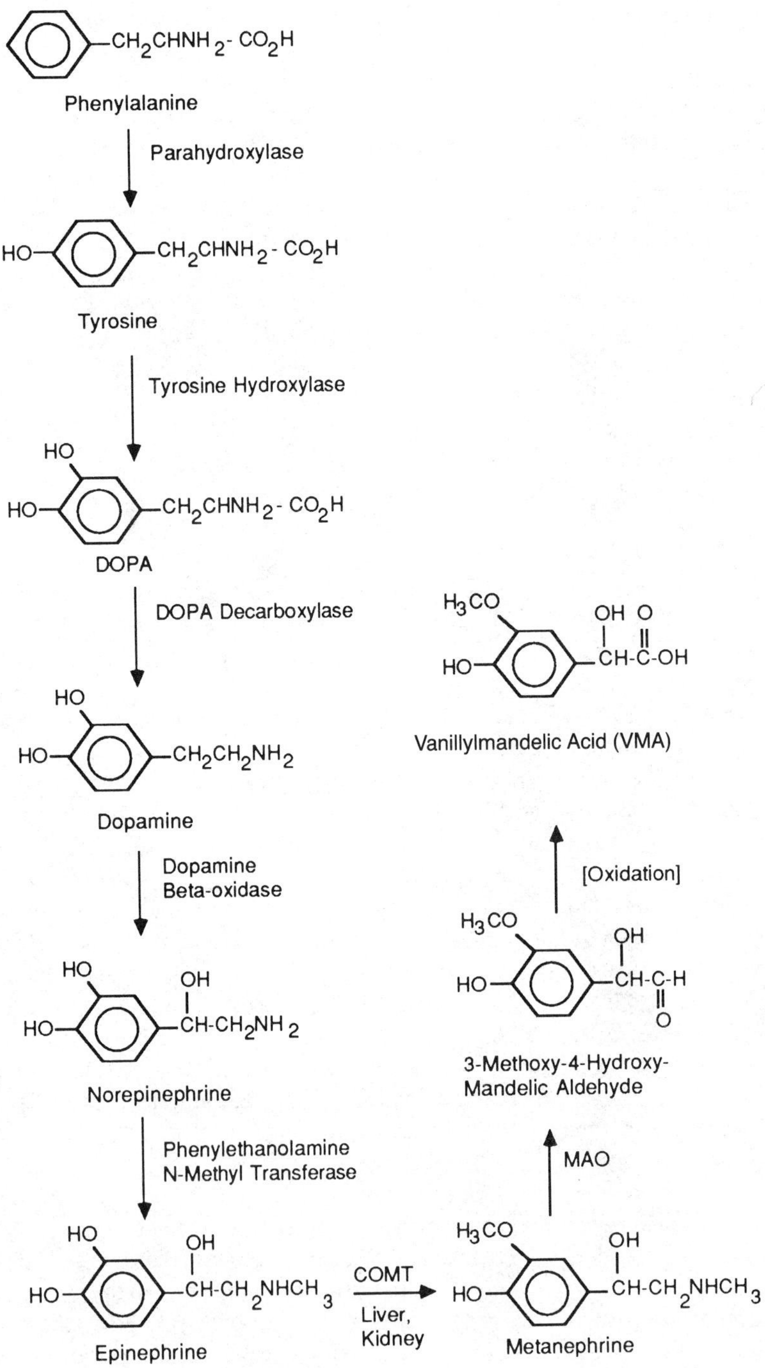

Figure 4-3 Biosynthesis and metabolism of catecholamines.

malities such as bicuspid aortic valve, ventricular septal defect, patent ductus arteriosus, mitral valve abnormalities, and berry aneurysms of the carotid circulation.[22] The hypertension may be caused by the constriction itself or result from a form of renal arterial hypertension. The diagnosis is most evident from clinical and routine x-ray findings.[23, 24]

Toxemia of Pregnancy (See also Chap. 40)

In the United States, approximately one-fifth of all maternal deaths and 25,000 stillbirths and neonatal deaths are a direct result of hypertension during pregnancy.[25] A sustained increase in pressure of 30/15 mm Hg or any level exceeding 140/90 mm Hg is considered hypertensive. Hypertension during pregnancy can be defined by four different forms of pregnancy-related elevations of blood pressure: (1) acute hypertension in pregnancy and preeclampsia-eclampsia (pregnancy-induced hypertension [PIH]), (2) chronic hypertension during pregnancy, (3) chronic hypertension during pregnancy with superimposed acute hypertension (preeclampsia), and (4) transient hypertension in pregnancy that occurs during labor or immediately postpartum and then subsides.

Acute hypertension during pregnancy is a condition most often associated with toxemia of pregnancy and preeclampsia-eclampsia.[2] PIH is the most current terminology for this form of hypertension. Typically, after the 24th week of gestation a mild preeclampsia patient develops overt edema of the face, hands, or feet, blood pressure over 140/90 mm Hg, and proteinuria. There are no other typical clinical signs. In 90% of patients, the sequential development of *edema, hypertension,* and *proteinuria* clearly identifies mild preeclampsia. The mild forms of pregnancy-induced hypertension are treatable but not preventable. The development of PIH consists of mild preeclampsia progressing to severe preeclampsia and then to eclampsia. The patient with severe preeclampsia is seriously ill and must be hospitalized, with her blood pressure continuously monitored and controlled. The severe forms of hypertension have a maternal mortality of 10% and a perinatal mortality of greater than 30%. The cause of preeclampsia is unknown, and extensive research is in progress to identify a "factor" or group of chemicals that may be responsible for the disease.[8]

Chronic hypertension during pregnancy is defined as hypertension usually recorded *before* the pregnancy or *before the 24th week* of gestation. It appears that pregnancy often unmasks hypertension; it is seen most often in multigravida women. Chronic hypertension of pregnancy is divided into primary and secondary types. The former is not related to any specific disease state and comprises 95% of the chronic hypertensive pregnancies. As in other forms of hypertension, secondary hypertension can be associated with an underlying disease process.

Drug- and Diet-Induced Hypertension

Many types of drugs can precipitate abnormally high blood pressure leading to stroke and cardiac arrest. For example, numerous deaths associated with high blood pressure and arrhythmias have been reported in the national news media recently, related to use by athletes of illicit drugs such as cocaine. The drug-induced hypertension most commonly reported, however, is associated with use of oral contraceptives by young and middle-aged women.

Oral Contraceptives Thorough studies of large populations of women show that, with prolonged usage, hypertension develops in approximately 5% of the women taking oral contraceptives. In addition, there appears to be a threefold risk of developing hypertension when oral contraceptives are used for more than 5 years. Oral contraceptives appear to increase renin production, angiotensin-II, aldosterone secretion, and salt and water retention. The increase in angiotensin-II may increase vasoconstriction, leading to hypertension.

The hypertension morbidity reported with oral contraceptives appears to be associated with cardiovascular effects that include thromboembolism, stroke, and myocardial infarction. Myocardial infarctions appear to be most closely correlated with cigarette smoking.[25] In addition, oral contraceptives appear to increase serum very-low-density lipoproteins, blood glucose, and platelet aggregation factors (prostaglandins). Estrogen-related steroids, used to treat postmenopausal women, have also been associated with elevated blood pressure.

Other Pharmacologic Agents An adverse reaction leading to hypertensive crisis can be observed in patients who receive monoamine oxidase (MAO) inhibitors (drugs prescribed for depression) and whose diet is high in tyramine from such sources as cheese, wines, herring, and liver.[1, 8] These drugs prevent the degradation of tyramine and tyrosine (biological precursors for catecholamines), alter the chemical balance of catecholamines in tissues, and markedly enhance their physiological effects (see Fig. 4-3). Other drugs that mimic catecholamines (*e.g.*, amphetamine, cocaine) have been reported to elevate blood pressure significantly. Finally, drugs used to combat inflammation (*e.g.*, indomethacin and other prostaglandin-synthesis inhibitors) have been associated with hypertension. The actual mechanism for this effect is not clearly known; however, these drugs may alter the balance between prostacyclins, thromboxanes, and prostaglandins in blood vessels. The display at upper right lists drugs known to cause hypertension.

Drugs Known to Cause Hypertension

1. Corticosteroids
2. Oral contraceptives
3. Sympathomimetic amines or combinations of:
   Phenylpropanolamine
   Methyldopa
   Guanethidine
   Reserpine
4. Vasopressin (Pitressin)
5. Oxytocin
6. Pentazocine (Talwin)
7. Carbenoxolone
8. Nitroglycerin
9. Drugs of abuse (*e.g.*, nicotine, PCP, cocaine)

Foods Interestingly, excessive licorice ingestion (50 to 100 g/day) can produce hypertension and hypokalemia due to the compound glycyrrhizic acid, which exhibits mineralocorticoid action.

CLINICAL MANIFESTATIONS

Blood Pressure

Any blood pressure reading with a value greater than 140/90 mm Hg suggests possible hypertension.[24] A family history of hypertension and reported episodes of labile hypertension usually point to primary hypertension. Elevated blood pressure before the age of 35 or after the age of 50 is usually associated with secondary hypertension. A history of repeated urinary tract infections (UTIs) with proteinuria, kidney stones, significant side pains, or use of steroids or oral contraceptives is very significant in the diagnosis of secondary hypertension.[8, 12] Nocturia and polydipsia with hypertension usually indicate endocrine disease. A history of significant weight loss points to pheochromocytoma. In contrast, weight gain associated with a round face reflects Cushing's syndrome. Inappropriate development of muscle strength or weakness in the extremities along with differences in pulse pressures suggests coarctation of the aorta. Detailed examination of the ocular fundi is mandatory to identify the duration of and prognosis for the hypertension.

Detailed examination of the heart and lungs is also essential, to identify unique sounds that point to ventricular hypertrophy, cardiac decompensation, murmurs, rales, and bruits in the cardiovascular system. Palpitation of the abdomen may reveal aneurysms or enlarged kidneys. Neurologic examination points to cerebral vascular accidents (CVAs) or other pathological events.

Symptomatology

In the majority of cases of primary hypertension, patients are unaware of their elevated blood pressure. The hypertension can persist for decades with no apparent symptoms to warn of future difficulties. Some persons may complain of fatigue, nervousness, dizziness, palpitation, insomnia, weakness, and headaches. When hypertension is left untreated, strokes, myocardial infarctions, and chronic renal failure are the major problems that result. Only with malignant hypertension will a patient possibly be aware of some underlying problem.[1] Severe throbbing headaches, vomiting, visual disturbances (including blindness), paralysis, angina pectoris, convulsions, stupor, or blackout periods are typical events that alert a patient to malignant hypertension.[26] Clinical findings in secondary hypertension are related to the underlying disease process responsible for the hypertensive state.

LABORATORY ANALYSES AND DIAGNOSIS

A variety of laboratory tests aid in determining the degree and type of hypertension.[4, 6, 8, 10, 12, 27] Because primary hypertension has no clearly identifiable etiology, most of the diagnostic procedures performed in the clinical laboratory center on secondary hypertension. Generally the diagnostic procedures include routine laboratory studies, common ancillary tests, and special tests (Figs. 4-4 and 4-5).

Evaluation of renal status is carried out with urinalysis, urine culture, determinations of serum creatinine level, and a rapid-sequence intravenous pyelogram. This approach will identify the majority of patients with renal disease and will point to those with renal arterial or parenchymal lesions. If parenchymal lesions are found, it may be difficult to ascertain whether the disease causes or results from hypertension. The display on page 48 highlights the clinical laboratory and other tests most useful for the diagnosis and differentiation of hypertension.[28]

Renin-Angiotensin System (See also Chap. 37)

It is now well established that assessment of renin production by each kidney is a useful diagnostic test.[1] The test can be performed on peripheral blood or differentially on renal vein plasma obtained by direct catheterization of the two renal veins under fluoroscopic control.

Renin activity is measured indirectly by the ability of the patient's plasma to generate angiotensin-I from angiotensinogen by renin (see Fig. 4-1). The value obtained is expressed as nanograms of angiotensin-I produced per milliliter of plasma per hour (μg/L/hr). Radioimmunoassay techniques are used, and normal values depend on the particular laboratory used. These values are subject to the patient's sodium and potassium levels, posture, and exposure to drugs.[28] Table 4-1 lists the normal values of plasma renin. Typically the values decrease with age and are slightly lower in women than in men.

The PRA assay is initiated with blood drawn into a tube containing Na-EDTA (1 mg/mL) and not K-EDTA. Table 4-2 indicates how renin activity is related to various disease states.[4]

Drugs can affect the PRA levels.[1] Drugs that tend to elevate renin include chlorthalidon, diazoxide, ethacrynic acid, oral contraceptives, estrogens, furosemide, guanethidine in sodium-depleted patients, hydralazine, spironolactone, and thiazide diuretics. Drugs that tend to lower PRA values are carbenoxolone, clonidine, deoxycorticosterone, glycyrrhiza, guanethidine in patients with normal sodium levels, methyldopa, prazosin, and propranolol. Patients should not receive drugs that affect renin for one week before PRA assays.[29]

(Text continues on page 48)

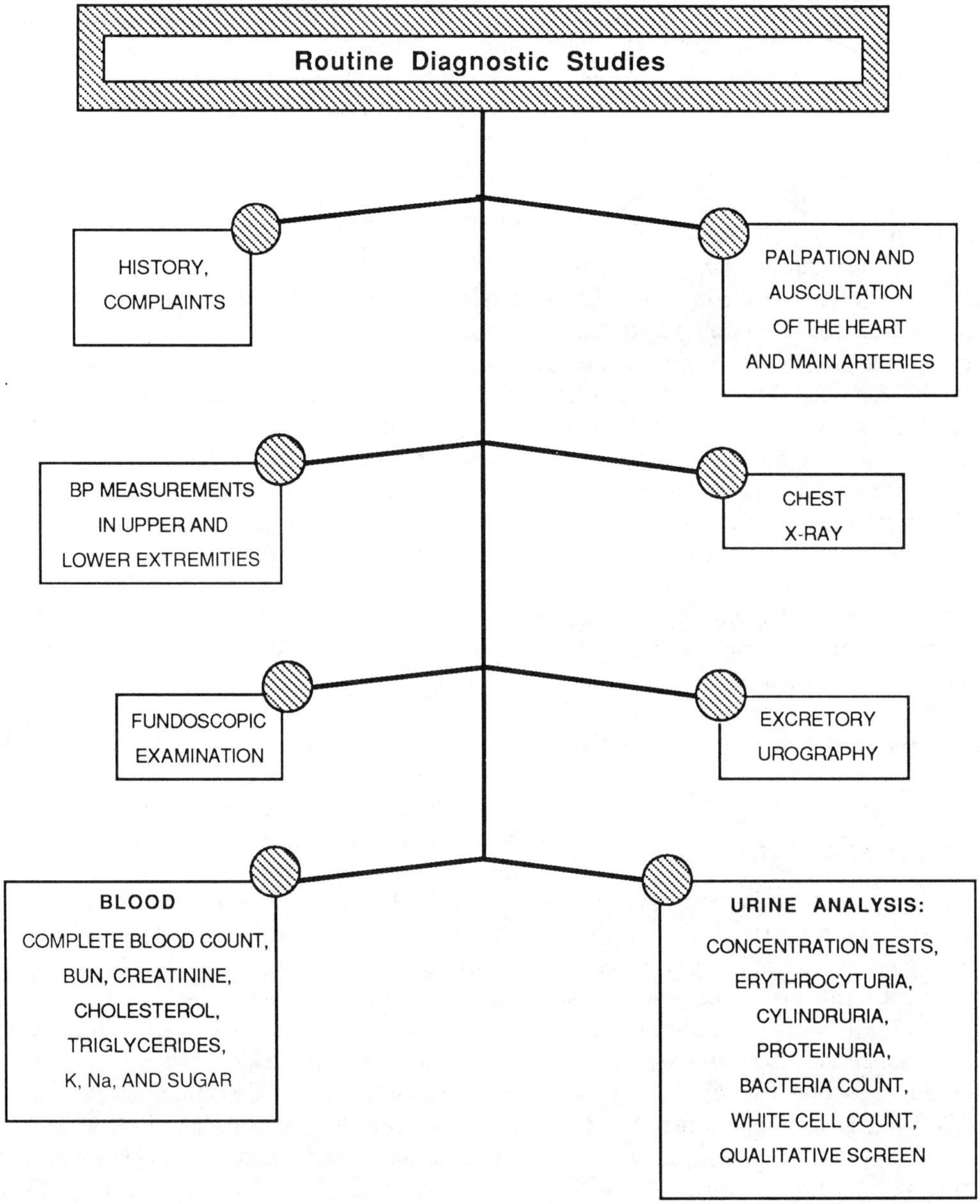

Figure 4-4 **General approach to the hypertensive patient.**

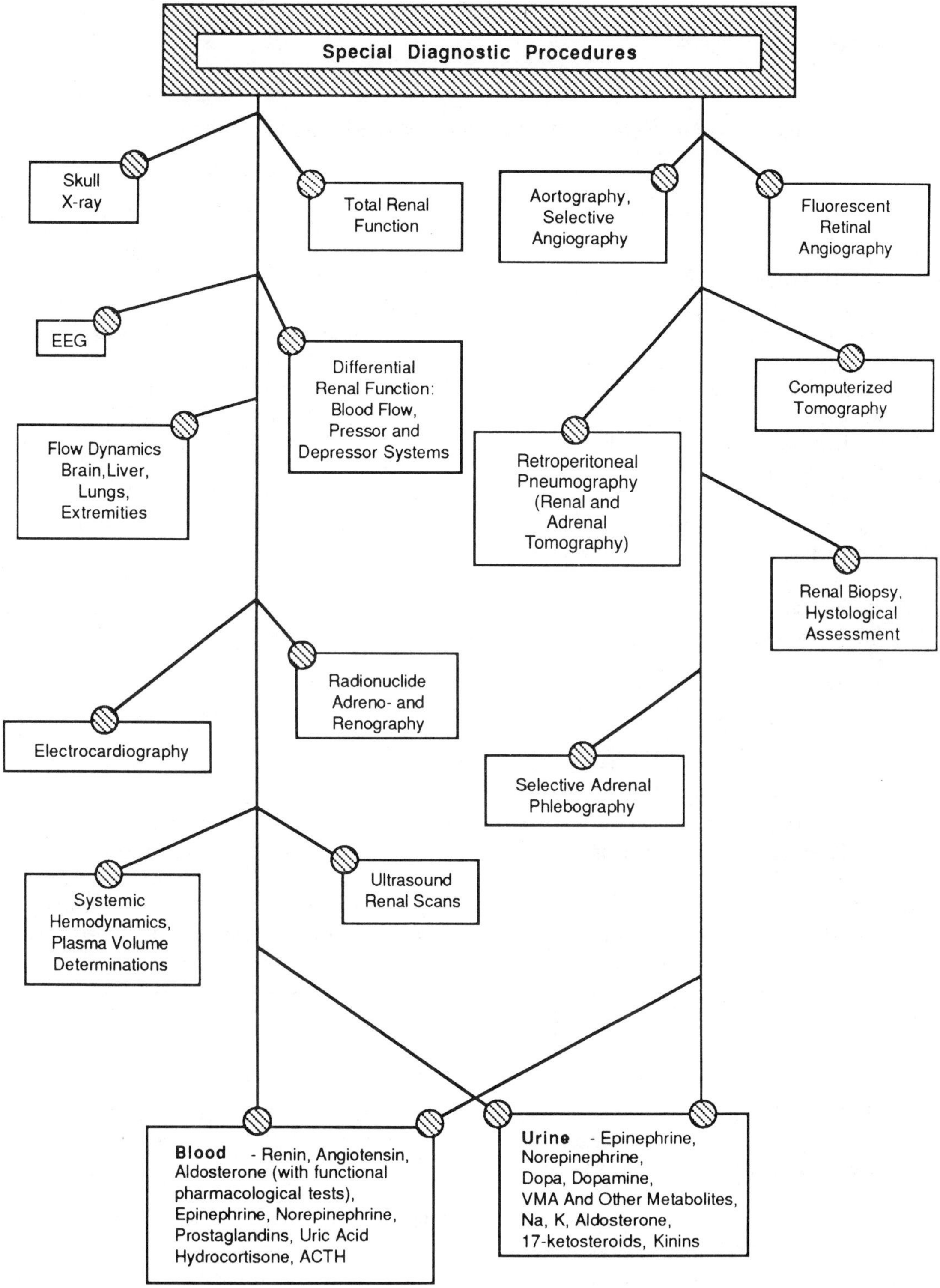

Figure 4-5 Special diagnostic procedures.

Tests and Special Studies Useful for the Evaluation of Hypertension

1. Urinalysis
   - (a) Glucose
   - (b) Protein
   - (c) Sediment
     - (1) Red blood cells
     - (2) White blood cells
   - (d) Urine culture
   - (e) 24-hour urine catecholamines, metanephrine, or vanillylmandelic acid
2. Blood
   - (a) Hemoglobin
   - (b) Urea nitrogen
   - (c) Creatinine
   - (d) Uric acid
   - (e) Fasting sugar and 2-hour postprandial sugar
   - (f) Sodium
   - (g) Potassium
   - (h) Calcium
   - (i) Triglycerides
   - (j) Thyroxine
   - (k) Carbon dioxide
3. Other tests
   - (a) Electrocardiogram (ECG)
   - (b) Posteroanterior chest x-ray
   - (c) Rapid-sequence intravenous pyelogram
4. Special tests
   - (a) When Cushing's syndrome is suspected
     - (1) Plasma cortisol (A.M. and P.M.)
     - (2) 24-hour urine 17-hydroxy or 17-keto-steroid measurements
     - (3) Dexamethasone suppression test
   - (b) When intravenous pyelogram suggests renal artery stenosis
     - (1) Radioisotope renogram (adrenal scintigraphy, computed tomography [CT] scan, ultrasound, split renal function tests)
     - (2) Renal arteriogram
     - (3) Renal vein plasma renin activity
     - (4) Ureteral catheterization studies
   - (c) When hypokalemia points to aldosteronism
     - (1) Plasma renin activity with sodium restriction
     - (2) Plasma aldosterone measurements
     - (3) 24-hour urine aldosterone with sodium loading
     - (4) Adrenal venography
     - (5) Adrenal vein aldosterone
   - (d) Angiotensin-II antagonist test: blood pressure measurements during rapid infusion of saralasin (polypeptide)

FUROSEMIDE STIMULATION TEST

Plasma renin activity will vary significantly depending upon a patient's levels of hydration and sodium intake.[30] The administration of furosemide, an effective diuretic, can be used to ascertain the response to dehydration and production of plasma renin (see Chap. 37). Patients with suppressed renin values would be considered for primary aldosteronism and should be studied further. Patients with very high renin values may have renal artery stenosis or pheochromocytoma.

DIFFERENTIAL RENAL VEIN RENIN

In patients with renovascular hypertension, the plasma renin activities will be higher on the involved side. A differential renal vein renin test can be performed on patients who initially have been on a low-sodium, high-potassium diet and on diuretic medications 3 to 4 days prior to the test.[2, 18] During percutaneous catheterization under fluoroscopic guidance, blood is obtained from both renal veins and inferior vena cava for later determinations of renin activities. Ratios of renin activity (affected side compared to unaffected side) greater than 1.5 suggest significant renovascular disease.

The display on page 50 shows factors resulting in high or low plasma renin activities.[28]

Table 4-1 ***Plasma Renin Activities: Formation of Angiotensin-I***

Age (Yr)	ng/mL/hr
2–4	2.37 ± 0.57
5–6	1.48 ± 0.17
7–9	2.13 ± 0.44
10–11	1.96 ± 0.36
14–15	1.18 ± 0.28
16–17	1.08 ± 0.25
Normal sodium diet: supine	1.6 ± 1.5
standing	4.5 ± 2.9
Low sodium diet: supine	3.2 ± 1.1
standing	9.9 ± 4.3

Convert to SI units as follows:
ng/mL/hr × 1 = μg/L/hr

PHARMACOLOGIC DIAGNOSTIC TESTS

A pharmacologic procedure, useful for identifying defects in angiotensin-II production, is based on the infusion of the antagonist, saralasin, 1-(N-methylglycine) - 5 - L - valine-8 - L - alanineangiotensin II. A reduction of 7 to 10 mm Hg in diastolic pressure in response to a rapid infusion of saralasin indicates a positive response. This test correlates well with renovascular hypertension.[4, 8]

Another pharmacologic diagnostic test is the infusion of angiotensin-II. In theory, hypertensive patients with renovascular hypertension will show very little response from preexisting high levels of endogenous circulating angiotensin-II.[1] However, due to many variables this test often generates inconsistent results.

Table 4-2 ***Renin Activity in Various Disease States***

Elevated	Depressed
Secondary aldosteronism	Adrenal cortical disease
Malignant or severe hypertension	Primary aldosteronism
Unilateral renal disease	Adrenal carcinoma
Renal parenchymal disease	Adrenal enzyme defects
Renin-secreting tumors	Steroid excess
Oral contraceptive induced	Without cortical disease
Edematous normotensive states	Liddle's syndrome
Cirrhosis of the liver	Licorice ingestion
Nephrosis	Mineralocorticoids
Congestive heart failure	Normotensive patients
Hypokalemic normotensive states	Renal parenchymal
Bartter's syndrome (JG cell)	Autonomic disorders
Kidney disease (Na and K release)	Postural hypertension
Electrolyte loss (alimentary route)	Uninephrectomized patients
	Adrenergic blockers
	Hyperkalemia

Factors in Plasma Renin Activity

High plasma renin activity is observed in

1. Primary hypertension (5%–10%)
2. High salt intake
3. Adrenergic hypertension
   (a) Pheochromocytoma
   (b) Hyperthyroidism
4. Renal hypoperfusion
   (a) Renovascular disease
   (b) Heart failure
   (c) Malignant hypertension
5. Renal Compression
   (a) Tumors (JG Cell or Wilms's tumor, hypernephroma, hematoma, cysts)
   (b) Scars, bands (Ask-Upmark kidney, perinephritis, radiation nephritis)
6. Miscellaneous
   (a) Renal failure
   (b) Glomerulonephritis
   (c) Hydronephrosis

Low plasma renin activity is observed in

1. No mineralocorticoid excess
   (a) Essential hypertension (20%–25%)
   (b) Race (40%–45% black persons hypertensive)
   (c) Reduced renal mass or responsiveness
   (d) Reduced sympathetic activity
      (1) Idiopathic
      (2) Adrenergic inhibitors
         (a.) Beta-blockers
         (b.) Methyldopa
         (c.) Clonidine
         (d.) Rauwolfia derivatives
2. Mineralocorticoid excess
   (a) Aldosterone excess
      (1) Primary hyperaldosteronism
      (2) Idiopathic hyperaldosteronism
      (3) Congenital hyperaldosteronism
      (4) Adrenal carcinoma
   (b) Desoxycorticosterone (DOC) excess
      (1) Adrenal adenoma
      (2) Ectopic ACTH-producing tumors
      (3) 17-alpha-hydroxylase deficiency
      (4) 11-beta-hydroxylase deficiency
      (5) 18-hydroxy-DOC excess
      (6) Licorice (glycyrrhizic acid)

ANGIOTENSIN ASSAY

The arterial blood concentration of angiotensin-II is 2.4±1.2 ng/dL (24.0±12 ng/L) and venous blood is typically 50% to 75% of the arterial blood concentration.[28] The plasma concentration of angiotensin-I is 11–88 pg/mL (11–88 ng/L). Both polypeptides are measured with radioimmunoassay. As with many immunoassay procedures the antisera used for angiotensin determinations often lack specificity, and reagents crossreact with many types of polypeptides. The lower limit of sensitivity is 10 pg/sample using commercial antisera. Active proteinases may destroy angiotensin following a phlebotomy, although it has been found that Fuller's earth can minimize this problem. Its protective capability is probably due to the attraction and denaturing of specific enzymes on its surface that otherwise would degrade angiotensin. Drugs, such as captopril or saralasin, that influence plasma renin activity will also influence the levels of angiotensin.

Adrenal Hypertension (see also Chap. 37)

Because of the biological activity of steroids and their importance in the sex characteristics, many clinical symptoms are apparent in persons with hypertension associated with mineralocorticoid abnormalities due to enzyme deficiencies and adrenal hyperplasia.[17] Depending upon which hydroxylase is missing, various deficiencies and excesses are also noted in the hypertensive individual.[31] Table 4-3 outlines these effects.

Diagnosis of excess mineralocorticoid production is based not only on the levels of steroids in the urine and blood, but also on *how the secretion rates change with volume increases or decreases.* These tests can be performed following salt restriction or ingestion of large amounts over several days.

STEROID MEASUREMENTS

The literature concerning the analysis of steroids in body fluids is extensive.[7, 14, 17] An approach for the analysis is based on the choice of specimen, levels encountered, accuracy needed, and method of analysis. Urinary and plasma cortisol determinations appear to be useful for the assessment of adrenal cortical function and have found useful application in clinical practice. Although other steroids and metabolites can be measured, cortisol measurements are the key to evaluating suspected abnormalities of glucocorticoid production (see Fig. 4-2). (See Chap. 37 for additional tests.)

Table 4-3 ***Types of Metabolic Blocks in Adrenal Hyperplasia***

Missing Enzyme	Deficiency	Excess	Phenotype
Desmolase	All steroids	Lipids in adrenals	Adrenal insufficiency
3-Beta-ol-dehydrogenase	Corticoids Aldosterone	Dehydroepiandrosterone	Salt loss, male: hypospadias; Female: mild virilism
17-Hydroxylase	Androgens Estrogens Cortisol Androsterone	Corticosterone, 11-Deoxycorticosterone	Immature female Hypertension Low potassium Alkalosis
21-Hydroxylase	Aldosterone Corticoids	Androgens	Masculinization
11-Hydroxylase	Corticoids Aldosterone	Androgens, 11-Deoxycorticosterone	Masculinization Hypertension
18-Hydroxylase	Aldosterone	Corticosterone	Salt-loser

In addition to the procedures discussed in Chapter 37, the differentiation of primary aldosteronism (adenoma or hyperplasia of the adrenals) from the secondary form can also be made following the administration of 400 mg (orally) per day of spironolactone.[8] Primary aldosteronism is controlled within three to five weeks, whereas the hypertension of the secondary form of aldosteronism is not. Spironolactone probably displaces aldosterone competitively from specific receptors and interferes wtih the normal reabsorption of sodium. Patients with adenomas are distinguishable from those with hyperplasia because the former appear to have higher aldosterone secretion rates, higher sodium and bicarbonate, and lower potassium and plasma renin activities.[7]

Pheochromocytoma

Patients with hypertension secondary to pheochromocytoma manifest cyclic hypertension and the absence of obesity. Hypertension with obesity is most often associated with Cushing's syndrome (see Chap. 37). It has also been observed that more than 95% of pheochromocytomas are located in the abdomen, and 90% are in one or both adrenals. Multiple pheochromocytomas are more common in children. The definitive diagnosis of pheochromocytoma is made through measurements of urine catecholamines and their metabolites. Urinary excretion of catecholamines is elevated in more than 95% of patients with pheochromocytoma, regardless of the effect on blood pressure. Any stress may exacerbate the excretion of catecholamines in normotensive persons and may lead to false positive results. If the excreted catecholamines contain less than 20% epinephrine, then the tumor is still in the adrenals.[28]

CATECHOLAMINE MEASUREMENT

Plasma

Due to the fact that blood catecholamines are present at very low concentrations, clinical methods of analysis are often performed at their limit of sensitivity.[2, 28] More specific methods that also possess high sensitivity and good selectivity have been employed recently. These are high pressure liquid chromatography (HPLC) with electrochemical detection, gas chromatography (GC) with electron capture detectors, and colorimetric assays that utilize fluorometric methods. New radioenzymatic methods are also available for the detection of low levels of catecholamines in blood and other body fluids.

In order to obtain valid laboratory results, an indwelling IV line is required for the collection of blood samples. This procedure eliminates patient stress, which may cause transitory increases in circulating catecholamines. The posture of the patient must be correctly maintained to obtain accurate catecholamine baseline values. Finally, cooled blood samples must be centrifuged immediately and the plasma quickly separated to obtain accurate catecholamine levels that otherwise may be depressed due to red blood cell metabolism. Using enzymatic, double-labeled isotope assays, plasma catecholamine levels have been accurately measured. Values of 5 mg per liter for pheochromocytoma patients are typical, compared to 0.24 mg per liter for normal patients.

Urine

Urine catecholamines and their metabolites can be quantitatively measured using chemical reactions that generate fluorescent products,[17, 18] although this approach involves many analytical problems. Drugs that can be made to be or are fluorescent (*e.g.*, ampicillin, methyldopa, promethazine, protamine, aspirin, sulfonamides, vitamin B complex), beverages (*e.g.*, those containing cocoa, coffee, or tea), and foods (*e.g.*, bananas, vanilla extract, citrus fruits) can often interfere with the fluorometric assays. In addition, laboratory lighting can photochemically degrade catecholamines and their fluorescent products, fluorophors. Brown or red glassware or subdued laboratory lighting can be employed to reduce analytical variability.

Increased sensitivity can also be achieved in urine assays by the hydrolysis of glucuronide and sulfate conjugates. Significant amounts of catecholamine-related compounds are excreted as conjugates.

Metanephrine

Most authorities recommend the measurement of urinary metanephrine as the first test for pheochromocytoma.[28] Very few false negative results are observed, and only rarely are false positive tests encountered. False positive tests are seen most often in severely stressed patients. In these individuals, false positive tests can be ruled out if catecholamines are measured at a later time when the patient is relaxed. The urinary values of metanephrine are expressed in relation to creatinine. A normal value (metanephrine/creatinine ratio) is less than 1.2 μg metanephrine/mg creatinine (0.69 nmol/mol).

Clonidine Suppression Test

Clonidine is a drug that significantly suppresses the production of catecholamines in normal subjects, but not in patients with pheochromocytoma.[31] Clonidine is given orally to a recumbent patient and plasma catecholamine levels are measured before and three hours after the oral administration of clonidine. Plasma norepinephrine levels that remain constant or are elevated at three hours strongly point to pheochromocytoma.

Vanillylmandelic Acid (VMA) and Other Metabolites

In certain patients with pheochromocytoma, the production and metabolism of catecholamines may be intermittent, or the uptake and degradation of catecholamines (half-life approximately two minutes) may be so great that normal or near-normal levels of catecholamines will be observed in the blood or urine. In these patients, however, metabolites of catecholamines are elevated and point to the underlying disease state. The principal end product of norepinephrine and epinephrine is vanillylmandelic acid (VMA). This metabolite reflects total rather than specific catecholamines.[28] In addition, although urinary VMA measurements are more specific, they are less sensitive and more subject to diet and drugs than metanephrine/creatinine determinations. The display on page 54 outlines values for catecholamines.

The urinary excretion of norepinephrine precursors, dopa, dopamine, and metabolites (homovanillic acid and 3-methoxytyramine) is more commonly identified with neuroblastomas. Malignant pheochromocytomas also often secrete dopa, dopamine, and their metabolites. Benign tumors in adults do not secrete these compounds.

Pharmacologic Approaches

A pharmacologic approach can also be applied to the diagnosis of pheochromocytoma. This approach is somewhat dangerous because it either blocks the action of circulating catecholamines or enhances the release of catecholamines from tissue reserves.[8] Phentolamine is an alpha-adrenergic blocking drug given intravenously to reduce blood pressure. A very small dose will produce a profound effect in pheochromocytoma patients. A drop in blood pressure of 35/25 mm Hg lasting four minutes or longer is considered a positive phentolamine test. A simultaneous fall in blood glucose and rise in insulin are also noted as a positive response.

Another pharmacologic approach is the administration of histamine, which releases catecholamines from nerve endings, or glucagon, which stimulates glycogenolysis in tissue stores. A rise in blood pressure of 50/25 mm Hg is highly indicative of pheochromocytoma. Urinalyses to determine the ratio of epinephrine and norepinephrine are very useful in ascertaining tumor location. If norepinephrine is greater than 80% of the two, then the tumor *is not* on the adrenals. Urinary vanillylmandelic acid/catecholamine ratios are also valuable to ascertain the size of catecholamine-secreting tumors. If the ratio favors epinephrine and norepinephrine, the tumor is newly active and typically less than 50 grams. Large tumors are able to metabolize more of the catecholamines and generate more metabolite, and the ratio of products favors vanillylmandelic acid.

Normal (Abnormal) Ranges of Catecholamines and Metabolites

1. Urine—Norepinephrine: 10–70 μg/24 hr
   Epinephrine: 0–20 μg/24 hr
   (Total catecholamines: >250 μg/24 hr)
   Normetanephrine plus metanephrine: <1.3 mg/24 hr
   Vanillylmandelic acid: 1.8–9.0 mg/24 hr
   (metabolite: >10 mg/24 hr)
   Dopamine: <200 μg/24 hr
2. Blood (Plasma)—Catecholamines: <1000 pg/mL
   Norepinephrine: 104–548 pg/mL
   Epinephrine: <88 pg/mL
3. Adrenal medulla—Norepinephrine: 0.04–0.16 mg/g tissue
   Epinephrine: 0.22–0.84 mg/g tissue

Conversion to SI units is as follows:
Norepinephrine—μg/24 hr × 5.91 = nmol/24 hr; pg/mL × 5.91 = pmol/L
Epinephrine—μg/24 hr × 5.46 = nmol/24 hr; pg/mL × 5.46 = pmol/L
Metanephrine—mg/24 hr × 5.07 = μmol/24 hr
VMA—mg/24 hr × 5.05 = μmol/24 hr
Dopamine—μg/24 hr × 6.53 = nmol/d

TREATMENT

Primary Hypertension

The prognosis for patients with primary hypertension is very good if the disease does not progress to the malignant form. No known therapy can correct and reverse the course of the disease, although long-term reduction of blood pressure does appear beneficial. It is now well established that exercise, avoidance of emotional stress, and control of overeating or intemperate drinking can lower the blood pressure of many persons with primary hypertension.[1, 14, 32] Restriction of sodium chloride intake to less than one gram per day significantly lowers the blood pressure in over one-third of primary hypertensive patients. In addition, thiazide diuretics can be used successfully for patients who do not comply with low-sodium intake instructions.

Secondary Hypertension

The successful treatment of secondary hypertension is based on the identification and treatment of the underlying disease.[2]

RENOVASCULAR HYPERTENSION

The prognosis for the disease depends on the age of the patient, extent of the renovascular disease, duration of the hypertension, and selection of the appropriate surgical approach. Surgery is usually employed for endarterectomy, bypass grafts utilizing synthetic grafts or the patient's own veins, and complete revascularization of the affected areas. Nephrectomy is the treatment of choice only in advanced parenchymal disease secondary to vascular problems. In one study, long-term observations of a large group of patients who underwent unilateral nephrectomy in connection with arterial hypertension revealed a 73% remission of arterial hypertension and a return to normal and/or improvement in the course of the disease. Arterial hypertension continued in 18% of the cases studied, and death occurred in 9%, in the first six years following nephrectomy. Partial nephrectomy is also beneficial in partially cystic and infarcted kidneys.

ARTERIOLAR NEPHROSCLEROSIS

Kidney lesions involving the small glomerular arterioles are often associated with hypertension. Although the kidney is affected, the patient is usually asymptomatic.[13] Death usually results from cardiac failure or cerebral hemorrhage with uremia. Benign nephrosclerosis is usually seen in adults from 35 to 55 years of age. In these persons, *hypertension is recorded prior to any urinalysis changes.* This contrasts with glomerulonephritis, in which the *urinalysis changes are observed before any hypertension is noted.* Typically, treatment is similar to that for primary hypertension. Normal renal function is desired to aid in the repair of the sclerotic tissue. No treatment other than the control of the hypertension is required.

PHEOCHROMOCYTOMA

Once catecholamines are identified as the underlying cause of the hypertension, surgical procedures are utilized (except in malignant cases). During surgery, hypertension may be significant. It can be controlled with phenoxybenzamine, phentolamine mesylate, or a tyrosine hydroxylase inhibitor. Propranolol or acebutolol can be used for potential arrhythmias. Following surgery for tumor removal, volume expansion with blood, plasma, or albumin obviates the need for pressor agents. Persistent hypotension may be observed following surgery, and can be controlled with norepinephrine.

OTHER DISEASES

Treatment for glomerulonephritis, nephrotic syndrome, and pyelonephritis is discussed in Part IV (Chaps. 14, 17, and 19 respectively). Treatment for hyperparathyroidism and Cushing's syndrome is discussed in Chapters 36 and 37.

CASE STUDY

A 43-year-old man presented to the hospital emergency room in a confused state. He was unable to move the left side of his body, his skin was cold and moist, and the blood pressure in both arms was 240/195 mm Hg. His pulse was 140 and regular, and his temperature was 101.6°F. Funduscopic examination revealed Grade 2 hypertensive retinopathy that changed rapidly with the development of necrotizing arteriolitis.

The patient was admitted and treated intitially with reserpine; however, after the second 1-mg injection, the blood pressure dropped to zero. He remained cold and clammy, output of urine was negligible, and venous pressure was also low. An infusion of 500 mL of dextran restored the blood pressure to 160/110. On the second day of admission, his blood pressure varied from 180/120 to 240/140 mm Hg and was unresponsive to injections of reserpine. An injection of 5 mg of phentolamine lowered the pressure to 98/60 mm Hg. Dibenzyline was administered by mouth, but did not control the blood pressure. With intermittent phentolamine injections, blood pressure was controlled and, on the third day, the neurologic symptoms cleared. A renal arteriogram was normal. Laboratory findings are listed in Table 4–4.

The patient was discharged with a blood pressure of 140/100 mm Hg. His medications consisted of 100 mg of hydrochlorothiazide and 150 mg of hydralazine daily. He returned to the hospital frequently with acute hypertension. One minute after his hands and wrists were immersed in ice water, blood pressure would rise dramatically. He would go into shock following small doses of pharmacological agents or when a minimum of blood was removed.

This patient was finally diagnosed as having sudden (paroxysmal) hypertension,[30] with clinical, hemodynamic, and metabolic hypersensitivity and

Table 4-4 ***Laboratory Findings***

Blood	
Hematocrit	60%
WBC	$20 \times 10^3/mm^3$ (85% neutrophils)
BUN	60 mg/dL
Creatinine	4.4 mg/dL
Glucose	114 mg/dL
Na	145 mEq/L
K	3.7 mEq/L
Chloride	110 mEq/L
PRA	normal
Cortisol	normal
Urine	
Sp. Gr.	1.020
Protein	3+
Microscopic	few coarsely granular casts/hp field
VMA	normal range
Catecholamines	normal range

Conversion to SI units is as follows:
BUN—mg/dL × 0.357 = mmol/L
Creatinine—mg/dL × 88.4 = μmol/L
Glucose—mg/dL × 0.0555 = mmol/L
Na—mEq/L × 1 = mmol/L
K—mEq/L × 1 = mmol/L
Chloride—mEq/L × 1 = mmol/L

possible signs of sympathoadrenal discharge. He was finally controlled with guanethidine and a diuretic.

Questions

1. Do the laboratory findings support the diagnosis of primary hypertension with an underlying hemodynamic etiology?
2. Why were laboratory studies apparently not ordered immediately when the patient presented to the emergency room?

Discussion

1. Yes, the laboratory findings do not indicate primary or secondary hypertension of renal origin, nor do the cortisol catecholamine and VMA results indicate adrenal hypertension or pheochromocytoma.
2. The clinical findings in this patient indicated a hypertensive emergency: malignant hypertension with rapid funduscopic changes. In this situation the patient must be stabilized before differential diagnostic studies can be performed.

REFERENCES

1. Nies AS: Hypertension. In Melmon K, Morelli HF (eds): Clinical Pharmacology, 2nd ed, Section I, Cardiovascular Disorder, pp 155–209. New York City, Macmillan, 1978
2. Conn R: Current Diagnosis-7, pp 386–392. Philadelphia, WB Saunders, 1985
3. Hypertension in the USA and USSR: Basic, Clinical, and Population Research. NIH Publication No. 80-2016: Second USA–USSR Joint Symposium, Williamsburg, VA, May 14–16, 1979. Bethesda, National Institute of Health, 1979
4. Chobanian AV: Hypertension. In Clinical Symposia, Vol 34, No. 5. Summit, NJ, CIBA Pharmaceutical, 1982
5. Heymans C (ed): The Pathogenesis of Essential Hypertension: Proceedings of the Prague Symposium. New York City, Macmillan, 1962
6. Philips T, Distler A: Hypertension: Mechanism and Management. New York City, Springer-Verlag, 1980
7. Chattoraj SC, Watts NB: Endocrinology. In Tietz N (ed): Textbook of Clinical Chemistry, pp 997–1171. Philadelphia, WB Saunders, 1986
8. Bauer J: Differential Diagnosis of Internal Diseases. New York City, Grune & Stratton, 1967
9. Nies AS: Shock. In Melmon K, Morrelli HF (eds): Clinical Pharmacology, 2nd ed, pp 210–224. New York City, Macmillan, 1978
10. Smith L, Wyngaarden J (eds): Review of General Internal Medicine: A Self-Assessment Manual. Philadelphia, WB Saunders, 1980
11. Muehrcke RC et al: Biopsy of the kidney in the diagnosis and management of renal disease. N Engl J Med 253:537–546, 1955
12. Kruppe MA et al: Physician's Handbook, 21st ed, pp 60–61. Los Altos, CA, Lange Medical Publications, 1982
13. Imber I, Clymer RH: Obstruction of the renal ar-

tery producing malignant hypertension. N Engl J Med 253:537–546, 1955
14. Marable SA et al: Treatment of hypertension associated with the solitary ischemic kidney. N Engl J Med 275:1278–1282, 1966
15. Fruchtman M, Caldwell JR: Hypertension due to renal infarction. N Engl J Med 263:907–909, 1960
16. Margolin EG, Merrill JP, Harrison JH: Diagnosis of hypertension due to occlusions of the renal artery. N Engl J Med 256:581–588, 1957
17. Howanitz P, Howanitz J: Evaluation of endocrine function. In Henry J (ed): Clinical Diagnosis and Management of Laboratory Methods, 17th ed, pp 299–305. Philadelphia, WB Saunders, 1984
18. Brunjes S: Catecholamine metabolism in essential hypertension. N Engl J Med 271:120–124, 1964
19. Masland RP et al: Hypertensive vascular disease in adolescence. N Engl J Med 255:894–897, 1956
20. Epstein FH et al: Hypercalcemia, nephrocalcinosis, and reversible renal insufficiency associated with hyperthyroidism. N Engl J Med 258:782–785, 1958
21. Shaw RS: Acute dissecting aortic aneurysm. N Engl J Med 253:331–333, 1955
22. Agress C, Estrin M: Biochemical Diagnosis of Heart Disease. Springfield, IL, Charles C Thomas, 1963
23. Silber EN, Katz LN: Heart Disease, pp 172–191. New York City, Macmillan, 1975
24. Hurst JW (ed): The Heart, 6th ed, Vol II, pp 1038–1104. New York City, McGraw-Hill, 1986
25. Rayburn W, Zuspan F (eds): Drug Therapy in Obstetrics and Gynecology, 2nd ed. Norwalk, CN, Appleton-Century-Crofts, 1986
26. Costrini N, Thomson WM: Manual of Medical Therapeutics, 22nd ed, pp 125–134. Boston, Little, Brown & Co, 1979
27. Collins RD: Illustratred Manual of Laboratory Diagnosis, p 275. Philadelphia, JB Lippincott, 1968
28. Tietz NW (ed): Clinical Guide to Laboratory Tests. Philadelphia, WB Saunders, 1983
29. Hoffman WS: The Biochemistry of Clinical Medicine, 4th ed. Chicago, Year Book Medical Pub, 1973
30. Cohn JN: Paroxysmal hypertension and hypovolemia. N Engl J Med 275:643–646, 1966
31. Holvey DN (ed): The Merck Manual of Diagnosis and Therapy. Rahway, NJ, Merck and Co, 1972
32. Krupp MK, Chatton MJ, Werdegard D: Current Medical Treatment, pp 201–211. Los Altos, CA, Lange Medical Publications, 1985

BIBLIOGRAPHY

Blaschke TF, Melmon KL: Antihypertensive Agents and the Drug Therapy of Hypertension. In Gilman AG, Goodman LS, Gilman A (eds): The Pharmacological Basis of Therapeutics, 6th ed, pp 793–818. New York City, MacMillan, 1980

Ticktin HE, Fazekas JF, Evans JM: Ammonia intoxication in a patient with congestive heart failure receiving ammonium chloride orally. N Engl J Med 255:905–907, 1955

Chapter 5

Atherosclerotic Heart Disease

Michael Sealfon

ETIOLOGY AND PATHOPHYSIOLOGY

Cardiovascular disease remains the chief cause of death in the United States and Western Europe, and atherosclerosis, the principal cause of myocardial and cerebral infarction, accounts for the majority of these deaths.[1] Atherosclerosis is the deposition of lipids in blood vessels resulting in narrowing of their lumina. It is believed to be a lifelong process beginning with the "fatty streak" found in the aorta of all infants by the age of 1 year and the coronary arteries by age 10. The fatty streak is a lipid-rich lesion consisting of both macrophages and smooth muscle. The basic lesion of atherosclerosis is called an *atheroma* or fibrous plaque and is composed of increased intimal smooth-muscle cell surrounded by connective tissue matrix and containing variable amounts of intracellular and extracellular lipid. At the arterial lumens, this lesion is generally covered by a dense fibrous cap of smooth muscle and connective tissue. Many atheromas eventually undergo a variety of complications such as calcification, ulceration, thrombus formation, and aneurysmal dilation.

The incidence of atherosclerosis in the elderly is 46% by the sixth decade of life and 84% by the ninth decade. Atherosclerosis of the coronary artery is ten times more common among men than among women under 45 years of age. Sex preference falls off rapidly between 45 to 60 years of age, although males in this group still suffer twice as many heart attacks as females. In the very elderly, the incidence is about the same for both sexes.

Plaque Formation

The aorta is the most common site for the atherosclerotic plaque (lesion), followed by other major arteries. Elderly populations have more fibrous material in plaques with marked calcification of their vessels. Recent studies have shown that plaque formation is a complex process involving (1) smooth-muscle cells and macrophages, (2) hypercholesterolemia, and (3) chemoattractants. Macrophages predominate in the early fatty streaks, which may represent a form of inflammatory response. The atherosclerotic lesions may, in effect, represent a defense mechanism that progresses to a pathological response. Diet-induced hypercholesterolemia leads to changes in the endothelial lining of the vessels as well as in increased monocyte adherence, subendothelial migration, accumulation of lipid to form foam cells, and gradual accumulation of smooth muscle to form fatty streaks. At some sites, endothelial cells may separate, exposing foam cells, which in some cases may interact with platelets to form mural thrombi. Such interactions appear to lead to relatively rapid smooth-muscle proliferation. All four principal cells involved in atherosclerosis—endothelium, smooth muscle, platelets, and monocyte/macrophages—either contain substances such as platelets or can synthesize and release chemoattractants and growth factors.

Biochemically, the atherosclerotic plaques are associated with a predominant lipid fraction, the low-density lipoprotein (LDL). The cholesterol in the LDL fraction is blocked from reesterification, and localized cellular removal does not occur. The lipids deposited in the atherogenic lesions are not easily removed by normal cellular clearing mechanisms and begin to accumulate.

Continued research concerning the etiology of atherosclerotic heart disease has identified a number of factors associated with an increase in the likelihood that a person will suffer a heart attack late in life. These factors, which directly correlate with the presence of coronary artery disease, are classified as "risk factors." Certain of these factors are unavoidable, such as a genetic or racial predisposition. Others, however, can be modified and include high blood pressure, cigarette smoking, diabetes, and elevated serum cholesterol. Several recent developments focusing on cellular receptors for LDL cholesterol have given new impetus to the prevention of coronary artery disease.[2]

Transport of Cholesterol

The relationship between *transport of cholesterol* and coronary artery disease can best be understood through the lipoprotein system (Fig. 5-1). Dietary cholesterol enters the body combined with chylomicrons. Chylomicron triglycerides are hydrolyzed, and residual particles, called *chylomicron remnants*, are rapidly removed by the liver. The liver also secretes triglyceride-rich lipoproteins called very-low-density lipoproteins (VLDLs), which are degraded into smaller VLDL remnants. The latter can be removed by the liver or converted to LDL. The LDLs are the major cholesterol-carrying lipoproteins in plasma. The major pathway for removal of LDLs is by way of LDL receptors on liver cells, although to a lesser extent, LDLs can be cleared by extrahepatic tissues. Finally, high-density lipoproteins (HDLs) may accept cholesterol from extrahepatic tissues and other sources and transfer it to VLDLs and LDLs. Cholesterol carried on these latter lipoproteins can be removed by the liver.

It has been shown that the LDL particle is

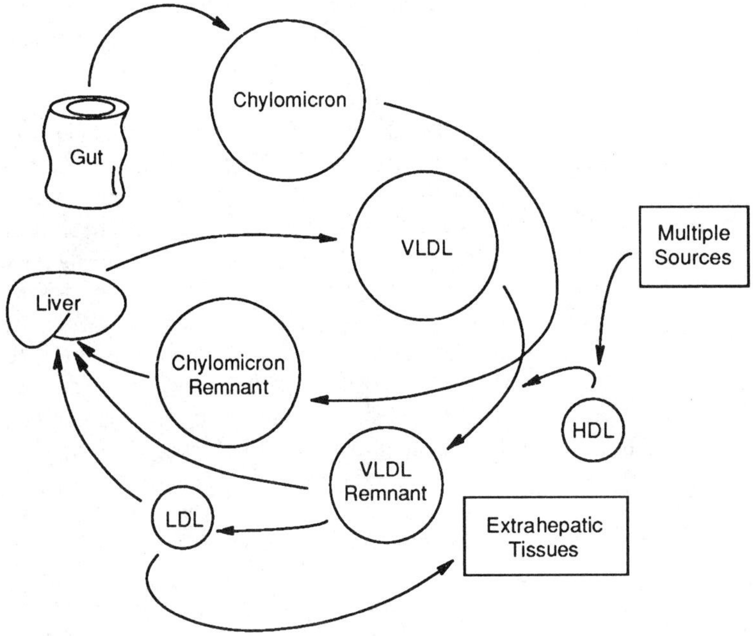

Figure 5-1 **Pathways for lipoprotein metabolism.**

engulfed by the LDL-specific cell in the liver after the phenomenon of receptor site recognition. Up to 45% of circulating LDL is used by hepatic cells per day. Breakdown of the normal mechanisms for LDL use by cells can quickly lead to increased circulating LDL concentrations. Studies of familial hypercholesterolemia (FH) homozygotes have shown that the absence of cell receptor sites can lead to increase in LDL concentrations 6 to 8 times the normal range.[2] Such affected individuals are prone to premature coronary artery disease. The incidence of the less severe form (heterozygous) of FH is one in every 500 persons, and these individuals carry a cholesterol level twice the normal reference interval.[2]

Risk of Coronary Artery Disease

Numerous studies have suggested that the rates of coronary artery disease are relatively constant for cholesterol values up to 200 to 220 mg/dL, (5.2 to 5.7 mmol/L) but above this threshold range the risk for coronary artery disease increases as the cholesterol concentrations rise.[2] A linear relationship has been proposed that links severity of coronary artery disease with the percentage of coronary artery surface covered with atherosclerotic lesions. Pathological studies indicate that when about 60% of the surface is covered with raised plaque, one enters a critical phase of substantially increased risk.[2]

Thus a significantly increased risk of coronary artery disease can be correlated with high total serum cholesterol values. Currently hypercholesterolemia is defined as plasma values exceeding 240 mg/dL (6.2 mmol/L), which corresponds to an LDL value of greater than 175 mg/dL (4.5 mmol/L). Hypercholesterolemia has been linked to three processes: (1) the synthesis of LDL receptors, which is under feedback regulation responsive to the concentration of cholesterol in hepatic tissue; (2) the ability of hepatocytes to transport LDL receptors to the cell surface; and (3) the increased conversion of VLDLs to LDL, which appears to be modulated by diet.

Diet appears to be a significant factor for a large

segment of the population. Certain individuals may be overly sensitive to excess dietary cholesterol, saturated fatty acids, or total calories and may respond with an unusually marked increase in their LDL values.

One of the most striking features of the effects of dietary cholesterol is the variability in response; some individuals show appreciable increases in plasma cholesterol and LDL-cholesterol levels when dietary cholesterol is raised, while others have little or no increase. It has been shown that saturated fatty acids definitely raise plasma cholesterol concentrations, seemingly by suppressing the activity of LDL receptors. Polyunsaturated fatty acids of the omega-6 variety (*e.g.*, linoleic acid), have been shown to have a cholesterol-lowering action. Recent studies have focused on the effects of dietary modification and increased exercise to reduce total cholesterol concentrations, and subsequently reduce the prevalence of coronary artery disease.

CLINICAL MANIFESTATIONS

The clinical effects of atherosclerosis are complications that accompany a critical decrease in blood volume to a coronary vessel. In addition to myocardial infarction and angina pectoris, ischemic heart disease is a common indicator of the presence of atherosclerosis.[3]

LABORATORY ANALYSES AND DIAGNOSIS

In addition to total serum or plasma cholesterol, several other lipid measurements have been preferred at various times to assess risk associated with premature coronary artery disease. Such determinations include the percentage of esterified cholesterol, the ratio of cholesterol to phospholipids, and the concentration of total lipids, triglycerides, LDL and HDL cholesterol, HDL phospholipids, and HDL_2 and HDL_3 cholesterol or total mass. Some of these measurements have fallen into disuse because of the cumbersome nature of the test or because often there have not been adequate prospective studies to establish potential usefulness. Most clinical laboratories now offer total cholesterol, total triglycerides, and HDL cholesterol as routine studies. Recent evidence indicates that concentrations of plasma apolipoprotein A-I, the major HDL protein, and apolipoprotein B, the major LDL protein, are better predictors of coronary artery disease than HDL cholesterol or LDL cholesterol respectively. Current research suggests that when age and apolipoproteins A-I, A-II, and B are all considered, their sensitivity for prediction is only 81% and the specificity is 58%.[4]

Cholesterol Measurement

Currently the measurement of total cholesterol is the single most important laboratory test for assessing the risk of cardiovascular disease. The accurate measurement of HDL cholesterol can be particularly important for the calculation of the total cholesterol : HDL ratio, yet the variation in precision and accuracy associated with the measurement of this analyte has been shown to exceed current acceptable clinical limits. For example interlaboratory precision during 1986 proficiency survey testing was reported to exceed 16.0%.[5] The majority of laboratories participating in the College of American Pathologists 1986 Chemistry Surveys used dextran sulfate (MW 50,000)/magnesium sulfate precipitation of all lipoproteins other than HDL followed by determination of the cholesterol remaining in the supernatant. The Lipid Research Clinic recommends a standard deviation (SD) of less than 3 mg/dL (0.08 mmol/L) for acceptable intralaboratory precision.[6]

The use of automated chemistry analysis has done much to increase the precision of currently available methods for total cholesterol determination, yet differences in reagent composition have biased several methods above or below the target values established by the reference method of Abell-Kendall.[7] Most authors agree that intermethod bias can be reduced by (1) use of calibrators that have been standardized using the Abell-Kendall method (2) use of more reliable enzymatic methods to reduce the effects of interferences, and (3) more efficient instrumentation with increased precision. The suggested goal for the coefficient of variation (CV) for total cholesterol determinations within a laboratory should be 3% or less.[6]

Most authors recommend that total cholesterol and HDL cholesterol values no longer be reported to include "normal" ranges but should reflect severity of cardiovascular risk (Table 5-1). The Consensus Conference on Lowering Blood Cholesterol to Prevent Heart Disease recommends that four categories of risk be established: (1) desirable reference range for the population (40th percentile or a total cholesterol value of 200 mg/dL [5.2 mmol/L]); (2) a mildly increased risk category from the 40th to 75th percentile or a total cholesterol value of from 200 to 240 mg/dL (5.2 to 6.2 mmol/L); (3) a moderately increased risk category from the 75 to 95th percentile representing a total cholesterol value of from 240 to 265 mg/dL (6.2–6.9 mmol/L); and (4) a high-risk category for individuals >95th percentile with a total cholesterol value exceeding 265 mg/dL (6.9 mmol/L).

TREATMENT

The efficacy of cholesterol-lowering bile acid sequestering or competitive inhibitors of 3-hydroxy-3-methylglutaryl coenzyme A reductase when combined with an appropriate diet can have a significant impact on the 15% to 20% of the population currently classified as hypercholesterolemic and thus at risk for premature cardiovascular disease.

The ideal suggested cholesterol range for the general population has been proposed to be from 130 to 190 mg/dL (3.4–4.9 mmol/L). If the cholesterol level of most Americans could be reduced to this range the rate of coronary artery disease could be reduced by 30% to 50%.

CASE STUDY

An obese 60-year old man presented to the hospital outpatient clinic with shortness of breath and concern over a family history of death in the fifth/sixth decades due to heart disease.

Patient history indicated that the patient was 30 pounds overweight, smoked at least one package of cigarettes per day, and worked at a sedentary desk job.

This specific history suggested the need for a lipid-cardiac risk profile. The results of this profile as performed by microcomputer are shown in Table 5-2.

Table 5-1 ***Risk Categories for Cardiovascular Disease***

Risk Category	Plasma Cholesterol	Population Percentile
Desirable range	<200 mg/dL	<40th
Mildly increased risk	200–240 mg/dL	40–75th
Moderately increased risk	240–265 mg/dL	75–95th
High risk	>265 mg/dL	>95th

Conversion to SI units is as follows:
cholesterol mg/dL × 0.0259 = mmol/L

Table 5-2 ***Lipid Phenotype***

Accn. or SSN: 2678
Age: 60

	Reference Range
Chlyomicrons present: None	
Cholesterol value: 275 mg/dL	171–259
Triglyceride value: 150 mg/dL	68–235
HDL value: 29 mg/dL	34– 69
LDL value: 222 mg/dL	106–188
Cholesterol-HDL ratio: 9	Reference range: 5.5

2 × Risk ASHD

Conversion to SI units is as follows:
mg/dL × 0.0259 = mmol/L

Questions

1. What parameters most likely suggest an increased risk of cardiovascular disease?
2. How are normal reference intervals obtained for each of the analytes?
3. What therapeutic regimen, if any, is available to reduce the risk of cardiovascular disease?

Discussion

1. The parameters suggesting increased risk of cardiovascular disease include elevated LDL cholesterol, decreased HDL cholesterol, and an elevated cholesterol-HDL ratio.
2. The normal reference values were obtained from age- and sex-adjusted ranges that represent the upper 75th percentile of the study population.
3. An initial therapeutic regimen might consist of initiation of a low fat/low cholesterol diet with reduced caloric intake. A graduated exercise program with cessation of smoking is also indicated. Drug therapy for reduction of total serum cholesterol is only indicated when diet and exercise cannot significantly reduce the value to an acceptable level.

REFERENCES

1. Russell R: The pathogenesis of atherosclerosis—An update. N Engl J Med 314:488–499, 1986
2. Schaefer EJ, Levy RI: Pathogenesis and management of lipoprotein disorders. N Engl J Med 312:1300–1312, 1985
3. Bierman, EL: Atherosclerosis and other forms of arteriosclerosis. In Petersdorf RG, Adams RD, Braunwald E et al (eds): Harrison's Principles of Internal Medicine, 10th ed, pp 1469–1475. New York, McGraw-Hill, 1983
4. Frantz ID: Cardiovascular risk—What should be measured? Mayo Clin Proc 61:396–398, 1986
5. College of American Pathologists: Chemistry Survey CD86. Skokie, IL, 1986
6. Grundy SM: A symposium: Laboratory lipid values. Am J Cardiol 56:23J, 1985
7. Blank DW, Hoag JM, Kroll MH, Riddel ME: The method of determination must be considered in interpreting blood cholesterol levels. JAMA 256:2867–2870, 1986

BIBLIOGRAPHY

Gorman LS: Advances in understanding heart disease. J Med Tech 3:21–23, 1986

Grundy SM: Cholesterol and coronary heart disease. JAMA 256:2849–2858, 1986

Naito HK: Disorders of lipid metabolism. In Kaplan LA, Pesce AJ (eds): Clinical Chemistry—Theory, Analysis, and Correlation, pp 589–593. St. Louis, CV Mosby, 1984

Chapter 6

Heart Failure

Linda Gorman

Heart failure is a clinical condition resulting from failure of the heart to maintain adequate circulation of blood. Pumping abnormalities result from failure of the right or left ventricle, or both. Heart weakness or fragility leading to heart failure results from biochemical changes in the tissue.

Heart failure may become the killer that myocardial infarction has been during recent decades. Patients classified as having *congestive heart failure (CHF)* have increased from 150,000 in 1970 to 500,000 in 1983. Presently heart failure, detected and undetected, is thought to affect 2 to 3 million persons.[1] The slow, often undetectable, changes that lead to full-blown heart failure make it prudent to prevent the disease as well as to ensure early diagnosis and treatment.

Age is one factor in heart failure. Because many confirmed heart failure patients are over 60 years of age, there is a general belief that heart failure does not begin until middle age or beyond. Patients between the ages of 25 and 45 years do not usually exhibit the symptoms of heart failure, but are a prime group for which to begin measures to reverse early indicators of heart disease.

ETIOLOGY AND PATHOPHYSIOLOGY

The etiology of heart failure involves either heart weakness or pumping abnormalities. Some of the conditions leading to congestive heart failure are displayed on the opposite page. Heart fragility or weakness can be induced by endogenous or exog-

Conditions That May Precipitate Heart Failure

1. Discontinuation of digitalis or diuretics
2. Excessive sodium intake
3. Hemorrhage and anemia
4. Infections
5. Myocardial infarction
6. Pulmonary embolism
7. Systemic hypertension
8. Tachy- or bradyarrhythmias
9. Undue physical exertion or emotional stress

enous substances. For example, changes in the body's hormonal balance can lead to myocardial weakness, as can ingestion of toxins or a lack of essential nutrients.

The pumping abnormalities that lead to heart failure have been studied extensively. Because these abnormalities are often the first manifestation of trouble, many physicians are aware of heart failure in the context of left and/or right ventricular failure. Left ventricular failure in particular leads to increased blood pressure and congestion of pulmonary veins and capillaries. Right ventricular failure exhibits increased blood pressure with congestion of systemic veins and capillaries.[2]

The pathophysiology of heart failure includes ischemia, which can be common to both myocardial weakness and pumping disorders. Hypertrophy as compensation for deficiencies can also occur. Cellular changes of the myosin, actin, and cytoplasmic areas may be the first signs of heart failure.

Myocardial Weakness

Myocardial weakness and associated diseases fall into three groups: (1) various cardiomyopathies caused by the adverse effects on myocardial tissue of endogenous or exogenous substances, (2) problems involving ischemia of the tissues, and (3) myocarditis due either to infection or to immunological problems.

CARDIOMYOPATHIES

Increases in potassium level caused by primary disease of the kidneys or endocrine glands can result in toxicity of the heart cells. Potassium toxicity leads to myocardial limpness and to stretched and flabby tissue.[3] Loss of tone by the myocardium weakens the heart's ability to perform complete strokes. Incomplete strokes lead to blood volume problems and circulation deficiencies.

Endocrine disorders upset hormonal balance and can adversely affect heart function. Thyroid imbalances with unrestrained thyroxine (T_4) and triiodothyronine (T_3) activity can cause the heart to pump vigorously without restraint. Adrenal hormones play an integral part in heart function. The effects of the catecholamines and their part in the development of systemic hypertension are discussed in Chapter 4.

Nutritional influence on cardiac function is being reexamined in light of new nutritional information. Doses of toxic vitamins can significantly alter the biochemistry of body cells, and the myocardial cells are not immune to these effects. In addition to the typical toxicity patterns reported, vitamin B_6 deficiencies have been implicated in cardiomyopathies. Vitamin B_6 deficiency leads to deterioration of cardiac muscle fibers and their replacement with fibrous strands. The contractility of heart muscle fibers is weakened when fibrosis replaces the bendable muscle fibers. This is one example of the infiltration of viable heart tissue by materials that hinder pumping and weaken cardiac function. Other infiltrates of bacterial or drug origin or metal toxins can also render the heart muscle unable to perform normally. Hemochromatosis, the infiltrate of iron into tissues, can adversely affect heart muscle and lead to loss of contractility and muscle function. Iron is probably the best known metal infiltrate, but other metals such as arsenic, lead, or magnesium, have been implicated, especially when abnormal amounts are found in the patient's environment.

Drug toxicity, as with heart medications like digitalis, can lead to (1) loss of heart muscle contraction, (2) increased volume loads, and (3) relaxation of muscle tone. Toxicity from poisons that upset the biochemical functions of myocardial cells obviously leads to myocardial weakness. Poisons that inhibit sodium-potassium ATPase activity and/or the movement of calcium to and from muscle fibers will adversely affect the contraction and relaxation of heart muscle.

Alcohol is particularly harmful to cardiac function, as is shown in cases involving chronically alcoholic patients. At least one fourth of all alcoholics suffer from an alcohol cardiomyopathy.[3] Alcoholism has been associated with nonatherogenic heart disease and, when linked with cardiovascular disorders, appears to be the cause of significantly higher mortality rates. Ethanol metabolism to acetaldehyde and acetate reduces myocardial cellular oxidation of fatty acids, which esterify and become fat droplets within the cardiac muscle cells. As more ethanol is ingested there is a further reduction in mitochondrial function, with decreasing oxygen respiration leading to reductions in ATP production.[1] Ethanol depresses cellular enzymes of sodium-potassium ATPase, acetyl Co-A synthetase, and ornithine carboxylase. The fatty esters and ethyl esters, formed by excessive ethanol ingestion, may also bind to the mitochondria and uncouple oxidative phosphorylation. These biochemical changes weaken the heart muscle and adversely affect blood flow, pumping pressures, and tissue tone.[1] Many heavy drinkers develop hypertension because alcohol dilates skin surface blood vessels but constricts arterioles.[1] This arteriolar constriction plays a part in the peripheral edema and pulmonary problems often seen in persons with alcoholic cardiomyopathies.

Acceleration of the heart rate with an increase in catecholamine levels has been seen in normal subjects with an ethanol concentration of 70 to 138 mg/dL (15–30 mmol/L).[1] At this level of ethanol there is a depression of myocardial function, with an increase in right atrial pressure and a decrease in perfusion pressure.[1] Regional blood flow at an ethanol concentration of 122 to 143 mg/dL (26–31 mmol/L) is decreased through ischemic areas and increased through normal tissue areas.[1]

MYOCARDIAL ISCHEMIA

Myocardial weakness due to myocardial ischemia is not often severe enough to precipitate an acute myocardial infarction (AMI). Probably because the biochemistry of cellular metabolism is a dynamic process, there are many ischemic events during the life of a heart. When the ischemic events begin to prevent the heart from performing either at rest or with increased exercise, the characteristic signs of ischemia are noticeable. Angina pectoris, a term for pain due to the imbalance between resting and work-oriented oxygen needs of the heart, can be caused by transitory ischemic events. The constricting pain lasts for only a few minutes, which distinguishes it from the prolonged pain of pericarditis, inflammation of pleural membranes, or chest wall spasms.[3]

Atherosclerosis of myocardial blood vessels can also lead to ischemia of tissues. The occlusion of vessels forces the blood-poor tissue to use anaerobic metabolism. If this continues for more than a few minutes, the anaerobic products damage the cells of the tissue. Necrosis sets in, leading to loss of viable cardiac muscle fibers. A decrease in the muscle mass increases the load carried by the remaining viable tissue. Ischemia as a process causes viable active muscle to be replaced with fibrous material that is unable to perform or function properly.

MYOCARDITIS

Myocarditis as a myocardial weakness leading to heart failure can be caused by infections, immunological injury to the tissues, or idiopathic diseases. A number of bacteria produce toxins that adversely affect heart tissue, causing a break up of the normal cellular biochemistry. Viruses and parasites can also damage heart tissue directly. The more indirect immunological injury seen in rheumatic fever is the type of myocarditis that could occur with many infections. In rheumatic fever, the bacterial antigens cross-react with circulating antibodies to form complexes that deposit in the myocardium.[3] As a result, there is destruction of tissue, which leads to myocardial weakness and loss of cardiac wall tone. The patient often has symptoms of weakness, fever, and/or joint pain that mask the myocardial damage of the infection. Inflammation of the pericardium causes a fluid build up in the pericardial space.[4] This fluid can press on the heart muscle and alter stroke volumes of the heart. Resolution of the inflammatory process may leave adhesions between the visceral and the parietal membranes of the pericardium. The immunological response to inflammation leads to the development of adhesions between these membranes. The adhesions formed restrict the contraction of heart muscle and interfere with the pumping function of the heart. The restrictive characteristics of myocarditis are also seen in the idiopathic states. Most common is the development of pericarditis after myocardial infarction that involves areas adjacent to the pericardium. A fibrous build-up occurs with correction of the pericarditis. This complicates the recovery from MI and often leads to congestive heart failure.

Increased Afterload

Increased afterload (tension in the ventricular wall during ejection)[4] causes pumping problems that, with time, will resemble congestive heart failure. The sluggish or incomplete movement of blood leads by degrees to congestive heart failure. A progression to pumping abnormalities requires physician intervention at the earliest stages to avert chronic problems. Heart failure originating from left or right ventricle pumping malfunction must be pinpointed and relieved if at all possible.

LUNG EFFECTS

Left ventricle problems can precipitate pulmonary congestion and edema. The edema will lead to stiffening of lung tissues and, if unchecked, will reduce the surface area available for exchange of oxygen and carbon dioxide. The accompanying dyspnea may first present as paroxysmal nocturnal dyspnea (in which fluid collects in the spaces only at night) or orthopnea (in which fluid collects in the spaces when the patient is lying down).[3]

Increases in blood pressure may cause rupture of small pulmonary blood vessels, resulting in areas of hemorrhage and secondary infection in the patient with congestive heart failure. The continued lag of left ventricle function increases the demand on the right ventricle to handle excessive volumes of blood. The back pressure harms the right atrium as well, leading to a three-chamber hypertrophy characteristic of cardiomegaly. Pooling of blood in the circulation causes systemic congestion and edema, especially in lower body limbs due to gravity. The systemic congestion and pressure build up lead to hepatic congestion and hepatomegaly. The pressure causing hemorrhagic damage to liver cells results in fibrotic replacement of connective tissue and loss of liver function. Disruption of the hepatic portal system causes changes in intestinal absorption and may lead to splenomegaly.[3]

Alterations in blood flow also affect kidney function and contribute to the edema seen in congestive heart failure. The increase in renal sympathetic nerve discharge caused by a decrease in renal blood flow increases the efferent arteriole vasoconstriction and increases the filtration function of the kidney. Increases in renal venous blood pressure lead to increases in renal lymph and in lymphatic flow to the thoracic duct. The increased discharge of the sympathetic nerves augments the kidney release of renin and stimulates the renin-angiotensin system to increase blood pressure.[2] The kidneys, trying to improve renal blood flow, contribute additional problems to imbalances in pressure in the patient with congestive heart failure (CHF). The hormonal imbalance that results when an increase in renin leads to an increase in aldosterone does not totally explain the electrolyte problems seen in CHF patients.[2] Recent evidence suggests that an atrial natriuretic factor (ANF) released from secretory granules of the heart atrials is responsible for increasing glomerular filtration rates and increasing solute excretion by the kidneys.[5] The action of ANF in inhibiting vasopression further suggests that ANF is released to counteract many of the fluid problems a CHF patient may develop. Because ANF levels are elevated in patients with untreated CHF,[6] perhaps ANF is released because of cardiac filling pressures and not because of decreases in renal blood flow. ANF is helpful in overcoming the effects of aldosterone changes in the kidney, but kidney influence on the heart is not reciprocal. Prorenin is thought to be a cardiotropic hormone that promotes myocardial cellular growth and contributes to the hypertrophy seen in congestive heart failure.[7] An increase in vascular resistance of the renal blood vessels seems to promote an increase in prorenin circulation, with uptake by the heart influencing myocardial contraction, blood pressure, and tissue perfusion rates. At least 58% of the circulating prorenin is extracted by the heart during a single passage through the coronary circulation.[7]

Many heart failure diseases involve problems of increased or decreased blood volume. Blood volume problems involve the right heart and are often precipitated by events in the lungs, blood pressure, or conduction circuitry of the heart.

Two mechanisms are thought to be associated with lung disease as the primary ailment causing secondary heart failure or *cor pulmonale.*[3]

1. Respiratory disease caused by hydrostatic blood pressure, which increases the right heart load
2. Hypoxemia and/or respiratory acidosis leading to respiratory malfunction and reduction in the ability of the myocardium to cope with normal blood volumes

The primary lung diseases of emphysema and chronic bronchitis alter pulmonary tissues in such a way that pulmonary blood pressure increases. The first mechanism of cor pulmonale can increase the blood volume load on the right heart, resulting in right heart hypertrophy and failure. Often there is a lack of pulmonary congestion or dyspnea until the right and left heart become involved.[3] The lack of respiratory gas exchange in the second mechanism of cor pulmonale quickly increases the level of toxic metabolites, preventing the myocardium from perfusing and performing its function. Normal blood volumes high in lactic acid and carbon dioxide hinder myocardial respiration. Toxic metabolites increase heart workload and reduce myocardium effectiveness.

HYPERTENSION

Just as heart failure can be caused by primary lung disease, so too can volume problems develop due to blood pressure changes unrelated to cardiac function. Hypertension can put added pressure on the heart and lead to heart failure. The increase in blood pressure increases the resistance that the left ventricle must overcome to maintain cardiac volumes[3] (see Chap. 4).

VALVULAR DISEASE

Valvular malfunction also alters the blood volume that the heart tries to regulate. Valves that remain only partially open precipitate flow back-up into heart and lung circulation. Valves that remain partially closed throughout pumping promote inappropriate ventricular filling and emptying. The endocarditis of rheumatic fever and the stenosis of other infections have been discussed. Valvular damage in a patient with myocardial infarction can be precipitated by rupture of the capillary blood vessels.[3] The valve may retain partial function, but no longer closes completely or opens sufficiently. Such patients will progress to cardiac failure as the blood volume changes alter blood load for ventricles and atrials.[8, 9] The progression to congestive heart failure in these patients depends on severity of valvular damage and on time sequence. With blood pressure changes and factors such as hypertension, ischemic areas, or increases in immunological complexes, the development of thrombi that either remain within the ventricle or pass through it also poses a risk for reducing blood output and increasing back pressure. Thrombi obstructing valve openings prevent blood flow and increase the risk of heart failure.

RESTRICTIONS IN PUMPING

Arrhythmias, or disruptions in the cardiac conduction system, appear to be caused by ischemia, infarction, infiltrates, electrolyte imbalances, or chemical toxins. The loss of a steady heart beat concerns the patient and is often the reason for admission to the emergency room. Tachycardia of more than 160 beats/minute causes rapid contractions; ventricular filling becomes inadequate, and diastolic volume, stroke volume, and cardiac output are reduced. Paroxysmal tachycardia may be attributed to stress or to emotional causes. Ischemia involving tachycardia can lead to a vicious cycle of increased oxygen demand, leading to electrical instability and increased contraction with further oxygen demands. Recognition of the ischemia and corrective measures are called for to alleviate tachycardia. Arrhythmias directly involving loss of sinoatrial (S-A) node control and/or atrioventricular (A-V) node stimulation present problems involving heart failure. The irregular cardiac rhythms, seen when the S-A node is not controlling myocardial muscle depolarization,[3] precipitate heart congestion and alteration of heart chamber filling capacities. These changes can increase pressure problems as well as inefficiencies of blood flow. Arrhythmias involving the A-V node often cause a slow or unresponsive depolarization of the A-V node to the S-A stimulus. Without A-V node response, an uncoordinated contraction occurs between the atrial and ventricular chambers. This inefficiency of heart pumping can be caused by fibrous deposits that isolate the A-V node from the heart conduction system.

CLINICAL MANIFESTATIONS

Heart failure that leads to congestive heart failure is detectable if it involves a patient with myocardial infarction or one with angina, pulmonary problems, or arrhythmias.[9] Episodes of pain or tachycardia can be alarming and usually cause the patient to seek medical attention. Hormonal disorders involving the thyroid or feelings of fatigue and weakness may also cause a patient to see a physician, but not specifically for heart failure. The question of how to detect possible heart failure early is a difficult one. Vigilant attention to patient histories and thorough physical examination involving up-to-date radiological examinations and laboratory testing can alter the situation.[10] Most patients with congestive heart failure present to the physician with symptoms of hypertension and/or edema. Many are already experiencing pulmonary congestion and have had frequent bouts with pulmonary infection. The signs and symptoms associated with congestive heart failure are listed below and additional criteria are listed on page 70.

LABORATORY ANALYSES AND DIAGNOSIS

Laboratory involvement in cases of heart failure is concerned primarily with the results of heart failure, such as lung congestion and kidney failure, as well as the monitoring of drug therapy. Radiological testing (e.g., chest x-rays) is the primary means for diagnosing heart failure.

Radiological Testing

The chest x-ray offers an opportunity for examining pulmonary blood vessels. The electrocardiogram (ECG) with multiple leads is a noninvasive

Signs and Symptoms of Congestive Heart Failure

1. Weakness and fatigue
2. Pulmonary congestion, breathlessness, dyspnea
3. Edema in lower portions of body
4. Cardiomegaly
5. Systemic congestion
6. Hepatomegaly
7. Splenomegaly
8. Abdominal discomfort

Criteria for Cardiac Failure

Major Criteria
Paroxysmal nocturnal dyspnea
Neck vein distention
Rales
Cardiomegaly
Acute pulmonary edema
S_3 gallop
Increased venous pressure (>16 cm water)
Hepatojugular reflux

Minor Criteria
Ankle edema
Night cough
Dyspnea on exertion
Hepatomegaly
Pleural effusion
Vital capacity reduced 1/3 from maximum
Tachycardia (>120)

Major or Minor
Weight loss 4.5 kg over 5 days
in response to treatment
Patients with two of the major criteria or one of the major and two of the minor criteria are prime candidates for a diagnosis of cardiac failure.

Data from reference number [2]

measure of the electrical impulse through the heart, and thus an aid for diagnosis of arrhythmias and possibly ischemia. The ability of the ECG to pinpoint the cause of congestive heart failure is minimal when applied to most causes of congestive heart failure, but the ECG is invaluable for detecting conduction changes found in the abnormal patient. The echograph, angiograph, and fluoroscope are more definitive techniques for pinpointing heart problems.

Clinical Laboratory Analyses

Clinical laboratory assessment of heart failure may be helpful in the early detection of disease in cases with lung congestion or edema. Blood gases are useful in determining the acid-base status of the patient. Respiratory acidosis with elevated PCO_2 levels is seen in patients with emphysema or lung congestion. The patient with edema will develop electrolyte and osmolality changes as a consequence of fluid build-up and ionic redistribution. An increased excretion of potassium and decrease in urinary sodium may be an early indicator of these imbalances. Serum electrolyte determinations (including sodium, potassium, chloride, and total CO_2) are important to monitor diuretic and drug therapy in patients with treated heart failure.[11]

The laboratory's role in detecting secondary causes of heart failure is also valuable. The patient who has secondary heart failure due to thyroid dysfunction can be identified by performing a typical thyroid profile of thyroxine (T_4), thyroid-stimulating hormone (TSH), and perhaps triiodothyronine (T_3). The first sign of chest pain usually suggests a need for performing cardiac enzyme profiles to eliminate the possibility of myocardial infarction.[11]

A patient suspected of congestive heart failure should be screened for kidney and liver involvement as well as lung congestion. Blood urea nitrogen (BUN) and creatinine levels are useful in assessing kidney function. The patient with heart failure who has an elevated creatinine has probably already developed some kidney complications. An elevated BUN is an early indicator of uremia in the congestive heart failure patient. Liver profiles of aspartate aminotransferase (AST), alanine aminotransferase (ALT), alkaline phosphatase, and total bilirubin show elevations in patients with chronic right ventricular failure.[11] The gamma glutamyl transferase (GGT) value in these patients is usually twice the value of the upper limit of the normal range. This suggests that liver congestion is occurring progressively.

The routine complete blood count (CBC) is important for detecting anemias, infections, and early signs of congestion. Hemolysis may indicate needed testing for hemoglobinuria and myoglobinuria, indicators of cardiovascular damage and myocardial disease. An increase in WBCs may indicate pericarditis, endocarditis, or other valvular infections. If kidney dysfunction has occurred, an anemia due to uremia may develop, and may be indicated on the WBC differential examination by red cell fragments. Alterations in hemoglobin concentration and hematocrit determinations can be helpful when following drug therapy to correct for congestive heart failure.[12]

The infections associated with pericarditis, endocarditis, and valvular problems should be identified by microbiology cultures. Blood cultures can be used but often will not pick up an infection located in the spaces around the heart. Collection of material from the pericardium and endocardium should be performed after suspicion has been raised by radiological testing[12] (see Chap. 3).

TREATMENT

The laboratory's part in monitoring the drug therapies used for heart failure is invaluable because many drugs have very narrow therapeutic ranges and can alter electrolyte balance. Procainamide, given to regulate arrhythmias, must be monitored for patient compliance and to prevent toxicity. Glycosides, particularly digoxin, are used to increase the contractility of the heart and slow the conduction impulses. Digoxin has a narrow therapeutic range, is strongly bound to protein, and depends on kidney function for elimination. In monitoring digoxin levels in the heart failure patient, attention must be paid to the drug level, the BUN/creatinine ratios, and the potassium level, especially if the patient is on diuretics.[13] If quinidine has also been given to regulate an arrhythmia, the mixture of digoxin and quinidine will heighten the digoxin effect to the detriment of the patient.[13] Diuretics like thiazides, furosemide, and ethacrynic acid should be monitored because they can induce hypokalemia and cardiac arrhythmia.[13] Kidney function tests of BUN, creatinine, and uric acid should be monitored in a patient on diuretics. The beta-blocker drugs used to lower blood pressure are seldom monitored as often as they should be.[13] Alterations in lipids and other analytes indicate that the beta blockers may have wide systemic influences.

The laboratory role in treatment of heart failure extends to the use of blood components, particularly when surgical intervention is needed. Bypass grafts, correcting valvular defects, and other surgical procedures to correct heart failure involve the use of fresh whole blood during the operation and blood components during the patient's recovery.

CASE STUDY

A 55-year-old man with a history of alcohol abuse was admitted to the hospital with shortness of breath and hyperventilation. His history revealed a chronic cough, edema of the feet and legs, and fatigue. The physical examination revealed moderate respiratory distress along with 160/90 blood pressure, a pulse rate of 70, and hepatomegaly.

Laboratory assessment revealed changes from normal reference ranges as follows:

LABORATORY FINDINGS

Electrolytes

Sodium:	Decreased
Potassium:	Increased
Chloride:	Increased
Total CO_2	Increased

Blood Gases

*p*H:	Increased
PCO_2:	Decreased
PO_2:	Decreased
O_2 saturation:	Normal

Liver Enzymes

AST:	Increased
ALT:	Increased
ALP:	Increased
GGT:	Increased × 2

Other Values

BUN:	Increased
Creatinine:	Increased
Bilirubin:	Increased
Hct:	Slightly decreased
CBC:	Normal
Microbiology cultures:	Negative

Questions

1. What physiological condition do the blood gas results and the patient's symptoms suggest?
2. What kind of heart failure is probably involved?
3. What are the implications of the other abnormal laboratory values?

Discussion

1. The physiological condition indicated is respiratory alkalosis due to hyperventilation.
2. CHF due to alcohol cardiomyopathy is probably involved. Increased blood pressure suggests right ventricular failure.
3. Liver enzymes and hepatomegaly suggest liver damage. The liver may be congested due to right ventricular failure and may be damaged due to alcohol abuse. BUN and creatinine values suggest kidney involvement.

REFERENCES

1. Unverfeith DV (ed): Dilated Cardiomyopathy. Mount Kisco, New York, Futura Publishing, 1985
2. Brest AN (ed): Congestive Heart Failure. New York City, Medcom Press, 1975
3. Emes, Nowak: Introduction to Pathophysiology—Basic Principles of the Disease Process, p 119. Baltimore, University Park Press, 1983
4. Petersdorf RG, Adams RD et al: Harrison's Principles of Internal Medicine, 10th ed. New York City, McGraw-Hill, 1983
5. Dillingham MA, Anderson RJ: Inhibition of vasopressin action by atrial natriuretic factor. Science 231:1572, March 28, 1986
6. Burnett JC et al: Atrial natriuretic peptide evaluation in congestive heart failure in the human. Science 231:1145, March 7, 1986
7. Skinner SL, Thatcher RL, Whitworth J, Horowitz JD: Extraction of plasma prorenin by human heart. Lancet 8488(Vol I):995, May 3, 1986
8. Harvey, Johns, Owens, Ross (eds): Principles and Practice of Medicine, 19th ed, pp 201–435. New York City, Appleton-Century-Crofts, 1976
9. Braunwald E, Mock MB, Watson J (eds): Congestive Heart Failure: Current Research and Clinical Application. New York City, Grune & Stratton
10. Cutler P (ed): Problem-Solving in Clinical Medicine: From Data to Diagnosis, 2nd ed. Baltimore, Williams & Wilkins, 1985
11. Tietz NW (ed): Textbook of Clinical Chemistry, 2nd ed. Philadelphia, WB Saunders, 1986
12. Henry JB: Clinical Diagnosis and Management by Laboratory Methods, 17th ed. Philadelphia, WB Saunders, 1984
13. Kaplan LA, Pesce AJ: Clinical Chemistry Theory, Analysis, and Correlation, p 490. St Louis, CV Mosby, 1984

Part III

PULMONARY DISORDERS

Marie Pezzlo, Associate Editor

The primary function of the respiratory system, in concert with the circulatory system, is to maintain optimal concentrations of oxygen and carbon dioxide throughout the body's tissues. As with the cardiovascular diseases, disruption of ventilation and respiratory functions can be immediately life-threatening, requiring emergency measures. The chronic pulmonary disorders are no less life-threatening, although more progressive in nature.

The respiratory system includes the nasal cavity, pharynx, larynx, trachea, bronchi, and lungs (see illustration on page 76). The lungs (and the heart) are contained in the thoracic cavity, which extends from just below the collarbone to the diaphragm. The right, and larger, lung is composed of three lobes, while the left lung is divided into two parts. The diaphragm is a muscular partition that separates the thoracic from the abdominal cavity. Each lung is enveloped in a double-folded membrane (*mesothelium*) that consists of the parietal and visceral pleura.

Under normal conditions, air enters the nasal passages and passes through the trachea into the bronchi, which subdivide into smaller airways known as *bronchioles.* These eventually end in even smaller sacs, the *alveoli.* Gases are exchanged by diffusion between air in the alveoli and blood in the capillaries of the lung.

Respiratory, radiologic, and clinical laboratory tests are vital in the evaluation and management of pulmonary diseases. Evaluation must take into consideration many factors, including those of extrapulmonary origin. The chapters in this section focus on both acute and chronic pulmonary disorders that are likely to require clinical laboratory assistance in the diagnosis or management of the disease.

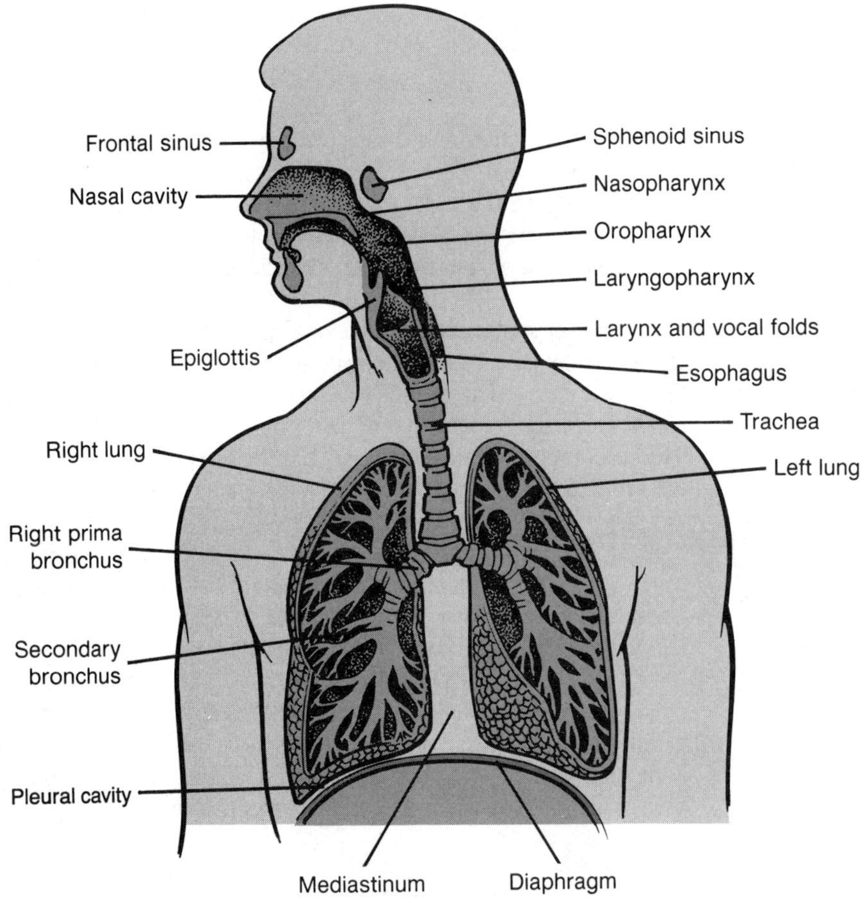

The respiratory system. (From Patrick ML, Woods SL, Craven RF et al: Medical-Surgical Nursing, p 298. Philadelphia, JB Lippincott, 1986)

Chapter 7

Acute Respiratory Failure

Kevin D. Fallon

ETIOLOGY AND PATHOPHYSIOLOGY

Respiratory failure, or acute respiratory insufficiency, is a term applied to a variety of problems in which the pulmonary system fails to provide the body with oxygen for tissue metabolism and to remove carbon dioxide as an end-product.[1] It results in a condition in which the PaO_2 (arterial oxygen tension) is below the predicted normal range for the patient's age without another defined cause, such as left-to-right shunt, and the $PaCO_2$ (arterial CO_2 tension) is above 50 mm Hg, not caused by compensation for metabolic alkalosis.[2]

Pulmonary causes of respiratory insufficiency can be classified as hypoventilation, inadequate diffusion, shunting, and perfusion to ventilation mismatches.[3] Nonpulmonary causes of respiratory failure are listed in Table 7-1.

Hypoventilation is movement of an inadequate amount of air into and out of the alveoli. One cause might be a partial or total block of the airway caused by material such as mucus or by constriction of the muscles of the bronchial tree. Another cause is a decrease in mechanical action resulting in movement of inadequate volumes of air. This is often seen in trauma, fractured ribs, abdominal pain, and fatigue. Another significant cause of hypoventilation is neurologic in nature, caused by injury to the brain, changes in neuromuscular transmission, or drugs. Drugs can affect both brain

Table 7-1 ***Examples of Causes of Respiratory Failure Nonpulmonary in Origin***

Nervous System	Neuromuscular	Thorax	Cardiovascular
Brain injury	Drugs	Broken ribs	Edema
Poliomyelitis	Electrolytes	Obesity	Embolism
Drugs	Infections	Trauma	Shock
Cord injury			

sensitivity to CO_2, which controls the signals to the respiratory muscles, and also the transmission at the neuromuscular junction.

Inadequate diffusion, the second class of respiratory failure, can result from an impairment in diffusion at the alveolar–capillary interface. This is caused most frequently by pulmonary edema, which has a variety of causes.

Shunting, or ventilation to perfusion inequality, is characterized by a percentage of the cardiac output that does not participate in gas exchange in the alveoli. This is caused by an anatomic connection between the venous and arterial circulation other than in the lungs, or it occurs because areas of the lung are not being ventilated but are being perfused, usually due to mucus plugs in the lower bronchi.

Perfusion to ventilation inequality, conversely, results in increased dead space, *i.e.*, volumes of air in the lungs that do not exchange with the blood. This condition is characterized by areas of the lung that are ventilated adequately but not perfused. Causes of the decrease in perfusion include emboli in the pulmonary circulation that block the flow of blood, and levels of arterial pressure inadequate to overcome the resistance provided by the pulmonary microcirculation. The latter condition can result from a severe drop in arterial pressure, or from an increase in resistance to blood flow caused by fluid buildup in lung areas as a result of immobility. Proper nursing care calls for frequent turning of the patient who has pain or is medicated, in order to prevent hypoventilation in areas of the lung that can result in mucus plugging, pneumonia, and respiratory failure. In this situation the weakened patient has to expend a lot of energy to ventilate unused lung by increasing both the rate and the volume of breathing.

The *adult respiratory distress syndrome (ARDS)* continues to be one of the most lethal conditions treated in surgical and medical intensive care units. Mortality rates of 50% have been reported in recent reviews in spite of many years of progress in critical care management.[4, 5] ARDS is acute respiratory failure caused by diffuse alveolar injury, and is considered the end stage of multiple insults such as accidental and surgical trauma, hemorrhage, sepsis, atelectasis, smoke inhalation, and many other conditions that result in direct damage to the alveolar–capillary interface.[6] ARDS is common, affecting more than 150,000 people each year, and is a common cause of acute respiratory failure,[7, 8] It is estimated that more than 75% of patients who require inspired oxygen concentrations above 50% to achieve reasonable blood oxygen content will die.[9]

ARDS is characterized by severe hypoxemia refractory to high inspired oxygen concentrations with diffuse interstitial or alveolar infiltrates that are generally bilateral on chest x-ray. There is a decrease in thoracic compliance (loss of elasticity) due to edema and abnormal airways.[10] The ratio of arterial to alveolar PO_2 is generally less than 0.3, and there is increased pulmonary microvascular permeability.[11] Proper management and monitoring of respiratory failure is necessary to prevent serious morbidity and even mortality. Although ARDS is often impossible to prevent, it is easier to prevent than to cure.

The physiologic response to ARDS is extremely complicated. It can be characterized by ventilation to perfusion mismatches, reduced functional residual capacity (useable lung volume), and diminished compliance that leads to hypoxemia. There is a massive response in the release of hormones and other agents that lead to cellular and functional changes in the lung.[12] ARDS involves diffuse lung injury, leading to pulmonary edema. This is not to be confused with cardiogenic pulmonary edema, although respiratory failure can result from both. Frequently the use of a pulmonary artery catheter with a thermistor for determining cardiac output by means of thermal dilution is required to ascertain the status of the heart and to distinguish between pulmonary and cardiogenic edema.

Although the term used for this syndrome is respiratory distress, the problem is actually ventilatory in nature. Ventilation occurs in the lungs, while respiration is carried out at the tissue level.

Prior to approximately 1950, respiratory failure was not recognized frequently because necessary laboratory analyses were not available.[13] Determination of arterial oxygenation was performed by volumetric analysis (Van Slyke method), which required more than 30 minutes for a single determination and therefore could not be of more than academic benefit to the patient.

Fewer people actually die from acute respiratory failure now because diagnosis is quick and treatment relatively effective. One study reported that only 16% of patients in an ARDS group died from respiratory failure. Most early deaths were due to the original trauma, and 73% of the group died later from sepsis. Large numbers of people survive the ventilation crisis only to succumb to other complications associated with long-term illness, such as sepsis, stress ulcers with hemorrhage, and heart and/or renal failure.[14]

Sepsis is the major cause of death in ARDS patients who survive the initial trauma. If the infection precedes the development of ARDS, the source is usually in the abdomen, while infection occurring after ARDS develops is usually pulmonary in origin.[15] Another study reported a mortality rate of 40% for uncomplicated acute lung injury, and of 81% when the injury was complicated by multisystem failure. When associated with acute renal failure, respiratory failure has a mortality rate of 89%[16] (see Table 7-2). As in other disorders, a major cause of morbidity and mortality associated with long-term ARDS-related illness is starvation.[17]

Not all acute episodes of respiratory insufficiency necessarily deteriorate into ARDS. There are numerous causes of respiratory arrest that are transient and, if properly managed, are resolved within a short time. ARDS usually is preceded by a

Table 7-2 ***Some Nonpulmonary Complications Associated with ARDS***

Nutritional	Hematologic	Infection
Starvation	Anemia	Sepsis
Fatty liver	Thrombocytopenia	Septic shock
Electrolyte imbalance	DIC	
Cardiovascular	**Renal**	**Gastrointestinal**
Shock	Renal failure	Peritonitis
Emboli	Fluid balance problems	Stress ulcers
Arrhythmias		Hemorrhage

catastrophic event, such as multiple trauma, occurring in an otherwise healthy individual.[18]

Among the causes of *transient respiratory insufficiency* are drugs, both controlled and uncontrolled. Narcotics affect the opiate receptors in the brain stem and can cause respiratory depression. Morphine has been linked to delayed respiratory suppression when injected into the epidural space for local anesthesia.[19] Almost any of the arsenal of drugs used by anesthesiologists will, in sufficient dose, cause respiratory depression through any one of several mechanisms (*e.g.*, impairment in chemoreceptor function, interference with neuromuscular transmission, or changes in metabolism).[20, 21] Properly managed, these situations are resolved by short-term ventilation support. Delays in treatment, frequently associated with overdoses of street drugs, can cause the patient's condition to deteriorate to the point that more aggressive therapy may be required.

Pain caused by abdominal incisions, broken ribs, and similar trauma can elicit shallow breathing (hypoventilation). The deep breath, or sigh, becomes too painful and periodic reinflation of the alveoli stops, which results in atelectasis, edema, and infection. If not managed aggressively at an early stage, this condition will deteriorate into ARDS.

Obesity is another cause of hypoventilation.[22] The added weight creates pressure and a need for increased ventilation to support the metabolism of the added tissue mass. As a result there are alterations in respiratory mechanics so that the work of breathing increases significantly. Morbidly obese people often underventilate and actually are prone to apnea.

CLINICAL MANIFESTATIONS

The symptoms of respiratory failure include tachypnea, dyspnea, an ashen-gray appearance, cyanosis, agitation, and anxiety. There are two types of failure: one exhibits *hypoxemia* (low O_2 with either *eucapnia* [normal CO_2] or *hypocapnia* [low CO_2]), while the second exhibits hypoxemia with *hypercapnia* (high CO_2). The first is usually associated in adults with ARDS resulting from acute lung injury. Stiff or noncompliant lungs are generally observed in these cases, along with sepsis.[23] In the second type of respiratory failure, patients generally have chronic problems superimposed on an acute episode. Some patients have been seen to exhibit both types of problems during an illness.[24] In many of these patients it is necessary to use a pulmonary artery catheter to determine whether the edema is caused by a cardiogenic or fluid overload problem or is pulmonary in origin.

LABORATORY ANALYSES AND DIAGNOSIS

Respiratory Failure

The primary concern in the support of the patient with acute respiratory failure is maintenance of respiration. This involves adequate ventilation of the lung and maintenance of cardiac output so that adequate oxygen is delivered to the tissues.

For proper management, arterial blood gas analyses must be available at all times. These provide the following crucial information:

1. *PaO_2*. Arterial oxygen tension indicates respiratory failure when the PaO_2 falls below 50 mm Hg. Oxygenation of the tissues is inadequate.
2. *$PaCO_2$*. Alveolar ventilation is determined by $PaCO_2$. An elevated $PaCO_2$ indicates hypoventilation and respiratory failure.
3. *Acid-base state.* This is determined by the $PaCO_2$, *p*H, and bicarbonate concentration.

A combination of ventilation/perfusion mismatching, alveolar hypoventilation, and occasionally abnormalities in respiratory drive will produce significant hypoxemia ($PaO_2 < 50$ mm Hg). In previously healthy patients, the $PaCO_2$ may be low initially as the patient hyperventilates to compensate; however, as the respiratory muscles tire, *hypercarbia* ($PaCO_2 > 50$ mm Hg) and *acidemia* ($pH < 7.35$) occur. In patients with chronic hypoventilation, the $PaCO_2$ may be high initially. In any case, as the concentration of CO_2 rises, acidemia results[25, 26] (see Table 7-3).

Table 7-3 ***Laboratory Results in Acute Respiratory Failure***

Cause	PaO_2	$PaCO_2$	pH
Nervous system	↓	↑	↓
Neuromuscular	↓	↑	↓
Thorax	↓	↑	↓
Cardiovascular	↓	↓	N or ↑
ARDS			
Early	↓	N ↓	N or ↑
Late	↓	↑	↓

Data from reference numbers[27, 28]

Because acid-base disorders result in compensatory responses of the lungs and kidneys, clinical assessment of patients' laboratory findings is difficult at first because the physician does not know if the findings represent an initial or a compensated situation.[29] Frequent blood gas values must be obtained, therefore, and aggressive ventilatory support provided. Because the goal is always to remove the patient from the ventilator as quickly as possible, laboratory data are consulted carefully to determine the most aggressive course possible for weaning the patient from the ventilator. The precision and timeliness of the laboratory work, starting with obtaining the sample and continuing through the analysis, are critical to this process. Small changes, if reliable, can confirm a trend and accelerate further modifications in therapy.

ARDS

In ARDS the PaO_2 falls despite oxygen enrichment of inspired gas.[30] It is possible that some time (days) can elapse after the insult before frank ARDS develops.[31] Because ARDS is such a complicated condition and is usually compounded by other serious conditions in the patient, it is necessary to assess a large number of biochemical variables in ARDS patients.

Fluid and electrolyte management has high priority. Even small changes in serum electrolyte concentrations may represent fluid-electrolyte shifts that can delay or prevent recovery.[32] Resuscitation of trauma victims will often require large amounts of blood and other fluids. Hormonal changes or kidney or cardiac problems associated with the trauma may prevent the excretion of the excess fluid.[33] Proper management of fluid-electrolyte problems involves a consideration of three dimensions: (1) the total amount of the electrolyte (concentration and volume of distribution), (2) body balance (rate of movement into and out of the body), and (3) body composition (movement into and out of body compartments). This requires serum electrolyte determinations.[34]

Coagulation problems, particularly disseminated intravascular coagulation (DIC), have been found to be common in patients with ARDS, so evaluation of the patient's coagulation status is often indicated. Modig[35] reports that coagulation tests such as fibrinogen, platelet count, activated partial thromboplastin time, ethanol gelation test, thrombotest, normotest, and fibrin degradation products are less predictive than antithrombin III, plasminogen (low values), or factor VIII (higher values) in assessing coagulation disorders in these patients. The platelet count seemed to be the most sensitive indicator and should be considered when transfusions are part of the overall therapy.[36] A plasma complement profile has been proposed as an early warning of the impending coagulopathy.[37]

Sepsis syndrome is specifically defined by clinical signs and laboratory tests, and can be a warning of impending ARDS.

A low serum protein concentration, disturbed renal function, and a low PaO_2/F_IO_2 (O_2 concentration of inspired air) in drowning victims indicate a greater risk for developing ARDS. Aggressive therapy is required from the start.[38]

The white blood count has a potential predictive value for patients who have a high risk for developing ARDS.[39] Counts below $5.0 \times 10^3/mm^3$ associated with respiratory failure indicate the onset of ARDS.

A strong correlation between immunoreactive trypsin and both ARDS and sepsis has been found,[40] suggesting that proteinases are implicated in the development of ARDS.

Because of the variety of pathologic conditions that result from trauma and other conditions that lead to or result from ARDS, the involvement of the laboratory in the treatment of these patients is very extensive. There is need for very aggressive management of pulmonary function, which involves blood gas analyses, co-oximetry (including total hemoglobin), and related calculated parameters. Cardiac output is correlated with these values to ensure that adequate oxygen is being carried to the tissues. Hemoglobin concentrations must be adequate, and the affinity of hemoglobin must provide for adequate oxygen delivery.

Fluid volumes must be maintained so that cardiac output is adequate. Dilution of all electrolytes is a potential hazard, so constant monitoring of these concentrations is required.

Kidney failure is not uncommon, and therefore constant evaluation of creatinine, urea nitrogen, and other renal function indicators is routine.

Liver function is carefully monitored using serum enzymes and other analytes that may indicate any changes in this organ.

Because, as described above, infections are the most common problem in these patients, proper identification of the causative agent so that specific antibiotic selection can be made is crucial for survival. Nutritional status is determined by a variety of methods, many of which are of marginal value. Currently 24-hour urine nitrogen, albumin, and transferrin tests are used by clinicians to follow the patient's nutritional status. Several new tests are being examined, but it is likely that actual caloric consumption by means of indirect calorimetry will become standard in the near future.[41]

TREATMENT

Treatment for respiratory distress centers on achieving adequate oxygenation of the tissues. Oxygen therapy is necessary but must be administered carefully and monitored, because toxicity or depression of the ventilatory response can occur in some patients. Moreover, decisions to intubate are always made with care because a number of complications can ensue. Alteration of the rate and volume of ventilation as well as diuresis are also mechanisms used to improve the respiratory status of the patient. ARDS is particularly difficult to treat because it represents a complicated mix of syndromes that are not well understood at this time.[25] Blood gas analyses are essential in monitoring the effectiveness of treatment. The responsibility of the laboratory is to produce useful, accurate information in a timely manner.

CASE STUDY

A 22-year-old man involved in a motor vehicle accident was brought to the emergency room and admitted to the surgical intensive care unit with multiple traumatic injuries. The patient was conscious and breathing spontaneously. The next day the patient became tachypneic and complained of difficulty in breathing (dyspnea).

Two days after admission, the chest x-ray showed diffuse infiltrates. Laboratory findings during the course of the hospital stay are listed opposite. On day 3, x-rays showed increased pulmonary edema. On day 5, the patient developed a fever (39.2° C).

Questions

1. Given the laboratory results, explain the development of the patient's condition by day 3 and the steps that should be taken.
2. What would you expect the blood and tracheal aspirate cultures taken on day 5 to show?
3. What analyses would the laboratory be performing on a frequent basis?
4. Given the laboratory findings later in the hospital stay, what is the prognosis for this patient?

Discussion

1. The patient developed respiratory failure subsequent to trauma. Given that the PaO_2 has fallen even though the F_IO_2 had increased, ARDS is likely unless aggressive treatment is

LABORATORY FINDINGS

Admission + 1½ days		2 days	3 days	4 days	7 days	9 days
PaO_2	75 mm Hg	70 mm Hg	50 mm Hg	70 mm Hg	80 mm Hg	95 mm Hg
$PaCO_2$	30 mm Hg	33 mm Hg	ND	40 mm Hg		
***p*H**	7.47	7.44	7.43	7.39		
F_IO_2	NA	40%	50%	60%	50%	40%
Culture	NA	NA	NA	NA	Blood + Trachea +	
WBC		$15 \times 10^3/mm^3$	ND	$21 \times 10^3/mm^3$ Shift to the left		

undertaken. In this case the patient was intubated and was ventilated with PEEP (positive end expiratory pressure). A pulmonary artery catheter was placed for determining cardiac output by thermal dilution and for obtaining blood for frequent blood gas analyses.

2. Because sepsis is a frequent complication of respiratory failure, especially ARDS, the cultures would be expected to be positive. The presence of fever and the high WBC with a shift to the left support the suspicion of infection. In this case the blood culture and tracheal aspirate grew *S. aureus*. Appropriate antibiotic therapy was instituted.

3. Blood gases and co-oximeter panels were determined four or more times per day to guide aggressive respiratory management. Electrolytes were also carefully watched.

4. Because oxygen concentration increased while F_IO_2 decreased, the prognosis is good. Once weaned from the respirator, the patient will probably do well breathing on his own.

REFERENCES

1. Balk R, Bone R: Classification of acute respiratory failure. Med Clin North Am 67:551, 1983
2. Pantoppodan H, Geffin B, Lowenstein E: Acute Respiratory Failure in the Adult, p 2. Boston, Little, Brown & Co, 1973
3. D'Alonso G, Dantzker D: Respiratory failure, mechanism of abnormal gas exchange, and oxygen delivery. Med Clin North Am 67:557, 1983.
4. Norwood S, Civetta J: Ventilatory support in patients with ARDS. Surg Clin North Am 65:895, 1985.
5. Bernard G, Brigham K: Pulmonary edema: Pathophysiologic mechanisms and new approaches to therapy. Chest 89:594, 1986
6. Shoemaker W: Circulatory pathophysiology of ARDS and its fluid management. In Shoemaker W, Thompson W, Holbrook P (eds): Textbook of Critical Care, p 310. Philadelphia, WB Saunders, 1984
7. Bernard G, Brigham K: Pulmonary edema: Pathophysiologic mechanisms and new approaches to therapy. Chest 89:594, 1986
8. Norwood S, Civetta J: Ventilatory support in patients with ARDS. Surg Clin North Am 65:895, 1985
9. Balk R, Bone R: The adult respiratory distress syndrome. Med Clin North Am 67:685, 1983
10. Norwood S, Civetta J: Ventilatory support in patients with ARDS. Surg Clin North Am 65:895, 1985
11. Bernard G, Brigham K: The adult respiratory distress syndrome. Annu Rev Med 36:195, 1985
12. Shoemaker W: Circulatory pathophysiology of ARDS and its fluid management. In Shoemaker W, Thompson W, Holbrook P (eds): Textbook of Critical Care, p 310. Philadelphia, WB Saunders, 1984
13. Balk R, Bone R: Classification of acute respiratory failure. Med Clin North Am 67:551, 1983

14. Montgomery A, Stager M, Carrico C, Hudson L: Causes of mortality in patients with the adult respiratory distress syndrome. Am Rev Respir Dis 132:485, 1985
15. Norwood S, Civetta J: Ventilatory support in patients with ARDS. Surg Clin North Am 65:895, 1985
16. Gillespie D, Marsh H, Divertie M, Meadows: Outcome in patients requiring prolonged (greater than 24 hrs) mechanical ventilation. Chest 90:364, 1986
17. McKone T, Davis A, Dean R: Fibronectin: A new nutritional parameter. Am Surg 51:336, 1985
18. Norwood S, Civetta J: Ventilatory support in patients with ARDS. Surg Clin North Am 65:895, 1985
19. Bromage P: Spinal opiate analgesia: Its present role and future in pain relief. Ann Chir Gynaecol 75:183, 1984
20. Kafer E, Marsh H: The effects of anesthetic drugs and disease on the chemical regulation of ventilation. Int Anesthesiol Clin 15:1, 1977
21. Rigg J, Isley A, Vedig A: Relationship of ventilatory depression to steady-state blood pethidine concentrations. Br J Anaesth 53:61, 1981
22. Brodsky J: Anesthetic management of the morbidly obese patient. In Racz G (ed): Problems and Advances in Respiratory Therapy, p 93. Boston, Little, Brown & Co, 1986
23. Balk R, Bone R: Classification of acute respiratory failure. Med Clin North Am 67:551, 1983
24. Balk R, Bone R: Classification of acute respiratory failure. Med Clin North Am 67:551, 1983
25. Fishman C et al: Medicine, p 85. Philadelphia, JB Lippincott, 1981.
26. Bone R: Acute respiratory failure: Classification, differential diagnosis, and introduction to management. In Burton GC, Hodgkin JE (eds): Respiratory Care, pp 844–845. Philadelphia, JB Lippincott, 1984
27. Lake KB: Adult respiratory distress syndrome (high permeability pulmonary edema). In Burton GC, Hodgkin JE (eds): Respiratory Care, p 860. Philadelphia, JB Lippincott, 1984
28. Bone R: Acute respiratory failure and chronic obstructive lung disease: Recent advances. Med Clin North Am 65:563, 1981
29. Levinsky NG: Acidosis and alkalosis. In Petersdorf RG, Adams RD, Braunwald E et al (eds): Harrison's Principles of Internal Medicine, p 235. New York, McGraw-Hill, 1983
30. Shoemaker W: Circulatory pathophysiology of ARDS and its fluid management. In Shoemaker W, Thompson W, Holbrook P (eds):L Textbook of Critical Care, p 310. Philadelphia, WB Saunders, 1984
31. Bernard G, Brigham K: The adult respiratory distress syndrome. Annu Rev Med 36:195, 1985
32. Shoemaker W: Fluids and electrolytes in the acutely ill adult. In Shoemaker W, Thompson W, Holbrook P (eds): Textbook of Critical Care, p 614. Philadelphia, WB Saunders, 1984
33. Wilson R: Trauma. In Shoemaker W, Thompson W, Holbrook P (eds): Textbook of Critical Care, p 877. Philadelphia, WB Saunders, 1984
34. Shoemaker W: Fluids and electrolytes in the acutely ill adult. In Shoemaker W, Thompson W, and Holbrook P (eds): Textbook of Critical Care, p 614. Philadelphia, WB Saunders, 1984
35. Modig J, Borg T, Wegenius G, Bagge L, Saldeen T: The value of variables of disseminated intravascular coagulation in the diagnosis of adult respiratory distress syndrome. Acta Anaesthesiol Scand 27:369, 1983
36. Watkins J, Wild G: The early diagnosis of impending coagulopathies following surgery and multiple trauma. Klin Wochenschr 63:1019, 1985
37. Montgomery A, Stager M, Carrico C, Hudson L: Causes of mortality in patients with the adult respiratory distress syndrome. Am Rev Respir Dis 132:485, 1985
38. Kaukinen L: Clinical course and prognostic signs in near drowned patients. Ann Chir Gynaecol 73:34, 1984
39. Thommasen H, Russell J, Boyko W, Hogg J: Transient leucopenia associated with adult respiratory distress syndrome. Lancet 1(8381):809, 1984
40. Deby-Dupont G, Haas M, Pincemail J, Braun M, Lamy M, Deby C: Immunoreactive trypsin in the adult respiratory distress syndrome. Intensive Care Med 10g:7, 1984
41. Grant J: Nutritional assessment in clinical practice. Nutr Clin Prac 1:3, 1985

BIBLIOGRAPHY

Balk, R, Bone R: Classification of acute respiratory failure. Med Clin North Am 67:551, 1983

Burrows B: An overview of obstructive lung diseases. Med Clin North Am 65:455, 1981

Cherniak R, Cherniak L, Naimark A: Respiration in Health and Disease. Philadelphia, WB Saunders, 1972

Fulmer J: An introduction to the interstitial lung diseases. Clin Chest Med 3:457, 1982

Macklem P: Obstruction in small airways: A challenge to medicine. Am J Med 52:721, 1972

Thurlbeck W: Overview of the pathology of pulmonary emphysema in the human. Clin Chest Med 4:337, 1983

Chapter 8

Asthma

Michael Boroch / Laura Martin Rahlfs / Jon O. Nilsestuen

Bronchial asthma is classified as an obstructive lung disease because the disease process interferes with the flow of gas through the lung. Asthma has several predominant characteristics, which include bronchial hyperreactivity or bronchoconstriction, swelling of bronchial mucosa, excessive secretion of viscous mucus, and secondary pulmonary hyperinflation. The hyperinflation occurs because of the constriction of small airways and resultant air trapping. These characteristics, while severe during asthmatic episodes, may completely disappear following a remission of the asthma attack (see Fig. 8-1).

The clinical spectrum of asthma ranges from intermittent mild forms of bronchospasm to very severe, unremitting, and life-threatening episodes known as *status asthmaticus*. Changes in the severity of asthma may occur spontaneously or as a result of therapy. Statistics indicate that the asthma death rate has risen in recent years from 0.8/100,000 in 1977 to 1.6/100,000 in 1984.[1] Because of this significant trend, it is important for

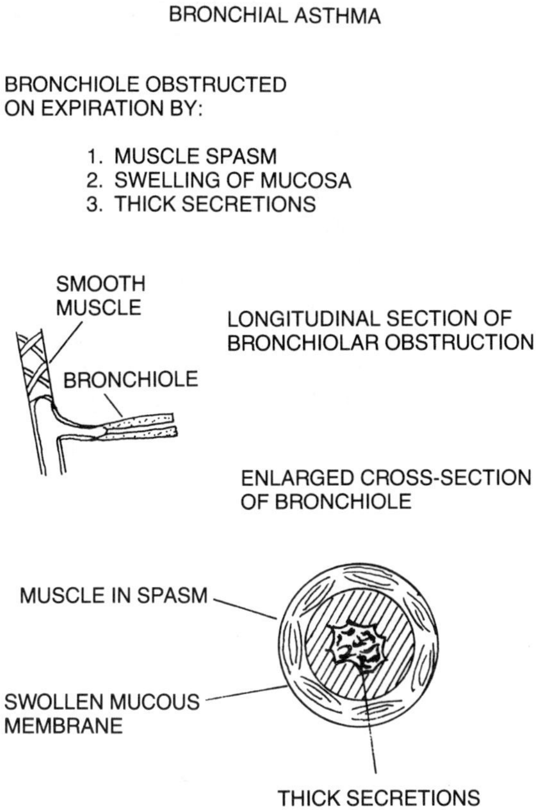

Figure 8-1 **Mechanism of bronchial asthma.**

patients presenting with asthma to be carefully monitored.

ETIOLOGY AND PATHOPHYSIOLOGY

Asthma occurs in 3% to 4% of the general population, although incidence among children is higher, 5% to 10%.[2, 3] In adults asthma is slightly less common in men, but in children it is 1½ to 2 times more common in boys than in girls. Onset of asthma before the age of 10 occurs in 50% of cases, but asthma may occur at any age.[4]

Asthma can be divided into two groups, depending on the nature of the factor that precipitates the attack:[5, 6] the first, *extrinsic asthma,* involves an antigen–antibody reaction. The second, *intrinsic asthma,* is the result of irritants or other factors that cause airway reactivity in the absence of an antigen–antibody reaction. This distinction between the two types of asthma is important when instituting preventive measures against future attacks, but the distinction has little value in the acute treatment of the disease because both forms require very similar therapy.[7]

Tables 8-1 and 8-2 list the common features and stimuli that provoke acute episodes of both groups of asthma.

Asthma can also be classified according to the mechanism or principal stimulus that causes bronchial hyperreactivity. Several mechanisms are postulated to explain the causes of bronchial hyperreactivity observed with asthma.[8, 9, 10] The mechanisms for both types of asthma, allergic and nonallergic, are probably interrelated (see Fig. 8-2). Both the mechanism for smooth muscle contraction and the mechanism for activation and release of chemical mediators are controlled by the adenyl cyclase AMP system.

Extrinsic Asthma

Extrinsic asthma is the result of an immunologic response that causes an antigen-antibody-induced bronchospasm. Initially, upon exposure to aerosolized antigens, IgE antibodies are formed that are capable of binding to and sensitizing mast cells, basophils, and lung tissue.[11] Following formation of the IgE antibodies, reexposure to the specific antigen results in the formation of an antigen–antibody complex on the surface of the mast cell, causing the mast cell to release primary (granule-associated substances that are stored preformed) or secondary chemical mediators[12] (see also Chaps. 53 and 54).

The release of chemical mediators from mast cells causes bronchoconstriction by decreasing the intracellular levels of cAMP (cyclic adenosine monophosphate) in the bronchial smooth muscle. Bronchoconstriction in conjunction with increased capillary permeability, increased mucosal edema, and hypersecretion of bronchial mucosa results in

Table 8-1 ***Extrinsic Asthma***

Synonyms	Stimuli That Provoke Acute Episodes of Asthma	Common Features
IgE-mediated asthma Allergic asthma Atopic asthma Reagin-mediated asthma	Exposure to external or environmental antigens (allergens) that cause an immunologic response. Common offenders include Pollens (grass, trees, flowers, etc.) Feathers House dust Dander from cats, dogs, and horses Dermatophagoides Mold spores (*e.g.*, Aspergillus) Ingested materials such as dairy products, chocolate, fish, and alcohol (less common)	• Best understood form of asthma • Personal and/or family history of allergic diseases • Asthmatic attacks less frequent with time, and may disappear in adulthood • Most often observed in children and young adults (<35 years old) • Frequently seasonal unless antigens are present in environment continuously • Increased serum levels of IgE

Table 8-2 ***Intrinsic Asthma***

Synonyms	Stimuli That Provoke Acute Episodes of Asthma	Common Features
Nonallergic asthma Nonatopic asthma Idiosyncratic asthma	Infections—most often respiratory tract Exercise Emotional stress Air pollution Drugs	• Negative personal and/or family history of allergic diseases • Disease usually more severe than extrinsic and may become worse with time • Typically appears later in life (>35 years old) • Normal serum levels of IgE

increased airway resistance, air trapping, and secondary pulmonary hyperinflation (see Fig. 8-3).

Intrinsic Asthma

Intrinsic asthma may be triggered by many factors; however, the mechanisms involved are related to the autonomic control of the airways according to the neurogenic theory. Stimuli, including upper respiratory infections, exercise, emotional stress, and many forms of air pollution and drugs, activate sensory fibers of the vagus nerve (irritant receptors) in the lining of the upper and lower airways. This initiates a reflex arc, which

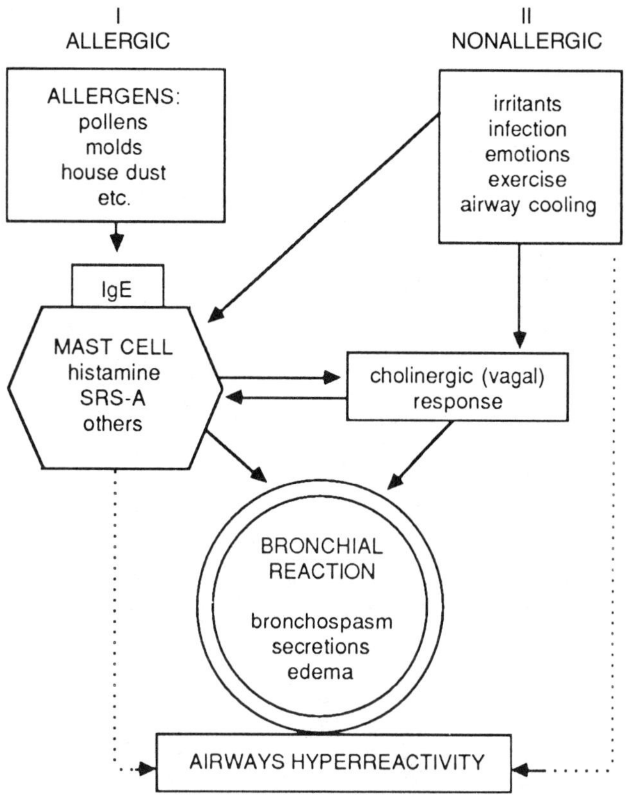

Figure 8-2 **Pathogenic mechanisms of asthma in allergic and nonallergic forms. Note their close interrelationship.**

results in an increase in airway resistance and bronchial secretions. In addition, this parasympathetic response also indirectly increases airway resistance and bronchial secretions by facilitating the degranulation of mast cells.[13]

In another approach, the beta adrenergic theory, the sympathetic nervous system is classically divided into alpha-receptors and beta-receptors, subgroups of which cause smooth muscle contraction (alpha) and cardiac stimulation and bronchodilation (beta).[14, 15] Evidence exists suggesting that a beta$_2$-receptor defect involving the pulmonary, hematologic, and metabolic response plays a part in severe asthma.[16–21] Normally, stimulation of the beta$_2$-receptor causes an increase in cAMP and a decrease in cyclic guanosine monophosphate (cGMP), resulting in bronchodilation. With the impairment of the beta$_2$-receptors, when cAMP levels decrease the cGMP levels increase, and bronchoconstriction results.

Catecholamine stimulation of the beta-receptors increases adenyl cyclase activity. The events that modulate cAMP in "target" cells (tissue mast cells, bronchial smooth muscle cells) are diagrammed in Figure 8-4.

CLINICAL MANIFESTATIONS

The clinical symptoms of bronchial asthma include wheezing, dyspnea, productive cough of thick tenacious mucus, sensation of tightness in the chest, night attacks of asthma, agitation, and, in the more

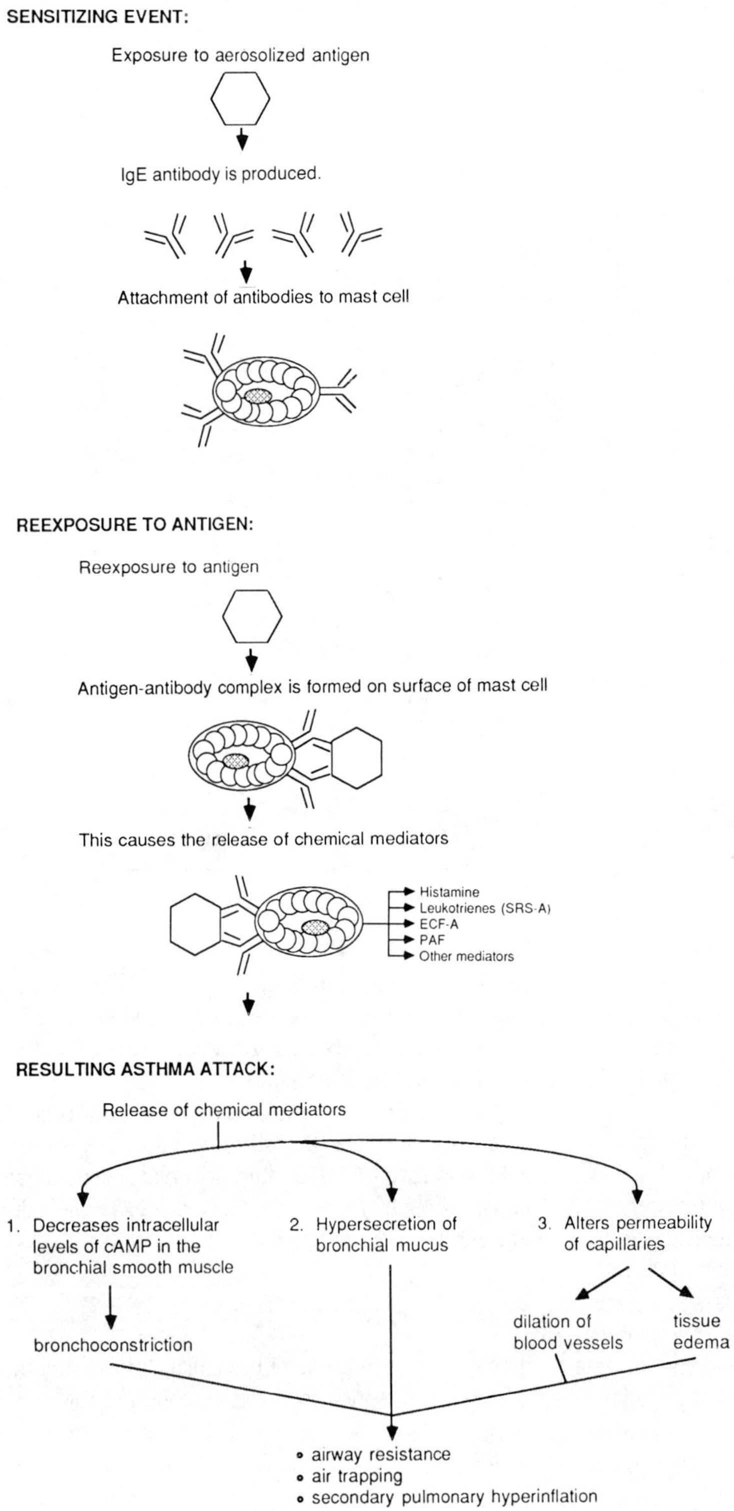

Figure 8-3 Mechanism of extrinsic asthma.

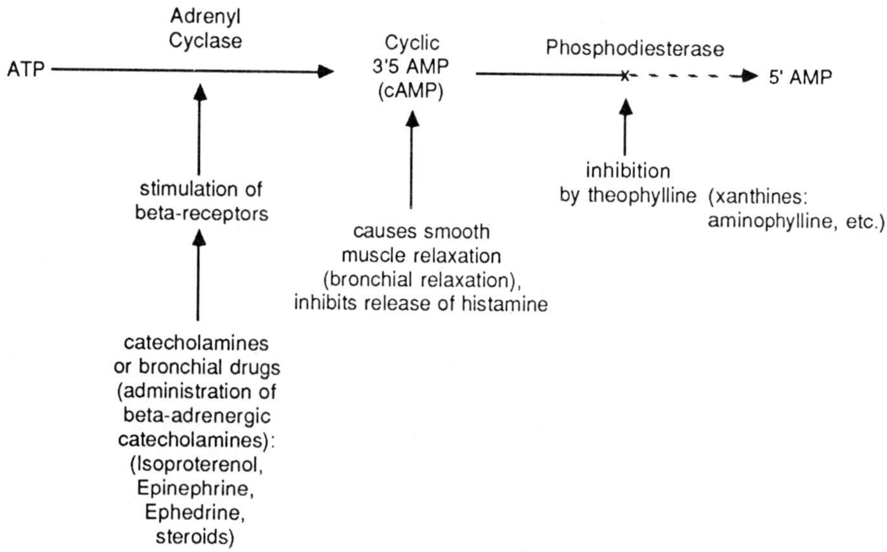

Figure 8-4 ATP mechanism. (Adapted from reference numbers[22, 23])

severe stages, inability to talk. The more common findings on physical examination are the result of increased airway resistance and air trapping. These mechanical changes produce a shuntlike effect (perfusion in excess of ventilation), and result in a decreased arterial PO_2 and hypoxemia. The hypoxemia causes tachypnea through stimulation of the peripheral chemoreceptors. Frequently patients use their accessory muscles because of the increase in the work of breathing.

The cardiovascular consequences of hypoxemia include increased heart rate, increased cardiac output, and increased blood pressure. In addition, during more severe stages where the work of breathing is greatly increased, there are associated changes in blood pressure that are cyclic in nature and follow the respiratory pattern. During inspiration, the pressure in the chest decreases significantly and results in a drop in the patient's systolic blood pressure of 10 mm Hg or more. During expiration, these pressures are reversed and result in an increase in blood pressure. This cyclic pattern of increasing and decreasing blood pressure associated with the respiratory cycle is called *pulsus paradoxus*. Finally, in the later stages of asthma, cyanosis or severe hypoxemia occurs.

LABORATORY ANALYSES AND DIAGNOSIS

Clinical Laboratory Tests

Patients with status asthmaticus who present to an emergency room are often severely compromised and approaching or already in a state of acute respiratory failure. In these cases there may be little time for more than measurement of arterial blood gases and a complete blood count (CBC) in order to confirm the diagnosis and determine whether to initiate mechanical ventilation. When patients present in a less severe state, however, there is more time to undertake a more thorough laboratory investigation and differential diagnosis. Clinical laboratory tests that are often ordered and their expected results are listed below in Table 8-3.

Additional considerations with respect to blood gases can be found in Table 8-4, and other clinical laboratory findings are listed in Table 8-5.

(*Text continues on page 94*)

Table 8-3 ***Laboratory Test Results in Asthma***

Test	Value				Comments/Reference Ranges
	Acute Attack			*Status Athmaticus*	
	Mild	*Moderate*	*Severe*	*(Very severe)*	
Blood gases					
*p*H	Nl.*	Inc.*	Nl.*	Dec.	7.38–7.44 (arterial) 7.36–7.41 (venous)
$PaCO_2$	Nl.	Dec.	Nl.	Inc.	35–40 mm Hg (arterial) 40–45 mm Hg (venous)
PaO_2	Nl.*	Dec.**	Very dec.**	Extremely dec.	95–100 mm Hg (arterial)
HCO_3	Nl.*	Dec.*	Dec.*	Dec.	Plasma: 21–28 mEq/L
Oxygen saturation	Dec.	Dec.	Dec.	Dec.	94–100%
Wheezing	Noisy	Noisy	Absent	Absent	
CBC					
WBC	Nl. to slightly inc.				$4.5–11.0 \times 10^3/mm^3$
Hemoglobin	Nl. to slightly inc.				Men 13.5–18.0 g/dL Women 12.0–16.0 g/dL
Hematocrit	Nl. to slightly inc.				Men 40–54% Women 38–47%
Eosinophil Count	Inc.				Absolute counts are recommended to monitor therapeutic effect.
Sputum Cytology	Eosinophils increased				May also be seen in acute bronchitis
	Curschmann's spirals				
	Charcot-Leyden crystals (eosinophil-laden secretions)				Rarely found in sputum
	WBCs present in acute episodes				
	Cellular debris				
	Creola bodies (large, compact clusters of ciliated columnar cells that may be vacuolated)				Large or increasing numbers are a poor prognostic sign Seen almost exclusively in the sputum of asthmatic patients
Eosinophil Smear	Hypersecretory goblet cells increased				

Conversion to SI units is as follows:
Hemoglobin: g/dL × 0.155 = mmol/L
Bicarbonate: mEq/L × 1 = mmol/L

* Secondary to the normal or decreased $PaCO_2$
** Develops from V/Q ratio (V/Q mismatching)
Data from reference numbers[24–36]

Table 8-4 ***Arterial Blood Gases***

Synonyms	What is Evaluated	Specimen Collection	Causes for Rejection
Arterial gases ABGs	1. *p*H 2. PCO_2, ($PaCO_2$)—PCO_2 measurements reflect respiratory disturbances. 3. PO_2 (PaO_2)	1. Arterial blood 2. Air-free	1. Improper collection 2. Air in sample
	4. The existence of dangerous levels of hypoxemia or hypercarbia or the severity of acute asthma may be indicated by arterial blood gas tests.	3. Heparinized glass syringe (needle-stoppered) 4. Specimen should be placed in a slurry of chipped ice and water.	3. Sample not heparinized 4. Specimen not submitted in ice
	5. Calculated: oxygen saturation, oxygen content, hemoglobin, carbyhemoglobin, methemoglobin, total CO_2, bicarbonate (HCO_3); used in evaluation of fixed-base, calculations for HCO_3 are based on the Henderson-Hasselbalch equation; standard bicarbonate, base excess.	5. Unless specimen is taken immediately to lab (in ice), it should be cooled to 0°C.	5. Improper ratio of blood to heparin

Special Interpretive Factors

Patient should remain in a "steady state" so as to prevent respiratory alkalosis due to hyperventilation.

For samples drawn from an indwelling arterial "line" (catheter), care must be taken to prevent dilution with flush solution.

100% A hemoglobin is assumed in O_2 saturation calculation. Hemoglobins with different dissociation curves may give misleading values.

A body temperature of 37°C is commonly assumed for calculations.

Plastic syringes can exchange gas with a blood sample, and a sample with a high PO_2 will fall, while a sample with a low PO_2 will rise.

Blood cells in samples with a very high white count respire more than normal. If the specimen is not collected in ice properly, the PO_2 will fall (especially if over 150 mm Hg), and the PCO_2 will rise, with a corresponding change in pH.

Immediately prior to analysis, the specimen should be adequately mixed to prevent a possible pH error caused by sample separation. The plasma is more alkaline than are the red cells.

Halothane and nitrous oxide (anesthetic gases) are potential contaminants, causing the traditional PO electrode to read the PO higher than it actually is.

High serum levels of lipids or lipidlike substances (*e.g.*, fat-emulsion-based hyperalimentation, perfluorocarbon-based blood substitutes, endogenous disease) may cause sample contamination.

Greatly elevated levels of serum proteins may cause the PO_2 and PCO_2 to be artificially lowered because of protein coating of electrode membranes.

Data from reference numbers[37–44]

Table 8-5 ***Other Clinical Laboratory Test Results***

Test	Type Specimen	Value	Comment
2,3-Diphosphoglycerate	RBC	Increased	In acute untreated attacks
Anti-smooth muscle	Serum	Increased	In 20% of cases
Antidiuretic hormone	Serum	Increased	In status asthmaticus
Aminotransferase	Serum	Increased	In 90% of acute untreated asthma patients
C4	Serum	Decreased	Usually normal
Chloride	Sweat	Increased	High concentration found in sweat of chronic asthmatics and their relatives
Cortisol	Plasma	Decreased	
Creatinine kinase	Serum	Increased	Increases correlate w/severity of symptoms (subjective) and objective measurement of airway obstruction. High in 38% of acute untreated asthma patients.
ESR (Erythrocyte sedimentation rate)	Blood	Normal to increased	
Glucose	Serum	Increased	May be due to epinephrine or corticosteroids
LD-1,2,3,4	Serum	Increased	LD-1 and LD-2 unaltered. LD-3 activity arises from lung involvement.
LD-5	Serum	Increased	LD-5 activity arises from the liver.
Lactic acid	Serum	Increased	In some patients, lactic acid, pyruvic acid, and the lactic/pyruvic ratio are increased.
Phosphorus, inorganic	Serum	Decreased	Decrease at initial hospitalization in 40% of 107 patients
Potassium	Serum	Decreased	May be found in corticosteroid-treated patients
Uric acid	Serum	Increased	Thought to be a consequence of the excessive level of sympathomimetic drugs

Other Tests

Other tests typically performed outside of the clinical laboratory include pulmonary function tests, chest x-rays, and electrocardiographic studies. These additional tests are important in the differential diagnosis and in the prescription for treatment of asthma. Findings in pulmonary function studies are outlined in Table 8-6.

Radiographs of the chest are nondiagnostic for asthma but may be helpful in ruling out other conditions such as lung tumor, emphysema, or lung infection and complications of asthma such as pneumothorax pneumomediastinum.

TREATMENT

Although there is no cure for asthma, some patients may recover spontaneously as they mature into adulthood. Treatment is aimed at relieving the symptoms of the existing attack, and varies from patient to patient as well as for the individual patient. Patients and their families must be educated about the causes of the disease in order to prevent recurrent exposure to either the antigen or the inhaled irritant. In addition, they must be educated about assessment, treatment (including proper use of an inhaler), and control of the disease.[47]

Table 8-6 ***Pulmonary Function Studies in Asthma***

Specific Test	Finding	Comments
TLC (total lung capacity)	Increased	TLC = VC + RV; temporary elevation may be observed when other symptoms absent
RV (residual volume)	Increased	Caused by air trapping
RV/TLC ratio	Increased	Proportionately greater increase
FRC (functional residual capacity)	Increased	FRC = RV + ERV
VC (vital capacity)	Decreased	VC = IRV + Vt + ERV
ERV (expiratory reserve volume)	Decreased	
Diffusion capacity	Normal	Significantly reduced in emphysema
IRV (inspiratory reserve volume)	Decreased	
Vt (Tidal volume)	Increased	
FEV (second forced expiratory volumes)	Decreased	Bronchoconstriction reflected, useful in day-to-day assessment of airway resistance changes
FEV_1 (timed forced expiratory volume)	Decreased	
FVC (forced vital capacity)	Decreased	
FEV_1/FVC ratio	Decreased	Useful in day-to-day assessment of airway resistance changes
PEFR (peak expiratory flow rate)	Decreased	Changes parallel those seen in FEV_1
MMF (maximum mid-expiratory flow)	Decreased	Also called forced expiratory flow, 25%–75%, bronchorestriction reflected
MVV (maximum volume vent)	Decreased	

Data from reference numbers[45, 46]

Extrinsic Asthma

Several preventive steps are available for patients known to have extrinsic asthma. These include (1) the elimination or avoidance of asthma-causing allergens; (2) hyposensitization (also called desensitization or immunotherapy), in which the patient is repeatedly exposed to small doses of the antigen (usually limited to those extrinsic asthma patients in whom specific asthma-causing allergens have been identified and who fail to respond to specific therapy); and (3) the administration of cromolyn sodium (sodium cromoglycate). Cromolyn sodium is a prophylactic agent that, with long-term treatment, reduces the intensity and number of attacks in allergic and exercise-induced asthma and acts by inhibiting degranulation of mast cells. It is also sometimes effective in reducing the level of corticosteroids needed to treat asthmatics. Cromolyn sodium is a dry powder and on inhalation may cause coughing or mild throat irritation.[48]

General Asthma

The prevention and treatment of general asthma is primarily reliant on the use of five categories of drugs.

Sympathomimetics, also known as adrenoceptor agonists or adrenergic stimulants. These are the most effective group of bronchodilators, having the added benefit of inhibiting the release of chemical mediators from the mast cell.[2] The adrenergic compounds include catecholamines such as epinephrine (adrenaline), isoproterenol, and isoetharine; resorcinols such as metaproterenol and terbutaline; saligenins such as salbutamol; and ephedrine.

Menthylxanthines, among the most common agents used in the prevention and treatment of asthma. They include theophylline and its salts. These compounds act through inhibition of phosphodiesterase and thus cause an increase in the amount of cAMP.

Anticholinergics, bronchodilators that act by inhibiting the action of acetylcholine or through inhibition of the parasympathetic nervous system.

Glucocorticoids, used when symptoms are not relieved by other methods. Their exact mechanism of action is not known; however, they are known to have some associated deleterious side-effects (see Chap. 37).

Miscellaneous. Two other methods of therapy are commonly used in the treatment of an acute asthma attack. The first is oxygen administration, used in the treatment of hypoxemia and to reduce the work of breathing. The second is mobilization and removal of bronchial secretions. Methods include hydration (6 to 10 glasses of water a day), nebulization, and suctioning if necessary.

CASE STUDY

A 35-year-old black man presented to the emergency room complaining of shortness of breath. Respirations were 46 breaths per minute (normal = 12–20) and auscultation of the chest indicated bilateral wheezing. Patient's blood pressure was 130/94 mm Hg and the heart rate was 120 per minute (normal = 60–100).

Laboratory results upon admission and 24 hours later on nasal oxygen follow.

LABORATORY FINDINGS

	Admission	24 Hours Later
*p*H	7.50	7.41
$PaCO_2$	29 mm Hg	41 mm Hg
PaO_2	79 mm Hg	72 mm Hg

Questions

1. What physical findings particularly suggest asthma as a diagnosis?
2. Explain the low $PaCO_2$ found on admission.
3. What precautions must be taken after blood gases apparently return to normal?

Discussion

1. Dyspnea and wheezing suggest asthma. This patient was admitted with bronchial asthma and was treated with bronchial dilators and oxygen therapy.
2. The patient was hyperventilating upon admission, secondary to the restricted airways and hypoxemia. Twenty-four hours later the arterial blood gases indicated a normal *p*H and a normal CO_2 with a slightly below normal oxygen level at 72 mm Hg.
3. Patients with asthma are anxious, hyperventilate, and often have some level of hypoxemia. They are working very hard to move air in and out of the airways, and can eventually tire. One indication of significant exhaustion of an asthma patient is when the carbon dioxide level stays in the mid- or low 30s. The level should be watched very carefully and the patient checked for alertness and monitored very closely during such a situation.

REFERENCES

1. Sly M: Asthma deaths increasing. Science News 129: 11, 1986
2. Farzan S: A Concise Handbook of Respiratory Diseases, p 97. Reston, VA, Reston Publishing, 1985
3. Schonell M, Campbell I (eds): Respiratory Medicine, p 113. New York City, Churchill Livingstone, 1984
4. Burrows B, Knudson RJ, Quan SF, Kettle LJ: Respiratory Disorders—A Pathophysiologic Approach, pp 168–169. Chicago, Year Book Medical Pub, 1983
5. Rachemann FM: Studies in asthma: I. A clinical survey of 1074 patients with asthma followed for two years. J Lab Clin Med 12: 1185–1197, 1927
6. Messer JW, Peters GA, Bennett WA: Causes of death and pathologic findings in 304 cases of bronchial asthma. Dis Chest 38: 616, 1960

7. Collins JV, Jones D: Corticosteroid mechanisms and therapeutic schedules. In Weiss EB (ed): Status Asthmaticus, p 235. Baltimore, University Park Press, 1978
8. Brenner BE, Yanos J: Asthma. In Brenner BE: Comprehensive Management of Respiratory Emergencies, pp 315–316. Rockville, MD, Aspen Systems, 1985
9. Reed CF: Mechanisms of hyperreactivity of airways in asthma. Eur J Respir Dis 63 (Suppl 117): 88, 1982
10. Empey D: Mechanisms of bronchial hyperreactivity. Eur J Respir Dis 63 (Suppl 117): 33, 1982
11. Schatx M, Patterson R, Fink J: Immunologic lung disease. N Engl J Med 300: 88, 1979
12. Austen KF, Orange RP: Bronchial asthma: The possible role of the chemical mediators of immediate hypersensitivity in the pathogenesis of subacute chronic disease. Am Rev Respir Dis 112: 423, 1975
13. Giola FR, Rogers MC: The hospital management of asthma. In Current Reviews in Respiratory Therapy, Lesson 9, Vol 1, p 68. Miami, FL, Current Reviews in Respiratory Therapy, 1980
14. Hoffman BB, Lefkowitz RJ: Alpha-adrenergic receptor subtypes. N Engl J Med 302: 1390–1396, 1980
15. Lands AM, Arnold A, McAuliff JP et al: Differentiation of receptor systems activated by sympathomimetic amines. Nature 214: 597–598, 1967
16. Grieco MH, Pierson RN Jr, Pi-Sunyer FX: Comparison of the circulatory and metabolic effects of isoproterenol, epinephrine, and methoxamine in normal and asthmatic subjects. Am J Med 44: 863–872, 1968
17. Inoue S: Effects of epinephrine on asthmatic children. J Allergy 40: 337–348, 1967
18. Kirkpatrick CH, Keller C: Impaired responsiveness to epinephrine in asthma. Am Rev Respir Dis 96: 692–699, 1967
19. Tsuchiya Y, Bukantx SC: Studies on status asthmaticus in children: I. Capillary blood *p*H and pCO_2 in status asthmaticus. J Allergy 36: 514–522, 1965
20. Alston WC, Patel KR, Kerr JW: Response of leukocyte adenyl cyclase to isoprenaline and effect of alpha-blocking drugs in extrinsic bronchial asthma. Br Med J 1: 90, 1974
21. Grieco MH, Pierson RN Jr: Mechanism of bronchoconstriction due to beta-adrenergic blockade: Studies with practolol, propranolol, and atropine. J Alergy Clin Immunol 48: 143, 1971
22. Middleton E: Antiasthmatic drug therapy and calcium ions: Review of pathogenesis and role of calcium. J Pharm Sci 69: 243–251, 1980
23. Norn S, Geisler A, Skov SP et al: Pathophysiologic mechanisms in bronchial asthma. Ugeskr Laeger 140: 5–8, 1977
24. Sokol WN, Beall GN: Asthma. In Conn HF, Conn RB Jr: Current Diagnosis 4, p 832. Philadelphia, WB Saunders, 1974
25. Orange RP, Rose B: Bronchial asthma: Clinical course and treatment. In Samter M, Austen DK: Immunological Diseases, p 873. Boston, Little, Brown & Co, 1978
26. Zilva JF, Pannal PR: Clinical Chemistry in Diagnosis and Treatment, p 104. Chicago, Year Book Medical Pub, 1975
27. Senior RM, Lefrak SS, Korenblat PF: Status asthmaticus. JAMA 231: 1277, 1975
28. Rees HA, Millar JS, Donald KW: A study of the clinical course and arterial blood gas tension of patients in status asthmaticus. Q J Med 37: 541–561, 1980
29. Zussman BM: Surveillance of ambulatory asthmatics by means of total circulating eosinophil count. Ann Allergy 40: 195–199, 1978
30. Horn BR, Robin ED, Theodore J, Van Kessel A: Total eosinophil counts in the management of bronchial asthma. N Engl J Med 292: 1152, 1975
31. O'Connell JM, Baird LI, Campbell AH: Sputum eosinophilia in chronic bronchitis and asthma. Respiration 35: 65–72, 1978
32. Epstein RL: Constituents of sputum: A simple method. Ann Intern Med 77: 259–265, 1972
33. Welsh RA: The genesis of the Charcot-Leyden crystal in the eosinophilic leukocyte of man. Am J Pathol 35: 1091–1103, 1959
34. Stevenson DD, Mathison DA, Tan EM et al: Provoking factors in bronchial asthma. Arch Intern Med 135: 777–789, 1975
35. Rebuck AS, Read J: Assessment and management of severe asthma. Am J Med 51: 788–798, 1971
36. Naylor B: The shedding of the mucosa of the bronchial tree in asthma. Thorax 17: 69–89, 1964
37. Mueller RG, Lang GE, Beam JM: Bubbles in samples for blood gas determination: A potential source of error. Am J Clin Pathol 65: 242–249, 1976
38. Eichhorn JH: Inaccuracy in blood gas/*p*H measurements caused by the blood sample. J Med Tech, Vol 2, 1: 24, Jan 1985
39. Restall RVF, Miller SE, Hahn CEW et al: Plastic or glass syringes: A comparison of the changes in

oxygen tension when blood or water samples are stored in iced water. Br J Anaesth 47: 636–637, 1975

40. Hess CW, Nichols AB, Hunt WB et al: Pseudohypoxemia secondary to leukemia and thrombocytosis. N Engl J Med 301: 361–363, 1979
41. Dent JG, Netter KJ: Errors in oxygen tension measurements caused by halothane. Br J Anaesth 48: 195–197, 1976
42. Severinghans JW, Weisbopp RB, Nishimura M et al: Oxygen electrode errors due to polarographic reduction of halothane. J Appl Physiol 31: 640–642, 1971
43. Alberry WJ, Brooks WN, Gibson SP et al: An electrode for PN_2O and PO_2 analysis in blood and gas. J Apply Physiol 45: 637–643, 1978
44. Evans MC, Cameron IR: Oxygen electrodes sensitive to nitrous oxide. Lancet 2: 1371, 1978
45. Blackhall MI, Jones RS: Lung volume and its subdivisions in normal and asthmatic males. Thorax 28: 89, 1973
46. Meisner P, Hugh-Jones P: Pulmonary function in bronchial asthma. Br Med J 1:470, 1968
47. Lourenco RV, Cottomanes E: Clinical aerosols: I. Characterization of aerosols and their diagnostic uses. Arch Intern Med 142: 2163–2172, 1982
48. Konig P: Conflicting viewpoints about treatment of asthma with cromolyn: A review of the literature. Ann Allergy 43: 293–296, 1979

BIBLIOGRAPHY

Allen WG: Management of Status Asthmaticus. In Current Reviews in Respiratory Therapy, Lesson 12, Vol 3. Miami, FL, Current Reviews in Respiratory Therapy, Inc, 1981

Cameron I, Bateman N (eds): Respiratory Disorders. Baltimore, University Park Press, 1983

DesJardins TR: Clinical Manifestations of Respiratory Disease. Chicago: Year Book Medical Pub, 1984

Eastham RD: A Laboratory Guide to Clinical Diagnosis, 5th ed. Bristol, Wright Publishing, 1983

Ferguson GG: Pathophysiology Mechanisms and Expressions. Philadelphia, WB Saunders, 1984

Fraser RG, and Pare JAP: Diagnosis of Diseases of the Chest, Vol 3. Philadelphia, WB Saunders, 1979

Friedman RB, Anderson RE: Effects of disease on clinical laboratory tests. Clin Chem 26:379D–385D, 1980

Jacobs DS, Kasten BL, Demott WR, Wolfson WL: Laboratory Test Handbook With DRG Index. St Louis: Mosby/Lexicomp, 1984

Kissane JF (ed): Anderson's Pathology, Vol 2, 8th ed. St Louis, CV Mosby, 1985

Kravis TC, Warner CG: Emergency Medicine: A Comprehensive Review. Rockville, Maryland, Aspen Systems, 1983

Krupp MA, Chatton MJ, Tierney LM Jr (eds): Current Medical Diagnosis and Treatment. Los Altos, CA, Lange Medical Publications, 1986

Lessof MH: Immunological and Clinical Aspects of Allergy. Philadelphia, JB Lippincott, 1981

Ogilvie AC: Asthma: A study in prognosis of 1,000 patients. Thorax 17:183, 1962

Rachemann FM, Edwards MC: Asthma in children: A follow-up study of 688 patients after an interval of twenty years. N Engl J Med 246:815, 858, 1952

Rebuck AS: Antiasthmatic drugs II: Therapeutic aspects. Drugs 7:370–390, 1974

Robbins: Pathological Basis of Disease, 3rd ed. Philadelphia: WB Saunders, 1984

Schonell M, Campbell I (eds): Respiratory Medicine. New York City, Churchill Livingstone, 1984

Sheldon H: Boyd's Introduction to the Study of Disease, 9th ed. Philadelphia, Lea & Febiger, 1984

Simmons DH: Current Pulmonology, Vol 4. Chicago, Year Book Medical Pub, 1982

Simmons DH: Current Pulmonology, Vol 6. Chicago, Year Book Medical Pub, 1984

Speicher CE, Smith JE: Choosing Effective Laboratory Tests. Philadelphia, WB Saunders, 1983

Sterling GM (ed): Integrated Clinical Science Respiratory Disease. London, William Heinemann, 1984

Young DS, Pestaner LC, Gibberman V: Effects of drugs on clinical laboratory tests. Clin Chem 21:1D–432D, 1975

Chapter 9

Pulmonary Thromboembolism

Michael Boroch / Laura Martin Rahlfs / Jon O. Nilsestuen

Pulmonary thromboembolism (PTE) is a group of disorders comprised of pulmonary embolism and pulmonary infarction. *Pulmonary embolism* is a secondary disease that results from the occlusion of the main pulmonary artery or its branches. Pathological changes that occur in the lung after pulmonary embolism are termed *pulmonary infarction.* Fewer than 10% of pulmonary emboli result in pulmonary infarction or cellular damage caused by oxygen debt.[1]

ETIOLOGY AND PATHOPHYSIOLOGY

Pulmonary embolism is one of the most common causes of acute death in the United States (exceeded only by heart attacks and strokes).[2] Yearly in the U.S. there are 600,000 to 700,000 cases of pulmonary embolism.[3, 4] Deaths in the U.S. caused by pulmonary embolism range from 20,000 to 50,000.[5, 6]

Origin

More than 90% of the clinically significant pulmonary emboli originate in the deep leg veins, pelvic veins, or inferior vena cava.[5, 7–11] Other sources of thrombus formation include the right heart chamber and any systemic vein. Virchow first suggested that venous stasis, hypercoagulability, and abnormal (damaged) vessel walls are the three factors primarily responsible for deep venous thrombosis (DVT). Because most pulmonary emboli originate in the deep veins, pulmonary embolism should be viewed as a complication of DVT. When a thrombus dislodges, in part or whole, it becomes a freely moving embolus that flows through the venous system to the right heart, and then usually on to the pulmonary arterial circulation.

Pulmonary embolus may be broadly classified into three categories: (1) massive pulmonary emboli, (2) pulmonary infarction, and (3) recurrent thromboembolism. If the embolus lodges in one of the main pulmonary arteries or spans the bifurcation of the main pulmonary trunk (saddle embolus) a *massive pulmonary embolism* occurs. Sudden death may ensue. A *pulmonary infarction* occurs if the embolus occludes one of the branches of the major pulmonary artery, causing inadequate circulation in the surrounding area and subsequent tissue death. This leads initially to necrosis and eventually to fibrous scarring. Third, the emboli may be so small that they flow through the pulmonary vasculature until they lodge in small pulmonary arteries or arterioles. If small emboli are recurrent and numerous, pulmonary hypertension results. This situation is known as *recurrent obstructive pulmonary thromboembolism* or *obliterative pulmonary hypertension.*

Primary Predisposing Factors for DVT

As Virchow identified, venous stasis, hypercoagulability, and damaged vessel walls are the primary predisposing factors for DVT.

Poor circulation and *venous stasis* can be caused by several factors, including prolonged bedrest, immobilization, prolonged sitting, prolonged standing, congestive heart failure, arterial fibrillation, and morbid obesity.[12, 13]

Hypercoagulation disorders that increase the likelihood of thrombus formation include pregnancy, childbirth, and puerperium; estrogen therapy, including birth control pills; polycythemia vera; sickle cell disease or trait; leukemia; malignancy; cardiac myxoma, multiple myeloma, malignant neoplasm, uterine malignancies, carcinoma of the pancreas (may be due to the release of thromboplastins); hemolytic anemias; antithrombin III deficiency; homocystinuria; nephrotic syndrome; fracture of the lower extremities; hemoglobinopathy; and dehydration.[14–21]

Abnormal or damaged blood vessel walls are predominantly the result of four conditions: vascular trauma, vasculitis, postoperative surgery, and heart disease. Vascular trauma leading to DVT may be a result of trauma to the lower extremities, criminal abortion, long bone fractures, fracture of the hip, burns, shunted hydrocephalus, myocardial infarction, vascular catheters, or popliteal venous aneurysm.[2, 22–25] The most common surgeries predisposing to PTE include cardiac surgery, surgery of the lower extremities, and prostatic, pelvic, biliary, and gastric surgery.

CLINICAL MANIFESTATIONS

Extreme variability in symptoms occurs depending on the size and location of the embolus and the patient's preexisting cardiopulmonary status. It is important to note that symptoms may be clinically silent following the vascular insult; however, many symptoms that are suggestive of the diagnosis may be clinically apparent and commonly reflect the consequences of the PTE on the pulmonary and cardiovascular systems.[26]

Related pulmonary symptoms include sudden onset of dyspnea, bronchospasm, wheezing (rare), sudden onset of chest pain (most commonly pleuritic), tachypnea, cough, hemoptysis, and exercise dyspnea.[27–31]

Cardiovascular findings on physical examination may reveal tachycardia and abnormal heart sounds. PTE may develop as a result of a preexisting cardiopulmonary or cardiac disorder. Signs of shock (pallor, diaphoresis, rapid pulse with low blood pressure) may occur with severe embolization; however, sudden cardiac death as a result of PTE is rare.[32]

Other associated symptoms may include profound apprehension, fever of unknown origin, confusion, and lightheadedness.[27] Concurrent thrombophlebitis is clinically suggestive of PTE and is often manifested by pain, swelling, ankle edema, cyanosis, as well as by tenderness of the affected limb.

LABORATORY ANALYSES AND DIAGNOSIS

Differential Diagnosis

Among the conditions that should be considered in the differential diagnosis of PTE are acute myocardial infarction, angina pectoris, pneumonia, asthma, paradoxical embolism (rare), primary pulmonary hypertension, congestive heart failure, pulmonary edema, undiagnosed sickle cell trait, spontaneous pneumothorax, bronchial carcinoma, and atelectasis.[33–37]

Clinical Laboratory Tests

No clinical laboratory test is diagnostic; however, other tests, such as a lung perfusion scan and pulmonary angiogram, will confirm the presence of pulmonary embolism. The laboratory tests most useful in the diagnosis of PTE are the arterial blood gases (see Chapter 8). These usually indicate a low $PaCO_2$ with an elevated *p*H due to hyperventilation. There is usually a low PaO_2 as well because of the arterial hypoxemia that results in PTE, although the PaO_2 result may be normal.[38] Other common laboratory test results may be seen in Table 9-1, although they are nonspecific and may not contribute materially to the diagnosis of PTE.[39]

Other Laboratory Tests

Other tests are more useful in the diagnosis of PTE, particularly the lung perfusion scan. Perfusion studies that display the distribution of blood flow are commonly performed in conjunction with ventilation scans (V/Q scans). The specificity of the test in resolving ventilation perfusion abnormalities is greatly enhanced when the two studies are performed simultaneously. The lung scan is an excellent screening test for pulmonary embolism.[40, 41] If the scan produces normal multiview findings, the diagnosis of pulmonary embolism can be ruled out.[42–44] Abnormal findings on the lung scan, however, are nonspecific;[45, 46] consequently, a ventilation scan and a plain chest film are ordered simultaneously. Lung-scanning defects caused by emphysema, chronic bronchitis, and asthma generally show concurrent areas of hyperaeration when viewed on the plain chest film. Similarly, scanning defects caused by parenchymal or pleural lesions (*e.g.*, neoplasm, atelectasis, pneumonitis, emphysematous bullae) are likely also to produce lesions on the plain chest film. When viewed together, the various types of scan patterns allow the determination of a probability estimate for pulmonary embolism.[47–49]

The chest x-ray is not definitive for the diagnosis of PTE, but is very helpful when used in conjunction with the history, clinical signs, and other clinical tests (ventilation-perfusion scan and pulmonary angiography). Frequently the chest film is normal or only minimally changed.

The pulmonary angiogram is an expensive, uncomfortable, and invasive procedure requiring experienced personnel;[50, 51] on the other hand, the test has a high degree of specificity and sensitivity and is the "gold standard" for the conclusive diagnosis of pulmonary embolism. The angiogram should be performed as soon as possible after symptoms appear, preferably within 48 hours.[51] However, it is only indicated when the other diagnostic tests (perfusion scan, x-ray) are inconclusive and accurate diagnosis is necessary.

The electrocardiograph (ECG) is nonspecific as a diagnostic test for PTE because a large percent-

Table 9-1 ***Common Laboratory Test Results in Pulmonary Embolism and Infarction***

Laboratory Test	Value	Pathophysiologic Factors
Chemistry (Serum)		
Bilirubin, total	↑	Unconjugated type originating from degraded erythrocytes
Calcium, total	—	
Carbon dioxide	—	
Chloride	—	
Cholesterol	—	
Creatine phosphokinase	↑	Unlikely to have arisen from lung tissue, but CPK-BB is present in lung tissue
Creatinine	—	
Glucose	↑	Elevated in 45% of patients at time of hospitalization; possibly related to stress
Lactic dehydrogenase	↑	From degraded erythrocytes, LD-1 or LD-2; or from the liver if there is heart failure, LD-4, or LD-5
Phosphatase, alkaline	↑	Originates from damaged vascular endothelium and proliferating vascular endothelial cells during healing
Phosphorus, inorganic	—	
Potassium	—	
Proteins, total	—	
Proteins, albumin	—	
Sodium	—	
Aspartate amino transferase	↑	Prevalence of elevation 0 to 30%. Originates from degraded erythrocytes and from the liver if there is heart failure
Urea nitrogen	—	
Uric acid	↑	Related to necrosis of lung tissue and increase in cell turnover from this lesion
Hematology (Blood)		
Hemoglobin	—	
Hematocrit	—	
Leukocyte count, total	↑	Usually normal in pulmonary embolism and elevated with pulmonary infarction
Platelet count	↑	May be increased as a predisposing cause for thrombosis

Key: — = No change; ↑ = can be increased; ↓ = can be decreased.
Based on information from Friedman RB, Anderson RE, Entine SM et al: Effects of diseases on clinical laboratory tests. Clin Chem 26:1D–476D, 1980; Wolf PL: Interpretation of Biochemical Multitest Profiles: An Analysis of 100 Important Conditions. New York City, Masson Publishing USA, 1977. Adapted with permission from Speicher CE, Smith JE: Choosing Effective Laboratory Tests. Philadelphia, WB Saunders, 1983.

age of pulmonary embolism cases present with normal ECG findings. More severe cases, however, present with ECG evidence of the acute strain on the right heart.[52, 53]

Pulmonary function findings are nonspecific for pulmonary embolism.

Laboratory tests for deep vein thrombosis (DVT) include radiocontrast venography, the most diagnostically useful of the techniques for detecting venous thrombosis. In the absence of positive findings, however, DVT cannot be ruled out.[54, 55]

Impedance plethysmography (IPG) is being

used more widely and is currently the noninvasive procedure of choice for detection of proximal DVT.[56] Interpretation of test results may be difficult; when accurately interpreted, however, the technique has a high degree of sensitivity and specificity (90%).[8]

Other techniques used include venous doppler examination, radioactive fibrinogen leg scanning, and radionuclide venography.

TREATMENT

Prophylactic Treatment

Coumadin therapy is the most effective prophylactic treatment. The drug is effective in preventing recurrent venous thromboembolism in patients with a recent episode of proximal venous thrombosis. The drug has a significant hemorrhagic complication rate, however, and therefore must be used with caution.[56]

Low-dose subcutaneous heparin is the modality most widely used for prevention of venous thrombosis.[5] It is very cost-effective in the prevention of pulmonary embolism in high-risk surgical patients,[57] but it is not effective in preventing pulmonary embolism in patients with major long bone fractures or in those undergoing above-the-knee amputation or hip surgery.[58]

Mechanical devices used to prevent PTE include custom-fitted leg stockings, external pneumatic compression (EPC) devices, and electrical stimulation.

Treatment After Diagnosis of PTE

Goals of therapy for PTE include inhibition of the growth of thromboemboli, resolution of the thromboemboli, and prevention of recurrence. Anticoagulant therapy after diagnosis is similar to that described above for prophylaxis.

Fibrolytic agents are administered to bring about clot lysis by activating plasminogen to form plasmin. Fibrinolytic agents have been shown to allow a more complete resolution of emboli than heparin therapy alone.[17] However, thrombolytic therapy does not replace the use of conventional anticoagulants. In lesions below the popliteal vein, thrombolysins are not effective.[59] The expense of thrombolytic therapy may be justified when compared to the costs of treating sequelae. Specific agents used include streptokinase, although it is contraindicated in patients with a recent history of streptococcal pharyngitis or a high titer of antistreptococcal antibody.[59] Urokinase, produced in the renal parenchymal cells, is more expensive than streptokinase, but is an effective alternative to streptokinase if needed. Dextran, a plasma expander, has also been used experimentally in the treatment of massive pulmonary embolism.[60]

Continuous monitoring of clotting studies is not necessary; furthermore, the value of coagulation tests in guiding alterations in dose or monitoring heparin effect has not been clearly established.[58]

CASE STUDY

A 56-year-old white woman was having a routine recovery from coronary artery bypass surgery. On her third day of postoperative care, she was stable and was discharged from the cardiovascular intensive care unit to the general care floor. At 2:00 a.m. the nurse caring for the patient took vital signs and noticed that the patient had rapid breathing/hyperventilation. Her nail beds and lips were cyanotic, and she was perspiring. Her blood pressure was checked and was slightly elevated at 148/92 mm Hg.

LABORATORY FINDINGS

	2nd Day Post-Op	*3rd Day Post-Op*
PaO_2	87 mm Hg	54 mm Hg
$PaCO_2$	39 mm Hg	28 mm Hg
*p*H	7.43	7.51

Questions

1. Correlate physical and laboratory findings on the 2nd day post-op.
2. Do the history and the physical and laboratory findings support a diagnosis of PTE?
3. What other procedures should be performed to confirm the diagnosis?

4. What therapy and subsequent monitoring are appropriate?

Discussion

1. Low oxygenation is evidenced by cyanosis, hyperventilation, and PaO_2. Hyperventilation leads to low $PaCO_2$ and increased *p*H.

2. Cardiac surgery is a primary predisposing factor for PTE. Clinical and lab findings are consistent with PTE.

3. Pulmonary angiography was performed to confirm the presence of pulmonary embolism.

4. Because results of the angiogram were positive and the patient did have a pulmonary embolism, the patient was immediately placed on 60% oxygen and arterial blood gas analyses were repeated and monitored to keep the oxygenation at adequate levels. Heparin was administered intravenously as an anticoagulant to treat the embolism. The patient was already receiving cardiotonic drugs to reduce heart strain. Constant ECG monitoring was occurring and the patient was moved back into the intensive care unit. Streptokinase to treat the pulmonary embolism was considered, but the patient's arterial oxygenation was restored to normal levels without such action. The heparin level was monitored closely to minimize the risk of bleeding.

REFERENCES

1. Soloff LA, Rodman T: Acute pulmonary embolism: I. Review. Am Heart J 74:710–724, 1967
2. Dalen JE, Alpert JS: Natural history of pulmonary embolism. Prog Cardiovasc Dis 17:257, 1975
3. Sharma GVRK, Tow DE, Parisi AF, Sasahara AA: Diagnosis of pulmonary embolism. Ann Rev Med 28:159–166, 1977
4. Gallus AS: Venous thromboembolism: Medical and clinical risk factors. In Madden JL, Hume M (eds): Venous Thromboembolism: Prevention and Treatment, pp 1–32. New York City, Appleton-Century-Crofts, 1976
5. Moser KM: Pulmonary embolism. Am Rev Respir Dis 115:829–852, 1977
6. Freiman DG, Suyemoto J, Wessler S: Frequency of pulmonary thromboembolism in man. N Engl J Med 272:1278–1280, 1965
7. Kakkar VV, Howe CT, Flanc C, Clarke MB: Natural history of postoperative deep-vein thrombosis. Lancet 2:230–232, 1969
8. Sasahara AA, Sharma GVRK, Tow DE et al: Pulmonary embolism: The target organ. In Madden JL, Hume M (eds): Venous Thromboembolism: Prevention and Treatment, pp 91-102. New York City, Appleton-Century-Crofts, 1976
9. Lopez-Majano V, Leininger B, Friedman F: Incidence of pulmonary embolism in deep venous thrombosis. Respiration 36:223–227, 1978
10. LeQuesne LP: Relation between deep vein thrombosis and pulmonary embolism in surgical patients. N Engl J Med 291:1292, 1974
11. Rosenow EC, Osmundson PJ, Brown ML: Pulmonary embolism. Mayo Clin Proc 56:161, 1981
12. Kent DC, Reid D: Pulmonary embolism in active duty servicemen. Arch Environ Health 12:509–517, 1966
13. Coon WW, Willis PW III: Deep vein thrombosis and pulmonary embolism: Prediction, prevention, and treatment. Am J Cardiol 4:611–621, 1959
14. Byrd RB, Divertie MB, Spittell JA Jr: Bronchogenic carcinoma and thromboembolic disease. JAMA 202:1019–1022, 1967
15. Amundsen MA, Spittell JA Jr, Thompson JH Jr et al: Hypercoagulability associated with malignant disease and with the postoperative state: Evidence for elevated levels and anti-hemophilic globulin. Ann Intern Med 58:608–616, 1963
16. Wilson JE III: Pulmonary embolism: Diagnosis and treatment. Clin Notes Respir Dis 19 (Spring):3–11, 1981
17. Sharma GVRK, Burleson VA, Sasahara AA: Effect of thrombolytic therapy on pulmonary-capillary blood volume in patients with pulmonary embolism. N Engl J Med 303:842–845, 1980
18. Shen VS, Pollak EW: Fatal pulmonary embolism in cancer patients: Is heparin prophylaxis justified? South Med J 73:841–843, 1980
19. Gore JM, Appelbaum JS, Greene HL et al: Association between pulmonary embolism and occult malignancy. Ann Intern Med 96:556, 1982
20. Keenan DJ, Morton P, O'Kane HO: Right atrial myxoma and pulmonary embolism: Rational basis for investigation and treatment. Br Heart J 48:510–512, 1982

21. Hunter JH, Ferrech A, Ridley W et al: Familial antithrombin III deficiency. Q J Med 51:373–375, 1982
22. Bauer G: Thrombosis following leg injuries. Acta Chir Scand 90:229–248, 1944
23. DesJardins TR: Clinical Manifestations of Respiratory Disease, p 228. Chicago, Year Book Medical Pub, 1984
24. Schonell M, Campbell I: Pulmonary thromboembolism: Pulmonary embolism and pulmonary infarction. In Schonell M, Campbell I (eds): Respiratory Medicine, p 153. New York City, Churchill Livingstone, 1984
25. Chantre, Cornund F, Bouckama A et al: Thrombosis as a complication of pulmonary-artery catheterization by the internal jugular vein: A prospective evaluation by phlebography. N Engl J Med 306:278, 1982
26. Williams JW, Eikman EA, Greenberg S: Asymptomatic pulmonary embolism: A common event in high risk patients. Ann Surg 195:323–327, 1982
27. Bell WR, Simon TL, DeMets DL: The clinical features of submassive and massive pulmonary emboli. Am J Med 62:355–360, 1977
28. Mack I, Beall AC Jr, Griffith GC et al: Salvaging the patient with acute massive pulmonary embolism. Dis Chest 42:584, 1962
29. Urokinase pulmonary embolism trial. Circ Res 47(Suppl 2):86–90, 1973
30. Goodall RJR, Greenfield LF: Clinical correlations in the diagnosis of pulmonary embolism. Ann Surg 191:219–223, 1980
31. Murray HW, Ellis GC, Blumenthal DS et al: Fever and pulmonary thromboembolism. Am J Med 67:232–235, 1979
32. Cobbs BW Jr, Logue RB, Dorney ER: The second heart sound in pulmonary embolism and pulmonary hypertension. Am Heart J 71:843, 1966
33. Boshour T, Lindsay J Jr: Hemoglobin S-C disease presenting as acute pneumonitis with pulmonary angiographic findings in two patients. Am J Med 58:559–562, 1975
34. Boyer NH, Curry JJ: Bronchospasm associated with pulmonary embolism: Respiratory failure. Arch Intern Med 73:403–409, 1944
35. Gurewich V, Thomas D, Stein M et al: Bronchoconstriction in the presence of pulmonary embolism. Circulation 27:339–345, 1963
36. Jewett JF: Asthma, emboli, and cardiac arrest. N Engl J Med 288:265–266, 1973
37. Dalen JE, Haynes FW, Hoppin FG Jr et al: Cardiovascular responses to experimental pulmonary embolism. Am J Cardiol 20:3–9, 1967
38. Levy SE, Stein M: Pulmonary embolism and infarction. In Burton GG, Hodgkin JE (eds): Respiratory Care, pp 819–830. Philadelphia, JB Lippincott, 1984
39. Speicher CE, Smith JE: Choosing Effective Laboratory Tests. Philadelphia, WB Saunders, 1983
40. Wagner HW, Tow DE: Radioisotope scanning in the study of pulmonary circulation. Prog Cardiovas Dis 9:382, 1967
41. Wagner HN Jr, Sabiston DC, McAfee JG et al: Diagnosis of massive pulmonary embolism in man by radioisotope scanning. N Engl J Med 271:377, 1964
42. Barner HB, DeWeese JA: An evaluation of the sphygmomanometer cuff pain test in venous thrombosis. Surgery 48:915–924, 1960
43. Biello DR, Mattar AG, McKnight RC et al: Ventilation-perfusion studies in suspected pulmonary embolism. AJR 133:1033–1037, 1979
44. Kipper MS, Moser KM, Kortman KE et al: Long-term follow-up of patients with suspected pulmonary embolism and a normal lung scan: Perfusion scans in embolic suspects. Chest 82:411–415, 1982
45. Rosen RJ, Goodman LR: Occult bronchogenic carcinoma masquerading as recurrent pulmonary embolism. AJR 132:133–135, 1979
46. Maynard CD, Cowan RJ: Role of the scan in bronchogenic carcinoma. Semin Nucl Med 1:195–205, 1971
47. Sostman HD, Ravin CE, Sullivan DC et al: Use of pulmonary angiography for suspected pulmonary embolism: Influence of scintigraphic diagnosis. AJR 139:673–677, 1982
48. McNeil BJ: Ventilation-perfusion studies and the diagnosis of pulmonary embolism. J Nucl Med 21:319–323, 1980
49. Cheely R, McCartney WH, Perry JR et al: The role of noninvasive tests versus pulmonary angiography in the diagnosis of pulmonary embolism. Am J Med 70:17–22, 1983
50. Fowler NO, Schaffer-Black B, Scott RC, Gueron M: Idiopathic and thromboembolic pulmonary hypertension. Am J Med 40:331, 1966
51. Ormond RS, Galf HH, Drake EH, Gahagan T: Pul-

monary angiography and pulmonary embolism. Radiology 86:658, 1966
52. McGinn S, White PD: Acute cor pulmonale resulting from pulmonary embolism: Its clinical recognition. JAMA 104:1473, 1935
53. Durant TM, Ginsburg I, Rossler H: Transient bundle branch block and other electrocardiographic changes in pulmonary embolism. Am Heart J 17:423, 1939
54. Rosenow EC III, Osmundson PJ, Brown ML: Pulmonary embolism. Mayo Clinic Proc 56:161–178, 1981
55. Hull RD, Hirsh J, Carter CJ et al: Pulmonary angiography, ventilation lung scanning, and venography for clinically suspected pulmonary embolism with abnormal perfusion lung scan. Ann Intern Med 98:891–899, 1983
56. Moser KM, LeMoine: Is embolic risk conditioned by location of deep venous thrombosis? Ann Intern Med 94:439–444, 1981
57. Hull RD, Hirsh J, Sackett DL et al: Cost-effectiveness of primary and secondary prevention and fatal pulmonary embolism in high-risk surgical patients. J Can Med Assoc 127:990–995, 1982
58. Moser KM: Pulmonary thromboembolism. In Petersdorf RG, Adams RD et al (eds): Harrison's Principles of Internal Medicine, p 1562. New York City, McGraw-Hill, 1983
59. Elliot J: Greater use of fibrinolytic agents urged. JAMA 243:2275–2276, 1980
60. Hauser C, Shoemaker W: Volume loading in massive acute pulmonary embolus. Crit Care Med 7:304, 1979

BIBLIOGRAPHY

Brenner BE: Comprehensive Management of Respiratory Emergencies. Rockville, MD, Aspen Systems, 1985

Cameron I, Bateman N (eds): Respiratory Disorders. Baltimore, University Park Press, 1983

Eastham RD: A Laboratory Guide to Clinical Diagnosis, 5th ed. Bristol, Wright Publishing, 1983

Eichhorn JH: Inaccuracy in blood gas/*p*H measurements caused by the blood sample. J Med Tech, Vol 2, 1:23, Jan 1985

Farzan S: A Concise Handbook of Respiratory Disease, 2nd ed. Reston, VA, Reston Publishing, 1985

Fraser RG, Pare JAP: Diagnosis of Diseases of the Chest, Vol. 3. Philadelphia, WB Saunders, 1979

Friedman RB, Anderson RE: Effects of disease on clinical laboratory tests. Clin Chem 26:379D–385D, 1980

Griner PF, Mayewski RJ, Mushlin AI et al: Selection and interpretation of diagnostic tests and procedures: Principles and applications. Ann Intern Med 94:575–579, 1981

Gitnick GL: Current Medicine, Vol 3. Chicago: Year Book Medical Pub, 1986

Jacobs DS, Kasten BL, Demott WR, Wolfson WL: Laboratory Test Handbook With DRG Index. St Louis, Mosby/Lexicomp, 1984

Kissane JF (ed): Anderson's Pathology, Vol 2, 8th ed. St Louis, CV Mosby, 1985

Kravis TC, Warner CG: Emergency Medicine: A Comprehensive Review. Rockville, MD, Aspen Systems, 1983

Krupp MA, Chatton MJ, Tierney LM Jr (eds): Current Medical Diagnosis and Treatment. Los Altos, CA, Lange Medical Publications, 1986

Robbins: Pathological Basis of Disease, 3rd ed. Philadelphia, WB Saunders, 1984

Sheldon H: Boyd's Introduction to the Study of Disease, 9th ed. Philadelphia, Lea & Febiger, 1984

Simmons DH: Current Pulmonology, Vol 4. Chicago: Year Book Medical Pub, 1982

Simmons DH: Current Pulmonology, Vol 6. Chicago: Year Book Medical Pub, 1984

Speicher CE, Smith JE: Choosing Effective Laboratory Tests. Philadelphia, WB Saunders, 1983

Sterling GM (ed): Integrated Clinical Science Respiratory Disease. London, William Heinemann, Wolfe EG, Sabiston DC Jr: Pulmonary Embolism. Philadelphia, WB Saunders, 1980, 1984

Wolfe EG, Sabiston DC Jr: Pulmonary Embolism. Philadelphia, WB Saunders, 1980

Young DS, Pestaner LC, Gibberman V: Effects of drugs on clinical laboratory tests. Clin Chem 21:1D–432D, 1975

Chapter 10

Respiratory Tract Infections

Marie Pezzlo

The most common infections in the United States occur in the respiratory tract, and may be divided into upper and lower tract infections. The upper respiratory tract (URT) includes the larynx, nasopharynx, oropharynx, nose, sinuses, and middle ear. Infections at these sites are usually caused by viruses, although certain bacteria such as *Streptococcus pyogenes* (Lancefield group A, beta-hemolytic streptococci) are also pathogenic.

A major portion of the upper respiratory tract, especially the oropharynx, is colonized with large numbers of normal microbial flora comprised of aerobic, facultatively anaerobic, and obligately anaerobic bacteria. These microorganisms are present in large numbers, and often the anaerobes exceed the aerobes. Nasal washings, saliva, tooth surfaces, and gingival scrapings have been shown to contain as many as 10^9 colony-forming units (CFU)/ml of bacteria.[1] Viruses are not considered to be part of the normal flora, although they may be isolated from asymptomatic patients with subclinical disease.[2]

The lower respiratory tract (LRT) includes the trachea, bronchi, bronchioles, and lungs. Infections of these areas are caused by a variety of etiologic agents including bacteria, viruses, fungi, and parasites. The lower respiratory tract is usually the primary site for pathogens such as the Legionnaires' disease agent, mycoplasma, mycobacteria, and pneumocystis. The organisms responsible for causing lower respiratory disease are those that colonize the URT and the gastrointestinal tract. Their presence is often dependent on many factors, including the age of the patient, immunosuppression, long-term hospitalization, travel history, other underlying diseases, and antimicrobic or cytotoxic therapy.

ETIOLOGY AND PATHOPHYSIOLOGY OF UPPER RESPIRATORY TRACT (URT) INFECTIONS

The Common Cold

The common cold is an acute self-limited syndrome caused by an infection that is generally viral. Complications are rare, but sinusitis, otitis media, or lower respiratory tract infection may follow. The common cold is the most common infectious disease in humans and the leading cause of absenteeism from work.[3]

Rhinoviruses are the most important etiologic agents of the common cold, causing approximately 25% of adult colds and 10% of colds in children. Other viral agents implicated in the common cold are coxsackie, echovirus, influenza, parainfluenza, respiratory syncytial virus (RSV), coronaviruses, and adenoviruses.[4]

The incubation period is usually 2 to 3 days, and most colds last for approximately one week. The infection is spread by person-to-person contact, and there is an increased incidence during the cold-weather months. Children become infected more often than adults, especially during the early school years, with approximately three to eight infections per year.[5]

Pharyngitis

Acute pharyngitis is an inflammatory disease of the mucous membranes of the throat, sometimes involving the uvula, nasopharynx, and soft palate.

The most common cause of bacterial pharyngitis is *Streptococcus pyogenes* (group A streptococci). Uncommon bacterial pathogens that may involve the pharynx include *Corynebacterium diphtheriae, Candida albicans,* and *Neisseria gonorrhoeae.* There is no convincing evidence that *Hemophilus influenzae, Streptococcus pneumoniae,* or *Neisseria meningitidis* are pharyngeal pathogens.[2] The presence of *Pseudomonas aeruginosa* and members of the *Enterobacteriaceae* usually represents colonization rather than infection. The viruses that cause the common cold have also been implicated as infectious agents in pharyngitis. Herpes simplex virus (HSV), Epstein-Barr virus (EBV), and measles virus are additional causes of pharyngitis. Adenoviruses are a common cause of primary pharyngitis, especially when associated with conjunctivitis. Pharyngitis is also associated with infectious mononucleosis and measles.

Laryngitis

Acute laryngitis is an inflammation of the larynx and is usually associated with the common cold or the influenza syndrome.[4] Children are more susceptible than adults.

The common causes of laryngitis are rhinoviruses, adenoviruses, influenza and parainfluenza viruses.

Laryngotracheobronchitis (Croup)

Acute laryngotracheobronchitis or croup is commonly caused by parainfluenza viruses and occurs in young children between the ages of 3 months and 3 years.[6] Parainfluenza type 1 causes a majority of croup cases, and the outbreaks usually occur in the fall.[7] Outbreaks that occur during the winter months and spring are thought to be caused by influenza A virus. Less common causes of croup include RSV, adenoviruses, rhinoviruses, and *Mycoplasma pneumoniae.* The infection can spread and eventually include the lower respiratory tract.

Epiglottitis

Epiglottitis is a form of croup caused by *H. influenzae* type B rather than by a virus as in the other form of croup. Young children are susceptible as hosts. The infection can progress rapidly to toxicity, prostration, severe dyspnea, and cyanosis. The infection is life-threatening and may be fatal.[8]

Sinusitis

Sinusitis, a common infection of the upper respiratory tract, is characterized by inflammation of the paranasal sinuses. Acute sinusitis is usually a bacterial infection that follows a viral infection of the upper respiratory tract. The mucosal lining of the sinuses becomes inflamed and swollen. Noninfectious sinusitis may be caused by allergic rhinitis, a deviated nasal septum, a nasal tumor, or foreign bodies.[9]

The common causes of acute infectious sinusitis include *S. pneumoniae* and *H. influenzae.* Anaerobes have also been associated with acute infection; however, they are usually isolated in patients with dental disease. Less common causes include *Staphylococcus aureus, S. pyogenes, P. aeruginosa, Klebsiella pneumoniae,* and *Escherichia coli.*[10] Sinusitis is more common in adults than in children, and fewer than 1% of upper respiratory infections are complicated by this syndrome. Infections of the frontal and ethmoidal sinuses may result in brain abscesses, meningitis, and osteomyelitis of the frontal bone of the skull.

Otitis Media and Otitis Externa

Otitis media is an infection of the middle ear caused by *Branhamella catarrhalis, S. pneumoniae, H. influenzae,* and *S. pyogenes.* Other organisms such as members of the family *Enterobacteriaceae* and *S. aureus* are less common causes.[11] The infection occurs most often in young children and results from an accumulation of fluid in the middle ear. Otitis media may also be caused by an allergy or anatomic defect of the middle ear or eustachian tube; however, the acute bacterial infection is the most common.

Otitis externa, also known as "swimmer's ear," is a superficial infection of the external ear canal commonly caused by *P. aeruginosa.* A more severe form is known as *malignant external otitis,* also caused by *P. aeruginosa.*[12] It occurs primarily in elderly diabetics. Serious complications include osteomyelitis, facial nerve palsy, cranial nerve involvement, and even death. Early diagnosis and antibiotic therapy are essential to prevent serious complications.

OTHER INFECTIONS

DIPHTHERIA

Diphtheria is an intoxication caused by toxigenic strains of *C. diphtheriae.* The infection occurs in the pharynx where the organisms multiply and produce toxin. A diphtherialike disease also due to an intoxication is caused by *Corynebacterium ulcerans.* This organism may also be part of the normal pharyngeal flora; therefore, it is important to differentiate it from *C. diphtheriae.*

Since the introduction of immunization programs, the incidence of the disease has declined sharply. Fewer than 100 cases are reported each year in the United States. The disease occurs predominantly in nonimmune individuals. It is transmitted by droplets from upper respiratory secretions of persons incubating the disease or from healthy carriers.

The upper respiratory tract is the common site; however, *C. diphtheriae* has also been isolated from mucous membranes of the eye and genitals, cutaneous ulcers, burns, and wounds.[13] Although the organism is noninvasive, the toxin is lethal for a variety of cells. Some of the more serious complications that result from absorbed toxin include myocarditis, kidney tubular necrosis, and neuritis.

PERTUSSIS

Pertussis, also known as *whooping cough,* is an acute infection of the tracheobronchial tree caused by *Bordetella pertussis.* The disease is less commonly caused by *B. parapertussis* and *B. bronchiseptica.* This disease has also shown a sharp decrease since the introduction of a potent vaccine in the mid-1940s. Neonates and young infants are susceptible to this disease, as are other nonimmunized individuals.

INFECTION OF THE ORAL CAVITY

Thrush (oral candidiasis) is a fungal infection of the mouth, oropharynx, and tongue caused by *C. albicans.* The infection usually occurs in immunosuppressed patients receiving antimicrobial therapy. The organism may be part of the normal upper respiratory flora in small numbers; however, following antimicrobial therapy it multiplies rapidly.

Vincent's angina is a mild pharyngitis caused by *Borrelia vincentii* and *Fusobacterium* species. The infection usually follows dental extraction or occurs because of poor oral hygiene. The etiologic agents are organisms of the oral flora such as anaerobes and spirochetes, which are present in high numbers below the gingival surfaces and tooth crevices. The infection may also spread to the tonsils, producing an acute pharyngitis.

The *canker sore* (aphthous stomatitis) is a common disease of the oral mucosa. The patient may have one or more lesions appearing throughout the oral cavity. The ulcers associated with this infection may be confused with herpes simplex virus lesions; however, the etiology of the canker sore is unknown.

Other infections of the oral cavity caused by oral flora include dental, facial, and cervical space infections and deep space infections.[14] A variety of preexisting conditions predispose the host to these infections. Viral infections of the oral cavity include primary herpetic gingivostomatitis caused by herpes simplex virus, and infections caused by herpes zoster virus and coxsackievirus. *Rubeola,* the measles virus, causes the characteristic Koplik's spots on the buccal mucosa at least two days before the appearance of the skin lesions.[14] Oral lesions are also associated with smallpox virus (variola) and chicken pox (varicella).

Actinomycosis, a chronic infection that may occur in the lower jaw following dental extraction, is caused by *Actinomyces* spp. The infection has also been called "lumpy jaw" because of the hardening of the tissues or presence of granulomas.

Other infections that may have associated oral lesions include syphilis *(Treponema pallidum),* yaws *(Treponema pertenue),* anthrax *(Bacillus anthracis),* glanders *(Pseudomonas mallei),* botryomycosis *(S. aureus),* scarlet fever *(S. pyogenes),* and a variety of fungi and parasites.[14]

ETIOLOGY AND PATHOPHYSIOLOGY OF LOWER RESPIRATORY TRACT (LRT) INFECTIONS

Acute Bronchitis/Tracheobronchitis

Acute bronchitis, a disease of all ages, is usually preceded by an upper respiratory tract infection. Acute bronchitis involves the airways between the larynx and the bronchioles, and *S. pneumoniae, S. aureus, H. influenzae, B. pertussis,* and *M. pneu-*

moniae are common bacterial causes. Of those infections with a viral etiology, RSV is the most common cause in young children.[4] Parainfluenza virus type 3 is the second most common cause, followed by adenovirus type 7, influenza A, and measles. Although these viruses also cause infections in adults, the influenza viruses are more common to adults. Individuals with allergies, poor nutrition, emphysema, and tuberculosis are more susceptible to acute bronchitis. Air pollution and rapid temperature changes may also result in infection.[15] Acute bronchitis is more prevalent in the winter months, a peak season for acute respiratory infections.

Acute tracheobronchitis, caused by the influenza virus, is characterized by a sudden onset. Often referred to as the "flu," it is usually uncomplicated and resolves within one week. Epidemics can occur during the winter months and are usually caused by type A or type B viruses. Infections may become complicated by a secondary infection with *S. aureus*. Pneumonia may develop in the older or debilitated patient.

Chronic Bronchitis

Chronic bronchitis is associated with a chronic or recurrent cough and results from cigarette smoking, air pollution, and infection. These factors are irritants to the airway of most patients, so the syndrome is not uncommon. Approximately 50% of all heavy cigarette smokers have chronic bronchitis, as do 6% to 10% of nonsmokers.[16] Other factors that predispose the patient to this disease are a history of frequent respiratory infections, a family history of respiratory disease, or exposure to pollutants. Chronic bronchitis is not associated with certain pulmonary diseases such as cystic fibrosis, bronchiectasis, tuberculosis, and malignancy.[15]

Bacteria do not cause the disease, except in the patient with a history of frequent respiratory infections, but they may perpetuate it.[17] The bronchi are normally sterile sites; however, in chronic bronchitis, microorganisms may be recovered. It appears that these organisms colonize the airways and the sputum and then cause infection. The organisms commonly associated with chronic bronchitis include *H. influenzae* and viruses, including influenza, parainfluenza, RSV, rhinovirus, and coronavirus.[18]

Bronchiolitis

Bronchiolitis is an acute viral respiratory infection of young infants. The most common cause of this infection is RSV, followed by parainfluenza virus type 3 and, less commonly, by adenovirus, rhinoviruses, influenza A and B, and enteroviruses.[19] These infections may be associated with pneumonia, otitis media, mild conjunctivitis, and diarrhea. Severe cases may require hospitalization.

Pneumonia

Pneumonia is an inflammation of the lungs caused by a variety of microorganisms, including bacteria, viruses, fungi, and parasites. When the lung defense mechanisms become compromised, the patient becomes susceptible to infection.[20] The factors that interfere with host defense mechanisms include aspiration as a result of consciousness impaired by a stroke, anesthesia, alcohol or drugs, and sleep, cigarette smoking, pollutants, immunosuppression, and mechanical obstruction.[21] Many factors are involved with pneumonia and its pathogenesis. These include the status of the host defense mechanisms, the type of infiltrate or anatomic type, the place of acquisition of the infection, and, finally, the infecting agents themselves.

The upper respiratory tract is colonized by both aerobic and anaerobic organisms as discussed above. These organisms may inhibit the colonization of more virulent organisms. Below the larynx, coughing helps to limit colonization by pathogens and maintain sterility of the respiratory bronchioles.[22] Other defenses include cellular and humoral immunity by lymphocytes, phagocytosis by macrophages and neutrophils, and complement-mediated cell lysis.[23] Alteration in any one of these defense mechanisms predisposes an individual to infection.

Almost any organism can cause pneumonia, and characteristic infiltrates or patterns occur with different types of organisms. These characteristic patterns or pulmonary infiltrates are observed radiologically. *Alveolar (lobar) pneumonia* is characterized by an extensive, homogeneous density. The most common organism associated with this type of infiltrate is *S. pneumoniae.* The organism gains access to the alveoli, which results in large amounts of fluid accumulation. A second type is *bronchopneumonia (lobular).* The organisms penetrate the lung through bronchi and bronchioles and cause an inflammatory response in airways, which results initially in a patchy infiltrate that may then become confluent. An *interstitial pneumonia* results when the organism causes infection in the connective tissue. Usually agents of atypical pneumonias cause an interstitial infiltrate, *e.g.*, viruses, mycoplasma, and the Legionnaires' disease agent. In addition to these three types of pneumonias, necrotizing and abscess-forming pneumonias can occur. These are caused primarily by anaerobes; however, other organisms may also be the cause of infection.

The etiology of the infection varies with the situation as well as with the place of acquisition. For example, patients with congestive heart failure, diabetes, chronic pulmonary disease, or alcoholism have a high incidence of pneumonia.[21] Also, certain microorganisms have been associated with certain diseases. "Place of acquisition" refers to whether the pneumonia is community-acquired or hospital-acquired (see Chap. 60). *S. pneumoniae* and *M. pneumoniae* are the two most common causes of *community-acquired pneumonia.*[22] Gram-negative pneumonias are uncommon causes of community-acquired pneumonias in otherwise healthy individuals. Other causes include influenza viruses A and B, adenoviruses, *Legionella pneumophila, H. influenzae, S. aureus,* and gram-negative bacilli in patients with chronic obstructive pulmonary disease (COPD). *Chlamydia trachomatis* has also been reported as a community-acquired pneumonia in infants.[24] These less common infections are often associated with other underlying clinical conditions or syndromes. *L. pneumophila* is associated with Legionnaires' disease, and staphylococcal pneumonias often follow influenza epidemics.[25] Patients with chronic pulmonary disease have a higher incidence of *S. pneumoniae* and *H. influenzae,* as previously described for chronic bronchitis. Cystic fibrosis patients develop pneumonia caused by *P. aeruginosa* and staphylococci.[26] *P. carinii* has become a common cause of pneumonia in AIDS patients.

Hospital-acquired (nosocomial) pneumonias occur in approximately 5% of hospitalized patients; however, the organisms responsible for these infections have changed over the last few decades.[22, 23] During the 1950s, the organisms commonly causing infection included *S. pneumoniae, H. influenzae,* and *S. pyogenes.* During the 1960s, *S. aureus* was a common cause, followed by the *Enterobacteriaceae* and *P. aeruginosa* in the 1970s and 1980s.[22] In the immunosuppressed or compromised patient, viruses, fungi, and parasites predominate regardless of the place of acquisition (see Chap. 61).

BACTERIAL PNEUMONIAS

Bacterial pneumonias remain the leading cause of death due to infectious diseases. *S. pneumoniae, K. pneumoniae, S. aureus,* and *S. pyogenes* are the causative agents in a majority of cases,[24] although pneumonia deaths due to *H. influenzae* and *L. pneumophila* are increasing.[27]

Streptococcus pneumoniae pneumonia occurs throughout the year, with a peak during the winter months. Persons with previous viral infections, alcoholism, chronic bronchitis or emphysema, immunoglobulin insufficiency, or absence of a spleen, or those younger than 5 years or older than 50 years are susceptible to *S. pneumoniae* pneumonia.

Hemophilus influenzae pneumonia is similar to pneumococcal pneumonia, and the infiltrates may be alveolar or bronchopneumonialike in the lower lung fields. Predisposing factors include chronic lung disease, alcoholism, and age. Patients usually have had a previous upper respiratory infection followed by fever and a productive cough.

Staphylococcal pneumonias cause approximately 5% to 10% of hospital-acquired pneumonias.[22, 23, 27] Patients with a history of drug abuse, diabetes mellitus, COPD, renal failure, or immunosuppression are more likely to develop pneumonia caused by Staphylococcus.

Klebsiella pneumoniae and other gram-negative bacilli are common causes of community-acquired infections among the elderly and nursing home patients.[28] The infection is also seen in chronically alcoholic men as well as in other debilitated hosts.

Klebsiella pneumoniae also causes hospital-acquired pneumonias, as do other aerobic gram-negative bacilli. These infections are usually associated with the use of inhalation therapy equipment, with postoperative patients, and with patients on antimicrobial therapy. It has been reported that, within 24 hours of admission to the hospital, 22% of patients in an intensive care unit become colonized with gram-negative enteric flora.[29] Within 1 week, the colonization rate is 45%. The presence of these organisms in sputum must be correlated with clinical symptoms in order to establish infection.

In 1976, a fastidious gram-negative bacillus was isolated from several individuals attending an American Legion convention in Philadelphia. The organism responsible for the epidemic that followed is now known as *Legionella pneumophila.* There are two forms of the disease, Pontiac fever and Legionnaires' disease. *Pontiac fever,* the nonpneumonic form, causes a benign infection and results in a spontaneous recovery. *Legionnaires' disease,* a more serious infection, causes an atypical pneumonia. The infection peaks in summer or fall and is usually associated with contaminated ventilation or air-conditioning systems. The infection occurs more frequently in alcoholics and heavy smokers, and affects two to four times more men than women.

ATYPICAL PNEUMONIA

Mycoplasma pneumoniae (primary atypical pneumonia), also known as *Eaton agent,* is responsible for approximately 20% of all pneumonias.[22] These often resolve spontaneously. Infections occur in crowded areas such as prisons and military camps.[30] Other organisms causing atypical pneumonias are *Coxiella burnetii* (Q fever) and *Chlamydia psittaci* (psittacosis).

VIRAL PNEUMONIAS

Viruses should be considered as causative agents of pneumonia, especially in children and in adults with COPD. Viral pneumonia in adults is uncommon except for influenza and adenovirus infections. The clinical picture is similar to that for *Mycoplasma* pneumonia, including cough and shortness of breath. Children become infected with RSV, influenza viruses A and B, and parainfluenza viruses.

Other respiratory viral infections associated with the immunocompromised host include cytomegalovirus (CMV), adenoviruses, and orthomyxo- and paramyxoviruses. *CMV,* a common infection in the compromised host, causes fatal interstitial pneumonitis in patients with renal transplants or bone marrow transplants, patients with malignancies, AIDS patients, and premature infants who have received multiple transfusions.[31, 32] Possible sources include blood products, the engrafted organ or bone marrow, sexual transmission, and reactivation of the latent virus.[4] CMV pneumonia suggests infection with other respiratory pathogens.[33]

Adenoviruses also cause severe pulmonary infection in the immunocompromised patients described above under CMV infection.[34] The organisms may cause interstitial pneumonitis, pleural effusion, or necrotizing bronchiolitis. Orthomyxo- and paramyxoviruses include influenza A, RSV, and parainfluenza viruses. These organisms cause pneumonia in younger patients and are associated with severe disease. Severe pneumonia is also a serious complication of *measles* (rubeola). *VZV* (varicella-zoster virus), *EBV* (Epstein-Barr virus), and *HSV* (herpes simplex virus) can also cause an interstitial pneumonitis in congenitally- or neonatally-infected infants.[4] Viral pneumonias occur in 2.4% of all children under 1 year of age.[35]

CHRONIC PNEUMONIA

Chronic pneumonia is an inflammation of the lung parenchyma that lasts for weeks to months (acute pneumonia lasts only for days). The radiological patterns are more helpful in the diagnosis than the symptoms. The group of organisms that cause patchy infiltrates and bronchopneumonia includes Actinomyces, Norcardia, and certain fungal agents such as Blastomyces, Cryptococcus, and Paracoccidioides. Microorganisms causing pulmonary cavitation include Mycobacteria, Histoplasma, Coccidioides, Sporothrix, Aspergillus, and certain parasites including Paragonimus and Echinococcus.

Nocardiosis is primarily a pulmonary infection, but infection may occur in other parts of the body. The organism *Nocardia* spp. (usually *N. asteroides*) is present in soil and enters the human host as a result of trauma or by inhalation. The infection begins as a pneumonitis that may result in tissue necrosis and abscess formation. In severe cases, the infection may spread into the pleural cavity and out through the chest wall, forming a draining sinus.

Actinomycosis is a chronic granulomatous disease that manifests itself as cervicofacial (lumpy jaw), gastrointestinal, or pulmonary. The pulmonary form presents as a low-grade pneumonitis with cough, empyema, and sinus formation. The organism most commonly associated with this syndrome is *Actinomyces israelii.*

PULMONARY TUBERCULOSIS

Mycobacterium tuberculosis is the most common mycobacterial infection of the lung, followed by *M. avium* and *M. intracellulare.* Primary tuberculosis is transmitted to the nonimmune host by aerosolized droplets. The course of the disease may be uncomplicated, and cases that are not treated may result in cure. Usually the infection is limited and the lesions heal. If the infection spreads to the pulmonary lymph nodes, however, complications may result. The organisms may then enter the blood stream and be carried to other parts of the body *(miliary tuberculosis)*. A hypersensitivity reaction may occur, leading to tissue necrosis. Organisms may persist for years and eventually cause *reactivation tuberculosis* (secondary tuberculosis).

Nontuberculous mycobacterial disease occurs in patients with underlying lung disease, malignancies, and chronic aspiration. The disease is similar to tuberculosis, but more indolent. Treatment is dependent upon the organism isolated.

PULMONARY MYCOSES

Three major pulmonary mycoses, coccidioidomycosis, histoplasmosis, and blastomycosis, occur in the immunocompromised host (see Chap. 61). Other common fungal infections include aspergillosis, candidiasis, and cryptococcosis.

Coccidioidomycosis, also known as *valley fever,* is caused by *Coccidioides immitis.* The organism is acquired by inhalation of arthrospores. Following inhalation of spores, an inflammatory response occurs. Within 48 to 72 hours the arthrospores evolve into spherules, which eventually rupture and liberate endospores. Chronic cavities, nodules, or abscesses may then develop. Pneumonia is a complication of primary infection. Cavities associated with pneumonia may grow rapidly, resulting in bronchopleural fistulas.

Histoplasmosis is caused by *Histoplasma capsulatum,* a soil-based organism acquired by inhalation of spores. Chronic pulmonary histoplasmosis is usually a complication of COPD, especially emphysema. Although pneumonia resolves spontaneously, it recurs frequently, and causes cavitary disease similar to chronic pulmonary tuberculosis.

Blastomycosis, caused by *Blastomyces dermatitidis,* occurs in the south central and Great Lakes regions of the United States and is also acquired by inhalation of spores. The pulmonary form of the disease resembles histoplasmosis and is usually self-limited. Radiological examination reveals patchy infiltrates that are not diagnostic. Blastomycosis, coccidioidomycosis, and histoplasmosis usually occur in normal hosts rather than in immunocompromised patients.

The fungi responsible for pulmonary disease in the immunocompromised patient include *Aspergillus* species, *Cryptococcus neoformans, Candida* species, and the phycomycetes (*i.e., Absidia, Mucor, Rhizopus* species). Patients usually have altered cell-mediated immunity or granulocyte defect due to leukemia or transplants.

Aspergillosis presents as a variety of conditions ranging from hypersensitivity with bronchospasm to invasive disseminated disease. The organism enters the respiratory tract and colonizes the bronchi or pulmonary cavities. It then invades the walls of the bronchi and bronchioles, producing an acute necrotizing pneumonitis. One of the manifestations of the disease is pulmonary mycetoma.

Cryptococcus neoformans has been associated with infections in patients with Hodgkin's disease, sarcoidosis, and other altered cell-mediated immunity conditions. Acquisition is through inhalation of yeast cells. Meningitis is a common complication of this infection. *Candida* species are common saprophytes of the upper respiratory tract, and cause pulmonary infection in the compromised host in rare instances. *Candida albicans* is the organism responsible for many of these infections.

The phycomycetes are being recognized as serious pathogens in the debilitated patient. Species of *Rhizopus, Mucor,* and *Absidia* have been implicated in invasive disease, and should be considered when evaluating infections in the immunocompromised patient. These organisms are widespread in nature, and colonization and mild localized infections are common in otherwise healthy individuals. They do not cause epidemics and are not transmitted from person to person.

PARASITIC PNEUMONIAS

Pneumocystis carinii has received attention as a pathogen in the immunocompromised patient, and the incidence of infection has increased with the increase in AIDS patients. It is the most common treatable infection in these patients, and it is present in more than 60% of AIDS cases at the time of diagnosis.[36] The infection presents as a diffuse interstitial (plasma cell) pneumonia. The alveoli are filled with an exudate containing many organisms.

Other parasites associated with pulmonary infections include *Toxoplasma gondii, Strongyloides stercoralis, Paragonimus westermani* (lung fluke), *Ancylostoma duodenale,* and Schistosoma. Most of these are associated with a recent history of travel. *Echinococcus granulosus* is associated with animal contact (see Chap. 58).

Other Pulmonary Infections

Aspiration pneumonia results from aspiration of saliva into the trachea or bronchi, carrying large numbers of microorganisms into the lungs. These include both aerobic and anaerobic flora of the upper respiratory tract. If gastric contents are aspirated, food particles enter the lung and cause a granulomatous response.[22] Patients with altered mental status due to coma, alcoholism, anesthesia, epileptic seizure, or drug overdose have a diminished cough reflex and are susceptible to aspiration pneumonia.[27] The infections that result range from a simple pneumonia that can be treated easily to necrotizing pneumonitis, lung abscess, and empyema.

Lung abscess, a complication of aspiration pneumonia, usually results from necrotizing pneumonia. A majority of these infections are anaerobic. The anaerobes most often involved in necrotizing pneumonia and lung abscess are *Bacteroides melaninogenicus, Fusobacterium nucleatum,* various anaerobic cocci (Peptococcus and Peptostreptococcus), and *Bacteroides fragilis.*[37]

Empyema may be confused radiologically with lung abscess; however, purulent fluid is present in the pleural space in empyema. The presence of fluid in the pleural space without large amounts of pus or neutrophils is a pleural effusion. Empyemas persist for a long time if they are not drained. Organisms associated with empyema include both gram-positive and gram-negative aerobes and anaerobes.

CLINICAL MANIFESTATIONS

Upper Respiratory Tract Infections

The typical manifestations of the *common cold* are rhinitis, pharyngitis, and rhinorrhea, and most patients are self-diagnosed. The problem for the physician is to be able to distinguish patients with the uncomplicated cold from the low percentage (2.5%) of those with secondary bacterial sinusitis and otitis media.[4] Inflammation of the pharynx, nasal cavity, ears, and sinuses suggests URT infection.

The most characteristic symptom of *pharyngitis* is a sore throat. The inflammation is characterized by a reddening with ulceration and possibly the presence of exudative lesions. Pharyngitis may also be accompanied by fever, chills, headache, myalgia, hoarseness, and cough.[38] In young children (<7 years old), gingivostomatitis (swollen gums) and herpangina (grayish white vesicles on the tonsils) may also accompany nonbacterial infections. The duration of the illness is usually 3 to 4 days, with complete recovery within 1 week.

In *laryngitis,* diagnosis is confirmed by examination of the larynx, which appears reddened with ulcerations. The symptoms include a barking cough, hoarseness, fever, dyspnea (difficulty in breathing) and, in severe, rare cases, cyanosis and suffocation.

Croup is characterized by inflammation of the nasopharynx and nasal passages. The classic stridor (vibratory sounds), hoarseness, and cough are always associated with the disease. The infection usually persists for 3 to 4 days; however, during that time, the symptoms may worsen in the evening.

Epiglottitis is characterized by an acute onset of fever, sore throat, hoarseness, and barking cough. The throat is very inflamed and the epiglottis is red, swollen, and stiff.

The symptoms associated with *acute sinusitis* include headache, facial pain, purulent nasal discharge, nasal-sounding noise, and alteration of the sense of smell. Other symptoms may occur, depending on which of the paranasal sinuses is infected: maxillary, frontal, ethmoidal, or sphenoidal. For example, swelling of the eyelids and tearing occur with ethmoid sinusitis.[9]

Otitis media is characterized by a severe, throbbing pain in the ear, and may be associated with fever, dizziness, nausea, vomiting, and hearing loss. The ear drum appears red and thickened, and bulges. Excessive pressure can cause the drum to rupture, releasing blood and purulent exudate into the outer ear. In *otitis externa* "cottage cheese"-like exudate is usually present.

The incubation period of *diphtheria* is from 2 to 5 days. The infection begins with pharyngitis, fever, a nonproductive cough, cervical lymphadenopathy, and soft-tissue swelling of the neck that may result in airway obstruction. The pharynx often exhibits a grayish pseudomembrane that is not pathognomonic for diphtheria, but is highly suggestive of this disease.

The incubation period of *pertussis* is from 10 to 16 days, and there are three stages of the disease, each lasting approximately 2 weeks.[39] The catarrhal stage, the most contagious, includes symptoms of a common cold, sneezing, night cough, and infected conjunctivas. The paroxysmal stage is characterized by frequent, paroxysmal cough with a distinctive whoop. Other complications include nose bleed, swelling around the eyes, conjunctival hemorrhages, and vomiting. During the convalescent stage, the symptoms resolve, but paroxysmal coughing may occur for many months.

Among infections of the oral cavity, *thrush* is characterized by white patches and exudate throughout the infected area. In *Vincent's angina,* ulcers appear on the pharynx and are covered with a grayish yellow pseudomembrane that can be confused with the membrane of diphtheria.[2] In *actinomycosis,* multiple draining abscesses often result.

Lower Respiratory Tract Infections

Acute bronchitis is characterized by fever and a cough sufficiently unusual to facilitate diagnosis.

Acute tracheobronchitis (flu) is characterized by fever, headache, malaise, and myalgia.

Bronchiolitis in infants is characterized by expiratory wheezing, nasal flaring, irritability, grunting, and dehydration.[40]

Bacterial pneumonias are associated with shaking chills and fever, weakness, chest pains, muscle aches, and vomiting. Patients present with an alveolar infiltrate usually confined to one lobe. The sputum is thick, purulent, and brownish, and may be bloody.

The patient with *Legionnaires' disease* has chills, fever, and malaise. Diarrhea and altered mental status may also be present. Unlike with other bacterial infections, the patient has a nonproductive cough.

Patients with *atypical pneumonia* usually have an upper respiratory tract infection. Radiologically they have an interstitial pneumonia, accompanied by a dry, persistent cough. Chills, fever, and headache are usually present.

In *nocardiosis,* the patient presents with chills, fever, chest pain, weight loss, and a productive cough. Neurological abnormalities occur in about one-third of the infected cases.

Only 5% of patients with *pulmonary tuberculosis* infections manifest clinical symptoms. These symptoms are those of chronic cavitary disease, and include fatigue, weight loss, fever, night sweats, blood sputum, chest pain, and shortness of breath.

Coccidioidomycosis patients present with fever, malaise, dry cough, night sweats, weight loss, and headache.

The symptoms of *histoplasmosis* and *blastomycosis* are those associated with chronic cavitary disease, described above.

Symptoms of *lung abscess* include recurrent fever and large amounts of sputum production. Radiologically there is evidence of cavitation, and the diagnosis may be confirmed by ultrasound.

LABORATORY ANALYSES AND DIAGNOSIS

Upper Respiratory Tract Infections

A throat specimen submitted for routine culture should be examined for beta-hemolytic streptococci only. *H. influenzae, S. pneumoniae, S. aureus,* and gram-negative bacilli commonly colonize the throats of adults and are of no clinical significance.[2] Their presence may indicate lower respiratory infection, but throat cultures should not be used to determine the status of the lower respiratory tract. These organisms should not be reported in throat cultures of children, because it has not been established that they cause pharyngitis. On occasion it may be necessary to report these organisms in the immunosuppressed patient; however, this should occur based on discussion with the clinician.

When a specific diagnosis such as Vincent's angina, thrush, or peritonsillar abscess is made, or a specific organism such as *N. gonorrhoeae, C. diphtheriae,* or *B. pertussis* is suspected by the clinician, this information should be communicated to the laboratory. Isolation and identification of these pathogens require specialized media and techniques and are not generally part of the routine throat culture. If a laboratory does not have the facilities or personnel to isolate these organisms, the specimens should be submitted to a reference laboratory.

It should be noted that the diagnosis of epiglottitis should be made by physical examination. Cultures are contraindicated for two reasons: manipulation of the epiglottis may pose a real threat to the patient by causing respiratory obstruction, and, although isolation of *H. influenzae* may suggest infection, it may also represent normal flora.[2] Approximately 50% of children with epiglottitis are septicemic, and the organisms may be recovered from blood cultures.

MICROSCOPIC EXAMINATION

Gram-stained smears of routine throat cultures are not recommended because large numbers of streptococci are present normally in the oral flora and cannot be distinguished from pathogenic strains *(S. pyogenes).* Gram-stained smears are helpful, however, to rule out thrush and Vincent's angina. The diagnosis of thrush or oral candidiasis is based on the demonstration of yeast cells in the Gram stain of material taken from whitish patches of exudate on the buccal mucosa, oropharynx, or tongue. The diagnosis of Vincent's angina is made by observing white blood cells, spirochetes, and fusiform bacilli swabbed from pharyngeal ulcers covered by a grayish yellow pseudomembrane. These organisms are best seen microscopically when stained with dilute carbolfuchsin.[2]

Other microscopic methods for demonstrating fungal elements include use of 10% KOH preparations or calcofluor white stain.[41] Direct fluorescent-antibody stains are also available. Direct smears of the pharynx or nasopharynx for diphtheria are not recommended.[2]

Examination of the "sulfur granules" often present in the pus of the draining sinuses of actinomycosis will demonstrate gram-positive branching rods in a sunburst formation.

Direct fluorescent-antibody stains are also available for detection of parainfluenza viruses 1 and 3; however, direct antigen detection for parainfluenza type 2 is not as sensitive a method as viral isolation.[42] Direct detection by immunologic methods of RSV in respiratory samples is preferred over viral isolation.[43] Antibodies to HSV-1 and HSV-2 permit direct detection of HSV antigen in clinical specimens by either immunofluorescence or immunoperoxidase stains.[44] The Tzanck preparation may also be used to identify HSV by demonstrating the presence of multinucleated giant cells; however, it is not specific for type 1 or type 2. Electron microscopy may also be employed for HSV, but it also is not specific for either type.

Immunofluorescent staining for VZV (*varicella-zoster* virus) is specific for this organism and is more sensitive than culture.[45] Adenovirus, the most common cause of acute pharyngitis in children, may also be detected directly from throat swabs by a commercially available immunofluorescent stain.

CULTURE METHODS FOR ISOLATION OF UPPER RESPIRATORY TRACT PATHOGENS

The culture result is dependent upon the quality of the specimen. Most upper respiratory pathogens, especially *S. pyogenes,* are not evenly distributed in the throat, and for that reason a thorough swabbing is required to prevent false-negative cultures.[46] Throat swabs should be plated onto media containing sheep blood, which is preferred because it lacks V-factor. The absence of this factor inhibits the growth of hemolytic *Hemophilus* species *(H. hemolyticus* and *H. parahemolyticus),* which may be part of the normal throat flora.[2] Growth of these organisms may cause confusion with colonies of beta-hemolytic streptococci, since they are similar morphologically. The use of selective media for group A streptococci has been suggested; however, there are conflicting reports regarding their performance.[47, 48] The optimal atmosphere for incubation of routine throat cultures has also been studied, with equivocal results.[49–51]

Rapid identification of group A beta-hemolytic streptococci is important to help prevent the noninfectious sequelae that may occur. Nonetheless, the use of bacitracin disks on primary culture plates has generally been discouraged because of the low rate of success of this method.[52] If a bacitracin disk is used to differentiate group A from non-group A, an 0.04 unit disk should be employed on pure cultures of the organism being tested. Use of the 10-unit bacitracin susceptibility disk is unacceptable. Identification of uncommon isolates of the upper respiratory tract requires the appropriate specialized media for isolation and/or identification. Several of these are discussed briefly below.

Bordet-Gengou (BG) is a selective medium that has been used for isolation of *B. pertussis,* but the use of a cough plate for isolation of this organism is no longer recommended.[2] Because *B. pertussis* is somewhat fastidious and is susceptible to drying, it is recommended that throat swabs be transported in an enriched medium and processed within three hours. Suspicious colonies should be confirmed with immunofluorescent staining.

Specialized media for isolation of *C. diphtheriae* include Loeffler's or Pai medium and cystine-tellurite agar. Confirmation of *C. diphtheriae* biochemically is not sufficient to determine pathogenicity; demonstration of toxin production is required.

URT specimens requesting *N. meningitidis* screen require selective media for isolation; however, such requests are made to detect carriers. Because these are usually associated with an epidemiological problem, a public health reference laboratory should be consulted prior to processing of the specimens.

The preferred specimens for isolation of viruses from the upper respiratory tract include throat washings or swabs and nasopharyngeal washings. For isolation of adenovirus, HeLa and HEp-2 cells are commercially available and less expensive than human embryonic kidney cells. Viral isolation in cell culture (human diploid cells) is diagnostic for rhinovirus.[4] Although direct fluorescent-antibody detection may be used for detection of parainfluenza viruses 1 and 3, cell culture is more sensitive for parainfluenza 2. Detection of viral growth on human embryonic kidney or monkey kidney cell lines is made by hemadsorption. Influenza viruses A and B may also be isolated in monkey kidney cell cultures or embryonated hen eggs.[53]

NONCULTURE METHODS FOR DETECTION OF UPPER RESPIRATORY PATHOGENS

Rapid methods for direct antigen detection have recently become available for the identification of group A streptococci from throat specimens. Approximately 30 commercial kits have been introduced for use in diagnostic laboratories and physicians' offices. These antigen detection methods are very specific; however, they range in sensitivity from 60% to >95%.[54] In order to replace the culture method, these kits should have a sensitivity and positive predictive value of at least 95%.[55] When these criteria are met, direct antigen detection can be a rapid alternative to cultural detection of *S. pyogenes*. Similar tests are being developed for other pathogens of the upper respiratory tract.

Lower Respiratory Tract Infections

Laboratory diagnosis of lower respiratory tract infection is also dependent upon the quality of the sample submitted for evaluation. Specimens from the lower respiratory tract are sterile under normal conditions, but they can be contaminated easily by upper respiratory flora. Contamination with normal flora is unavoidable when sputum is expectorated, or if aspirates are collected from the nasopharynx, or if unprotected bronchoscopic brushes are used. There is also no guarantee that invasive procedures used to collect samples will produce specimens of good quality lacking oropharyngeal contamination. Specimens submitted for evaluation of lower respiratory tract pathogens include expectorated sputum, bronchoscopy specimens, tracheostomy and endotracheal tube aspirates, transtracheal aspirates, lung aspirates, and lung biopsies.

MICROSCOPIC EXAMINATION

The most useful procedure for evaluating the quality of a sputum specimen is the Gram stain. It should be used routinely on specimens submitted for bacterial cultures to determine the acceptability of the specimen, based on the presence or predominance of leukocytes and the virtual absence of squamous epithelial cells. Microscopic screening of sputum specimens to determine the quality should be reserved for sputum bacteriology only.[56]

Acid-fast smears (Ziehl-Neelsen or Kinyoun carbolfuchsin) may be used to demonstrate mycobacteria, and modified acid-fast smears will demonstrate *Nocardia*. A fluorescent auramine or rhodamine-auramine stain may also be used to detect acid-fast organisms.

A calcofluor white stain is a rapid fluorescent method for detecting fungi. Fungal elements may also be observed under phase contrast microscopy with 10% KOH. Yeasts may be seen easily with the Gram stain.

P. carinii may be identified using a modified Gomori methenamine silver stain or a more rapid toluidine blue-O stain.[57] *N. asteroides* may also be observed with toluidine blue-O stain as filamentous branching structures that are also gram-positive by the Gram stain.[56] Intranuclear inclusions of herpes simplex and CMV may be observed in H and E stained permanently fixed sections. A modified Dieterle stain may be used for the Legionnaires' disease agent.[58]

Direct fluorescent-antibody stain is commonly used for detection of *Legionella* species, including all serotypes. A DNA probe is also commercially available. Direct fluorescent-antibody stains are also available for a wide variety of viruses, including herpes, CMV, RSV, and adenovirus, as described above. Immunofluorescent reagents may also be used to detect *Bacteroides* species and chlamydia infections. A fluorescein-conjugated monoclonal antibody test system is both sensitive and specific for direct detection of the chlamydia antigen.[57]

CULTURE METHODS FOR ISOLATION OF LOWER RESPIRATORY TRACT PATHOGENS

Most of the organisms causing bacterial pneumonias may be isolated on routine laboratory media. Chocolate agar should always be included with blood and MacConkey agars in the routine processing of lower respiratory specimens, since *H. influenzae* is a common pathogen. Anaerobic cultures of expectorated sputum are not recommended, but transtracheal and percutaneous lung aspirates may be processed for anaerobes. Cultures for *Legionella* species should be inoculated onto an appropriate selective medium.

Specimens requiring mycobacterial studies should be decontaminated prior to inoculation of selective media. Expectorated or induced sputum, bronchial aspirates, and lavages are all acceptable for mycobacterial cultures. Gastric aspirates may be submitted if the patient is unable to produce sputum or has swallowed it.[57] Recently, a rapid radiometric method has been introduced for detection of mycobacteria that yields results in approximately half the time of conventional methods.

Fungal cultures should also be plated onto appropriate specialized media and should be incubated at 30° C. Yeast isolated from expectorated sputum should be screened for *C. neoformans* only.[59]

M. pneumoniae may be cultured, but serology is presently the preferred method.[60] *C. trachomatis* may be isolated; isolation procedures for viruses have been described above. A throat swab or washings may be used to isolate viruses from patients with a typical lower respiratory tract infection. Most viruses causing lower respiratory tract infections may be isolated on cell cultures, but most are fragile and should be placed in a buffered fluid transport medium with a high protein content and stored at 4° C until cultured.

NONCULTURE METHODS FOR DETECTING LOWER RESPIRATORY PATHOGENS

Many methods have been described that enable rapid detection of lower respiratory pathogens. Many of these methods offer an alternative to conventional, time-consuming culture methods, and are especially helpful and practical for detection of viral, chlamydial, and mycoplasmal antigens. For example, *Chlamydia* antigens may now be detected by an enzyme-linked immunosorbent assay (ELISA). This test eliminates the need for cell culture and fluorescence microscopy required by the direct fluorescent-antibody test. A similar type of test has also been introduced for *B. pertussis*.

DNA probe techniques are being introduced into the diagnostic laboratory and may eventually replace some of the very costly conventional methods with results that are available in minutes, rather than in the hours and days required for most present-day microbiology procedures.

TREATMENT

In general, respiratory tract infections caused by bacteria and fungi are treated with antimicrobials chosen in accordance with the principles outlined in Chapter 63. In some instances antiviral agents are also available.

Upper Respiratory Tract Infections

Treatment of the *common cold* usually involves decongestants, cough suppressants, and gargles. Handwashing and care to avoid contamination by nasal secretions may help limit the spread of infection. Antibiotics have no effect, and the ingestion of large doses of vitamin C is questionable.[61]

It is important to distinguish bacterial (streptococcal) *pharyngitis* from viral pharyngitis because of treatment. Streptococcal pharyngitis is usually treated with penicillin to prevent the occurrence of rheumatic fever. Acute viral pharyngitis may be treated with aspirin or gargles to relieve some of the symptoms.[3, 38]

Because of the viral etiology of laryngitis, antibiotics have no effect unless the condition is associated with streptococcal pharyngitis. Resting the voice and inhalation of moist air may give some relief.

There is no treatment for croup; however, significant clinical improvement has been reported in hospitalized children with croup who were receiving racemic epinephrine.[8] Use of a vaporizer may provide some relief in the home.

Because of the potentially high mortality rate of *epiglottitis,* antibiotic treatment is generally instituted immediately. Although ampicillin is the antibiotic of choice, the prevalence of ampicillin-resistant strains of *H. influenzae* requires that chloramphenicol be used as well until ampicillin sensitivity is established.[62]

Antibiotics may be used to treat *sinusitis* because of the bacterial etiology of this infection. Nasal decongestants and nose drops may also be used, as well as anti-pain medication for headaches and facial pain. Inhalation of warm air and application of moist heat may also help relieve the symptoms. Promoting drainage as well as correction of a nasal septal defect or removal of polyps may also be useful.

Appropriate antibiotic therapy for *otitis media* should be initiated following tympanocentesis (aspiration of the fluid). Because *otitis externa* is a superficial infection, a topical treatment may be used.

Since *diphtheria* is an intoxication, antitoxin therapy is essential in order to neutralize the toxin produced by the organism. Antimicrobial therapy is also administered. Active immunization using toxoid prevents the disease. Preschool-age children are immunized in the United States; however, immunity is not lifelong.

Antimicrobial therapy for *pertussis* should be administered for 10 to 14 days. Immunization should be given early in life (6 to 12 weeks of age), followed by two additional monthly injections. Boosters at ages 1, 3, and 5 years will help prevent the disease.

More severe infections of *Vincent's angina* may be treated with antimicrobials. Most infections of the oropharynx associated with pain or discomfort may be relieved with mouthwashes or anesthetics.

Actinomycosis is usually treated with appropriate antimicrobials, but drainage of the lesions is often required as well.

Lower Respiratory Tract Infections

Bacterial pneumonias require appropriate antibiotic therapy. In pneumonias due to *S. pneumoniae,* immediate therapy with penicillin is required because the mortality rate is around 10%.[27]

For pneumonia due to *H. influenzae,* as in *epiglottitis,* ampicillin has been the drug of choice for treatment but many strains have developed resistance. For resistant strains, chloramphenicol or cefamandole have been used.

In *staphylococcal pneumonia,* oxacillin or nafcillin are drugs of choice because most strains are resistant to penicillin. Patients with allergies to penicillin may be treated with a cephalosporin. Vancomycin is reserved for oxacillin/nafcillin-resistant organisms.

K. pneumoniae infections require an aminoglycoside or a second- or third-generation cephalosporin. Erythromycin is the drug of choice for *Legionnaires' disease* and for *primary atypical pneumonia.* In the latter case, erythromycin has been found to relieve symptoms but not eradicate the organism.

Sulfonamides have been used to treat *nocardiosis*. Treatment of *tuberculosis* varies. High-risk-group patients have been treated with isoniazid (INH) to prevent infection. The purpose of treatment is to stop the disease progression and to limit contagion.[22] Other more commonly used drugs given in combination or alone include streptomycin, ethambutol, and rifampin.

Treatment for most *systemic fungal diseases,* such as those causing pulmonary infections, is Amphotericin B. Treatment for *pneumocystis* includes Trimethoprim-sulfamethoxazole (Bactrim) or pentamidine isethionate.

CASE STUDY

A 54-year-old unemployed man with a past history of alcohol abuse and cirrhosis arrived at the emergency room with a chief complaint of shortness of breath and a persistent cough of 5 days' duration.

On physical examination, the patient presented as a moderately malnourished, middle-aged caucasian, appearing older than his stated age. He was in moderate respiratory distress with rapid, shallow breathing and a cough productive of thick, greenish yellow mucoid sputum with flecks of blood.

His vital signs included a temperature of 100.5° F, a heart rate of 100/minute at rest, and a labored respiratory rate of 25/minute. The significant findings on physical examination included bilateral chest rales and increased breath sounds. Chest x-ray showed bilateral pulmonary infiltrates.

Laboratory tests included a white blood cell (WBC) count of $16.2 \times 10^3/mm^3$ with 88% leukocytes (PMNs). A test for cold agglutinins was negative, as was a TB skin test. Gram stain of sputum revealed large numbers of PMNs and gram-positive lancet-shaped diplococci. Large numbers of alpha-hemolytic, mucoid colonies appeared on the culture. The growth was observed on blood and chocolate agars, but not on MacConkey agar.

Questions

1. What is the probable diagnosis?
2. What should be considered in the differential diagnosis prior to obtaining laboratory test results?
3. What is the significance of the macroscopic appearance of the sputum?
4. Are the results of the cold agglutinins and TB skin test important?
5. What is important about the results of the microscopic examination of the sputum?

Discussion

1. The probable diagnosis is acute bilateral bronchopneumonia caused by *Streptococcus pneumoniae.*
2. Other possible causes would include *Mycoplasma pneumoniae, Mycobacterium tuberculosis,* viral pneumonia, and bacterial pneumonia due to other agents. The patient's history of alcoholism is helpful in making the diagnosis of bacterial pneumonia, especially pneumococcal pneumonia.
3. The appearance of the sputum along with large numbers of PMNs also suggests a bacterial pneumonia.
4. The negative cold agglutinins exclude *Mycoplasma* pneumonia, and a negative TB skin test may exclude *Mycobacterium tuberculosis.*
5. The Gram stain is characteristic of pneumococci and is supported by the culture, which

suggests *S. pneumoniae.* The Gram stain excludes gram-negative pneumonia and the culture excludes *Staphylococcus aureus,* another cause of gram-positive bacterial pneumonia. The large numbers of PMNs seen confirm that the sputum was an acceptable sample for laboratory evaluation.

REFERENCES

1. Hoeprich PD: Etiologic diagnosis of lower respiratory tract infections. Calif Med 112:1, 1970
2. Bannatyne RM, Clausen C, McCarthy LR: Laboratory diagnosis of upper respiratory tract infections. In Duncan IB (ed): Cumitech 10. Washington, DC, American Society for Microbiology, 1979
3. Gwaltney JM: The common cold. In Mandell GL, Douglas RG, Bennett JE (eds): Principles and Practice of Infectious Diseases, p 429. New York City, John Wiley & Sons, 1979
4. Greenberg SB, Krilov LR: Laboratory diagnosis of viral respiratory disease. In Drew WL, Rubin SJ (eds): Cumitech 21. Washington, DC, American Society for Microbiology, 1986
5. Cherry JD: Upper airway infections—The common cold. In Feigin RD, Cherry JD (eds): Textbook of Pediatric Infectious Disease, p 97. Philadelphia, WB Saunders, 1981
6. Downham MAPS, McQuillan J, Gardner PS: Diagnosis and clinical significance of parainfluenza virus infections in children. Arch Dis Child 49:8, 1974
7. Hall CB: Acute laryngotracheobronchitis, croup. In Mandell GL, Douglas RG, Bennett JE (eds): Principles and Practice of Infectious Diseases, p 442. New York City, John Wiley & Sons, 1979
8. Wesley CR, Cotton EK, Brooks JG: Nebulized racemic epinephrine by IPPB for the treatment of croup. Am J Dis Child 132:484, 1978
9. Gwaltney JM: Sinusitis. In Mandell GL, Douglas RG, Bennett JE (eds): Principles and Practice of Infectious Diseases, p 458. New York City, John Wiley & Sons, 1979
10. Hamory BH, Sande MA, Snydor A, Searle DL, Gwaltney JM: Etiology and antimicrobial therapy of acute maxillary sinusitis. J. Infect Dis 139:197, 1979
11. Bluestone CD, Shurin PA: Middle ear disease in children: Pathogenesis, diagnosis, and management. Pediatr Clin North Am 21:379, 1974
12. Chandler JR: Malignant external otitis: Further considerations. Ann Otol 86:417, 1977
13. Goldstein E, Hoeprich PD: Diphtheria. In Hoeprich PD (ed): Infectious Diseases: A Modern Treatise of Infectious Processes, p 247. Hagerstown, MD, Harper & Row, 1977
14. Meyers BR, Lawson W: Infections of the oral cavity. In Mandell GL, Douglas RG, Bennett JE (eds): Principles and Practice of Infectious Diseases, p 466. New York City, John Wiley & Sons, 1979
15. Liu C: Bronchitis and bronchiolitis. In Hoeprich PD (ed): Infectious Diseases: A Modern Treatise of Infectious Processes, p 264. Hagerstown, MD, Harper & Row, 1977
16. Reynolds HY: Chronic bronchitis and acute infectious exacerbations. In Mandell GL, Douglas RG, Bennett JE (eds): Principles and Practice of Infectious Diseases, p 484. New York City, John Wiley & Sons, 1979
17. Leeder SR: Role of infection in the cause and course of chronic bronchitis and emphysema. J Infect Dis 131:731, 1975
18. Tager I, Speizer FE: Role of infection in chronic bronchitis. N Engl J Med 292:563, 1975
19. Hall CB, Hall WJ: Bronchiolitis. In Mandell G, Douglas RC, Bennett JE (eds): Principles and Practice of Infectious Diseases, p 390. New York City, John Wiley & Sons, 1985
20. Johanson WD Jr, Gould KG Jr: Lung defense mechanisms. Basics of RD 6:1, 1977
21. Donowitz GR, Mandell GL: Acute pneumonia. In Mandell GL, Douglas RC, Bennett JE (eds): Principles and Practice of Infectious Diseases, p 489. New York City, John Wiley & Sons, 1979
22. Miller LG, Kazemi H: Pneumonia. In Manual of Clinical Pulmonary Medicine, p 137. New York City, McGraw-Hill, 1983
23. Lerner AM, Jankauskas K: The classic bacterial pneumonias. Disease-A-Month, February, 1975
24. Rosenow EC: Pneumonia: Clinical challenge in cardiopulmonary medicine. Am Coll Chest Phys 3:4, 1982
25. Martin CM, Kunin CM, Gottlieb LS et al: Asian Influenza A in Boston 1957–58. II. Severe staphylococci pneumonia complicating influenza. Arch Intern Med 103:532, 1959
26. Sprunt K: Infection in the chronic lung disease. Bull NY Acad Med 48:698, 1972
27. Pechere JC, Joly J: Acute pneumonias in adults. In

Pechere JC (ed): Infections: Recognition, Understanding, and Treatment, p 77. Philadelphia, Lea & Febiger, 1984

28. Ebright JR, Rytel MW: Bacteria pneumonia in the elderly. J Am Geriatr Soc 28:220, 1980
29. Johanson WG, Pierce AK, Stanford JP, Thomas GD: Nosocomial respiratory infections with gram-negative bacilli. Ann Intern Med 77:701, 1972
30. Mogabgab WJ: *Mycoplasma pneumoniae* and adenovirus respiratory illness in military and university personnel 1959–1966. Am Rev Respir Dis 97:345, 1968
31. Starr SE: Cytomegalovirus. Pediatr Clin North Am 26:283, 1979
32. Meyers JD, Fluornoy N, Thomas ED: Nonbacterial pneumonia after allogenic marrow transplantation: A review of ten years' experience. Rev Infect Dis 4:1119, 1982
33. Abdallah PS, Mark JBD, Merigan TC: Diagnosis of cytomegalovirus pneumonia in compromised hosts. Am J Med 61:326, 1976
34. Zahradnik JM, Spencer MJ, Porter DD: Adenovirus infection in the immunocompromised patient. Am J Med 68:725, 1980
35. Glezen WP: Viral pneumonia as a cause and result of hospitalization. J Infect Dis 147:765, 1983
36. Centers for Disease Control: Update: Acquired immunodeficiency syndrome—United States. MMWR 34:245, 1985
37. Bartlett JG, Gorbach SL, Tally FP, Finegold SM: Bacteriology and treatment of primary lung abscess. Am Rev Respir Dis 109:510, 1974
38. Liu C: Nonbacterial pharyngitis. In Hoeprich PD (ed): Infectious Diseases: A Modern Treatise of Infectious Processes, p 230. Hagerstown, MD, Harper & Row, 1977
39. Morse SI: Whooping cough. In Hoeprich PD (ed): Infectious Diseases: A Modern Treatise of Infectious Processes, p 277. Hagerstown, MD, Harper & Row, 1977
40. Wohl MEB, Chernick V: Bronchiolitis. Am Rev Respir Dis 118:759, 1978
41. Hageage GJ Jr, Harrington BJ: Use of calcofluor white in clinical mycology. Lab Med 15:109, 1984
42. McIntosh K, Clark JC: Parainfluenza and respiratory syncytial viruses. In Lennette EH, Balows A, Hausler WJ Jr, Shadomy HJ (eds): Manual of Clinical Microbiology, 4th ed, p 763. Washington, DC, American Society for Microbiology, 1985
43. Friedman HM, Forrer CB: Diagnosis of viral respiratory infections in the 1980s. Clin Lab Med 2:383, 1982
44. Schmidt NJ, Dennes J, Devlin V, Gallo D, Mills J: Comparison of direct immunofluorescence and direct immunoperoxidase procedures for detection of herpes simplex virus antigen in lesion specimens. J Clin Microbiol 18:445, 1983
45. Schmidt NJ: Varicella-zoster virus. In Lennette EH, Balows A, Hausler WJ Jr, Shadomy HJ (eds): Manual of Clinical Microbiology, 4th ed, p 720. Washington, DC, American Society for Microbiology, 1985
46. Ross PW: Throat swabs and swabbing technique. Practitioner 207:791, 1971
47. Kurzynski TA, Meise CK: Evaluation of sulfamethoxazole-trimethoprim blood agar plates for recovery of group A streptococci from throat cultures. J Clin Microbiol 9:189, 1979
48. Dykstra MA, McLaughlin JC, Bartlett RC: Comparison of media and techniques for detection of group A streptococci in throat specimens. J Clin Microbiol 9:236, 1979
49. Murray PR, Wold AD, Schreck CA et al: Effects of selective media and atmosphere of incubation on the isolation of group A streptococci. J Clin Microbiol 4:54, 1976
50. Liberten CR, Wold AD, Washington JA II: Effects of trimethoprim-sulfamethoxazole and incubation atmosphere on isolation of group A streptococci. J Clin Microbiol 18:680, 1983
51. Randolph MF, Redys JJ, Cope JB: Evaluation of aerobic and anaerobic methods for recovery of streptococci from throat cultures. J Pediatr 104:897, 1984
52. Murray PR, Wold AD, Hall S, Washington J: Bacitracin differentiation for presumptive identification of group A beta-hemolytic streptococci: Comparison of primary and purified plate testing. J Pediatr 89:576, 1976
53. Frank AL, Couch RB, Griffis CA, Baxter BD: Comparison of different tissue cultures for isolation and quantitation of influenza and parainfluenza viruses. J Clin Microbiol 10:32, 1979
54. Kellogg JA, Manzella JP: Detection of group A streptococci in the laboratory or physician's office. JAMA 255:2638, 1986
55. Radetsky M, Wheeler RL, Roe MH et al: Comparative evaluation of kits for rapid diagnosis of group A streptococci disease. Pediatr Infect Dis 4:274, 1985

56. Bartlett JG, Brewer NS, Ryan K: Laboratory Diagnosis of Lower Respiratory Tract Infections. In Washington JA II (ed): Cumitech 7. Washington, DC, American Society for Microbiology, 1978
57. Finegold SM, Baron EJ: Bailey and Scott's Diagnostic Microbiology, 7th ed, p 253. St Louis, CV Mosby, 1986
58. Van Orden A, Greer P: Modifications of the Dieterle spirochete stain. J Histotechnol 1:51, 1977
59. Murray PR, Van Scory RE, Roberts GD: Should yeasts in respiratory secretions be identified? Mayo Clin Proc 52:42, 1977
60. Clyde WA Jr, Kenny GE, Schachter J: Laboratory diagnosis of chlamydial and mycoplasmal infections. In Drew WL (ed): Cumitech 19. Washington, DC, American Society for Microbiology, 1984
61. Schwartz AR, Togo Y, Hornick RB et al: Evaluation of the efficacy of ascorbic acid in prophylaxis of induced rhinovirus 44 infection in man. J Infect Dis 128:500, 1973
62. Smith, DH: Hemophilus infections. In Petersdorf RG et al (eds): Harrison's Principles of Internal Medicine, 10th ed, p 969. New York City, McGraw-Hill, 1983

Chapter 11

Emphysema

Michael Boroch / Laura Martin Rahlfs / Jon O. Nilsestuen

The term *chronic obstructive pulmonary disease* (COPD) is often used to describe collectively the occurrence of three different pulmonary diseases—emphysema, asthma, and chronic bronchitis—since all three cause airflow limitation. Emphysema may occur by itself as primary or idiopathic emphysema, the cause of which is not completely understood, or in conjunction with chronic bronchitis. Approximately 60% of emphysema patients present with symptoms of both emphysema and chronic bronchitis. Generally, symptoms associated with emphysema are not present if less than 20% of the lung is involved.

ETIOLOGY AND PATHOPHYSIOLOGY

Most patients with emphysema present between the fourth and sixth decades of life, with the exception of the genetic form known as alpha$_1$-antitrypsin deficiency.

Definition

Emphysema has been defined as a condition of the lung characterized by "abnormal permanent enlargement of the air spaces distal to the terminal bronchiole, accompanied by destruction of their walls."[3, 4] With the destruction of the alveolar walls, adjacent alveolar capillaries also break down, causing the alveoli to coalesce into enlarged structures called *bullae* that contain less surface area for gas exchange. In addition, the small airways that were once held open by the elastic fibers of the surrounding alveoli begin to collapse, resulting in air trapping or wasted ventilation.

Emphysema is defined morphologically according to the portion of the acini it involves. Consequently, precise diagnosis during life is difficult.

Classification

Classifications of emphysema are determined according to the area of destruction within the acinus (also known as the secondary lobule),[2] which consists of the respiratory bronchiole and its subdivisions. The first group is known as *selective emphysemas* because the destruction occurs within a specific area in the acinus: These include alveolar duct emphysema, centrilobular emphysema (CLE), and paraseptal emphysema. The second group is known as *unselective emphysemas* because the destruction occurs throughout the acinus. Panlobular emphysema is an example of this particular type. The two most common types of emphysema are centrilobular and panlobular; these are illustrated in Figure 11-1.

(Centrilobular) centriacinar emphysema (CLE) is the most common variety of emphysema. The disease is frequently associated with a long history of cigarette smoking and is rarely found among nonsmokers.[6, 7] It is often seen in patients with both emphysema and chronic bronchitis. CLE usually affects the respiratory bronchioles and the alveolar ducts by causing dilation of these areas. The disease process usually begins in the superior and apical segments[8, 9] of the upper lobes and becomes more severe with time. Initially the respiratory bronchioles are selectively involved and, seen microscopically, can be described as having a punched-out appearance, usually containing dark (black) pigment, and varying in severity from one part of the lung to another even within the same lobule.[10]

(Panlobular) panacinar emphysema (PLE) is distinguished from other emphysema types because the disease process involves the entire acinus, including the respiratory bronchiole, alveolar duct, alveolar sac, and alveoli. These gradually become overdistended and degenerated. PLE occurs most often in middle-aged cigarette smokers[9] and is the characteristic form of emphysema associated with alpha$_1$-antitrypsin deficiency.[11–13] The destruction of lung tissue that occurs with the disease process begins in the lower lungs in the anterior margin and is more uniformly distributed than is centrilobular emphysema.[8–10] Unilateral emphysema, also known as *McLeod's syndrome,* is generally of the panlobular type.

Paraseptal (distal acinar) emphysema is synonymous with superficial periacinar (when it occurs subpleurally) or linear emphysema. Paraseptal emphysema commonly occurs adjacent to areas of scarring, atelectasis, or fibrosis and may be associated with CLE. It is usually more severe[1] in the upper half of the lungs, and often predisposes patients to pneumothorax. Typically, however, patients are asymptomatic and the affected area, as long as it is an isolated finding, is not associated with COPD.

Irregular (paracicatricial) emphysema is an irregular involvement of the acinus and is almost invariably associated with scarring; thus the term *scar emphysema.* Usually patients are asymptomatic; however, extensive irregular emphysema usually presents as a result of other diseases such as granulomatous diseases of the lung, healing of tuberculosis, or longstanding sarcoidosis.

Mixed unclassified emphysemas are "end stage" emphysemas and are classified as mixed if more than one type of emphysema is found. Frequently the lesions are atypical or the disease process is so

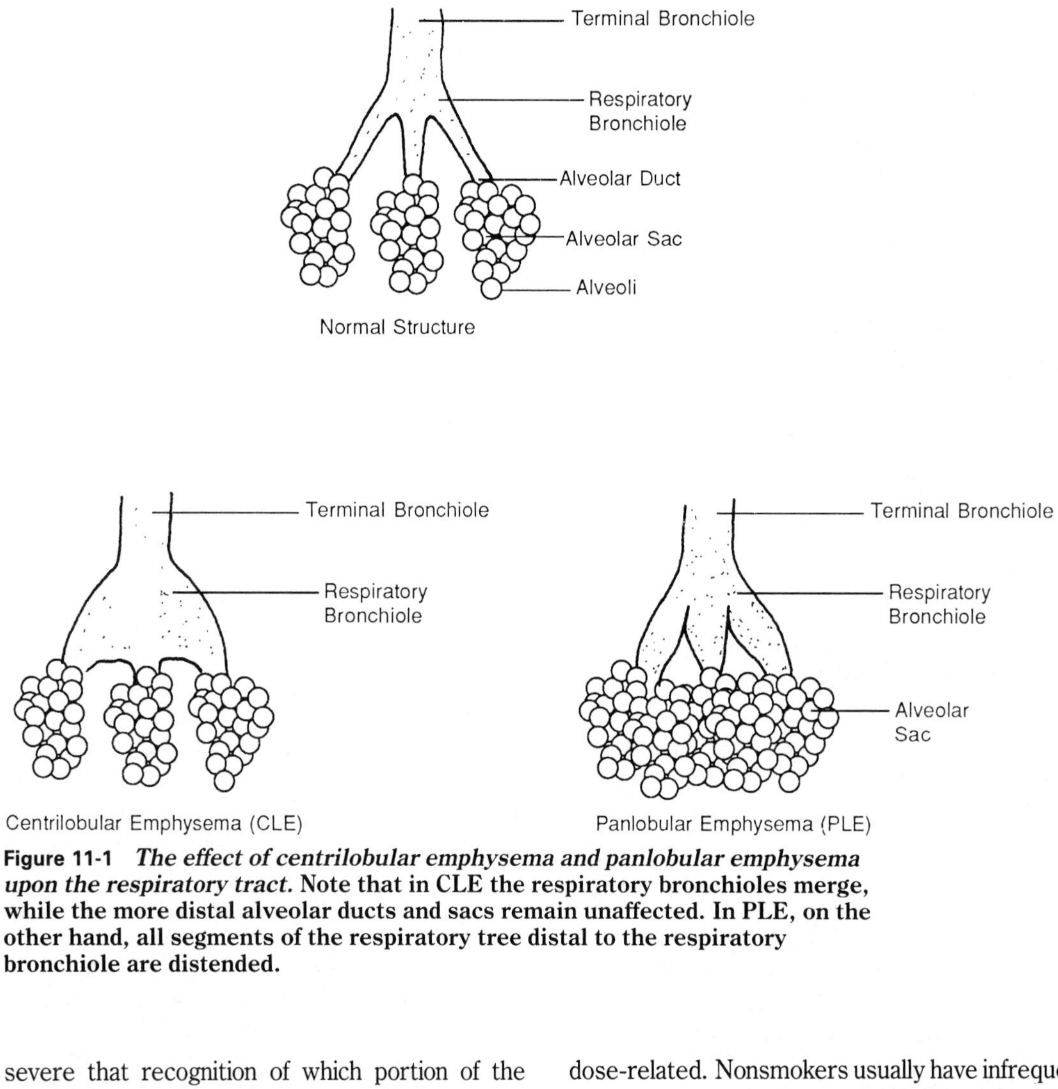

Figure 11-1 ***The effect of centrilobular emphysema and panlobular emphysema upon the respiratory tract.* Note that in CLE the respiratory bronchioles merge, while the more distal alveolar ducts and sacs remain unaffected. In PLE, on the other hand, all segments of the respiratory tree distal to the respiratory bronchiole are distended.**

severe that recognition of which portion of the acinus was initially involved is impossible.

Contributory Factors

Although there is an incomplete understanding of the pathogenesis and etiology of emphysema, the single most recognized cause is *cigarette smoking.*[14] Moreover, cigarette smoking is known to be the most common factor leading to the development of chronic airways obstruction. The severity of emphysema caused by cigarette smoking is dose-related. Nonsmokers usually have infrequent and low-grade emphysema, while heavy smokers develop a more severe and extensive disease. There are some exceptions to the above classifications, however, and there is an indication that other factors may determine individual susceptibility[2] or may work additively in the development of the disease.

Alpha$_1$-antitrypsin deficiency also can result in the development of emphysema. Alpha$_1$-antitrypsin is a serum glycoprotein, synthesized and secreted by the liver, that inactivates trypsin, thus preventing the breakdown of lung elastic fibers. When it is deficient, the digestive activity of trypsin is left unimpeded.

Characteristics of alpha$_1$-antitrypsin deficiency include[13, 15–18] a family history of emphysema, an equal effect on both sexes (although it is found more often in whites than in blacks), a disease onset compounded by smoking, and usually the eventual development of COPD. Patients also have absent or deficient levels of alpha$_1$-antitrypsin in the serum because they are unable to release it from the liver. In fact, emphysema is frequently found in association with other liver disorders, including neonatal hepatitis, hepatoma, cirrhosis, and chronic active hepatitis. The deficiency is inherited as an autosomal codominant recessive gene, and it is accentuated on the lower lobes of the lung of homozygous A_1AT-deficient individuals. There is early onset (30–40 years of age) of severe panlobular emphysema.

A third factor contributing to the development of emphysema is recurrent *infections*. Repeated childhood respiratory infections have been indirectly linked to permanent airway damage and the development of COPD in later life.[19] In addition, severe viral pneumonia, if contracted early in life, has been shown to lead to the development of small airways disease and COPD.[20]

A fourth factor contributing to the development of emphysema is *inhaled irritants* such as particulate matter, sulphur dioxide (SO_2), ozone, and possibly nitrogen oxide (NO_2). The heavily industrialized areas of the country that are known to have higher levels of air pollution are frequently associated with the increased incidence of the disease and increased morbidity rates.

CLINICAL MANIFESTATIONS

Symptoms associated with emphysema are generally nonspecific and variable; however, the symptoms occur with increasing frequency as the disease state progresses. Patients usually present with unremitting dyspnea that is often described as insidious in onset and steadily progressing. One of the characteristic observations is a pattern of breathing with a very slow, forced expiration that is laborious and may sometimes be associated with the use of pursed lip breathing. Another sign associated with this pattern of breathing is the distention of the neck veins during the expiratory period and their immediate collapse upon inspiration. The chest is frequently overexpanded because of the loss of elastic recoil in the lung, resulting in the characteristic barrel chest.

Tachypnea is common, with increased use of accessory muscles during the inspiratory cycle. Coughing may be minimal, with expectoration of only a scant amount of mucoid sputum. The chest is hyperresonant to percussion because of the general overexpansion, and breath sounds are usually diminished and faint. High-pitched wheezes are sometimes heard toward the end of expiration when the airways are beginning to close.

Cyanosis of the lips, earlobes, skin, and fingernail beds is often seen in advanced stages of emphysema and is associated with the developing hypoxemia. Other observations during the advanced state include clubbing of the fingertips and, possibly, weakness and weight loss.

Cardiovascular signs are indicative of the body's attempt to compensate for the hypoxemia, and include increased cardiac output, heart rate, and blood pressure, and abnormal heart sounds.

LABORATORY ANALYSES AND DIAGNOSIS

Differential Diagnosis

The respiratory diseases that must be differentiated from emphysema are bronchial asthma, chronic bronchitis, lung infection (pneumoconiosis, tuberculosis), or lung tumors, and coronary artery disease.

General Laboratory Tests

The most useful laboratory analyses in the differential diagnosis of emphysema are blood gas analyses and antitrypsin deficiency tests. Tests frequently used to evaluate emphysema include arterial blood gases, sputum cytology, serum alpha$_1$-antitrypsin, electrolytes, digoxin, serum theophylline, histopathology, and red cell mass. The arterial blood gas and hematology results in emphysema will reflect the severity of the respiratory acidosis caused by emphysema and the degree of hypoxemia being experienced by the patient (see Table 11-1).

Alpha$_1$-antitrypsin Deficiency

If alpha$_1$-antitrypsin deficiency is suspected, then a serum protein electrophoresis may be run, but it is imperative that qualitative and quantitative tests be used to confirm the diagnosis. Such tests include estimation of alpha$_1$-antitrypsin by radial immunodiffusion, nephelometry, or electroimmunodiffusion techniques. In addition, phenotyping may be indicated. Laboratory results for an alpha$_1$-antitrypsin-deficient patient may be found in Table 11-2.

Other Diagnostic Tests

Pulmonary function studies are helpful in evaluating emphysema, but chest x-rays do not particularly contribute.[22]

TREATMENT

There is no cure for emphysema because damage to the lungs is irreversible. Education of patients

Table 11-1 ***Blood Gas and Hematology Results***

Arterial Blood Gases	Advanced Emphysema
PaO_2	Decreased < 60 mm Hg
$PaCO_2$	Increased
*p*H	Normal or decreased
HCO_3	Increased
Oxygen saturation	Decreased
Hemoglobin	Increased
Hematocrit	Increased
WBC	Increased

Table 11-2 ***Laboratory Findings in Alpha$_1$-antitrypsin Deficiency Laboratory Results***

Test	Results
Total bilirubin	Increased; related to liver disease
Total calcium	Decreased; related to decreased albumin
Chloride	Decreased; suggests chronic hyperventilation
Cholesterol	Decreased; related to liver disease
Lactic dehydrogenase	Increased; related to liver disease
Alkaline phosphatase	Increased; related to liver disease
Potassium	Decreased; with coexisting metabolic acidosis
Total proteins	Increased; polyclonal gammopathy with cirrhosis
Albumin	Decreased; decreased synthesis of liver disease
Hemoglobin	Increased; polycythemia secondary to hypoxemia Decreased; hypersplenism and/or high incidence of peptic ulcer with COPD
HCT	Increased; polycythemia secondary to hypoxemia Decreased; hypersplenism and/or high incidence of peptic ulcer with COPD
RBC	Increased; polycythemia secondary to hypoxia
WBC	Increased; lung inflammation Decreased; hypersplenism
Platelet count	Decreased; hypersplenism

Data from reference number[21]

and/or their families about preventive measures is among the more important aspects of management. Treatment centers on the prevention or alleviation of symptoms.

Prevention and Management

Important preventive measures include the cessation of smoking and avoidance of infections and irritants.

Exercise programs will *not* improve lung function but can increase endurance as well as improve sense of well-being. These programs may be contraindicated in patients with concomitant cardiac disorders. To be effective, the pulmonary rehabilitation exercise program should be task-specific (goal-oriented).

Proper nutrition is very important for patients who have significant lung disease. Some patients may require a high-protein diet, with six to eight small meals a day supplemented with vitamins, because the work of breathing is so great. Obese patients must lose weight (obesity causes an excessive demand for oxygen).

Medications

Mobilization of bronchial secretions is essential in order to improve gas exchange and prevent recurrent infection. The choices for mobilization are the same as those for asthma, and include aerosol treatment coupled with postural drainage and percussion.

Drug therapy is primarily symptom-related. Bronchodilators usually produce only slight improvement in emphysema patients unless they have significant airway reactivity. Three major types of *bronchodilators* may be considered: the anticholinergics, methylxanthines, and sympathomimetics (see Chap. 8). *Mucolytics* are used when liquefaction of secretions by water alone is insufficient. Their action is to liquify mucus and promote expectoration. Acetylcysteine is a common agent used to break up thick secretions. *Antibiotics* are used to prevent secondary respiratory tract infections, especially *Streptococcus pneumoniae* and *Hemophilus influenzae.* Prophylactic use of antibiotics may be indicated in patients with frequent bacterial respiratory tract infections.

Supplemental oxygen is indicated for patients with severe and persistent hypoxia who meet certain clinical criteria. Although it has been shown that a significantly lower mortality rate is associated with continuous O_2 administration, oxygen therapy should be carefully administered and titrated for patients with severe dyspnea because overuse can depress normal respiration.[23]

Digitalis may be prescribed for emphysema patients whose progressive disease has led to increased pulmonary vascular resistance and subsequent right ventricular failure.

CASE STUDY

History and Findings

A 62-year-old white male was admitted to a hospital emergency room complaining of shortness of breath. The physical examination revealed bilateral wheezing in both lung fields, a barreled chest, and a very long expiratory phase during the breathing cycle. The patient's color was greyish, and the patient indicated that he had been coughing up copious amounts of very thick, tenacious sputum.

LABORATORY FINDINGS

*p*H 7.36
PaO_2 55 mm Hg
$PaCO_2$ 64 mm Hg
Sputum Gram stain—gram-negative bacilli

Questions

1. Do the physical findings support a diagnosis of emphysema?
2. What probably triggered this episode?
3. Do the laboratory findings support these conclusions?
4. What precautions must be taken in oxygenating and following this patient?

Discussion

1. Yes. The age range and dyspnea with barrel chest are characteristic, as is a long expiratory phase.
2. This patient has chronic obstructive pulmonary disease with an exacerbation secondary to infection of gram-negative rods.
3. From a laboratory testing standpoint, one should first be concerned about whether the blood gas values as shown might indicate that the sample is venous rather than arterial.
4. Of significant importance for patients with advanced chronic obstructive pulmonary disease is the fact that they are usually sensitive to oxygen and breathe on a hypoxic drive. This means that these patients normally live on an arterial PO_2 of 60 mm Hg. If such a patient is given too much oxygen, respirations will slow down or stop, and thus the partial pressure of the carbon dioxide will rise and the patient could have respiratory and cardiac arrest. Therefore, both the PaO_2 (approximately 60 mm Hg in these patients) and the acid-base balance should be monitored closely. The acid-base situation in these patients usually shows a normal *p*H with a carbon dioxide level of between 50 and 60 mm Hg.

REFERENCES

1. Miller MJ: Pathophysiology: Principles of Disease, p 245. Philadelphia, WB Saunders, 1983
2. Millard M: Lung and mediastinum. In Kissane JM (ed): Anderson's Pathology, Vol 1, p 900. St Louis, CV Mosby, 1985
3. American Thoracic Society Committee on Diagnostic Standards for Nontuberculous Respiratory Diseases: Definitions and classification of chronic bronchitis, asthma, and pulmonary emphysema. Am Rev Respir Dis. 85:762, 1962
4. Definition and diagnosis of pulmonary diseases with special reference to chronic bronchitis and emphysema. In Chronic Cor Pulmonale: Report of an Expert Committee. Geneva, World Health Organization, Tech Rep Ser 213:15, 1961
5. Thurlbeck WM: Chronic Airflow Obstruction in Lung Disease, p 220. Philadelphia, WB Saunders, 1976
6. Thurlbeck WM, Henderson JAM, Fraser RG, Bates DV: Chronic obstructive lung disease: A comparison between clinical, roentgenologic, functional, and morphologic criteria in chronic bronchitis, emphysema, asthma, and bronchiectasis. Medicine 49:81–145, 1970
7. Anderson AE Jr, Hernandez JA, Holmes WL, Foraker AG: Pulmonary emphysema: Prevalence, severity, and anatomical patterns in macrosections, with respect to smoking habits. Arch Environ Health. 12:556–577, 1966
8. Anderson AE Jr, Foraker AG: Centrilobular emphysema and panlobular emphysema: Two different diseases. Thorax 28:547, 1973
9. Thurlbeck WM: Chronic obstructive lung disease. Pathol Annu 3:367, 1968.
10. Bates DV, Machlem PT, Christie RV: Respiratory Functions in Disease, p 159. Philadelphia, WB Saunders, 1971
11. Martelli NA: Lower-zone emphysema in young patients without alpha$_1$-antitrypsin deficiency. Thorax 29:237, 1974
12. Gough J: The pathogenesis of emphysema. In Liebow AA, Smith DE (eds): International Academy of Pathology, Monographs in Pathology, The Lung, Vol 8, pp 109–133. Baltimore, Williams & Wilkins, 1968
13. Eriksson S: Studies in alpha$_1$-antitrypsin deficiency. Acta Med Scand 177 (Suppl 432):1, 1965
14. Spain DM, Siegel H, Bradess VA: Emphysema in apparently healthy adults: Smoking, age, and sex. JAMA 224:322, 1973
15. Ferguson GG: Pathology Mechanisms and Expressions, p 216. Philadelphia, WB Saunders, 1984
16. Speicher CE, Smith JW Jr: Choosing Effective Laboratory Tests, p 283. Philadelphia, WB Saunders, 1983
17. Greenberg SD et al: The lungs in homozygous alpha$_1$-antitrypsin deficiency. Am J Clin Pathol 60:581, 1973
18. Carrell RW et al: Structure and variation of human alpha$_1$-antitrypsin. Nature 298:329, 1982
19. Des Jardins TR: Clinical Manifestations of Respiratory Disease, p 135. Chicago, Year Book Medical Pub, 1984
20. Ingram RH Jr: Chronic bronchitis, emphysema, and airways obstruction. In Petersdorf RG, Adams RD et al (eds): Harrison's Principles of Internal Medicine, 10th ed, p 1546. New York City, McGraw-Hill, 1983
21. Friedman RB, Anderson RT, Entire SM et al: Ef-

fects of diseases on clinical laboratory tests. Clin Chem 26:1D, 476D, 1980

22. Thurlbeck W, Simon G: Radiographic appearance of the chest in emphysema. AJR 130:429–440, 1978
23. Ingram RH Jr: Chronic bronchitis, emphysema, and airways obstruction: Diffuse lung disease. In Petersdorf RG, Adams RD et al (eds): Harrison's Principles of Internal Medicine, 10th ed, p 1547. New York City, McGraw–Hill, 1983

BIBLIOGRAPHY

Brenner BE: Comprehensive Management of Respiratory Emergencies. Rockville, MD, Aspen Systems, 1985

Burrows B, Knudson RJ, Quan SF, Kettle LJ: Respiratory Disorders, A Pathophysiologic Approach, 2nd ed. Chicago, Year Book Medical Pub, 1983

Cameron I, Bateman N (eds): Respiratory Disorders. Baltimore, University Park Press, 1983

Eastham RD: A Laboratory Guide to Clinical Diagnosis, 5th ed. Bristol, Wright Publishing, 1983

Eichhorn JH: Inaccuracy in blood gas/*p*H measurements caused by the blood sample. J Med Tech, Vol 2, 1:23, Jan 1985

Farzan S: A Concise Handbook of Respiratory Diseases, 2nd ed. Reston, VA, Reston Publishing, 1985

Ferguson GG: Pathophysiology Mechanisms and Expressions. Philadelphia, WB Saunders, 1984

Fraser RG, Pare JAP: Diagnosis of Diseases of the Chest, Vol 3. Philadelphia, WB Saunders, 1979

Gitnick GL: Current Medicine, Vol 3. Chicago, Year Book Medical Pub, 1986

Griner PF, Mayewski RJ, Mushlin AI et al: Selection and interpretation of diagnostic tests and procedures: Principles and applications. Ann Intern Med 94:575–579, 1981

Jacobs DS, Kasten BL, Demott WR, Wolfson WL: Laboratory Test Handbook With DRG Index. St Louis, Mosby/Lexicamp, 1984

Kissane JF (ed): Anderson's Pathology, Vol 2, 8th ed. St Louis: CV Mosby, 1985

Kravis TC, Warner CG: Emergency Medicine: A Comprehensive Review. Rockville, MD, Aspen Systems, 1983

Krupp MA, Chatton MJ, Tierney LM Jr (eds): Current Medical Diagnosis and Treatment. Los Altos, California, Lange Medical Publications, 1986

Lessof MH: Immunological and Clinical Aspects of Allergy. Philadelphia, JB Lippincott, 1981

Robbins: Pathologic Basis of Disease, 3rd ed. Philadelphia, WB Saunders, 1984

Schonell M, Campbell I: Respiratory Medicine, 2nd ed. New York, Churchill Livingstone, 1984

Sheldon H: Boyd's Introduction to the Study of Disease, 9th ed. Philadelphia, Lea & Febiger, 1984

Simmons DH: Current Pulmonology, Vol 4. Chicago, Year Book Medical Pub, 1982

Simmons DH: Current Pulmonology, Vol 6. Chicago, Year Book Medical Pub, 1984

Sterling GM (ed): Integrated Clinical Science Respiratory Disease. London, William Heinemann, 1984

Young DS, Pestaner LC, Gibberman V: Effects of drugs on clinical laboratory tests. Clin Chem 21:1D–432D, 1975

Wanner A: Management of Acute Respiratory Failure in COPD. Lesson 21, Vol 1: Current Reviews in Respiratory Theory. Miami, FL: Current Reviews in Respiratory Therapy, 1979

Chapter 12

Lung Cancer

Sharon S. Ehrmeyer

The great majority of primary carcinomas of the lung are bronchogenic in origin, and thus primary lung cancer is synonymous with bronchogenic carcinoma. Lung cancer occurs most frequently between the ages of 45 and 70 years, with peak incidence in the sixth and seventh decades. It is the most common malignancy and cause of death from cancer in males. In 1987 it surpassed breast cancer to become the number one cause of cancer death in females in the United States.[1, 2] Only 13% of lung cancer patients survive for more than 5 years after diagnosis.[1] Survival is directly related to early diagnosis and treatment; however, early detection is often difficult. Lung cancer is of particular interest because most cases could be prevented by eliminating smoking.

ETIOLOGY AND PATHOPHYSIOLOGY

Cigarette smoking is considered the primary cause of lung cancer, accounting for 90% of all cases.[3, 4] The risk of lung cancer increases in direct proportion to the number of cigarettes smoked per day, the degree of inhalation of the smoke, and the duration of the habit.[5–7] The risk diminishes with increasing years of abstention. The disease is present at a very low rate in nonsmokers, which further substantiates that smoking is the primary cause of lung cancer. The risk for cigar and pipe smokers is not increased appreciably, perhaps because these products are rarely inhaled. Additional evidence is required before a link can be confirmed between lung cancer and passive inhalation of cigarette smoke by nonsmokers.[8]

A small proportion of lung cancer is caused by occupational exposure to certain substances. These include asbestos, ionizing radiation, nickel, chromates, coal products, mustard gas, arsenic, beryllium, polyvinyl chloride, iron oxides, and bischloromethyl ether.[9, 10] It must be recognized, however, that many occupationally exposed workers are also heavy smokers and that certain substances, *e.g.*, asbestos and uranium, may act synergistically with the effects of tobacco smoke.[11, 12]

Although industrial atmospheric pollution has been implicated in causing lung cancer, it is unclear whether this type of pollution alone impacts on the incidence of lung cancer.[13] While the concentration of cancer-causing agents may be increased in "urban" air, the concentration of these carcinogens is much less than that found in cigarette smoke.

Finally, previous pulmonary scarring, resulting from such conditions as scleroderma, granulomatous infection, and wounds, has been associated with pulmonary carcinoma. The reasons for this are unknown, and the tumors are usually adenocarcinomas.[14]

There are four major histologic types of lung cancer: squamous cell, adenocarcinoma, small cell, and large cell undifferentiated.[15] Table 12-1 shows the incidence, growth rate, metastatic potential, and 5-year survival rate for each type. A histologic examination is necessary to confirm the diagnosis and to determine the cell type and the extent of the disease, as well as to help plan the appropriate therapeutic regimen. Thorough tissue evaluation is necessary, because many lung tumors are composed of more than one histologic pattern.

Squamous Cell Carcinoma

Squamous cell carcinoma is the most common form of lung cancer, arising from altered epithelium of the bronchi. The majority of cases are located centrally, near the hilum of the lung and at the points of bifurcation of the large bronchi. Histologically the cells can vary from well-differentiated to poorly-differentiated. Growth of the tumor into the bronchial lumen may cause obstruction. Local metastases can involve the mediastinum and the superior vena cava. Peripheral lesions may invade the chest wall. Lymphatic spread to the hilar nodes and blood-borne metastasis to the adrenal glands, liver, bone, and brain occur frequently, especially with poorly-differentiated squamous cell car-

Table 12-1 ***Bronchogenic Cancer: Histologic Type, Incidence, Growth Rate, Metastatic Potential, and 5-Year Survival Rate***

Histologic Type	Incidence	Growth Rate	Metastatic Potential	5-Year Survival Rate*
Squamous cell	38%	slow	moderate	25%
Adenocarcinoma	23%	fast	high	12%
Small cell	29%	fast	high	1%
Large cell	9%	fast	high	13%

* Without treatment
Data from reference number[16]

cinoma. The majority of patients do not experience symptoms until the disease has advanced considerably.

Adenocarcinoma

Adenocarcinomas are tumors that form glandular structures. These tumors may arise from surface epithelial cells or from bronchial mucous glands within the respiratory tract. Adenocarcinoma occurs more peripherally than centrally, and it is frequently associated with pulmonary fibrosis or scars. The cause and effect relationship between smoking and this type of tumor is suspected but has not been established. These tumors tend to grow more rapidly than do squamous cell tumors, and blood-borne metastasis may occur early.

Small Cell Carcinoma

Small cell carcinoma is a highly malignant, aggressive tumor characterized by rapid growth and early metastasis via the lymphatics and blood. Patients with this type of tumor are much more likely to have widespread and early disseminated disease with metastasis to the central nervous system, liver, bone, bone marrow, lymph nodes, and adrenal glands. It is the form least amenable to surgery. This carcinoma may arise in any part of the bronchial tree, but most occur centrally. There is a strong correlation between small cell carcinoma and cigarette smoking.

It has been suggested that small cell carcinomas originate in the endocrine cells (Kulchitsky cells) of the lung. Some of the lymphocytelike tumor cells show dense-core neurosecretory granules similar to those seen in other neuro-endocrine tumors of the amine precursor uptake and decarboxylation (APUD) system.[16] Many small cell carcinomas are associated clinically with paraneoplastic syndromes caused by ectopic hormone secretion such as ADH (antidiuretic hormone) and ACTH (adrenocorticotropic hormone). The symptoms of inappropriate hormone secretion may precede pulmonary problems. Some small cell carcinomas have been associated with deletion of the short arm of chromosome 3.[16]

Large Cell Carcinoma

The tumor cells in the large cell form of bronchogenic carcinoma are poorly differentiated. Special stains and ultramicroscopic studies may show that some large cell carcinomas are, in reality, adenocarcinomas or squamous cell carcinomas. They usually arise peripherally and metastasize frequently to the mediastinal lymph nodes, pleura, adrenals, central nervous system, and bone.

CLINICAL MANIFESTATIONS

Bronchogenic carcinoma manifests in a variety of ways, but it is not uncommon for the diagnosis to be made when an asymptomatic mass is discovered on a chest x-ray ordered as part of a routine physical examination. Patients presenting with asymptomatic tumors that are localized and resectable have a better prognosis. As symptoms become evident, the lung cancer is usually advanced, unresectable, and often incurable.

Pulmonary Symptoms

Early symptoms often mimic other pulmonary conditions. Cough is the most common first symptom of bronchogenic cancer.[17] Because most of its victims are smokers, patients may initially consider the cough as a consequence of their habit and ignore it. Hemoptysis is also a common complaint, occurring in 35% to 45% of lung cancer patients.[17, 18] Bleeding may result from invasion of the bronchial wall and vessels by cancer or from chronic bronchitis associated with smoking.

Other pulmonary symptoms correlate with extension of the bronchogenic tumor within the chest. The cough may worsen, and the production of sputum may increase. New onset of wheezing or dyspnea is highly suggestive of bronchial obstruction. Depending on the specific location of the local extension, hoarseness, chest pain, pericardial involvement, and/or superior vena cava obstruction may occur.

Extrapulmonary Manifestations

Bronchogenic carcinoma commonly metastasizes widely, and no part of the body is exempt. Extrapulmonary manifestations may be seen before the primary cancer produces symptoms. Weight loss and general malaise may be the only evidence that a problem exists. Involvement of the central nervous system can cause the initial manifestation. Ten to twenty percent of patients with bronchogenic carcinoma have neurologic symptoms due to tumor metastasis to the brain.[16] Hepatic metastases are found in 35% of patients with bronchogenic carcinoma, and bone metastases occur in 10% to 35%.[17] Metastatic spread to the kidneys, adrenals, and remaining lung tissue is common.[19, 20] A variety of symptoms associated with disease of the organs involved can be expected.

Other Manifestations

Paraendocrine syndromes represent various unusual clinical manifestations associated with malignancies, particularly bronchogenic carcinoma.[21] The symptoms are due to the inappropriate production and release of biologically active hormones or hormonelike substances. Identification of these substances can aid in the monitoring of the malignancy.

Cushing's syndrome is a rare manifestation resulting from corticotropinlike (ACTH) substances secreted primarily by small cell tumors. Symptoms include hypokalemic, hypochloremic alkalosis; weakness; muscle wasting; and hyperglycemia.[19] Ectopic ADH production, also seen with small cell carcinoma, inhibits diuresis.

A common manifestation of lung cancer is hypercalcemia due to the excessive secretion of parathyroid hormonelike substances from squamous cell carcinoma, but it may also result from the osteolytic activity of bone metastases. Symptoms are directly related to the calcium level. Other hormonelike substances (*e.g.*, insulin, calcitonin, TSH, prolactin, renin, glucagon) have also been reported to be secreted by tumor cells.[22]

Venous thrombosis and migratory thrombophlebitis are found in 3% to 30% of patients with bronchogenic carcinoma. Nonbacterial thrombotic endocarditis is occasionally associated with mucin-producing adenocarcinoma.[19, 22]

In older patients, bronchogenic carcinoma can manifest as *acanthosis nigricans* (thickening and darkening of the basal skin layer) and *dermatomyositis* (inflammation and degeneration of the skin, subcutaneous tissue, and muscle).[23]

LABORATORY ANALYSES AND DIAGNOSIS

The diagnosis of bronchogenic carcinoma is primarily established by radiological techniques. The imaging techniques of chest x-ray and computerized tomography (CT scans) are commonly used to detect the pulmonary tumor, and are useful in the staging of the tumor for prognostic and treatment purposes. Mediastinoscopy assesses tumor extension to the mediastinal lymph nodes.[19, 24]

Cytologic examination of sputum, bronchial secretions and washings, and pleural fluid is useful in the diagnosis of lung cancer. Bronchoscopy is the most common method of obtaining tissue for microscopic diagnosis when the tumor is centrally located. Transthoracic needle aspirations, thoracentesis, and pleural biopsies are also used, as well as axillary and supraclavicular node biopsies to determine metastases.[19]

Bone marrow aspiration and biopsy are essential, especially with small cell carcinoma, to determine the extent of metastasis. Other conditions have to be considered for the patient showing a shadow on x-ray film and suspected of having a lung tumor. These include tuberculous and other granulomatous lesions and infections. Microbiologic studies are needed to differentiate these active and chronic bacteriological processes from malignancies.

Hematologic, chemical, and microbiologic procedures, depending on the specific situation, are sometimes useful in evaluating the lung cancer patient. General laboratory procedures are helpful in screening for abnormalities. A CBC evaluates the patient's general condition. A mild anemia (hemoglobin of 10 gm/dL [1.55 mmol/L] or less) is seen in about one-fifth of patients with bronchogenic carcinoma. Leukocytosis may reflect complications such as pneumonia, but may occur without evidence of infection.[19] A chemistry panel with electrolytes may detect abnormalities due to inappropriate hormone secretion and metastatic lesions. Ectopic ADH production results in hyponatremia, hypochloremia, decreased serum osmolality, and elevated urine osmolality.[22] There are also increased calcium levels in some patients. Microbiologic testing is necessary to monitor infections caused by obstructions from the tumor.

Depending on the specific situation, additional laboratory tests may be warranted. Arterial blood gas and oxygen saturation analyses may be performed when a patient is being considered for surgery. A patient with poor oxygen exchange and inadequate oxygen saturation is not considered a good surgical candidate. Coagulation studies may be necessary to diagnose and monitor coagulopathies that develop. Hypercoagulation and shortened thrombin times associated with disseminated intravascular coagulopathy and thrombocytopenic purpura occur less frequently.

TREATMENT

Many factors influence the treatment of and prognosis for bronchogenic carcinoma. The histologic cell type, duration and type of symptoms, age and sex of the patient, presence of other disease, growth rate, and stage of the tumor are all considerations. Of these, the histologic cell type and stage are the two most important factors. *Stage of the tumor* refers to the anatomic extent of the tumor at the time of detection. It describes the location and size of the primary tumor, the presence of or absence of spread to the regional lymph nodes, and the presence or absence of metastases to distant lymph nodes and other parts of the body.[25] The patient workup determines whether the cancer is the type and stage suitable for surgical resection. The treatment of choice for localized, nonsmall carcinomas is surgery. However, the vast majority of patients with bronchogenic carcinoma have tumor spread and are treated primarily by radiation, with or without adjuvant chemotherapy.[1]

Laboratory tests are primarily used to evaluate the well-being of the patient. The chemistry panel and electrolytes assist in detecting metastatic lesions causing damage to certain organ systems, in detecting recurrence of inappropriate hormone production, and in assessing the patient's general metabolic state. The CBC is useful in identifying early signs of wasting. Carcinoembryonic antigen (CEA), a tumor-related antigen marker, may be useful in monitoring the effectiveness of therapy. CEA is not useful in screening for small lesions or to differentiate between types of malignancies.[26]

CASE STUDY

A 72-year-old caucasian man, a retired bank clerk, was admitted to the hospital with a chief complaint of muscle weakness, with intermittent episodes of confusion and frequent falls within the past 2 to 3 months. His past medical history included chronic obstructive pulmonary disease (since 1978) and a 35 pack/year (one pack a day for 35 years) smoking history.

Physical examination revealed an elderly man with thin atrophic skin and numerous scattered ecchymoses. BP was 136/90, pulse 90/minute, respirations 18/minute, and the patient was afebrile. Bilateral pitting edema of the extremities was evident. The neurological examination revealed generalized weakness and muscular atrophy, and proximal weakness greater than distal.

Blood chemistries included: serum potassium of 2.8 mEq/L (2.8 mmol/L), plasma cortisol (0800 h) of 45 μg/100 mL (1.3 μmol/L), and plasma ACTH (0800 h) of 400 pg/mL (400 ng/L).

Chest x-ray film showed an enlarging right lower lung infiltrate. A bone marrow test done one week prior to death revealed metastatic malignant cells compatible with small cell carcinoma. Chemotherapy was begun 5 days prior to death with cytoxan, lomustine (CCNU), and methotrexate. The patient subsequently became more confused and lethargic with development of fever and hypotension. Several blood cultures grew *S. aureus* and enterococci. Despite antibiotics, the patient's condition deteriorated with worsening pneumonia and hypotension. A chest x-ray film just prior to death showed extensive changes consistent with pneumonia and adult respiratory distress syndrome.

The diagnosis was small cell carcinoma, metastatic, with ectopic ACTH production.

Questions

1. How is muscle weakness related to the underlying bronchogenic carcinoma?
2. What is the relationship of chronic obstructive pulmonary disease (COPD) to bronchogenic carcinoma?
3. Why does this patient have a positive blood culture?

Discussion

1. Muscle weakness is due to two factors. Cancer patients not eating properly often develop a negative nitrogen balance. Also, the metabolic derangement due to ectopic hormone production produces hypokalemia.
2. Most lung cancers develop in patients with a history of chronic bronchitis, usually precipitated by smoking. Often the cough and pulmonary symptoms associated with COPD and smoking delay the diagnosis.
3. Bronchogenic carcinomas often partially obstruct the bronchus, which results in an increased susceptibility to infection beyond the obstruction.

REFERENCES

1. 1987 Cancer Facts and Figures, pp 3–9. New York, American Cancer Society, 1987
2. Silverberg E, Lubera J: Cancer statistics 1987. Ca 37:1–2, 1987
3. Smoking and Health: A Report of the Surgeon General. Washington, DC, U.S. Dept of Health, Education, and Welfare, Public Health Service, 1979
4. Frank AL: The epidemiology and etiology of lung cancer. Clin Chest Med 3:219, 1982
5. Hammond EC, Horn D: Smoking and death rates: Report on 44 months of follow-up of 187,783 men. JAMA 166:1159, 1294, 1958
6. Hammond EC: Smoking in relation to the death rate of one million men and women. Natl Cancer Inst Monogr 19:127, 1966
7. Wynder EL: Etiology of lung cancer: Reflections on 2 decades of research. Cancer 30:1332–1339, 1972
8. Wynder EL: The etiology, epidemiology, and prevention of lung cancer. Semin Respir Med 3:137–139, 1982
9. Fraumeni JF Jr (ed): Persons at High Risk of Cancer: An Approach to Cancer Etiology. New York, American Cancer Society 1975
10. Israel L, Chahinian A: Lung Cancer: Natural History, Prognosis, and Therapy. New York City, Academic Press, 1976
11. Strauss MJ (ed): Lung Cancer: Clinical Diagnosis and Treatment. New York, Grune & Stratton, 1977
12. Selikoff IJ et al: Asbestos-associated disease in United States shipyards. Ann NY Acad Sci 330:295, 1979
13. Wynder EL, Hoffmann D: Tobacco. In Schottenfeld D, Fraumeni JF (eds): Cancer Epidemiology and Prevention. Philadelphia, WB Saunders, 1982
14. Robbins S et al: Basic Pathology. Philadelphia, WB Saunders, 1981
15. International Histologic Classification of Tumors, Nos 1–20. Geneva, World Health Organization, 1978
16. Brower M, Carney D: Lung cancer: The latest on diagnosis and therapy. J Respir Dis 5:13–14, 19, 1984
17. Hyde L, Hyde CI: Clinical manifestations of lung cancer. Chest 65:299, 1974
18. LeRoux BT: Bronchial carcinoma. Thorax 23:136, 1968
19. Andersen H, Prakash U: Diagnosis of symptomatic lung cancer. Semin Respir Med 3:165–175, 1982
20. Rassam JW, Anderson G: Incidence of paramalignant disorders in bronchogenic carcinoma. Thorax 30:86, 1975
21. Bhattacharya SK, Sealy WC: Paraneoplastic syndromes. Curr Probl Surg May:3, 1972

22. Umsawasdi T, Valdivieso M: Paraneoplastic syndromes in lung cancer. Semin Respir Med 3:200–209, 1982
23. Gautam HP: Malignant acanthosis nigricans associated with squamous cell carcinoma of bronchus. Ann Thorac Surg 7:418, 1969
24. Carlens E, Larsson S: Mediastinoscopy in lung cancer. Semin Respir Med 3:176, 1982
25. Staging of Lung Cancer/1979 American Joint Committee for Cancer Staging and End Results Reporting. Chicago, Task Force on Lung, 1978
26. Vincent R: Biologic markers in lung cancer. Semin Respir Med 3:187–188, 1982

BIBLIOGRAPHY

Weiss W: Lung Cancer. In Kahn SB et al (eds): Concepts in Cancer Medicine, p 421. New York, Grune & Stratton, 1983

Chapter 13

Pleural Effusions

Herb Miller

Pleural fluid, an ultrafiltrate of the blood plasma, is formed continuously in the pleural cavity. This cavity, normally containing from 1 to 10 milliliters of fluid, is formed by the parietal pleura lining the chest wall and the visceral pleura covering the lung.[1] Each lung is enveloped by this double-folded membrane of contiguous mesothelial layers.

Pleural fluid acts as a natural lubricant for the contraction and expansion of the lungs during respiration. It is reabsorbed by the lymphatics and the venules in the pleura. Regulatory mechanisms involve hydrostatic pressure (blood pressure), colloid osmotic (oncotic) pressure, intrapleural pressure, permeability/constriction of the capillaries, and lymphatic reabsorption.

Under normal conditions the colloid pressure remains constant on both sides of the pleural membrane. The colloid pressure, primarily because of the presence of large-molecular-weight proteins in the blood plasma, prevents water from being filtered. This colloid pressure is an opposing pressure to filtration across the parietal pleura. Hydrostatic pressure is greater at the parietal pleura and favors filtration. At the visceral pleura the hydrostatic pressure is decreased, allowing the fluid to pass out of the pleural cavity and to be reabsorbed by the capillaries and lymphatic system.[2, 3] Figure 13-1 illustrates the normal filtration and reabsorption of pleural fluid. *Thoracentesis,* removal of pleural fluid, is performed for diagnostic reasons, for relief of symptoms associated with the fluid accumulation, or to introduce medication.

ETIOLOGY AND PATHOPHYSIOLOGY

Formation

A pleural effusion is an accumulation of serous fluid in a pleural cavity. Disturbances that interfere with hydrostatic pressure, protein concentration in the blood (oncotic pressure), normal dilation/contraction of the vessels (vasomotion), or blockage of the lymphatic drainage system or other disease states of the lungs result in accumulation of increased amounts of serous fluid in the pleural cavities. Pleural effusions can be referred to alternatively as *thoracentesis fluid* or *empyema fluid* (pus in the pleural fluid).

Vasomotion, which affects the normal filtration of blood plasma into the pleural cavities, refers to the dilation/contraction of the capillaries. During dilation water leaves the capillary, and during contraction water enters the capillary. Inflammation is a cause of increased dilation, while decreased cardiac output and thrombosis are causes of constriction.[4] *Capillary permeability,* the degree to which the capillary blocks the loss of protein, is a third important factor.[5] Damage to the capillary increases the loss of protein, which decreases the oncotic effect and thereby enhances the transfer of

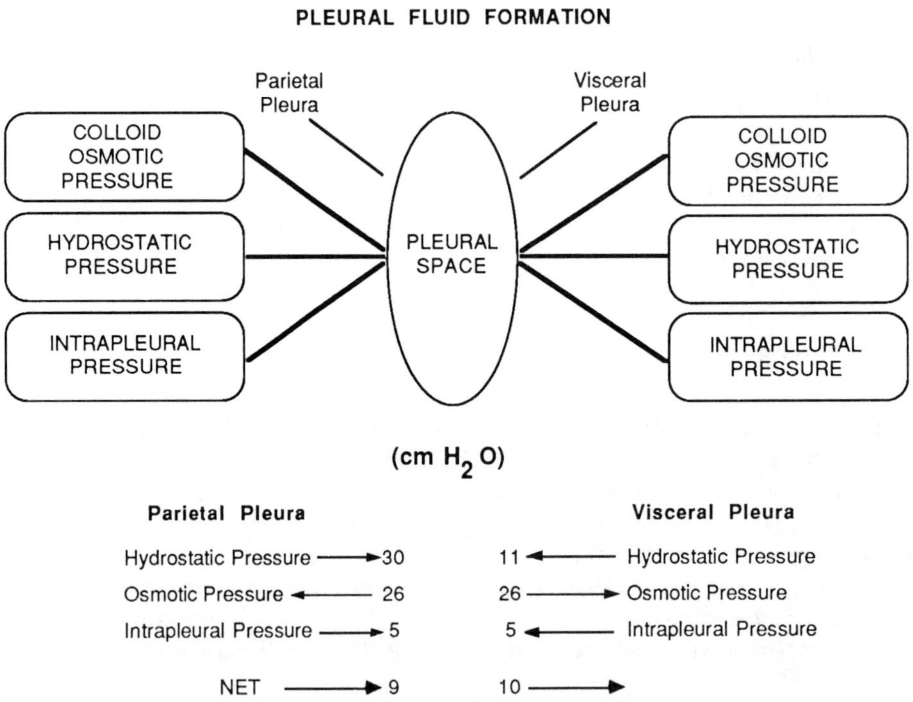

Figure 13-1 **Normal filtration and reabsorption of pleural fluid.**

water. Adequate lymphatic drainage of the pleural fluid is also important.[6] Any disruption of lymphatic flow, such as that caused by a neoplasm or other disease process of the lungs, will decrease the drainage and enhance the accumulation of fluid.

Effusions are generally classified into two main categories, transudates or exudates. A *transudate* is an effusion caused by systemic diseases outside the pleural cavity itself, while an *exudate* results from a disease state within the pleural cavity or lungs.[7] Classification of a pleural effusion as to type is based on clinical laboratory findings and involves various chemical, microbiologic, immunologic, and cytologic tests.

Terminology

Physical and radiological examination usually precedes the removal of pleural fluid and subsequent clinical laboratory testing. It is important for the clinical laboratory scientist to have a basic understanding of the medical terms and abbreviations used in reporting both the physical and the radiological results, in order to ensure adequate communication with the physician and other medical personnel. Terms and abbreviations commonly used include those found in Table 13-1.

Table 13-1 ***Medical Terms: Definitions and Abbreviations***

Medical Terms	Definitions
Atelectasis:	An incomplete expansion of the lungs
Auscultation:	Listening to sounds within the body
Dyspnea:	Difficult or labored breathing
Hemithorax:	One side of the pleural cavity or chest
Hemothorax:	The presence of blood in the pleural cavity
Lobectomy:	The removal of a lobe of a lung
Opacification:	Opaque to radiation
Percussion:	The act of striking with sharp, short blows to aid in diagnosis by sound
Pneumonectomy:	The removal of a lung
Pneumothorax:	A collapsed lung
Rales:	An abnormal rattling sound heard on auscultation
Thoracotomy:	Cutting into the pleural cavity
Common Abbreviations	
A & P:	Auscultation and percussion
ARDS:	Adult respiratory distress syndrome
COPD:	Chronic obstructive pulmonary disease
CXR:	Chest x-ray
SOB:	Shortness of breath
RUL, RLL:	Designate right upper and right lower lobes of the lung
LUL, LLL:	Designate left upper and left lower lobes of the lung

Data from reference number[8]

The disease states responsible for pleural transudates that are encountered most often are congestive heart failure, hepatic disease, and nephrotic disease.[9–11] In *congestive heart failure,* there is an increase in hydrostatic pressure; in *hepatic disease* there is a decreased production of protein; and in *nephrotic disease,* there is an increased loss of protein. These three systemic conditions affect the pressure gradients, causing fluid accumulation in the pleural cavity.

Exudates, caused by disease states of the pleural cavity or lungs, are usually encountered in cases of inflammation, which increases the capillary permeability, and in cases of tumor obstruction, which decreases lymphatic drainage.[12, 13] Examples of such diseases include bacterial, viral, and fungal infections, pulmonary infarctions, trauma, systemic lupus, rheumatoid arthritis, and neoplasms.[14] Postmyocardial exudate effusions (Dressler's syndrome) and effusions secondary to drug reactions from nitrofurantoin, dantrolene, methysergide, bromocriptine, procarbazine, or methotrexate are also encountered.[15]

CLINICAL MANIFESTATIONS

Patients with pleural effusions usually present with pleuritic pain. This may be mild to severe, and is described as sharp or cutting. Dyspnea is often a presenting symptom. A nonproductive or slightly productive cough is also frequently present. In infectious effusions a fever is usually present, but fever can also be encountered in pulmonary infarction and neoplastic or collagen diseases.[16] Typical physical findings include grunting respiration, splinting of the affected chest, shortness of breath, increased abdominal breathing, stifling of deep respiration, coughing, and impaired resonance on percussion. A shifting of the area of impaired resonance with changes in body position is virtually pathognomonic of a pleural effusion.[17]

LABORATORY ANALYSES AND DIAGNOSIS

Pleural fluid specimens are usually of large volume and are collected by needle aspiration. It is important to collect anticoagulated, sterile, and nonanticoagulated specimens.[18] The anticoagulated tube is used for cell counts, the sterile tube is used for microbiologic examination, and the nonanticoagulated tube is observed for spontaneous clotting and chemical testing. Before performing cytologic and microbiologic tests on large-volume samples, it is important to concentrate the specimen by centrifugation.[19]

Transudates vs. Exudates

It is necessary to classify effusions accurately as either transudates or exudates in order to understand and treat the actual disease process involved. As described above, *transudates* are effusions caused by systemic disorders. *Exudates* are effusions that result from a disease process directly involving the pleural cavity membranes, seen in infections, malignancies, or actual damage to the lungs. If a patient has a transudative pleural effusion, it can be treated and the pleural surface can be ignored. If the patient has an exudative pleural effusion, further investigation should be directed toward the pleura in order to discover the etiology of the disease.[20]

Gross evaluation of a pleural fluid can reveal information useful in classifying the fluid as either a transudate or an exudate. Color, turbidity, and the presence of clotting are valuable in this regard. Transudates are usually pale yellow, clear, with no clot formation, while exudates are usually cloudy, are dark in color, and tend to clot due to the presence of fibrinogen. Blood in specimens may be caused by a traumatic tap, malignancy, pulmonary infarction, trauma, pancreatitis, or tuberculosis.[21] Traumatic taps must be distinguished from hemorrhagic specimens. In true hemothorax, the hematocrit of the specimen will be similar to that of peripheral blood, while with a traumatic tap the amount of blood will diminish as the aspiration continues and the hematocrit will be lower. There will also be uneven distribution of blood throughout the specimen.[22] Icteric or hemolysed fluid on a centrifuged hematocrit tube containing the specimen usually indicates a true hemothorax.

Chylous Effusions

Chylous is a third classification used to denote effusions that appear milky white to greenish. A true chylous effusion is rare, and is usually caused by leakage from the thoracic ducts or by lymphatic obstruction. Complications from thoracic surgery, cancer, thrombosis of the great veins, or filariasis can also be a cause of chylous effusions.[23] Chylous effusions are characterized by a large amount of chylomicrons. Pseudochylous effusions, appearing whitish to greenish, are seen in cases of tuberculosis and rheumatoid arthritis. These do not contain large amounts of chylomicrons but exhibit high levels of cholesterol, with cholesterol crystals often found.[24]

Physical and Chemical Tests

Specific gravity tests are useful for classifying effusions. Exudates exhibit an increased specific gravity. Total protein measures are also helpful. Values over 3 gm/dL (30 gm/L) are seen most commonly with exudates. Lactate dehydrogenase (LD) and LD isoenzymes have been used, with greater activity seen in exudates. Malignancies have been shown to exhibit both increased and normal LD-4 and LD-5 levels.[25, 26] Glucose levels are expected to be decreased in cases of increased utilization, as seen in malignancies and bacterial infections, and *p*H values are decreased in exudates. These laboratory findings are helpful but must be considered together before a definite classification can be made. Table 13-2 summarizes the laboratory tests most often performed to differentiate pleural transudates from exudates.

All specimens should be examined as soon as possible. Prolonged standing can interfere with test results, especially glucose, *p*H, and cytologic parameters.

Cytologic Studies

Red and white blood cell counts are generally performed on pleural fluid using a hemocytometer. Increased red blood cells (RBC) can indicate a hemothorax, traumatic tap, or malignancy. Increased white blood cells (WBC) are indicative of inflammation. It is beneficial to utilize a cytocentrifuge in preparing the specimen for a cell differential. Traditional Wright's stain, Papanicolaou's stain, and hematoxylin-eosin stain are used in the cytospin preparations. Enumeration and cytologic evaluation of the cells after cytospin concentration have allowed the laboratory to detect early malignancies and to classify the various white blood cell types seen in different transudates and exudates. For example, a moderately increased count with a predominance of lymphocytes is seen in tuberculosis, while higher counts with a predominance of neutrophils (PMNs) are seen in bacterial infections. It has been suggested that the presence of eosinophils is a good prognostic sign, because such fluids seldom become infected.[30] Table 13-3 summarizes the most common cytologic parameters helpful in differentiating pleural transudates and exudates.

Microbiologic Studies

Microbiologic studies on pleural fluid for aerobic and anaerobic bacteria are an important part of a pleural fluid work-up. Mycobacterial (acid-fast ba-

Table 13-2 ***Pleural Transudates Versus Exudates***

	Transudates	Exudates
Color/transparency	Clear/pale yellow	Cloudy/dark
Spontaneous clotting	No	Yes
Total protein	<3 gm/dL	>3 gm/dL
LD	<200 IU/L	>200 IU/L
Specific gravity	<1.015	>1.015
*p*H	7.3–7.4	<7.3 Below 6 seen in esophageal rupture
Glucose	Similar to serum	Normal to decreased
Amylase		Elevated in pancreatitis, malignancies, and esophageal rupture
Carcinoembryonic antigen (CEA)		Exudates only

Conversion to SI units is as follows:
Protein—gm/dL × 10 = gm/L LD—IU/L × 1 = U/L

Data from reference numbers[27–29]

Table 13-3 *Cytologic Laboratory Tests*

	Transudates	Exudates
WBC	<1000/μL	>1000/μL
RBC	Few	>10,000/μL
Differential		
Mesothelial	Variable	Increases seen in pneumonias, infarctions, and malignancies; scarce in pyogenic diseases
PMN	Variable	Predominate in bacterial pneumonia and infarctions
Lymphocytes	Variable	Predominate in TB and malignancies
Mononuclear	Variable	Variable

Data from reference numbers[31–33]

cilli), fungal, and parasitologic studies may also be performed. Fluid appearing purulent or seropurulent often yields *Streptococcus pneumoniae* and other streptococci, *Staphylococcus aureus, Hemophilus influenzae,* or various anaerobes such as *Bacteroides melaninogenicus, Fusobacterium nucleatum,* and anaerobic and microaerophilic cocci on culture.[34] Systemic fungi such as Histoplasma, Blastomyces, and Coccidioidomyces are very dangerous and usually enter through the lungs before spreading throughout the body. Pulmonary candidiasis, cryptococcosis, aspergillosis, and *Pneumocystis carinii* are opportunistic infections encountered.[35] Rarely, *Echinococcus granulosis, Entamoeba histolytica,* and *Paragonimus westermani* will be found.[36, 37]

TREATMENT

Resolution of or improvment in the underlying cause of the effusion generally results in its disappearance. If the etiology of the effusion is unknown or if there is dyspnea, however, aspiration will be performed. Hemothorax usually improves upon draining the pleural space; however, thoracotomy is sometimes necessary if bleeding continues. Neoplastic effusions often reaccumulate rapidly after aspiration. To avoid the necessity of multiple aspirations, sclerosing compounds are sometimes instilled to reduce the rate of liquid accumulation.[38]

CASE STUDY #1[39]

A 41-year-old caucasian man was admitted to the hospital confused but responsive. He complained of shortness of breath (SOB), urinary incontinence, and bleeding per rectum for four days. He had a temperature of 102.6° F, respiration rate of 20/minute, and blood pressure (BP) of 124/82. Liver function tests showed an elevated alkaline phosphatase of 157 IU/L (157 U/L), lactic dehydrogenase (LD) of 124 IU/L (124 U/L), and serum aspartate transaminase (AST) of 47 IU/L (47 U/L). An oral examination revealed candidiasis. Chest x-ray (CXR) film results showed complete opacification of the left hemithorax with pleural effusion. One hundred fifty cc of pleural fluid were removed by needle aspiration. On examination, the fluid was dark in color, was cloudy, and had a specific gravity of 1.022. Chronic inflammatory cells including lymphocytes, plasma cells, macrophages, and eosinophils were found. *Pneumocystis carinii* and Candida species were noted. *Enterobacter aerogenes* grew in thioglycolate broth. The specimen was negative for malignancy, viral inclusions, and acid-fast bacilli.

Case 1: Questions

1. Given the physical and laboratory findings, is this an exudative or a transudative effusion?
2. What is the significance of the chronic inflammatory cells?

3. What is the significance of the opportunistic organisms found?
4. Is the presence of eosinophils important?
5. What is the probable diagnosis?

Discussion

1. The effusion is an exudate.
2. Inflammatory cells are seen in a number of infectious diseases.
3. *Pneumocystis carinii* infection is often a complication in AIDS patients, as is candidiasis.
4. Eosinophilia is nonspecific and seen in a number of disorders.
5. The diagnosis is Acquired Immune Deficiency Syndrome (AIDS) with acute bronchopneumonia.

CASE STUDY #2[39]

A 30-year-old black woman presented with painful micturition, polyuria, and periorbital, peritibial, and generalized edema. She had a blood pressure (BP) of 220/90, respiration rate of 28/minute, and shortness of breath (SOB). Urinalysis revealed massive proteinuria with a variety of renal casts, oval fat bodies, and renal epithelial cells. Clinical chemistry results indicated a blood creatinine of 8.1 mg/dL (716 μmol/L), a blood urea nitrogen (BUN) of 80 mg/dL (29 mmol/L), and a decreased total protein and albumin. Chest x-ray (CXR) film results revealed that the right and left lower lungs (RLL, LLL) showed diffuse opacification. Thoracentesis analysis revealed pale, clear, acellular effusion with no microorganisms found.

Case 2: Questions

1. Is this an exudative or transudative effusion? What is the significance of the proteinuria, renal casts, and oval fat bodies?
2. What is the significance of the elevated serum creatinine and BUN?
3. What is the significance of the effusion being acellular?

Discussion

1. and 2. The urine and blood findings indicate nephrotic disease, and that the fluid is a transudate. Loss of protein due to kidney damage (nephrosis) reduces oncotic pressure, enhancing movement of water into tissues and serous cavities.

3. Effusions caused by nephrosis are transudative and present with very few lymphocytes or other cellular components.

REFERENCES

1. Kjeldsberg CR, Knight JA: Body Fluids: Laboratory Examination of Cerebrospinal, Synovial, and Serous Fluids: A Textbook Atlas, pp 28–42. Chicago, American Society of Clinical Pathologists Press, 1982
2. Glasser L: Evaluation: Serous fluids. Diagn Med 3:80, 1980
3. Strasinger SK: Urinalysis and Body Fluids: A Self-Instructional Text, pp 169–170. Philadelphia, FA Davis, 1985
4. Valtin H: Renal Function: Mechanisms Preserving Fluid and Solute Balance in Health, 2nd ed, p 35. Boston, Little, Brown & Co, 1983
5. Valtin H: Renal Dysfunction: Mechanisms Involved in Fluid and Solute Balance, pp 65–66. Boston, Little, Brown & Co, 1979
6. Kjeldsberg CR, Knight JA: Body Fluids: Laboratory Examination of Cerebrospinal, Synovial, and Serous Fluids: A Textbook Atlas, p 28. Chicago, American Society of Clinical Pathologists Press, 1982
7. Glasser L: Evaluation: Serous fluids. Diagn Med 3:79–90, 1980
8. Chabner D: The Language of Medicine, pp 309–334. Philadelphia, WB Saunders, 1985
9. Strasinger SK: Urinalysis and Body Fluids: A Self-Instructional Text, p 172. Philadelphia, FA Davis, 1985
10. Kjeldsberg CR, Knight JA: Body Fluids: Laboratory Examination of Cerebrospinal, Synovial, and Serous Fluids: A Textbook Atlas, p 29. Chicago, American Society of Clinical Pathologists Press, 1982
11. Glasser L: Evaluation: Serous fluids. Diagn Med 3:80, 1980

12. Kjeldsberg CR, Knight JA: Body Fluids: Laboratory Examination of Cerebrospinal, Synovial, and Serous Fluids: A Textbook Atlas, p 29. Chicago, American Society of Clinical Pathologists Press, 1982
13. Glasser L: Evaluation: Serous Fluids. Diagn Med 3:80, 1980
14. Kjeldsberg CR, Knight JA: Body Fluids: Laboratory Examination of Cerebrospinal, Synovial, and Serous Fluids: A Textbook Atlas, pp 28–29. Chicago, American Society of Clinical Pathologists Press, 1982
15. Light RW, Management of pleural effusions. In Chretien J, Bignon J, Hirsch A (eds): The Pleura in Health and Disease, p 804. New York City, Marcel Dekker, 1985
16. Lowell JR: Pleural Effusions: A Comprehensive Review, p 17. Baltimore, University Park Press, 1977
17. Lowell JR: Pleural Effusions: A Comprehensive Review, p 19. Baltimore, University Park Press, 1977
18. Strasinger SK: Urinalysis and Body Fluids: A Self-Instructional Text, p 170. Philadelphia, FA Davis, 1985
19. Strasinger SK: Urinalysis and Body Fluids: A Self-Instructional Text, p 170. Philadelphia, FA Davis, 1985
20. Light RW: Management of pleural effusions. In Chretien J, Bignon J, Hirsch A (eds): The Pleura in Health and Disease, p 791. New York City, Marcel Dekker, 1985
21. Kjeldsberg CR, Knight JA: Body Fluids: Laboratory Examination of Cerebrospinal, Synovial, and Serous Fluids: A Textbook Atlas, p 29. Chicago, American Society of Clinical Pathologists Press, 1982
22. Kjeldsberg CR, Knight JA: Body Fluids: Laboratory Examination of Cerebrospinal, Synovial, and Serous Fluids: A Textbook Atlas, p 30. Chicago, American Society of Clinical Pathologists Press, 1982
23. Lowell JR: Pleural Effusions: A Comprehensive Review, p 136. Baltimore, University Park Press, 1977
24. Kjeldsberg CR, Knight JA: Body Fluids: Laboratory Examination of Cerebrospinal, Synovial, and Serous Fluids: A Textbook Atlas, p 30. Chicago, American Society of Clinical Pathologists Press, 1982
25. Kjeldsberg CR, Knight JA: Body Fluids: Laboratory Examination of Cerebrospinal, Synovial, and Serous Fluids: A Textbook Atlas, p 40. Chicago, American Society of Clinical Pathologists Press, 1982
26. Ross DL, Neely AE: Textbook of Urinalysis and Body Fluids, pp 279–280. Norwalk, Connecticut, Appleton-Century-Crofts, 1983
27. Ross DL, Neely AE: Textbook of Urinalysis and Body Fluids, pp 276–278. Norwalk, Connecticut, Appleton-Century-Crofts, 1983
28. Strasinger SK: Urinalysis and Body Fluids: A Self-Instructional Text, pp 172–173. Philadelphia, FA Davis, 1985
29. Kjeldsberg CR, Knight JA: Body Fluids: Laboratory Examination of Cerebrospinal, Synovial, and Serous Fluids: A Textbook Atlas, p 29. Chicago, American Society of Clinical Pathologists Press, 1982
30. Light RW: Management of pleural effusions. In Chretien J, Bignon J, Hirsch A (eds): The Pleura in Health and Disease, p 793. New York City, Marcel Dekker, 1985
31. Ross DL, Neely AE: Textbook of Urinalysis and Body Fluids, pp 276–278. Norwalk, Connecticut, Appleton-Century-Crofts, 1983
32. Strasinger SK: Urinalysis and Body Fluids: A Self-Instructional Text, pp 172–173. Philadelphia, FA Davis, 1985
33. Kjeldsberg CR, Knight JA: Body Fluids: Laboratory Examination of Cerebrospinal, Synovial, and Serous Fluids: A Textbook Atlas, p 29. Chicago, American Society of Clinical Pathologists Press, 1982
34. Finegold SM, Martin WJ: Diagnostic Microbiology, 7th ed, pp 315–316. St Louis, CV Mosby, 1986
35. Rippon JW: Medical mycology: The pathogenic fungi and the pathogenic actinomycetes. In Freeman BA: Burrows's Textbook of Microbiology, 22nd ed, pp 874–937. Philadelphia, WB Saunders, 1985
36. Kjeldsberg CR, Knight JA: Body Fluids: Laboratory Examination of Cerebrospinal, Synovial, and Serous Fluids: A Textbook Atlas, p 41. Chicago, American Society of Clinical Pathologists Press, 1982
37. Lowell JR: Pleural Effusions: A Comprehensive Review, p 10. Baltimore, University Park Press, 1977
38. Ingram RH: Diseases of pleura, mediastinum, and diaphragm. In Petersdorf RG et al (eds): Harrison's Principles of Internal Medicine, 10th ed, pp 1581–1582. New York City, McGraw-Hill, 1983
39. Balchum OJ, Jung RC: Chest Diseases Case Studies. Flushing, New York, Medical Examination Publishing Company, 1973

Part IV

RENAL DISORDERS

Marie Pezzlo, Associate Editor

The organs of the urinary system include the kidneys, ureters, urinary bladder, urethra, and, in males, prostate (see the accompanying illustration). The kidneys secrete urine and the ureters or collecting tubes allow urine to flow into the bladder, where it is temporarily stored until it passes through the urethra and is eliminated from the body.

The kidneys are in large part responsible for maintaining the constancy of the body's internal environment. They accomplish this feat not only by excreting waste products of metabolism, other solutes, and excess water, but also by selective reabsorption of these various constituents in time of deficit.

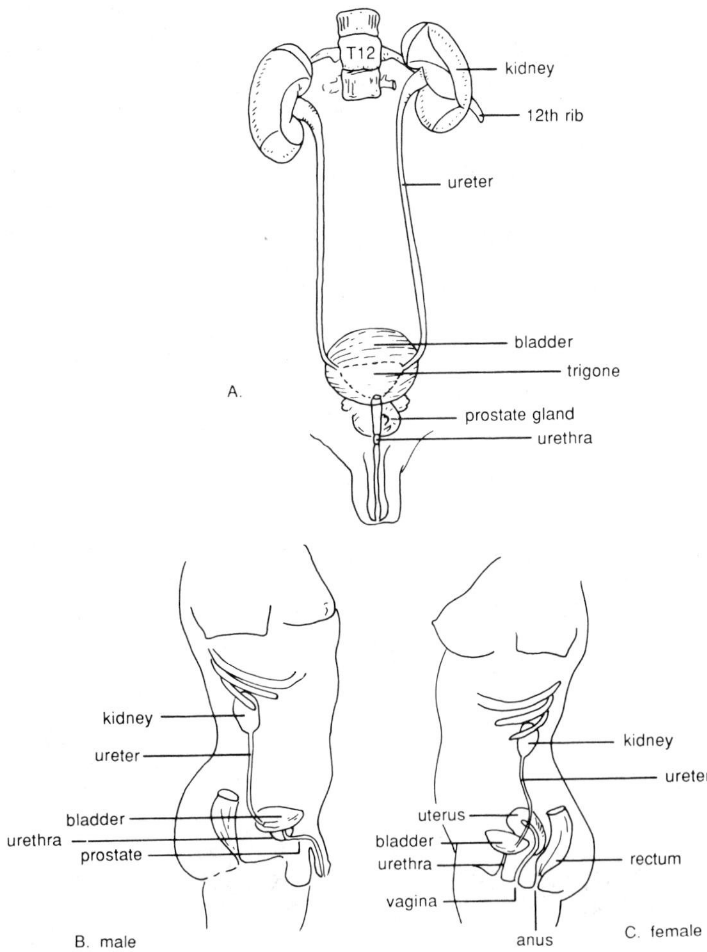

The urinary tract.

The functional unit of the kidney is the *nephron,* which consists of a renal corpuscle made up of a tuft of parallel capillaries (the *glomerulus*) surrounded by a tubule known as *Bowman's capsule.* These structures, together with the proximal and distal tubules, make up the *cortex* or outer portion of the kidney. The inner portion, the *medulla,* consists of Henle's loop and the collecting duct. Blood is supplied to the kidney through the renal artery. (See the illustration opposite.)

The kidneys adjust the volume and composition of all extracellular fluid to the body's continual needs. Although the renal arteries deliver approximately 20% of the total output of the blood from the heart to the two kidneys, normal excretion of urine per day is only about 1.5 liters because most of the glomerular filtrate is reabsorbed (see the illustrations below and on page 154).

The glomerular filtrate is an ultrafiltrate of the blood plasma containing only small-molecular-weight solutes. Blood cells and large molecules, such as protein, do not cross the normal glomerular membrane. Urine, which obtains its normal straw color from bile pigments, is thus a result of two processes: filtration and reabsorption.

In the clinical laboratory diagnosis of renal disorders, the chemical and microscopic analyses of urine are among the procedures useful in guiding further diagnostic inquiry. The diagram on page 155 outlines various disease states associated with urinalysis findings.

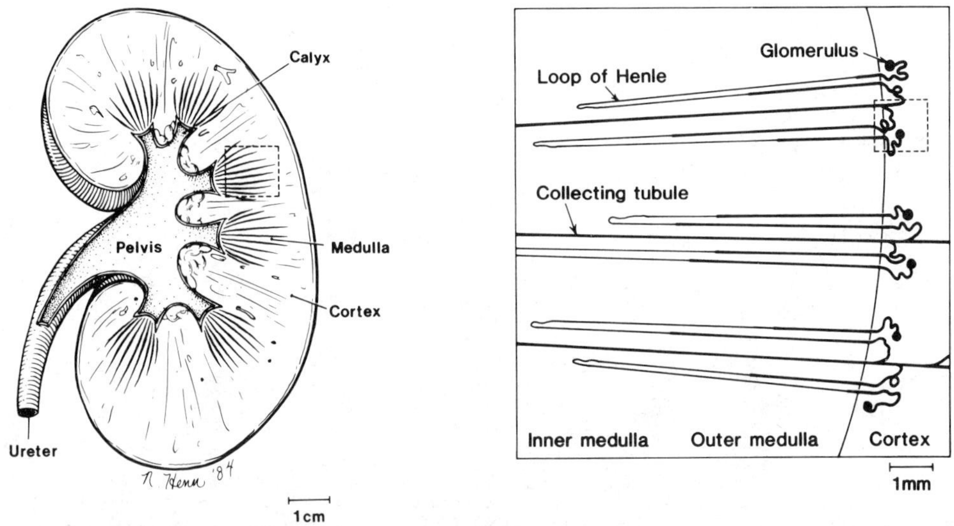

The kidney. (From Bishop ML, Duben-Von Laufen JL, Fody EP: Clinical Chemistry, p 428. Philadelphia, JB Lippincott, 1985)

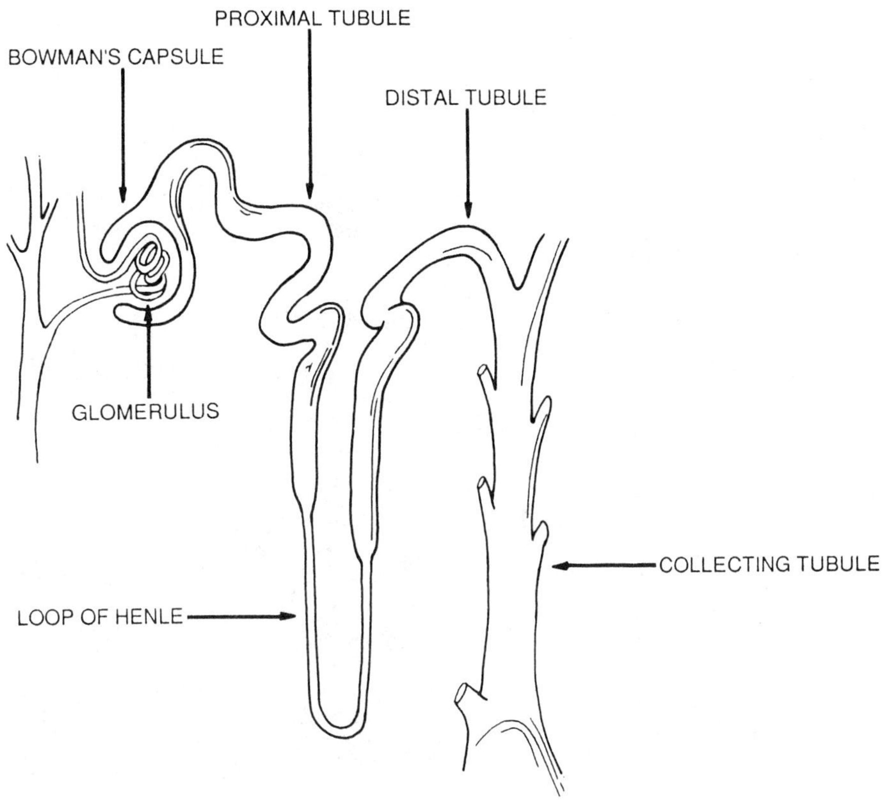

The nephron. (Modified from Bishop ML, Duben-Von Laufen JL, Fody EP: Clinical Chemistry, p 429. Philadelphia, JB Lippincott, 1985)

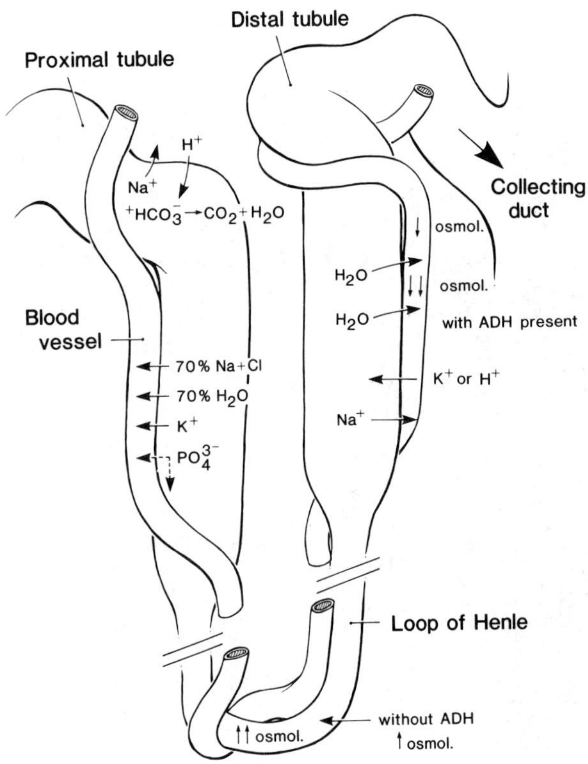

Simplified summary of electrolytes in the renal tubules. (From Bishop ML, Duben-Von Laufen JL, Fody EB: Clinical Chemistry, p 286. Philadelphia, JB Lippincott, 1985)

- Chemical
  - pH
    - <6
      - Acidosis
      - Diarrhea
      - High protein diet
      - Starvation
      - Uncontrolled diabetes mellitus
    - >6
      - Renal failure
      - Urinary tract infection
      - Renal tubular acidosis
      - Vegetarian diet
  - Protein
    - Nephrotic syndrome
    - Glomerulonephritis
    - Pyelonephritis
    - Renal TB
    - Glomerulosclerosis
  - Glucose
    - Renal tubular disease
    - Diabetes mellitus
    - Low renal threshold
  - Hgb
    - Cystitis
    - Polycystic kidney
    - Renal calculi
    - Bladder tumor
    - Renal TB
    - Glomerulonephritis
    - Urinary tract trauma
    - Intravascular hemolysis
    - Bleeding disorders
- Microscopic
  - Microorganisms
    - Bacteria
    - Fungi
    - Parasites
  - RBC
    - (See Hgb)
  - Casts
  - Crystals ($pH < 7$)
    - Tyrosine
    - Leucine
    - Cystine
    - Bilirubin
    - Cholesterol
    - Sulfonamide
    - X-ray media

Casts:

	Hyaline	WBC	RBC	Epithelial	Granular	Fatty	Waxy
Strenuous exercise	++++	0	0	++	+++	0	0
Acute glomerulonephritis	++	++	++++	++	++	+	+
Nephrotic syndrome	++	++	++	++++	++	++++	++
Acute pyelonephritis	++	++++	0	0	0	0	0
Chronic renal disease	++	++	++	++	+++	++	+++
Diabetic nephropathy	++	0–+	0–+	+	++	++	++
Acute renal failure	++	0	0	++	+++	0	0

Abnormal urinalysis findings and various disease conditions

Chapter 14

Glomerulonephritis

Martha Savage Payne

Glomerulonephritis refers to an inflammatory process affecting the renal glomerulus. About two thirds of all patients with chronic renal failure have some form of glomerular disease.[1] These include both the primary glomerular diseases, in which the glomeruli are the sole or predominant tissue involved, and those associated with many systemic diseases.

The nomenclature of glomerular disease is constantly undergoing revision as new clinicopathologic entities emerge, based on studies using various sophisticated techniques. Renal biopsy has become a very important tool in the diagnosis of glomerular disease, and there are terms commonly used to describe pathological lesions seen in renal biopsy. *Focal* has been used to indicate changes present only in some glomeruli, whereas *generalized* means that all the glomeruli are involved. *Segmental* means that changes are present only in part of the glomerulus while other parts are spared. For example, most focal lesions are also segmental. *Diffuse,* on the other hand, means changes involving most or all of the glomeruli in their entirety. *Membranous* refers to the thickening of the glomerular capillary wall that may result from the development of immune deposits in the glomerular structures. In electron microscopy, deposits are described by their location. *Subendothelial deposits* are between the endothelial cell and the capillary basement membrane. *Intramembranous deposits* are within the basement membrane, and *subepithelial* deposits are outside the basement membrane underneath the epithelial cell (see Fig. 14-1).

A *crescent* is a sickle-shaped collection of epithelial cells and macrophages along the inside wall of Bowman's capsule but external to the glomerular capillaries. It is believed that the leakage of fibrin into the capsule causes this inflammatory response. The finding of crescents on renal biopsy indicates severe glomerular injury.

Proliferative changes in a glomerulus refers to an increased number of endocapillary or extracapillary cells. The endocapillary cells may be either endothelial or mesangial cells. The extracapillary cells may be either epithelial cells or blood-derived cells such as neutrophils or macrophages.

ETIOLOGY AND PATHOPHYSIOLOGY

The etiology of most glomerular disease is unknown. Present theory, based on experimental animal models, clinical observation, and immunohistochemical detection of IgG and mediators such as complement, suggests that most, if not all, forms of human glomerulonephritis are mediated by an immunologic mechanism.[2] Most cases of glomerulonephritis are associated with some form of immune deposits. These may be antibodies to circulating antigens that form soluble immune complexes in the circulation and are subsequently trapped in the glomerulus, or may be antibodies to antigens that have been trapped nonimmunologically in the glomerulus. In other cases they may be antibodies to portions of the glomerular basement membrane itself. These deposits may damage the glomeruli and may also activate other portions of the immune system such as the complement system, leukocytes (neutrophils, monocytes, and T-lymphocytes), coagulation factors, and possibly kinins and prostaglandins. All of these can become involved in an inflammatory reaction that damages the glomeruli, resulting in the hematuria, proteinuria, decreased renal function, and edema and/or hypertension associated with the glomerular diseases.

The glomerular capillary wall normally permits a high rate of fluid filtration but markedly restricts the passage of macro molecules, such as protein; therefore, the urine of a normal individual contains very little protein. Experimental evidence suggests that this results from a discrete structural barrier of the glomerulus as well as a charge-selective characteristic of the capillary wall.[3] Negatively-charged component(s) of the capillary wall may result in an electrostatic hindrance to circulating, negatively-charged proteins. The large size and shape of the proteins are also factors in their restricted passage through the small pores of the glomerular membrane. In glomerular disease, such as minimal change lesion, little structural damage is noted in the glomerulus, but massive amounts of negatively-charged albumin are excreted. Experimental evidence suggests that this is due to loss of glomerular fixed-negative charges.[3] No evidence exists for change in the structural barrier or pore size of the glomerulus. In more severe inflammatory diseases of the glomerulus, greater structural damage occurs within the glomerulus and large, protein-perme-

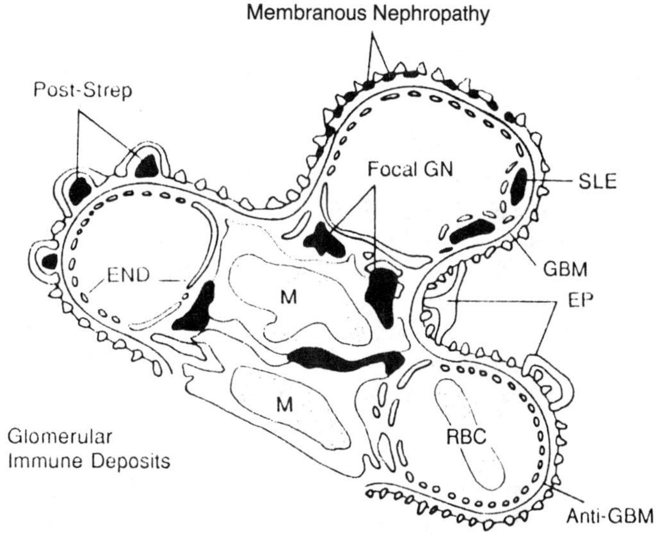

Figure 14-1 **Diagrammatic representation of three glomerular capillary loops and a mesangial area (dark shading) illustrating the types of immune deposits seen in glomerulonephritis. Deposits in the mesangium and along the subendothelial surface of the basement membrane may result from trapping of circulating immune complexes. They are characteristic of focal nephritis (mesangial deposits) or of diffuse proliferative lupus nephritis and type I mesangiocapillary glomerulonephritis (subendothelial deposits). The linear deposits by immunofluorescence seen in anti-GBM antibody disease, the finely granular deposits on the subepithelial surface of the capillary wall characteristic of membranous nephropathy, and the subepithelial humps of poststreptococcal glomerulonephritis probably form locally. END = endothelial cell; EP = epithelial cell; GBM = glomerular basement membrane; M = mesangium; RBC = red blood cell; SLE = systemic lupus erythematosus. (Modified from Latta H. In Geiger SR, Orloff J, Berliner RW (eds): Handbook of Physiology, Sec. 8: Renal Physiology, p. 19. Washington, DC, American Physiological Society, 1973)**

able pores develop. A size- and charge-dependent flux of protein ensues, evidenced by large amounts of both albumin and large proteins such as IgG.[3]

The hematuria of glomerulonephritis is also associated with the immunologically damaged glomerular membrane barrier. Marked disruption in its integrity allows red cells to be pushed through these gaps in the glomerular basement membrane because of the pulsatile capillary hydraulic pressure and the deformability of the red cell.[4]

The reduction in total kidney glomerular filtration rate (GFR) is a result of the alteration in the filtering surface area and/or intrinsic hydraulic conductivity of the capillary wall of the glomerulus or the loss of entire nephron units in a focal manner.

The edema and/or hypertension is a manifestation of the salt and water retention that leads to the expansion of extracellular fluid volume in the peripheral capillary circulation.[5]

Glomerular diseases may be grouped together into patterns primarily based on clinical onset, progression, and pathology shown on renal biopsy. These include acute glomerulonephritis, rapidly progressive glomerulonephritis, chronic glomerulonephritis, recurrent or primary hematuria with few or no symptoms, and nephrotic syndrome.[5] These syndromes may appear with primary glomerular disease or in association with various multisystem, infectious, drug-induced or hereditary diseases.

Acute *poststreptococcal glomerulonephritis (PSGN)* is related to a recent group A beta-hemolytic streptococcal infection of the skin or the pharynx.[6] Only certain strains of group A beta strep are capable of inducing nephritis. M type 12 is the nephritogenic strain most commonly encountered, but more than ten others have been identified.[7] The latent period between the pharyngitis and the ensuing nephritis is usually 1 to 2 weeks, with the attack rate being less than 5%. In the skin infection with group A beta-hemolytic streptococcal infection, the latent period is usually longer (3 weeks) and the attack rate can be 25% to 50%.[6] Children are most commonly affected, but PSGN can occur at any age.

The exact mechanism of the pathogenesis of poststreptococcal glomerulonephritis is unknown. The latent period between infection and onset of nephritis, the granular immune deposits in glomeruli seen on renal biopsy, and the hypocomplementemia suggest an immune complex disease. However, the identification of antigen from nephritogenic streptococci in the glomeruli of such patients has not been very successful. It has been suggested that nephritogenic streptococci release an enzyme capable of altering IgG to the extent that these patients develop antibody to their own altered IgG. These immune complexes may be involved in the pathogenesis of the disease.[8] The exact role of these mechanisms is still unclear and will only be resolved by further investigation.

Although renal biopsies are not usually performed when poststreptococcal glomerulonephritis is the presumptive diagnosis, much has been learned of the pathology of PSGN from percutaneous renal biopsies that have been done on a widespread basis in the last several decades. Early in the course of the disease a typical picture emerges. On tissue sections using light microscopy, all the glomeruli are uniformly involved and appear bloodless and hypercellular as a result of proliferation of mesangial and endothelial cells as well as infiltration of neutrophils, monocytes, and sometimes eosinophils in the glomerular capillaries.[9] In a few cases cellular crescents may form from extensive accumulation of cells in Bowman's capsule. This is the exception rather than the rule, and may be associated with a more grave prognosis.

Electron microscopy shows discrete electron-dense, dome-shaped deposits projecting outward from the epithelial side of the basement membrane (see Fig. 14-1). With immunofluorescence, bright diffuse granular staining for IgG and/or C3 is found along the glomerular basement membrane and in early glomerulonephritis in mesangial deposits.[1]

While PSGN is the most common postinfectious glomerulonephritis, its incidence has significantly decreased in developed countries, making other forms of postinfectious glomerulonephritis relatively more common in those countries. Infections associated with glomerulonephritis are listed at left on page 161. In the majority of cases, kidney involvement is mild and reversible. Occasionally, however, progression to renal failure occurs even when the infection is controlled.[10]

Rapidly progressive glomerulonephritis (RPGN), also referred to as subacute glomerulonephritis or extracapillary proliferative glomerulonephritis, is a term used to refer to a clinical syndrome that presents with an abrupt or insidious onset of acute nephritis accompanied by a rapid and progressive decline in renal function. Without treatment, this syndrome will progress to end stage renal disease in a short period of time (weeks or months).[1] This syndrome may accompany a number of infectious diseases or multisystem dis-

Infectious Agents/Syndromes Associated with Acute Glomerulonephritis

Bacterial

Group A streptococci
Viridans streptococcus
Pneumococcal infections
Klebsiella pneumoniae
Hemophilus influenzae
H. aphrophilus
Shunt infections with *Staphylococci, diphtheroids, Corynebacterium bovis, Propionibacterium acnes*
Brucellosis
Typhoid fever
Legionnaires' disease

Viral and Mycoplasmal

Hepatitis B
Mumps
Measles
Varicella-zoster
Echovirus
Coxsackie
Infectious mononucleosis
Dengue hemorrhagic fever
Mycoplasma pneumoniae

Fungal

Candida albicans

Protozoal

Plasmodium malariae
Plasmodium falciparum
Toxoplasma gondii

Heminthic

Schistosoma mansoni

Spirochetes

Treponema pallidum (syphilis)
Leptospirosis

eases, such as Goodpasture's syndrome, or be a primary (idiopathic) renal disease. The diseases that have been associated with RPGN are listed below. Idiopathic RPGN, which is a primary glomerular disease, affects older persons and has a male predominance of 2 : 1.[1] No consistent antecedent event, such as toxic exposure or viral prodrome, has been identified.

One type of RPGN is associated with Goodpasture's syndrome, which is clearly mediated by antibodies directed against the glomerular basement membrane (GBM). In addition to the glomerulonephritis there is lung hemorrhage. In order to be considered Goodpasture's syndrome, all three ele-

Disorders Associated with Rapidly Progressive Glomerulonephritis

In Primary Glomerular Diseases

Primary rapidly progressive glomerulonephritis with crescent formation
  Antiglomerular basement membrane disease
  Immune complex disease
Mesangiocapillary glomerulonephritis
Membranous nephropathy with crescents
IgA nephropathy (Berger's disease)
Focal and segmental glomerulosclerosis

After Infectious Diseases

Poststreptococcal glomerulonephritis
Bacterial endocarditis
Visceral abscesses
Shunt nephritis
Other infections (*e.g.*, hepatitis B)

In Association With Multisystem Diseases

Systemic lupus erythematosus
Henoch-Schönlein syndrome
Goodpasture's syndrome
Cryoglobulinemia
Polyarteritis and other vasculitides
Wegener's granulomatosis
Lung cancer, lymphoma

ments must be present: (1) nephritis, (2) antiGBM antibody, and (3) pulmonary hemorrhage.[11]

Renal biopsy reveals extensive extracapillary proliferation or crescent formation (50% or more of the glomeruli) in Bowman's capsule.[12] The infiltrated cells that, along with fibrin, form the crescents are probably macrophages derived from blood monocytes. These cells undergo proliferation and epitheloid transformation upon exposure to the fibrinogen and fibrin polymers that have escaped into Bowman's capsule.

The variability of the immunofluorescence findings reflects the variation in the underlying mechanisms of this disease syndrome.[13] In one third of the cases, linear deposits of IgG and C3 indicate involvement of antiglomerular basement membrane (antiGBM) antibodies (see Fig. 14-1). Circulating antiGBM antibodies are also found in these patients. Another one third of the cases will have granular deposits of immunoglobulin (IgG and/or IgM, sometimes with C3), which suggests an immune-complex-mediated disease. Another third have no immunoglobulin deposits, linear or granular, which suggests a nonimmunological or possibly a cell-mediated basis for the disease. This group of patients is generally older, except when their disease is associated with Goodpasture's disease, for which the typical patient is 30 to 40 years of age and male.

Chronic glomerulonephritis is a vague, all-inclusive term referring to progressive diminished renal function that often has an insidious onset and, over a 5- to 10-year or longer course, leads to end stage renal disease. Thus, chronic glomerulonephritis is not a disease entity, but can be caused by many glomerular diseases and results in persistent and usually deteriorating renal functional abnormalities.[7] If it is detected early by routine screening, the only manifestations may be abnormal urine sediment, proteinuria, and mildly reduced renal function. The final stage of this syndrome is total renal failure with uremia.

The basic initiating process may subside, but the progressive loss of renal function through destruction of the glomerular capillary bed may persist.[14] The exact mechanism is unknown, but may be related to the adaptive hemodynamic events arising from the initial loss of filtering surface area, which include increase in glomerular capillary pressure and flow. This process may then damage the remaining capillaries and set up a vicious cycle of destruction of the glomerular capillary beds.

Recurrent or primary hematuria is a clinical syndrome characterized by persistant or recurrent hematuria (gross or microscopic) that is caused by glomerular capillary hemorrhage. This occurs in the absence of systemic diseases involving renal tissue, lesions within the lower urinary tract, and other major signs of renal disease. Proteinuria may be present, and is mild. Renal biopsy is probably unnecessary in the evaluation of every patient with primary hematuria, but when it is performed, many patients (30%–50%) with recurrent hematuria of a glomerular origin are found to have focal glomerulonephritis.[15] This term refers to the finding of inflammatory changes in some of the glomeruli while adjacent glomeruli appear normal. These changes are also seen in association with such systemic diseases as systemic lupus erythematosus, polyarteritis nodosa, Wegener's granulomatosus, subacute bacterial endocarditis, Henoch-Schönlein syndrome, and early Goodpasture's syndrome.[7] These diseases must be ruled out in recurrent hematuria by clinical and laboratory data. About 20% to 50% of hematuria patients reveal a diffuse mesangial proliferation sometimes resembling poststreptococcal glomerulonephritis.[7] The remaining patients reveal more advanced lesions, such as diffuse proliferative glomerulonephritis with variable crescentic involvement.

The immunofluorescence patterns have also been variable. Some patients may have IgM and/or IgG with C3 deposits.[7] Some studies have shown that as many as 50% of patients have extensive granular deposits of IgA in the mesangium, usually in association with IgG and C3. This syndrome is referred to as *IgA mesangial nephropathy* or *Berger's disease.* Other patterns of IgG and/or C3 deposits may be seen, or, in some cases, no IgG or C3 deposits are seen at all.

IgA nephropathy (Berger's disease) is a primary renal disease in which IgA is the principal glomerular immunoglobulin. Renal biopsy usually reveals a focal and segmental proliferative glomerulonephritis. Electron microscopy usually reveals homogeneous electron-dense deposits in the mesangium of the glomeruli (see Fig. 14-1). The diagnostic immunofluorescence pattern is granular deposits of IgA in the mesangium.[16] In a high percentage of the biopsies, IgG is found in the same pattern as IgA, leading some to call the entity IgA/IgG nephropathy.[17] Also, IgM, C3, properdin, and fibrin deposits have been found in the mesangial areas. The pathogenesis is unknown; however, the presence of IgA and C3, but not early-acting C components, suggests that it is a circulatory immune-complex-mediated disease involving prominent activation of the alternate C pathway.

Henoch-Schönlein syndrome is characterized by multiorgan involvement: dermal (skin purpura), gastrointestinal (colic and bleeding), articular (arthritis of the ankles and knees), and renal (IgA nephropathy). The renal biopsy reveals findings similar to those for IgA nephropathy (Berger's disease).[32]

Hereditary nephritis (Alport's syndrome) occurs in families by variable modes of inheritance. Renal failure seems to be preferentially linked with the X chromosomes.[18] Men are involved more frequently and with more severe disease than are women. The glomerular alterations by light microscopy are nondescript, and immunofluorescence studies are generally negative. The electron microscopy picture is the most diagnostic, with thinning, splitting, and a moth-eaten appearance of the glomerular capillary basement membrane.[18] Table 14-1 outlines characteristics of several inflammatory glomerulonephritis conditions.

CLINICAL MANIFESTATIONS

Acute glomerulonephritis, or the *nephritic syndrome,* is typified by the sudden onset over a matter of hours to days of hematuria, oliguria, hypertension, proteinuria, and symptoms of uremia. All five abnormalities do not have to be present to establish the diagnosis, but hematuria is necessary in combination with at least one of the other four abnormalities. The syndrome of acute renal failure may supervene, and systemic complications of

Table 14-1 ***Inflammatory Glomerulonephritis, Hematuria, Red Blood Cell Casts, Proteinuria***

Primary	Age	Renal Function at Presentation	Serum C3	Serum C4	Prognosis	Other
Acute post-streptococcal	Childhood	Sl ↓	↓ for 2–12 weeks	↓ to Nl	Good	ASO or antiDNase B usually positive
Idiopathic crescentic glomerulo-nephritis	Young males > female	↓	Nl or ↓	Nl or ↓	Poor; 80% progress to renal failure	Antiglomerular basement membrane antibody
Recurrent hematuria (IgA nephropathy)	Young males > female	Nl	Nl	Nl	Good; 15% progress to renal failure	
Hereditary nephritis (↓ hearing)	Young adults	Variable	Nl	Nl	Renal failure in men	

azotemia and hypertension may occur, such as congestive heart failure, salt and water retention, edema, central nervous system manifestations, and electrolyte and acid-base disturbances. These complications are not unique to glomerular diseases, and can result from any form of renal injury sufficient to produce acute renal failure. When the signs and symptoms develop over a 4- to 8-week period, the resulting syndrome is often referred to as *subacute* or *rapidly progressive renal failure.*

A number of patients may present with persistent hematuria (with or without proteinuria). The individuals may have mild renal insufficiency that may ultimately progress and result in a nephrotic or a nephritic syndrome or in a relentless progressive deterioration in renal function ultimately ending in end stage renal failure.

Poststreptococcal glomerulonephritis classically presents with an abrupt onset of hematuria (microscopic or gross), proteinuria (less than 3.0 grams per day in 80% of cases), edema, hypertension, and varying degrees of renal dysfunction.[7] However, a broad range of severity of disease exists, from entirely asymptomatic cases detected by the incidental finding of microscopic hematuria to oliguric acute renal failure. The patient usually reports a low amount of urine (oliguria) and a smoky or rusty appearance to the urine (hematuria). Dysuria may be present in a few cases with gross hematuria, but severe loin or abdominal pain is generally not a presenting symptom. Since there is considerable variability in the presenting features of acute poststreptococcal glomerulonephritis, anyone presenting with edema, oliguria, hypertension, and circulatory congestion should have a urine sediment examination and urine protein quantitation.

Clinically, *RPGN* presents with a 4- to 8-week or sometimes more abrupt onset of severe oliguria or even anemia. The presenting complaints usually relate primarily to the uremia and/or fluid retention. Fever, myalgia, and abdominal pain are other features that are sometimes present. Hypertension is typically mild. The RPGN associated with Goodpasture's syndrome includes lung hemorrhage as a clinical finding, in addition to the symptoms associated with the glomerulonephritis.

In *recurrent hematuria,* the patient presents with either persistent or recurrent hematuria with or without mild proteinuria. Other primary renal diseases and systemic diseases that involve the kidney and lower urinary tract bleeding must be excluded by the laboratory and by radiological and endoscopic examination.

IgA nephropathy occurs most commonly in young patients from the ages of 16 to 35 years. The man-to-woman ratio of occurrence of this disease is 2 : 1.[19] Berger's disease is one of the most common of the primary glomerular diseases.

The most common clinical presentation of IgA mesangial nephropathy is recurring episodes of gross (macroscopic) hematuria immediately following or concurrent with upper respiratory infections, which may confuse the initial diagnosis with PSGN. Low-grade fever along with a loin pain or dysuria may accompany the hematuria; therefore, bacterial hemorrhagic cystitis must be ruled out. Blood pressure is usually normal but may be elevated, especially in advanced disease. Reversible acute renal failure may occur with episodes of macroscopic hematuria.

Most patients with Berger's disease have a chronic course, with recurrent episodes of gross and/or microscopic hematuria that may last for years. A certain percentage (up to 25%) of patients show a progressive loss of renal failure over several years. It has been estimated that 1% to 2% of patients will enter end stage renal failure each year from time of diagnosis.[7] Clinical features that indicate a poorer prognosis include older age, decreased GFR at time of onset, hypertension, and nephrotic range proteinuria.

LABORATORY ANALYSES AND DIAGNOSIS

The laboratory findings in acute glomerulonephritis include hematuria, red blood cell (RBC) casts in urine sediment, proteinuria, decreased clearances due to a diminished GFR, and imbalance in serum electrolytes due to sodium and fluid retention. The renal dysfunction involving sodium and water retention probably reflects a reduction in glomerular function with intact tubular function. Clinically, this results in edema and, in severe cases, massive fluid retention with circulatory overload and congestive heart failure. The urinary sodium and calcium are reduced. The patient may exhibit a mild dilutional hyponatremia and hyperchloremia and acidosis with mild hyperkalemia. The blood urea nitrogen (BUN) may be increased disproportionately to the serum creatinine (see Chap. 20).[7]

The presence of RBCs in the urine (hematuria) is a necessary diagnostic sign of the nephritic syndrome. Although hematuria may be associated with many other urinary tract abnormalities, if red cell casts are found, the RBCs are known to have a renal origin (see Chap. 20 for discussion of cast formation). An inflammatory glomerulonephritic urine that contains RBCs, especially with RBC casts, is said to have an *active sediment* because these findings suggest an active inflammatory process in the kidney. The combination of RBCs, RBC casts, and proteinuria is also commonly called a *nephritic sediment.* It should be noted that, to best identify RBC casts on urine microscopic examination, a large aliquot of urine should be spun lightly and the sediment gently resuspended. It is best if the sample is very fresh and the urine *p*H is acidic. Scanning along the edge of the coverslip will also facilitate the important finding of RBC casts. Several authors have noted that the RBCs in acute glomerulonephritis are dysmorphic (fragmented, distorted, and poorly hemoglobinized)[20, 21] because of the shearing stresses to their surfaces when they are forced through the gaps in the GBM of the immunologically damaged glomerulus. This finding can be important, especially in primary recurrent hematuria, because it helps to establish that the RBCs are of glomerular origin rather than from the lower urinary tract.

Most patients with glomerulonephritis present with proteinuria caused by increased permeability of the glomerulus. In selective proteinuria with mostly albumin in the urine, the cause is probably the loss of glomerular fixed charge. In unselective proteinuria, both albumin and large-molecular-weight proteins are in the urine due both to loss of the glomerular fixed charge and to the existence of large pores developed because of the damage to the glomerulus. There may be moderate amounts of protein lost (less than 3.0 grams per day) or heavy proteinuria (greater than 3.5 grams per day), which is seen in the nephrotic syndrome[1] (see Fig. 14-2).

In *PSGN,* throat cultures will be positive in only 50% of those patients appearing with nephritis, but many will have elevated antistreptolysis-O (ASO) titers (above 200 Todd units in about 90% of patients).[22] Patients with streptococcal skin infections may have elevated ASO titers, and may have other streptococcal antibodies such as antistreptokinase, antihyaluronidase, and antiDNase B and antiNADase.[23] The Streptozyme test (Wampole Laboratories) may also be used. It detects five antibodies to extracellular breakdown products of the organism. Although less specific, it is more sensitive to streptococcal infection than any of the above tests used alone.

A very important laboratory parameter in the investigation of acute glomerulonephritis is the serial estimation of complement (C) components. In PSGN, serum C3 levels are very depressed. However, Clq, C4, and C2 are only slightly decreased or normal. Properdin levels are decreased in about 60% of cases. This pattern suggests complement activation by the alternate pathway. The serum C3 levels are depressed for from 2 to 12 weeks, and then usually return to normal levels.[24] If C3 levels do not return to normal, this suggests a poor prognosis or possibly a different glomerular disease such as membranoproliferative glomerulonephritis. The degree of depression of C3 levels is not related to disease severity or prognosis. Elevation of cryoglobulins and immune complexes is frequently detectable,[25] and may play a role in the pathogenesis of the disease.

The patient with acute glomerulonephritis usually has a slight normocytic, normochromic anemia and hypoalbuminemia, probably as a result of the retention of fluid and circulatory congestion. About

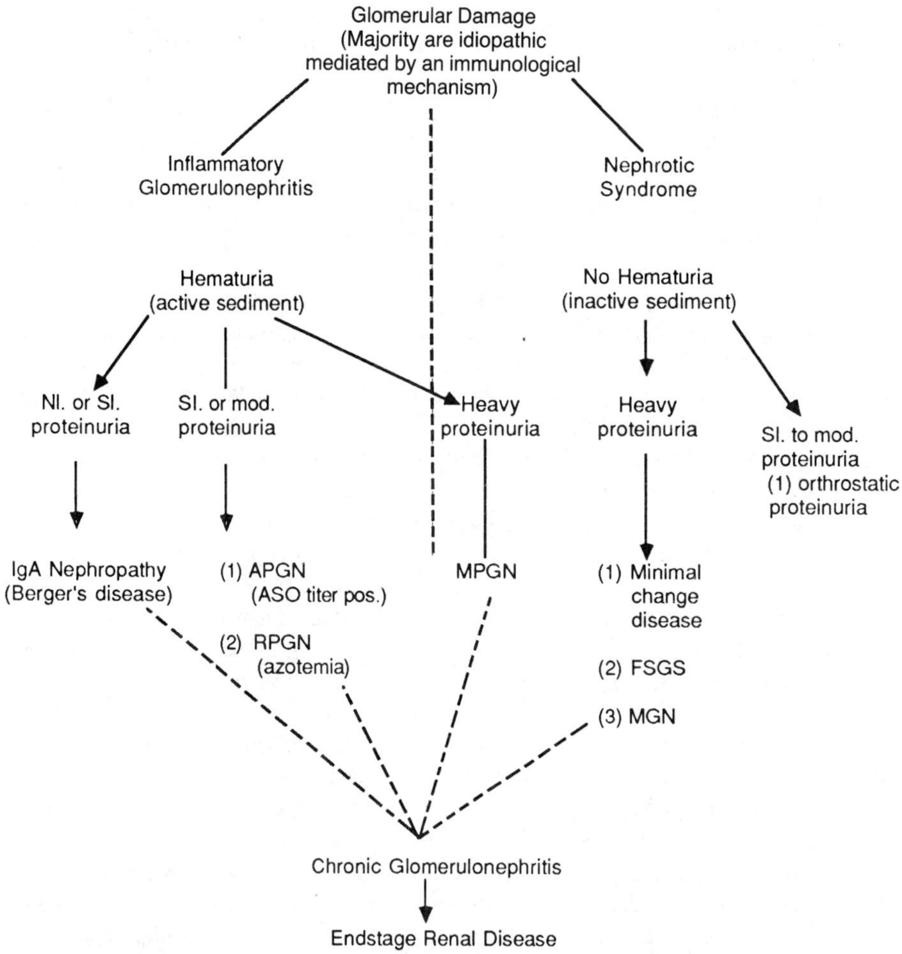

Figure 14-2 **Glomerular disorders. NL = normal; SL = slight; APGN = acute poststreptococcal glomerulonephritis; RPGN = rapidly progressive glomerulonephritis; FSGS = focal and segmental glomerulosclerosis; MGN = membraneous glomerulonephritis; MPGN = mesangial proliferative glomerulonephritis; broken line = from disorders indicates they may lead to chronic glomerulonephritis.**

20% of patients with acute poststreptococcal glomerulonephritis who have a case severe enough to require hospitalization have a frank nephrotic syndrome.[7] They may also exhibit hyperlipemia, seen in nephrotic syndrome for a short time.

In *RPGN,* the urinalysis reveals a nephritic (active) sediment with hematuria, dysmorphic red blood cells, and RBC casts. Proteinuria, which is nonselective, is a consistent finding but usually is not in the nephrotic range. Azotemia develops early in the course of the disease and increases at a rapid rate. Goodpasture's syndrome has similar laboratory findings.

Early in the course of *chronic glomerulonephritis,* when there are no clinical symptoms, routine laboratory screening test abnormalities (urinalysis and chemistry profile) are the only detectable manifestations of the disease. Any combination of abnormal urine sediment with RBCs and RBC casts, proteinuria, or mildly reduced renal function with elevated creatinine or BUN may be present. The final stage of this syndrome is total renal failure with uremia (see Chap. 20).

Laboratory findings in *IgA mesangial nephropathy* (Berger's disease) reveal recurrent macroscopic hematuria, usually with persistent microscopic hematuria. Dysmorphic erythrocytes may be seen in the urine.[26] Proteinuria is absent or mild, with excretion of less than 1 gram per day in 60% of cases. The GFR is usually normal on presentation but, in the majority of cases, shows a slowly progressive decline over many years.[27]

Serological studies (cryoglobulins, rheumatoid factor, and antinuclear factors) are usually normal. In 50% of patients there is an increased IgA concentration in the serum.[28] Complement component levels are typically normal or elevated. Skin biopsy usually reveals dermal capillary deposits of IgA, C3, properdin, and fibrin, which are similar to the pattern seen in the renal biopsy.[29]

The laboratory findings related to the renal involvement in *Henoch-Schönlein syndrome* include hematuria and proteinuria.[32]

Laboratory Monitoring

The laboratory plays a key role in both diagnosis of glomerulonephritis and also follow-up of glomerular disease syndromes. Laboratory monitoring is needed to monitor the severity of renal impairment and to manage fluid and electrolyte disorders. To help in identifying the clinical syndromes, the laboratory data base should include a complete urinalysis, complete blood count, and the following analyses of blood or serum: urea nitrogen, creatinine, sodium, potassium, chloride, CO_2, phosphorus, calcium, and uric acid.[30] Supplemental data should include a 24-hour protein excretion, urine protein electrophoresis, urine cultures, and serial measurements of serum creatinine or GFR and of 24-hour urine volume.[30] The serial estimation of complement components is a very important laboratory parameter utilized in the investigation of patients with glomerulonephritis.

Diagnosis of glomerular disease is made by history and physical examination along with the data provided by the laboratory. Selected laboratory tests including urea nitrogen, creatinine, and electrolyte analyses are used to follow the progress of the disease and to evaluate when supportive therapy such as hemodialysis is needed.

SECONDARY GLOMERULAR DISEASES THAT PRESENT WITH A NEPHRITIC PICTURE

Many diseases have a renal component and have manifestations of glomerular disease, but the renal involvement is only one part of the total clinical picture. Sometimes the renal involvement may be subtle, or it may be responsible for the presenting symptoms. Thus it is very important to consider the possibility of these disorders when a patient presents with renal abnormalities, and appropriate laboratory tests such as antinuclear antibodies for systemic lupus erythematosus, blood cultures for bacterial endocarditis, and cryoglobulins should be performed to facilitate the differential diagnosis.

Systemic Lupus Erythematosus (SLE)

Renal involvement in SLE can present in several different clinicopathologic ways. It is clearly immunologically predicated, with the antigen being DNA (see also Chap. 55). Immune complexes composed of DNA and antibodies to DNA are localized in glomerular capillaries, where they bind and activate complement via the classic pathway initially. When glomerular injury is intense, a typical "nephritic urine sediment" of RBC and RBC casts will occur, frequently accompanied by proteinuria, hypertension, and varying degrees of renal failure.[18]

Several histologic types of lesions are seen on renal biopsy. Focal proliferative glomerulonephritis of SLE is characterized by areas of focal and segmental cellular proliferation, with or without polymorphonuclear leukocyte infiltration. Diffuse proliferative glomerulonephritis is a much more serious disorder, with a high mortality rate unless reversed either spontaneously or by intervention with immunosuppressive agents. The membranous form of SLE glomerulonephritis is discussed in Chapter 19. Immunofluorescence demonstrates variable results, usually with any combination of the immunoglobulins being present. Electron microscopy shows large, dense deposits that are usually subendothelial in location[18] (see Fig. 14-1).

Renal failure is the leading cause of death from lupus nephritis, even though the course is highly variable and is sometimes punctuated by spontaneous remissions and exacerbations. Many patients respond dramatically to the use of high doses of corticosteroids.

Necrotizing Vasculitis

Vasculitic disorders occur in several distinct clinical forms, including polyarteritis nodosa, microscopic polyarteritis (hypersensitivity angitis), Wegener's granulomatosis, or with mixed cryoglobulins.[28] All types may have an associated glomerulonephritis, with the typical clinical findings of a nephritic urine sediment and elevated BUN and creatinine. The histologic appearance is often characterized by the presence of numerous crescents, and the patient's condition often progresses rapidly to uremia.[18] About 50% of cases demonstrate immune deposits by immunofluorescence.[18] Aggressive treatment with corticosteroids and cyclophosphamide may produce dramatic improvement, especially in the small vessel types.[18]

Bacterial Endocarditis

Bacterial endocarditis produces several types of vessel injury. These range from gross infarctions, secondary to emboli, to renal abscesses, focal and segmental glomerular injury, and diffuse proliferative glomerulonephritis.[31] The last two forms of glomerulonephritis both result from immune complex injury and are associated with reduced levels of serum complement. Each of the forms of glomerulonephritis are accompanied by variable degrees of renal impairment, which is usually less severe in the focal segmental form. Each of these will respond to irradication of the bacterial antigen by appropriate antibiotic therapy.

TREATMENT

The therapy for most of the glomerulonephritis syndromes is predominantly supportive and directed toward prevention and management of the potentially lethal complications of uremia, hyperkalemia, hypertensive encephalopathy, and pulmonary edema.[33] The laboratory provides the data (serum potassium and urea nitrogen) to monitor the first two complications.

The treatment for PSGN and other infective types of glomerulonephritis is primarily symptomatic and supportive. Appropriate antibiotic therapy is given if persistent infection is present. Sodium restriction is critical in managing hypertension, congestive heart failure, and edema. Temporary dialysis may be required if the renal failure is severe enough.

The prognosis, especially in children, is quite favorable, with 95% recovering normal renal function within 2 months. Some, however, may exhibit minimal hematuria and proteinuria for more than 2 years, and, rarely, a patient may develop end stage renal failure. The more severe cases usually occur in older patients. The vast majority of patients experience a spontaneous diuresis accompanied by resolution of circulatory congestion, edema, and hypertension within a week of onset. Prolonged oliguria or anuria exceeding 1 week's duration is observed in only 5% to 10% of patients.[33] No therapeutic maneuver will influence the severity of renal dysfunction or promote histologic healing.

In the case of RPGN, the prognosis is not good, with 50% to 70% of the patients requiring maintenance hemodialysis within 6 months of onset of symptoms. Various treatments, including intermittent "pulse" high-dose steroids, plasma exchange, cytotoxic agents, and anticoagulant therapy, have been tried with varying success. Current evidence seems to indicate a favorable role for the use of plasmapheresis and immunosuppression in the RPGN of Goodpasture's syndrome.[34]

No specific therapy is indicated for patients who have recurrent hematuria or IgA nephropathy, because most patients do not have the progressive form of the disease. Treatment for this syndrome is supportive only.

CASE STUDY

A 54-year-old man was admitted to the hospital with marked cellulitis of the left knee. Five to six weeks prior to admission the patient had traumatized ("scraped") his left knee. This was followed by minimal erythema and tenderness, progressing to a more widespread area over the next 4 weeks. One week prior to admission the patient developed fever, chills, and progressive edema. He was found to be oliguric and in acute renal failure. His blood pressure was 70/50.

The patient was started on acute dialysis on 7/12. His urine volume increased on 8/6, and acute hemodialysis was stopped. He was discharged 4 weeks after admission, when the acute renal failure had resolved. Pertinent laboratory data follow:

LABORATORY FINDINGS (REFERENCE RANGES)

	7/11	*7/12*	*7/30*	*8/6*	*8/12*
BUN (10–20 mg/dL)	135	153	88	72	41
Creatinine (0.7–1.5 mg/dL)	8.6	9.0	9.2	7.4	3.0
Sodium (135–145 mEq/L)	131	133	131	135	141
Potassium (3.5–5.0 mEq/L)	4.9	5.0	5.1	4.0	3.6
Chloride (95–105 mEq/L)	86	91	99	66	112
Culture of fluid from wound	negative				
WBC (5–10.0 × 10^3/mm^3)	37.3	51.5	13.6	10.5	8.6
Urine blood (neg)	large	large	mod	small	neg
Urine RBC (2–3 RBC/HPF)	40–50	100–150	15–20	2–4	neg
RBC Casts (0/LPF)	1–2	2–4	0	0	0
Urine albumin (neg)	4+	4+	2+	1+	neg
ASO (0–166 Todd units)	333				
Streptozyme (0–100 STZ units)	300				
Complement (C3) (83–177 mg/dL)	87.2	–	99.0	–	–

Conversion to SI units is as follows:
BUN—mg/dL × 0.357 = mmol/L
Creatinine—mg/dL × 88.4 = μmol/L
Sodium—mEq/L × 1 = mmol/L
Potassium—mEq/L × 1 = mmol/L
Chloride—mEq/L × 1 = mmol/L
Complement—mg/dL × 10 = mg/L

Questions

1. What is the most probable cause of acute renal failure?
2. Is the negative culture on the fluid from the wound unexpected?
3. Is the patient's presenting blood pressure unexpectedly low?
4. What is the patient's prognosis?
5. Is it likely that the patient will experience acute renal failure from this cause again?

Discussion

1. The most probable cause of acute renal failure is acute poststreptococcal glomerulonephritis.
2. The negative culture on the fluid from the wound is not unexpected. In group A beta-hemolytic streptococcal skin infections, the latent period is usually 3 weeks. The positive Streptozyme and ASO titer give evidence of a streptococcal infection.
3. Hypertension is usually present. However, when this patient first was admitted to the hospital he was very ill and in acute distress. His blood pressure was somewhat elevated at a later time.
4. The patient's prognosis is favorable. However, because he is older and his renal function did not improve until 4 weeks after admission, his renal function status should be followed with periodic urine proteins and microscopic examination of the urine sediment.
5. Patients do not usually experience poststreptococcal glomerulonephritis a second time. However, the first episode may damage the kidney and possibly begin a chronic process in a small percentage of patients.

REFERENCES

1. Couser WG, Salant DJ, Magda MS: Glomerulonephritis. In Flamenbaum W, Hamburger RJ (eds): Nephrology, pp 265–301. Philadelphia, JB Lippincott, 1982
2. Couser WG, Salant DJ: In situ immune complex formation and glomerular injury. Kidney Int 17:1, 1980
3. Myers B, Okarma T, Friedman S et al: Mechanisms of proteinuria in human glomerulonephritis. J Clin Invest 70:732, 1982
4. Lin JT, Wada H, Maed H et al: Mechanism of hematuria in glomerular disease: An electron microscopic study in the case of diffuse membranous glomerulonephritis. Nephron 35:68, 1983
5. Glassock RJ: Glomerular diseases. In Massry S, Glassock RJ (eds): Textbook of Nephrology, pp 63–67. Baltimore, Williams & Wilkins, 1983
6. Nissenson AR, Baraff LJ, Fine RN et al: Poststreptococcal acute glomerulonephritis: Fact and controversy. Ann Intern Med 91:76, 1979
7. Glassock RJ, Adler SG, Ward HJ et al: Primary glomerular diseases. In Brenner BM, Rector FC Jr (eds): The Kidney, 3rd ed, p 930. Philadelphia, WB Saunders, 1986
8. Rodriguez-Iturbe B, Silva-Beauperthory Y, Parra G et al: Skin window immune response to normal human IgG in patients with rheumatoid arthritis and acute poststreptococcal glomerulonephritis. Am J Clin Pathol 76:270, 1981
9. Sagel I, Treser G, Ty A et al: Occurrence and nature of glomerular lesions after Group A streptococcal infections in children. Ann Intern Med 79:492, 1973
10. Quadracci L, Stricker G: Glomerulonephritis due to other infections. In Massry S, Glassock R (eds): Textbook of Nephrology, pp 6.19–6.26. Baltimore, Williams & Wilkins, 1983
11. Teague C, Doak P, Simpson I et al: Goodpasture's syndrome: An analysis of 29 cases. Kidney Int 13:492, 1978
12. Glassock R: A clinical and immunopathologic dissection of rapidly progressive glomerulonephritis. Nephron 22:253, 1978
13. Morrin P, Hinglais N, Nabarra B et al: Rapidly progressive glomerulonephritis: A clinical and pathologic study. Am J Med 65:446, 1978
14. Brenner BM: Hemodynamically-mediated glomerular injury and the progressive nature of kidney disease. Kidney Int 23:647, 1983
15. Hendler E, Kashgarian M, Hayslett J: Clinicopathological correlation of primary hematuria. Lancet 1:458, 1972
16. Berger J: IgA glomerular deposits in renal disease. Transplant Proc 1:939, 1969
17. Zimmerman SW, Burkholder PM: Immunoglobulin A nephropathy. Arch Intern Med 135:1217, 1975
18. McDonald FD, Briggs WA, Stephen DM: The kidney in systemic conditions. In Flamenbaum W, Hamburger RJ (eds): Nephrology I, pp 391–417. Philadelphia, JB Lippincott, 1982
19. Clarkson AR, Woodroffe AJ, Bannister KM et al: The syndrome of IgA nephropathy. Clin Nephrol 21:7, 1984
20. Fairley KF, Birch DF: Hematuria: A simple method for identifying glomerular bleeding. Kidney Int 21:105, 1982
21. Fassett RG, Horgan BA, Mathew TH: Detection of glomerular bleeding by phase-contrast microscopy. Lancet 1:1432, 1982
22. Rodriguez-Iturbe B, Costillo L, Valbeuna R et al:

Acute poststreptococcal glomerulonephritis: A review of recent developments. Pediatrician 8:307, 1979

23. Dillon HC: Pyoderma and Nephritis. Ann Rev Med 18:207, 1967
24. Sjoholm AG: Complement components and complement activation in acute poststreptococcal glomerulonephritis. Int Arch Allergy Appl Immunol 59:3, 1979
25. Yoshizawa N, Treser G, McClung JA et al: Circulating immune complexes in patients with uncomplicated Group A streptococci pharyngitis and patients with acute poststreptococcal glomerulonephritis. Am J Nephrol 3:23, 1983
26. Kincaid-Smith P, Nicholls P: Mesangial IgA nephropathy. Am J Kidney Dis 3:90, 1983
27. Droz D, Kramar A, Nawar T et al: Primary IgA nephropathy: Prognostic factors: Contrib Nephrol 40:202, 1984
28. McPhaul JJ Jr: IgA-associated glomerulonephritis. Am Rev Med 28:37, 1977
29. Lamperi S, Carozzi S: Skin-muscle biopsy in patients with various nephropathies. Nephron 24:46, 1979
30. Rock R, Walker WG, Jennings CD: Nitrogen metabolite and renal function. In Tietz NW (ed): Fundamentals of Clinical Chemistry. Philadelphia, WB Saunders, 1987
31. Glassock RJ, Cohen AH, Adler SG et al: Secondary glomerular diseases. In Brenner BM, Rector FC Jr (eds): The Kidney, 3rd ed, p 930. Philadelphia, WB Saunders, 1986
32. Ballard HS, Eisinger RP, Gallo G: Renal manifestations of the Henoch-Schönlein syndrome in adults. Am J Med 49:328, 1970
33. Kassirer J: The treatment of acute poststreptococcal glomerulonephritis. Kidney 4:1–6, 1971
34. Erickson S, Kurtz S, Donadio J et al: Use of combined plasmapheresis and immunosuppression in the treatment of Goodpasture's syndrome. Mayo Clin Proc 54:714, 1979

Chapter 15

Transplants

Cynthia Karr

The annual number of renal transplants in the United States is increasing dramatically, and for many persons renal transplant is considered the preferred therapy.[1, 2, 3, 4] Transplantation practices, including laboratory procedures, are continually developing. This chapter will consider current indications for transplantation and pre- and posttransplantation patient monitoring, with emphasis on immunologic testing.

PRETRANSPLANTATION MONITORING

General Assessment

There are many types of renal diseases that are predisposing conditions for renal transplantation. These include glomerulonephritis, pyelonephritis/interstitial nephritis, multisystem disease such as systemic lupus erythematosus, and cystic kidney disease. At least ten criteria must be considered in assessing the transplant candidacy of an individual. Laboratory analyses play a significant role in determining a patient's renal, cardiovascular, gastrointestinal, hepatic, hematologic, immunohematologic, and infectious status. The need for any special pretransplantation therapy, such as blood transfusion to treat anemia or antibiotics for infection, may be identified as well.[5]

Immunologic Assessment

In addition to these general considerations, a major factor in renal transplantation is the "passing" of certain immunologic tests. Major procedures performed involve the major human histocompatibility antigens ABO and class I and class II HLA (human leukocyte antigen) antigens, and the determination of the presence of any recipient antibodies to donor antigens. Incompatibility of these antigens between donor and recipient represents strong immunogenic stimuli that could result in graft rejection. *ABO grouping* is accomplished by direct tests in which the antigens are detected on erythrocytes, and indirect tests in which the opposing serum antibodies are detected by agglutination procedures. Grafting is not generally performed across ABO barriers; if the donor kidney possesses antigens to which the recipient has preformed antibodies, hyperacute allograft rejection would result.

Complement-dependent cytotoxicity testing (CDC) for HLA antigens, as commonly performed using the lymphocytotoxicity test (LCT), constitutes a major immunologic test for donor/recipient selection. It enables the identification of antigens determined by alleles of the class I A, B, C and class II DR loci. The method commonly used is the NIH microlymphocytotoxicity test. Newer molecular biologic procedures are more specific, but less practical.[6] Technical problems include obtaining sufficient numbers of suitable cells uncontaminated by other cells. Required time may be up to six hours, especially if DR typing is included, precluding the typing of cadavers. Errors may arise based on the available specificities and strength of typing sera. Although antigens such as DRw6 are extremely difficult antigens to define, DRw6-positive patients have exhibited poor graft survival in some studies, and optimal DR matching for these individuals is recommended.[7]

A number of factors must be considered in the interpretation of these results. Strict matching requirements have been relaxed and frequently ignored since the introduction of cyclosporine A (Cys A) as an immunosuppressive agent.[2, 5, 6, 8, 9] Nevertheless, reports from both North America and Europe show that A and especially B matching are important for graft survival, and that choosing the best possible match is the best course of action.[2, 5, 8] Matching may be more important in children receiving a cadaver kidney than in adults.[3] Haplotype identity is desirable because this nearly always means that other influential antigens are also shared, and there seems to be a matching dosage effect with two shared haplotypes.[3, 5] DR matching has the effect of A and B matching combined.[1] If individuals can be matched at both DR loci, A and B matching makes no difference; however, if this cannot be done, at least a two-antigen A and B match should be sought.[10] Most transplant units agree that A and B or DR mismatches should not be repeated on subsequent grafts, since the chance of rejection is often increased. One study reported survival at 6 months as 55% and 64% respectively for the worst and best matched kidneys. At 4 years, however, these figures were 18% and 44%, and patients with good matches had lower serum creatinine levels and less glucocorticoid steroid use.[1, 2]

Screening tests are used to detect preformed cytotoxic antibodies. Approximately one-third of potential recipients develop antibodies to antigens of prospective donors. Individuals who possess antibodies that react with a majority of randomly selected panel cells are poor recipient prospects, because they are likely to have a positive crossmatch with the majority of possible donors. Testing a single serum against cells with all HLA antigens can substitute for the performance of multiple crossmatches with all available sera. Cumulative lists of antigens to which the recipient has responded can be used to exclude some donors so that a final crossmatch may be performed with donors lacking these antigens.

Potential recipient sera are usually obtained and tested monthly to expedite selection of a well-matched recipient for any available kidney, since antibodies may persist, disappear, or be newly formed. In the case of a person who has rejected a kidney, serial serum samples must be collected in the immediate postnephrectomy period to aid in the selection of a subsequent graft. Autoantibodies, recognized by their ability to react with all cell panels while at the same time failing to react or giving weak reactions with the B cells of chronic lymphocytic leukemia, are not involved in graft rejection, but they may coexist with anti-HLA antibodies.

Crossmatches are performed to detect the presence of lymphocytotoxic antibodies to donor cells that could mediate graft rejection. The test method of choice is some form of the LCT. Some transplant centers test both T and B cells, and will not transplant when a current positive test is obtained with T cells, B cells, or both.[3] Antibodies reactive with B cells alone, however, may play no role in graft rejection (*e.g.*, autoantibodies), or may be involved in graft rejection (*e.g.*, DR antibodies), or may actually enhance graft survival (*e.g.*, those directed against surface immunoglobulin or even D antigens).[5, 8] Endothelial-monocyte antibodies appear to have a stronger association with irreversible rejection than those directed against B cells, but monocyte crossmatches are not practical. Testing performed with spleen or lymph node cells from cadaveric donors may give weak positive crossmatch results with B cell antibodies. These antibodies may actually be enhancing if there are no anti-HLA class I antibodies also present.

Cold reactive antibodies to B or T cells do not appear to be clinically significant.[1, 3] Antibodies reactive at room temperature or at 37° C may not be harmful; however, warm antibodies to B cells are harmful.[1, 3] An anti-human globulin phase can be added to the classic LCT test to make it more sensitive.[3] Use of chromium-labeled cells may increase sensitivity, as may flow cytometry.[11] Flow cytometry is said to have other advantages, including speed, lack of need for B- and T-cell separation, and ability to detect humoral and cell-mediated lymphocytotoxicity.[11] At an absolute minimum, current sera should be crossmatched, but some centers also test all historically positive sera and some selected past sera.[1, 3, 12] Definitions of "current" sera may vary, from sera obtained in the past 4 to 6 months to sera obtained up to 12 months previously.[1, 13]

Immunologic testing may be less relevant if the recipient is treated with Cys A.[11] Moreover, there is a lack of complete correlation between the positive cytotoxic crossmatch and graft rejection confirming that the interplay between humoral and cellular factors in rejection is still unclear.[5]

In *mixed lymphocyte culture (MLC)* or mixed lymphocyte response, intensity of the reaction of responder T cells to the HLA-D antigens on stimulator cells may be assessed. Compatibility of these class II HLA antigens is critical to graft survival.[3] Because the testing requires up to 7 days, it is of use only in choosing between living related donors who each share only one haplotype identity with the recipient. Alternatively, DR typing may be performed, especially with cadaver donors, since this locus is close to the MLC-stimulating region.[8]

Other *in vitro* and *in vivo* tests may be performed in an attempt to predict the chance of graft rejection. These are research procedures primarily, and for the most part assess the potential recipient's cellular immune responsiveness. Hyporesponsiveness in tests like cell-mediated lympholysis (CML), lymphocyte-mediated cytotoxicity (LMC), and antibody-dependent cell-mediated cytotoxicity (ADCC) tends to indicate the likelihood of long-term graft survival.[5]

POSTTRANSPLANTATION MONITORING

Posttransplantation testing for renal status must take into account immunologic, infectious, urologic, and toxic conditions. Ideally, test procedures should fulfill the following set of criteria: (1) the tests should be sensitive enough to detect evidence of rejection, recurrent renal disease, drug toxicity, and/or infection before irreversible damage is done, so that appropriate preventive measures may be taken; (2) they should be specific enough to allow for a differential diagnosis of the patient's status, because presenting symptoms often overlap; (3) they should be adaptable to the routine rather than to research laboratory situation, with results that are available on the day that the specimen is obtained, and procedures that are inexpensive to allow for multiple testing, are well-standardized, and are quality-controlled; and (4) sufficient specimen should be readily available.

No one test procedure fulfills all these criteria,

but serum creatinine levels are the tests most commonly performed and considered the most useful by some.[14] There are other methods, however, that may be used to help achieve the ultimate goal of maintenance of graft function.

Renal Status

Graft status is of obvious concern during the posttransplantation period. Various clinical stages designated according to their time of occurrence and highlighted by various types of graft rejection may be observed. Since there are still gaps in our knowledge of immunologic mechanisms, biochemical parameters must often be relied on for necessary testing and differential diagnosis.

Hyperacute graft rejection is mediated by preformed antibodies to ABO or HLA antigens on allograft endothelial cells, and it is almost always preventable by adequate pretransplantation screenings.[3] Its occurrence in the first few days posttransplantation is marked by anuria and its most sensitive indication is a decreased platelet count.

Accelerated rejection occurs within the first week and, according to some experts, is most likely antibody-mediated.[3] Marked oliguria or even anuria is present, with an increased BUN and an unchanged or slightly decreased serum creatinine observed in the first 2 days posttransplantation.

Acute rejection is most common and is seen in recipients of all cadaver kidneys, generally within the first 4 months depending upon the type of immunosuppression used. Chances of reversal are good if treatment is instituted early. Diagnosis is dependent upon general monitoring tests of renal function. Increases in the BUN and serum creatinine, a decrease in renal output, and the presence of proteinuria indicate rejection.[15]

Chronic rejection represents a nonreversible process that occurs over months or years and may be seen any time after the first month. Proteinuria, mild azotemia, and a gradual decline in glomerular filtration rate (GFR) as well as decline in other renal function tests signal its presence. Of the available methods to determine GFR, creatinine clearance is probably the most accurate and the most practical for routine clinical use.[15] Diagnosis and differentiation of this and the other types of rejection from recurrent kidney disease, drug toxicity, and infection are often difficult, if not impossible, and are dependent upon not only these tests but histologic and microbiologic findings as well.

Immunologic Testing

By far the greatest difficulty to be overcome with respect to immunologic monitoring is determination of the mechanism(s) of acute and chronic allograft rejection. A specific marker of graft rejection is as yet unknown, so there are a variety of specific assays for various parameters of humoral and cell-mediated responses as well as for nonspecific markers. It is also difficult to compare studies in which there have been nonstandardized tests run on individuals receiving different immunosuppressive regimens.

Looking first at the *humoral immune system,* conflicting results have been obtained regarding the usefulness of immunoglobulin and complement monitoring. One study, however, demonstrated a significant increase in C3d levels in recipients with cytomegalovirus (CMV) infection, in contrast with levels in those undergoing rejection.[16] There is general agreement both that the presence of circulating immune complexes has no significance in acute rejection and that their presence is closely associated with the occurrence of chronic rejection.[17] Lymphocytes capable of lysing erythrocytes, that is, plaque-forming cells, have been associated with rejection, but they also may be seen in infections.[18]

Many investigations have centered around analysis of the cells and processes involved in *cellular responses.* Depending on the type of immunosuppression used, determination of subpopulations of cells—particularly the helper: suppressor (4:8) populations—but not total T-cell quantitation may be useful in certain patients such as diabetics.[1, 4, 12, 19] A 4:8 ratio of less than one may indicate a nephrotoxic condition caused by Cys A or a viral infection.[23] A ratio of less than 1:3 would rule out a diagnosis of rejection unless the patient is receiving antilymphocyte globulin (ALG). While a consistently low ratio may be useful in predicting continued graft function, an increased ratio correlates with rejection for at least 3 weeks following surgery.[4, 20] Results obtained using flow cytometry rather than fluorescent microscopy are more accurate and reproducible.[21] Spontaneous blastogenesis as determined by radioactive thymidine incorporation increases with both infections and rejection, but flow cytometry results on pure lymphocytes in one series predicted more than three-quarters of acute rejection episodes prior to clinical diagnosis.[22, 23] While a negative MLC is no guarantee of graft survival, inhibition of the donor-specific response by recipient serum is bad prognostically, whereas blockage of a positive pretransplantation reaction by recipient lymphocytes is a good sign. Although ADCC and NK analyses are not predictive, the former may aid in determining usefulness of steroids as immunosuppressives.

Nonspecific markers such as B_2 microglobulin (B_2M), C-reactive protein (CRP), and serum amyloid protein (SAA) may also be present in severe infections. Testing for B_2M can be used as a supplemental test, because levels are affected by immune activity and the GFR but are affected to a lesser degree by acute tubular necrosis (ATN) than by serum creatinine changes that are seen later.[24–29] Daily monitoring of CRP levels may be a simple way to predict the severity of rejection, since changes occur only in acute rejection. Monitoring of SAA may likewise be used; it may be performed on anuric or oliguric patients because it is not a renal function test.[30]

Serum creatinine remains the major post-transplantation monitoring test at most institutions, although it is neither as sensitive nor specific as immunologic testing.[14] An elevation of more than 25% suggests allograft rejection, but further evaluation is required. False positive reactions may be seen in hyperglycemia, infection, arterial stenosis, recurrence of the original disease, ureteral obstruction, and lymphocele, although other laboratory tests can rule out the first four possibilities.[31]

Infection

Although the incidence of infection in transplant recipients has decreased, the diagnosis and treatment of infection is very important. Most common are urinary and respiratory tract infections. Viruses are responsible for half of the infections, followed by bacteria, mixed infections, and fungi. The monitoring and differential diagnosis of infections requires that the physician be attuned to unexplained fever and other signs of possible infection. Appropriate laboratory followup would include culturing of specimens for both routine and nonroutine organisms, determining suitable antimicrobial therapy, monitoring hematologic parameters such as white cell counts, and serodiagnosis.

Transplant recipients are particularly predisposed to infections if they are leukopenic, hyperglycemic, over age 40, recipients of a cadaver kidney, and/or receiving high doses of corticosteroids or ALG.[32] There is a decreased incidence of infections in general and CMV infections in particular in recipients on Cys A.[3, 33] Determination of nonresponder status to concanavalin A in a test for migration inhibition factor production may allow for reduction in immunosuppressive drugs.[32]

Blood cultures are important in suspected infections, especially if there are no obvious foci. Fresh, uncontaminated urine should be cultured for urinary tract infections. False negatives may result from forced diuresis, previous antibiotic therapy, low urine *p*H, and/or contamination with antiseptics.[34] Definitive diagnosis of pulmonary infections is based on microbiological techniques. Transtracheal aspirations are preferable to sputum specimens. Bronchial brushings or washings or transbronchial biopsy can be obtained for diffuse lesions, and needle aspirations can be obtained from localized lesions. Counterimmunoelectrophoresis gives rapid results in the detection of pneumococcal antigen in sputum.

Bacterial infections are the most common cause of infection in the first month posttransplantation, with the urinary and respiratory tracts and wound and vascular access sites most frequently involved. Septicemia may follow. Common bacteria are regularly recovered, in contrast to unusual organisms observed in later infections. At the later time, differential diagnosis becomes more difficult because more specialized media, procedures, and technical expertise are required, so the laboratory should be informed of any clinical suspicions. *Listeria monocytogenes* meningoencephalitis, although uncommon, is the infection seen most frequently. Diagnosis of atypical mycobacteria, *Legionella,* and *Nocardia* infections poses other diagnostic problems.

Viruses, especially herpesviruses, either reactivated or introduced in blood transfusions or in the graft, are often implicated in viral infections. In the first month posttransplant, self-limiting herpes simplex infections, rapidly diagnosed by direct tissue immunofluorescence, are the most common. Later, more severe CMV and herpes zoster (HZ) infections are seen. Cellular immune competence can be further suppressed by CMV, leading to an increased risk of other infections. Leukopenia, thrombocytopenia, and temporarily impaired renal function may be seen. Prior testing of recipients would allow for use of kidney and blood seronegative donors in like patients. Epstein-Barr virus (EBV) infections may result in the development of B-cell lymphomas. Although hepatitis B is not associated with impaired graft function, HBsAg-positive recipients frequently have chronic hepatitis, which is associated with increased mortality. Increased aspartate aminotransferase and alanine aminotransferase levels are seen in these individuals. A similar situation may exist with non-A, non-B hepatitis, for which no specific diagnostic laboratory tests exist. Papovaviruses BK and JC may cause ureteric obstruction, with diagnosis being obtained by culture and histologic examination of tissue respectively.

Fungal infections are uncommon. *Candida* should be suspected, especially if the patient is a leukopenic diabetic on steroids. *Cryptococcus* is the second most common cause of late infections. Rapid serodiagnostic antigen detection permits treatment before culture results are available. *Coccidioides immitis, Histoplasma capsulatum,* and *Aspergillus* species may be recovered. Careful interpretation of serodiagnostic antibody tests for the dimorphic fungi is necessary, especially if the patient comes from an endemic region.

Parasites such as *Leishmania donovani, Schistosoma* species, and *Strongyloides stercoralis* should be considered, particularly if the patient comes from an endemic area. Bone marrow, urine, and feces may be screened and routinely checked if warranted. *Toxoplasma gondii* infections may be detected serologically or by demonstration of diagnostic forms in tissue.

Antimicrobial therapy requires laboratory guidance. Use of broad-spectrum antimicrobials could result in the development of resistant organisms. Septicemia, bacterial pneumonia, and neutropenia with fever, however, should be treated aggressively even prior to susceptibility testing. Therapy in septicemia should be reviewed frequently, because failure is common. Nephrotoxic drugs such as amphotericin B, whose efficacy may be affected by dialysis and bone marrow suppressive agents, require more stringent monitoring.

Urologic Parameters

Urologic parameters can be used for determination of rejection, prognosis, type and dosage of immunosuppressive agents, and need for and the monitoring of dialysis. Cells present in the kidney itself have been studied, using traditional renal and fine-needle aspiration biopsy. The presence of the DR antigen on renal tubular cells may be increased during their regeneration, possibly making them more prone to a cellular immune attack. Although subject to sampling error, biopsy is still a powerful diagnostic and prognostic tool that may also uncover evidence of recurrent renal disease and other disorders. Urine output coupled with plasma creatinine levels indicates the need for dialysis, especially in those suffering from hypercalcemia. Assessment of tubular epithelial cells in urine sediment, using immunofluorescence, is not affected by ATN, and may be useful in the early determination of rejection. False-positive results stand at about 20%, and false-negative results may occur if mucus, casts, microorganisms, and other cells interfere.[35]

Tubular cell enzymes such as gamma-glutamyltranspeptidase, N-acetyl B-D-glucose-aminidase, alanine aminopeptidase, and alkaline phosphatase have been reported to be increased in urine in rejection.[22] Preliminary studies using ELISA tests of sera have detected antigen from renal proximal tubule epithelial cells prior to the clinical diagnosis of rejection or drug toxicity.[36]

Immunosuppressive Agents

Since rejection mechanisms are not completely understood, various agents are used in an attempt to counteract the immune system's response to an allogeneic graft. Effects are complex, but primarily these agents interfere with lymphocyte proliferation and/or function, and may also affect the inflammatory response. Levels must be carefully monitored to prevent generalized immunosuppression below safe limits and other side-effects, such as bone marrow depression and nephrotoxicity, that may be confused with graft rejection.

Azathioprine and *prednisone,* as the mainstays of conventional therapy, are the cause of the majority of complications. The former leads to the suppression of leukocyte production, severe oliguria, and proteinuria.[3] Steroids are ideally suited to treat rejection crises, but a few individuals develop diabetes, and the hyperparathyroidism resulting from dose reduction may complicate renal failure.

Antilymphocyte globulin results in thrombocytopenia in up to 50% of patients.[37] Immune complex-based serum sickness is difficult to monitor using any one procedure; however, analysis of peripheral blood lymphocytes with OKT 3 monoclonal antibody is useful, because classic E rosette results tend to be inaccurate, especially in leukopenic patients.

Cyclosporine A (Cys A) has rapidly gained acceptance in transplantation communities because this agent, which primarily inhibits helper T-cell activity, is up to 20% more effective than standard therapy.[2, 9] Unfortunately, this spectacular benefit is marred by side-effects, including hepatotoxicity, hyperuricemia, hyperkalemia, increased incidence of lymphoma and opportunistic infections, and, of the greatest concern, nephrotoxicity.[2, 3, 9] Nephrotoxicity makes early management especially difficult, since a balance must be achieved among immunosuppression, toxicity, and ATN.[9, 38] Monitoring of blood or plasma levels is not reliable in the control of rejection or the avoidance of nephrotoxicity, but it does indicate absorption and facilitate dosage adjustment.[6, 39] It appears that the most effective levels of Cys A are 150 to 400 ng/mL of plasma.[15, 40] Increased serum creatinine and BUN levels, especially if they are rising rapidly during the first 3 months posttransplantation, are likely to signal rejection with Cys A values at or below the lower end of the scale. Higher values observed after this time are usually associated with nephrotoxicity.[3, 37, 38] Both radioimmunoassay (RIA) and high-performance liquid chromatography (HPLC) assays are used. HPLC is more accurate, since RIA detects metabolites, but RIA is simpler and more sensitive.[38] Results should be interpreted at the nadir if the drug is given twice daily,[38] and hyperkalemic and hyperuricemic patients should be carefully watched. Hepatotoxicity generally disappears with dose reduction.

CASE STUDY

A 56-year-old diabetic man with chronic renal failure had been on hemodialysis for the past 2 years. At the end of the first year, he had his name placed on a waiting list as a candidate for a cadaver transplant. During the second year, he had received three blood transfusions from random donors and had had his blood screened monthly. Shortly after the start of his third year on dialysis, a donor kidney became available, and after a final crossmatch was done the patient was transplanted.

Following transplantation the patient, who was receiving both azathioprine and prednisolone, was monitored closely with daily serum blood urea nitrogen and serum creatinine tests. His recovery was unremarkable until the third week, when he displayed an elevated temperature, slight oliguria, and an elevated BUN of 30 mg/dL (10.7 mmol/L), along with a serum creatinine of 2.0 mg/dL (177μmol/L). *Escherichia coli* was isolated from his urine. The patient recovered after treatment with an appropriate antibiotic and an alteration in his immunosuppressive regimen to reverse any coexisting rejection crisis.

For the next 2 years he did well until symptoms such as those previously seen reappeared, along with a declining glomerular filtration rate. Fine-needle biopsy of the kidney revealed evidence of chronic rejection. Nephrectomy of the transplanted kidney was performed a short time later.

Questions

1. Laboratory tests evaluating the status of various body systems are critical in pretransplantation testing. Which are the most important immunological procedures?
2. Symptoms are often overlapping in post-transplant recipients. Laboratory procedures aid in determining the differential diagnosis from among what common possibilities?
3. Should the patient's initial crisis have been anticipated?

Discussion

1. Ensuring ABO compatibility by determining the ABO group of both the potential donor and the recipient is probably the most critical test. After that, periodic screens of the patient serum should be performed to determine if cytotoxic antibodies have been formed, most often as the result of blood transfusions. The final cross-match is needed to ensure that the patient possesses no lymphocytotoxic antibodies specifically directed against the donor's HLA antigens.
2. In the posttransplantation followup of a kidney graft recipient, it is necessary to be able to distinguish among symptoms caused by rejection and those caused by recurrent disease, drug toxicity, or infection so that appropriate and timely treatment may be instituted.
3. Given the patient's age, diabetic history, kidney transplant source, and immunosuppressive regimen, it is not surprising that the patient developed a urinary tract infection with a common bacterial etiologic agent. Patients should also be stringently monitored for the development of other infections, especially those of the respiratory tract. Unusual microorganisms should not be omitted from consideration. Pretransplantation serological testing may aid in the avoidance of certain infections and/or their diagnosis.

REFERENCES

1. Monaco AP: Clinical kidney transplantation in 1984. Transplant Proc 17: 5, 1985
2. Najarian JS: Transplantation. In Schwartz SI (ed): Yearbook of Surgery, p 137. Chicago, Year Book Medical Pub, 1985
3. Sheldon CA, Najarian JS, Mauer SM: Pediatric renal transplantation. Surg Clin North Am 65: 1589, 1985
4. Delmonico FL, Cosimi AB, Jaffers GJ et al: Immunologic monitoring of diabetics and nondiabetic recipients of renal allografts. J Surg Res 35: 271, 1983
5. Solinger AM: Organ transplantation and the IR gene: Clinical correlations and donor requirements. In Corman LC, Katz P (eds): The Medical Clinics of North America, p 565. Philadelphia, WB Saunders, 1985
6. Calne RY: Clinical transplantation summary. Transplant Proc 17: 1599, 1985
7. Donnelly PK, Proud G, Shenton BK et al: Are DRw6-positive patients high responders? Transplant Proc 16: 1153, 1984
8. Benvenisty A, Cohen DJ, Hardy MA: Tissue typing in renal transplantation: The impact of cyclosporine. Transplant Proc 18: 19, 1986
9. Fine RN (mod): Renal transplantation update. Ann Intern Med 100: 246, 1984
10. Corry RJ, Schulak JA, Goeken NE et al.: The effect of HLA A, B, and DR matching and blood transfusion in first cadaver kidney transplantation. Transplant Proc 17: 756, 1985
11. Keman R, Van Buren CT, Fletcher S et al.: Correlation of visual ^{51}Cr release and flow cytometry cross-match results and graft survival. Transplant Proc 16: 1430, 1984

12. Norman DJ, Barry JM, Wetzsteon PJ: Successful Cadaver Kidney Transplantation in Patients Highly Sensitized by Blood Transfusions. Transplantation 39: 253, 1985
13. Falk JA, Cardella CJ, Halloran P et al.: Transplantation can be performed with positive (noncurrent) crossmatch. Transplant Proc 17: 1530, 1985
14. Howard FJ: Definition, diagnosis, and treatment of acute kidney rejection—the first 30 days. Transplant Proc 18: 92, 1986
15. Carpenter CB, Lagarus IM: Dialysis and transplantation in the treatment of renal failure. In Petersdorf RG et al (eds): Harrison's Principles of Internal Medicine, p 1626. New York City, McGraw-Hill, 1983
16. Van Son WJ, Vanderwoude FJ, Vanderhem GK et al: Complement activation associated with active cytomegalovirus infection in renal transplant patients, and its absence in transplant rejection episodes. Transplantation 39: 510, 1985
17. Fukuda M: Evaluation and clinical significance of circulating immune complexes after renal transplantation. Transplantation 36: 155, 1983
18. McNaughton DC, White DJG: Measurement of immune activity in transplant recipients. Transplant Proc 17: 669, 1985
19. Bishop GA, Hall BM, Duggin GG et al: Immunopathology of renal allograft rejection analyzed with monoclonal antibodies to mononuclear cell markers. Kidney Int: 708, 1986
20. Mohanakuman T, Ellis TM, Reinitz ER et al: Daily monitoring of T cell subpopulations in renal allograft recipients: High-resolution measurement of T cell kinetics. Transplant Proc 16: 1490, 1984
21. Ganghoff O, Gross U, Whitley T et al: Factors in the accuracy and reproducibility of T cell and T cell subset measurements in transplant patients. Transplantation Proc 17: 640, 1985
22. Kahan BD: Immunologic monitoring: Utility and limitations. Transplant Proc 17: 1537, 1985
23. Tanimura S, Taguchi Y, Kunori T et al: Monitoring of *in vivo* blastogenic response in kidney transplant patients by flow cytometry. Transplantation Proc 17: 652, 1985
24. Vernon WB, DeLong ER, Briner WH et al: Renal transplant monitoring with serum B_2 Microglobulin and creatinine. Transplant Proc 17: 646, 1985
25. Woo KT, Lee EJC, Lau YK et al: Beta-2-microglobulin in the assessment of renal function of the transplanted kidney. Nephron 39: 223, 1985
26. Maury CPJ, Teppo AM: Comparative study of serum amyloid-related protein SAA, C-reactive protein, and B_2 microgloublin as markers of renal allograft rejection. Clin Nephorol 22: 284, 1984
27. Maury CPJ, Teppo AM, Ahonen J et al: Evaluation of serum amyloid A protein as a marker of allograft rejection in patients with initially nonfunctioning renal transplants. Transplant Proc 18: 86, 1986
28. Fields BL, Sollinger HW, Glass NR et al.: Beta-2-Microglobulin versus creatinine as the sole indicator of rejection in renal transplants. Transplant Proc 16: 1591, 1984
29. Barnes RM, Alexander LC, West CR: B_2-Microglobulin and renal graft rejection: Relationship of plasma creatinine during stable transplant function and graft rejection. Transplant Proc 16: 1613, 1984
30. Maury CPJ, Teppo AM, Eklund B et al: Serum amyloid A protein: A sensitive indicator of renal allograft rejection in humans. Transplantation 36: 501, 1983
31. Matas AJ, Simmons RL, Kjellstrand CM et al: Pseudorejection: Factors mimicking rejection in renal allograft recipients. Ann Surg 186: 51, 1977
32. MacSween JM, Cohen AD, Rajaraman K et al: The influence of pretransplant immune responsiveness on the incidence of infection after renal transplantation. Transplant Proc 18: 148, 1986
33. Cunningham TR, Ascher NL: Effect of prerenal transplant OKT 4-OKT 8 Ratio and imunosuppression protocol on posttransplant viral infections. Transplant Proc 17: 633, 1985
34. Freedman LR: Inflammatory and infectious disorders of the kidney: A special form of interstitial nephritis. In Bricker NS, Kirschenbaum MA (eds): The Kidney: Diagnosis and Management. New York City, John Wiley & Sons, 1984
35. Madras PN, Simpson MA, Monaco AR: Monitoring the renal allograft by immunofluorescence of tubular epithelial cells in the urine sediment. Transplant Proc 16: 1583, 1984
36. Shen SY, Weir MR, Litkowski L et al: Enzyme-linked immunosorbent assay for serum renal tubular antigen in kidney transplant patients. Transplantation: 642, 1986
37. Morris PJ: Immunosuppression in renal transplantation. Transplant Proc 17: 1153, 1985

38. Diethelm AG: Clinical diagnosis and management of the renal transplant recipient with cyclosporine nephrotoxicity. Transplant Proc 18: 82, 1986
39. Matas AJ, Tellis VA, Quinn T et al: Definition, diagnosis, and management of rejection in the second to sixth months posttransplant—an overview. Transplant Proc 18: 141, 1986
40. Drakopoulos S, White DJG, Merion RM et al: An assessment of the clinical value of monitoring cyclosporine plasma levels. Transplant Proc 17: 1258, 1985

BIBLIOGRAPHY

Morris PJ (ed): Kidney Transplantation Principles and Practice, 2nd ed. New York City, Grune & Stratton, 1984

Chapter 16

Urinary Obstructive Disorders

Catherine Conley Downs

Obstruction can occur anywhere in the urinary tract between the renal tubules and the distal urethra. Obstruction of the urinary tract is an important clinical problem because, when the normal flow of urine is impeded by an obstructive lesion, the potential exists for impairment of renal function and urinary tract infection.[1] The patient's clinical presentation and the degree of renal function impairment will vary depending on the location of the obstruction, whether it is acute or chronic, partial or complete, unilateral or bilateral, and whether an infection is present.[2] Urinary tract obstruction requires early diagnosis and prompt, appropriate treatment in order to minimize the structural and functional changes that the obstruction may produce in the kidneys. If uncorrected, the obstruction may lead to complete, irreversible loss of renal function.[3]

ETIOLOGY AND PATHOPHYSIOLOGY

Terminology and Classification

Obstructive uropathy is a general term used to describe the obstruction of urinary flow. Initially, obstructive uropathy results in dilatation of the ureter, renal pelvis, and calyces with urine. This dilatation is referred to as *hydronephrosis*. If uncorrected, obstructive uropathy may lead to *obstructive nephropathy,* a term that refers to the functional and histological changes in the kidney resulting from obstruction of urinary flow. It should be noted that the definition of these terms may vary from author to author.[1]

Urinary tract obstructions are described using three classifications. These are: (1) *duration,* as acute (having short duration and abrupt onset), subacute (lasting from days to weeks), or chronic (months to years); (2) *degree,* as total (complete) or partial (incomplete); and (3) *location,* which may be in the renal tubule, upper urinary tract, or lower urinary tract. Upper urinary tract obstruction is most frequently unilateral and may involve the renal pelvis, the ureter, or its junction with the pelvis (ureteropelvic) or bladder (ureterovesical). Obstruction involving the bladder or urethra is described as lower urinary tract obstruction and thus is bilateral, affecting the upper urinary tract of both kidneys.[4]

Various causes of urinary tract obstruction appear in Table 16-1. Urinary tract obstruction can result from intrinsic (intraluminal or intramural) or extrinsic causes. The obstructive lesion may occur in the renal tubule or the upper or lower urinary tract. Depending on the age and the sex of the individual, the predominant cause of urinary tract obstruction will vary.

Intraluminal Causes

Intraluminal obstruction is caused by a mechanical obstruction of the lumen at any level of the urinary

Table 16-1 ***Various Causes of Urinary Tract Obstruction***

	Intrinsic Causes	Extrinsic Causes
Upper Urinary Tract Obstruction	Calculi Sloughed papillae Ureteropelvic dysfunction Ureteral tumor Ureteral stricture	Pregnancy Pelvic malignancies Ureteral ligation Retroperitoneal fibrosis
Lower Urinary Tract Obstruction	Posterior urethral valve Neurogenic bladder Urethral stricture	Prostatic obstruction

tract.[2] The deposition of uric acid crystals in the tubules, seen most commonly in hematologic malignancies, is a common cause of intraluminal obstruction arising within the renal parenchyma. Patients with multiple myeloma may also develop intraluminal obstruction caused by the deposition of Bence Jones protein in the renal tubule. Renal failure is a common cause of death in these patients; however, controversy exists as to whether the renal insufficiency results from toxic effects or from obstructive effects of Bence Jones protein.[4]

Urinary tract calculi are a predominant cause of intraluminal obstruction, especially in the young adult male. Most stones are comprised of one or more of the following substances: calcium oxalate, calcium phosphate, uric acid, cystine, or magnesium ammonium phosphate (struvite). Those comprised of calcium oxalate are the most common stones encountered. A multitude of factors are probably responsible for stone formation, including reduction in urine volume, increased urinary excretion of the relatively insoluble substances listed above, urine *p*H, and the absence of inhibitors to precipitation of these insoluble agents.[5]

Sloughed papillae resulting from necrosis of renal papillae may also cause intraluminal obstruction. Papillary necrosis is associated with a number of conditions, including analgesic abuse, sickle cell disease or trait, diabetes mellitus, and severe pyelonephritis. In addition, blood clots and fungus balls have been known to obstruct the ureter.[4]

Intramural Causes

Intramural obstruction can be caused by either functional or anatomical abnormalities of the ureter, bladder, or urethra. These can be the result of congenital conditions, seen most commonly in children, or acquired conditions, which occur most frequently in adults. In childhood, posterior urethral valves and anomalies of the ureteropelvic junction are two conditions that produce obstruction.

Neurogenic bladder dysfunction is a common cause of an acquired functional obstruction. It occurs as the result of metabolic and neurologic disorders or of injuries to the spinal cord. A significant number of individuals with diabetes mellitus or multiple sclerosis develop neurogenic bladder dysfunction.[4]

Examples of anatomical alterations that lead to obstruction are ureteral strictures (as a consequence of surgical procedures in the retroperitoneum, complication of radiation therapy in cervical carcinoma, or treatment of tuberculosis that has directly involved the ureter) and urethral strictures (secondary to chronic instrumentation and surgery, or, in men, following gonococcal infections). In addition, urinary tract obstruction may result from tumors of the renal pelvis, ureter, or bladder.[4]

Extrinsic (Extramural) Causes

Extrinsic causes of urinary tract obstruction are the result of pressure from masses or of processes extrinsic to the urinary tract. In elderly men, benign prostatic hypertrophy and carcinoma of the prostate are the most common causes of obstruction of the urinary tract. In women, pregnancy and pelvic malignancies account for the most common causes of obstruction. Accidental ureteral ligation during surgery can also result in obstruction. Retroperitoneal fibrosis, a chronic inflammation of unknown etiology, can also cause ureteral compression.[4]

Increased Pressure

When the urinary tract is obstructed, there is an increase in pressure throughout the urinary tract proximal to the obstruction as the formation of urine continues. The pressure increase is transmitted to the kidney, where its initial effects are on distal tubule function, and thus an early manifestation may be inability to concentrate the urine. Inability to acidify the urine then follows.[6]

Elevated pressure also results in a decreased glomerular filtration rate and a reduction in renal blood flow, although in the initial period following obstruction renal blood flow may increase.[6]

Renal Damage

The longer the obstruction persists, the more likely it is that renal damage will occur.[7] Obstruction that is not relieved will result in ischemic atrophy of the kidney and subsequent renal failure. Unilateral obstruction will result in destruction of only one kidney, with the remaining kidney able to maintain normal excretory function. Bilateral obstructive disease, if uncorrected, leads to progressive renal failure, uremia, and possibly death. If the obstruction is prolonged, permanent damage to the kidneys may result, although renal function may significantly improve or at least stabilize if the obstruction is relieved prior to this stage of irreversible damage.[2, 8] Studies have shown that glomerular filtration rate will improve over a period of 1 to 4 weeks if obstruction is of recent onset.[1]

Diabetes Insipidus

A syndrome of vasopressin-resistant diabetes insipidus may arise secondary to the obstructive disorder.[9] Acquired nephrogenic diabetes insipidus may be the presenting manifestation of the obstructive disorder in these patients. The mechanism whereby the nephron does not respond to vasopressin is unknown.[1]

Infection

Although obstruction alone may injure the kidney, an additional risk is the predisposition of the urinary tract to infection. Urinary tract infection superimposed on the obstruction inevitably contributes to the increased rate of nephron destruction.[1] Infection, once established in the obstructed urinary tract, is difficult to eliminate and may contribute significantly to morbidity.[2]

CLINICAL MANIFESTATIONS

The clinical manifestations observed in urinary tract obstruction will depend on the duration, location, and degree of obstruction. They can be nonspecific, although some signs and symptoms, when they exist, are sufficiently definitive to suggest to the physician that an obstructive disorder is the most likely diagnosis.[4]

Pain

Patients with urinary tract obstruction most commonly seek medical attention because of pain caused by distention of the renal capsule or urinary collecting system. The intensity of the pain, however, is influenced more by how rapidly the distention develops than by the degree of distention. Thus, chronic obstruction may not produce pain, or it may be associated with only mild discomfort. The severe pain experienced with acute urinary tract obstruction due to renal calculi is referred to as *renal colic.* This pain often radiates from the flank into the groin.[3, 4]

Changes in Urinary Output

Total anuria or urine volumes that fluctuate from oliguria to polyuria are highly suggestive of an obstructive disorder. Total anuria may result if obstruction is complete and bilateral. Urine output may be normal if the obstruction is partial, although polyuria may occur as a result of the kidney's impaired concentrating ability. This concentrating defect may also result in nocturia as an early symptom when there is significant obstruction. If the patient is hospitalized, it is wise to determine the pattern of urinary output. Recognition of abrupt changes, gradual decline, or fluctuation may aid in the diagnostic process. Sudden cessation of voiding may point to a bladder outlet obstruction.[1, 4]

Recurrent Urinary Tract Infections

The presence of a urinary tract obstruction must be investigated in any patient who presents with a history of repeated urinary tract infections or resistance of the infection to normal antibiotic therapy. In these patients it may be extremely difficult to clear the infection as long as the obstruction continues.[4]

Renal Failure

Acute or chronic renal failure can result from bilateral obstruction or from unilateral obstruction in patients with only one functioning kidney.[2] It is therefore important to suspect urinary tract obstruction in patients presenting with signs and symptoms of renal failure. This is especially true when there is no previous history of renal disease and routine urinalysis results are negative, or when there is sudden deterioration of renal function for no reason in a patient with known renal disease.[4]

Urolithiasis

The stasis resulting from obstruction of the urinary tract may encourage stone formation.[3]

Hypertension

Elevated blood pressure may be present in patients with acute unilateral obstruction due to increased renin secretion. Abnormal salt and water retention appears to be responsible for the hypertensive state in cases of chronic, bilateral hydronephrosis.[2]

Gross Hematuria

Gross hematuria may be associated with specific etiologies of urinary tract obstruction, such as urinary tract stones, neoplasms, or infection.

Polycythemia

The polycythemia manifested in a few instances of obstructive disorders is believed to be caused by abnormal erythropoietin production by the obstructed kidney. This belief has been supported by the resolution of the erythrocytosis once the obstruction is relieved.[2]

Presenting Symptoms

The diagnostic approach to a patient presenting with possible urinary tract obstruction will vary depending on initial symptoms.[4] Obstruction at or below the bladder is commonly associated with complaints of hesitancy, urinary frequency, overflow incontinence, and postvoid dribbling.[3] Evidence of recurrent urinary tract infections should lead to the suspicion of urinary tract obstruction. These patients will present with the typical symptoms of fever, flank tenderness, and dysuria. In addition, gastrointestinal symptoms of nausea, vomiting, and abdominal fullness will occur frequently.[1]

As mentioned before, pain in the flank, groin, or lower abdomen is often the presenting symptom that causes the patient to seek medical advice. It is important to remember, however, that with chronic, low-grade obstruction pain may be nonexistent. Symptoms may be totally absent until kidney damage is so severe that renal failure becomes the initial manifestation of the obstructive disorder.

Obstructive disorders generally represent treatable causes of renal failure. Therefore, timely diagnosis is a major goal.[10] Urinary tract obstructions may be caused by such a wide variety of lesions that, in order to make a diagnosis, consideration must be given to the entire urinary tract. Certain preliminary information is important in the diagnostic process and in the choice of laboratory and radiological tests. In addition to comprehensive review of all presenting symptoms, these preliminaries should include patient history and a thorough physical examination.

Patient History

A thorough patient history may reveal background etiologic factors that may aid in the diagnostic process. The patient may have experienced similar symptoms in the past. There may be a history of previous stone disease or recurrent urinary tract infection. Family history of renal disease or renal stones is also important in the screening process. It is essential to evaluate drug ingestion and recent surgery. Other medical problems, including diabetes mellitus or neurologic disturbances, must also be investigated for their obvious role in the presenting problems.[4]

Physical Examination

The physical examination is very important for the detection of abdominal or flank masses involving the urinary tract. A distended bladder may be apparent on palpation of the abdomen. Lesions responsible for urinary tract obstruction may be revealed by careful flank and abdominal palpation, as well as on prostate examination in men and on pelvic examination in women.[8]

LABORATORY ANALYSES AND DIAGNOSIS

Once the patient history, presenting symptoms, and physical examination results have been compiled, further assessment of the patient's condition will then proceed along two lines. One involves assessment by clinical laboratory evaluation of urine and blood samples. The results from these tests may suggest an obstructive disorder, although it is the second line of assessment, involving radiological evaluation of the urinary tract, upon which a diagnosis is generally based.[7]

Several laboratory tests are generally considered particularly useful in evaluating urinary tract obstruction; however, laboratory evaluation of possible systemic conditions or diseases (*e.g.*, hypercalcemia or multiple myeloma) that predispose the patient to obstructive disorders is also important to consider.[11]

Urine Studies

A complete urinalysis that includes microscopic evaluation of the urinary sediment can be a helpful tool for assessing urinary tract obstruction. The results are generally nonspecific, but may occasionally be diagnostic, as in the observation of fragments of necrosed renal papillae or bladder tumor in the urinary sediment. The urinalysis may even be completely normal, especially in complete unilateral obstruction in which abnormal urine cannot reach the bladder.[1]

The finding of hematuria without other positive findings may suggest renal calculi, papillary necrosis, or a tumor as the cause of obstruction.[4] Hematuria has been found to occur consistently when stones are present, even asymptomatically.[12] With the presence of bacteria and leukocytes, urinary tract infection should be suspected, and urine culture and sensitivity testing performed. The presence of crystals in the urinary sediment may also offer diagnostic clues. For example, the identification of uric acid crystals may suggest the possible source for urinary tract obstruction. The presence of urinary crystals such as cystine and calcium oxalate can also provide important information regarding the etiology of urinary tract stones.

Urinary *p*H measurement, on a fresh sample from a patient in a fasting state, may be valuable in determining the kinds of crystals precipitating the urolithiasis. Calcium oxalate forms stones at a *p*H of less than 7.5, calcium phosphate at 6.0 to 6.5, and uric acid at 5.3. Magnesium ammonium phosphate forms stones (struvite or infection stones) at an alkaline *p*H. These stones are produced when there is an infection from urea-splitting organisms, such as *Proteus* species, which cause alkalinization of the urine. Twenty-four hour urine chemistry measurements of calcium, phosphorus, uric acid, and oxalate along with screening for cystine are important in assessing the metabolic basis for stone development.[12] Patients should eat a customary diet during this evaluation process, because controlled diet could obscure abnormalities.[13]

Urinary cytology studies, although not part of the routine urinalysis, may offer useful diagnostic information in patients with bladder tumors.[14]

Evaluation of renal concentrating ability can be estimated with the measurement of urinary specific gravity and/or osmolality, osmolality being the preferred measurement. Urine concentration varies widely depending on several factors, especially water intake. Therefore, a random urine concentration measurement provides little information about renal concentrating ability unless a period of water deprivation of from 18 to 24 hours precedes the sample collection. A urine osmolality greater than 900 mOsm/kg and/or a urine specific gravity greater than 1.023 (in the absence of glucose, protein, or contrast dyes) would be indicative of a normal renal concentrating mechanism.[15]

Information about the kidney's ability to acidify the urine, which may be impaired in urinary tract obstruction, can be obtained by measuring the lowest urinary *p*H obtained when the patient is in a state of metabolic acidosis. The acidosis may be either spontaneous or induced with administration of ammonium chloride. An abnormal response is indicated when the urinary *p*H will not drop below 5.4[16]

Observations of urine volume output, as discussed above, can be an important diagnostic tool. Therefore, measurement of 24-hour urine volume may be indicated. Additionally, bladder catheterization to measure residual urine volume after voiding may be helpful in diagnosing lower urinary tract obstruction, which is suggested by the presence of increased residual urine in the bladder.[2] This form of obstruction may also be observed with post-voiding radiological films of the bladder.[17] Urine culture may be indicated to ensure the absence of infection.

Assessment of Renal Function

To assess renal function, blood urea nitrogen (BUN) and serum creatinine levels should be measured. These levels will vary depending on the extent of the obstruction, but may be elevated when obstruction is severe enough to have compromised renal function. The BUN/creatinine ratio can be an important clue to diagnosis in that it is often elevated in disease caused by urinary tract obstruction. The normal ratio is between 10:1 and 20:1, but in postrenal azotemia (resulting from obstructive disorders) the BUN rises out of proportion to the serum creatinine, due to the increased reabsorption of urea that occurs with a low rate of urine flow.[1]

An additional evaluative tool is measurement of the glomerular filtration rate to estimate the number of functioning nephrons. There is no ideal material of endogenous origin used to measure glomerular filtration rate, but the performance of a creatinine clearance is overall the most useful and convenient indicator of glomerular filtration rate. A clearance test using an exogenous substance such as inulin is the method of choice when a more accurate assessment of glomerular filtration rate is required.[16] Again, results will be variable depending on the etiology of the urinary tract obstruction, and thus will reflect the extent of renal function impairment induced by the obstruction.

Other Blood Studies

Information regarding underlying metabolic disorders may be obtained by performing a chemistry profile. The results should be evaluated for indications of abnormalities that may give rise to obstructive disorders, such as hypercalcemia, gout, and diabetes. In evaluating obstruction due to disorders of the prostate, acid phosphatase is important. Protein abnormalities present in multiple myeloma should be considered as a cause of urinary tract obstruction.

Analysis of Urinary Tract Calculi (Stones)

Analysis of urinary calculi is essential for establishing etiology and for prevention of their recurrence in the future. A number of physical and chemical techniques have been used to analyze the composition of urinary tract stones. Among these are x-ray diffraction and infrared spectroscopy, which are specialized techniques usually performed in commercial reference laboratories. These analyses provide quantitative data regarding stone composition and offer the most complete and accurate analysis.[18] They are gradually replacing the less specific qualitative chemical methods that only assess elemental composition of the calculi.[11] Separate analyses can also be performed on the center of the stone and on the rim. This aids in identifying the factors contributing to stone formation.[19]

Radiological Evaluation

Once urinary tract obstruction is suspected, the diagnosis is usually confirmed by intravenous pyelography (IVP). Because of the complications associated with the IVP (*e.g.*, allergic reactions to the iodinated contrast material and renal failure), the noninvasive technique of ultrasonography is often used as an alternative diagnostic tool. More complex procedures may then be used to further assess the obstruction.[8, 16]

TREATMENT

The primary goals of therapy are to relieve the symptoms of obstruction, control or prevent infection, and preserve renal function. The specific medical (nonsurgical) or surgical intervention to relieve the obstruction must be determined on an individual basis. Among other things, the general status of the patient, the specific etiology and location of the obstruction, whether the procedure is an emergency or elective, and the state of renal function in the obstructed kidney must all be taken into consideration by the physician prior to making a decision about appropriate intervention.[6] The severely ill patient may, on occasion, need to be treated with dialysis or temporary drainage of urine through nephrostomy or other bypass procedures.[17] Furthermore, management of the complications of obstruction such as pain, infection, and stones will also be necessary.

Many urinary tract stones will be relieved by spontaneous passage of the stone. High fluid intake, to ensure a minimum urine volume of 2 liters per day, can help the stone pass. Stones larger than 0.5 to 1.0 cm in diameter usually require surgical intervention, although new, less invasive techniques based on *lithotripsy* (stone fragmentation) have been introduced. Lithotripsy utilizes either shock waves or ultrasonic energy to fragment the stone, with subsequent passage of the stone fragments. In one of these techniques, extracorporeal shock wave lithotripsy, an electrode is discharged in the bottom of a water bath in which the patient is submerged. This technique is emerging as the treatment of choice for removal of most simple upper urinary tract stones.[20] Prevention of further stone formation is the primary aim in treatment. Dietary modifications, forcing of fluids, and acidification or alkalinization of the urine may constitute an appropriate treatment regimen, along with management of underlying conditions that contribute to stone formation (*e.g.*, primary hyperparathyroidism, cystinuria, gout).

A syndrome of postobstructive diuresis may be observed after relief of bilateral urinary tract obstruction. This is caused by the unloading of retained water and solute, and the osmotic effect of excretion of retained urea. The diuresis is usually transient, but careful monitoring of the patient's fluid and electrolyte balance is necessary to determine if fluid and salt replacement are required.[4]

The prognosis for the patient with urinary tract obstruction depends largely on whether irreversible renal damage has occurred before treatment is begun. Serial measurements of the various kidney function tests may be useful in evaluating the patient's course.[10] The duration and completeness of the obstruction and the presence or absence of infection will greatly influence the degree of renal damage and thus the prognosis. The ultimate course of the patient may also be dependent on the underlying condition that has led to the obstruction.[7, 8]

CASE STUDY

A 31-year-old white man presented to the emergency room with the chief complaint of a steady and continuous flank pain radiating to the groin. The patient reported feeling fine until an hour before, when the pain began and gradually increased in severity, forcing the patient to seek medical attention. A urinalysis was ordered, and the results indicated a urine *p*H of 6.5 and the presence of a microscopic hematuria (20–30 rbc/hpf); all other results appeared normal.

Questions

1. What additional test should be performed to determine the patient's diagnosis?
2. If the test reveals an obstruction in the urinary tract, what would be the most common cause, given the age, sex, and presenting symptoms and signs of this patient?
3. If an obstruction due to urinary tract calculi were found in this patient, what additional laboratory tests should be performed?
4. What would be the appropriate treatment for the prevention of further stone formation?

Discussion

1. Diagnosis of a urinary tract obstruction is generally based on the results of radiological examination of the urinary tract, that is, IVP.
2. Urinary tract calculi are a predominant cause of intraluminal obstruction, especially in the young adult male.
3. Serum and urine (24-hour) calcium, phosphorus, uric acid, and creatinine measurements should be performed. Tests for urinary oxalate and citrate may also be indicated. Some patients with urinary tract calculi have underlying metabolic disorders that cause stone formation. These can be detected by chemical analyses performed on serum and urine. In addition, analysis of the composition of any stones that might pass spontaneously should be performed to help establish etiology and define appropriate treatment.
4. No matter what disorder(s) is/are found, the patient should be instructed to avoid dehydration and to increase water intake. Dietary modification, acidification/alkalinization of the urine, or use of medications will depend on stone type. This patient had a calcium phosphate stone and the cause was identified as idiopathic hypercalciuria (normal serum calcium, unexplained hypercalciuria—urine calcium greater than 300 mg/24-hr). A thiazide diuretic agent was prescribed as the appropriate treatment to prevent further stone formation.

REFERENCES

1. Beck LH, Stein JH, Earley LE: Obstructive uropathy. In Early LE, Gottschalk CW (eds): Strauss and Welt's Diseases of the Kidney, 3rd ed, pp 877–879, 887–889. Boston, Little, Brown & Co, 1979
2. Rector FC: Obstructive nephropathy. In Wyngaarden JB, Smith LH (eds): Cecil Textbook of Medicine, 17th ed, pp 604–607. Philadelphia, WB Saunders, 1985
3. Brenner BM, Humes HD: Urinary tract obstruction. In Isselbacher KJ, Adams RD, Braunwald E et al (eds): Harrison's Principles of Internal Medicine, 9th ed, pp 1353–1354. New York City, McGraw-Hill, 1980
4. Klahr S, Buerkert J, Morrison A: Urinary tract obstruction. In Brenner BM, Rector FC Jr (eds): The Kidney, 3rd ed, pp 1444–1448, 1467–1469, 1477, 1482. Philadelphia, WB Saunders, 1986
5. Pak CYC: Renal calculi. In Wyngaarden JB, Smith LH (eds): Cecil Textbook of Medicine, 17th ed, p 628. Philadelphia, WB Saunders, 1985
6. Wright FS, Howards SS: Obstructive injury. In Brenner BM, Rector FC Jr (eds): The Kidney, 2nd ed, p 2026. Philadelphia, WB Saunders, 1981
7. Muldowney FP: Obstructive nephropathy. In Beeson PB, McDermott W, Wyngaarden JB (eds): Cecil Textbook of Medicine, 15th ed, pp 1447–1450. Philadelphia, WB Saunders, 1979
8. Boyd JC, Boyce WH: Obstructive nephropathy. In Conn RB (ed): Current Diagnosis, 7th ed, pp 1114–1115. Philadelphia, WB Saunders, 1985
9. Yarger WE, Harris RH: Urinary tract obstruction. In Seldin DW, Giebisch G (eds): The Kidney: Physiology and Pathophysiology, p 1964. New York City, Raven Press, 1985
10. Lytton B, Epstein FH: Obstructive uropathy. In Thorn GW, Adams RA, Braunwald E et al (eds): Harrison's Principles of Internal Medicine, 8th ed, pp 1421–1423. New York City, McGraw-Hill, 1977
11. Rock RC, Walker WG, Jennings CD: Nitrogen metabolites and renal function. In Tietz NW (ed): Textbook of Clinical Chemistry, pp 1309, 1314. Philadelphia, WB Saunders, 1986

12. Bradley M, Schumann GB: Examination of urine. In Henry BH: Clinical Diagnosis and Management by Laboratory Methods, 17th ed, pp 436–437. Philadelphia, WB Saunders, 1984
13. Coe FL: Clinical and laboratory assessment of the patient with renal disease. In Brenner BM, Rector FC Jr (eds): The Kidney, 2nd ed, p 1174. Philadelphia, WB Saunders, 1981
14. Rowland RG, Garrett RA: Tumors of the ureter and urinary bladder. In Conn RB (ed): Current Diagnosis, 7th ed, p 1128. Philadelphia, WB Saunders, 1985
15. Kassirer JP, Gennari FJ: Laboratory evaluation of renal function. In Earley LE, Gottschalk CW (eds): Strauss and Welt's Diseases of the Kidney, 3rd ed, p 62. Boston, Little, Brown & Co, 1979
16. Dennis VW: Investigations of renal function. In Wyngaarden JB, Smith LH (eds): Cecil Textbook of Medicine, 17th ed, pp 510–512. Philadelphia, WB Saunders, 1985
17. Stein MF: The kidney. In Taylor RB (ed): Family Medicine: Principles and Practice, pp 878–879. New York City, Springer-Verlag, 1983
18. Mandel, Neil: Urinary tract calculi. Lab Med 17: 450–451, 1986
19. Resnick MI, Freidland GW: Urinary stone disease. In Resnick MI, Older RA (eds): Diagnosis of Genitourinary Disease, pp 309–311. New York City, Thieme-Stratton, 1982
20. Health and Public Policy Committee, American College of Physicians: Lithotripsy. Ann Intern Med 103:626, 1985

Chapter 17

Urinary Tract Infections

Marie Pezzlo

The second most frequently occurring infections in the United States involve the urinary tract. Although many infections are acute or asymptomatic and may respond to single-dose antimicrobial therapy,[1] they can also cause major clinical problems. These include serious infections in the newborn associated with pyelonephritis as well as decreased survival of the elderly.[2, 3, 4] The urinary tract is normally free of microorganisms and, under normal conditions, urine should be a sterile fluid. Any interruption or disorder of the urinary tract may cause microorganisms to multiply. If the microbial count exceeds 100,000 ($>10^5$) colony-forming units (CFU)/ml or if white blood cells (WBC) are present, an infection usually exists. The microorganisms that cause infection include bacteria, fungi, protozoa and viruses; the majority of infections are caused by bacteria. The presence of bacteria in the urinary tract is referred to as *bacteriuria,* and the presence of white blood cells as *pyuria.* Urinary tract infections (UTI) include a wide range of clinical entities from asymptomatic bacteriuria to serious symptomatic infections that may result in renal damage and failure. These infections may be acute or chronic, and they may recur (relapse) or the patient may become reinfected.

ETIOLOGY AND PATHOPHYSIOLOGY

Mechanisms of Invasion

Bacteria can invade and spread throughout the urinary tract by three routes: ascending, hematogenous, and lymphatics. The usual route of infection is *ascending.* Bacteria from the feces, the skin, and the vagina enter the urethral meatus and ascend into the bladder, where they multiply and cause infection. Bacteria may also ascend into the ureters and kidneys. Massage of the female urethra and sexual intercourse introduce bacteria into the bladder.[5, 6] Ascending infection in association with instrumentation is common in both sexes. For most catheter-associated infections, especially in women, bacteria migrate from the rectum, colonize the urethra, and ascend between the catheter and the urethral mucosa.[7] It is now known that adherence to the uroepithelial cells of the bladder can initiate the colonization.[8] In men, the length of the urethra and the antibacterial properties of prostatic secretions act as defense mechanisms against infection.

The *hematogenous* route occurs less commonly than the ascending route; however, it is an important source of infection of the kidney. Large volumes of blood flow through the kidney, and any systemic infection can seed the organ. *Staphylococcus aureus, Candida* species, and *Mycobacterium* species are common agents that infect unobstructed kidneys, causing hematogenous pyelonephritis.[9] The pathogenesis of staphylococcal perinephric abscess is also via the hematogenous route. The *lymphatic* route seems to have very little significance in urinary tract infection,[10] although it may play a role in prostatitis.

The urethra is normally colonized by organisms such as gram-negative bacilli, staphylococci, streptococci, lactobacilli, and diphtheroids. These organisms may contaminate urine specimens; however, they are usually present in low numbers. The anatomy of the female urethra is of particular importance in the pathogenesis of urinary tract infection. Colonizing organisms may be easily inoculated into the urethra and bladder following minor trauma associated with instrumentation or sexual intercourse, causing cystitis or acute urethral syndrome. Conditions that interfere with the flushing action of urine outflow predispose the urinary tract to infection. Increased pressure on the bladder forces urine into the urethra. Urine may then flow back into the bladder once the pressure returns to normal, washing urethral organisms along with the flow. This can occur in normal women during coughing. The presence of these organisms in the bladder may result in infection. Other risk factors include obstruction to urine flow or stasis as a result of congenital abnormalities, renal calculi, or ureteral occlusion. Residual urine in the bladder as a result of a neurogenic bladder, urethral stricture, or prostatic hypertrophy also predisposes the host to infection. Instrumentation associated with catheterization, urethral dilatation, and cystoscopy also greatly increases the risk of infection. The loss of urethral peristalsis in pregnancy makes it easier for microorganisms to ascend to the kidney, accounting for the high incidence of pyelonephritis during pregnancy.[11]

Bladder Defense Mechanisms

There are three mechanisms the bladder uses to defend itself against infection.[12] Bacteria are removed from the bladder by repeated voiding. This is known as the *primary* bladder defense mechanism. Bacterial counts will be greatly reduced with a high fluid intake and frequent voiding. The *secondary* bladder defense mechanism is the effect of the bladder mucosa on the remaining bacteria. The *tertiary* bladder defense mechanism includes the antimicrobial properties of urine, such as organic acids, low *p*H, and high concentrations of urea.

Table 17-1 ***Incidence of Infection***

Age Group	Male–Female Ratio
Newborns	4:1
Preschool	1:15
School-age	1:30
Young adults	1:>30
Elderly	1:2
Catheter-related	1:1

Special Patient Groups

All individuals are susceptible to urinary tract infections, but the prevalence of infection differs with age and sex as well as with certain predisposing factors (see Table 17-1). Infections can begin as early as the first few days of life and may continue throughout life. The incidence of infection peaks at certain times during life and is associated with both age and sex. The overall prevalence of bacteriuria is approximately 1% during the first decade of life, and seems to increase by at least 1% with each subsequent decade.

NEWBORNS

The first peak of incidence occurs during the first few months of life; at this time, bacteriuria is more common in males than in females. Moreover, the incidence of infection in premature infants is higher than in full-term babies.[13] A septic or febrile infant who fails to thrive should be screened for a possible urinary tract infection.

PRESCHOOL AND SCHOOL CHILDREN

Symptomatic urinary tract infections in preschool children are not uncommon. They are seen more frequently in girls than in boys with a ratio of approximately 15:1. The ratio increases to 30:1 among school-age children. Approximately 5% of all girls will have at least one episode of urinary tract infection prior to completion of high school.[9]

ADULT WOMEN

The most common infection among adult women is urinary tract infection. Interviews of women between the ages of 20 and 40 years have revealed that as many as 25% to 35% have had a urinary tract infection.[9] Approximately 25% to 40% of these persons develop a spontaneous cure; however, as many as 50% of them may become reinfected within one year.[14, 15, 16] The association between sexual intercourse and subsequent urinary tract infection contributes to the increased incidence of both infection and recurrence in young adult women.[17]

Bacteriuria during pregnancy occurs in 2% to 5% of women. The incidence increases with age, and can result in serious infection of both the mother and the fetus.[18] Undetected asymptomatic bacteriuria is of great concern because, if left untreated, it can lead to acute infection and symptomatic pyelonephritis, which usually occurs during the third trimester.[9] Women who have had urinary tract infections as children have a much higher incidence of infection during pregnancy.[17] These women have 26 times the attack rate of pyelonephritis in pregnancy, and are more likely to have low-birth-weight deliveries and perinatal deaths.[19] Pyelonephritis during pregnancy is the most frequent cause of hospitalization during this period and is associated with increased perinatal mortality, more frequent premature deliveries, and deficient infant development.[20, 21]

MEN

After infancy, bacteriuria in males is uncommon before the age of 50. Prostatic obstruction and instrumentation become the major cause of infection among middle-aged and older men.[9] Inability to empty the bladder completely and seeding of the urinary stream with organisms from the prostate cause persistent or recurrent infection. After age 70, the incidence of infection in men approaches or exceeds that in women, and therapy is neither necessary nor effective for asymptomatic bacteriuria.[22] The most commonly isolated organisms in men are *Proteus* species. In women, *Escherichia coli* is the most common cause of acute urinary tract infection.

ELDERLY

Bacteriuria in the elderly population occurs frequently in both men and women. The prevalence of infection in elderly men ranges from 5% to 30% and from 10% to 50% in women. Elderly patients with obstruction, poor bladder emptying, dementia, stroke, diabetes mellitus, and cardiovascular disease are more likely to have bacteriuria than patients in the same age group without these abnormalities.[23] There is also an increase in mortality among elderly patients with bacteriuria.[2, 4]

CATHETER-ASSOCIATED PATIENTS

The risk of acquiring a urinary tract infection associated with catheterization ranges from 1% to 5% after a single brief catheterization to 100% with an indwelling urethral catheter draining into an open system for longer than 4 days.[24, 25] Use of a closed system decreases the risk of infection to approximately 20%.[26]

Infectious Agents

Bacteria are by far the most frequent cause of urinary tract infections, and aerobic gram-negative bacilli predominate (see Fig. 17-1). *E. coli* is responsible for at least 90% of initial infections among the outpatient population; however, this organism is isolated less frequently from outpatients with recurrent infections or from hospitalized patients. *Proteus mirabilis* is the second most common isolate among the outpatient population, followed by the *Klebsiella-Enterobacter* group and gram-positive cocci. *Pseudomonas aeruginosa* is rarely isolated in outpatient populations. Although the same organisms are isolated from hospitalized patients, their frequency of isolation differs greatly. The frequency of isolation of *E. coli* decreases to <50% among hospitalized patients, and the isolation rates of both *P. aeruginosa* and *Streptococcus faecalis* (Enterococcus) greatly increase, especially in

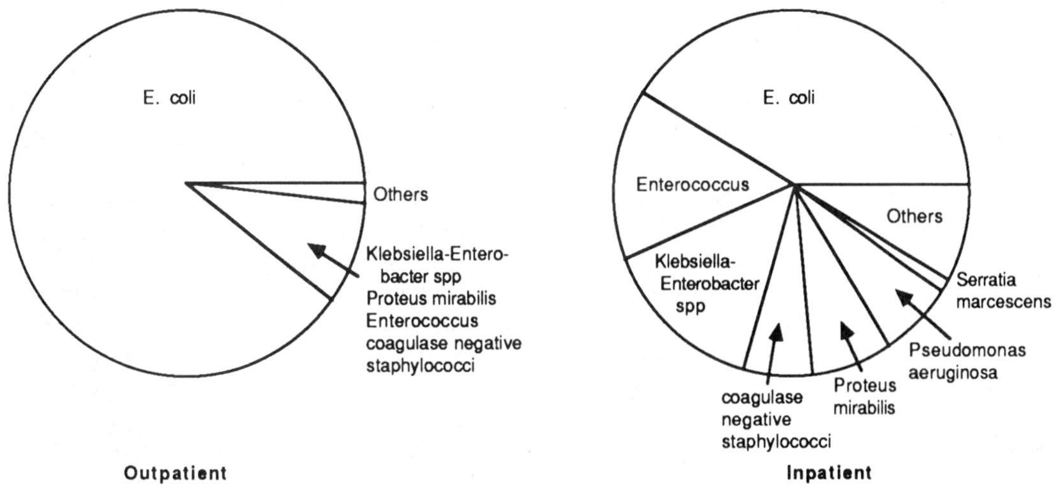

Figure 17-1 **Organisms causing urinary tract infections.**

catheterized patients. This is largely due to the use of broad-spectrum antimicrobials, allowing more resistant organisms to cause infection. Resistant organisms also occur with long-term catheterization and chronic infections following multiple courses of antimicrobial therapy. These facultative organisms, primarily members of the *Enterobacteriaceae,* staphylococci, and enterococci, comprise the normal flora of the intestinal tract, the skin, and the vagina. They are successful as urinary tract pathogens because they colonize the urethra and periurethral area, can readily grow and multiply in urine, have the ability to adhere to urogenital epithelial surfaces, and are pathogenic.

Although the majority of bacteria causing infections among all patient populations are gram-negative bacilli, gram-positive cocci contribute to large numbers of infections among hospitalized and institutionalized patients and certain other patient groups. Enterococcus is a common cause of nosocomial urinary tract infections, especially in men. Its rate of isolation has been second only to that of *E. coli* in catheterized patients, regardless of antimicrobial therapy. This organism has also been associated with renal transplant rejection.[27] *Streptococcus agalactiae* (group B streptococci), although an uncommon cause of urinary tract infection, is responsible for approximately 5% of infections in pregnant females.[28] Infection in the mother predisposes the newborn infant to infection with this same organism. In recent years, group B streptococci infections of the newborn have become more common than *E. coli* infections.[29]

The significance of infections with staphylococci has been recognized in recent years. Although *S. aureus* has usually been considered pathogenic, coagulase-negative staphylococci were often interpreted as contaminants or colonizers. The incidence of urinary tract infection with these organisms is increasing, and their pathogenicity has been recognized.[30] *S. aureus* is not a common nosocomial pathogen; however, there is an increased incidence of infection with this organism in association with urinary tract obstruction, neoplasm, and manipulation.[31] Elderly men undergoing urologic procedures are also at risk. The source is the intestinal tract; the organism is also present in the vagina of approximately 10% of women. *Staphylococcus saprophyticus* is now recognized as a pathogen, especially in the young adult female population.[32] The incidence of infection may be as high as 30% in young female outpatients between the ages of 16 and 25. There also appears to be a seasonal association, with peaks in late summer and early fall.[33] Pyelonephritis is a complication, but septicemia is rare. *S. saprophyticus* has also been implicated as a possible cause of nongonococcal urethritis.[34] The source of the organism is thought to be the skin, vagina, or urethra. The coagulase-negative staphylococci (previously referred to as *Staphylococcus epidermidis*) have been increasing as agents of infection.[35] The patients at risk include men undergoing urologic procedures, patients with underlying urinary tract pathology, and catheterized patients. The organism is part of the normal flora of the vagina, perineal skin, and urethra. During catheterization the bladder becomes colonized; if certain predisposing factors are present, infection with this organism may result.

Anaerobes play a very minor role in urinary tract infections. If routine aerobic cultures are negative and there is reason to suspect anaerobic bacteriuria, a suprapubic bladder aspiration may be evaluated.

After *E. coli, Chlamydia trachomatis* is the second most common infectious agent associated with the urethral syndrome in young adult women.[36] This organism has also been established as a cause of nongonococcal urethritis in men,[37] and has been isolated in a majority of patients with chronic prostatitis and in women with cystourethritis.[38] Mycoplasmas and ureaplasmas can also cause urinary tract infections. *Mycoplasma hominis* causes upper urinary tract infection, and has been the causative agent in approximately 9% of patients with pyelonephritis.[39, 40] *Ureaplasma urealyticum* has been isolated in cases of chronic prostatitis.[39] Urinary tract infections caused by *Mycobacterium* species are not common, but can be very serious when they occur. The kidney becomes infected from a primary site in the lung, and the organism spreads via the hematogenous route.[41] The infection causes stricture formation in the kidney and frequency, pain, and hematuria. If the infection is very severe, kidney failure and death may result.

Although fungi are not common causes of urinary tract infections, the incidence of infection with these microorganisms increases with catheterization, pyelonephritis, and symptomatic female patients.[42] The organisms causing funguria include *Candida albicans, Torulopsis (Candida) glabrata,* and *Candida parapsilosis.* The viruses associated with urinary tract infections include cytomegalovirus (CMV) and herpesvirus (HSV-2). These organisms have been isolated in acute urethral syndrome, but neither WBC nor bacteria are present in the urine. CMV is shed in the urine of young females ($\leq$14 years old), but this stops by age 30.[43] The shedding of HSV-2 in women increases slightly with age. The protozoan *Trichomonas vaginalis* is a common cause of sexually-transmitted disease and has been isolated from the urinary tract,[44] although it has not been established that this organism is a urinary tract pathogen.

Other Complications

Urinary tract infections can *relapse.* This term refers to instances in which the organisms disappear during treatment and reappear sometime after therapy is discontinued. The condition may result from structural abnormalities, renal involvement, or chronic prostatitis.[10] *Reinfection* or *recurrence* refers to the reappearance of infection whether as soon as 1 month after therapy or as long as once every 2 to 3 years. If the same organism is reisolated, the infection has relapsed. However, if a different organism is isolated, it may be a reinfection. The incidence of relapse and reinfection is high (20% to 30%) in chronic pyelonephritis following treatment.[11] In young women, symptomatic reinfections are associated with sexual activity.[45] If reinfection occurs while the patient is on therapy, the antimicrobial must be changed because this indicates that the organism is resistant to the prophylactic agent.

Perinephric abscess is an uncommon complication of urinary tract infection. The symptoms are similar to pyelonephritis, with fever and flank pain. The infection is always secondary to another disease, usually obstruction of an infected kidney, and it effects both men and women with equal frequency. It is a purulent process within the connective tissue external to the kidney capsule.[46]

CLINICAL MANIFESTATIONS

Infections of the urinary system may involve either the upper or the lower tract, and may or may not produce symptoms.

Upper Urinary Tract Infection

The *upper urinary tract* includes the kidneys, renal pelvis, and ureters, and its infections are usually characterized by flank pain, chills, fever, nausea, and vomiting. The patient may experience dysuria (painful, burning, difficult urination) and frequency.

Acute pyelonephritis may be associated with mild to severe flank pain and tenderness, chills, fever, nausea, and vomiting. Examination of the urine usually demonstrates the presence of $\geq 10^5$ bacteria/ml along with large numbers of white blood cells and white blood cell casts. There is also tissue invasion by white blood cells. These findings are often associated with obstruction, stones, and neurological damage. Acute pyelonephritis may be associated with more serious conditions such as septicemia, shock, toxemias of pregnancy, diabetes mellitus, pregnancy, hypertension, and stone formation.[18] The frequency of pyelonephritis increases with age, multiple births, urinary tract instrumentation, and catheterization.

Chronic pyelonephritis is a term used to describe a prolonged infection associated with the presence of bacteria or the presence of lesions in the absence of active disease. The symptoms may range from those of an acute infection to those of a mild infection accompanied by malaise, or the patient may be completely asymptomatic. The presence of bacteriuria and pyuria indicates infection. These patients may also experience nocturia and frequency, and may produce only dilute urine.[9, 11] Presumptive diagnosis may be based on the patient's clinical history and symptoms as well as on specific laboratory findings.

Lower Urinary Tract Infection

Lower urinary tract infections involve the bladder, the urethra, and in men the prostate. Symptoms associated with lower tract infections include dysuria, increased frequency of urination, and suprapubic pain. The most common symptomatic infection is *acute cystitis,* also called "honeymoon cystitis" or "acute urethral syndrome."[47] Its symptoms include dysuria and frequency with small amounts of urine that may be turbid and bloody. Unlike in upper tract infection, fever is usually absent. If the infection is in the bladder (cystitis), large numbers of bacteria, $\geq 10^5$ CFU/ml, are usually present.[24] Dysuria and frequency may be associated with infection of the urethra only; however, routine cultures may be negative (acute urethral syndrome).[47]

Included in this group of patients with symptomatic lower tract infections are those who have no recognizable pathogen but have acute dysuria and pyuria (dysuria-pyuria syndrome).[48] It is important for the physician to distinguish between *urethritis* and *vaginitis,* because in the case of vaginitis urine cultures and urinalysis are not necessary for detection of the etiologic agent. Patients with vaginitis have a vaginal discharge and dysuria, but increased frequency of urination is uncommon.

Prostatitis

Prostatitis may be an acute or a chronic disease. *Acute prostatitis* may be accompanied by symptoms of tenderness and fever, chills, and back pain, as well as dysuria and pyuria.[13] The prostate gland is swollen, and prostatic fluid contains many white blood cells and gram-negative bacilli, usually enteric organisms. Pyelonephritis, bacteremia, and prostatic abscess are some of the complications that may result from infection of the prostate gland. *Chronic bacterial prostatitis,* a common affliction in men, results from infection by organisms commonly causing urinary tract infection. It is also a common cause of relapsing urinary tract infections in men with normal upper urinary tracts, and is difficult to cure.[49] Patients with chronic bacterial prostatitis may be asymptomatic, with normal prostate glands, or may experience urgency, frequency, back pain, and low-grade fever. (See Fig. 17-2.)

LABORATORY ANALYSES AND DIAGNOSIS

Laboratory analyses of a urinary tract infection may involve localization of the infection and/or detection and identification of the microorganism(s) causing it. Laboratory testing usually includes routine urinalysis as well as cultural studies. Although the urinalysis results may suggest an infection, they are not confirmatory; for this reason, microbiologic testing is necessary. A microbiologic examination should be performed on urine specimens from patients with the following conditions: in the presence of acute symptoms of infection, as a followup to treatment, as part of a septic workup, to monitor urinary catheters, for prostatitis, when symptoms of dysuria and frequency are present, and to determine the possible cause for blood and protein in the urine.

Localization of Infection

The presence of characteristic symptoms may be very helpful in distinguishing upper tract from lower tract infection. The presence of WBC casts suggests tissue invasion associated with pyelonephritis. The presence of antibody-coated bacteria suggests kidney invasion and prostatitis. Nonspecific serologic responses related to inflammation or tissue invasion as a result of acute pyelonephritis include C-reactive protein, elevated

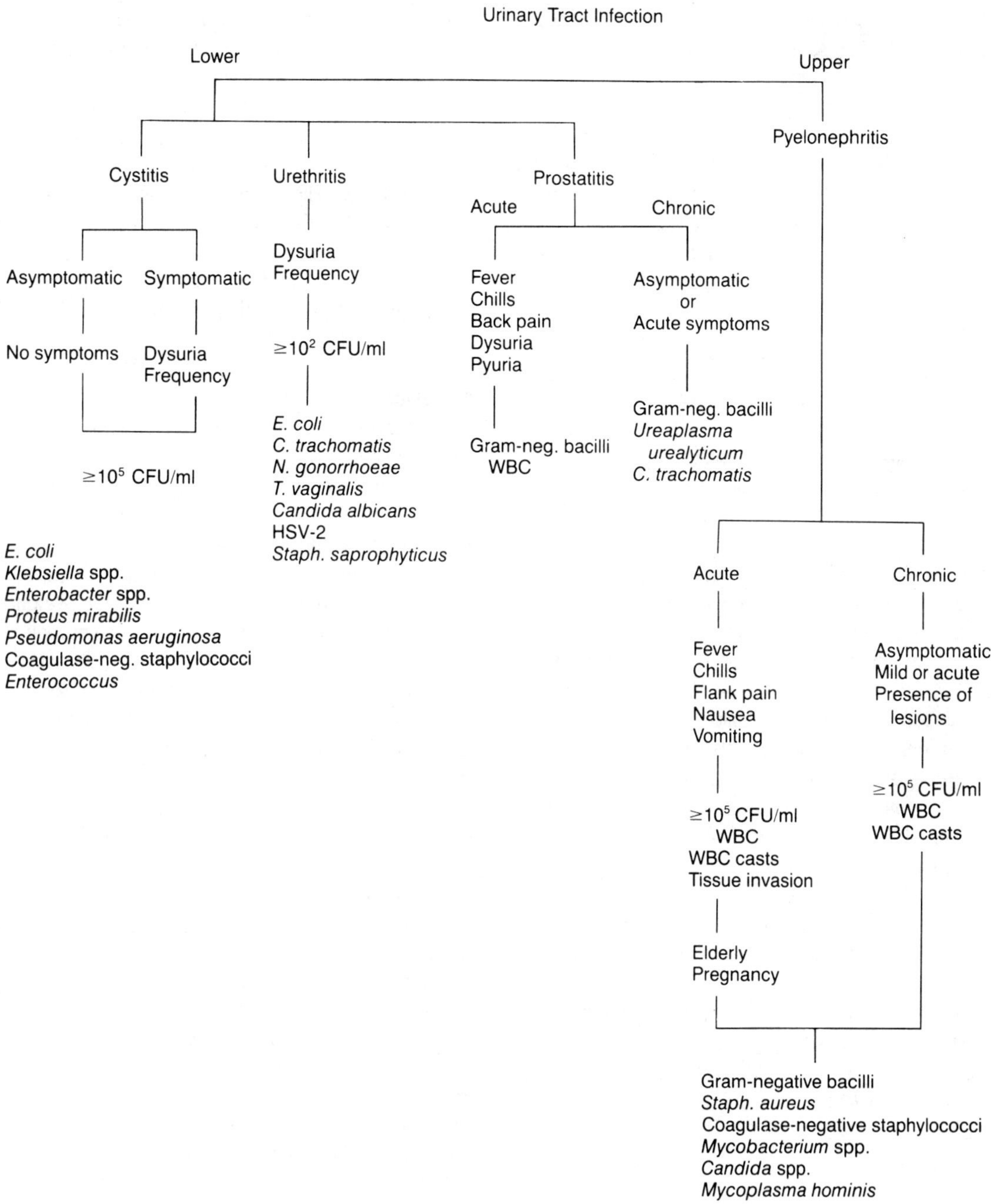

Figure 17-2 Clinical manifestations and etiology of urinary tract infections.

sedimentation rate, and antibodies to Tamm-Horsfall protein. Creatinine clearance also aids in the diagnosis of renal disease.

Specific gravity and *p*H do not provide useful information unless the *p*H is 8.0, suggesting infection with *Proteus* species, one possible reason for an alkaline *p*H. Glycosuria, proteinuria, and hematuria may be associated with bacteriuria; however, they may also be present with other clinical entities.

Specimen Collection and Transport

Specimen collection and transportation are important considerations in the evaluation of a urinary tract infection. Urine is normally a sterile fluid, but during collection it can be contaminated easily with microorganisms from the feces, perineum, vagina, and urethra. Detailed instructions on collection should be provided to the patient by trained persons. Cleaning of the male genitalia prior to collection of a voided specimen may not be necessary.[50] The first voided morning specimen should be collected whenever possible. If this is not possible, urine should be allowed to incubate in the bladder for as long as possible prior to collection, in order to increase the number of organisms per mL and thereby provide more accurate test results. Collection of the specimen from infants by means of a strap-on bag device may provide unreliable culture results. For this reason, urine obtained by suprapubic bladder aspiration is recommended when evaluating infants for a possible urinary tract infection.

Proper evaluation of the specimen by the microbiology laboratory requires information regarding the method of collection, clinical diagnosis, and antimicrobial therapy.

Detection of Bacteriuria

The methods available for detection of bacteriuria include microscopic, chemical, culture, and automated techniques (see Table 17-2). The semiquantitative plate culture method has been the approach most widely used,[51] but within the last decade many screening methods have been introduced that enable more rapid detection. Although the classic overnight culture method allows for isolation and enumeration of the causative agents of infection, it does not provide for rapid reporting of negative specimens. Rapid elimination of negative specimens allows the microbiologist to spend more time on those that are positive. Rapid screening followed by culture for positive specimens provides same-day results on negative specimens and makes possible more cost-effective and timely care of the patient.

Microscopic Methods

Microscopic examination of uncentrifuged urine demonstrating the presence of $\geq$8–10 WBC/mm^3 and at least one microorganism per oil immersion field on Gram stain suggests significant pyuria and bacteriuria. A culture should contain $\geq 10^5$ CFU/ml of a single species, a finding in 96% of patients with symptomatic pyelonephritis.[52] In chronic pyelonephritis, however, more than one organism may be present.[11] Use of uncentrifuged urine for microscopic evaluation is considered more accurate and correlates better with infection.[53] Although red blood cells (RBC) may be present, they may be due to other disorders such as renal calculi, tumor, vasculitis, glomerulonephritis, or renal tuberculosis.[10] It is important to note that these microscopic and culture findings may be present not only in pyelonephritis, but also in infections of the lower urinary tract. The presence of leukocyte (WBC) casts along with significant bacteria ($\geq 10^5$ CFU/ml) suggests pyelonephritis. The antibody-coated bacteria test has been suggested to distinguish upper from lower tract infection. A positive test may also indicate prostatic infection or invasive bladder infection. Because of the high false-negative findings (17%) and the need for a fluorescent microscope, the test has been recommended for epidemiologic or research purposes rather than for clinical use.[54, 55]

The *Gram stain* is a rapid, reliable, and inexpensive procedure for the detection of significant bacteriuria.[51] The presence of at least one organism per oil immersion field from uncentrifuged urine

Table 17-2 ***Laboratory Methods for Detection of Urinary Tract Infections***

Method	Detection Time	Approximate Cost($)/Test*	Comment
Microscopic			
Gram stain	2 min	0.50	Sensitivity at $\geq 10^5$ CFU/ml
Chemical	2 min	0.35	May detect bacteriuria and pyuria
Catalase			
Glucose oxidase			
Leukocyte esterase			
Nitrite			
Leukocyte esterase + nitrite (LN)			LN detects bacteriuria and pyuria
Culture	18 hr	1.50†	Results available next day
Automation			
Colorimetric filtration			Detects bacteriuria and pyuria
Bac-T-Screen (Marion Labs)	2 min	0.95	
Bioluminescence			Detects bacteriuria
Lumac (3M)	35 min	1.45	
Monoscreen (Analytical Luminescence Lab)	15 min	1.35	
Growth-Dependent Photometry			Requires expensive equipment Negatives require 5–13 hr.
Autobac (Organon Teknika Corp)	1–6 hr	0.60	
AMS (Vitek Systems)	4–13 hr	1.25	AMS provides colony count and identity
Advantage (Abbott Laboratories)	1–5 hr	0.60	

* Includes estimated technical time
† Cost of semiquantitative loop method

has a sensitivity of 85% when correlated with 10^5 CFU/ml.[24] This method should be available upon request because it provides the Gram reaction and morphology of the organism, which can be used in initial selection of appropriate antimicrobial therapy. However, it should be noted that specimens with $<10^5$ CFU/ml may appear negative. Use of acridine-orange-stained smears will detect $\geq 10^4$ CFU/ml,[56] but this procedure requires a fluorescent microscope.

Large numbers of polymorphonuclear leukocytes are present in prostatic fluid, which may be observed on Gram stain. The infecting organism may be cultured from urine, since most patients also have an associated bacteriuria. Prostatic massage is discouraged because it may result in bacteremia.[49]

Chemical Methods

The chemical tests that are available as dipsticks are rapid, inexpensive, and easy to perform. The most widely used are *catalase, glucose oxidase, nitrite (Griess's test),* and *leukocyte esterase.* These tests should not be used alone as bacteriuria screens because of the large number of false-positive and false-negative results. False-positive results occur because cells other than bacteria may contain the enzymes being tested. Although catalase is present in many organisms causing urinary tract infection, it is also present in both red and white blood cells and in kidney cells. False-negative results occur because the concentration of enzyme tested is lower than is detectable by the method employed. For this reason, to obtain accurate results urine should be allowed to incubate in the bladder for at least four hours and preferably overnight. Both glucose oxidase and nitrite tests give false-negative results with low concentrations of enzyme. Leukocyte esterase is an enzyme present in WBC. Use of this test as a dipstick detects the presence of pyuria. In combination with nitrite it is a rapid and inexpensive method for detection of bacteriuria and pyuria. The combination of leukocyte esterase and nitrite has increased the sensitivity beyond that of either test alone. The sensitivity of this test combination is <95% for pure pathogens, but it is inexpensive, simple to perform, and can easily be used in combination with another rapid detection method.[57, 58]

Culture Methods

The calibrated loop method for counting bacteria is the technique most widely used for detection of a urinary tract infection, which is evaluated based on the number of CFU/ml. The loop method is semiquantitative, and many variables exist that interfere with its accuracy.[59] However, it is an acceptable, widely used culture method for detection of bacteriuria.

Significant bacteriuria refers to the presence of $\geq 10^5$ CFU/ml in most patients, although young adult women with *acute dysuria* may have as few as 10^2 CFU/ml.[24, 60] Several factors may contribute to low bacterial counts, even when infection is present. These include early infection, dilute urine due to forced fluids, rapid urine flow, low *p*H (<5), and the presence of antimicrobic agents.[24] For this reason, the "gold standard" of $\geq 10^5$ CFU/ml as the definition of significant bacteriuria may not be applicable to all patient groups. Therefore, one of two alternative definitions should be used, depending upon the prevalence of disease. Use of $\geq 10^5$ CFU/ml is acceptable when screening the asymptomatic population in which the prevalence of disease is low;[24] however, if the prevalence of disease is high, as seen in the symptomatic population, then the interpretation criterion should be dropped to 10^2 CFU/ml.[61]

Patients with *perinephric abscesses* also have colony counts of $\geq 10^5$ CFU/ml in urine specimens. Common organisms associated with this infection include *S. aureus, Streptococcus* species, gram-negative bacilli, *Mycobacterium tuberculosis,* and anaerobes. Perinephric abscess is a life-threatening infection if undiagnosed and untreated.

The tube dilution pour plate method is the most definitive culture method for counting bacteria,[62] but it is not practical for routine use. Dipsticks or dipslides are available commercially and are used primarily in the physician's office rather than in a hospital diagnostic laboratory. These devices make it possible for physicians to rule out negative specimens and submit positive results to a diagnostic laboratory for identification and antimicrobial susceptibility testing; however, these devices are not accurate below 10^3 CFU/ml, and should not be used when there is a possibility of low-count bacteriuria (10^2 CFU/ml). Use of these techniques may be necessary when transport to a laboratory is delayed and refrigeration is not available.

Although the etiologic agent of acute prostatitis can be determined from a urine culture alone, cultures of the urethra, urine, midstream urine, and prostatic secretions are necessary to confirm the diagnosis of chronic bacterial prostatitis. A quantitative localization technique has been described for making the bacterial diagnosis.[49] The specimens must be cultured immediately after collection, and small numbers of organisms should be quantified.

Automated Methods

Automated methods were developed as a result of the need for rapid urine screening (see Table 17-2), and have been reviewed extensively.[63] There are a number of rapid, accurate, cost-effective bacteriuria screens that allow positive urines to be detected within time periods that range from 2 minutes to 13 hours. More important, many of these instruments can detect bacteriuria at $<10^5$ CFU/ml, a significant finding in the symptomatic patient. Additionally, some instruments have the ability to detect pyuria rapidly and easily along with bacteriuria, therefore providing more meaningful information.

Detection of Pyuria

Significant pyuria, the presence of $\geq$8–10 WBC/mm^3 in urine, is an important finding in the presence of low-count or negative bacteriuria. Also, the presence of pyuria in the absence of symptoms may suggest infection rather than colonization. Use of the urinary sediment is not a reliable method unless the procedure is well-defined and standardized regarding volume of urine centrifuged, resuspended, and examined as well as speed and time of centrifugation.[53, 64] A method using uncentrifuged urine in a hemocytometer chamber has been described.[64] The presence of at least 8–10 WBC/mm^3 correlates with a leukocyte excretion rate of >400,000 WBC/hour. Other alternative methods for detecting pyuria are listed in Table 17-2.[57] Significant pyuria in the absence of bacteriuria may alert the physician and the laboratory to investigate such pathogens as *C. trachomatis, Neisseria gonorrhoeae,* or *M. tuberculosis,* or possible other pathologic conditions such as tumor or stones.

Certain practices should not be followed when processing urine specimens for bacteriuria and/or pyuria because they provide inaccurate or unreliable results. These include inoculation of the urine specimen into a broth, culture of the urine sediment, routine cultures for anaerobes, antimicrobial susceptibility testing directly from the urine specimen, inoculation of multiple media (>3), allowing the urine to remain at room temperature for longer than 2 hours without refrigeration, and culturing of Foley catheter tips.[65]

TREATMENT

Many antimicrobials have been used for treatment of urinary tract infections. Treatment regimens range from single-dose oral drugs for acute, symptomatic infections of the outpatient population without complicating urologic abnormalities to parenteral prolonged therapy (7 days to 6 weeks) for more serious urinary tract infections. Oral chemotherapeutic agents that have been used for treatment of acute urinary tract infections include ampicillin, amoxicillin, cephalexin, cephradine, nitrofurantoin, sulfisoxazole, tetracycline, and trimethoprim-sulfamethoxazole.[66] Asymptomatic infections may be treated similarly. If the patient relapses after appropriate therapy, this may indicate renal involvement, a urologic abnormality, or chronic bacterial prostatitis. These infections may be cured with extended therapy for as long as 2 to 6 weeks if there are no structural abnormalities.[67] The treatment for structural abnormalities may be surgery. Prolonged therapy (>6 weeks) should be reserved for patients who are at great risk for renal damage. For patients who develop reinfections, long-term therapy should be considered if the infections are frequent.

Single-dose therapy has been shown to be as effective as a 1- to 2-week course in patients who have lower urinary tract infections.[1, 68, 69] Amoxicillin, sulfisoxazole, and trimethoprim-sulfamethoxazole have been effective as single-dose oral therapy. Single-dose therapy has the advantages of development of fewer side-effects, better compliance, less chance of development of resistant organisms, and lower cost.[68] On the other hand, the disadvantages include a higher rate of reinfection and an increase in pyelonephritis if an upper urinary tract infection is mistaken for a lower tract infection. There appears to be less chance of relapse in women with acute dysuria when a 10-day course of trimethoprim-sulfamethoxazole is given instead of a single dose of the drug.[70] Similar regimens may be used during pregnancy; however, tetracycline should be avoided and sulfonamides should not be used during the last few weeks of gestation.[10]

Patients with acute bacterial prostatitis respond dramatically to antimicrobial therapy, but patients with chronic prostatitis do not. It is felt that most antimicrobics are unable to penetrate prostatic fluid, although trimethoprim-sulfamethoxazole appears to be the most effective therapy for chronic prostatitis.[71]

All symptomatic patients should be treated, regardless of age. Bacteriuria should disappear or be greatly reduced within 48 hours of therapy. If bacteria persist, they are most likely resistant to the chemotherapeutic agent. Urine cultures should be obtained after 3 or 4 days of therapy to demonstrate the effectiveness or failure of therapy. It is sometimes possible to demonstrate moderate resistance with antimicrobial susceptibility testing, although the patient seems to have responded to therapy. The reason is that most antimicrobics are excreted in the urine, and the concentrations are much higher than those used in antimicrobial susceptibility testing. However, if the patient has not responded, the antimicrobial should be changed.

Repeat urine cultures should be performed 48 hours after initiation of therapy, soon after discontinuation of therapy, and after 6 months. The 48-hour followup culture will determine the efficacy of the therapy, a followup culture after the discontinuation of therapy will detect a relapse, and a culture after 6 months will detect reinfection.

CASE STUDY

A 24-year-old woman presented to her physician with symptoms of 3 days' duration of dysuria, frequency, and urgency. She appeared otherwise healthy and had recently returned from a 2-week honeymoon trip to Hawaii.

Physical examination revealed a healthy, well-developed woman with suprapubic pain but no flank pain or fever. The patient had no previous history of kidney stones, diabetes, urologic abnormalities, recent antimicrobial therapy, or pregnancy. The pelvic examination appeared negative for genital herpes, *Candida, Trichomonas,* and nonspecific vaginitis. This was confirmed by examination of the vaginal fluid, performed in the physician's office.

Urinalysis findings included positive nitrite and leukocyte esterase tests as well as hematuria and proteinuria. The microscopic examination of centrifuged urine sediment contained 15 leukocytes per high-power field. *E. coli* was isolated from the urine culture, with a colony count of 54,000 CFU/ml.

Questions

1. What conditions should be included in the differential diagnosis?
2. Are the urinalysis findings helpful?
3. Is a colony count of $<10^5$ CFU/ml significant?
4. Are the leukocyte findings significant?
5. What is the probable diagnosis?

Discussion

1. Although this case is apparently one of a lower urinary tract bacterial infection that may have previously been referred to as "honeymoon cystitis," recent evidence suggests that "cystitis" may actually include any one of five different clinical conditions that must be differentiated because each is managed differently. These include subclinical pyelonephritis, chlamydial urethritis, vaginitis, dysuria without urinary tract or vaginal infection, and lower urinary tract bacterial infections (LTI).
2. The distinction between these conditions is made primarily from clinical findings and urinalysis demonstrating significant pyuria. Chlamydial urethritis may be excluded in this case because of the absence of mucopurulent endocervical secretions and the occurrence of hematuria and proteinuria.
3. Although most patients with lower tract bacterial infection have greater than 100,000 bacteria/mL of urine, a large majority of symptomatic women with pyuria may have between 100 and 100,000 CFU/mL of pure cultures. *E. coli* and *S. saprophyticus* are the two urinary pathogens found most frequently in women with lower urinary tract infection.
4. In cases of vaginitis, pyuria and hematuria are absent. Patients with subclinical pyelonephritis have findings similar to those of patients with lower urinary tract infections, in that the symptoms persist for a long time (>10 days). These

patients may have a history of childhood infections, diabetes, recurring infection, and acute pyelonephritis within the past year. None of these findings had occurred in this case. Lastly, patients with dysuria without a recognizable pathogen do not have pyuria. Thus, the finding of pyuria may be the most helpful information in this case. Determination of pyuria may be performed on uncentrifuged or centrifuged urine. The presence of eight or more leukocytes/mm^3 in uncentrifuged urine corresponds to that of two to five leukocytes/HPF in centrifuged urine sediments. The isolation of $>10^2$ CFU/mL of a pure pathogen from the culture in a symptomatic patient confirms the diagnosis.

5. The probable diagnosis is lower urinary tract infection.

REFERENCES

1. Fang LST, Tolkoff-Rubin NE, Rubin RH: Efficacy of single-dose and conventional amoxicillin therapy in urinary-tract infection localized by the antibody-coated bacteria technic. N Engl J Med 298:413, 1978
2. Dontas AS, Kasviki-Charvati P, Chem L et al: Bacteriuria and survival in old age. N Engl J Med 304:939, 1981
3. Kass EH: Bacteriuria and pyelonephritis of pregnancy. Arch Intern Med 105:194, 1960
4. Nordenstam GR, Branberg CA, Oden AS et al: Bacteriuria and mortality in an elderly population. N Engl J Med 314:1152, 1986
5. Bran JL, Levison ME, Kaye D: Entrance of bacteria into the female urinary bladder. N Engl J Med 286:626, 1972
6. Buckley RM, McGuckin M, MacGregor RR: Urine bacterial counts after sexual intercourse. N Engl J Med 298:321, 1978
7. Daifuku R, Stamm WE: Association of rectal and urethral colonization with urinary tract infection in patients with indwelling catheters. JAMA 252:2028, 1984
8. Daifuku R, Stamm WE: Bacterial adherence to bladder uroepithelial cells in catheter-associated urinary tract infection. N Engl J Med 314:1208, 1986
9. Kunin CM: Detection, Prevention, and Management of Urinary Tract Infections. Philadelphia, Lea & Febiger, 1979
10. Kaye D, Santoro J: Urinary tract infection. In Mandell GL, Douglas RG, Bennett JE (eds): Principles and Practice of Infectious Disease, p 537. New York City, John Wiley & Sons, 1979
11. Pazin GJ, Braude A: Pyelonephritis. In Hoeprich PD (ed): Infectious Diseases: A Modern Treatise of Infectious Processes, p 462. Hagerstown, MD, Harper & Row, 1977
12. Kunin CM: In defense of the bladder. West J Med 137:237, 1982
13. Edelmann CM, Ogwo JE, Fine BP et al: The prevalence of bacteriuria in full-term and premature newborn infants. J Pediatr 82:125–132, 1972
14. Kass EH, Savage W, Santamarina BAG: The significance of bacteriuria in preventive medicine. In Kass EH (ed): Progress in Pyelonephritis, pp 3–11. Philadelphia, FA Davis, 1965
15. Asscher AW, Sussman M, Waters WE et al: The clinical significance of asymptomatic bacteriuria in the nonpregnant woman. J Infect Dis 120:17–21, 1969
16. Mabeck CE: Uncomplicated urinary tract infection in women. Postgrad Med J 47 (Sept Suppl):31–35, 1971
17. Davison JM, Sprott MS, Selkon JB: The effect of covert bacteriuria in schoolgirls on renal function at 18 years and during pregnancy. Lancet 2:651–655, 1984
18. Kass EH: Horatio at the orifice: The significance of bacteriuria. J Infect Dis 138:546, 1978
19. Platt R: Quantitative definition of bacteriuria. Am J Med 75:44–52, 1983
20. Harris RE: Infections of the urinary tract during pregnancy. South Med J 69:1429, 1936
21. Kass EH: Bacteriuria and pyelonephritis of pregnancy. Arch Intern Med 105:194, 1960
22. Nicolle LE, Bjornson J, Harding GKM et al: Bacteriuria in elderly institutionalized men. N Engl J Med 309:1420, 1983
23. Yoshikawa TT: Unique aspects of urinary tract infection in the geriatric population. Gerontol 30:339, 1984
24. Kass EH: Asymptomatic infections of the urinary tract. Trans Assoc Am Phys 69:56, 1956
25. Turck M, Goffe B, Petersdorf RG: The urethral catheters and urinary tract infection. J Urol 88:834, 1962

26. Garibaldi RA, Burke JP, Dickman ML et al: Factors predisposing to bacteriuria during indwelling urethral catheterization. N Engl J Med 291:215, 1974
27. Byrd LH, Cheigh JS, Stenzel KH et al: Association between *Streptococcus faecalis* urinary infections and graft reject in kidney transplantation. Lancet 2:1167
28. Wood EG, Dillon HCL: A prospective study of group B streptococcal bacteriuria in pregnancy. Am J Obstet Gynecol 140:515, 1981
29. Pass MA, Gray BM, Dillon HC: Puerperal and perinatal infections with group B streptococci. Am J Obstet Gynecol 143:147, 1982
30. Bailey RR: Significance of coagulase-negative *Staphylococcus* in urine. J Infect Dis 127:179, 1973
31. Demuth PJ, Gerding DN, Crossley K: *Staphylococcus aureus* bacteriuria. Arch Intern Med 139:78, 1979
32. Gillespie WA, Sellin MA, Gill P et al: Urinary tract infections in young women, with special reference to *Staphylococcus saprophyticus.* J Clin Pathol 31:348, 1978
33. Wallmark G, Arremark I, Telander B: *Staphylococcus saprophyticus:* A frequent cause of acute urinary tract infection among female outpatients. J Infect Dis 14-38:791, 1978
34. Hovelivs B, Thelin I, Mardh PA: *Staphylococcus saprophyticus* in the etiology of nongonococcal urethritis. Br J Vener Dis 55:369j, 1979
35. Shrestha TL, Darrell JH: Urinary infection with coagulase-negative staphylococci in a teaching hospital. J Clin Pathol 32:299, 1979
36. Stamm WE, Wagner KF, Amsel R et al: Causes of acute urethral syndrome in women. N Engl J Med 303:409, 1980
37. Holmes KK, Handsfield HH, Wang SP et al: Etiology of nongonococcal urethritis. N Engl J Med 292:1199, 1975
38. Bruce AW, Chadwick WS, Willett WS et al: The role of *Chlamydiae* in genitourinary disease. J Urol 126:625, 1981
39. Brunner H, Weidner W, Schiefer HG: Studies of the role of *Ureaplasma urealyticum* and *Mycoplasma hominis* in prostatitis. J Infect Dis 147:807, 1983
40. Thomsen AC: Occurrence of mycoplasmas in urinary tracts of patients with acute pyelonephritis. J Clin Microbiol 8:84, 1978
41. Riddle PR: Urinary tuberculosis. Nurs Times 70:1976, 1974
42. Krautz G, Bernhardt H, Dutz W et al: Mycotic urinary tract infection in pyelonephritic patients. Proc Eur Dial Transplant Assoc 17:678, 1980
43. Knox GE, Pass RF, Reynolds DW et al: Comparative prevalence of subclinical cytomegalovirus and herpes simplex virus infections in the genital and urinary tracts of low-income urban women. J Infect Dis 140:419, 1979
44. Dans PE, Klaus B: Dysuria in women. Johns Hopkins Med J 138:13, 1976
45. Vosti KL: Recurrent urinary tract infections: Prevention by prophylactic antibiotics after sexual intercourse. JAMA 231:934, 1975
46. Finegold SM: Perinephric Abscess. In Hoeprich PD (ed): Infectious Diseases: A Modern Treatise of Infectious Processes, p 474. Hagerstown, MD, Harper & Row, 1977
47. Gallagher DJA, Montgomerie JZ, North JDK: Acute infections of the urinary tract and the urethral syndrome in general practice. Br Med J 1:622, 1965
48. Komaroff AL, Friedland G: The dysuria-pyuria syndrome. N Engl J Med 303:452, 1980
49. Meares EM: Bacterial prostatitis and recurrent urinary tract infections. In Hoeprich PD (ed): Infectious Diseases: A Modern Treatise of Infectious Processes, p 437. Hagerstown, MD, Harper & Row, 1977
50. Lipsky BA, Inui TS, Plorde JJ et al: Is the clean-catch midstream void procedure necessary for obtaining urine culture specimens for men? Am J Med 76:257, 1984
51. Pezzlo MT, Tan GL, Peterson EM et al: Screening of urine cultures by three automated methods. J Clin Microbiol 15:468, 1982
52. Kass EH: Bacteriuria and the diagnosis of infections of the urinary tract, with observations on the use of methionine as a urinary antiseptic. Arch Intern Med 100:709, 1957
53. Brumfitt W: Urinary cell counts and their value. J Clin Pathol 18:550, 1965
54. Stamm WE: Recent developments in the diagnosis and treatment of urinary tract infections. West J Med 137:213, 1982
55. Matuscak RR, Pasculle AW, Barnhart L et al: Slide method for detection of antibody-coated bacteria in urine sediments. J Clin Microbiol 12:761, 1980

56. Hoff RG, Newman DE, Staneck JL: Bacteremia screening by use of acridine-orange-stained smears. J Clin Microbiol 21:513, 1985
57. Pezzlo MT, Wetkowski MA, Peterson EM et al: Detection of bacteriuria and pyuria within two minutes. J Clin Microbiol 21:578, 1985
58. Pfaller MA, Koontz FP: Laboratory evaluation of leukocyte esterase and nitrite tests for the detection of bacteriuria. J Clin Microbiol 21:840, 1985
59. Albers AC, Fletcher RD: Accuracy of the calibrated-loop transfer. J Clin Microbiol 18:40, 1983
60. Stamm WE, Counts GW, Running KR et al: Diagnosis of coliform infection in acute dysuric women. N Engl J Med 307:463, 1982
61. Bartlett RC, Galen RS: Predictive value of urine culture. Am J Clin Pathol 79:756, 1983
62. Hoeprich PD: Culture of the urine. J Clin Lab Med 56:899, 1960
63. Pezzlo MT: Detection of bacteriuria by automated methods. Lab Med 15:539, 1984
64. Stamm WE: Measurement of pyuria and its relation to bacteriuria. Am J Med 75:53, 1983
65. Clarridge JE, Pezzlo MT, Vasti KL: Laboratory diagnosis of urinary tract infections. In Weissfeld AL (ed): Cumitech 2A. Washington, DC, American Society for Microbiology, 1987
66. Levison ME, Kaye D: Management of urinary infection. In Kaye O (ed): Urinary Tract Infection and Its Management, p 188. St Louis, CV Mosby, 1972
67. Turck M, Ronald AP, Petersdorf RG: Relapse and reinfection in chronic bacteriuria: II. The correlation between the site of infection and pattern of recurrence in chronic bacteriuria. N Engl J Med 278:422, 1968
68. Komaroff AL: Acute dysuria in women. N Engl J Med 310:368, 1984
69. Slade N, Crowther ST: Multicentre survey of urinary tract infections in general practice: Clinical trial of single dose treatment with sulfametopyrazine (Kelfizine-W). Br J Urol 44:105, 1972
70. Schultz HJ, McCoffrey LA, Keys TF et al: Acute cystitis: A prospective study of laboratory tests and duration of therapy. Mayo Clin Proc 59:391, 1984
71. Meares EM: Long-term therapy of chronic bacterial prostatitis with trimethoprim-sulfamethoxazole. Am Med Assoc J 112:225, 1975

BIBLIOGRAPHY

Asscher AW: Covert infections. In The Challenge of Urinary Tract Infections, p 52. New York City, Grune & Stratton, 1980

Bartlett RC: Urine screening—to screen or not to screen. Clin Microbiol Newsl 6:29, 1984

Meares EM: Prostatitis: A review. Urol Clin N Am 2:3, 1975

Pezzlo MT, Conway S, Jacobson M et al: Effect of the B-D Urine Culture Kit on an automated bacteriuria screen. J Clin Microbiol 20:1207, 1984

Thomas V, Shelokov A, Forland M: Antibody-coated bacteria in urine and the site of urinary-tract infection. N Engl J Med 290:588, 1974

Chapter 18

Renal Hypertension

Martha Savage Payne

ETIOLOGY AND PATHOPHYSIOLOGY

Essential or Primary Hypertension

Hypertension as defined in Chapter 4 is characterized by systolic and diastolic blood pressures exceeding 140/90 mm Hg. Hypertension, in the vast majority of patients, has no identified specific etiology; this form is classified as primary, or essential hypertension. Current authorities recognize that essential hypertension is a complex problem, and the mosaic theory of factors has evolved.[1] This theory considers hypertension to be a disease of regulation in which several of the mechanisms that control blood pressure, lipid metabolism, or collagen synthesis are disordered or reset. There are many variables that control and regulate blood pressure, and near the center of the schema is the kidney. The kidney produces both vasopressor and vasodepressor materials, and is the excretory organ for sodium. The kidney may be damaged by elevated blood pressure, even to the point of renal failure.

There are three major mechanisms through which the kidney can effect blood pressure: (1) production by the kidney of the hormone renin, which helps maintain blood pressure; (2) the effector mechanism for the control of sodium and fluid volume; (3) production by the kidney of prostaglandins, which may have vasodepressor or blood pressure-lowering properties.[2] Any disease, either primary in the kidney or one to which the kidney may be responding, can cause hypertension.

Renin is a proteolytic enzyme that is synthesized, stored, and secreted by the kidney. It is a highly specific proteolytic enzyme that cleaves a decapeptide from an α_2-globulin synthesized by the liver to produce angiotensin I. This is converted to angiotensin II, an octapeptide, by a converting enzyme located primarily in the lung. Angiotension II is both a potent vasoconstrictor and a stimulus to aldosterone production (see Fig. 4-1, Chap. 4). Renin release is the rate-limiting step in angiotensin production. This release is subject to feedback control, by angiotensin II directly and indirectly through the effect of angiotensin on blood volume, blood pressure, and sodium balance. The renin-angiotensin system is complex, and interrelates with various other systems for the control of vascular volume and resistance. The measurements of renin activity are made by using specific, precise, and reproducible radioimmunoassays for angiotensin I and II. These tests can be used to identify significant renal artery stenosis and categorize patients with other forms of hypertension (see Chap. 4).

The second group of mechanisms through which the kidney can influence blood pressure are the factors that control sodium excretion. Epidemiologic studies have demonstrated a direct correlation between the level of sodium intake and the incidence of hypertension in population groups.[3] The factors that control sodium excretion in the kidney are glomerular filtration rate, aldosterone, and the peritubular capillary Starling forces.[2] Under normal circumstances, the sodium balance in humans is not regulated by variation in the glomerular filtration rate (GFR). In renal failure, however, the GFR may be so depressed that it is the rate-limiting step for sodium excretion. Sodium and water retention will therefore produce a volume-dependent hypertension. Aldosterone, a corticoid steroid produced in the adrenals, facilitates sodium reabsorption and potassium excretion by the distal tubules. Sodium depletion, potassium excess, and elevated angiotension II stimulate aldosterone secretion. Aldosterone can participate in hypertensive disease either by primary adrenal overproduction or secondarily in response to renal renin secretion (see Chap. 4). The third factor controlling sodium excretion is the Starling forces in the peritubular capillaries. An increase in the pressure will inhibit sodium reabsorption and enhance sodium excretion. This may not be a cause of hypertension, but rather a mechanism to achieve sodium homeostasis. When patients with renal failure are unable to excrete sodium equivalent to their intake due to a low GFR, volume-expansive hypertension will increase peritubular capillary pressure and facilitate sodium excretion.

Prostaglandins produced by the renal medulla (PGE_2 and possibly PGA_2) may have the capacity to lower blood pressure by dilating peripheral arteries. It has also been postulated that these compounds may influence sodium and water reabsorption by redistribution of blood flow within the kidney.[4] The relevance and importance of these compounds in hypertension in humans are not clearly understood.

Essential hypertension seems to involve the kidney or some aspect of renal function, but the exact mechanism in most cases is elusive. Changes in arterial pressure involve changes in vascular resistance. The development of hypertension is associated with vasoconstriction, while cardiac output remains relatively unchanged. It has been shown that vascular smooth muscle responds to both local conditions and systemic neural and humoral signals. The local response is called *autoregulation of blood flow,* and normal blood flow and elevated vascular resistance might be expected in hypertension. It is difficult to connect autoregulation with the general contention that the kidneys dominate blood pressure control. One explanation to connect the renal involvement with autoregulation is that salt and water are retained when the excretory load exceeds the kidney's excretory capability. Some of this retained fluid that is in the circulation tends to increase venous return and cardiac output. Elevated cardiac output increases arterial pressure while also triggering autoregulatory vasoconstriction. Rising pressure facilitates salt and water excretion and helps reestablish salt and water balance. The eventual hemodynamic picture is one of sodium balance, elevated arterial pressure, vasoconstriction, and normal cardiac output.[5]

It is not clearly understood which is the cause and which is the result in the relationship between arteriolar nephrosclerosis and hypertension. Evidence exists that can be used to support the view that hypertension is responsible for nephrosclerosis.[2] However, some of the same evidence can be interpreted differently to be consistent with the view that hypertension is secondary to arteriolar nephrosclerosis. At this time evidence is not conclusive.

Renal Artery Stenosis

Renal artery stenosis (RAS) can cause hypertension. Some authors have estimated that approximately 5% of all the hypertension population have RAS.[2] Many lesions can produce RAS, with atherosclerosis being more common in older men and fibromuscular dysplasia more common in women whose average age is 40 years.[6] The altered pressure-flow relationships within the kidney due to renal artery stenosis activate compensatory mechanisms that produce the hypertension and metabolic and physiological abnormalities. Total renal blood flow is reduced by the stenosis when the diameter of the renal artery is reduced by 60% or more. This leads to an increase in angiotensin II via renin production, with a subsequent increase in peripheral vascular resistance. Aldosterone secretion is increased also by the angiotensin, which favors potassium excretion and sodium and water retention. The other normal kidney excretes the sodium and water, decreasing plasma volume. The flow and pressure are not restored to the affected kidney, and renin secretion continues.

Hypertension Associated With Other Forms of Renal Disease

All forms of chronic renal disease and acute renal failure may be associated with an increased incidence of hypertension. Chronic glomerulonephritis, chronic pyelonephritis, vascular lesions such as in polyarteritis nodosa and lupus erythematosus, polycystic disease, and renal carcinoma can cause hypertension. Obstructive uropathies, analgesic abuse, and renal calculi can also cause hypertension. Acute renal failure can cause rapid elevation of blood pressure, especially in fluid overloaded patients.

Patients without kidneys or those in terminal renal failure with very low GFR values are extremely sensitive to changes in salt and water balance. Plasma renin and angiotensin are usually low. This form of hypertension must be managed by salt and water restriction and elimination of excess by dialysis.

CLINICAL MANIFESTATIONS

Clinically it is very difficult to distinguish essential hypertension from renal artery stenosis hypertension. Patients with RAS usually have hypertension of short duration that is severe and accelerated in nature. Renal artery stenosis frequently occurs in patients younger than age 25 or older than 50. In general, those with RAS caused by fibromuscular hyperplasia are younger and those with RAS caused by atherosclerosis are older than patients with essential hypertension. However, truly distinctive clinical features of RAS versus essential hypertension have not been found in many studies.[6]

Those patients with hypertension secondary to renal disease have the characteristic clinical findings of the individual disorders.

LABORATORY ANALYSES AND DIAGNOSIS

The diagnostic evaluation in patients with hypertension should help to stage organ damage, to identify factors that will affect treatment and prognosis, and to identify any correctable etiology. Renal artery stenosis comprises more than half of the correctable causes. The majority of the other correctable causes may be strongly suspected based on initial history and physical examination (*e.g.*, pheochromocytoma). The decision is usually whether to carry out the diagnostic studies for renovascular hypertension (see Chap. 4 for discussion of these studies). Each of these studies should be done only after the risks are assessed in relation to the specificity and sensitivity of the study. If renovascular hypertension is the diagnosis, then surgical or medical therapy must be chosen. If the patient is known to be an unsuitable candidate for surgery, then the expensive diagnostic evaluation is of little use and not cost-effective. As is discussed in Chapter 4, the first step in diagnosis is the history, followed by routine laboratory tests (urinalysis, blood chemistries) and then by special tests such as rapid sequence excretory urogram, selective renal angiograms, renal vein renin determinations, and saralasin infusion tests.

In hypertension secondary to specific renal disease, the laboratory values will correspond to the particular disease entity.

The reader is referred to Chapter 4 of this text for a major discussion of hypertension, with suggested treatment and representative case study.

REFERENCES

1. Mendlowitz M: Some theories of hypertension: Fact and fancy. Hypertension 1:435, 1979
2. Dougherty JC: Hypertension and the kidney. In Farland M (ed): Nephrology. New Hyde Park, NY, Medical Examination Publishing, 1983
3. Tobian L: Salt and hypertension. Ann NY Acad Sci 304:178, 1978
4. Zins GR: Renal prostaglandins. Am J Med 58:14, 1975
5. Coleman TG, Hull JE, Norman RA: Regulation of arterial blood pressure in hypertension. In Brenner BM, Stein JH: Contemporary Issues in Nephrology. New York City, Churchill Livingstone, 1981
6. Simon N, Franklin SS, Bleifer KH et al: Clinical characteristics of renovascular hypertension. Mayo Clin Proc 46:161, 1971

Chapter 19

Nephrotic Syndrome

Martha Savage Payne

ETIOLOGY AND PATHOPHYSIOLOGY

Nephrotic syndrome, one of the major clinical syndromes of glomerular disease, can be associated with many different pathogenic mechanisms both of primary renal disorders and of systemic disease (see the listing on the opposite page).

Nephrotic syndrome is primarily a noninflammatory defect of the glomeruli that causes abnormal leaking of albumin and other macromolecules

Classification of the Disease States Most Commonly Associated With Nephrotic Syndrome

Primary Glomerular Diseases

Membranous

Proliferative and focal

- Acute (poststreptococcal) glomerulonephritis (rare)
- Rapidly progressive glomerulonephritis
- Focal segmental glomerulosclerosis

Membranoproliferative, including dense deposit disease

Minimal lesion

Other Disorders

Medications and drugs

- Mercury
- Gold
- Penicillamine
- "Street" heroin
- Probenecid
- Captopril
- Paramethadione

Allergens

- Bee sting
- Pollens

Infections

- Bacterial endocarditis and shunt infections
- Malaria
- Syphilis
- Hepatitis B
- Schistosomiasis

Neoplasia

- Solid tumors (lung, colon, stomach, breast)
- Leukemia and lymphoma (Hodgkin's)

Multisystem disease

- Diabetes mellitus
- Systemic lupus erythematosus
- Amyloidosis
- Polyarteritis
- Henoch-Schönlein purpura
- Cryoglobulinemia

Pregnancy-associated

Chronic renal allograft rejection

across the glomerular filtration barrier. Nephrotic syndrome can be associated with many clinical entities, and by definition is manifested by massive proteinuria and lipiduria with a tendency toward edema, hypoalbuminemia, and hyperlipiduria.[1] In the Western world, the most common causes of nephrotic syndrome are diabetes mellitus, systemic lupus erythematosus (SLE), childhood minimal change renal disease, and the idiopathic glomerulonephritides, including idiopathic membranous nephropathy, focal glomerulosclerosis, and proliferative and membranoproliferative glomerulonephritis. Nephrotic syndrome may also follow exposure to certain nephrotoxins. Heroin nephropathy, which is being seen more often as heroin use increases, is characterized by focal glomerular sclerosis on renal biopsy and a nephrotic syndrome with progressive azotemia.[2]

The patient with nephrotic syndrome usually presents with generalized edema, which is caused by reduced plasma oncotic pressure resulting from the loss of serum albumin to the urine. There is a resultant translocation of fluid to the interstitium of body tissue, a reduced effective circulating volume, and a secondary sodium retention.

If the protein in the urine is primarily albumin (*selective proteinuria*), it is the result of a loss of net negative charge on the capillary wall of the glomerulus. Normally this is one of the mechanisms preventing albumin from passing across the glomerular filtration barrier.[3] (see Chap. 14). Other diseases associated with nephrotic syndrome that have extensive capillary wall immune deposits, such as membranous nephropathy, or disorders of basement membrane biochemistry or structure, such as diabetes, result in increased filtration of all serum proteins. This is called *nonselective proteinuria*[3] and is the result of damage to the structural barrier and possibly of increased pore size in the glomerular membrane.

Additionally, in nephrotic syndrome the effects of drugs bound to plasma albumin will be altered because with lower plasma albumin levels less drug will be bound. This will leave a greater amount of active free drug in the plasma to cause potential overdose problems after ordinary therapeutic doses.[4]

There may also be changes in coagulation system proteins. Reduction of plasma albumin levels apparently stimulates the liver to increase synthesis of many proteins. Some very large-molecular-weight proteins such as fibrinogen, Factor V, and Factor VIII may be increased not only because of increased synthesis but also because they are retained in the plasma and not excreted into the urine. At the same time anticoagulant and antifibrinolytic factors such as antiplasmin, α_1-antitrypsin, and plasminogen activators may be decreased. The increased levels of procoagulant factors and decreased levels of anticoagulant factors lead to hypercoagulability in nephrotic syndrome, resulting in a high incidence of thromboembolic problems (10%–40%).[5] Reduced levels of antithrombin III and antiplasmin also occur, as does increased platelet aggregation. The incidence of renal vein thrombosis appears to be particularly high in patients with nephrotic syndrome due to membranous nephropathy and membranoproliferative glomerulonephritis.[4]

As mentioned above, hyperlipidemia is common in nephrotic syndrome. It is inversely proportional to the serum albumin concentration. The state of hypoalbuminemia stimulates the liver to synthesize low-density lipoproteins (LDL) and very-low-density lipoproteins (VLDL).[6] See Fig. 19-1.

Minimal Change Disease

The patient presenting with nephrotic syndrome due to *minimal change disease,* also called *minimal lesion nephrotic syndrome* or *lipoid nephrosis,* will show swelling of the epithelial cell foot processes on renal biopsy. Under light microscopy, there is little alteration of the glomerular membrane or the glomerulus itself.[7, 8] Tubular changes, however, seen on light microscopy include vacuolization, and accumulation of hyaline droplets and lipids in the tubular lumina, which led Munk in 1913 to call the disease *lipoid nephrosis.*[1] With electron microscopy, the characteristic glomerular lesion was identified and consists of swollen foot processes of the glomerular epithelial cells (*podocytes*), with fusion over the surface of the basement membrane. Mesangial cell proliferation, inflammatory infiltrate, and fibrosis or fibrin deposits are not evi-

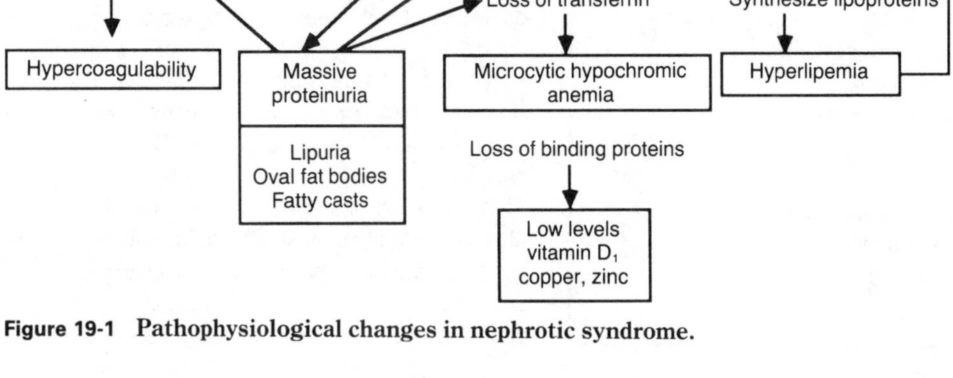

Figure 19-1 **Pathophysiological changes in nephrotic syndrome.**

dent.[8] It is not known if the increased permeability is caused by the swelling of the epithelial cells or by the excessive filtration of plasma proteins. Immunofluorescence microscopy findings are noteworthy for showing the absence of deposition of IgG and complement in the glomeruli.[8] The cause of the minimal change lesion is entirely unknown. Because patients with Hodgkin's disease, in whom nephrotic syndrome is present, have an identical lesion, a role of lymphocytes has been suggested in its pathogenesis.[9]

Mesangial Proliferative Glomerulonephritis (MPG)

Mesangial proliferative glomerulonephritis (MPG) is a rather rare glomerular lesion that is associated with nephrotic syndrome. Light microscopy shows glomeruli characterized by variable degrees of increased cellularity of the mesangium.[10] Electron microscopy shows epithelial foot processes diffusely swollen and effaced. Immunofluorescence frequently shows IgM deposits, primarily in the mesangium.[10] This type of lesion with IgA deposits is classified as *IgA nephropathy* or Berger's disease. (see Chap. 14).

Focal and Segmental Glomerulosclerosis (FSG)

This condition is classified as such because of a characteristic lesion seen on renal biopsy that consists of sclerosis and hyalinization of some but not all glomeruli (focal) and not involving the whole glomerulus (segmental). These patients may initially present with minimal lesion nephrotic syndrome but later develop hypertension and increasing impairment of renal functions. In this group of patients there is generally a poor response to steroid therapy. In some patients, these characteristic lesions first develop in the juxtamedullary region and progressively involve glomeruli farther outward in the cortex. The remaining glomeruli may appear normal as in minimal change disease or may reveal diffuse mesangial proliferation.[11] By electron microscopy, most of the glomeruli show diffuse or segmented foot process alterations.[11] IgM, Clq and C3 deposits may be seen by immunofluorescence, but only in association with the focal sclerotic lesions.[11] The cause of this disorder is unknown, but the mesangial deposits of immunoglobulin suggest an immune complex disease.[1] A high incidence of similar lesions occurs in the allograph following transplantation. Most of the patients who present with FSG will demonstrate a progressive decline in glomerular filtration rate (GFR), hypertension, and persistent proteinuria.[11]

Membranous Glomerulonephritis (MGN)

The most common cause of idiopathic nephrotic syndrome in adults, MGN accounts for 30% to 50% of cases. It occurs less frequently in childhood, accounting for 10% of cases.[4] The term *membranous* refers to the characteristic pathologic lesion of diffuse thickening of the glomerular capillary wall.[1] Membranous glomerulonephritis may be a primary glomerulonephritis (idiopathic) or secondary to various underlying diseases. A very strong association exists with solid tumors (6%–11% of patients with MGN), especially carcinoma of the lung, colon, stomach, or breast.[4] The malignancy may be overt at presentation of MGN or occult in as many as 30% of cases at the time of discovery of the nephrotic syndrome.[4] Thus a differential diagnosis must be made between MGN that is idiopathic and MGN that is secondary to other entities. MGN may also be the initial manifestation of an infection such as chronic hepatitis B or a multisystem disease such as SLE.

The characteristic light microscopic finding in MGN is a diffuse and uniform thickening of the capillary wall, usually without significant proliferation of endothelial, mesangial, or epithelial cells.[12] This finding may be absent early in the course of the disease, but it enables easy diagnosis of advanced MGN. On silver stain, basement membrane spikes may be seen projecting toward the urinary space.[12] The findings on electron microscopy are consistent with the light microscope finding. Early in the disease small, dense, discrete, subepithelial deposits appear at the level of the slit pore membrane. In more advanced cases the deposits increase in number and projections of basement membrane extend between deposits, corresponding to the silver positive spikes seen by light microscopy.[12] Immunofluorescence findings are typical of MGN, with IgG nearly always present in a uniform granular distribution outlining all of the capillary loops.[1] C3 usually is present in a pattern and intensity similar to those of IgG.[1]

The cause of MGN is unknown, but HLA studies suggest that a genetic basis of susceptibility exists.[13] It has been suggested that immune deposits on the capillary wall form from reaction of circulating antibodies with either exogenous or endogenous antigens previously localized on the epithelial surface of the capillary.[1] Some antigens have been identified in association with secondary MGN due to hepatitis and tumors.[1] The lesion is noninflammatory, as evidenced by the lack of neutrophils. Experimental evidence suggests that the C3 deposits may play a role in the increased glomerular permeability.[12]

Mesangiocapillary Glomerulonephritis (MCGN)

Also known as membranoproliferative glomerulonephritis, MCGN is characterized by a lesion with a prominent increase in mesangial cellularity and the segmental capillary wall changes that lead to a thickened and reduplicated ("tram track") capillary wall as seen by light microscopy.[14] Mesangiocapillary glomerulonephritis may be a primary renal disease or a manifestation of a multisystem disease such as SLE. The primary forms are heterogeneous, and two main pathologic varieties of MCGN have been identified: type I is typified by subendothelial electron-dense deposits suggestive of an immune complex disease, and type II characteristically shows dense deposits within the glomerular basement membrane.[14] The clinical features of both are quite similar.

The pathologic hallmarks of this group of glomerular lesions are pronounced abnormalities of mesangial areas and the peripheral capillary walls. There is diffuse glomerular cell proliferation, and frequently the glomeruli contain numerous polymorphonuclear leukocytes.[14] Silver methenamine-stained sections demonstrate thickened capillary walls, resulting in a "double contoured" or "tram track" appearance due to the extension and interposition of the mesangial matrix.[14] A few cases of MCGN are complicated by the formation of cellular crescents in Bowman's space. By electron microscopy, both types of MCGN show an extension of the mesangial cell cytoplasm and mesangial matrix between the basement membrane and the endothelial cell, which accounts for the splitting of the basement membrane seen on light microscopy. In type I MCGN, discrete subendothelial electron-dense deposits are seen along some of the capillary loops. In type II MCGN, the basement membranes are widened by ribbon-like, continuous, dense intramembrane deposits (which is the reason this disease received its common name, *dense deposit disease*). The immunofluorescent findings vary widely and are not very specific. C3 is usually present, and may be accompanied by variable amounts of IgG or IgM.

The pathogenesis of MCGN is unknown. The depression of serum complement and subendothelial deposits in type I suggest an immune complex disorder. However, there is no direct link of the hypocomplementemia to the renal disease, and part of this phenomenon may be related to decreased synthesis as well as to increased activation. Although evidence of recent streptococcal infection may be found in some cases, its importance in the pathogenesis of MCGN is unknown. There is a high incidence of recurrent disease in transplanted kidney patients with MCGN, which suggests a circulating factor as the genesis of the glomerular lesion.[4]

CLINICAL MANIFESTATIONS

The patient with nephrotic syndrome usually presents with generalized edema. The edema is usually manifested by puffiness around the eyes in the mornings and ankle swelling when the patient is up and walking about. As the condition progresses, massive fluid retention (anasarca) may result, and swelling of the genitals, ascites, and pleural effusion may develop. Symptoms such as dyspnea and orthopnea do not occur until anasarca is marked or pleural effusion is present. Venous pressure is usually normal. Common physical complaints are anorexia and fatigue.

Minimal change disease occurs predominantly in young children, with peak occurrences between ages 2 and 6 years.[8] In fact, 80% to 90% of the nephrotic syndrome in children is of the minimal change variety. Conversely, in adults, only 15% to 20% of cases of nephrotic syndrome are due to minimal change disease.[8] Males predominate by about 2 : 1 in cases of children, while in adult cases the ratio is closer to 1 : 1.[8] The onset of symptoms sometimes immediately follows an upper respiratory viral infection. The illness often presents suddenly, and a full-blown nephrotic syndrome with heavy proteinuria, hypoalbuminuria, and hyperlipidemia is the rule. The edema is frequently massive and may be accompanied by ascites and pleural effusion. Gross hematuria and hypertension are uncommon.[8]

Mesangial proliferative glomerulonephritis (MPG) can affect any age, but older children and young adults are most frequently represented. There is a slight male to female predominance. Hematuria is present in the majority of cases. Mild hypertension is present in 30% of the cases. Clinically, this entity is very difficult to separate from minimal change disease.

Patients with *focal glomerular sclerosis (FSG)* are usually older than the typical minimal change disease patient. Overall FSG is found in 7% to 15% of children and 15% to 20% of adults with nephrotic syndrome.[1] Hypertension and microscopic hematuria occur more frequently and severely. Patients run a progressive course to renal failure without responding to steroid therapy.

Idiopathic *membranous glomerulonephritis (MGN)* presents with a nephrotic syndrome in 80% of cases, and in the remaining cases as an asymptomatic proteinuria. Occurrence of MGN is unusual in children, with about 80% to 90% of patients being over age 30 at time of diagnosis (mean age 40–50).[12] A male predominance is usually reported. Renal function is usually normal at presentation, with azotemia occurring late in the course of the disease. Overt diabetes mellitus appears to be more common than might be expected by chance alone, and some authors have suggesed a common underlying phenotype related to susceptibility to both disorders.[13]

The course of idiopathic MGN is variable, but usually is indolent and slowly progressive. Patients may have both clinical remissions and relapses of the nephrotic syndrome.[13] The overall prognosis in children is good. However, 40% to 60% of MGN patients who present with nephrotic syndrome have progressive deterioration of renal function over a 3-to-10-year period.[4]

The majority of patients with *mesangiocapillary glomerulonephritis (MCGN)* have the onset of the disease after age 5 and before age 30.[1] There is a slight predominance of females in type I and a nearly equal sex ratio in type II.[14] MCGN is the most common proliferative lesion seen in children with idiopathic nephrotic syndrome.[14]

The initial clinical presentation is quite varied. From 40% to 50% of patients present with a well-developed nephrotic syndrome; from 30% to 40% present with asymptomatic proteinuria or hematuria; and another 20% to 30% present with features of an acute nephritic syndrome.[14] About 30% of patients present with hypertension and azotemia, which is associated with a poor prognosis. The course of MCGN is slowly progressive, with the majority of cases culminating in end stage renal failure within 10 to 15 years. Once azotemia develops, deterioration toward end stage disease generally occurs within 1 to 2 years.

LABORATORY ANALYSES AND DIAGNOSIS

When a patient presents with massive proteinuria on the screening reagent strip, and a history and physical by the physician indicate probable renal abnormalities, the following laboratory data should be obtained: 24-hour urine collection for quantitative protein excretion, blood urea nitrogen (BUN), serum creatinine, glucose, electrolytes, creatinine clearance and protein electrophoresis, and a complete blood count. In addition, the physician may perform a renal biopsy and order additional serological tests such as streptozyme, antinuclear antibodies (FANA), total complement, VDRL, hepatitis B surface antigen, and cryoglobulins to facilitate the differential diagnosis of the multiple causes of nephrotic syndrome (see the classification of disease states associated with nephrotic syndrome listed at the beginning of this chapter).

The most prominent laboratory changes in nephrotic syndrome are massive proteinuria, hypoalbuminemia, and hyperlipidemia (increased triglycerides and cholesterol). Other changes in protein levels in the serum include increased α_2- and β- globulins with normal to slightly decreased α_1-globulins. IgG levels may be significantly decreased, while other immunoglobulins are usually normal. Factor B of the alternative pathway of complement (C) may be significantly decreased.[1] These factors, especially in children, may lead to an increased susceptibility to infection with such organisms as *Streptococcus pneumoniae.*[1] Other complement components are not significantly decreased. Hypercholesterolemia and elevated phospholipids are the consistent laboratory abnormalities, but increased levels of LDL and VLDL may be present.[6]

Serum levels of several binding proteins including transferrin, transcortin, and thyroxine-binding globulin are decreased. These serum abnormalities in turn affect other laboratory tests such as total iron binding capacity, total serum iron, and total T_3 and T_4.[15, 16] A microcytic hypochromic anemia that is resistant to iron therapy may develop because of the decreased levels of transferrin.[16] In addition, nephrotic syndrome patients may have reduced concentrations of various vitamins and minerals due to loss of their respective binding proteins. These include vitamin D, copper, and zinc.[1]

The urine from a patient with nephrotic syndrome shows heavy proteinuria and an abnormal urinary sediment. Lipuria occurs and is seen in the urine sediment as free fat, oval fat bodies (renal tubular epithelial cells containing cholesterol esters), and fatty casts. (See Chap. 20 for discussion of cast formation). All of these exhibit a Maltese cross pattern under polarizing light. A positive stain with Sudan IV on the sediment will also occur with the fat. Lipuria parallels the level of urine protein excretion rather than serum lipid levels.[4]

In children with *minimal change disease,* the usual findings are a highly selective type of heavy proteinuria containing mostly albumin, a normal or near normal glomerular filtration rate (GFR), a normal serum C3 concentration, and an unremarkable urine sediment. Microscopic hematuria is seen in only 15% to 20% of cases.[8] Serum albumin levels are low. Serum creatinine may be mildly increased in as many as one-third of cases at the time of initial presentation. Serum sodium may be decreased.[8] Hematocrit and hemoglobin may be increased if plasma volume is greatly reduced. Platelet counts are modestly increased. The erythrocyte sedimentation rate is increased.[1] Total cholesterol, triglycerides, and VLDL and LDL levels are increased. High-density lipoprotein (HDL) levels may be increased as well.[1]

IgG levels may be profoundly depressed during relapse, and this may account for the susceptibility of such children to infection with pneumococci. The complement fractions, C3, C4, and properdin levels are usually within normal limits. IgM levels are modestly increased during both remission and relapse.[1]

In *MPG,* the typical nephrotic syndrome features are present. Proteinuria is nonselective. Hematuria is frequently present. Renal function tests are decreased in about 25% of patients.[1] IgG levels may be modestly reduced, and complement levels are most often normal.

In *FSG,* heavy proteinuria that is nonselective

is nearly always present. Hematuria is common.[11] C3 levels are nearly always normal, whereas IgG levels may be significantly depressed.[17] Tubular malfunctions are more common in this syndrome than in other causes of nephrotic syndrome. This may be evidenced by pyuria, glycosuria, aminoaciduria, and phosphaturia.[18]

Proteinuria in *MGN* is usually, but not always, nonselective, and is in the nephrotic range of greater than 3.5 gm/day in more than 80% of cases. Proteinuria of more than 20 gm/day has been reported.[17] Microscopic hematuria is common.[12] The C3 level and other complement components are usually normal in idiopathic MGN.[12] The urinary sediment and GFR are usually normal in the early course of the disease.

Proteinuria and microscopic hematuria are almost universal features of *MCGN*. In about 50% of cases, the proteinuria is in the nephrotic range.[14] Urine protein selectivity is usually moderate or poor.[1] In about 90% of cases, an important diagnostic marker for MCGN is the depression of hemolytic complement activity of serum, accompanied by the lowering of the C3 component.[14] This is an important differential diagnostic feature, because both the serum hemolytic complement activity and the C3 component are lowered in acute postinfectious glomerulonephritis but characteristically return to normal within 3 to 8 weeks. The failure of C levels to return to normal within 2 months of onset of an acute nephritic syndrome is highly suggestive of underlying MCGN. In general, type I MCGN is associated with a depressed serum C3 concentration, accompanied by low levels of Clq, C4, and C2, which are early complement components. This is suggestive of activation of the classic complement pathway. In type II disease, some patients have a heat-stable factor called *C3 nephritic factor* (C3NF) that is capable of cleaving C3 in fresh normal plasma. C3NF is an IgG autoantibody to the C3 convertase of the alternate C pathway. It apparently stabilizes this converting enzyme, resulting in the continuous degradation of native C3.[19]

The GFR in MCGN is frequently decreased but may be normal. Normocytic, normochromic anemia is found in more than 50% of cases, and may be severe and out of proportion to the degree of azotemia.[1]

SECONDARY GLOMERULAR DISEASES THAT PRESENT WITH A "NEPHROTIC" PICTURE

Diabetic Nephropathy

This condition usually presents with asymptomatic proteinuria, which frequently increases to the nephrotic range. The patient has usually had insulin-dependent diabetes mellitus for at least 10 to 15 years.[20] The disease progresses from the onset of proteinuria to the development of end stage renal failure in a relatively short period of time, from 1.5 to 6 years.[20] The glomerular lesion is a nodular glomerulosclerosis in about 20% of diabetic patients.[20] Glomerulosclerosis with an increase in mesangial matrix and a decrease in mesangial endothelial and epithelial cells is the rule.[20] These patients characteristically do more poorly in chronic hemodialysis than do patients with other forms of renal failure, probably because of the systemic nature of the diabetes and the widespread atherosclerosis that usually accompanies this disorder.

Amyloidosis

In adulthood, *amyloidosis* accounts for up to 12% of cases of nephrotic syndrome.[21] Both primary and secondary amyloidosis can involve the kidney. The patient with amyloidosis presents with a relatively sudden onset of nephrotic syndrome. The primary form of amyloidosis is much more common in elderly patients and is frequently associated with other organ involvement such as hepatomegaly and restrictive cardiomyopathy with congestive heart failure.[21] The secondary form of amyloid renal involvement can be seen with any longstanding chronic inflammatory process such as tuberculosis, bronchiectasis, rheumatoid arthritis, chronic urinary tract infections, or osteomyelitis, or in patients with multiple myeloma.[21] There is no satisfactory evidence that any form of treatment ameliorates either the proteinuria or the development of renal failure that usually occurs in a period of a month to 1 to 2 years.[21] The renal disease appears to be secondary to deposition of amyloid protein within the kidney. Light microscopy shows infiltration, with the amyloid glycoprotein replacing the mesangial matrix of the glomeruli and obliterating the capillary loops. Amyloid substances may also be noted in vessel walls and interstitium. Electron microscopy shows that the deposits contain fibrils with characteristics specific for amyloid.[21]

Multiple Myeloma

Nephrotic syndrome in *multiple myeloma* most commonly represents an "overflow" proteinuria, that is, the presence in the urine of light chains that are easily filtered by the glomerulus.[22] These are usually picked up in quantitative determinations of proteinuria by the sulfosalicylic acid test, but may be missed with the reagent strip test that reacts with albumin. There are no characteristic glomerular abnormalities in multiple myeloma, as the glomerulus tends not to be primarily involved and the myeloma is more a tubulointerstitial disease in the form of acute renal failure.

Pregnancy-Induced Hypertension (Toxemia of Pregnancy)

Nephrotic syndrome is a part of the systemic state of pregnancy-induced hypertension (*toxemia of pregnancy*). It is usually accompanied by significant edema and hypertension in the third trimester of pregnancy. As seen by light microscopy, the glomerular lesion is predominantly characterized by endothelial cell swelling, which is thought to be a response to fibrin deposition in the glomerular capillaries.[22] The lesion usually undergoes complete remission following termination of pregnancy.

Systemic Lupus Erythematosus

As discussed in Chapter 14, renal involvement in *systemic lupus erythematosus (SLE)* can present in several different clinicopathologic ways. Renal involvement develops in approximately 75% of patients with SLE (see Chap. 55). This is an immunologically-mediated form of renal disease. One form of the lupus nephritis is diffuse membranous glomerulonephritis, a form that is clinically and pathologically very difficult to differentiate from the idiopathic form of membranous glomerulonephritis. Its clinical manifestations are predominantly those of proteinuria and nephrotic syndrome, with variable degrees of hypertension, hematuria, and renal insufficiency.[21] The serologic parameters of SLE are frequently helpful in making the differential diagnosis, as are the systemic features of this disorder. This lesion may evolve in the absence of striking extrarenal manifestations of SLE. Evidence of active complement consumption is less common in the membranous form of lupus than it is in other forms of lupus nephritis. By light microscopy, this lesion in SLE is indistinguishable from idiopathic membranous glomerulonephritis.[21] Immunofluorescence may demonstrate the presence of multiple immunoglobulins IgA, IgG, C3, and IgM, rather than the classical pattern of idiopathic membranous glomerulonephritis.[19] Electron microscopy usually shows a similar pattern. Corticosteroid therapy does not appear to alter the course of this form of lupus nephritis. Development of end stage renal failure usually occurs 8 to 12 years after onset of the disease (see Table 19-1).

TREATMENT

The course and treatment of the nephrotic syndrome varies with the particular lesion associated with it. The urine protein can be used as a measure of response to treatment. Laboratory data can also be used to monitor both kidney function and the biochemical abnormalities associated with deteriorating function.

Table 19-1 ***Nephrotic Syndrome***

Massive proteinuria
Hypoalbuminemia
Increased blood lipids
Active sediment with RBC and/or RBC casts

	Age	Renal Function at Presentation	Serum C3	Serum C4	Prognosis	Other
Primary						
Mesangiocapillary glomerulonephritis	Young usually	N1 or ↓	Often ↓	Often ↓	Renal failure in 70%–90%	C3 nephritic factor in serum of some
Multisystem						
Systemic lupus erythematosus	Young adults, usually female	N1 usually	↓	↓	Often responds to therapy if early SLE remission	

Massive proteinuria (>3.5 g/day in adult)
Hypoalbuminemia
Increased blood lipids
Minimal or no hematuria (inactive urine sediment)

	Age	Renal Function at Presentation	Serum C3	Serum C4	Prognosis
Primary					
Minimal change disease	Children more common but any age	N1	N1	N1	Good
Focal sclerosing glomerulonephritis	Children more common but any age	Usually N1	N1	N1	Renal failure in 70%–80%
Membranous glomerulonephritis	Adults usually	Usually N1	N1	N1	20% remission, renal failure in 80%; slowly progressive
Multisystem					
Diabetic glomerulo-nephropathy	Adults	Decreased	N1	N1	Very poor
Amyloidosis	Adults usually	Decreased	N1	N1	Very poor

Minimal change disease is characterized by a remitting and relapsing course. A large body of evidence indicates that corticosteroids enhance the natural tendency to undergo remission.[23] Most patients who respond to steroid therapy do so within 4 weeks.[1] The long-term prognosis for idiopathic nephrotic syndrome with minimal change lesions is excellent. Most patients, given time, will undergo spontaneous remission. Chronic renal failure is a rare outcome, and is usually associated with the development of a glomerular lesion of focal and segmental glomerulosclerosis.

Among *MPG* patients, the progression to renal failure does occur, especially in those with well-developed nephrotic syndrome, failure to respond to glucocorticoids, and the development of superimposed focal and segmental sclerosis. However, 50% or more of patients do respond to glucocorticoid therapy and develop a complete remission of proteinuria.[1] Most of the patients who present with *FSG* will demonstrate a progressive decline in GFR, hypertension, and persistent proteinuria.[11] At present, no therapy has definitely been shown to benefit patients with focal and segmental glomerulosclerosis. The course of idiopathic *MGN* is variable, but usually is an indolent and slowly progressive one. Patients may have both clinical remissions and relapses of the nephrotic syndrome.[13] The overall prognosis in children is good. In adults, however, 40% to 60% of patients who present with nephrotic syndrome have progressive deterioration of renal function over 3 to 10 years.[4] Steroid therapy studies have suggested a long-term beneficial effect in membranous nephropathy.[1] The course of *MCGN* is slowly progressive, with the majority of cases culminating in end stage renal failure within 10 to 15 years.[1] Once azotemia develops, deterioration toward end stage disease generally occurs within 1 to 2 years. No form of treatment has proven to be beneficial, although steroids, immunosuppressants, anticoagulants, and indomethacin have been used.[1] Recurrent disease in renal allographs is common, perhaps universal in type II MCGN and occurring commonly in type I MCGN.[4]

CASE STUDY

A 22-year-old man with a history of acute glomerulonephritis, type unknown, was admitted to the hospital to have a renal biopsy because of continued proteinuria. His blood pressure was 130/84. Extremities revealed no edema. The biopsy revealed some mesangial proliferative glomerulosclerosis, which was thought to be related to his previous glomerulonephritis.

LABORATORY FINDINGS (Reference Ranges)

Urine blood	Neg
Urine albumin	4+
24-hour urine protein (0–150 mg/24 hr)	15 mg/24 hr
Creatinine clearance (97–137 cc/min)	115 cc/min

One year later the patient returned for a followup visit. He had no complaints. His blood pressure was normal and his extremities revealed no edema.

LABORATORY FINDINGS:

Urine blood	Neg
Urine albumin	4+
24-hour urine protein (0–150 mg/24 hr)	1577 mg/24 hr
Creatinine clearance (97–137 cc/min)	95 cc/min

The patient did not come for followup until 5 years later. At this time the patient presented with edema, which had been present less than 1 year. His blood pressure was 137/80. Pertinent laboratory data is shown. Another renal biopsy was performed and revealed focal segmental glomerulosclerosis.

Urine blood	Small
Urine albumin	4+

Urine electrophoresis

Fraction		
Albumin	(6.28–8.48 mg/dL)	4.60
Alpha-1	(0.11–0.25 mg/dL)	0.17
Alpha-2	(0.32–0.76 mg/dL)	0.93
Beta	(0.53–0.92 mg/dL)	0.90
Gamma	(0.43–1.30 mg/dL)	0.29

Total protein	(6.28–8.48 mg/dL)	4.60
A/G ratio		1.00
24-hr protein	(0–150 mg/24 hr)	10,462
Creatinine clearance	(97–137 cc/min.)	90
Cholesterol	(125–245 mg/dL)	483

Conversion to SI units:
Quantitative proteins—mg/dL × 10 = mg/L

The physician discussed in detail with the patient his diagnosis and therapeutic options. Although this glomerular process is not known for its response to steroids, both physician and patient agreed that a trial of steroids should be given, considering the severity of the nephrotic state. After a 2-month trial of steriods, the patient's protein was 6090 mg/24 hr and his creatinine clearance was normal. He was still experiencing edema, and was also experiencing recurrent upper respiratory infections, which were treated with antibiotics.

Questions

1. What abnormal laboratory values in this patient are consistent with a nephrotic syndrome?
2. What type of urine sediment would be expected in this patient?
3. Could the recurrent respiratory infections be related to the nephrotic syndrome?
4. What is the patient's prognosis?

Discussion

1. The very high 24-hour urine protein value, the hyperlipidemia (high cholesterol value), and the low serum albumin values are consistent with a nephrotic syndrome.
2. The patient would probably have free fat, oval fat bodies, and fatty casts. These would exhibit a Maltese cross pattern under polarizing light.
3. Yes; IgG levels are decreased, which may lead to increased susceptibility to infections.
4. Patients with focal segmental glomerulosclerosis usually run a progressive course to renal failure without responding to steroid therapy.

REFERENCES

1. Glassock RJ, Adler SG, Ward HJ et al: Primary glomerular diseases. In Brenner MB, Rector FC Jr (eds): The Kidney, 3rd ed, p 930. Philadelphia, WB Saunders, 1986
2. Friedman EA, Rao TK, Nicastri AD: Heroin-associated nephropathy. Nephron 13:421, 1974
3. Myers BD, Okarma TB, Friedman S et al: Mechanisms of proteinuria in human glomerulonephritis. J Clin Invest 70:732, 1982
4. Coggins CH: Nephrotic syndrome. In Flamenbaum W, Hamburger RJ (eds): Nephrology, p 302. Philadelphia, JB Lippincott, 1982
5. Harrington JT, Kassiner JP: Renal vein thrombosis. Ann Rev Med 33:255, 1982
6. Newmark SR, Anderson CF, Donadio JV Jr et al: Lipoprotein profiles in adult nephrotics. Mayo Clin Proc 50:359, 1975
7. Jao W, Pollack VE, Norris VE et al: Lipoid nephrosis: An approach to the clinicopathologic analysis and dismemberment of idiopathic nephrotic syndrome with minimal glomerular changes. Medicine 52:445–468, 1973
8. Grupe WE: Minimal change disease. Semin Nephrol 2:241, 1982
9. Sherman RL, Susin M, Weksler ME et al: Lipoid nephrosis in Hodgkin's disease. Am J Med 52:699, 1972
10. Cohen AH, Border WA: Mesangial proliferative glomerulonephritis. Semin Nephrol 2:228, 1982
11. Hoyer JR: Focal segmental glomerulosclerosis. Semin Nephrol 2:253, 1982
12. Coggins CH, Frommer JP, Glassock RJ: Membranous nephropathy. Semin Nephrol 2:264, 1982
13. Rao KV, Crosson JT: Idiopathic membranous glomerulonephritis in diabetic patients. Arch Int Med 140:624, 1980
14. Donadio JV Jr, Holley KE: Membranoproliferative glomerulonephritis. Semin Nephrol 2:214, 1982
15. Feinstein EI, Kaptien EM, Nicoloff JT et al: Thyroid function in patients with nephrotic syndrome and normal renal function. Am J Nephrol 2:70, 1982
16. Hancock FE, Onstad JW, Wolf PL: Transferrin loss into the urine with hypochromic, microcytic anemia. Am J Clin Pathol 65:73, 1976
17. Gingiacomo J, Cleary TG, Cole BR et al: Serum immunoglobulins in the nephrotic syndrome. Pediatrics 56:598, 1975
18. Bouisson F, Barthe P, Pieragi MTH: Severe id-

iopathic nephrotic syndrome with tubular dysfunction. Clin Nephrol 14:135–141, 1980

19. Curtis JJ, Wyatt RJ, Bhathena D et al: Renal transplantation for patients with Type I and Type II membranoproliferative glomerulonephritis: Serial complement and nephritic factor measurements and the problem of recurrent disease. Am J Med 66:216, 1979
20. Takacs FJ, Finkle RM: Diabetic nephropathy. In Flamenbaum W, Hamburger RJ (eds): Nephrology, p 351. Philadelphia, JB Lippincott, 1982
21. Glassock RJ, Cohen AH, Adler SG et al: Secondary glomerular diseases. In Brenner BM, Rector RC Jr (eds): The Kidney, p 1014. Philadelphia, WB Saunders, 1986
22. McDonald WA, Briggs SD, Migdol SD: The kidney in systemic conditions. In Flamenbaum W, Hamburger RJ (eds): Nephrology, p 391. Philadelphia, JB Lippincott, 1982
23. White RHR, Glasgow IEF, Mills RJ: Clinicopathological analysis of nephrotic syndrome in childhood. Lancet 1:1353, 1970

Chapter 20

Renal Failure

Martha Savage Payne

ETIOLOGY AND PATHOPHYSIOLOGY

Acute Renal Failure (ARF)

This condition *(acute renal failure)* can be defined as a *rapid deterioration of the renal function of filtration,* and is associated with the accumulation of nitrogenous wastes in the body *(azotemia)* that are normally excreted by the kidney.[1] The azotemia of acute renal failure is usually, but not always, accompanied by *oliguria,* defined as a *urine volume of less than 400 mL/24 hours.* This definition includes many different parenchymal renal diseases as well as several extrarenal disorders. These disorders may be divided into three groups: (1) prerenal azotemia, caused by renal hypoperfusion, which can be reversed immediately upon restoration of renal blood flow with no structural damage in the kidney; (2) acute intrinsic renal failure, resulting from renal hypoperfusion or a nephrotoxin, and associated with tubular cell damage; and (3) postrenal azotemia (obstructive uropathy), resulting from obstruction in the urinary collecting system. Other syndromes such as acute interstitial nephritis, acute glomerulonephritis or vasculitis, and acute renovascular disease resulting from obstruction of the renal artery or vein of both kidneys or of one kidney functioning alone can cause acute renal failure.

The diagnosis of acute renal failure must be a diagnosis of exclusion, because both prerenal and postrenal factors can lead to the deterioration of renal function, resulting in azotemia and oliguria. The differential diagnosis is extremely important because, in contrast to acute intrinsic renal failure, prerenal and postrenal azotemia are immediately reversible when the initiating disturbance is eliminated. This is accomplished by modifying the causative factors external to the kidney, such as instituting volume repletion therapy or removing obstructions in the urinary tract. If the situation is managed properly and expeditiously, no renal damage results. Intrinsic renal failure, in which there is actual tubular cell damage, however, continues from 1 to several weeks before renal function is restored, while tubular cells regenerate.[2]

Prerenal azotemia results from events leading to a decrease in renal perfusion pressure and/or an increase in renal vascular resistance. Either can decrease the glomerular filtration rate (GFR) to such a degree that the daily endogenous load of

Prerenal Azotemia
(Decrease in GFR, resulting in renal hypoperfusion)

Intravascular Volume Depletion

Excessive diuresis (diuretic use)
Hemorrhage (postpartum, gastrointestinal, surgical)
Gastrointestinal losses (vomiting, diarrhea, dehydration)
Major trauma, burns, crush syndrome
Pancreatitis, peritonitis
Hypoalbuminemia

Cardiac and Vascular Disorders

Congestive heart failure
Acute myocardial infarction
Pericardial effusion with tamponade
Pulmonary hypertension, massive pulmonary embolism
Renal artery: emboli, thrombosis, stenosis, dissecting aneurysm, vasculitis
Renal vein: thrombosis, compression

Peripheral Vasodilatation

Sepsis
Antihypertensive medications (norepinephrine, ergotamine)

Increased Renal Vascular Resistance

Surgery
Anesthesia
Hepatorenal syndrome
Prostaglandin inhibitors (aspirin, indomethacin, ibuprofen)

nitrogenous wastes cannot be excreted.[3] (See the listing displayed on the opposite page). This azotemic state is not associated with structural damage in the kidney, and can be corrected if the extrarenal circumstances causing the renal ischemia are reversed. Prerenal azotemia accounts for the vast majority of patients with acute azotemia. Improvement in renal function may involve increasing the extracellular fluid volume, enhancing cardiac output, or correcting the cause of systemic vasodilation, such as bacteremia or excessive use of antihypertensive drugs.[4] Improvement after anesthesia or surgical trauma may reverse a state of prerenal azotemia. Since some of the same factors that cause prerenal azotemia can lead to intrinsic acute renal failure, distinguishing between these two disease states may become possible only after seeing the outcome of therapy. If a patient immediately improves, then prerenal azotemia was present.

Postrenal azotemia occurs subsequent to urine formation and as a result of obstruction to the elimination of urine from the urinary tract.[3] Common causes of postrenal azotemia are displayed at right. Postrenal azotemia is immediately reversible when the obstructive lesion is corrected—again, in contrast to acute renal failure (see Chap. 16).

Postrenal Azotemia

Urethral Obstruction
Congenital valve
Stricture
Phimosis
Tumor

Bladder Neck Obstruction
Stones
Clots
Prostatic hypertrophy or malignancy
Bladder carcinoma
Bladder infection
Autonomic neuropathy or ganglionic blocking agents

Ureteral Obstruction (bilateral, or unilateral functional kidney)
Intraureteral
- Stones
- Blood clots
- Pyogenic debris or sloughed necrotic papillae
- Edema (following retrograde pyelography)
- Fungus balls
- Sulfonamide and uric acid crystals

Extraureteral
- Prostatic, bladder, cervical cancer
- Endometriosis
- Periureteral fibrosis
- Accidental ureteral ligation or trauma during pelvic surgery
- Retroperitoneal hemorrhage

The diagnosis, therefore, of *acute intrinsic renal failure* must be a diagnosis of exclusion. Primary renal disturbances that result in actual renal damage, causing acute azotemia, cannot be immediately changed by volume repletion, removal of urinary tract obstructions, or changing other factors outside the kidney. Numerous clinical situations can be associated with acute intrinsic renal failure. Those that are unassociated with primary glomerular or vascular disorders have been referred to as *acute tubular necrosis*. However, although proximal tubular necrosis is often present, it is not consistently present in patients with acute intrinsic renal failure and the terms should not be used interchangeably.[4] The categories and specific disorders that cause acute intrinsic renal failure are shown on page 228.

Ischemic disorders predispose to the development of acute renal failure because of reduced blood flow to the kidneys.[2] The loss of blood supply has its greatest impact upon the proximal tubule, resulting in the death of tubular epithelium.[5] It is seen most commonly in postsurgical patients, following trauma, and following muscle damage (crush syndrome with myoglobinuria).[1]

Myoglobinuria is being recognized with greater frequency, and may account for many cases of acute renal failure previously classified as "etiology

Acute Intrinsic Renal Failure
(Decrease in GFR, resulting from renal hypoperfusion or a nephrotoxin associated with tubular cell damage)

Ischemic Disorders
Complications of surgery
Hemorrhage
Trauma
Sepsis
Postpartum hemorrhage
Pancreatitis
Myoglobinuria

Nephrotoxic Disorders
Antibiotics
- Aminoglycosides (neomycin, kanamycin, gentamicin, tobramycin, amikacin, netilmicin, and streptomycin)
- Cephalosporins
- Tetracyclines
- Sulfonamides
- Amphotericin B
- Polymyxins
- Bacitracin
- Pentamidine

Iodine-containing x-ray contrast media
Heavy metals (arsenic, lead, cadmium, mercury, bismuth, uranium)
Organic solvents
Glycols (ethylene glycol [antifreeze] and diethylene glycol)
Carbon tetrachloride and other halogenated hydrocarbons
Toluene
Hydrocarbons (gasoline, kerosene, turpentine, paraphenylene diamine [hair dye])
Anesthetics (methoxyflurane, enflurane)
Analgesics (aspirin, ibuprofen, indomethacin)
Antiulcer regimens (cimetidine)
Diuretics
Chemotherapeutic agents
Cyclosporin A
Poisons
Recreational drugs (heroin, amphetamines)

unknown." Various causes of myoglobinuria are *rhabdomyolysis* (an acute, fulminating, potentially fatal disease of skeletal muscle accompanied by myoglobinuria), crush injuries (with muscle damage), coma (lying in one position without moving for prolonged periods, especially after drug overdose or alcohol ingestion), and, in some normal individuals, very vigorous exercise.[6] In cases that present with acute azotemia, accompanied by brown urine with a positive hemoglobin test in the absence of intact red blood cells on the urine microscopic, myoglobin should be considered and more specific tests performed to identify the pigment.[7]

Nephrotoxic disorders are caused by the ingestion of certain chemicals or the administration of certain drugs (see the listing opposite). Because the kidneys are exposed to a large blood volume, they are exposed to higher concentrations of blood-borne substances than are most body tissues. The renal tubular cells are a prime target for these substances. In hospitalized patients, nephrotoxins have become a major cause of acute renal failure. Antibiotics, especially the aminoglycosides, are implicated frequently in acute renal failure. It has been estimated that 15% to 25% of all cases treated with aminoglycosides result in some degree of nephrotoxicity.[8, 9]

In some disease states, especially multiple myeloma and diabetes mellitus, intravenous x-ray contrast administration is a major cause of acute renal failure.[10] Many of these patients probably have preexisting renal insufficiency, proteinuria, and vascular disease.

Fluorinated anesthetic agents have occasionally been reported as causes of renal failure.[11] The combination of unrelated nephrotoxins may have an additive nephrotoxic effect on the kidney. In some experimental animal studies, aminoglycoside antibiotics are more nephrotoxic if given after the fluoride-containing anesthetic methoxyflurane.[12]

Various therapeutic agents also may cause interstitial nephritis. The primary area of the kidney affected is the interstitial space, which in acute interstitial nephritis is markedly edematous and infiltrated with white blood cells. The mechanism is mediated immunologically.[13] Loss of renal function from the drug sensitivities tends to be less severe than in classic renal failure. Recovery of renal function following withdrawal of the drug is sometimes slow and may be incomplete.[14]

Other causes of acute renal failure are primary renal diseases (*e.g.*, glomerulonephritis), systemic diseases (*e.g.*, Goodpasture's syndrome, systemic lupus erythematosus), and vascular diseases (*e.g.*, renal artery thrombosis, malignant hypertension). See the displayed material on page 230. The acute azotemia associated with these disorders is often only one of many serious complications of an underlying disease. In these disorders, the glomerulus is the primary site of injury and the tubules and interstitial areas are relatively uninvolved. In most cases fever, extrarenal systemic manifestations, and nephritic urinary sediment and composition help in the differentiation from other types of ARF[4] (see Chap. 14).

Chronic Renal Failure (CRF)

Chronic renal failure may result from many processes that have a prolonged downhill course with progressive loss of nephron mass. CRF is not a specific disease, therefore, but refers to any situation in which there is a permanent reduction of renal function, causing significant abnormal chemical findings in the blood of a patient. Although the condition usually begins with minor alterations in blood analytes, it is almost always a progressive process that eventually becomes life-threatening.[15]

Even as nephrons are destroyed by the processes, however, the surviving nephrons and the rest of the body adapt; an individual can survive even if 90% of the original nephron population is destroyed. In adults, the common causes of CRF are glomerulonephritis, polycystic kidney disease, interstitial nephritis, diabetic glomerulosclerosis, and hypertension (nephrosclerosis). In pediatric patients, common causes are also glomerulonephritis, polycystic kidney disease, and interstitial nephritis, but also include renal hypoplasia, obstruction in the urinary tract, and a variety of individually rare hereditary disorders. Some less frequent causes of CRF are amyloidosis, sickle cell anemia, tuberculosis, hemolytic uremic syndrome, and renal artery or vein occlusion.

End Stage Renal Disease (Uremic Syndrome)

The decline in renal function in a patient with chronic renal failure occurs over a long period of time and culminates in *end stage renal disease* with physiological symptoms of the *uremic syndrome.*

Primary Renal Systemic and Vascular Diseases That May be Associated With Acute Azotemia

Glomerular and Small Vessel Obstruction
Acute poststreptococcal glomerulonephritis
Rapidly progressive glomerulonephritis
Vasculitis
Pregnancy-induced hypertension (toxemia of pregnancy)
Hemolytic uremic syndrome
Disseminated intravascular coagulation
Malignant hypertension
Radiation injury

Renovascular Obstruction
Renal artery: atherosclerosis, embolism, thrombosis, dissecting aneurysm, vasculitis
Renal vein: thrombosis, compression

Other
Goodpasture's syndrome
Systemic lupus erythematosus
Subacute bacterial endocarditis
Postpartum renal failure
Multiple myeloma
Macroglobulinemia
Polycythemia

Many pathophysiologic adjustments are made by the kidney because of the progressive loss of nephrons. Other organ system problems also occur in response to renal failure. The patient becomes progressively less able to maintain electrolyte balance with deficiencies or excesses of salt, and hypertension usually develops. Calcium metabolism becomes impaired, leading to adverse adjustments by the parathyroid and skeletal systems. Anemia occurs, as do metabolic acidosis and the associated buffer-base depletion. The kidneys fail to maintain adequate excretory, regulatory, and endocrine function.[15]

CLINICAL MANIFESTATIONS

Acute renal failure usually presents with oliguria, fluid overload, acidosis, or frank uremia. Because hospital patients are monitored daily with many biochemical screenings, nonoliguric acute renal failure is now being recognized much more frequently, even before other symptoms appear. The early identification of patients at risk, with prompt elimination of potential insults, can save many lives.

The clinical course of acute renal failure can be divided into three phases: an oliguric phase, a diuretic phase, and a recovery phase. The oliguria may last from a few hours to several weeks or months—the longer the oliguric phase, the poorer the prognosis. The diuretic phase begins by an increase in urine flow to more than 400 mL/day. Sometimes there is profuse diuresis of several liters a day. Usually the BUN and creatinine levels continue to rise during the diuretic phase, and then plateau and begin to fall after several days of urine output greater than 1000 mL/day. In the diuretic phase, the patient is still in danger of complications because electrolyte and other biochemical abnormalities still persist. Both glomerular filtration and tubule function improve as diuresis progresses.

The prognosis of a patient with acute renal failure is dependent on the condition that precipitated the problem. About 50% of patients who develop acute renal failure after surgery, about 33% of medical cases, and about 15% of obstetrical cases will die in the course of the syndrome.[4] Those patients who are nonoliguric have the best prognosis. The primary causes of death are infectious, cardiovascular, and respiratory complications.[4] The majority of the patients who recover have nearly normal renal function.

In *chronic renal failure,* as a general rule, a patient with 25% or more of normal kidney function is likely to have few physical symptoms. However, as the nephron population decreases, the glomerular filtration rate (GFR) falls; the first chemical abnormalities noted are an increase in urea (azotemia) and creatinine in the blood. Early chronic renal disease is therefore often found incidentally by routine laboratory analyses of blood and urine. As the GFR decreases below 25% of normal, physical symptoms will appear. At this point, other solutes such as phosphate, sulfate, and urate that are normally either filtered, reabsorbed, or secreted may also be retained in body fluids. This may lead to bone disease, a well-recognized complication of chronic renal failure. The abnormal divalent ion metabolism plus increased parathyroid activity and disordered vitamin D metabolism can lead to many forms of skeletal abnormalities. However, patients usually manage quite well until renal function is reduced to about 10% of normal. At this level, the patient usually begins to experience symptoms of uremia, a toxic state caused by retention of waste products. The list of waste products includes organic acids, phenolic compounds, indoles, guanidines, various metabolic intermediates, and certain peptides. Many of these have a toxic potential and could possibly contribute to the symptoms of chronic renal disease.

Classic clinical signs of uremia include progressive weakness and easy fatigability, loss of appetite followed by nausea and vomiting, muscle wasting, tremors, abnormal mental function, frequent but shallow respirations, and metabolic acidosis. The patient progresses to a state of stupor, coma, and ultimately death unless dialysis or successful renal transplantation is provided.

LABORATORY ANALYSES AND DIAGNOSIS

The clinical laboratory is vital in the diagnosis of renal disease and in following the course of patients with both acute and chronic renal failure. Laboratory measurements needed to detect the various renal syndromes include urinalysis, measurement of serum creatinine and blood urea nitrogen (BUN), a chemistry profile including electrolytes, and a complete blood cell count.

Urinalysis

The *examination of urine* is one of the simplest yet most important procedures in detecting and monitoring renal parenchymal or urinary tract disease. Especially important for the diagnosis of these disorders are tests for protein and hemoglobin and the examination of the urinary sediment.

The screening test for protein is usually done with a reagent strip test, which shows a color change in the presence of albumin but does not react as well or at all with globulin or Bence Jones protein. The sulfosalicylic acid test, based on protein precipitation, should also be done to detect these other proteins, especially when renal disease is suspected.[16] Subsequent protein immunoelectrophoresis will confirm the presence of light chains (Bence Jones proteinuria).[16] Although Bence Jones proteinuria is most commonly associated with multiple myeloma, it may also be found in other malignancies. The urine protein test is the most important screening test for renal function because proteinuria signals chronic renal disease before symptoms appear or before serum creatinine or BUN levels become abnormal. A positive protein test may be the first indication that a patient will ultimately go into chronic renal failure. It should be remembered, however, that the presence of proteins in the urine may occur in healthy individuals. This *functional proteinuria* may result from such physiological processes as fever, strenuous exercise, emotional stress, salicylate therapy, or exposure to cold. In teenagers and in patients recovering from glomerular disease, *orthostatic (postural) proteinuria* should be considered. Orthostatic proteinuria is not usually associated wtih chronic renal failure.[17]

If all nonrenal causes for proteinuria and orthostatic proteinuria have been excluded, renal disease must be considered. A quantitative protein determination should be performed on a 24-hour sample and repeated three or four times to determine if the protein is persistent or intermittent. Intermittent proteinuria is usually associated with a benign course, whereas persistent proteinuria is associated with renal disease.[17]

Repeated measurements of protein excretion are a valuable guide in following the course of patients with renal disease (see Chaps. 14 and 19). A return to normal protein excretion indicates healing of the glomerular lesion, and conversion from persistent to postural proteinuria indicates a good prognosis. By contrast, persistence of proteinuria increases the likelihood that progressive renal insufficiency and renal failure will develop.[17] In lupus nephritis, an increase in protein excretion suggests heightened immunologic activity.

When proteinuria is greater than 2 g/day, *selectivity,* which determines if the protein is mainly albumin or is albumin and globulin, should be assessed by electrophoresis of the urine and comparison of clearance proteins of differing molecular weights, such as the IgG/albumin ratio. When selectivity is high (IgG/albumin ratio <0.16), as it often is in children with minimal lesion disease, treatment with corticosteroids is likely to be successful[17] (see Chaps. 14 and 19).

The methods for quantitation of urinary total protein all have some disadvantages. Recently, however, a dye-binding method using benzethonium chloride Ponceau dye reagent became available, and it is now the method of choice. The range for protein concentration is 1–14 mg/dL (10–140 mg/L).[18] The reference range for 24-hour (d) excretion is <100 mg/d (<150 mg/d in pregnancy).[18] The concentration may reach 300 mg/d in urine of healthy subjects after exercise.[18]

Hematuria is the second most important clue to the presence of kidney disease or diseases of the urinary tract. A positive reaction by a dipstick method can indicate the presence of free hemoglobin *(hemoglobinuria),* intact red blood cells *(hematuria),* or myoglobin *(myoglobinuria)* in the urine. Sediment from a fresh, concentrated urine sample with low *p*H should also be examined for the presence of red blood cells to confirm hematuria. If few or no intact red cells are found, hemoglobinuria or myoglobinuria should be suspected and may be the cause of acute renal failure. Hematuria along with red blood cell casts may indicate acute glomerulonephritis, which may also present as acute renal failure (see Chap. 14).

A urine microscopic examination provides invaluable information concerning renal disease. The finding of specific type casts, cells, or crystals in urine sediment is associated with various renal diseases and causes of renal failure, as outlined opposite. These characteristic urine sediments are discussed in detail in the chapters on the specific disorders; however, a general discussion will follow here. *Casts* are cylindrical formed elements found in urine sediment that were formed in the tubules. The major component of their matrix is Tamm-Horsfall protein, which is excreted in the urinary tract.[19] Because casts are formed in the renal parenchyma they are of particular significance, indicating intrinsic renal disorders.[20] The cellular composition inside casts may help indicate various processes occurring in the renal parenchyma.

Hyaline casts are transparent cylinders without cellular components. Increased excretion of these occurs after exercise, fever, or dehydration and in many settings in which protein excretion is increased. *Granular casts* are semitransparent cylinders containing fine refractile granules that are probably aggregates of serum proteins.[19] (This is contrary to the assumption made for many years

Characteristic Urine Sediments

Glomerular Inflammatory Diseases
(In association with 2 to 4+ proteinuria)
Nephritic (active sediment)
Hematuria
Red blood cell casts

Nephrotic Syndrome
(In association with 3 to 4+ proteinuria)
Nephrotic syndrome
Free fat
Fatty casts
Oval fat bodies

End Stage Chronic Renal Disease
(Degree of proteinuria varies)
Broad casts (with many inclusions)
Waxy casts
Increased numbers of white and red cells

Combination of Nephritic, Nephrotic, and Chronic Renal Failure Sediments (Telescoped Sediment) (seen in vasculitis, collagen vascular disease [SLE])
Hematuria
Red blood cell casts
Free fat
Oval fat bodies
Waxy casts
Broad casts

Acute Renal Failure (Acute Tubular Necrosis)
(In association with a 1 to 2+ proteinuria)
Many narrow, pigmented, granular (dirty brown) casts
Renal tubular epithelial cells
Epithelial cell casts
Hyaline casts

that granular casts consist of degenerating cellular material.) They are seen physiologically in the same setting as hyaline casts. Both of these are nonspecific and occur with proteinuria, so are common findings in many types of renal disease and in renal failure.[17]

White blood cells, red blood cells, and tubular epithelial cells may appear in urine sediment and be associated with various pathological processes. Increased red blood cells (normally zero to five per high power field) are associated with bleeding into the urine from various causes such as cystitis, renal tumors, calculi, and hemoglobinopathies and bleeding across the glomerular membrane in inflammatory glomerular disease, all of which may be involved in different causes of renal failure.[20] Increased numbers of tubular epithelial cells (normally less than one per high power field) may appear in the urinary sediment of acute renal failure from numerous causes, including drug nephrotoxicity and tubular interstitial inflammation. In the case of transplant patients, renal tubular epithelial cells are evidence for allograph rejection, which may lead to repeated renal failure for the patient.[21, 22]

Patients with acute renal failure often have many narrow, pigmented, ("dirty") brown, granular casts, and have renal tubular epithelial cells, free and in casts. Hyaline casts may also appear, along with increased red and white cells. The urine of chronic renal failure may exhibit granular and hyaline casts, but will usually also contain broad and waxy casts. In the nephrotic syndrome, oval fat bodies and fatty casts may be present. When nephritic, nephrotic, acute, and chronic elements are found together in a single sediment, the sediment is referred to as "telescoped." This usually indicates a rapidly progressive nephritis or a collagen vascular disease such as lupus erythematosus.

Renal Function Tests

The *glomerular filtration rate (GFR)* is the rate at which plasma water crosses all the glomeruli into the tubular system of the nephron. This can be measured by calculating the amount of various substances that are totally filtered across the glomeruli without being either reabsorbed from the tubules or secreted into the tubules. Inulin, para-aminohippurate (PAH), and iothalamate are such substances and are used in clearance tests. A clearance (Cx) is measured using the following formula:

$$\text{Cx}\,[\text{mL/min}] = \frac{\text{Ux} \times \text{V}\,[\text{mL/min}]}{\text{Px}}$$

Ux is the concentration of substance *(x)* in the urine, *Px* is the concentration of *x* in the plasma, and *V* is the rate of urine flow.

Although the clearance of any substance excreted by the kidney can be measured using the same formula, such clearances are equal to the GFR only when the substance is totally filtered across the glomeruli and not reabsorbed from the tubules. Although inulin, PAH, and iothalamate are good indicators of renal function, they are not products of human metabolism. Their use in clearance tests involves intravenous administration over a long period of time to maintain a stable blood concentration. This is very time-consuming and expensive.

As a compromise among convenience, expense, and accuracy in clinical situations, the creatinine clearance test has been used. Creatinine is a natural product of muscle metabolism produced in the body at a constant rate, and it is filtered easily through the glomeruli. It is eliminated from the body only through the kidney. For these reasons the creatinine clearance is often used in the clinical setting to provide an approximate measure of GFR. Some creatinine is also secreted by the renal tubules, resulting in creatinine clearances that are slightly higher than inulin clearances. This is not clinically significant until severe renal failure is present. The creatinine clearance is calculated by the following formula:

$$\text{Ccr(mL/min)} = \frac{\text{Ucr (mg/dL)} \times \text{V urine (mL/24 hr)}}{\text{Pcr (mg/dL)} \times 1440\ \text{min/24 hr}} = \text{GFR}$$

Ccr = creatinine clearance

V urine = volume of urine excreted in 24 hours

Ucr = concentration of creatinine in urine

Pcr = concentration of creatinine in serum

GFR = glomerular filtration rate

The reference ranges for creatinine clearance in persons of average body surface area are, for males, 97–137 mL/min/1.73m^2 (0.93–1.32 mL/s/m^2) and, for females, 88–128 mL/min/1.73m^2 (0.85–1.23 mL/s/m^2).[23] This decreases 6.5 mL/min/1.73m^2 per decade.

Other Chemical Analyses for Renal Function

These include analyses of urea and of creatinine. In renal disease, *urea,* a catabolic by-product of protein, increases in the plasma because more than 90% of urea is normally excreted through the kidney. Urea is neither actively reabsorbed nor secreted by the tubules, but is filtered freely by the glomerulus. In the normal kidney, 40% to 70% of the highly diffusible urea moves passively out of the renal tubule and reenters the plasma. More urea flows back when blood flow is slow; therefore, urea clearance underestimates GFR. Urea production is also very dependent on diet and synthesis by the liver; therefore, the blood level of urea is not a very good independent indicator of renal function. Other nonrenal factors such as mild dehydration, high protein diet, increased protein catabolism, muscle wasting, reabsorption of blood protein after a GI bleed, certain drugs (such as cortisol), and decreased renal perfusion can also cause increases in blood urea (azotemia). These factors cause prerenal azotemia. Postrenal azotemia is caused by obstruction of the flow in the urinary tract by renal stones, tumors of the bladder or prostate, or severe infection (see Chap. 16).

Although current methods for measurement of urea use serum or plasma, the measurement of urea was originally performed on a protein-free filtrate of whole blood and was based on the amount of nitrogen present. Thus, the assay was called a *blood urea nitrogen (BUN).* The term is still commonly used to denote this assay, although serum urea nitrogen (SUN) would be more appropriate. In the United States, urea assays are still reported as urea nitrogen, although the SI system recommends the use of urea expressed in mmol/L.

The reference range of urea nitrogen is 7–18 mg/dL or 2.5–6.4 mmol urea/L.[23]

The BUN can be used in conjunction with the measurement of plasma creatinine to help distinguish between prerenal and postrenal azotemia, by calculating the urea nitrogen/creatinine ratio.[12] For a normal individual on a normal diet, the ratio ranges between 12 and 20. Very low ratios usually denote acute renal failure, low protein intake, starvation, or severe liver disease (decreased urea synthesis). High ratios with normal creatinine levels may be seen with catabolic states of tissue breakdown, prerenal azotemia, and high protein intake, and following gastrointestinal bleeds. High ratios associated with elevated creatinine concentrations may denote either postrenal obstruction or prerenal azotemia superimposed on renal disease. The ratio may be affected by the degree of specificity of the laboratory method used to measure both urea and creatinine. This measurement should not be considered a precise quantity, because the urea nitrogen/creatinine ratio can show great variability.

Two analytical approaches have been used to assay for urea. The method involving hydrolysis of urea to ammonia and the subsequent measurement of NH_4^+ has the disadvantage of being very sensitive to ammonia contamination, and endogenous NH_3 must be removed from urine samples before assaying; however, this method demonstrates good specificity and sensitivity when done as a kinetic assay. The other approach measures the rate of increase in conductivity in the sample as the nonionic urea is hydrolyzed by urease to the ionic species NH_4^+ and HCO_3^-. Ammonia contamination is not a problem in this method. Direct condensation methods have the disadvantages of caustic chemical use and limited linearity.[24]

Creatinine is a by-product of muscle metabolism, and is excreted into the plasma at a relatively constant rate. It is continuously excreted, almost entirely by glomerular filtration. The excretion rate in any one individual, in the absence of renal disease, is relatively constant and parallels endogenous production. For these reasons, creatinine is used as a measure of GFR, as described above. The linear decrease of creatinine clearance over time as renal function fails has been thoroughly documented for several forms of chronic glomerulonephritis, diabetic nephropathy, chronic interstitial nephritis, and chronic pyelonephritis. It is used by physicians to estimate the severity of renal failure and to make decisions about dialysis. After its important initial use, creatinine clearance is a time-consuming and expensive index of glomerular function, and it has been shown that the creatinine clearance of a patient increases (or decreases) as the reciprocal of plasma creatinine increases (or decreases) linearly. This relation is shown in Figure 20-1. It has been suggested that plasma creatinine alone may be used as an index of glomerular function, especially after an initial clearance has been determined.[24] It should be noted, however, that at lower levels of serum creatinine a random error may greatly affect the serum creatinine and cause the estimated clearance to be unreliable. An estimated clearance should not be considered reliable when plasma creatinine is <2.5 mg/dL (<221 μmol/L), but might be acceptable when creatinine is 2.5–5.0 mg/dL (221–442 μmol/L), because the precision of plasma creatinine determination increases as the concentration rises.[23]

The methods used most frequently to measure creatinine are rather nonspecific and subject to interference by many compounds present in blood. Automated kinetic methods have been developed that eliminate some positive interferences, such as alpha keto acids often found in diabetic serum. Bilirubin in icteric serum samples, however, has been shown to give low creatinine results when measured by the kinetic Jaffe method.

Clinical laboratory scientists who serve active renal disease centers must recognize how the specificity of the method used in their facility af-

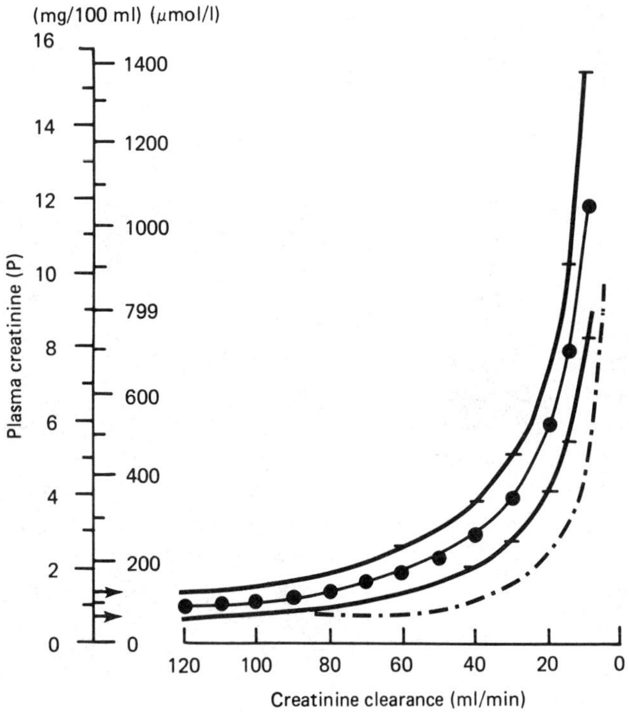

Figure 20-1 Relationship between plasma creatinine and creatinine clearance (mL/min). Continuous lines show the calculated relationship in young men as creatinine clearance falls (assuming UcrV is constant). The interrupted lines indicate the approximate extreme relationship that might be observed in healthy elderly men. (UcrV, urine volume.) (From Smith ST: Nonprotein nitrogen. In Bishop ML, Duben-Von Laufen JL, Fody EP [eds]: Clinical Chemistry. Philadelphia, JB Lippincott, 1985)

fects the clinical application of results. Reference ranges for creatinine clearance, the reciprocal of plasma creatinine concentration, and the urea nitrogen/creatinine ratio will vary depending on how specific the method is for creatinine that is used in the calculation. The more a method *overestimates* true creatinine, the greater the *underestimation* of creatinine clearance (see the formula at the top of the left-hand column, page 234.

Reference ranges for serum or plasma creatinine measured by methods similar to those discussed are 0.6–1.2 mg/dL (53–106 μmol/L) in men and 0.5–1.1 mg/dL (44–97 μmol/L) in women.[23] Other biochemical abnormalities present in renal failure can be seen in Table 20-1.

Laboratory Results in Acute Renal Failure

Acute renal failure is associated with a daily elevation of the BUN level of 10 mg per deciliter (3.6 mmol/L) (azotemia) and a daily elevation of the serum creatinine level of 0.5 mg per deciliter (44.2 μmol/L).[4] The creatinine value, as discussed above, reflects kidney function better than the urea level because urea production is altered by food intake, by tissue catabolism, and by the presence of blood in the intestines. Oliguria is commonly present, but the urine output may exceed this limit. Nonoliguric acute renal failure has increasingly been recognized in nephrotoxin-induced as well as hypoperfusion-induced disease. It is usually associated with a less severe insult to the kidney and with lower morbidity and mortality than oliguric acute renal failure.[4]

The differential diagnosis between prerenal azotemia and acute renal failure is facilitated by several laboratory tests. The urinary indices (see Table 20-2) show concentrated urine (specific gravity often higher than 1.010 and high osmolality) in prerenal failure, in contrast with lower specific gravity (approximately 1.010) similar to blood plasma in acute renal failure. The urine sodium is lower in prerenal than in acute renal failure,

Table 20-1 ***Biochemical Abnormalities in Renal Disease and Renal Failure***

	ARF	CRF	AGN	NS
Blood Urea Nitrogen	↑	↑	↑	NL
Serum Creatinine	↑	↑	↑	NL
Serum Potassium	↑	↑	↑ or NL	↑ or NL
Serum Phosphorus	↑	↑	↑ or NL	NL
Serum Calcium	↑	↑	NL	↑
Serum Uric Acid	↑	↑	NL	NL
Acidosis	P	P	Abs	Abs
Proteinuria	↑ or NL	↑	↑	↑ ↑ ↑ ↑
Hematuria	P	↑	↑ ↑	↑

ARF, acute renal failure; CRF, chronic renal failure; AGN, acute glomerulonephritis; NS, nephrotic syndrome
↑ = increased, P = present, Abs = absent, NL = normal

and the urine-to-plasma creatinine ratio is higher in prerenal azotemia.[4] It should be emphasized that diuretics may invalidate the use of these indices for up to 24 hours, and should not be used prior to collecting urine for these analyses.[4]

Patients with acute renal failure exhibit the biochemical abnormalities associated with uremic syndrome, but there is a more rapid onset of these abnormalities. The patient may be hyperkalemic even without an exogenous source of potassium, because of the catabolic release of potassium from tissues. Hyponatremia is present because of retention of water. Acidosis may occur as the kidneys lose their capacity to regulate the acid-base balance of the body. Metabolic alkalosis may also be a laboratory finding if the patient is losing large amounts of acidic gastric juice from vomiting.

Divalent ion disturbances are commonly seen in acute renal failure. Due to retention of the ions, hyperphosphatemia and hypermagnesemia are almost always present in oliguric acute renal failure.[4] Hyperphosphatemia (up to 20 mg/dL [6.5 mmol/L]) may be very severe in patients with renal failure, due to tissue breakdown or rhabdomyolysis. Patients with acute renal failure given magnesium-containing medications such as antacids or laxatives may have very high magnesium levels. Hypocalcemia in the range of 5 to 8 mg/dL (1.25–2.0 mmol/L) is also common.[4]

Anemia is common in acute renal failure, and may occur rapidly due to suppressed erythropoiesis, hemolysis, bleeding, and hemodilution. A low white count is usually the result of the precipitating illness. A bleeding problem may also exist, as in chronic uremia, because of platelet dysfunction and factor VIII dysfunction.

Table 20-2 ***Urinary Diagnostic Indices***

Index	Prerenal	ARF
U_{Na} mEq/L	<20	>40
U_{Cr} (mg/dL)/P_{Cr} (mg/dL)	>40	<20
U_{OSM} mOsm/kg H_2O	<350	>500
Renal failure index (RFI)		
$RFI = \frac{U_{Na}}{U_{Cr}/P_{Cr}}$	<1	>1
Fractional excretion of filtered sodium (Fe_{Na})		
$Fe_{Na} = \frac{U_{Na} \cdot P_{Cr}}{P_{Na} \cdot U_{Cr}} \times 100$	<1	>1
Urine specific gravity	>1.010	≈1.010

Conversion to SI units is as follows:
Sodium—mEq/L × 1 = mmol/L
Creatinine—mg/dL × 88.4 = μmol/L

U_{Na} = Urine sodium, U_{Cr} = Urine creatinine
U_{OSM} = Urine osmolality, RFI = Renal failure index
Fe_{Na} = Fractional excretion of filtered sodium
P_{Cr} = Plasma creatinine, P_{Na} = Plasma sodium

The microscopic evaluation of urine sediment is helpful in the diagnosis of acute renal failure. A sediment that contains renal tubular epithelial cell cellular debris and renal tubular epithelial cell casts supports the diagnosis of acute renal failure.[4] Sometimes there are only "muddy" brown granular casts, and there may or may not be accompanying free renal tubular epithelial cells. A few red blood cells and white blood cells per high power field may be present. A 1+ or 2+ proteinuria on a urinary reagent test strip is also compatible with acute renal failure. These results are in contrast to the large amounts of urine protein and numerous red blood cell casts found in acute renal failure secondary to renal disorders such as glomerulonephritis (see the listing on page 233). Hyaline casts in large numbers may be seen in prerenal azotemia. The absence of cellular elements and protein in the urine are most compatible with prerenal and postrenal azotemia. Numerous crystals such as uric acid, oxalate, or hippuric acid crystals may occur with ethylene glycol, methoxyflurane, or other chemical toxicity when the cause of acute renal failure is a nephrotoxic agent.[4, 25]

Myoglobinuria as the cause of the acute renal failure should be suspected when there has been muscle injury, prolonged periods of unconsciousness, alcohol or drug abuse, or seizures.[6] The urinary reagent test strip does not distinguish between myoglobin and hemoglobin. Myoglobin should be suspected, however, in a heme-positive urine in the absence of intact red cells and a normal color of the patient's blood serum, which would be pink if intravascular hemolysis had occurred. Myoglobin, a low-molecular-weight protein, is cleared from the circulation much faster than is hemoglobin. The patient with myoglobinuria will also have an elevated serum creatinine phosphokinase (CK) and aldolase. Precise identification of myoglobin depends on sophisticated absorption spectrophotometry, electrophoresis, or immunochemical methods.[7]

In acute drug-induced interstitial nephritis, the laboratory finding of a 10% to 60% eosinophilia usually accompanies the clinical symptoms of fever and maculopapular skin rash.[4] Also present will be a proteinuria, and urinary sediment abnormalities of casts, hematuria, and white blood cells, many of which may be eosinophils. A Wright's stain preparation on a sediment of freshly voided urine is useful in demonstrating the eosinophils.[14]

It must be kept in mind that a blood screen for toxic chemicals and drugs may give valuable information in cases of acute renal failure if no other causes can be detected from the patient's history and laboratory results.

Laboratory Results in Chronic Renal Failure

Chronic progressive renal disease that ultimately results in *chronic renal failure* can be divided into four stages that are associated with the following laboratory abnormalities. In the first stage, the only abnormalities present may be proteinuria and an abnormal urine sediment. The renal function (GFR) is usually nearly normal, and there is only a slight decrease in renal reserve. The second stage evolves with mild renal insufficiency. At least 50% of normal function must be lost before the concentration of urea nitrogen or creatinine rises above the normal range. In the third stage, frank renal failure develops. Anemia and acidosis are present, along with the biochemical abnormalities mentioned above. Development of end stage renal disease accompanied by the uremic syndrome is the fourth stage.

The characteristic physiological and laboratory findings are the same in end stage renal disease (the uremic syndrome), regardless of the initiating disease process. The most characteristic findings are increased concentrations of the nitrogen compounds, such as urea nitrogen and creatinine, as a result of reduced GFR and decreased tubular function. Retention of these compounds and of metabolic acids is followed by progressive hyperphosphatemia, hypercalcemia, and hyperkalemia. Hyperkalemia is potentially very dangerous because of possible cardiac arrest. Reduced endocrine function is manifested by inadequate synthesis of erythropoietin, resulting in anemia, and inadequate synthesis of vitamin D, resulting in osteomalacia. Hypertension is usually a problem because regulation of blood sodium is disordered (see Fig. 20-2).

TREATMENT

In *acute renal failure,* the treatment involves diagnosing and treating the underlying cause of renal failure, restoring fluid and electrolyte balance, preventing or delaying metabolic complications, and treating any infections promptly.[26] The clinical laboratory plays an important role in the management of these patients by performing daily serum electrolyte measurements. The management of electrolytes is concerned principally with sodium and potassium. Serum sodium concentrations should

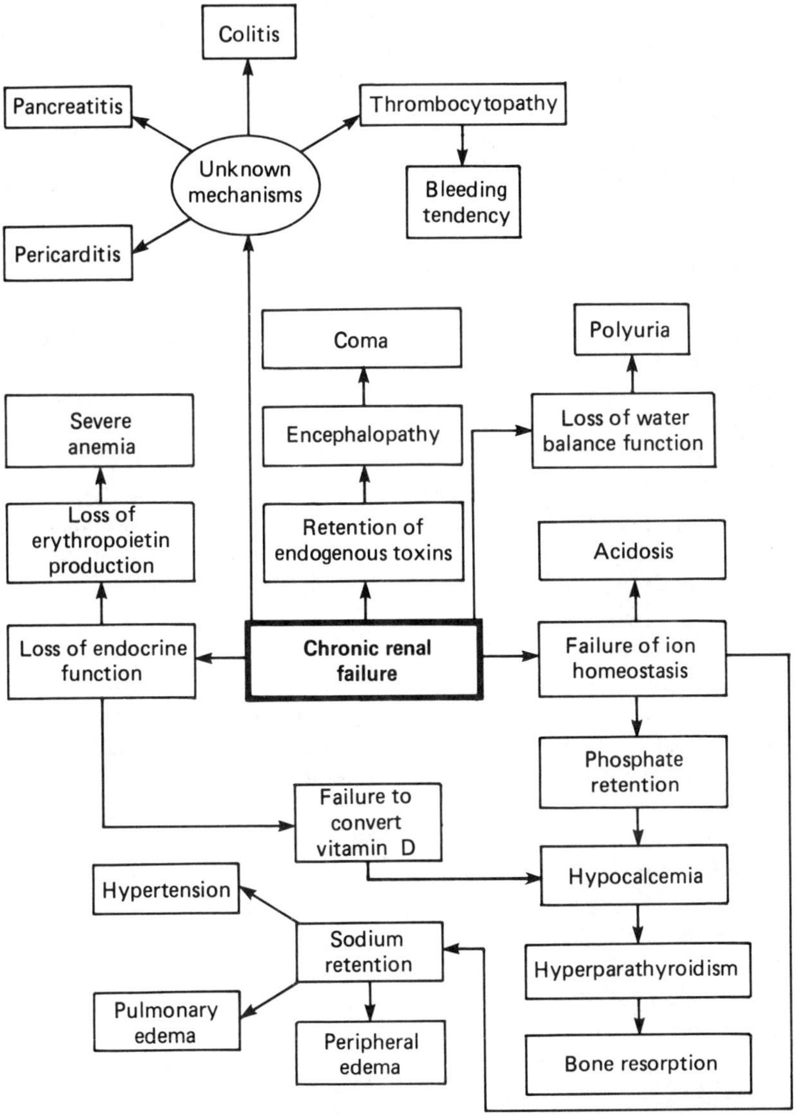

Figure 20-2 Pathophysiology of chronic renal failure. (From Uthman EO: Renal function. In Bishop ML, Duben-Von Laufen JL, Fody EP [eds]: Clinical Chemistry. Philadelpia, JB Lippincott, 1985)

remain in the range between 135 and 145 mEq/L (135–145 mmol/L). Changes in sodium concentrations indicate changes in water balance. A rising serum sodium is generally an indication of a water deficit, and a falling serum sodium is an indicator of excessive water administration. Hyperkalemia is one of the more common complications of renal failure, and can cause death through induction of cardiac arrhythmias. Usually potassium can be controlled with dialysis, which can also control fluid balance and correct other electrolyte abnormalities. Patients can be put on either peritoneal dialysis or hemodialysis. Even when patients enter the diuretic phase of acute renal failure, careful management is necessary because glomerular filtration rates remain low. Daily serum sodium and potassium concentration measurements remain imperative to good management of the patient.

In *chronic renal failure,* the abnormal laboratory results of proteinuria and, at a later stage, elevated BUN and creatinine levels may be the only indication of silent but progressive progress toward end stage renal disease. In managing any patient with renal insufficiency, the first goal is to identify and treat its underlying cause if possible. The laboratory plays an important role in this phase in that the abnormal laboratory parameters, rather than clinical symptoms, may be the first clue to renal disease. The second goal is to identify and treat any conditions that aggravate the underlying renal disease or have adverse effects in renal function. Some commonly found reversible contributions to deterioration of renal function that the laboratory can play a role in detecting are urinary tract infections, which can be detected and treated on the basis of culture and sensitivity. Sodium and water depletion are common causes of acute deterioration in renal function. Serum sodium should be checked periodically. Metabolic derangements such as electrolyte imbalance produced by anorexia and vomiting can aggravate renal failure. Metabolic acidosis can also adversely affect renal function and should be controlled. Patients who have chronic renal disease should have their phosphorus excretion monitored, because abnormalities of phosphorus excretion are central to the problems of uremic osteodystrophy. Both calcium and phosphorus levels are also important in the prevention and management of renal disease-induced bone problems.

When renal failure can no longer be managed through diet and medication, the treatment must involve dialysis to prolong life. Laboratory data is still vital in following and managing these dialysis patients. Renal transplantation may finally be considered in the management of some patients with chronic renal failure.

CASE STUDY

A 39-year-old Caucasian man with no significant past history presented to a small community hospital with a 2-day history of nausea and vomiting. He was found on initial examination to be moderately icteric. The patient had a history of chronic headaches and had been taking four to ten extra-strength Tylenol every day throughout the past year. Alcohol consumption consisted of three to four drinks of rum and Coke routinely on weekday evenings, with a higher intake on weekends.
The patient was transferred to a tertiary care hospital and admitted to the intensive care unit. He

LABORATORY FINDINGS

	Reference Ranges	Patient Values
AST	8–20 IU/L	>19,000 IU/L
ALT	8–20 IU/L	>6,000 IU/L
Prothrombin time	10–14 sec	20 sec
Creatinine	0.7–1.5 mg/dL	7.2 mg/dL
BUN	10–20 mg/dL	48 mg/dL
Urinalysis		
Protein	Neg	4+
Bile	Neg	Pos
Blood	Neg	Large amt. hemoglobin
Casts	Neg	8–11 coarsely granular casts

received 2 units of fresh-frozen plasma and 20 mg of vitamin K intravenously. His hepatitis profile was negative.

Urine output was initially only 300 mL/24 hours. Repeated renal parameters revealed that creatinine was increasing rapidly and was 14.3 mg/dL by the third day of hospitalization. Consultation with the Nephrology Service was obtained. Because of the severe nature of the liver insult, consultation was also obtained with the liver transplant team. However, liver function values began a slow descent toward normal. On the third day, acute dialysis was initiated and urine output began to increase. Creatinine returned toward the normal range. The patient was discharged on the 14th hospital day with the following laboratory results:

	Reference Ranges	***Patient Values***
AST	8–20 IU/L	19 IU/L
ALT	8–20 IU/L	16 IU/L
Creatinine	0.7–1.5 mg/dL	2.3 mg/dL
BUN	10–20 mg/dL	32 mg/dL

Conversion to SI units is as follows:
Creatinine—mg/dL × 88.4 = μmol/L
BUN—mg/dL × 0.357 = mmol/L

Questions

1. What is the diagnosis?
2. What is the cause of the renal failure?

Discussion

1. The patient was diagnosed as having severe hepatocellular necrosis secondary to Tylenol abuse and acute renal failure.
2. The renal failure possibly could be secondary to the Tylenol abuse and be a drug-induced interstitial acute renal failure. More likely, it is a volume depletion prerenal azotemia caused by the severe vomiting secondary to the liver problem. The patient responded promptly to fluids and acute hemodialysis. No renal biopsy was done, so interstitial nephritis was not definitely ruled out. The patient refused to come back at a later time for reevaluation of either renal function or liver status.

REFERENCES

1. Anderson RJ, Schrier RW: Clinical spectrum of oliguric and nonoliguric acute renal failure. In Brenner BM, Stein JH (eds): Acute Renal Failure (Contemporary Issues in Nephrology, Vol 6). New York City, Churchill Livingstone, 1980
2. Schrier RW: Acute renal failure: Pathogenesis, diagnosis, and management. Hosp Pract: 93–112, 1981
3. Rasmussen HH, Ibels LS: Acute renal failure: Multivariate analysis of cause and risk factors. Am J Med 73:211–218, 1982
4. Brezis M, Rosen S, Epstein FH: Acute renal failure. In Brenner BM, Rector FC (eds): The Kidney, p 735. Philadelphia, WB Saunders, 1986
5. Jones D: Ultrastructure of human acute renal failure. Lab Invest 46: 254, 1981
6. Honda N, Kurokawa K: Acute renal failure and rhabdomyolysis. Kidney Int 23:888, 1983
7. Markowitz H, Wobig GH: Quantitative method for estimating myoglobin in urine. Clin Chem 23:1689, 1977
8. Hou SH, Bushinsky DA, Wish JB et al: Hospital-acquired renal insufficiency: A prospective study. Am J Med 74:243–248, 1983
9. Smith CR, Lipsky JJ, Laskin OL et al: Double-blind comparison of the nephrotoxicity and auditory toxicity of gentamycin and tobramycin. N Engl J Med 302:1106–1115, 1980
10. D'Elia JA, Gleason RE, Alday M et al: Nephrotoxicity from angiographic contrast material: A prospective study. Am J Med 72:719–25, 1982
11. Hanthett MN, Lane W, Bennett WM: Non-oliguric renal failure and enflurane. Ann Intern Med 81:560, 1974
12. Cronin RE: Aminoglycoside nephrotoxicity: Pathogenesis and prevention. Clin Nephrol 11:251, 1979
13. Linton AL, Clark WF, Driedger AA et al: Acute interstitial nephritis due to drugs: Review of the literature with a report of nine cases. Ann Intern Med 93:735–741, 1980
14. Appel GB, Kunis CL: Acute tubulointerstitial nephritis. In Cotran RS, Brenner BM, Stein JH (eds): Tubulointerstitial Nephropathies, pp 151–185. (Contemporary Issues in Nephrology, Vol 10). New York City, Churchill Livingstone, 1983
15. Del Greco F, Krumlovsky FA: Role of the labora-

tory in management of acute and chronic renal failure. Ann Clin Lab Sci 11:283–291, 1981

16. Graff L: Chemical examination. In Graff L (ed): A Handbook of Routine Urinalysis, p 22. Philadelphia, JB Lippincott, 1983
17. Kassierer JP, Gennari FJ: Laboratory evaluation of renal function. In Earley LE, Gottschalk, CW (eds): Strauss and Welt's The Kidney, p 41. Boston, Little, Brown & Co, 1979
18. Silverman LM, Christensen RH, Grant GH: Amino acids and proteins. In Tietz NW (ed): Textbook of Clinical Chemistry, p 519. Philadelphia, WB Saunders, 1986
19. Rutecki GJ, Goldsmith C, Schreiner GE: Characterization of protein in urinary casts. N Engl J Med 284:1049, 1971
20. Graff L: Microscopic examination of the urinary sediment. In Graff L (ed): A Handbook of Routine Urinalysis, p 70. Philadelphia, JB Lippincott, 1983
21. Kesson AM, Talbott JM, Gyory AZ: Microscopic examinations of urine. Lancet 2:809, 1978
22. Schumann GB, Burleson RL, Henry JB et al: Urinary cytodiagnosis of acute renal allography rejection using the cytocentrifuge. Am J Clin Pathol 67:134, 1977
23. Rock RC, Walker GW, Jennings CD: Nitrogen metabolites and renal function. In Tietz NW (ed): Textbook of Clinical Chemistry, p 1254. Philadelphia, WB Saunders, 1986
24. Smith ST: Non-protein nitrogen. In Bishop ML, Guben-Von Laufen JL, Fody EP (eds): Clinical Chemistry, p 411. Philadelphia, JB Lippincott, 1985
25. Frommer JP, Ayus JC: Acute ethylene glycol intoxication. Am J Nephrol 2:1, 1982
26. Dougherty JC: Acute renal failure. In Forland M (ed): Nephrology, p 168. New Hyde Park, NY, Medical Examination Publishing, 1983

Part V

GASTROINTESTINAL DISORDERS

Sharon L. Zablotney, Associate Editor

The primary function of the gastrointestinal (GI) system is the digestion, absorption, and processing of nutrients used for the maintenance of the body's physiological functions. In fulfilling this function, the system articulates with the external environment, including the many potentially harmful agents associated with that environment. The resulting complexity of the gastrointestinal system makes it vulnerable to a diverse group of potential disorders. See the illustration on page 246 for anatomic landmarks of the GI tract.

This section is organized around those disorders commonly associated with the GI system, that is, malabsorption, ulceration, hemorrhage, diarrhea, malignancy, and inflammation. These abnormalities are not necessarily independent occurrences and, in fact, there is frequent overlap and often common etiology. Thus, an infectious agent may initiate an episode of diarrhea followed by bleeding that culminates in a chronic inflammation of the bowel. Chronic inflammatory bowel disease may actually be the result of immunological responses, infection, or dietary, psychosomatic, or genetic factors.

The value of the laboratory evaluation in diagnosis varies among these disorders. Obviously the identification of the infectious agent and initiation of appropriate antimicrobial therapy are central events in diarrheal disorders associated with an infectious process. On the other hand, the laboratory may play an initial, but vital, role in identifying a possible disease state but subsequently have little or no role in confirmation of the disorder. This situation occurs in the detection of GI bleeding through a screening test and subsequent diagnosis and confirmation of malignancy through sigmoidoscopy.

The chapters in this section provide an introduction to the variety of gastrointestinal disorders commonly encountered and to the concepts necessary for the clinical laboratory scientist to understand and facilitate the clinical and laboratory management of each.

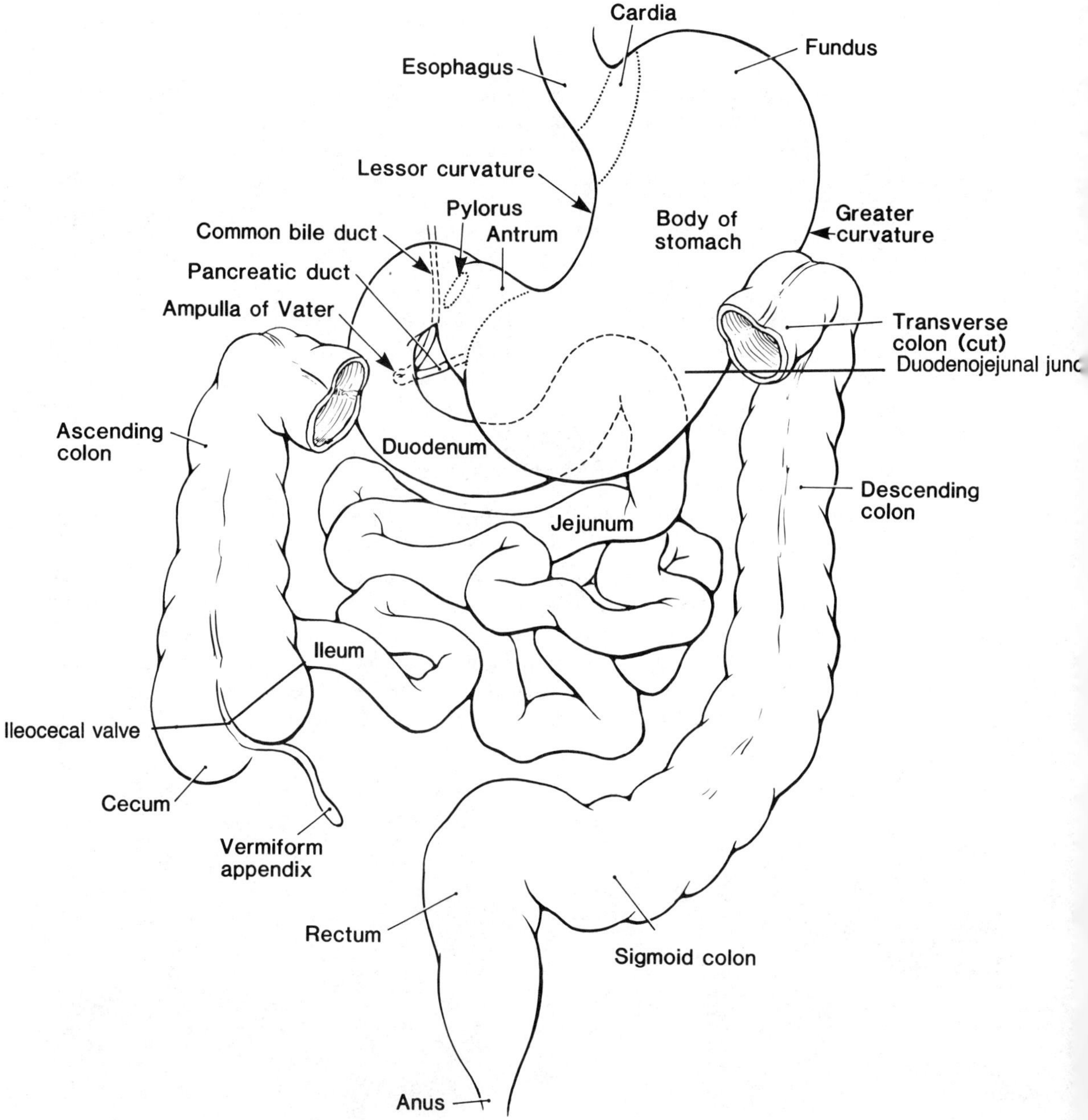

Anatomic landmarks of the gastrointestinal tract.

Chapter 21

Malabsorption

Larry Schoeff

Normal assimilation of food into the body occurs in three phases. The first two, the cephalic and gastric phases, are purely digestive processes that break down the food for subsequent absorption. The intestinal phase begins as these partially digested food substances traverse the duodenum, where gastrointestinal hormones and pancreatic enzymes effect further degradation. The digestive products then enter the jejunum and ileum for absorption. Carbohydrate, fat, and protein assimilation occurs in three stages within the small intestine: the intraluminal phase, the brush border phase and, finally, intracellular absorption.

Carbohydrate absorption begins with the action of salivary amylase on starch, and proceeds quickly to the duodenum, where pancreatic amylase essentially completes the hydrolysis of starch into di- and oligosaccharides. Hydrolases of the mucosal brush border further split these sugars into monosaccharides, which are absorbed intracellularly for delivery to the liver.[1]

Fat is assimilated less efficiently than are carbohydrates and protein, requiring more time for lipolysis in the duodenum and a greater surface area in the jejunum for absorption. Although dietary triglycerides are first hydrolyzed in the stomach by pharyngeal and gastric lipases, most hydrolysis occurs in the duodenum with pancreatic lipase.[2] A pancreatic factor, co-lipase, is also secreted to facilitate more efficient lipolysis by binding to lipid-bile salt surfaces.[3] Moreover, cholesystokinin release from the duodenal mucosa stimulates the pancreas and gallbladder to synchronize optimal mixtures of lipid, lipase, and bile salts for efficient lipolysis.[4] Liberated fatty acids and monoglycerides then solubilize with bile acids, forming micelles in the lumen. At the mucosal cell surface, bile salts dissociate and the lipids are absorbed, with the aid of a cytosol fatty acid-binding protein, into the jejunal mucosa. Within the cell they reassemble into triglycerides, which stimulate specific apoproteins and form chylomicrons. The chylomicrons are transported out of the cell in the systemic circulation via the lymphatic pathway.

Digestion of dietary protein begins in the stomach as the acidity and pepsin denature the protein, producing polypeptides. Protein digestion is more significant in the duodenum, where proteolytic proenzymes from the pancreas, including trypsinogen and chymotrypsinogen, are secreted to hydrolyze protein into small peptides and amino acids. Once in the duodenum, these proenzyme forms are activated by a brush border enzyme, enterokinase, which selectively acts on trypsinogen to form trypsin. Traces of trypsin in turn promote activation of the other proenzymes. Some of the resulting small peptides are hydrolyzed to amino acids at the brush border membrance by aminopeptidases. Amino acids, as well as di- and tripeptides, are absorbed intact into the mucosal cell, aided by several stereospecific transport systems.[5, 6] The peptides are rapidly hydrolyzed in the mucosa so that only amino acids are found in portal blood.

The water-insoluble vitamins A, D, E, and K depend on the formation of soluble lipid micelles in the intestinal lumen for adequate absorption. The water-soluble vitamins folic acid and vitamin B_{12} require specialized digestive and transport mechanisms for absorption. Dietary folate in the intestinal lumen must be hydrolyzed to free folate by a brush border enzyme before absorption occurs. It is then absorbed by diffusion and carrier-mediated transport. Cobalamin (B_{12}) competes with two different substances in the stomach for binding: intrinsic factor and a binding protein called R protein. The latter has a greater affinity for B_{12}. The difficulty with intestinal absorption is that only B_{12} that is bound to intrinsic factor can be absorbed. Since neither free B_{12} nor R protein-bound B_{12} is absorbable, a pancreatic protease is required to alter the R protein attached to B_{12} in such a way that intrinsic factor can bind to the B_{12}. Ultimately, intrinsic factor-bound B_{12} attaches to membrane receptors of the ileal mucosa for absorption.[7]

Sodium is absorbed by active transport involving the absorption of glucose and amino acids. Calcium uptake by the jejunal mucosa is facilitated by a calcium-binding protein, synthesis of which is regulated by vitamin D and parathyroid hormone. Iron absorption is regulated by ferritin and transferrin, working together in the mucosal cells to trap and transport the ferrous iron into body stores. When body iron stores are too high, mucosal cells with iron still inside are sloughed into the lumen.

ETIOLOGY AND PATHOPHYSIOLOGY OF DISORDERS OF ASSIMILATION

Maldigestion vs. Malabsorption

It is important to distinguish between maldigestion and malabsorption for etiological reasons. Although the absorptive process itself may be impaired, malabsorption may also be caused by inadequate digestion of the various nutrients before they reach the mucosal lining for assimilation. Maldigestion of nutrients may occur anywhere along the gastrointestinal tract after ingestion, but most commonly it is the result of some form of pancreatic insufficiency.

Disease Classification

Diseases that cause malabsorption syndrome are classified according to the stages of digestion and absorption where the pathophysiological processes occur in the gastrointestinal tract (see the classification in the opposite column).

In the digestive, or intraluminal stage, a deficiency of pancreatic enzymes or bile acids leads to malabsorption because nutrients in the lumen are not digested into an absorbable state. Defective secretion of pancreatic enzymes as a result of the diseases listed above causes maldigestion of carbohydrates, fat, and protein. Also, duodenal hyperacidity can inactivate pancreatic enzymes. Deficiency of bile acid secretion or activity in the intestinal lumen prevents digestion of lipids. This diminution may result from biliary obstruction, liver disease, or terminal ileitis (Crohn's disease).[8] Overgrowth of bacteria in the small intestine can inactivate bile acids, which also leads to lipid malabsorption.[9]

In the absorptive, or intestinal mucosal stage, defects at the brush border or impairment of the epithelium cause inadequate absorption. Genetic and biochemical abnormalities, such as deficiencies of brush border enzymes and defects in amino acid transport, and loss of absorptive surface area, as in short bowel syndrome, are examples of diseases that involve the absorptive phase.[10] Short bowel syndrome is a condition of malabsorption and malnutrition following a major resection of the small intestine.[5, 11, 12, 13] An example of infiltrative disease is Whipple's disease, a rare condition of intestinal lipodystrophy. Two chronic inflammatory disorders of malabsorption with unknown etiologies and potentially severe complications are ulcerative colitis and extensive regional enteritis (Crohn's disease)[8, 14] (see Chap. 26).

Malabsorption may also result from disturbances of the mucosal immune system.[15] These include immunodeficiency states, the most common of which is selective IgA deficiency, proliferation or malignant expansion of immune-related cells, as in primary intestinal lymphoma, and hypersensitivity reactions, such as celiac disease.[16, 17] Celiac disease, or gluten-sensitive enteropathy, is characterized by a severe allergy of the intestinal mucosa to the glycoprotein gluten, which is found in wheat and other cereal grains.[18, 19, 20] It is the water-insoluble gliadin frac-

Classification of Malabsorption Syndromes

Maldigestion — Intraluminal Stage

Deficiency of Pancreatic Enzymes

Chronic pancreatitis
Pancreatic carcinoma
Cystic fibrosis
Pancreatic resection
Duodenal hyperacidity states
Postgastrectomy syndrome

Deficiency of Bile Acids

Bile duct obstruction
Intrahepatic disease
Terminal ileitis (Crohn's disease)
Ileal resection
Bacterial overgrowth

Malabsorption — Intestinal Mucosal Stage

Defects at Brush Border

Deficiencies of oligosaccharidases
Deficiency of enteropeptidase

Impairment of Epithelium

Celiac disease (gluten-sensitive enteropathy)
Tropical sprue
Whipple's disease
Ulcerative colitis
Short bowel syndrome
Extensive regional enteritis (Crohn's disease)
Primary intestinal lymphoma
Radiation enteritis
Amino acid transport defects
Immunodeficiency states
Pernicious anemia
Food allergy
Parasitic infections
Amyloidosis
Lymphangiectasia
Abetalipoproteinemia

tion (single polypeptide) of gluten in wheat and other cereal grains that leads to the mucosal damage. This damage characteristically manifests as a flattened surface with no villi and infiltration of the lamina propria with lymphocytes and plasma cells.

Carbohydrate Malabsorption

Malabsorption of various ingested sugars can occur following mucosal injury caused by a number of diseases, including celiac disease, tropical sprue,[21] and gastroenteritis. Structural damage to and/or physiological dysfunction of the mucosa may decrease hydrolase enzymes along the brush border, or alter the active transport mechanism for monosaccharide absorption, or both. Disorders of intraluminal starch digestion are rare because of the excessive amylase normally secreted and the fact that total pancreatic insufficiency is required before the effect is significant. A normal exception to this is the transient physiological deficiency of amylase in the neonate. Although abnormal digestion of starch in the lumen is rare, abnormal digestion of oligosaccharides at the brush border is common. The most common disorder of carbohydrate malabsorption is lactose intolerance, caused by a deficiency at the brush border of lactase, which normally hydrolyzes the milk sugar into glucose and galactose. There are two distinct types of lactase deficiency—congenital and acquired.[18] Congenital lactase deficiency is rare, with mucosal levels low or absent at birth. The disease exhibits autosomal recessive inheritance, involving a structural mutation that prevents lactase synthesis. When suspected, it must be distinguished from glucose-galactose malabsorption and from developmental lactose intolerance in the newborn. Acquired or late-onset lactase deficiency occurs in many ethnic groups around the world. In fact, most adults in the world are lactase-deficient. In population groups that consume dairy products all their lives, the lactase mechanism typically persists into adulthood. However, in nondairy cultures, such as African and Asian groups, lactase levels tend to decline steadily through childhood and adolescence, and a high prevalence of lactose malabsorption exists (>65%).

Two other oligosaccharidase deficiencies are sucrase-isomaltase deficiency and trehalase deficiency. Sucrase-isomaltase, a major disaccharidase in the microvillus membrane, hydrolyzes sucrose and isomaltose. Its deficiency is inherited as an autosomal recessive trait, with symptoms appearing when sucrose-sweetened foods are consumed. Trehalase deficiency, a rare genetic disorder, is caused by ingestion of mushrooms that have a high content of the sugar trehalose.

Glucose-galactose malabsorption is a rare transport defect in which poor mucosal binding of glucose and galactose occurs. Fructose malabsorption occurs rarely, following the ingestion of fruit.

Fat Malabsorption

Conditions that are associated with malabsorption of lipids are classified as follows: impaired lipolysis, impaired micelle formation, and defective mucosal absorption. Defects in lipolysis may occur in postgastrectomy patients when rapid gastric emptying of fat into the small intestine is too excessive for lipase action. The fat may be delivered normally, but pancreatic insufficiency may prevent adequate secretion of lipase into the lumen. Diminished lipase secretion may also result if there is decreased release of cholecystokinin from a damaged duodenal mucosa, caused by celiac sprue or Crohn's disease. If none of these conditions exists, lipolysis may still be impaired by an altered luminal environment, such as a low *p*H from hypersecretion of gastric acid that spills into the duodenum; lipase is not effective in an acid environment. Co-lipase may be deficient from the lumen, which would limit lypolysis by preventing activation of lipase.

Defects in micellar solubilization of lipolytic products with bile salts involve synthesis, conjugation, delivery, or loss of bile salts. Without micellarization, lipids do not efficiently penetrate the microvillus membrane or diffuse into the mucosal cell. Intrahepatic cholestasis from cirrhosis or hepatitis causes decreased synthesis of bile salts, whereas bile duct obstruction causes decreased delivery to the lumen. The bile salt-binding drug cholestyramine and excessive intestinal bacteria, which deconjugate bile salts, both decrease the effective concentration of conjugated bile salts already in the lumen. Deconjugation renders them less capable of solubilizing the lipids. Ileal disease or resection causes a significant defect in the enterohepatic circulation of bile salts that can result in large fecal losses.

Mucosal diseases, such as celiac and tropical sprue or regional enteritis, cause decreased absorption of lipids. If lipids are absorbed into the mucosa, they are then dependent on the formation of chylomicrons for transport out of the cell and uptake by the lymphatic system. In the rare disorder abetalipoproteinemia, no synthesis of chylomicrons occurs because its major apolipoprotein B is absent. Whipple's disease causes decreased transport of chylomicrons through the lamina propria to the lymphatics because of "foamy" macrophages in the lamina propria that hinder the movement of chylomicrons. Finally, uptake by the lymphatics may be impaired by lymphatic obstruction, as in lymphoma or lymphangiectasia.

Protein Malabsorption

Although significant protein digestion by pepsin occurs in the stomach, it is not essential. There are no known malabsorption disorders from decreased pepsin. Total gastrectomy does not even alter protein metabolism significantly. The only maldigestive disorder of protein to be considered is trypsin deficiency, which may result from any cause of pancreatic insufficiency or from a deficiency of enterokinase. Without enterokinase in the duodenum, pancreatic trypsinogen is not activated to trypsin. Enterokinase deficiency may manifest as a rare primary disorder, or secondarily from congenital exocrine pancreatic insufficiency, in which a dependence of pancreatic secretions (trypsinogen) on enterokinase activity has been demonstrated.[10]

Decreased carrier-mediated transport of amino acids in mucosal cells may occur by a number of mechanisms. Mucosal diseases may cause reduced brush-border enteropeptidase activity, as well as reduced absorptive capability for amino acids. Segments of intestine that are specialized for absorption of certain amino acids or vitamins may be removed by surgical resection. Exudative loss of plasma proteins through inflamed or ulcerated mucosa may be a dramatic cause of protein malassimilation in protein-losing enteropathy.

Vitamins/Minerals Malabsorption[22]

The fat-soluble vitamins A, D, E, and K are dependent upon micellar solubilization for absorption. Therefore, deficiencies of these vitamins may be caused by similar disorders of fat malabsorption, in which formation of bile salt micelles is impaired. Folate and cobalamin deficiencies are common in intestinal disease. Patients most susceptible to folate deficiency are those who have a poor diet and those with malabsorption secondary to jejunal mucosal disease or drugs that interfere with the metabolism of folate.[23] Ileal resection is a common cause of cobalamin deficiency, because the ileal segment that absorbs the B_{12}-intrinsic factor complex by active transport is removed. Iron malabsorption is most significant in diseases that cause long-term blood loss, such as extensive Crohn's disease. Because calcium absorption is under the influence of vitamin D, which in turn is regulated by adequate dietary fat and plasma parathyroid hormone levels, decreased calcium absorption can occur by several mechanisms. Fat malabsorption leads to decreased vitamin D absorption; unabsorbed intestinal fat and certain drugs, such as steroids, can bind calcium and prevent absorption; any disruption of absorptive surface area decreases calcium absorption; hypoparathyroidism also decreases intestinal calcium absorption.

CLINICAL MANIFESTATIONS

The classic symptoms common to all diseases of malabsorption are weight loss and diarrhea, regardless of etiology (see Fig. 21-1). An increase in appetite following weight loss may be the only manifestation in early or mild cases. Anorexia may also be seen, as in celiac disease, although hyperphagia typifies pancreatic insufficiency. Weight loss is primarily due to the wasting of dietary calories, and is accompanied by malnutrition as the disorder progresses. The diarrhea of malabsorption disorders reflects the stimulus effect of unabsorbed bile acids and fatty acids on the colon, which results in water and electrolyte secretion in the stools.

The clinical hallmark from the laboratory perspective is *steatorrhea,* or pathological increase in stool fat. Steatorrhea tends to be a manifestation of almost all major causes of malabsorption, because the pancreas, bile, and mucosal integrity are all important in lipid digestion and absorption. The

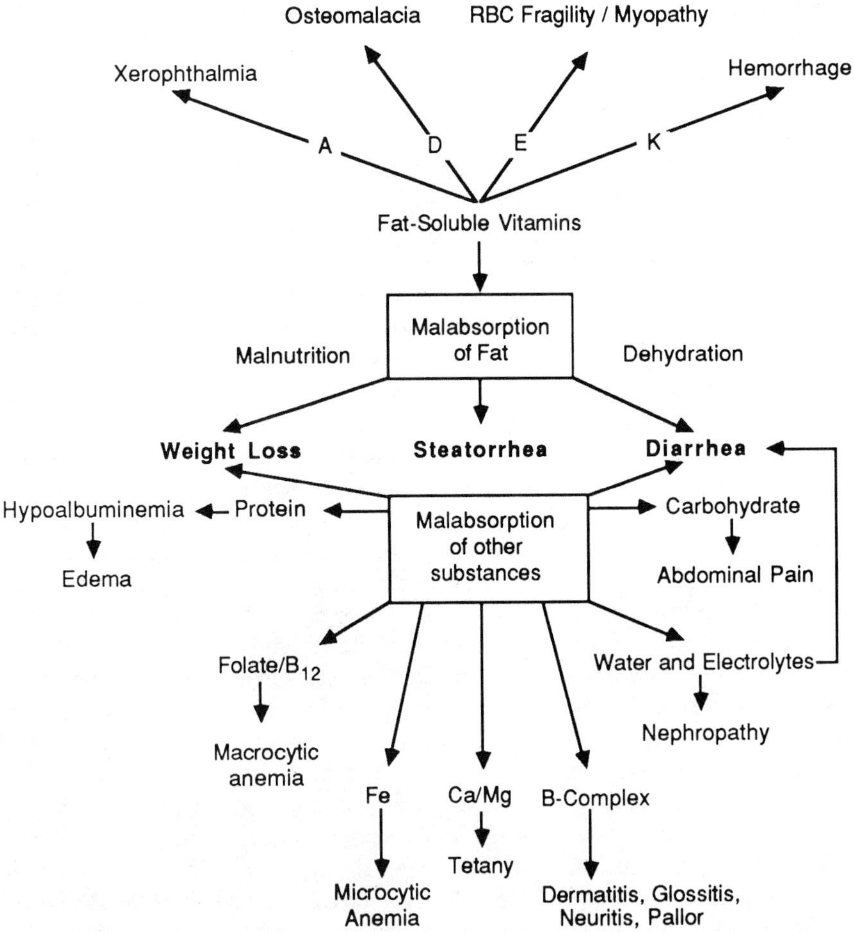

Figure 21-1 **Symptoms of malabsorption. (Adapted from Cerda J, Artnak E: Nutritional aspects of malabsorption syndromes. Compr Ther 9(11):35–46, 1983)**

physical findings in the malabsorption syndrome relate both to the underlying disease process and to malnutrition.

Malnutritional and abdominal symptoms are more specific in nature, reflective of the malabsorbed or deficient substance involved. Clinically, malabsorption of fat from pancreatic or mucosal disease occurs before carbohydrate or protein malabsorption, because of less efficient metabolism and dependence on intraluminal bile salt levels. In addition to steatorrhea, specific symptoms of fat malabsorption include those caused by subsequent deficiencies of the fat-soluble vitamins. Osteomalacia results from vitamin D and calcium malabsorption; susceptibility to hemorrhage occurs because of vitamin K malabsorption; xeropthalmia because of lack of vitamin A; and myopathy and red blood cell fragility because of lack of vitamin E.

Symptoms of carbohydrate malabsorption are abdominal distention and cramps, flatulence, and watery diarrhea. There is usually no steatorrhea present. Unabsorbed sugars in the intestinal lumen enter the colon, where bacteria ferment them into monosaccharides, short-chain fatty acids, hydrogen, and carbon dioxide. The watery diarrhea results from osmotic retention of water in the colon by the fatty acids and monosaccharides. The production of hydrogen and carbon dioxide gases and the colonic fluid accumulation cause the abdominal symptoms. Symptoms of sugar malabsorption may vary depending on the ingested sugar load, the colonic bacterial flora, and the compensatory capacity of the colon to absorb excess water and fatty acids.[1]

Dietary protein malabsorption or excessive intestinal protein loss leads to hypoalbuminemia, which in turn causes peripheral edema in association with proximal muscle wasting. If the protein deficiency or loss is severe enough, there may be some endocrine dysfunction of gastrointestinal and other hormones, as well as some osteoporosis from lack of protein-bound calcium. Folate and/or vitamin B_{12} malabsorption manifests as a megaloblastic (macrocytic) anemia, while iron deficiency produces a microcytic anemia. The symptoms of dermatitis, neuritis, glossitis, and pallor are seen as a result of deficiency of vitamin B complex. In addition to osteomalacia, symptoms of tetany are also produced by calcium deficiency, with or without diminished magnesium levels. Dehydration may be present in some malabsorption patients because of electrolyte imbalance and water loss.

LABORATORY ANALYSES AND DIAGNOSIS

The laboratory investigation of malabsorption usually begins with screening tests for malnutrition and steatorrhea to assess the symptoms of diarrhea and weight loss, and for symptoms related to nutritional deficiency, such as anemia or osteomalacia (see Fig. 21-2).[24, 25] A variety of common laboratory tests can be used to screen for nutritional deficiency. These include a complete blood count (CBC) with peripheral smear, serum levels of albumin, phosphorus, calcium, and cholesterol, and prothrombin time. Followup studies from the CBC might include serum iron, vitamin B_{12}, and red cell folate. Other followup studies may include protein electrophoresis, bone studies, and liver function tests. The simplest test used to detect steatorrhea is the Sudan III stain for fecal fat. This qualitative test may suffice as an alternative to the definitive test for fat malabsorption, which is a quantitative measurement of fat from a 72-hour collection of feces. Inspection for parasites may also be done at this time. Because of the difficulty of collection and unpleasantness of handling the specimen, other alternatives have been promoted. Among these are serum carotene or vitamin A assays and ^{14}C triolein breath tests. Low carotene (<50 μg/dL [0.93 μmol/L]) and vitamin A levels (<25 μg/dL [0.87 μmol/L]) are seen in 86% of patients with fat malabsorption. Serum carotene is more popular as a screening test, because vitamin A assays are more difficult to perform and the diagnostic ability of the two tests is not significantly different. Another screening procedure is a survey x-ray of the abdomen to detect pancreatic calcification. Invasive small bowel x-rays are not initial studies.

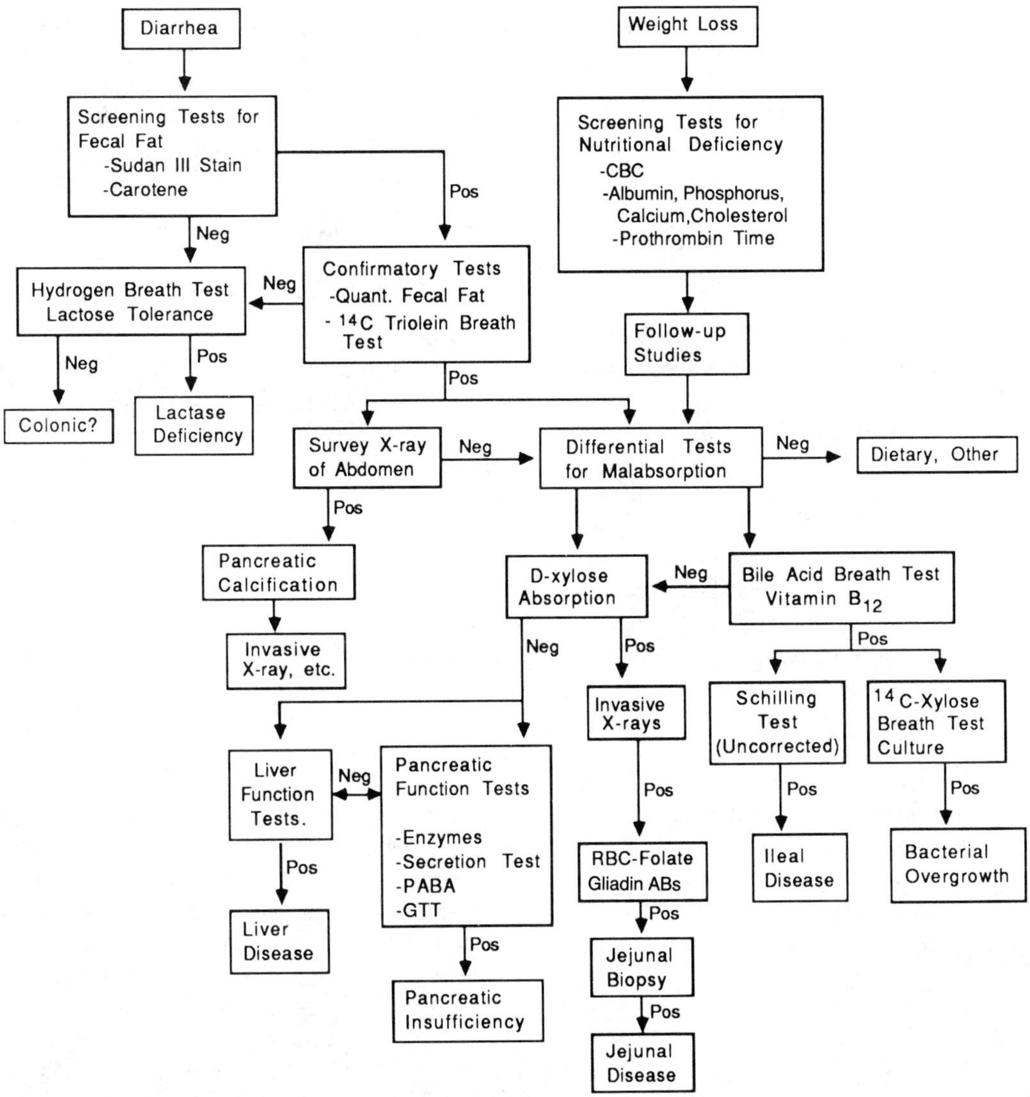

Figure 21-2 Laboratory evaluation of malabsorption.

Breath analyses may eventually be the best laboratory tests available to evaluate malabsorption, although their availability is not yet widespread.[26, 27] These tests offer the advantages of simplicity and convenience, and in most cases sensitivity and specificity. Specific uses of breath tests include direct detection of: fat malabsorption (^{14}C-triolein), carbohydrate malabsorption (H_2-lactose and H_2-sucrose), bile salt malabsorption (^{14}C-glycocholate), and bacterial overgrowth (^{14}C-xylose). In the ^{14}C-triolein breath test, the ^{14}C-labeled triglyceride is administered orally, with the absorbed fat ultimately metabolized to carbon dioxide and water. The radioactivity of $^{14}CO_2$ is measured in specimens of expired air with scintillation counters. Results are usually expressed as a percentage of the administered dose; low results indicate impaired fat absorption. A sensitivity of 100% and specificity of 96%, with a predictive value of approximately 90%, have been reported with this test.[28] Both the quantitative fecal fat and the ^{14}C-triolein breath test assess the degree of lipid malabsorption.

Once the suspicion of malabsorption raised by the presenting symptoms is confirmed by the screening tests, specific tests are employed to differentiate the diagnostic possibilities. Differential diagnosis of disorders should be directed toward three major organ systems: pancreatic insufficiency, liver disease, and impairment of the small intestine itself. Surgical alteration of the stomach and intestine should also be kept in mind for absorption problems. If the diagnosis has been narrowed to the small intestine, then further differentiation is required to identify jejunal disease, ileal disease, bacterial overgrowth, or lactose intolerance.

The D-xylose absorption test has been and still is widely used to distinguish malabsorption from maldigestion. Oral D-xylose does not require digestion and is normally absorbed directly by the jejunum only; therefore, ileal malabsorption will not be detected by this test. After absorption into the bloodstream, the amount of D-xylose excreted into the urine over a 5-hour period is closely correlated with the amount of D-xylose absorbed in the jejunum. Low urinary excretion of D-xylose (<25%) suggests jejunal disease, while normal results point to maldigestion, as in pancreatic disease. Low levels may also be seen in ascites, delayed gastric emptying, and kidney disease.

If D-xylose absorption is normal in the presence of steatorrhea, then pancreatic function should be evaluated. Testing for pancreatic disease may begin with serum levels of amylase, lipase, and trypsin. More precise studies are intubation tests, although they are more difficult to perform. Pancreatic and duodenal secretions are aspirated, after stimulation of the pancreas with secretin or Lundh meal, and tested for volume, bicarbonate concentration, and trypsin activity. Low results in all three parameters are highly indicative of pancreatic insufficiency. A tubeless stimulation test utilizes N-benzoyl-L-tyrosyl-*p*-aminobenzoic acid, which is hydrolyzed after ingestion by chymotrypsin. The hydrolysis product, *p*-aminobenzoic acid (PABA), is absorbed and ultimately excreted in the urine. Low urinary excretion of PABA suggests pancreatic disease; however, the test depends on normal absorption and liver function. A glucose tolerance test assesses the endocrine function of the pancreas. Finally, if an initial abdominal film showed pancreatic calcification, more sophisticated visualization techniques might be indicated (*e.g.*, CT scan, ultrasound).

If D-xylose is abnormal in the presence of steatorrhea, then confirmatory tests for jejunal disease are warranted. The diagnosis of celiac disease and other abnormalities of the jejunal mucosa is almost always confirmed by jejunal biopsy. The morphological examination of the intestinal tissue and histochemical tests for enzymes may be necessary to evaluate the nature and extent of mucosal damage. X-rays with contrast media and other visualization techniques may be required to demonstrate abnormal anatomic features or motility of the small bowel. The only definitive laboratory tests worthy of investigation are red blood cell folate levels and serum levels of gliadin antibodies. Folate deficiency is commonplace in celiac disease and tropical sprue. The determination of serum antibodies to dietary wheat gluten antigens by ELISA techniques[29] and fluorescent immunosorbent techniques[30] is highly sensitive and specific for adult and childhood celiac disease. Gliadin antibody titers could be used to screen for celiac disease, which must then be confirmed by biopsy. The titers are also a valuable adjunct in the followup of celiac disease, particularly in monitoring the clinical response to a gluten-free diet.

Ileal disease may be evaluated with tests for vitamin B_{12} and bile salts, because the ileum is the only small bowel segment capable of absorbing both substances. The test of choice is the bile acid breath test, in which radiolabeled ^{14}C-glycocholic acid is given orally. If the terminal ileum is diseased, the unabsorbed glycocholate will pass into the colon, where bacteria hydrolyze it to deconjugated bile salt and glycine. The ^{14}C-glycine is absorbed and metabolized to $^{14}CO_2$, which is measured in expired air in a manner similar to the triolein breath test for fat absorption. Positive results are also observed in bacterial overgrowth syndrome. The Schilling test for vitamin B_{12} absorption is the next best test for ileal dysfunction. Radioactive B_{12} is given orally with and without intrinsic factor, pancreatic enzyme extract, and antibiotics. B_{12} is normally absorbed and excreted in the urine. Low urinary B_{12} excretion implies one of four conditions, which are then differentiated by administering each of the substances listed above for correction of the abnormal urine levels. Correction with intrinsic factor indicates pernicious anemia; correction with pancreatic extract suggests pancreatic insufficiency; correction with tetracycline for several days before the next B_{12} dose points to bacterial overgrowth (bacteria metabolize the B_{12}). If B_{12} absorption is not corrected by any of these substances, then the patient has damaged ileal receptors, or has had an ileal resection. Biopsy and/or x-ray films may not be necessary for ileal dysfunction.

Culture of jejunal or duodenal contents is the definitive test for bacterial overgrowth syndrome, although it is not commonly performed. The bacteria are usually anaerobes, and multiply because of stasis of bowel contents in blind loops. Because the resulting malabsorption syndrome is very similar to ileal dysfunction, the bile acid breath test is also utilized for bacterial overgrowth. This test will not differentiate between the two conditions. A newer and more specific test for bacterial overgrowth is the ^{14}C-xylose breath test. When ^{14}C-xylose is given orally, subsequent measurement of $^{14}CO_2$ in the breath indicates that overgrowth flora catabolized xylose to CO_2 prior to absorption. This test is reported to be even more sensitive and specific than intestinal culture.[26] An alternative to laboratory testing may be a therapeutic trial of various antibiotics.

The diagnosis of lactose malabsorption has traditionally been made with the lactose tolerance test, in which oral lactose is converted to glucose by lactase and timed blood specimens are measured for glucose. The most reliable and now widely used test for lactose malabsorption is the hydrogen breath test.[31] Lactase-deficient patients will not absorb an oral dose of lactose, which is metabolized to hydrogen by bacteria in the colon, absorbed into the bloodstream, and eliminated in exhaled breath. The breath hydrogen is measured with a gas chromatograph. Patients may also be tested with a milk-free diet for a period of time. Peroral mucosal biopsy may be indicated to rule out secondary causes of lactose malabsorption. The hydrogen breath test is also useful in screening for other disaccharidase deficiencies.[32]

CASE STUDY

A thin 35-year-old man was admitted to the hospital with persistent diarrhea. His medical history from childhood revealed intermittent episodes of diarrhea and failure to thrive during the first decade of life. Gradual weight loss over several months was observed. He also reported an increasing sensitivity to milk, which had never previously affected him. He had foul-smelling, bulky stools, and slight edema was observed.

His admission CBC revealed a macrocytic anemia. A vitamin B_{12} assay was normal. A screening test for fecal fat was positive. A chemistry profile revealed below normal levels of albumin, calcium, phosphorus, and cholesterol. His prothrombin time was prolonged. A breath hydrogen test was elevated. A D-xylose absorption test was then ordered, and showed reduced urinary excretion (19%). At this point the presumptive diagnosis of celiac sprue was entertained. To confirm this, a peroral jejunal biopsy and x-ray filming of the small bowel with contrast media were performed. The biopsy showed a subtotal villous atrophy. The x-ray film showed thickening of mucosal folds, but was otherwise unremarkable. The diagnosis of adult celiac disease was confirmed. The patient was treated symptomatically for the diarrhea and anemia, and was started on a gluten-free diet. Significant improvement with steady weight gain was observed within six weeks.

Questions

1. How do you account for an apparent reemergence of sprue in adulthood?
2. What is the most likely explanation for the lactose intolerance?
3. What additional laboratory findings are significant, and what followup is recommended?

Discussion

1. It is not uncommon for patients with childhood celiac sprue to have a clinical remission as adolescents and to tolerate gluten ingestion without symptoms until the third decade of life.
2. Secondary lactose intolerance may develop as a result of the chronic irritation and subsequent injury to the brush border.
3. Additional laboratory studies to consider are red blood cell folate and serum gliadin antibodies. Because folate is absorbed by the jejunum, deficiency is common in celiac sprue. Assessment of serum antibodies to wheat gliadin is potentially useful in the followup of celiac disease, particularly with the clinical response to a gluten-free diet. Treatment requires life-long restriction of gluten from the diet.

REFERENCES

1. Ravich W, Bayliss T: Carbohydrate absorption and malabsorption. Clin Gastroenterol 12:335–356, 1983
2. Hamash M, Klaeveman H, Wolf R et al: Pharyngeal lipase and digestion of dietary triglyceride in man. J Clin Invest 55:908–913, 1975
3. Borgstrom B: On the interaction between pancreatic lipase and colipase and substrate, and the importance of bile salts. J Lipid Res 16:411–414, 1975
4. Glickman R: Fat absorption and malabsorption. Clin Gastroenterol 12:323–334, 1983
5. Newsholme E, Leech A: Biochemistry for the Medical Sciences. New York City, John Wiley & Sons, 1983
6. Tietz NW: Textbook of Clinical Chemistry. Philadelphia, WB Saunders, 1986
7. Ryan M, Olsen W: A diagnostic approach to malabsorption syndromes: A pathophysiological approach. Clin Gastroenterol 12:533–550, 1983
8. Donaldson R: Crohn's disease. In Sleisenger M, Fordtran J: Gastroentestinal Disease: Pathophysiology, Diagnosis, Management; 3rd ed. Philadelphia, WB Saunders, 1983
9. King C, Toskes P: Small intestine bacterial overgrowth. Gastroenterol 76:1035–1055, 1979
10. Rossi E, Lentze M: Clinical significance of enzymatic deficiencies in the gastrointestinal tract with particular reference to lactase deficiency. Ann Allergy 53(6):649–656, 1984
11. Gray D: Short bowel syndrome. Am Fam Physician 30(3):227–323, 1984
12. Morris J, Selwanov V, Sheldon G: Nutritional management of patients with malabsorption syndrome. Clin Gastroenterol 12(2):463–474, 1983
13. Weser E: Nutritional aspects of malabsorption: Short gut adaptation. Clin Gastroenterol 12(2): 443–461, 1983
14. Cello J: Ulcerative colitis. In Sleisenger M, Fordtran J: Gastrointestinal Disease: Pathophysiology, Diagnosis, Management, 3rd ed. Philadelphia, WB Saunders, 1983
15. Doe W, Hapel A: Intestinal immunity and malabsorption. Clin Gastroenterol 12(2):415–435, 1983
16. Eidelman S, Parkins R, Rubin C: Abdominal lymphoma presenting as malabsorption. Medicine 45:111, 1966
17. Koistinen J: Selective IgA deficiency in blood donors. Vox Sang 29:192–202, 1975
18. Cole S, Kognoff M: Celiac Disease. Ann Rev Nutr 5:241–266, 1985
19. Falchuk Z: Gluten-sensitive enteropathy. Clin Gastroenterol 12(2):475–493, 1983
20. Ferguson A, Ziegler K, Strobel S: Gluten intolerance (coeliac disease). Ann Allergy 53:637–642, 1984
21. Tomkins A: Tropical malabsorption: Recent concepts in pathogenesis and nutritional significance. Clin Sci 60:131–187, 1981
22. Cerda J, Artnak E: Nutritional aspects of malabsorption syndromes. Compr Ther 9(11):35–46, 1983
23. Gallagher N: Importance of vitamin B_{12} and folate metabolism in malabsorption. Clin Gastroenterol 12(2):437–441, 1983

24. Cerda J, Dobbins W, Rider J: Simplifying diagnosis of malabsorption. Patient Care 15(17):128–178, 1981
25. Theodozzi A, Gazzard B: Have chemical tests a role in diagnosing malabsorption? Am Clin Biochem 21(3):153–165, 1984
26. King C, Toskes P: The use of breath tests in the study of malabsorption. Clin Gastroenterol 12(2):591–610, 1983
27. West P, Levin G, Griffen G et al: Comparison of simple screening tests for fat malabsorption. Br Med J 282:1501–1504, 1981
28. Newcomer A, Hofmann A, DeMagno E: Triolein breath test: A sensitive and specific test for fat malabsorption. Gastroenterol 76:6–13, 1979
29. Scott H, Fausa O, Brandtzaeg E & P: Immune response patterns in coeliac disease: Serum antibodies to dietary antigens measured by an enzyme-linked immunosorbent assay (ELISA). Clin Exp Immunol 57:25–32, 1984
30. Burgin-Wolff A, Bertele R, Berger R et al: A reliable screening test for childhood celiac disease: Fluorescent immunosorbent test for gliaden antibodies. J Pediatr 102:655–660, 1983
31. Rosado J, Solomons N: Sensitivity and specificity of the hydrogen breath-analysis test for detecting malabsorption of physiological doses of lactose. Clin Chem 29(3):545–548, 1983
32. Newcomer A: Screening tests for carbohydrate malabsorption. J Pediatr Gastroenterol 3(1):6–8, 1984

BIBLIOGRAPHY

Sleisenger M, Brandborg L: Malabsorption. Philadelphia, WB Saunders, 1977

Green M, Greene H: The Role of the Gastrointestinal Tract in Nutrient Delivery. Orlando, FL, Academic Press, 1984

Gitnick G: Gastroenterology. New York City, John Wiley & Sons, 1983

Sleisenger M, Fordtran J: Gastrointestinal Disease: Pathophysiology, Diagnosis, Management, 3rd ed. Philadelphia, WB Saunders, 1983

Jeejeebhoy K: Gastrointestual Diseases: Focus on Clinical Diagnosis, 2nd ed. New Hyde Park, NY, Medical Examination Publishing, 1985

Nurse's Clinical Library: Gastrointestinal Disorders. Springhouse, PA, Springhouse Corp, 1985

Chapter 22

Ulcers

Linda Gorman

ETIOLOGY AND PATHOPHYSIOLOGY

Ulcers are lesions of the stomach or intestinal tract mucosa that are breaks in the protective lining of the affected organs. These breaks allow "foreign" substances to invade the epithelial cells of these organs. A disruption of these cells and cell fittings can disrupt the absorption of food, ions, and essential molecules. The disruption also allows the strong acids of the stomach and the digestive enzymes of the intestinal tract to act on cell linings of the stomach and intestines, exposing the inner organ bacterial flora to the body cavity.

The acute ulcer is precipitated by certain drugs and pathological conditions that induce stress. Ulcers are classified as initial erosions that break the mucosal lining and have minimal bleeding, and acute and chronic stages that are of increased diagnostic concern. The acute ulcer breaks through the mucosa and into the cellular layers.

The chronic ulcer breaks through the stroma of the organ and creeps toward perforation of the organ wall and exposure of the stomach and intestinal contents to the body cavity beyond.

Statistical evidence indicates that patients under age 30 rarely exhibit symptoms of ulcer unless experiencing extreme stress.[1] Women over age 55 with frequent pain made worse by food intake are prone to gastric ulcers. Men under age 55 with heartburn and relief of pain with food intake have the larger percentage of duodenal ulcers. Four factors are involved in the formation of ulcers:

1. Increases in acid and pepsinogen
2. Rupture of mucosal linings
3. Alterations in hormonal feedback mechanisms
4. Decreases in bicarbonate ion concentrations

Evidence[2] exists that increase in stomach acid is the culprit in ulcer development, but some authors[1, 3, 4] contend that the root cause is polarization of the mucosa that results in tight junction breaks susceptible to acid and enzyme digestion of the mucosa.

The development of ulcers, especially severe peptic ulcers, would appear to occur over an extended period of time. These chronic ulcer conditions may be brought on by a change in drug usage, by emotional stress, or perhaps by an aging mechanism that reduces the body's ability to cope with immunological insult. Acute ulcers referred to as *stress* ulcers can develop in patients with such conditions as severe burns, trauma, and cancer. The development of an ulcer is a serious matter regardless of the cause, because the ulcer is a break in the mucosal lining of the stomach or small intestine. Mucosal layers in these organs provide the more sensitive muscle layers with protection from the high acid and enzymatic contents that pass through. Some strong digestive enzymes, such as pepsin and trypsin, could digest the epithelial layers of the stomach and intestine were it not for the mucosa. One classification of ulcers[1] defines erosions, acute ulcers, and chronic ulcers as stages in an increasingly deep invasion of the mucosal and muscular layers of the organs affected (see Fig. 22-1). As each layer is exposed, the blood vessels in that area are damaged and bleeding occurs into the cavity. Continued acid and enzyme destruction widens the affected area and results in bleeding that erupts into epigastric pain and discomfort.

Although ulceration is invariably associated with increased acid output, other factors such as blood flow and ionic transport are also important. Normal defense mechanisms cannot overcome the fourfold attack seen in ulcer development:[1]

1. The breaking of the gastric mucosal barrier, with resulting back diffusion of hydrochloric acid (HCl) into the mucosa
2. The failure of intracellular metabolism to maintain normal ionic equilibrium
3. The local ischemia of the mucosa with necrosis
4. The failure of bicarbonate and mucus secretions to buffer the affected area

Peptic ulcers, because of their chronic nature[1] and deep invasion of the mucosal lining,[2] are of primary clinical importance. The peptic ulcer has a defined border, from 1 to 3 cm in diameter.[2] Peptic ulcers are often chronic and may occur in the stomach or, more frequently, in the duodenum. Duodenal peptic ulcers occur five to ten times more often than do gastric ulcers.[2] Major factors in the development of peptic ulcers are the concentration of hydrogen ions secreted and the integrity of the defense mechanisms of the mucosal lining. Adverse effects of hydrogen ions on cellular deoxyribonucleic acids (DNA) have shown protein turnovers that contribute to the cellular degeneration.[1] Epithelial cells of the mucosa have joining points, called *tight junctions,* that prevent a significant flow of hydrogen ions into the GI walls. Damage to these junctions is minimized by a constant replacement of the epithelial cells through normal defense mechanisms.[2] In gastric ulcers the defense system breaks down, acid damages the junctions, and erosion of the mucosal wall occurs. In duodenal ulcers the hypersecretion of acid overwhelms the buffering abilities of the defense mechanisms, causing ulceration. Duodenal ulcers show twice the

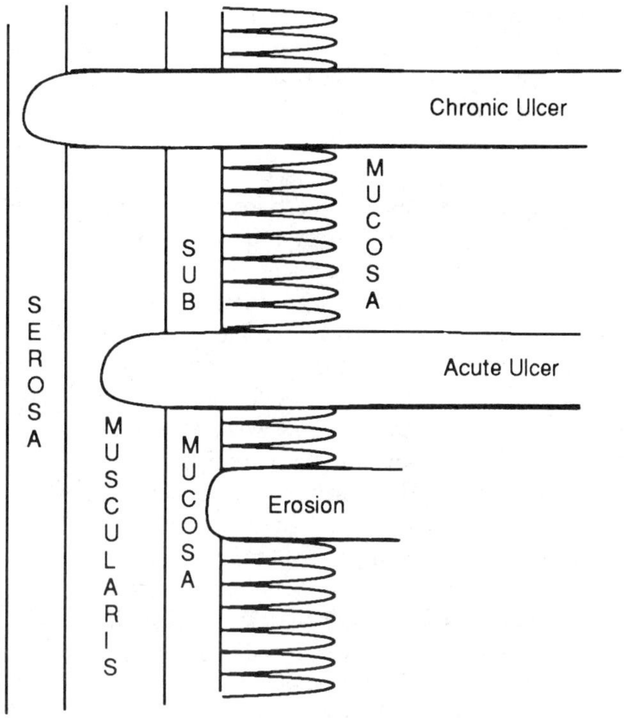

Figure 22-1 Differences in ulcer erosion. (Modified from Brooks FP, Cohen S, Soloway RD [eds]: Peptic Ulcer Disease. New York, Churchill Livingstone, 1985)

number of parietal-acid-secreting cells as does the normal duodenum, probably because of a defect in the feedback mechanism that the normal duodenum maintains. Irritants such as aspirin, coffee, and chronic alcohol intake can damage the mucosal lining and lead to breakdown in normal defense mechanisms.[1] Emotional stress may or may not[2] be a causative agent, but does precipitate an increase in hydrogen ion concentration in many patients.

Acute Peptic Ulcers

Acute peptic ulcers invade the mucosa to the muscularis and often result from the underlying causes of drugs, stress, or other disease trauma.[1]

Cushing's ulcer patients are persons who have experienced head injury and develop acid outputs of 100 to 150 mmol/hr.[2] The results of one study were that, of 47 head-injury patients, 36 developed ulcerative lesions: 32 in the stomach and 4 in the duodenum. Findings in another study[3] were that the hyperacid secretion in a group of head-injury patients lasted 4 to 5 days, accompanied by elevated serum gastrin levels.[5] There was a four-fold increase in gastric secretion volume. The use of steroids in head injuries may increase the risk of ulceration, but this has not been proven; in combination with cimetidine, steroids appear to decrease bleeding problems in Cushing's ulcer patients. The use of PGE prostaglandin in drug combinations has reduced the incidence of ulceration in animal experiments and has aided healing in cases involving erosion development.[1]

Patients with burns over one-third of the body appear at risk for the development of acute ulcers, called *Curling's ulcers.*[1] Often erosions appear within 24 hours after the burn, gastric ulcers within 96 hours, and duodenal ulcers by the fourth day.[1] In one study, 9 of 15 cases deteriorated from erosions to full ulcers. Of the nine ulcers, seven progressed to hemorrhage and two to perforation of the GI wall. Contributing factors in burn patients may be dehydration, sepsis, and reduction of gastric acid. The reduction in blood flow and ischemia accompanying burns probably lead to a decrease in mucus secretion and an increased risk of ulceration.[1]

Drug induced erosions and ulcerations may be of an acute nature, although more frequently they are of the chronic type. Aspirin, ethanol, and various over-the-counter medications can result in acute erosions and ulcerations.[1] Combinations of these drugs can compound the problem. Aspirin has the most severe effect on the antrum of the stomach, and even healthy persons can develop erosions in the stomach after 1 week of aspirin intake. Aspirin reduces the ion potentials across the stomach mucosa and can be especially harmful if ethanol is added. Aspirin can cross the lipid membranes of gastric mucosa as unionized compounds, increasing hydrogen ion and deoxyribonucleic acid (DNA) loss in the gastric wash. In this way aspirin reduces the pressure on the pyloric sphincter, reduces potential differences across the stomach wall, and increases duodenogastric reflux.[1] Kuo and Shamboar[6] found that aspirin inhibited mucosal transport of sodium and chloride ions by initially reducing the adenosine triphosphate (ATP) content of the mucosa. Prostaglandins, important to mucosal defense mechanisms, are also inhibited by aspirin.

Indomethacin, an anti-inflammatory agent, can also induce ulcers if exogenous prostaglandins (PGE_2) are not used.[1] Phenylbutazone, reserpine, and cinchophen are also linked to the development of acute gastric mucosal erosions,[1] although they appear to act on the central nervous system (CNS) rather than affecting the ionic potentials across the stomach or the intestine.

Large quantities of ethanol imbibed over short time periods can result in acute mucosal damage and thus erosions and ulceration. The effects of ethanol damage to the mucosa include the following:[1]

1. Increased protein loss from the stomach with hydrochloric acid present
2. An increase in cyclic adenosine monophosphate (cAMP) and adenyl cyclase activity
3. Decreased potentials and increased electrical resistance across stomach wall, causing direct inhibition of active transport
4. Increased permeability of the GI wall
5. Hemorrhage of the GI wall when large quantities of ethanol are ingested

Stress ulcers are associated with diseases such as respiratory failure, hypotension, sepsis, and jaundice. Cancer patients can develop stress ulcers, as can persons who undergo hepatic artery chemotherapy infusions. The acute erosions of stress ulcers often occur in the fundus and corpus of the stomach.[1] These ulcers often are difficult to detect because the increased gastric secretions cross the mucosal barrier and are not reflected in increased basal acid output (BAO) and maximum acid output (MAO) levels by Histalog stimulation. Stress ulcers may occur in both very young and elderly persons. In children under 12 years of age, acute ulcer situations arise with perforation and subsequent life-threatening hemorrhage. After 12 years of age, the clinical presentation is similar to that of adults. Elderly persons may present with an acute stress ulcer complicated by hemorrhage. After the acute episode, however, the ulcer often persists as a chronic ulcerative condition.

Chronic Peptic Ulcers

Chronic ulcers occur in both gastric and duodenal areas of the GI tract. Patients who have chronic ulcers experience episodes of healing and reoccurrence over extended periods of time. The pepsin and acid secretions interact to eat away the mucosa and then the underlying cell layers of the GI wall.

Chronic gastric ulcers occur in older persons and generally do not have acid output levels as high as seen in duodenal ulcers.[1, 4, 7] A chronic gastric ulcer may be located in the corpus or fundus of the stomach as well as in the antrum. Ulceration in these areas does not result in the acid output mechanisms seen in duodenal ulcers. Often an older person has another disease complication and the chronic ulcer may be due to ischemia in the stomach area or to medications such as aspirin. A patient history can be helpful in suggesting a chronic gastric ulcer, because it occurs 2 to 2½ times more frequently in patients who have relatives with gastric ulcers. Older patients with cardiovascular and/or pulmonary disease often present an added risk for development of chronic gastric ulcers. A Japanese study[8] reported that a majority of ulcers occur just proximal to the pyloric gland and fundus gland, making a 2.0-cm-wide zone in the mucosa. Abnormal gastric motility and disruption of the sphincter-closing mechanism appear to occur, resulting in a lack of acid response and entry of bile into the stomach. Increases in lysolecithin from bile in the stomach can harm the gastric mucosal layers. Emotional stress can lead to gastric ulcers, and removal of the strain can reduce or eradicate the ulcer.[1]

The *chronic duodenal ulcer* patient does not fit neatly into a single category because duodenal ulcers may be associated with a heterogenous mixture of underlying causes.[1] The patient may have a high or a normal acid output, with normal or elevated gastrin levels. The pepsinogen I levels appear higher in patients with recurrent chronic duodenal ulcers, and may have ulcerative properties. Somatostatin levels and the influence of gastric calcium also appear to play a part in some cases of duodenal ulcer. Epidemiological studies of patient populations suggest that, because of familial occurrence of duodenal ulcer, siblings of affected patients are three times more susceptible to ulcer development than are persons without such history. Persons with Group-O-type blood and nonsecretor status also have an increased risk of duodenal ulcers. Tissue-typing studies implicate HLA-B and HLA-B12 lines.

The influence of histamine on ulceration has prompted review of its metabolism in duodenal ulcer patients. Histamine release from mast cells occurs through gastrin and acetylcholine stimulation.[1] In duodenal ulcer patients a reduction of histamine methyl transferase, an enzyme for the catabolism of histamine, results in histamine effects that can continue for extended periods. Increased pancreatic bicarbonate and increased serum secretin are seen as beneficial in duodenal ulcer patients, but duodenal ulcer patients have a faster stomach-emptying process, which reduces buffering capacity.[1] Normally, somatostatin levels increase and work to suppress acid pepsin secretions. In duodenal ulcer patients, however, the somatostatin is not as effective in the inhibition of gastrin or acid secretion because there is a reduction in somatostatin-secreting cells of the antrum in these patients. Gastrin fractions, especially G-34 and G-17, may be normal in fasting states and then rise with meal intake. The gastrin content of the antrum of the stomach is higher in duodenal ulcer patients with a higher G-cell mass. Gastrin release after a meal differentiates groups of chronic duodenal ulcer patients.[1] Duodenal ulcer patients have increased parietal cell mass, reduced antrums, large transition zones between pyloric and fundic mucosae, and gastriclike changes in surface epithelium of the intestinal wall.

Duodenal ulcers in elderly persons appear more likely to develop bleeding episodes.[1, 4] It has been suggested that the immunological defenses of mucosa in the elderly are lacking; as a result, the severity of the ulcer increases and hemorrhage and perforation are more likely to occur. The elderly patient with diabetes and duodenal ulcers lacks the PGE prostaglandin response that would aid ulcer healing.

Of the various chronic ulcer diseases, it is the *Zollinger-Ellison (Z-E) syndrome* that spans the pathological barrier between ulcers and cancers.[1, 7] Zollinger-Ellison syndrome is a hormonally-induced peptic ulcer disease caused by unrestrained gastrin secretion from a pancreatic islet cell tumor. It is extremely rare, with fewer than 100 cases reported over a 30-year period. Many progressive ulcer disease patients with hypertension, an increased basal acid output/maximal acid output (BAO/MAO) ratio, and elevated serum gastrin levels are classed as duodenal ulcer patients but may actually have Zollinger-Ellison syndrome.

CLINICAL MANIFESTATIONS

It is not always easy to make an ulcer diagnosis, but the clinician who takes the time to obtain a complete history and description of the patient's symptoms has a head start in the diagnosis. Ulcers are painful, and most patients who have symptoms of distress during digestion will hurry to their doctor's office for relief. Unfortunately the patient will often go through several episodes of pain before its severity is recognized. Large ulcers are more difficult to heal, and medications are decreasingly effective the longer the disease remains untreated. In order to avoid alarming the patient unnecessarily, many physicians will prescribe antacids and wait before ordering laboratory confirmation of their suspicions.

Symptoms of peptic ulcer include anorexia, dyspepsia, and pain relieved by antacids and/or food. There is often a history of cigarette smoking, a family history of ulcers, or seasonal variation in the severity of symptoms.[1] The differentiation of gastric ulcers from duodenal ulcers is based on the type of patient (gender, age, and clinical presentation—see Fig. 22-2). Gastric ulcer patients are usually women over age 55 with frequent or daily pain that is increased by food intake. Duodenal ulcers are found more often in men under 55 years of age who experience heartburn and a relief of pain with food intake.

LABORATORY ANALYSES AND DIAGNOSIS

In laboratory testing for the diagnosis of ulcers, only a few confirmatory tests are useful in profiling possible ulceration. Initial screening after reviewing the patient's symptoms and history may already provide the physician with a high-percentage probability. First symptoms of diarrhea or abdominal pain would be indicators for a stool guaiac test and CBC.

Chemistry Tests

Because *acid output* is a measurable cause of most ulceration, performing gastric acid content analyses is helpful but uncomfortable for the patient. Although betazole and histamine have been used, stimulation with pentagastrin has fewer side-effects.[7] The initial basal acid output (BAO) should be less than 6 mmol/hr, with maximal acid output (MAO) less than 40 mmol/hr. Ratios of BAO to MAO should be less than 0.3. Gastric ulcers, whether acute or chronic, usually have BAOs greater than 10 mmol/hr with MAOs less than 40 mmol/hr, because gastric ulcer patients have normal or lower acid secretion.[7]

Duodenal ulcer patients have increased acid secretion and will have BAOs elevated but less than 15 mmol/hr, with 25% to 50% of these patients having MAOs greater than 40 mmol/hr.[7] Many of

Gastric Ulcer	Duodenal Ulcer
female	male
>55 years old	<55 years old
frequent or daily pain	heartburn
pain increases with food intake	pain decreases with food intake

Figure 22-2 General differentiation between gastric and duodenal ulcers.

the acute ulcers involving trauma, burns, and/or stress show varied BAO and MAO levels.[1] Seventy percent of patients with Zollinger-Ellison syndrome have BAOs of 15 mmol/hr or higher without stimulation. The BAO/MAO ratio in Z-E is 0.6 or greater, indicating a need for serum gastrin analysis.[7]

Gastrin analysis using totals and fractionated results can be helpful in diagnosing the various ulcer diseases. Gastric ulcers of the corpus have higher serum gastrin levels than normal, but ulcers of the antrum often show gastrin levels below normal.[4] Fractionation of gastrin can be helpful, because most gastric ulcers have an increase in the G-34 fraction.[1] Antral gastrin is usually the G-17 type.[4] Prostaglandins are reduced in gastric ulcers of the antral and corpus mucosae.

Burn patients with Curling's ulcer appear to have normal serum gastrin levels with modest basal acid output (8.53–4.96 mmol/hr) and a slightly better than 50% chance of a positive guaiac test for stool blood a week after the burn.

Provocative tests for gastrin stimulation, such as the feeding of a standard test meal or secretin or calcium infusions, have been suggested to follow gastrin increases and aid in diagnosis of Z-E. Fractionation of circulating gastrin shows that Z-E patients have 60% G-34, and 30% G-17, while the tumor has 75% G-17.

Diagnosis of stress ulcer is aided by measuring the *p*H of gastric juices and the partial pressure of carbon dioxide (P_{CO_2}). Duodenal ulcer patients fall into two groups. One group has a high gastrin output with normal acid output, a positive family history of dyspepsia, and an early-age onset of duodenal ulcer. A second group has normal gastrin levels with high acid output and gastrin release at a *p*H of 2.5 instead of the normal 3.5. The second group shows a failure to respond normally to the feedback mechanism for gastrin release inhibition.[1]

Supportive information can be obtained by performing serum analyses for albumin, total protein, fats, and electrolytes. Sophisticated analysis of serum and biopsy material for prostaglandins may prove useful in the future for predicting ulcerative disease.

Hematology

Patients with ulcers require constant monitoring of hematological indicators of bleeding and anemia. The initial screening of ulcer disorders involves complete blood counts (CBC) to ascertain the hemoglobin, hematocrit (Hct), and red blood cell count (RBC), along with occult blood tests (guaiac tests) to detect blood in feces. Occult blood tests are susceptible to erroneous results due to diet (red meat) and vitamin C (ascorbic acid).[7] Recent ingestion of these two substances causes false positives with occult blood reagents. Hemorrhage is a major concern in patients suffering from acute ulcer disorders.

The chronic ulcer patient must be monitored for anemia and iron deficiency. Modest blood loss through the gastrointestinal tract can result in an iron deficiency anemia that may endanger the patient's life in the event of an ulcer attack.

Radiological Examinations

Laboratory testing of bleeding ulcer patients is an emergency situation, and the utility of radiological exams is limited during the acute bleeding episode. For other nonactive ulcer or chronic ulcer patients, however, the radiological exam can confirm the physician's suspicions.

Prior to the advent of fiber optics and isotopic scans of the patient, physicians used barium contrast media for examining colon integrity and to detect ulcers.[7] Upper-GI x-rays of the stomach and duodenum with contrast media and air were used to locate lesions of possible ulcer origin in the stomach and duodenum. Both methods are still in use.[7]

Newer techniques enable gastroenterologists to observe lesions and take tissue samples for histological confirmation. These include proctoscopy, sigmoidoscopy, and fiber optic colonoscopy, and can be performed in the physician's office on an outpatient basis. Direct visualization using the proctoscope, sigmoidoscope, or fiber optic colonoscope is considered diagnostic for many of the nonbleeding acute and chronic ulcer disorders.

TREATMENT

Medication

Whether the ulcer is located in the stomach or in the duodenum, patients recover more quickly if acid secretions can be neutralized or inhibited. Both gastric and duodenal ulcers heal faster with histamine-receptor blocking drugs (H_2-receptor blocking drugs) such as cimetidine.[1] Patients maintained on such drugs can reduce recurrent episodes of ulcer flareup and heal more rapidly. However, the development of hematemesis and/or melena is a potential problem that should be monitored. Treatment of chronic gastric ulcers often involves stress reduction, drugs, and consideration of age factors and the size of the ulcer. Ulcers with defined margins and healthy blood flow have a better chance to heal, especially if they are small. Larger ulcers take longer and seem susceptible to further recurrence. Smoking and salicylates can hamper healing, along with increased age (>67 years of age). Bedrest in conjunction with H_2-receptor blocking drugs, low-dose antacids, and stress reduction can aid ulcer healing.[1] Drugs like carbenoxolone, derived from licorice, and tripotassium dicitratobismuthate do not alter mucosal secretion but do aid in ulcer healing.[1] Trimipramine aids in stress reduction.[1] Surgery for chronic gastric ulcers is controversial, but if medications cannot correct or control the problem some feel vagotomy is warranted.[1, 9]

Various drugs have been used to inhibit acid secretions in ulcer patients. The most successful is cimetidine (or Tagamet), which has been hailed as the cure-all for patients afflicted with ulcer disorders.[1, 2, 3, 4, 7, 9] Although helpful, cimetidine and the other drugs have their limitations. Cimetidine therapy results in increased mucosal histamine. Secretin's utility in retarding acid secretion and gastrin release is minimized in chronic duodenal ulcer patients because the stomach empties faster and the buffering capacity is lost.[1]

The hydrogen-potassium ATPase pump of parietal cells can be inhibited with benzimidazole or omeprazole. Antacids and nonacid inhibitors of carbenoxolone, colloidal bismuth, and cimetidine have also been effective. Sucralfate seems to help by binding to ulcerative surfaces and protecting against acid-pepsin digestion of the ulcer. Fifteen to twenty percent of patients do not respond well to medication, possibly because of smoking or lack of compliance with the therapeutic regimen. Males with abnormal acid secretion and large ulcers are particularly susceptible to duodenal ulcers of long-term duration. Surgery may be indicated to decrease acid secretions. Although proximal gastric vagotomy can reduce acid secretions and improve healing, persons with long ulcer histories and high preoperative BAO and MAO often have recurrence of ulcers.[1] Cimetidine and second surgeries have been used to treat such patients.[4]

Doses of cimetidine and prostaglandins that do not prevent secretion but modify acidity have been protective against stress ulcers. Altering the bicarbonate level has been shown to influence stress ulcer development more than altering blood flow.[1] Medications to inhibit acid secretion include cimetidine, ranitidine (Zantac) for patients experiencing estrogen excess, and anticholinergic drugs with cimetidine to avoid increasing cimetidine dosage to unsafe levels to control acidity. Omeprazole has successfully been used to make patients achlorhydric. When medication fails, vagotomy, pyloroplasty, and the H_2-blocking agents are used. Total gastrectomy is a final alternative if other treatments fail.

For the elderly ulcer patient, drug therapy is complicated by the presence of other diseases and/or medications. Duodenal ulcers with frequent bleeding episodes occur in elderly persons. The reduced immunological defenses of the elderly patient are blamed for the frequent episodes of hemorrhage. Cholecystokinin increases enhance ulcer healing but are lacking in many elderly ulcer patients.[1]

Surgery

The need for surgery arises when medications cannot inhibit hydrochloric acid (HCl) secretions in the stomach parietal region nor gastrin synthesis in the stomach antrum. The surgery involves cutting the vagus nerve that stimulates stomach secretions of HCl acid. The surgery, when successful, effectively limits HCl acid secretion into the stomach and intestinal tract, although mucosal histamine is increased. Vagotomy for elderly ulcer patients is risky, but necessary if bleeding cannot be curbed with medication.

CASE STUDY

A 62-year-old Caucasian man was admitted to hospital for evaluation after visiting his physician. One week prior to visiting his doctor, the patient had developed black tarry stools and an episode of hematemesis. He was afebrile, with a blood pressure of 120/79 supine, 114/75 sitting, and pulses of 61 and 73 respectively. The patient's skin was cool and moist and his heart and lungs appeared normal. Abdominal exam revealed active bowel sounds without masses or organomegaly. The rectal exam showed enlarged prostate and positive guaiac test on stool sample.

LABORATORY FINDINGS

Urinalysis—cloudy urine
*p*H 8.0
3+ amorphous urates
trace leukocytes

Hematology—WBC: $4.5 \times 10^3/mm^3$
RBC: $3.83 \times 10^6/mm^3$
Hemoglobin: 11.6 g/dL
Hematocrit: 34.4%

		Reference Ranges
Chemistry—	Triglycerides: 16/mg/dL	(50–165)
	BUN: 27 mg/dL	(5–20)
	Creatinine: 2.4 mg/dL	(0.7–1.9)
	Sodium: 137 mEq/L	(135–145)
	Potassium: 4.1 mEq/L	(3.5–5.2)
	Chloride: 119 mEq/L	(92–103)
	Total CO_2: 23 mEq/L	(20–28)
	Glucose: 103 mg/dL	(85–115)

Blood Bank—Transfused 6 units O-positive packed cells
1 unit plasma

Conversion to SI units is as follows:
Hemoglobin— g/dL × 0.155 = mmol/L
Triglycerides— mg/dL × 0.0113 = mmol/L
Creatinine— mg/dL × 88.4 = μmol/L
BUN— mg/dL × 0.357 = mmol/L
Sodium— mEq/L × 1 = mmol/L
Potassium— mEq/L × 1 = mmol/L
Chloride— mEq/L × 1 = mmol/L
Total CO_2— mEq/L × 1 = mmol/L
Glucose— mg/dL × 0.0555 = mmol/L

Questions

1. Given the laboratory results, what additional tests should be performed in the hospital to diagnose the patient's condition?
2. If the patient's tests reveal a duodenal ulcer, what additional laboratory studies should be performed?
3. A perforated duodenal ulcer is found in this patient through radiological and laboratory analysis. Which drug(s) might be administered to aid the healing process?

Discussion

1. Radiological upper and lower GI after bleeding is stopped
   Coagulation studies of PTT and PT
   Gastric acid analysis
2. Gastrin analysis
   Gastric *p*H
   Evaluation for surgery
3. Cimetidine
   Ranitidine

REFERENCES

1. Brooks FP, Cohen S, Soloway RD (eds): Peptic Ulcer Disease. New York City, Churchill Livingstone, 1985
2. Emes JH, Novak TF: Introduction to Pathophysiology. University Park Press, Baltimore, 1984
3. Catler P (ed): Problem-Solving in Clinical Medicine, 2nd ed, pp 363–397. Baltimore, Williams & Wilkins, 1985
4. Tietz NW (ed): Textbook of Clinical Chemistry, pp 1451–1459. WB Saunders, Philadelphia, 1986
5. Stremple JF, Molot MD, McNamara J et al: Post-traumatic gastric bleeding: Prospective gastric secretion composition. Arch Surg 105:17–185, 1972
6. Kuo Y-J, Shanbour LL: Mechanism of action of aspirin on canine gastric mucosa. Am J Physiol 230:762–767, 1976
7. Ravel R: Clinical Laboratory Medicine, 4th ed. Chicago, Year Book Medical Pub, 1984
8. Oi M, Oshida K, Sugimura S: The location of gastric ulcer. Gastroenterology 36:45–56, 1959
9. Zilva JF, Pannall PR (eds): Clinical Chemistry in Diagnosis and Treatment, 4th ed. Chicago, Lloyd-Luke Publications, distributed by Year Book Medical Pub, 1984

Chapter 23

Gastrointestinal Bleeding

Douglas W. Estry

Gastrointestinal hemorrhage can occur in a wide range of pathophysiologic disorders. The presence of blood within the gastrointestinal (GI) tract can arise from a diverse group of etiologic agents varying from ulcers, gastritis, and carcinomas to disorders of hemostasis involving either platelets or coagulation factors. Although the laboratory is limited in the number of diagnostic tools directly applicable to the detection of GI hemorrhage, the proper application of these tests can aid in the differentiation of upper and lower GI hemorrhage. They can also give some indication of the extent and severity of the hemorrhagic episode, particularly when evaluated in conjunction with the patient's clinical symptoms. In addition, once the etiology has been established, accurate, reproducible, and precise laboratory results provide an effective means of monitoring the course of bleeding.

ETIOLOGY AND PATHOPHYSIOLOGY

Terminology of Gastrointestinal Bleeding

In some cases the location of the GI lesion, and to some extent the severity of the bleeding, can be inferred based on the site of major blood loss. Terms that are descriptive of the specific sites of obvious bleeding are therefore important to an understanding of the diagnostic approach to GI hemorrhage.

Hematemesis, the vomiting or spitting up of blood without concomitant blood in the stool, localizes the bleeding to the upper GI tract. Anatomically, hematemesis localizes the primary bleeding site to an area proximal to the ligament of Treitz, which is located at the junction between the duodenum and the jejunum.[1, 2, 3] Overt bleeding is also noted in relation to *melena,* the passage of black, tarry, loose stools stained with blood pigments or altered blood. Melena, in either the presence or the absence of hematemesis, suggests that the hemorrhage is localized to the upper GI tract, as its presence results from the partial degradation of hemoglobin to acid hematin in the small bowel or stomach. It has been suggested that, in general, more rapid blood loss gives rise to hematemesis, whereas slower rates of blood loss result in melena.[4] The extent of bleeding associated with the presence of melena has been shown to vary from 100 to 200 mL/day in disease states, with as little as 50 mL required when blood is directly introduced into the stomach.[5]

The presence of *hematochezia* (bright or dark red blood in the stool) or grossly apparent rectal bleeding is usually associated with hemorrhage from the lower GI tract, either the anus, rectum, or colon, or possibly the distal portion of the small bowel. It should be noted, however, that in cases of extreme blood loss into the upper GI tract, bright red blood may be passed in the stool. In these cases, it has been demonstrated that the amount of blood lost into the upper GI tract is extensive enough to also result in the clinical signs associated with hypovolemia or hemorrhagic shock.[5]

In addition to the terminology used to describe the type and basic location of GI bleeding, certain terms are also applied to indicate the extent of the hemorrhage. *Massive hemorrhage* implies a significant loss of blood with signs of hypovolemic shock that requires extensive transfusion therapy. *Overt bleeding,* on the other hand, is not associated with clinical signs of shock, but presents with hematemesis and/or melena. Finally, *occult bleeding* implies that blood can only be detected by laboratory testing.

Upper Gastrointestinal Tract Bleeding

Disorders of the upper GI tract often present with more severe and life-threatening bleeding complications than do those lesions associated primarily with the large bowel. Table 23-1 lists some of the more common lesions associated with upper GI bleeding.

Among the various causes of upper GI bleeding, *peptic ulceration* is probably the most important of the gastrointestinal diseases[1] (see also Chap. 22). The etiology of this particular GI lesion, although somewhat obscure, is influenced by environmental, hereditary, and psychological factors. Peptic ulcers can occur in any section of the GI tract that is exposed to the action of acid-peptic juices. These sites vary from the esophagus to a Meckel's diverticulum in the ileum.[6] Two major forms of peptic ulcer include the *duodenal ulcer,* associated with increased exposure of the duodenal mucosa to acid and peptic secretions, and the *gastric ulcer,* associated with a decrease in the ability of the gastric mucosa to protect against the acid and pepsin secretions. Early clinical features related to GI bleeding include the presence of melena, associated with mild or less severe episodes. This is often followed by hematemesis and evidence of hypovolemic shock.

The *Mallory-Weiss syndrome* is associated with lacerations or tears in either the gastric or the esophageal mucosa. The syndrome was first described by Mallory and Weiss, and occurs primarily at the gastroesophageal junction because of an excessive rise in the intragastric pressure.[7] These lesions can occur from protracted retching or vomiting, coughing, or trauma to the abdomen. The Mallory-Weiss syndrome has been reported to occur in approximately 2% to 7% of patients with upper GI bleeding. An incidence of 15% among alcoholic patients presenting with acute bleeding has been reported,[8] and 50% of patients presenting with Mallory-Weiss tears were found to have a recent history of alcoholic consumption.[9]

Stress ulcers, Cushing's ulcers, and Curling's ulcers, although all related to physical trauma, have differing etiologies. *Cushing's ulcers* are associated with trauma that results in a rise in intracranial pressure, such as brain tumors or cranial surgery or trauma. The specific mechanism of mucosal damage in *stress ulceration* is somewhat obscure, but excessive secretion of gastric acid in Cushing's ulcers, not associated with the other forms of stress-induced gastric lesions, has been demonstrated.[10] *Curling's ulcers,* occurring following severe burns, may result in part from ischemic damage to the gastric mucosa due to the fluid loss and subsequent hypovolemic shock. The commonality among the various forms of stress ulceration lies in damage to the gastric mucosa, whether it occurs as a result of hypersecretion of gastric acid, of ischemic necrosis, and/or of thrombosis of the mucosal blood supply as a result of a gram-negative septicemia and disseminated intravascular coagulation.

Drug ingestion, particularly of aspirin, and the use of alcohol are related to the development of *acute gastritis.* The etiology of the gastric alterations and bleeding is varied. They include aspirin-induced alteration in platelet function, which is exacerbated by alcohol ingestion; alteration in prostaglandin metabolism, which may play a role in protecting the gastric mucosa;[14] and damage to the lipoprotein membrane of surface epithelial cells, which results in increased permeability of the gastric mucosa by hydrogen ions and an exfoliation of the surface cells.[15] Additional drugs shown to cause GI bleeding include indomethacin, adrenocortical steroids, and phenylbutazone.

Cancers are a relatively rare cause of massive GI bleeding. As indicated in Table 23-1, they account for only 2% to 3% of the cases of upper GI bleeding. Most of these are gastric cancer, discussed in Chapter 27.

The most common cause of *variceal hemorrhage*

Table 23-1 ***Common Upper Gastrointestinal Lesions Associated With Bleeding, and Their Relative Frequency***

Upper Gastrointestinal Lesion	Frequency		
	Larson & Farnell	*Middleton*	*Palmer*
Peptic Ulcer			
Duodenal Ulcer	25–29%	22.4%	27.7%
Gastric Ulcer	10–20%	24.4%	12.6%
Mallory-Weiss Syndrome	2–7%	4.1%	5.14%
Cancer	2%	2.4%	–
Variceal Hemorrhage	–	5.2%	18.7%

Data from reference numbers [11], [12], and [13]

is related to cirrhosis of the liver and the subsequent development of portal hypertension. The increase in pressure in the portal circulation produces dilated vessels within the esophageal plexus, known as *varices*. The rupture of these varices results in massive hematemesis. Although varices are a frequent complication of alcoholic cirrhosis, it should be kept in mind that massive hematemesis in the chronic alcoholic may also occur as a result of gastritis, peptic ulcer, or esophageal lacerations.[6]

Lower Gastrointestinal Tract Bleeding

Unlike bleeding from upper GI tract lesions, severe bleeding from the lower GI tract is uncommon. Gastrointestinal bleeding from this portion of the GI tract results in either melena or bright or dark red rectal blood. Because massive upper GI bleeding can result in rectal blood, nasogastric aspiration may be performed to rule out this possibility.

It has been found that carcinomas occurring in the distal colon and diverticular disease each accounted for approximately 31% of cases of lower GI bleeding.[16] Most other disorders, including inflammatory bowel diseases and polyps, are much less common, and rectal bleeding as a result of hemorrhoids or anal fissures is usually relatively apparent on initial examination by the clinician.

Disorders Other Than Primary Gastrointestinal Bleeding

Gastrointestinal bleeding can be the end-result or the presenting symptom of a wide variety of disorders. Much of the laboratory screening is aimed at ruling out disorders that are secondary to a defect not associated with a primary lesion of the GI tract but that result in GI bleeding. These could include various inherited disorders of coagulation, primary or secondary alterations in platelet function, anticoagulant therapy, or other inherited disorders such as hemorrhagic telangiectasia.

Physiological Responses to Gastrointestinal Bleeding

The physiological alterations in GI bleeding are associated with both the rate and the amount of blood lost. In cases of acute blood loss, the major concern is related to the development of hypovolemic shock. The metabolic alterations occurring as a result of hemorrhagic shock are well documented, and include acid-base imbalance resulting from cellular conversion to anaerobic respiration. The imbalance is exacerbated by increased ketone bodies arising from the metabolism of free fatty acids. In the case of less severe hemorrhage, this may be compensated for by hyperventilation. In addition to the acid-base alterations, there is a decrease in urinary output, related initially to the renin-angiotensin system and ultimately to ischemic necrosis of renal tubular cells. The patient with chronic GI blood loss will most likely present with chronic anemia or a recurrent iron-deficiency anemia.

CLINICAL MANIFESTATIONS

Clinical manifestations include obvious hemorrhage, such as hematemesis, melena, or rectal bleeding. Information related to protracted retching, alcohol consumption, drug ingestion, any concomitant diseases or disease history, anticoagulant therapy, foreign travel, and the potential for GI bleeding associated with parasitic infection is important to guide the choice of laboratory procedures. Dysphagia or anorexia and a history of abnormal weight loss, as possible indicators of cancer, are also important considerations.

Physical examination of the patient is directed at determining the extent and location of the hemorrhage. The patient's pulse, blood pressure, respiration, and reporting of excessive thirst and sweating can provide valuable initial information about the extent of blood loss. In addition, gastric aspiration, as a relatively simple and risk-free procedure, will provide important information about upper GI bleeding.

LABORATORY ANALYSES AND DIAGNOSIS

Laboratory testing in association with presenting symptoms of gastrointestinal bleeding varies over a wide range, including the initial evaluation and subsequent monitoring of the patient's hemoglobin and hematocrit. Additional testing should include specific serum enzyme levels, as indicators of both liver and pancreatic function. It should also include determination of electrolytes, blood urea nitrogen (BUN), and creatinine (as indicators of both the amount of blood loss and the site of the bleeding lesion), and the screening of the patient's hemostatic mechanism. The latter is an indicator of the ability to effectively promote coagulation, and may be a potential source of the bleeding problem. Testing of fecal samples for occult blood as an indicator of either cancerous or precancerous lesions is also important.

Complete Blood Count

Variations in the complete blood count (CBC) can occur as a result of either chronic or acute GI bleeding. The hemoglobin and hematocrit are usually considered to be important guides to the extent of blood loss occurring in most hemorrhagic disorders. Because time is required for hemodilution to occur, the hematocrit cannot be used as an effective monitoring device for the first 24 hours following an acute GI hemorrhage. It has been suggested, however, that blood replacement and the use of crystalloid solutions such as normal saline or Ringer's lactate can be guided by the need to maintain a hematocrit of greater than 30%.[16] A hematocrit that is reduced at the time of admission is a good indicator of chronic blood loss that may have progressed to an acute hemorrhagic episode. In addition, the presence of hypochromic, microcytic red cells is evidence of chronic blood loss and possible iron-deficiency anemia. Following the initial assessment of the patient's hematologic status, the hemoglobin and hematocrit provide useful tools for monitoring the course of the patient's bleeding episode.

Additional responses to acute blood loss that can be observed include a rise in both the white blood cell count and the number of platelets, which peaks several hours following the onset of blood loss. A reticulocytosis also occurs within the first 48 hours. Increases in the white blood count would also be expected in septic disorders, suggesting the possibility of disseminated intravascular coagulation.

Hemostatic Function Tests

It is unlikely that screening of hemostatic function will provide any information related to hereditary disorders of either platelets or coagulation that were not previously suspected by the clinician. However, because the most common disorders of hemostatic function are secondary either to drugs or to other metabolic abnormalities, it is essential to have an adequate assessment of both platelet function and coagulation. The primary hemostatic screening tests include the prothrombin time (PT), the activated partial thromboplastin time (APTT), the bleeding time, and the platelet count.

Specific disorders that might be expected to result in alterations in hemostatic function include aspirin ingestion, which will result in a prolonged bleeding time, particularly when the test is performed using a template bleeding method; liver cirrhosis, resulting in decreased coagulant protein production; disseminated intravascular coagulation, which affects numerous aspects of the hemostatic pathway; and malabsorption syndromes, resulting in decreased vitamin K and inadequate synthesis of factors II, VII, IX, and X. Finally, in acute hemorrhage requiring extensive replacement therapy, maintenance of normal platelet and coagulant levels is critical if hemostasis is to be promoted.

Liver Function Tests

The importance of liver screening tests is primarily related to the identification of possible cirrhotic liver diseases that result in portal hypertension

...l hemorrhage. Liver function testing ...nclude a determination of bilirubin and se-... albumin. In addition, elevation in specific se-...um enzymes, aspartate aminotransferase (AST), alanine aminotransferase (ALT), alkaline phosphatase (ALP), gamma-glutamyl transferase (GGT), or isocitrate dehydrogenase (ICD) would provide additional evidence of hepatocellular damage.

Pancreatic Function Tests

Pancreatitis may also play a role in the development of GI bleeding. Bleeding can result from an involvement of the duodenum in the inflammatory process, which occurs as a result of damage to pancreatic tissue and release of hydrolytic enzymes. If pancreatitis is suspected as an underlying cause, analysis of both serum amylase and lipase will aid in this diagnosis.

Blood Urea Nitrogen (BUN) and Creatinine Tests

Both the BUN and the creatinine tests can be used as indicators of the site and extent of GI bleeding. A BUN of greater than 40 mg/dL (14.3 mmol/L) in conjunction with a normal serum creatinine indicates a blood loss of at least 1 liter in the upper GI tract.[12, 17] The rise in BUN is due to a breakdown of hemoglobin in the intestinal tract. It may result, in addition, in an elevated serum bilirubin.[1]

Determination of Occult Blood

Much attention has been directed toward the use of occult blood testing as an early indicator of possible colorectal cancer in otherwise asymptomatic patients.[18, 19] Tests that have been used for determining occult blood include the guaiac test, Hemoccult™ slides, and the Hemotest™ tablets. However, these tests often result in an unacceptable number of both false positives and false negatives.[20] It has been demonstrated by one authority that the guaiac test and the hematest tablets yielded false-positive values of 49% and 27% respectively. The Hemoccult™ slide, on the other hand, did not result in false-positive reactions, but there was a 50% incidence of false-negative tests. Problems that have been described with this test include the variability in the amount of blood necessary to obtain a positive reaction (which appears to be related to the amount of fecal hydration), the extent of hemoglobin degradation in the intestinal tract (since the test is not sensitive to porphyrins), and the presence of interfering substances such as vitamin C and dietary red meat products.

Recently a new assay, HemoQuant™, has been tested as an alternative to the Hemoccult™ slide test.[21] This test is based on the detection of free porphyrin liberated by heating with a reducing acid. The Hemoquant™ assay appears to be a very sensitive indicator of fecal hemoglobin concentration, and does not appear to be affected by vitamin C, iron, or cimetidine, an inhibitor of basal gastric acid secretion from parietal cells. Degradation of hemoglobin in the GI tract will not result in false-negative reactions, as the test is based on the detection of porphyrins.[22]

Although initial studies have been conducted to compare the Hemoccult slide test to the HemoQuant assay, several variables need more thorough evaluation before the feasibility of introducing the HemoQuant test into the laboratory as a routine procedure can be determined.[23, 24] Among these variables is the increased cost of performing the test, although this may be considered negligible when viewed in terms of the potential for detecting a greater number of colorectal cancers at an early, curable stage in patients who are still asymptomatic.

Additional Diagnostic Tools

External to the laboratory, the clinician has available a battery of additional tests that will aid in determining the specific location of the bleeding lesion. These include endoscopy, which permits viewing of the esophagus and most of the stomach and duodenum, as well as an evaluation of the colon, angiography, barium contrast radiology, radionuclide imaging, and sigmoidoscopy.

TREATMENT

The initial treatment of the patient admitted for GI bleeding centers on providing adequate replacement therapy designed to maintain fluid volume, red cell mass, and an intact coagulation mechanism. Central to this process is the laboratory's role in providing the appropriate blood and blood products. The treatment of GI bleeding varies, depending on the site and extent of the bleeding. Beyond the use of transfusion therapy, various additional treatments are available.

In cases of esophageal varices, several nonsurgical methods have been used to stop the variceal bleeding. These include vasopressin, a drug that lowers the portal venous pressure, balloon tamponade, percutaneous transhepatic embolization, and injection sclerotherapy. Surgical treatment includes esophageal transection, ligation of varices, and portacaval shunts. Treatment in stress ulceration has been directed at a reversal of the events leading to ulcer formation, such as correction of hypotension or regulation of the acid-base imbalances that occur as a result of shock. Drugs such as cimetidine or antacids are also used to control gastric acids. If the bleeding is difficult to control, intraarterial administration of vasopressin has been used. A similar treatment protocol has been used in cases of both acute peptic ulcers and Mallory-Weiss syndrome, although in both cases surgical intervention may be required. Treatment for lower GI bleeding is much the same as that described for the upper GI tract; when the hemorrhage does not stop spontaneously, vasopressin, electrocoagulation, or surgical intervention such as segmental colectomy may be required.

CASE STUDY

A 74-year-old woman with a long history of alcoholism was admitted to the hospital because of confusion, shortness of breath, and hematemesis. Several years earlier, the patient had had a diagnosis of spontaneous portal vein thrombosis and, in the interim, had had several episodes of upper gastrointestinal bleeding secondary to esophageal varices. On several occasions during the course of her hospital stay, the patient developed right-sided hydrothorax, necessitating thoracentesis. The laboratory results are detailed below.

LABORATORY FINDINGS

AST	Increased
ALT	Increased
Albumin	Decreased
Alkaline phosphatase	Increased
Hemoglobin	8.7 gm/dL (1.35 mmol/L)
WBC	15.0×10^3/mm^3
Prothrombin time	Prolonged
BUN	20 mg/dL (7.1 mmol/L)
Total bilirubin	22 mg/dL (376 μmol/L)
Conjugated bilirubin	11 mg/dL (188 μmol/L)

Questions

1. Based on the patient's history and clinical findings, what is the underlying disorder most likely to be responsible for this episode of bleeding?
2. Based on the laboratory findings, what conditions should be considered? Given the clinical findings, what specific diagnosis is more likely?
3. Why is upper GI bleeding a common occurrence in this condition?
4. Given the laboratory findings, what are other clinical implications for this patient?

Discussion

1. From an evaluation of the relevant clinical laboratory data and knowledge of the patient's history, it is clear that the presenting symptoms of confusion, shortness of breath, and hematemesis, although manifestations of hemorrhage and upper GI bleeding, are secondary to an underlying liver disorder.
2. The laboratory profile suggests hepatocellular damage, viral hepatitis, alcoholic hepatitis/cirrhosis, or toxic liver damage. Based on the patient's history of chronic alcohol abuse, alcoholic cirrhosis would be expected. Any condition that leads to obstruction of portal blood flow can cause portal hypertension. Cirrhosis of the liver is the most common cause.

3. In cases of portal hypertension, the normal flow of blood from the coronary veins to the portal veins is reversed. Portal blood is shunted from the esophageal veins into the azygous system, and the increased pressure in the esophageal plexus results in tortuous dilated vessels called varices. The esophageal veins lie just under the mucosa and can rupture easily, resulting in hematemesis and, on occasion, melena.

4. Additional factors that impact on the overall implications for this patient include a decrease in the ability of the liver to manufacture protein (resulting in a decrease in specific coagulation factors and a prolongation of the clotting times) as well as alterations in the colloidal osmotic pressure due to a decrease in total protein, primarily albumin. In addition, an elevated ammonia would contribute to the confusion and result in marked alterations in acid-base regulation. Finally, possible common bile duct obstruction could further exacerbate the coagulation problem, based on a potential malabsorption of vitamin K related to the decreased presence of bile salts.

REFERENCES

1. Shearman DJC, Finlayson NDC: Gastrointestinal bleeding. In Diseases Of The Gastrointestinal Tract And Liver, p 192. New York City, Churchill Livingstone, 1982
2. Steer MI, Silen W: Diagnostic procedures in gastrointestinal hemorrhage. N Engl J Med 309(11): 646, 1983
3. Pingleton SK: Gastrointestinal hemorrhage. Med Clin North Am 67(6):1215, 1983
4. Kennedy T: Clinical evaluation of the bleeding adult. In Fiddiam-Green R, Turcotte J (eds): Gastrointestinal Hemorrhage. New York City, Grune & Stratton, 1980
5. Schiff I, Stevens RJ, Shapiro N et al: Observations on oral administration of citrated blood in man: Effect on stools. Am J Med Sci 203:109, 1942
6. Robbins SL, Cotran RS, Kumar V: The gastrointestinal tract. In Pathologic Basis of Disease. Philadelphia, WB Saunders, 1984
7. Mallory GK, Weiss S: Haemorrhages from lacerations of the cardiac orifice of the stomach due to vomiting. Am J Med Sci 178:506, 1929
8. Graham DY, Schwartz JF: The spectrum of the Mallory-Weiss tear. Medicine 57:307, 1978
9. Hasting PR, Peters KW, Cohn I Jr: Mallory-Weiss syndrome: Review of 69 cases. Am J Surg 137:47, 1979
10. Watts CC, Clark K: Gastric acidity in the comatose patient. J Neurosurg 30:107, 1969
11. Larson DE, Farnell MB: Upper gastrointestinal hemorrhage. Mayo Clin Proc 58:371, 1983
12. Middleton WRJ: Acute gastrointestinal bleeding. In Grant AK, Skyring A, Conn AO (eds): Clinical Diagnosis Of Gastrointestinal Disease. Oxford, Blackwell Scientific Publications, 1981
13. Palmer ED: The vigorous diagnostic approach to upper gastrointestinal tract hemorrhage: A 23-year prospective study of 1,400 patients. JAMA 207:1477, 1969
14. Robert A, Nezamis JE, Lancaster C et al: Cytoprotection by prostaglandins in rats: Prevention of gastric necrosis produced by alcohol, HCl, NaOH, hypertonic NaCl, and thermal injury. Gastroenterology 77:433, 1979
15. Croft DN: Aspirin and the exfoliation of gastric epithelial cells: Cytological and biochemical observations. Br Med J 2:897, 1963
16. Balint JA, Sarfeh IJ, Fried MB: Gastrointestinal bleeding: Diagnosis and management. In Clinical Gastroenterology Monograph Series. New York City, John Wiley & Sons, 1977
17. Pumphrey CW, Beck ER: Raised blood urea concentration indicates considerable blood loss in acute upper gastrointestinal haemorrhage. Br Med J 1:527, 1980
18. Simon JB: Occult blood screening for colorectal carcinoma: A critical review. Gastroenterology 88:820, 1985
19. Macrae FA, St John DJB: Relationship between patterns of bleeding and hemoccult sensitivity in patients with colorectal cancers or adenoma. Gastroenterology 82:891, 1982
20. Ostrow JD, Mulvany CA, Hansell JR et al: Sensitivity and reproducibility of chemical tests for fecal occult blood, with an emphasis on false-positive reactions. Am J Dig Dis 18:930, 1973
21. Schwartz S, Dahl J, Ellefson M et al: The "Hemo-Quant" test: A specific and quantitative assay of

heme (hemoglobin) in feces and other materials. Clin Chem 29:2061, 1983

22. Ahlquist DA, McGill DB, Schwartz S et al: HemoQuant, a new quantitative assay for fecal hemoglobin: Comparison with Hemoccult. Ann Intern Med 101:297, 1984
23. Ahlquist DA, McGill DB, Schwartz S et al: Fecal blood levels in health and disease: A study using HemoQuant. N Engl J Med 312:1422, 1985
24. Peterson WL, Fordtran JS: Quantitating the occult. N Engl J Med 312:1448, 1985

Chapter 24

Acute Diarrhea

Suzanne W. Conner

Diarrhea occurs when there is an interference with the transport of water and electrolytes through the intestinal wall, increasing the liquidity of the stool. Diarrhea is an abnormal increase in stool liquidity and daily stool weight of more than 200 grams.[1] There is often an increase in stool frequency to more than three per day with accompanying urgency, perianal discomfort, incontinence, or a combination of all three.

Under normal circumstances, the large and small intestine are presented daily with 7 to 9 liters of fluid derived from fluid intake as well as salivary, gastric, pancreatic, and biliary secretions.[2] Normal stool water excretion is approximately 100 to 200 mL per day. The human intestine is a highly efficient system and is able to absorb large amounts of fluid daily.

The jejunum absorbs 4 to 5 liters, the ileum 3 to 4 liters, and the colon .9 to 1.8 liters per day.[3] Water passively moves in both directions across the intestinal mucosa to maintain iso-osmolality between the gut and plasma. The primary function of the jejunum is to absorb nutrients. The ileum uses an active transport mechanism to absorb sodium and chloride and excrete hydrogen and bicarbonate ions.[3] The principle function of the colon is to absorb water and sodium through an active transport mechanism under the influence of aldosterone.

It is evident that there are fluid and electrolyte consequences of diarrhea. The excessive water loss may result in dehydration. Plasma potassium levels may be drastically reduced because of the loss through the stool and the inability of the kidney to conserve plasma potassium. There may be a shift in the acid-base balance, depending on the amount of bicarbonate, sodium, chloride, potassium, and water lost. Metabolic acidosis may result if the primary losses are water, salt, potassium, and bicarbonate. Alkalosis may result if sodium and potassium are lost in excess of bicarbonate, or if severe hypokalemia causes an intracellular exchange of hydrogen ion for depleted potassium.[4]

In the discussion that follows, general considerations of diarrheal mechanisms and laboratory analyses will be addressed before discussion of specific diarrheal disorders.

ETIOLOGY AND PATHOPHYSIOLOGY: GENERAL

There are four major pathophysiologic categories of diarrhea: osmotic, secretory, impaired absorption, and altered motility of the bowel. Many cases of diarrhea involve more than one of the four mechanisms of diarrhea.

Osmotic Diarrhea

Osmotic diarrhea occurs either when water is not absorbed normally and thus remains in the intestinal lumen or when excess water is pulled into the lumen from the extracellular fluid compartment to maintain the iso-osmolality between the plasma and intestinal contents. The latter may occur when hypertonic solutes accumulate in the intestine, causing excess water to be pulled into the lumen. Laxatives such as citrate of magnesia cause this phenomenon.[4] Other causes of osmotic diarrhea include ingestion of large amounts of mannitol and sorbitol. This is known as "chewing gum diarrhea" because of the use of mannitol and sorbitol as sweeteners in sugar-free gum.[5] The ingestion of lactose in lactase-deficient individuals also may cause osmotic diarrhea.[6]

A deficiency of the enzyme lactase is fairly common in adults, but may also occur in children. In this condition, lactose hydrolysis is reduced and lactose absorption is impaired. The lactose remaining in the intestinal lumen causes retention of water in the small intestine. The fecal flora of the colon ferment the unabsorbed lactose, producing hydrogen and small organic molecules such as lactate, butyrate, and others. These organic molecules increase the osmotic load and cause additional water to accumulate in the colon, producing diarrhea.[6]

In general, osmotic diarrhea is related to food ingestion and will stop when the patient fasts or stops ingesting the poorly absorbed solute.

Secretory Diarrhea

Secretory diarrhea is caused by a malfunction of the secretory cells lining the small intestine. These cells normally secrete, as well as absorb, electrolytes and water.[1] If these cells are stimulated to secrete large amounts of fluid, secretory diarrhea occurs. Often the increased secretion also causes decreased ion absorption.

In this form of diarrhea, the intestinal lumen and stool contain an excess of monovalent cations and water. The fecal water osmolality is essentially the same as plasma, in contrast to a higher fecal water osmolality in osmotic diarrhea.[1]

Secretory diarrhea may be caused by bacterial enterotoxins such as those produced by *Vibrio cholerae* and *Escherichia coli,* viral infections, parasites, neoplasms, and cathartics such as castor oil. Other causes include ulcerative colitis, various drugs, hyperthyroidism, and diabetes.[7] Because secretory diarrhea is independent of ingestion, it will persist even when the patient fasts.

Impaired Absorption

Impaired absorption causes decreased electrolyte and water absorption, and may be the cause of diarrhea. Reasons for impaired absorption include celiac and tropical sprue, exudation from inflammation and ulceration of the intestinal mucosa, congenital chloridorrhea, excess bile salts resulting from ileac resection, and the presence of lumen-dwelling parasites.[3]

Altered Motility

Altered motility is another mechanism of diarrhea. Hypomotility may allow bacterial overgrowth in the small intestine, resulting in diarrhea. This occurs because the metabolic products of bacterial activity inhibit water absorption or cause excessive water excretion.[4] Hypermotility in the small intestine may result in delivery to the colon of large amounts of fluid containing unabsorbed nutrients. This load may exceed the colon's absorptive capabilities. Diarrhea results from premature emptying of the colon because of the abnormality of its contents or because of irritability or inflammation in addition to the increased fluid volume.

CLINICAL MANIFESTATIONS: GENERAL

Acute diarrhea is an illness of short duration (usually less than 2 weeks) either because it is self-limited with spontaneous recovery or because it is easily diagnosed and treated. The diagnostic approach should include a history to gain information about travel, eating and drinking patterns, toxic and allergic reactions, and medications as well as the frequency and nature of the stools. Information about symptoms among other family members, groups of friends, or multiple patrons of an eating establishment may be helpful.

Lactase deficiency is characterized by abdominal distention, audible bowel sounds, and diarrhea after the ingestion of 50 grams of lactose.[7]

Passage of blood indicates an inflammatory infection or neoplastic disease. Passage of pus or white cells indicates inflammation or infection. Passage of nonbloody mucus is suggestive of irritable bowel syndrome. Frothy stools or oil-containing stools suggest malabsorption.[1]

The nature and duration of the diarrhea, history of vomiting, presence or absence of fever, and presence of abdominal cramps all give clues as to the etiology of acute diarrhea (see Table 24-1). The patient should be examined for dry mucous membranes, pulse that is weak, thready, or rapid, and low blood pressure—all signs of dehydration. Poor skin turgor and a weak cry in infants are signs of serious dehydration.[8]

LABORATORY ANALYSES: GENERAL

Because most acute diarrhea is self-limited and does not cause extreme morbidity and mortality, and the laboratory effort to detect all possible pathogens can be extremely costly and time-consuming, the clinician should use a selective approach in ordering laboratory tests.

Patients with a history that reveals a common source, such as seen in food poisoning, usually need no further workup. Patients without profuse diarrhea with dehydration, bloody stools, severe pain, or fever usually do not need further diagnostic tests if the symptoms resolve in 1 to 2 weeks. These patients do not benefit substantially from therapy.[9]

Patients with fever and severe or persistent symptoms, and debilitated patients, require prompt diagnosis so that specific therapy can be

Table 24-1 *Correlation of Clinical Symptoms with Infectious Agents of Diarrhea*

Symptom	Possible Cause
Profuse, watery diarrhea	*Vibrio*, ETEC, *Clostridium difficile, Cryptosporidium, Giardia*
Vomiting	Food poisoning organisms *Staphylococcus aureus, Clostridium perfringens, Bacillus cereus, Salmonella* species, Rotavirus, Norwalk virus
High fever	*Shigella, Salmonella* species, *Campylobacter, Yersinia, C. difficile,* Rotavirus, Norwalk virus
Severe abdominal cramps	Food poisoning, EIEC, *Shigella, Salmonella, Campylobacter, Yersinia, Cryptosporidium, Giardia, Blastocystis,* Norwalk virus
Bloody diarrhea	*Escherichia coli* (0157:H7), *Shigella, Campylobacter, Entamoeba histolytica*

initiated. Evaluation should include stool culture for *Salmonella, Shigella,* and *Campylobacter,* as well as examination for *Giardia.* A sigmoidoscopic examination may be done to detect pseudomembranous colitis. Observation of a pseudomembrane constitutes sufficient evidence to initiate appropriate treatment.[9] If these initial studies do not reveal any pathogens, more elaborate tests may be ordered such as viral studies, culture for *Yersinia enterocolitica,* assay for *Clostridium difficile* toxin, culture for *Vibrio* species, duodenal aspiration or intestinal biopsy for *Giardia* and *Entamoeba histolytica,* and special stain for *Cryptosporidium.*

Examination of the stool for leukocytes helps to distinguish between invasive and noninvasive infection, but it is not sensitive enough to obviate the need for stool culture. The invasive organisms that cause the appearance of numerous polymorphonuclear leukocytes (PMNs) in the stool include *Salmonella, Shigella, Campylobacter, Y. enterocolitica, C. difficile,* invasive *E. coli,* and *E. histolytica.* Figure 24-1 is an algorithm to aid in the determination of the cause of acute diarrhea.

If this series of diagnostic procedures does not reveal the cause of diarrhea and it persists more than 2 weeks, the patient should be evaluated for causes of chronic diarrhea such as malabsorption, endocrine disease, or bacterial overgrowth.

The clinician should become familiar with the battery of tests designated as "routine" in the various laboratories where services are obtained, as they may vary from laboratory to laboratory.

TREATMENT: GENERAL

The treatment of acute diarrhea first involves fluid replacement if the patient is dehydrated. Depending on the cause of the diarrhea, antimicrobial and/or antidiarrheal medications may be administered.

Agents available for treating diarrhea can be grouped into four categories: *antiperistaltic agents* such as codeine and paragoric, *absorbants* such as kaolin and aluminium hydroxide, *inhibitors of intestinal secretion* such as bismuth subsalicylate, and *antimicrobial agents.* The use of antiperistaltic agents is not recommended in patients with high fever, dysentery, or antibiotic-associated diarrhea because slowing peristalsis allows organisms to stay in contact with the mucosal surface longer. This may actually lead to potentiation of the infection.

Antimicrobial agents are not recommended for treatment of food poisoning, Rotavirus, Norwalk agent, or *Vibrio* infections. Antimicrobial agents are recommended if the diarrhea is severe or complications such as bacteremia occur with nontyphoidal *Salmonella, Campylobacter, Yersinia,* enterotoxigenic *E. coli,* or invasive *E. coli.* Antimicrobial agents should also be given if the infection is due to *Salmonella typhi, Shigella, E. histolytica,* or *Giardia lamblia,* or in colitis due to *C.*

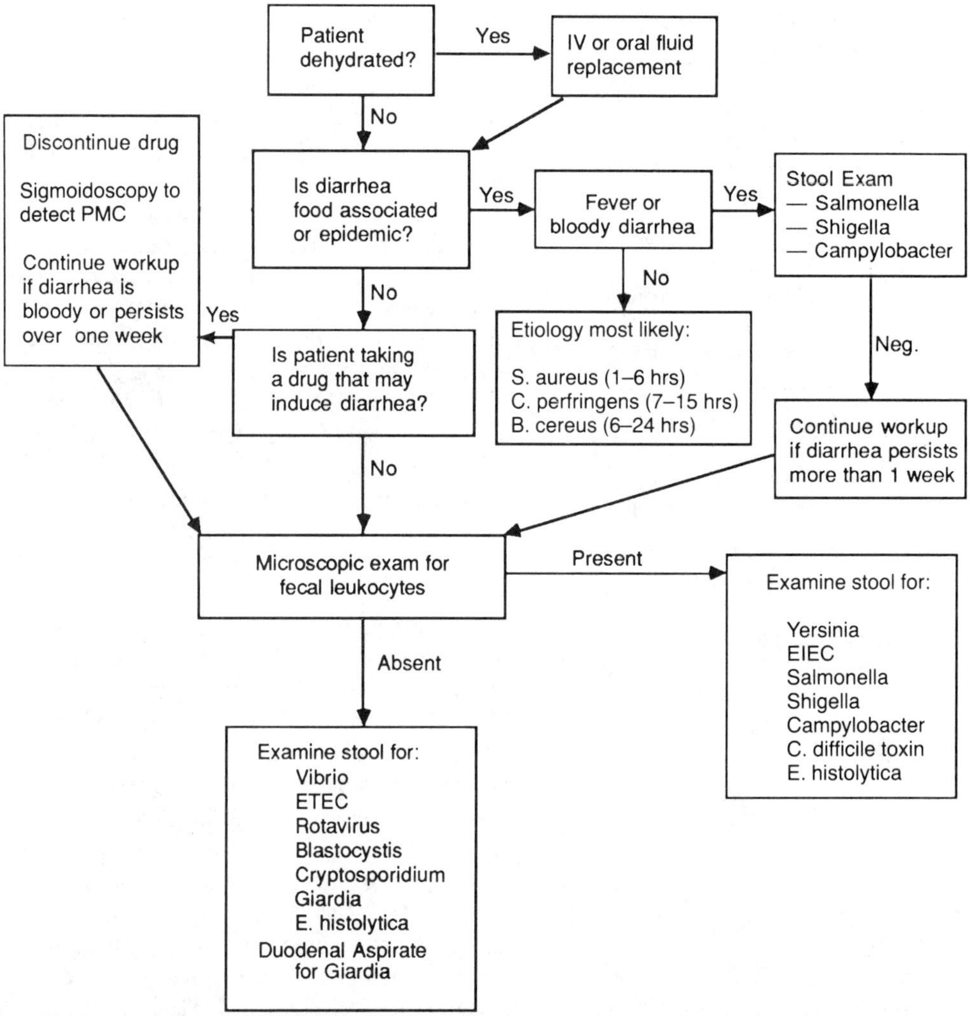

Figure 24-1 **Diagnostic procedures to determine cause of acute diarrhea.**

difficile. Guidelines for use of antimicrobial agents appear on the opposite page.

SPECIFIC DIARRHEAL DISORDERS

Bacterial Food Poisoning

Food poisoning may be caused by ingestion of bacteria that multiply in the gut or by ingestion of bacterial enterotoxins already in the food. Food poisoning caused by ingestion of preformed bacterial enterotoxins has a sudden onset with diarrhea, nausea, vomiting, and abdominal pain. The three organisms most commonly implicated in this type of food poisoning are *Staphylococcus aureus, Clostridium perfringens,* and *Bacillus cereus.*

S. aureus produces a heat-stable enterotoxin that is the most common cause of food poisoning in the western world.[10] If food contaminated with *S. aureus* is allowed to remain at an optimal temperature, the bacteria will multiply and elaborate toxin into the food. The toxin is ingested and, within 6

Antimicrobial Therapy for Infectious Diarrhea Caused by Specific Organisms

Antimicrobial agent not given
- *Staphylococcus aureus* (intoxication)
- *Clostridium perfringens*
- *Bacillus cereus*
- Rotavirus
- Norwalk virus
- *Vibrio cholerae*

Antimicrobial agent not given unless diarrhea is severe or complications such as bacteremia occur
- Nontyphoidal *Salmonella*
- *Campylobacter*
- *Yersinia*
- Enterotoxigenic *Escherichia coli*
- Invasive *E. coli*

Antimicrobial agent given when illness occurs
- *Salmonella typhi*
- *Shigella*
- *Entamoeba histolytica*
- *Giardia lamblia*
- *Clostridium difficile* colitis

hours after ingestion, the patient suddenly experiences nausea and abdominal cramps, with subsequent vomiting and diarrhea. This may be very serious in children and the elderly because of potential dehydration and electrolyte imbalance. In this population, intravenous fluids may be needed to restore liquid and electrolyte balance.[3] Usually the symptoms last only a few hours, rarely more than 24 hours, and recovery is spontaneous.[10] Foods commonly implicated in staphylococcal food poisoning are cream-filled pastries, custards, cheese, milk, ham, and cold meats. Sources of contamination are from the skin and nasopharynx of food handlers. Treatment may range from fluid replacement to antiemetics, and antispasmodics to relieve the symptoms.[3]

C. perfringens food poisoning usually results from ingestion of meat that has not been cooked sufficiently to kill the spores of the organism and has been allowed to sit at room temperature for several hours before being eaten. The spores germinate into vegetative cells that are ingested with the food. In the alkaline intestinal environment spores are formed from the vegetative cells, and an enterotoxin is given off in the process.[11] This enterotoxin causes symptoms of abdominal cramping and diarrhea 7 to 15 hours after ingestion of the contaminated food. Most patients are afebrile, and nausea and vomiting occur in fewer than one-third.[11] Patients usually recover in 2 to 3 days after onset of symptoms.

B. cereus food poisoning is associated with the ingestion of meats, sauces, and rice contaminated with the spores of the organism. There are two types of disease caused by the enterotoxins produced by *B. cereus*: an emetic type associated with rice, and a diarrheal type associated with meats and sauces.[12] The latter type is more common, and has an incubation period of 6 to 24 hours. The symptoms include watery diarrhea, abdominal cramps, and fever. Because the organism may be found in the stool of healthy individuals, its isolation from stool is not sufficient evidence for diagnosis. The disease is usually mild and self-limited.[12]

The diagnosis of individual cases of food poisoning caused by one of these three organisms is best made by history of food ingestion and symptoms. Since the organisms may occur in small numbers as part of the normal flora of the bowel, simple recovery of the organism in a stool culture is not diagnostic. When a large number of people become ill after eating a common food, epidemiological studies may be carried out that involve recovery of the organism from clinical specimens as well as from the suspected food. A protocol has been established by the American Public Health Association for carrying out testing in large outbreaks of foodborne illness.[13]

Infectious Bacterial Diarrhea

Infectious diarrheal disease still ranks high as a major cause of illness throughout the world.[14] In the gastrointestinal tract, multiplying bacteria cause disease by one of two mechanisms: (1) noninvasive, enterotoxigenic, or (2) invasive and/or destructive. A list of organisms, including bacteria, in each of these categories appears below.

The enterotoxigenic bacteria secrete an exotoxin that causes a rapid, profuse secretion of fluid across the mucosal surface of the small intestine, resulting in profuse, watery diarrhea *(secretory diarrhea)*. The invasive bacteria actually invade the epithelium of the intestinal mucosa, causing epithelial necrosis and an acute inflammatory response. This is manifested by pus and blood in the stool as well as tenesmus and abdominal cramps.[14]

Diarrheas caused by toxin-secreting bacteria that have colonized the small bowel are not associated with inflammation or fever. The resulting profuse, watery diarrhea results in saline depletion, acidosis, and potassium deficiency. *Vibrio cholerae* is the prototype organism in this category. Certain strains of *Escherichia coli* also may produce an enterotoxin that acts in the same manner.[14] These toxin-producing strains are called enterotoxigenic *E. coli* (ETEC).

Microbial Agents of Acute Diarrhea

Enterotoxigenic/Noninvasive
- *Staphylococcus aureus*
- *Clostridium perfringens*
- *Bacillus cereus*
- Enterotoxigenic *Escherichia coli*
- *Vibrio cholerae*

Invasive
- Enteroinvasive *E. coli*
- *Shigella*
- *Salmonella*
- *Yersinia*
- *Campylobacter*
- *Clostridium difficile*
- *Entamoeba histolytica*
- *Cryptosporidium*
- Rotavirus
- Norwalk virus

Other
- *Giardia lamblia*
- *Blastocystis hominis*

Cholera is the most severe of all the diarrheal diseases, but only 1% to 10% of persons infected develop the severe clinical syndrome.[15] Humans are the only known natural host of *V. cholerae*; therefore, water or food contaminated with human excreta must be ingested for the disease to occur. In the United States, the Gulf Coast of Texas and Louisiana are endemic areas.[16]

Symptoms begin abruptly, a few days after ingesting the organism, with the onset of painless, massive, watery diarrhea. Vomiting may also occur. The stools become very liquid and are often referred to as "rice water" stools. Fluid loss in an adult may reach a rate of 1 liter of isotonic fluid per hour at its peak.[17]

A diagnosis of cholera should be considered if the patient has the appropriate history or geographic exposure and has acute, afebrile, watery diarrhea. A Gram stain of the stool may reveal short, comma-shaped, gram-negative bacilli. Fluorescent antibody techniques are available for detection of the organism. The laboratory should be notified if cholera is suspected because the organism will not grow well on routine stool culture media and must be inoculated to special media.[15]

In the late 1940s, particular serotypes of *E. coli* were incriminated as etiologic agents of childhood diarrhea, especially in nurseries. These serotypes were referred to as "enteropathogenic *E. coli*" (EPEC). In the 1960s, investigators found that *E. coli* serotypes other than the previously-identified EPEC groups caused a secretory diarrhea in third world countries and in travelers to those areas. These strains produce one or both of two plasmid-mediated enterotoxins—heat-labile (LT) and heat-stable (ST)—and are enterotoxigenic *E. coli* (ETEC).[18] Many of the EPEC serotypes have since been found to be enterotoxin-producing strains.[15]

The patient suffering from ETEC gastroenteritis is usually afebrile and has moderate abdominal cramping and watery stools with no inflammatory exudate. Usually the patient with ETEC-associated diarrhea is not as ill as the patient with cholera.[14]

Enterotoxigenic strains of *E. coli* are indistinguishable from other *E. coli* by routine culture techniques. Demonstration of toxin production is not routinely performed in the clinical laboratory, as it now requires animal testing or cell culture techniques. Enzyme-linked immunosorbent assay (ELISA) and DNA hybridization techniques are under development and will be available commercially.[14] Due to a lack of readily available methods to test for ETEC, its importance as a cause of diarrhea in the United States is not yet clear. The development of these new enterotoxin detection methods should help clarify its role. Reagents for serotyping ETEC are not commercially available for routine testing in the clinical laboratory.[19]

In both cholera and ETEC secretory diarrhea, replacement of fluid losses and electrolytes is the primary element of therapy. In addition to intravenous therapy, oral glucose-electrolyte preparations are available. Oral therapy may be given as the sole treatment in mild cholera cases and ETEC cases. If an antibiotic is needed, tetracycline is the antibiotic of choice. A cholera vaccine is available.[14, 17]

Invasive bacteria that cause diarrhea include *Shigella, Salmonella, Yersinia, Campylobacter,* and some *E. coli.* These organisms invade the intestinal epithelium, where they multiply and cause mucosal cell death that leads to poor absorptive capability and inflammation. Mucosal cell death is responsible for the presence of blood and PMNs in the stool. The mechanism of this diarrhea is not completely understood, but it is most likely a process of acute inflammation and elaboration of enterotoxins.[18]

Invasive *E. coli* are implicated in clinical illness in Eastern Europe, but rarely cause acute diarrheal disease in the United States.[14] The symptoms include severe abdominal cramps and bloody diarrhea. These strains appear to belong to a limited number of serotypes that are different from ETEC and EPEC.

Enteroinvasive *E. coli* (EIEC) diarrhea must be diagnosed primarily from clinical and epidemiological data, because EIEC do not differ in their appearance on culture or biochemical reactions from normal intestinal flora. A Gram stain or methylene blue stain of a stool smear may reveal many PMNs. Specific serotypes have been associated with EIEC, but serotyping reagents are not commercially available for routine testing. The state health department laboratory may be able to serotype for EIEC in nursery or other outbreaks of diarrheal disease. In sporadic cases of diarrhea, it is not recommended that routine serotyping be performed.[15]

Recently, a new *E. coli*-mediated infection has been described. In 1982, two outbreaks of acute hemorrhagic gastroenteritis associated with eating beef occurred. Patients experienced severe abdominal cramps and watery diarrhea, followed by grossly bloody diarrhea.[10] The *E. coli* isolated was neither toxigenic nor invasive. The serotype of the implicated organism was 0157:H7.[20] This organism can be identified definitively by serotyping in a reference laboratory or a state department of health laboratory.

Shigellosis, or bacillary dysentery, is transmitted via the fecal-oral route. As few as 200 bacilli are capable of causing disease.[10] There are four species of *Shigella.* The most virulent, the Shiga bacillus, is *Shigella dysenteriae.*[17] The most common species in the United States is *S. sonnei,* which accounts for about 65% of all clinical isolates each year. *S. flexneri* accounts for nearly all the rest.[21] *S. dysenteriae* and *S. boydii* are rarely isolated in the United States, but may be isolated from travelers who have visited less developed areas of the world.

In the U.S., 12,000 to 15,000 cases of shigellosis are reported per year, most of which are in children.[21] Populations at high risk include those in custodial institutions, prisons, and daycare centers, and those on Indian reservations. Venereal transmission in homosexual men has also been well documented.

The symptoms, which occur after an incubation

period of 36 to 72 hours, include fever, abdominal cramps, and watery diarrhea.[17] In the subsequent 24 to 72 hours clinical dysentery appears, which is characterized by tenesmus, rectal urgency, and frequent loose bowel movements containing blood, mucus, pus, and unformed fecal material. Symptoms last less than a week in otherwise healthy adults. Morbidity and mortality are particularly high in young children, who may become dehydrated and develop electrolyte imbalance.[17]

Shigella infections are usually limited to the lining of epithelial cells and submucosa of the colon, and do not penetrate beyond the submucosa. As a result, extraintestinal infections and septicemia are rare.[10]

Shigella can be cultured and speciated in most clinical laboratories. The stool specimen submitted must be freshly passed and not allowed to stand at room temperature for more than 2 to 3 hours because the organism is quite sensitive to acid products and may die before the culture is performed.[15] Mucosal exudate obtained from proctoscopic examination usually produces a higher yield of organism than does a routine stool specimen.[1] A stool smear stained with methylene blue should reveal many PMNs. This finding is not specific for *Shigella* infection, as increased PMNs may occur with infection by any enteroinvasive organism.[17]

Antimicrobial treatment for shigellosis is controversial, as most patients recover spontaneously. However, the duration of bacterial shedding is shortened by administering antimicrobials.[22] It is recommended that children and adults with severe symptoms be treated with antimicrobials.[17] Plasmid-mediated resistance is common, and susceptibility testing should be performed on all isolates. Antidiarrheal agents such as Lomotil prolong the symptoms and the duration of fecal excretion, and for this reason are not recommended.[17] There is no vaccine available to prevent *Shigella* infection.

Salmonella species cause three different forms of infection in humans: enteric fever, gastroenteritis, and extraintestinal infection. DNA studies have shown that all *Salmonella* species and *Arizona* species belong to one species called *Salmonella choleraesuis*.[23] However, many laboratories still use the serotype as a species designation—for example, *S. typhi* or *S. typhimurium*. Typhoid fever caused by *Salmonella typhi* represents the classic enteric fever spread by contaminated food and water. *S. typhi* causes prolonged fever, bacteremia, and, finally, localization of infection in the submucosal lymphoid tissue of the small intestine before gastrointestinal symptoms appear. In *S. typhi* infection, constipation occurs as often as does diarrhea.[22] Unlike salmonella gastroenteritis, enteric fever is a prolonged and generalized infection that requires specific therapy.[22] The incidence of typhoid fever in the U.S. has been falling steadily since 1900, with only 384 reported cases in 1985.[24]

Gastroenteritis caused by *Salmonella* species varies from mild to severe, and may occasionally be associated with bacteremia. Sporadic cases and outbreaks are associated with contaminated foods, particularly powdered milk, meat products, powdered eggs, and poultry, as well as contact with infected animals. Chronic carriers are also a reservoir of infection.[17]

The incubation period for salmonella gastroenteritis is usually 8 to 48 hours. Symptoms include nausea and vomiting, followed by abdominal cramps and diarrhea. Diarrhea usually persists for 3 to 4 days. Temperature is elevated in about half of the cases, and usually returns to normal in 1 to 2 days. A temperature that remains elevated suggests bacteremia.[17]

Diagnosis of salmonella gastroenteritis can be made by recovering the organism in a stool culture. There are more than 1800 serotypes of *Salmonella* species, and most clinical laboratories can determine if an organism belongs to serogroups A to E, which are the most common groups occurring in the United States. Complete serotyping is important for public health reasons and is usually available through state health department laboratories. The Widal test, which measures antibodies directed against *Salmonella* O and H antigens, is not indicated for diagnosis of salmonella gastroenteritis because an antibody response does not occur in the acute or carrier state. The Widal test is only helpful in more invasive conditions such as enteric fever and extraintestinal infection (osteomyelitis).[17]

In mild cases of salmonella gastroenteritis, antimicrobials are not recommended unless diarrhea is severe or complications such as bacteremia occur. There is evidence that antimicrobial therapy prolongs the carrier state.[22]

Yersinia enterocolitica and *Yersinia pseudotuberculosis* both may cause intestinal disease. *Y. enterocolitica* causes diarrhea; *Y. pseudotuberculosis* causes purulent mesenteric adenitis with little or no diarrhea and will not be considered here.[10]

Y. enterocolitica occurs widely in the environment and has been recovered from raw milk and water supplies as well as from wild and domestic animals. Outbreaks associated with consumption of infected meat and other foods have occurred. The incubation period is 4 to 10 days.[25]

Y. enterocolitica causes intense inflammation of the terminal ileum that mimics appendicitis. Symptoms vary greatly in different age groups. Children younger than 5 years old usually present with diarrhea, fever, and abdominal cramps. They frequently have vomiting and bloody diarrhea. Older children and adults present with less severe diarrhea and colicky abdominal pain that often localizes in the right lower quadrant. Many patients exhibit joint pain for more than a month after infection.[17] Septicemia is rare.

Diagnosis can be made by recovery of the organism from stool, lymph node culture, and blood in bacteremia. If *Yersinia* infection is suspected, the laboratory should be notified because special culture techniques must be used for more rapid isolation and identification of the organism.[14] Increased PMNs will be found on a stool smear because of the invasiveness of the organism.[17] A serologic test for *Yersinia* antibody is available in some laboratories.

In uncomplicated gastroenteritis, the infection is usually self-limited and requires no antimicrobial treatment. In chronic or extraintestinal infection, antibiotic treatment is indicated.[25]

Many species of *Campylobacter* are capable of causing disease in humans. The most common cause of bacterial diarrhea is *Campylobacter jejuni.*[17] It is estimated that two million cases of *Campylobacter* infection occur in the United States each year.[26] The source appears to be food of animal origin or contaminated water supplies. Person-to-person transmission of *C. jejuni* has been documented between mothers and neonates as well as in day-care centers.[17]

The presence of blood and leukocytes in the stool suggests an enteroinvasive mechanism, but a secretory diarrhea also occurs, which suggests the elaboration of an enterotoxin.[26] The incubation period is 2 to 4 days.[17] Onset is sudden; the patient exhibits abdominal pain, nausea, anorexia, fever, malaise, and headache. The diarrhea is watery, and associated with eight to ten bowel movements per day. Gross blood is seen in about 30% of patients, and occult blood in an additional 30%.[17] Most cases recover in 3 to 5 days, but there have been reports of cases in which recurrent or relapsing diarrhea occurred for 9 months.[27] Bacteremia has been known to occur.

Campylobacter may be cultured from the stool in most laboratories. The stool specimen should be cultured within 2 hours of collection, or placed in transport media and refrigerated.[26] Special media and culture conditions are required, so it is helpful to advise the laboratory of the suspected diagnosis. Although many laboratories routinely culture all stool specimens for *Campylobacter* as well as *Salmonella* and *Shigella,* the clinician should inquire about routine protocols in the laboratory performing those tests. *Campylobacter* multiplies slowly on culture media, and isolation may take up to 72 hours.[26] Confirmatory identification may take an additional 1 to 2 days. Tests for blood in the stool and for increased fecal PMNs are usually positive.

Campylobacter enteritis is usually self-limited and does not require antimicrobial therapy, but in severe illness fluid replacement and antibiotic treatment may be necessary.[27]

Viral Diarrhea

Viral gastroenteritis is estimated to be one of the most common viral illnesses in the United States, second only to the common cold.[28] Symptoms include nausea, vomiting, and diarrhea. Infants and young children often require treatment for dehydration and electrolyte imbalance because of the severity of the vomiting and diarrhea. Rotavirus and the Norwalk group of viruses are the two most common causes of viral gastroenteritis.[28]

Rotaviral gastroenteritis usually occurs in the winter months, and primarily affects infants and children under 5 years of age; however, it has also caused outbreaks in school-age children and in geriatric patients.[29, 30] Mild cases have occurred in adult contacts of pediatric cases.[31] The transmission most likely occurs via the fecal-oral route. The virus directly infects and damages the intestinal epithelial cells, and the diarrhea is the result of repopulation of the intestinal epithelium with immature cells that cannot absorb well.[32]

The incubation period is 48 to 72 hours, with sudden onset that includes diarrhea and vomiting. Fever occurs in the majority of cases. Upper respiratory tract symptoms frequently occur. Diarrhea may last for 5 to 8 days, and causes dehydration in 40% to 83% of cases.[28]

Because the virus is shed in the stool for up to 8 days, the laboratory diagnosis is based on the direct detection of virus in the stool. Stool specimens to be submitted to another laboratory for identification or those to be stored should be frozen at $-70°$ C and shipped on dry ice.[33] Rotavirus may be identified by electron microscopy, but not all clinical laboratories have EM capability. Radioimmunoassay (RIA) and enzyme-linked immunosorbent assays (ELISA) procedures are available for virus detection in some hospital or reference laboratories.[28] The ELISA test has a 90% to 95% specificity, but a high incidence of false positives has been reported in infants under 3 months old.[34] The test is most useful in diagnosing gastroenteritis in children 6 months to 2 years old and in epidemiological studies. Children under 6 months of age are often asymptomatic but still shed Rotavirus. Therefore, a positive test in this age group should not preclude searching for other pathogens.[35]

The disease is usually self-limiting, and no treatment is required. However, children and debilitated patients may become dehydrated and require intravenous or oral fluid therapy.

Diarrhea caused by Norwalk virus is seen primarily in older children and adults. It is named after a public school epidemic in Norwalk, Ohio in 1968.[28] Approximately half of gastroenteritis epidemics are caused by Norwalk viruses, which occur worldwide. Norwalk antibodies have been found in 50% to 75% of American adults.[33] The antibody is not protective, but is an indication of previous exposure to the virus. Norwalk virus is spread by contaminated water and food such as shellfish.[33]

The incubation period is 18 to 48 hours, and symptoms last for 24 to 48 hours. The symptoms include mild to severe vomiting and diarrhea as well as abdominal cramps, headache, myalgia, and low-grade fever.[33]

The virus is shed in the stool for only a brief time, but it can be detected by electron microscopy. An RIA procedure to detect Norwalk virions in the stool is available in some reference laboratories but is not widely used. An ELISA test is not available. The development of a vaccine is unlikely, because the Norwalk virus cannot be grown *in vitro*. Treatment is rarely needed, except for debilitated patients who may need fluid therapy.

Parasitic Diarrhea

Diarrhea may be caused by heavy infection with protozoa, roundworms, and flatworms (tapeworms). The two most common causes of parasitic diarrhea are *Entamoeba histolytica* and *Giardia lamblia*.[10] Two additional protozoans, *Blastocystis hominis* and *Cryptosporidium*, have been reported increasingly over the past few years (see also Chap. 58).

Entamoeba Histolytica

Infection with *E. histolytica* is potentially the most serious infection caused by pathogenic intestinal protozoans, as it may cause liver abcess and even death. Amebiasis occurs worldwide in areas where poor sanitation and malnutrition exist. The prevalence in the United States is between 1% and 5%.[36] Humans become infected by eating or drinking food or water contaminated with amebic cysts. Excystation occurs in the small bowel, and the actively-feeding trophozoites that emerge inhabit the large intestine, where they may live in the lumen or invade the mucosal crypts and cause ulceration. This may give rise to amebic dysentery, but does not always do so; some patients may have extensive damage and yet be asymptomatic.[36] The laboratory diagnosis is made by demonstration of *E. histolytica* in a stool specimen. Multiple fresh stool specimens may need to be examined to find the cysts or trophozoites. Trophozoites are more likely to be found if the patient has diarrhea, and cysts are more likely to be found in a formed stool specimen.[10] Specimens obtained by sigmoidoscopy or biopsy may also be submitted. Freshly-obtained specimens should be delivered to the laboratory within 1 hour, as the trophozoites may rapidly deteriorate beyond recognition. Specimens that cannot be examined immediately should be refrigerated.[10] The following substances may cause interference with the recovery and identification of cysts and trophozoites: antimicrobials, antiprotozoal and antihelminthic drugs, barium, kaolin, magnesium hydroxide, soap, and salt enemas.[10] Stool samples for laboratory examination should be collected before any of the above are administered to the patient.

Many serologic tests are available, such as enzyme-linked immunosorbent assay (ELISA), complement fixation, and indirect hemagglutination (IHA). All of these are likely to be positive only in extraintestinal infection or in invasive amebiasis where the absence of trophozoites in stool is common.[36] A skin test is also available.

Drug regimens have been established for treatment of both asymptomatic and symptomatic amebiasis.[36] It is felt that asymptomatic cyst passers should be treated to prevent the spread of the organism.[10]

G. lamblia is a flagellated protozoan that may exist in a cyst or trophozoite form. Infection is transmitted by the oral ingestion of cysts in contaminated water. Excystation occurs in the lumen of the upper portion of the small intestine, where the trophozoites live closely attached to the mucosa.[36]

Many infected individuals are asymptomatic, but some have diarrhea, abdominal cramps, malaise, and weight loss. Spontaneous remission may occur, but treatment is usually necessary. The incubation period is 1 to 3 weeks, and acute watery diarrhea may last for 5 to 7 days.[10] Fever, vomiting, and abdominal distention may occur. Blood and mucus are not often found in the stool, which helps differentiate giardiasis from amebic dysentery and shigellosis.

Laboratory diagnosis can be made by demonstrating cysts or trophozoites in the stool. The organism is often passed only intermittently, so a stool should be examined for *Giardia* every other day on three or four occasions.[10] Examinations of duodenal material may be necessary if the organism cannot be detected in the stool and the index of suspicion remains high. An ELISA test for the detection of *Giardia* antigen in a stool has recently been developed.[37] A number of drugs are available for treating *Giardia* infection.[10]

Cryptosporidium causes enterocolitis in animals such as calves and lambs. It has been reported to cause a self-limited diarrhea of 1 to 2 weeks in persons who have had direct contact with infected animals. Transmission is through the fecal-oral route. Since 1982, an increase of cryptosporidiosis has been reported in immunocompromised patients, such as those with acquired immune deficiency syndrome (AIDS).[38] These patients have a longlasting, watery, frothy diarrhea with intense abdominal pain, anorexia, and weight loss. Diarrhea may last for months, and death may result.

The organisms live on the mucosal surface attached to the epithelial cell brush border. Development of the organism is under the surface membrane of the host cell and not in the cell proper.[38] Diarrhea is caused by impaired absorption. It is not clear whether the damage to the mucosa is mechanical, toxin-mediated, or due to hypersensitivity to parasitic antigen.

Diagnosis is based on detection of the organism in the stool, duodenal or jejunal aspirate, or biopsy.[39] Special techniques and stains are needed to detect *Cryptosporidium,* so the laboratory should be notified if this parasite is suspected.

Cryptosporidiosis in the immunocompetent patient is usually self-limiting, and treatment is not necessary. A variety of treatments have been tried in the immunocompromised patient with little success. Detection of *Cryptosporidium* in such a patient carries a poor prognosis.[40]

B. hominis has long been thought to be a nonpathogenic yeast found normally in the stool. Recently it was reclassified as a protozoan.[41] When it is present in large numbers in the absence of other parasitic, bacterial, or viral causes, it is thought to be the cause of diarrhea and cramps.

Diagnosis is made by ruling out other causes of diarrhea and also finding more than five organisms per high power microscopic field.[42] Antiprotozoal drugs are available for treatment.[43]

Antibiotic-associated Colitis

Antibiotic therapy may alter the intestinal flora and cause diarrhea. Often this condition is mild, and disappears when the therapy is discontinued. In some patients, however, severe diarrhea occurs, with the development of a thick mucosal exudate that resembles a membrane—hence the name *pseudomembranous colitis* (PMC).

PMC has been etiologically linked to *C. difficile* and the cytotoxins produced by this organism.[44] *C. difficile* is associated with a wide spectrum of symptoms, ranging from none in asymptomatic carriers to PMC with bowel perforation and death.[45] Patients with PMC have a rapid onset of watery diarrhea, and up to 10 to 20 stools per day.[45] Abdominal tenderness, fever, and leukocytosis are also usually present. Sigmoidoscopic findings include edema, hyperemia, and friability. In fully-developed cases, raised yellow plaques of exudate can be seen, which coalesce to form the pseudomembrane. Microscopic examination of the membrane reveals leukocytes, mucus, and sloughed epithelial cells.

Diagnosis can be made by observing the pseudomembrane during sigmoidoscopy, as this finding following recent exposure to antibiotics is diagnostic. However, the absence of a pseudomembrane does not exclude the diagnosis of *C. difficile* infection.[45]

C. difficile may produce two toxins, called A and B. Not all organisms produce both toxins. The organism may also be found as part of the normal intestinal flora.[45] Therefore, detection of toxin production by organisms is more diagnostic than a stool culture. Toxin may be detected by cell culture techniques and ELISA methods in some hospitals and in reference laboratories. Recently, a commercial latex agglutination test has been marketed for the rapid detection of toxin A; however, a recent study has shown that the test does not, in fact, detect toxin A but reacts with nontoxigenic strains of *C. difficile* as well.[46] Because the potential for false-positive results appears to be great, this test cannot be recommended at present.

Several oral antimicrobials are effective for treatment of *C. difficile* colitis in its various forms. The drug of choice is Vancomycin.[45] The use of antidiarrheal agents may prolong or worsen the symptoms.[41] Relapse occurs in 12% to 14% of patients.[45]

CASE STUDY #1

A well-nourished 30-year-old woman presented with abdominal cramps, fever of 102° F, and bloody diarrhea that had persisted for 36 hours. The symptoms had appeared approximately 1 week after the patient had returned from a Caribbean cruise. There were no signs of dehydration, and the patient had not been taking any medication.

Because the patient was febrile, a "routine" stool culture was ordered as well as a microscopic examination for fecal leukocytes. The culture report stated "No pathogens" and the fecal leukocyte report stated "12 leukocytes per high power field." Since the fecal leukocytes examination was positive, indicating an invasive process, and the culture revealed no pathogens, an Ova and Parasite test was ordered. A repeat stool culture was also done, specifically for *Yersinia* and *Campylobacter* as well as *Salmonella* and *Shigella*. No parasites were found, but the cultures revealed *Campylobacter jejuni*.

Questions

1. Why did the report of the routine stool culture indicate no pathogens?
2. What was the consequence of the lack of information about the laboratory protocol?
3. What steps could this laboratory have taken to avoid delay in diagnosis?

Discussion

1. The protocol for a "routine" stool culture in this particular laboratory included checking for *Salmonella* and *Shigella* only. Cultures for *Campylobacter* and *Yersinia* are only done upon special request. The clinician should become familiar with the battery of tests designated "routine" in the various laboratories where services are obtained, as they may vary from laboratory to laboratory.
2. Because the patient presented with bloody diarrhea, the request for *Campylobacter* culture on the initial stool specimen would have speeded the diagnosis and indicated specific treatment. The patient was placed on Erythromycin, and the symptoms subsided within 48 hours.
3. If the clinical laboratory scientist had had sufficient clinical information, a suggestion could have been made that *Campylobacter* culture be specifically requested initially.

CASE STUDY #2

A total of 17 students and instructors out of a group of 33 became ill with diarrhea after a graduation banquet. All 17 had nausea and vomiting, and 10 had severe abdominal cramps. All were afebrile. They all presented to a local emergency room within 2 to 6 hours after the banquet.

No stool cultures were ordered. The patients were given symptomatic treatment. Five were hospitalized due to dehydration, and the other 12 were sent home.

Questions

1. What is the most likely cause of these clinical symptoms, and what history and physical findings support this conclusion?
2. Why were no stool cultures ordered?

Discussion

1. Since all the patients had similar symptoms, all had attended the banquet, and all were afebrile, the diarrhea was thought to be food-associated. Histories revealed that all had eaten deviled eggs that had been prepared in a private home and had been stored for approximately 6 hours at room temperature before being served. Because the symptoms began within 2 to 6 hours, the most probable cause was *S. aureus*.
2. Culturing for the suspected agent, *S. aureus*, would contribute nothing to the diagnosis. Moreover, because a number of patients with a common food source presented themselves within a short span of time at the clinic, the decision not to order stool cultures saved much time and money. The patients all made an uneventful recovery with symptomatic treatment.

REFERENCES

1. Krejs GJ, Fordtran JS: Diarrhea. In Sleisenger MH, Fordtran JS (eds): Gastrointestinal Disease, pp 257–269. Philadelphia, WB Saunders, 1983
2. Binder JB: The pathophysiology of diarrhea. Hosp Pract 19:107, 1984
3. Jinich H, Hersh T, Swartz H: Physician's Guide to

the Etiology and Treatment of Diarrhea, pp 1–8, 17–19, 157–160. Oradell, NJ, Medical Economics Books, 1982
4. Haubrich WS: Diarrhea and constipation. In Buckus HL (ed): Gastroenterology, Vol 2, pp 918–936. Philadelphia, WB Saunders, 1976
5. Hyams JS: Sorbital intolerance. Gastroenterology 84:30, 1983
6. Phillips SF: Diarrhea. Postgrad Med 57:65, 1975
7. Gray GM: Acute diarrhea. In Scientific American Medicine 4:III. Gastroenterology 84:30, 1983
8. Woodward WE, Woodward TE: Management of dehydrating diarrhea. Hosp Pract 21:60, 1986
9. Griner PF et al: Clinical Diagnosis in the Laboratory, p 333. Chicago, Year Book Medical Pub, 1986
10. Youmans GP, Paterson PV, Sommers HM: Infectious Diseases, pp 496–537, 623. Philadelphia, WB Saunders, 1985
11. Allen SD: *Clostridium.* In Lennette EH (ed): Manual of Clinical Microbiology, 4th ed, p 434. Washington, DC, American Society for Microbiology, 1985
12. Doyle RJ, Keller KF, Wezzell JW: *Bacillus.* In Lennette EH (ed): Manual of Clinical Microbiology, 4th ed, p 214. Washington, DC, American Society for Microbiology, 1985
13. Speck ML (ed): Compendium of methods for the microbiological examination of foods, 2nd ed. Washington, DC, American Public Health Association, 1984
14. Carpenter CJ, Sack RB: Infectious diarrheal syndromes. In Isselbacher KJ, Adams RD et al (eds): Harrison's Principles of Internal Medicine, Update I, pp 209–229. New York City, McGraw-Hill, 1981
15. Sack RB, Tilton RC, Weissfeld AS: Laboratory Diagnosis of Bacterial Diarrhea. Cumitech 12, pp 1–16. Washington, DC, American Society for Microbiology, 1980
16. Johnston JM, Martin DL et al: Cholera on a gulf coast oil rig. N Engl J Med 309:523, 1983
17. Rubin RH: Infections due to gram-negative bacilli. In Scientific American Medicine 7:II: Infectious Disease, pp 1–16. New York City, Scientific American, 1985
18. Giannella RA: Pathogenesis of acute bacterial diarrheal disorders. Ann Rev Med 32:341–357, 1981
19. Merson MH, Rowe B et al: Use of antisera for identification of enterotoxigenic *E. coli.* Lancet 2:222–224, 1980
20. Pai CH, Gordon R, Sims HV et al: Sporadic cases of hemorrhagic colitis associated with *E. coli* O157:H7. Ann Intern Med 101:738, 1984
21. CDC: Current trends: Shigellosis—US. MMWR 34:600, 1985
22. Satterwhite TK, Dupont HL: Infectious diarrhea in office practice. Med Clin North Am 67(1):203, 1983
23. Farmer JJ et al: Biochemical identity of new species and biogroups of enterobacteriaceae isolated from clinical specimens. J Clin Microbiol 20:46, 1985
24. CDC: MMWR 34:777, 1986
25. Vantrappen G et al: *Yersinia* enteritis. Med Clin North Am 66(3):639, 1982
26. Morris GK, Patton CM: *Campylobacter.* In Lennette EH (ed): Manual of Clinical Microbiology, 4th ed, p 302. Washington, DC, American Society for Microbiology, 1985
27. Blaser MJ, Reller LB: *Campylobacter* enteritis. N Engl J Med 305:1444, 1981
28. Barnett B: Viral gastroenteritis. Med Clin North Am 67(5):1031–1058, 1983
29. Hara M, Mukoyama J et al: Acute gastroenteritis among school children associated with reovirus-like agent. Am J Epidemiol 107:161, 1978
30. Marrie TJ, Lee SHS et al: Rotavirus infection in a geriatric population. Arch Intern Med 142:313, 1982
31. Kim HW, Brandt CD et al: Human reovirus-like agent infection: Occurrence in adult contacts of pediatric patients with gastroenteritis. JAMA 238:404, 1977
32. Davidson GP, Gall DG et al: Human rotavirus enteritis induced in conventional piglets. J Clin Invest 60:1402, 1977
33. Blacklow NR, Cukor G: Viral gastroenteritis agents. In Lennette EH (ed): Manual of Clinical Microbiology, 4th ed, p 805. Washington, DC, American Society for Microbiology, 1985
34. Krause PJ et al: Unreliability of rotazyme ELISA test in neonates. J Pediatr 103:259, 1983
35. Bishop RF et al: Clinical immunity after neonatal rotavirus infection. N Engl J Med 309:72, 1983
36. Markel EK, Voge M, John DT: Medical Parasitology, pp 20–59. Philadelphia, WB Saunders, 1986
37. Ungar B, Yolken R, Nash T et al: Enzyme immunoassay for the detection of *G. lamblia* in fecal specimens. J Infect Dis 149:90, 1984
38. Current WL et al: Human cryptosporidiosis in immunocompetent and immunodeficient persons. N Engl J Med 308:1252, 1983

39. Garza D: Diarrhea caused by a coccidian parasite, *Cryptosporidium.* Lab Med 14:283, 1983
40. CDC: Cryptosporidiosis: Assessment of chemotherapy of males with acquired immune deficiency syndrome (AIDS). MMWR 31:589, 1982
41. Zierdt CH, Tan H: Endosymbiosis in *Blastocystis hominis.* Exper Parasitol 39:422, 1976
42. Phillips BP, Zierdt CH: *Blastocystis hominis:* Pathogenic potential in human patients' gnotobiotes. Exp Parasitol 39:358, 1976
43. Zierdt CH et al: In vitro response of *Blastocystis hominis* to antiprotozoal drugs. J Protozool 30:332, 1983
44. Bartlett JG, Chang TW, Gurwith M et al: Antibiotic-associated pseudomembranous colitis due to toxin-producing *Clostridia.* N Engl J Med 298:531, 1978
45. Trnka YM et al: *Clostridium Difficile* Colitis. In Tollerman GHS (ed): Advances in Internal Medicine, p 85. Chicago, Year Book Medical Pub, 1984
46. Lyerly DM, Wilkins TD: Commercial latex test for *C. difficile* toxin A does not detect toxin. Am J Clin Microbiol 23:622, 1986

Chapter 25

Pancreatitis

R. Lyle Christensen

ETIOLOGY AND PATHOPHYSIOLOGY

Classification

The 1963 Marseilles Conference on Pancreatitis suggested that pancreatic inflammation be classified according to the following categories: acute pancreatitis, recurrent acute pancreatitis, chronic pancreatitis, and recurrent chronic pancreatitis.[1] Acute and chronic pancreatitis were differentiated by the recovery of structural and functional integrity of the gland after the course of the disease. *Acute pancreatitis* results in complete recovery from the disease, with no deficiencies of the gland except those present before the attack. Acute pancreatitis can be subclassified as interstitial type (interstitial edema), hemorrhagic or necrotic type (release of pancreatic enzymes), and traumatic type. Conversely, *chronic pancreatitis* results in irreversible injury to the gland, leading to permanent necrotic or fibrotic changes. Differentiation between acute and chronic pancreatitis, especially in individuals with marginal loss of gland function, can be very subjective. *Relapsing* or *recurrent pancreatitis* of either variety results from conditions such as alcohol abuse that continue to damage the gland.

Etiology

The etiology of pancreatitis for most individuals with acute symptoms is unknown. The majority will, however, possess conditions known to be associated with acute pancreatitis (see list at right). The most common etiologic factors of pancreatitis are biliary tract disease (30%) and alcohol-induced disease (30%), with an additional 30% of cases without known cause (idiopathic).[2] The additional 10% present with the remaining etiologic factors listed above.

Etiologic Factors Associated with Acute Pancreatitis

1. *Mechanical factors*
   (a) Biliary tract disease and gallstones
   (b) Tumors of the pancreas
   (c) Duodenal obstruction
   (d) Endoscopic retrograde cholangiopancreatogram
2. *Tissue injury*
   (a) Infection
   (b) Toxins: alcohol, venom
   (c) Drugs
3. *Circulatory factors*
   (a) Atherosclerosis
   (b) Shock
   (c) Emboli
   (d) Vasculitis
4. *Endocrine factors*
   (a) Pregnancy
   (b) Hyperparathyroidism
5. *Metabolic factors*
   (a) Hypercalcemia
   (b) Hyperlipidemia
   (c) Hereditary pancreatitis
6. *Immunologic factors*
   (a) Hypersensitivity
   (b) Postrenal transplantation
7. *Trauma*
   (a) Postoperative states
   (b) Abdominal
8. *Idiopathic*

Pathogenesis

The predominant pathogenic theory of pancreatitis involves the autodigestion of the gland by the abnormal release of proteolytic proenzymes, and their subsequent conversion to active enzymes, presumably via trypsin-catalyzed cleavage. Virtually all of the etiologic factors listed above share a common ability to cause damage to acinar cells, resulting in pancreatic edema, proteolysis, hemorrhage, parenchymal damage, and fat necrosis. Autodigestion progresses until enzyme activation and cell damage abate.

CLINICAL MANIFESTATIONS

Symptoms

The dominant symptom of pancreatitis is abdominal pain (see Table 25-1). The character of this pain has been described as aching, twisting, stabbing, or knifelike, and it is felt most often in the mid-epigastrium and the left upper quadrant of the abdomen, with occasional generalization to the back.[3] The pain can range in intensity from mild to excruciating, and can last for as little as 24 hours or as long as several days. Nausea and vomiting are the second most common symptoms, and accompany abdominal pain in most cases. The remaining symptoms occur less frequently in pancreatitis but can be associated with an increased morbidity and mortality due to pancreatitis as well as other disorders.

Table 25-1 ***Incidence of Clinical Manifestations of Pancreatitis***

Symptoms	%	Signs	%
Pain	95	Abdominal tenderness	95
Nausea and vomiting	84	Tachycardia	80
Respiratory distress	40	Fever	60
Jaundice	17	Distention	50
Diarrhea	7	Hypotension-shock	44
Melena	4	Mass	5
Hematemesis	3	Xanthoma, Chvosteck, Cullen, Grey Turner	Rare

Data from reference numbers [3, 11, 15, 27]

Signs

The major sign present in mild acute pancreatitis may be only mild abdominal tenderness. The other signs listed in Table 25-1 are more often present in the more fulminant cases of pancreatitis, with tachycardia, fever, distention, and hypotension occurring more frequently. Other signs will be seen in rare cases.

LABORATORY ANALYSES AND DIAGNOSIS

Historically, the diagnosis of pancreatitis has been largely dependent on finding an increase in serum amylase to above the reference range, although such an elevation can result from several causes other than pancreatitis (see Table 25-2).[3] The diagnostic implication of this increase is dependent on the cutoff level chosen to discriminate between disorders, with diagnostic specificity studies often questioned due to the lack of an independent means of diagnosis, a "gold standard" for the disease.[4] Such nonspecificity has generated a lively controversy among investigators, leading to the exploration of alternate diagnostic tests that could improve the probability of correctly diagnosing pancreatitis. Table 25-2 outlines some of these tests and their applicability to the diagnosis of pancreatitis, as well as some of the other disorders that might lead to the elevation of these tests.

It should be noted that pancreatitis in conjunction with a normal serum amylase is very rare. Clinical suspicion of pancreatitis with a normal amylase result requires at least a repeat amylase analysis as well as patient followup to discern the cause of the signs and symptoms that led to the suspicion of pancreatitis. It should also be noted that an elevated serum amylase can occur in the absence of pancreatitis. As can be seen in Table 25-2, many disorders can result in an elevation of serum amylase without pancreatitis, especially macroamylasemia and certain salivary disorders. The analysis of pancreatic-specific isoenzyme, P-amylase, has been found to be useful in discriminating salivary causes of hyperamylasemia from other causes of hyperamylasemia.[5] Unfortunately, there is a high false-positive rate in cases of macroamylasemia as a result of slower clearance of the macroenzyme complex. Other amylase tests, urinary amylase and urinary amylase-to-creatinine ratio, have been found to have only limited utility in the diagnosis of pancreatitis.[6]

Serum lipase, on the other hand, is gaining favor for its reportedly lower false-negative rates and higher sensitivity than serum amylase for the diagnosis of pancreatitis,[7, 8] especially with the development of new test methodologies described below. Additionally, increased serum lipase can be observed for much longer periods of time than can increases in serum amylase, thereby making diagnosis possible well after the acute attack.[8, 9] Lipase

Table 25-2 *Tests for the Diagnosis of Pancreatitis*

Tests	Alternate Diagnoses	References
1. Amylase		
Serum amylase	Macroamylasemia, mumps, diabetic ketoacidosis, abdominal surgery, mesenteric thrombosis, perforated ulcer, drugs, tumors, acute cholecystitis, intestinal obstruction, ectopic pregnancy	3, 8, 9, 14, 15, 27, 28, 29
Urine amylase	Intestinal obstruction, acute biliary disease	3, 15, 30
Serum isoenzymes	Acute biliary disease, perforated peptic ulcer, intestinal obstruction	3, 5, 8, 15, 28, 31
Urine amylase/creatinine ratio	Diabetic ketoacidosis, severe burns and renal insufficiency, duodenal perforation, pancreatic cancer, pregnancy	3, 15, 27
2. Lipase		
Serum lipase	Acute cholecystitis, mesenteric infarction, peritonitis, pancreatic cancer	3, 5, 8, 9, 14
3. Immunoreactive trypsin	General pancreatic insufficiency, chronic vs acute pancreatitis, bowel disease, surgery, endoscopic examination	5, 7, 8, 15, 32, 33
4. Miscellaneous	(Generally nonspecific)	
Serum calcium	Nonspecific	16
Serum glucose	Diabetes	15
Hematocrit	Nonspecific	
Blood gases	Nonspecific	
Serum methemalbumin	Nonspecific indicator of hemoglobin breakdown	3, 6, 16
Activity of serum trypsin, elastase, etc.	Generally not available	
C-reactive protein	Index of inflammation	33
5. Future possibilities		
Serum RNase	Possibly indicate pancreatic necrosis or pancreatic cancer, burns, trauma, renal failure	6
Plasma fibrinogen	Not fully understood	16
6. Nonlaboratory procedures		
Endoscopic retrograde cholangiopancreatogram		
Computerized tomographic scan		
Magnetic resonance imaging scan		
Ultrasound		
Percutaneous transhepatic cholangiography		
Angiography		
Radiocontrast studies		

has been assayed by several methods, including turbidometric, spectrophotometric, and immunometric techniques.[10, 11, 12, 13] Maximal sensitivity and specificity can be attained for serum lipase by using an immunometric assay, or the turbidometric and spectrophotometric assays when performed in the presence of added colipase to overcome many of the edogenous lipase inhibitors present in the serum and the low concentration of endogenous serum colipase.[14] These modifications and refinements of the analysis of serum lipase have made it possible to improve the sensitivity and specificity of serum lipase, not to mention the ease of analysis. The evaluation of the utility of serum lipase, however, suffers from the same defect as the analysis of serum amylase—the lack of an established objective diagnosis or "gold standard" for pancreatitis.

A combination of both serum tests, amylase and lipase, coupled with temporal measurement of both enzymes should increase the probability of correctly diagnosing pancreatitis. There is evidence that urinary amylase should also be measured temporally in parallel with the serum tests to increase maximally the probability of diagnosing pancreatitis.[15] The major problems with this testing protocol are its as yet unproven efficacy and the extra cost of multiple analyses involved. Therefore, until the superiority of this protocol is established, only serum amylase and lipase should be performed periodically over the first 24 hours of hospitalization.

Other serum tests have also begun to gain favor for their potential for improving the differential diagnosis of pancreatitis. Of these, immunoreactive serum trypsin has shown the most promise as an additional test to assist in the diagnosis of pancreatitis.[5, 7, 8] Other laboratory tests and findings listed in Table 25-2 have been correlated with acute pancreatitis, although none of these shows the necessary improved specificity for pancreatitis.[16] The quest for better diagnostic tests has led to studies that show promise as improvements in specificity for pancreatitis as well as indicators of morbidity. Two such analyses are serum RNase[17] and plasma fibrinogen,[18, 19] but they have yet to be employed in the clinical laboratory.

Many nonspecific observations can also be made in patients with acute pancreatitis, and can be indicators of poor patient prognosis (see the observations displayed below). Increased methemalbumin can be consistent with severe disease, especially hemorrhagic disease,[20, 21] but can occur as a result of many other pathologies.[22] It should be emphasized that interpretation of methemalbumin levels may be dependent on method and time of analysis with respect to acute attack. Fluid sequestration can correlate with the degree of pa-

Indicators of Poor Prognosis in Acute Pancreatitis

1. *Initial observations*
   WBC > 16.0 × 10^3/mm^3
   Serum glucose > 200 mg/dL (11.1 mmol/L) (without diabetes history)
   LD > 2× normal
   AST > 5× normal
   Age > 55 y
   Chronic alcohol abuse > 10 y
   Previous diagnosis of pancreatitis
2. *Observations after 24-h hospitalization*
   Drop in hematocrit (>10%), calcium (to <4 mEq/L[2mmol/L]) and albumin (<3.2 g/dL [32g/L])
   Rise in serum urea and creatinine
   PO_2 < 60 mm
   Base deficit > 4 mEq/L
3. *Additional observations*
   Methemalbuminemia
   Hyperfibrinogenemia
   Fluid sequestration (>6L)
   Declining complement proteins (especially C3)
   Computerized tomographic scan and abdominal paracentesis

Data from reference numbers[1, 3, 15, 16, 29]

tient shock as well as with hemorrhagic pancreatitis.[23] Decline of complement proteins such as C3 has been thought to be correlated with severity of disease,[24, 25] although confirmation of this finding is still questioned.[25, 26] Additional nonlaboratory tests listed in Table 25-2 can also be used to judge severity of the disease as well as to detect possible additional or alternative organ involvement.

The final stage in the differential diagnosis of acute pancreatitis is to rule out malignant disease. Various tests have been used to determine the presence of malignant pancreatic disease, including carcinoembryonic antigen (CEA), alpha-fetoprotein (AFP), and pancreatic oncofetal antigen, among others.

TREATMENT

Treatment of acute pancreatitis usually consists of initial support for shock, reduction of food and fluids by mouth, and the necessary relief from pain.[27] Hypocalcemia with tetany should be corrected by the intravenous administration of calcium gluconate. Culture for possible infection should be taken prior to use of any antibiotic therapy. The patient should be watched closely, and periodic analyses of blood count, hematocrit, and serum amylase and/or lipase should be performed. These indices should return to within reference range upon resolution of the attack. Alternatively, further increases in the indices would indicate an extension of the attack, and require additional treatment. Conservative management is recommended, although severe or prolonged disease will require at least exploratory surgery to rectify the causative factor (*e.g.*, cholestatic liver disease, ulcer, hemorrhagic lesions, abscess, pseudocysts). The patient will be maintained on a low-fat diet and antacids until attacks subside.

The resolution of the disease can be followed by the return to reference range levels of the diagnostic indices described above. Disease resolution will depend on the cause and severity of the disease and the course of treatment pursued by the physician.

CASE STUDY

An 85-year-old man was seen in the emergency room after several hours of severe cramping, nonradiating, epigastric, and upper quadrant pain, nausea, and vomiting. There was no history of chills, cough, or diarrhea. The patient was observed to be cool and diaphoretic but otherwise unremarkable, with the exception of a diffusely tender abdomen, especially in the right upper quadrant. No rebound was evident, but a poorly defined mass was felt in the right upper quadrant.

Past medical problems included congestive heart failure, ischemic heart disease, type-II diabetes with hyperlipidemia, and organic brain disease, which have resulted in multiple hospital stays. The patient was taking the following medications: digoxin, lasix, nitrol paste, and nitroglycerin. He smoked (50 pack/year), but reportedly drank no alcohol. Initial laboratory findings revealed greatly elevated triglycerides, cholesterol, glucose, ALP (3 × normal), serum amylase ($2^1/_2$ × normal), lipase (3 × normal), LD (10 × normal), CK (4 × normal), with negative MB-CK. Urinary and serum ketones were moderately positive; blood urea nitrogen (BUN) was 21 mg/dL (7.5 mmol/L), and total bilirubin was 1.2 mg/dL (20.5 μmol/L). The patient underwent sonographic and x-ray studies that indicated the presence of a 6-mm pancreatic mass.

Questions

1. Given this patient's history, clinical findings, and laboratory results, what conditions probably exist?
2. What procedure might confirm a diagnosis in this case?

Discussion

1. In addition to acute pancreatitis and possibly chronic pancreatitis, an underlying familial lipid disorder appears to exist, along with probable coronary artery disease. The pancreatitis has apparently aggravated the ongoing diabetes.

2. A surgical procedure was performed in this case. Acute hemorrhagic pancreatitis and fibrotic chronic pancreatitis were found.

REFERENCES

1. Ranson JHC: Acute pancreatitis: Where are we? Surg Clin North Am: 55, 1981
2. Cruetzfeldt W, Schmidt H: Aetiology and pathogenesis of pancreatitis (current concepts). Scand J Gastroenterol (suppl 6):47–62, 1970
3. DiMagno EP, Bell JS: Acute pancreatitis and pancreatic injuries. In Gitnick G (ed): Handbook of Gastrointestinal Emergencies, pp 215–259. Gordon City, NY, Medical Examination Pub, 1982
4. Spechler SJ: How much can we know about acute pancreatitis? Ann Intern Med 102:704–705, 1985
5. Ventrucci M, Gullo L, Daniele C et al: Comparative study of serum pancreatic isoamylase, lipasc, and trypsin-like immunoreactivity in pancreatic disease. Digestion 28:114–121, 1983
6. Moosa AR: Diagnostic tests and procedures in acute pancreatitis. N Engl J Med 311:639–643, 1984
7. Steinberg WM, Goldstein SS, David ND et al: Diagnostic assays in acute pancreatitis. Ann Intern Med 102:576–580, 1985
8. Eckfeldt JH, Kolars JC, Elson MK et al: Serum tests for pancreatitis in patients with abdominal pain. Arch Pathol Lab Med 109:316–319, 1985
9. Hathaway JA, Kitt D, Wingate B: A comparison of currently used lipase and amylase procedures in the serial detection of enzyme elevations in acute pancreatitis. Clin Chim Acta 133:327–330, 1983
10. Orda R, Orda S, Baron J et al: Lipase turbidimetric assay and acute pancreatitis. Dig Dis Sci 29:294–296, 1984
11. Williamson T: The estimation of pancreatic lipase: A brief review. Med Lab Sci 33:265–279, 1976
12. Mayer AD, McMahon MJ, Holdsworth PJ et al: Screening for acute pancreatitis: A rapid assay for plasma lipase. Br J Surg 72:436–437, 1985
13. Moller-Petersen JT, Klaerke M, Dati F et al: Immunochemical qualitative latex agglutination test for pancreatic lipase in serum evaluated for use in diagnosis of acute pancreatitis. Clin Chem 31:1207–1210, 1985
14. Lott JA, Speicher CE, Nemesanszky E: Is serum amylase an obsolete test in the diagnosis of acute pancreatitis? Arch Pathol Lab Med 109:314–315, 1985
15. Lott JA: Inflammatory diseases of the pancreas. CRC Crit Rev Clin Lab Sci 17:201–228, 1982
16. Williamson RCN: Early assessment of severity in acute pancreatitis. Gut 25:1331–1339, 1984
17. Warshaw AL, Lee KH: Serum ribonuclease elevations and pancreatitis. Surgery 86:227–234, 1979
18. Berry AR, Taylor TV, Davies GC: Pulmonary function and fibrinogen metabolism in acute pancreatitis. Br J Surg 68:870–873, 1981
19. Ranson JHC, Lackner H, Berman IR et al: The relationship of coagulation factors to clinical complications of acute pancreatitis. Surgery 81:502–511, 1977
20. Winstone NE: Methaemalbumin in acute pancreatitis. Br J Surg 52:804–808, 1965
21. Lankisch PG, Koop H, Otto J et al: Pulmonary function and fibrinogen in acute pancreatitis. Scand J Gastroenterol 13:975–978, 1978
22. Mackie CR, Moosa, AR, Go VLW et al: Prospective evaluation of some candidate tumor markers in the diagnosis of acute pancreatitis. Dig Dis Sci 25:161–172, 1980
23. Overy RD, Evans M, Pollack AV: Fluid sequestration: An accurate index of severity in acute pancreatitis in man. Br J Surg 67:817, 1980
24. Foulas AK, Murray WR, Galloway D et al: Endotoxemia and complement activation in acute pancreatitis. Gut 23:656–661, 1982
25. Williamson RCN: Early assessment of severity in acute pancreatitis. Gut 25:1331–1339, 1984
26. Whicher JT, Barnes MP, Brown A et al: Complement activation and complement control proteins in acute pancreatitis. Gut 23:944–950, 1982
27. Krupp MA, Chatton MJ: Current Medical Diagnosis and Treatment, pp 405–408. Los Altos, CA, Lange Medical Publications, 1982
28. Pace BW, Bank S, Wise L et al: Amylase isoenzymes in the acute abdomen: An adjunct in those patients with elevated total amylase. Am J Gastroenterol 80:898–901, 1985
29. Blamey SL, Imrie CW, O'Neill J et al: Prognostic factors in acute pancreatitis. Gut 25:1340–1346, 1984
30. Holdsworth PJ, Mayer AD, Wilson DH et al: A simple screening test for acute pancreatitis. Br J Surg 71:958–959, 1984

31. Massey TH: Efficiency in the diagnosis of acute pancreatitis increases by improved electrophoresis of amylase isoenzyme P_3 on cellulose acetate. Clin Chem 31:70–75, 1985
32. Jacobson DG, Curington C, Connery K et al: Trypsin-like immunoreactivity as a test for pancreatic insufficiency. N Engl J Med 310:1307–1309, 1984
33. Mayer AD, McMahon MJ, Bowen M et al: C-reactive protein: An aid to assessment and monitoring of acute pancreatitis. J Clin Pathol 37:207–211, 1984

Chapter 26

Chronic Inflammatory Bowel Disorders

R. Lyle Christensen

Inflammatory bowel disorders (IBD) cannot at this time be diagnosed by specific biochemical, immunological, or microbiological features. The diagnosis of these diseases, therefore, is based on macroscopic and microscopic analyses of the bowel lesions, on clinical signs and symptoms, and on the exclusion of other disorders.

ETIOLOGY AND PATHOPHYSIOLOGY

Classification

Inflammatory bowel disease is classified as one of two important chronic disorders: either as Crohn's disease, first described in 1932,[1] or as ulcerative colitis. Both of these disorders progress from acute to chronic stages, with the majority of their symptoms appearing in the chronic phase. These diseases are classified and differentiated macroscopically as seen in Table 26-1. *Crohn's disease,* a form of regional enteritis, is characterized by transmural inflammation of the gastrointestinal tract in any location from the mouth to the anus, with anal lesions being very common. *Ulcerative colitis* involves the colon primarily, often presenting with pseudopolyps not common in Crohn's disease.

Table 26-1 ***Macroscopic Differences Between Ulcerative Colitis and Crohn's Disease***

Ulcerative Colitis	Crohn's Disease
Colonic involvement only	Mouth to anus at risk
Continuous disease	Discontinuous lesions
Rectum usually involved	Rectal sparing frequent (50%)
"Backwash" ileitis (2%–5%)	Terminal ileum involved (30%)
Rectal ulceration rare	Rectal ulceration common
Fistulae rare	Fistulae common (10%–20%)
Pseudopolyps common	Pseudopolyps rare
Anal lesions fairly common (20%)	Anal lesions very common (75%)

Data from reference number [2]

Etiology

The cause of IBD is not known. A number of observations and speculations have generated causative hypotheses. Among the possibilities suggested are abnormal immunologic responses and infection, as well as dietary, psychosomatic, and genetic factors.[2, 3, 4, 5] Additionally, there may be an interaction between any or all of these factors and responses.

Epidemiology

The incidence of the two diseases ranges from 1.0 to 6.0 per 100,000 for Crohn's disease, and from 3.2 to 7.6 per 100,000 for ulcerative colitis.[6] White populations are much more prone to both diseases than are other races, with American Jews having the highest incidence.[6] The age of onset peaks at approximately 20 years of age for both types of IBD.[6] It remains to be seen if there is a greater predisposition to the disorders in Western than in Eastern societies.

CLINICAL MANIFESTATIONS

Intestinal

The major intestinal manifestations of IBD are outlined in Table 26-2. The onset of symptoms may be more subtle in cases of Crohn's disease than in ulcerative colitis, with the type of symptom often dependent upon the lesion site.[5] The signs that appear in the two disorders are compared in Table 26-3. Crohn's disease commonly (>40% of the time) presents with signs of bloody diarrhea, abdominal mass, perianal disease, and malabsorption, in contrast to ulcerative colitis, which presents primarily as bloody diarrhea (>90% of the time), with only rare occurrence of the other signs seen in Crohn's disease.

Extraintestinal

The manifestations not directly involved with the intestine form the basis for the only laboratory observations that can be correlated with either type of IBD.[5] Table 26-2 lists many of these findings, none of which alone is pathognomonic for IBD.

LABORATORY ANALYSES AND DIAGNOSIS

The differential diagnosis of IBD, not to mention the subclassifications, is based primarily on exclusion. Ruling out virtually all of the disorders that might present as IBD is an exhaustive undertaking, in terms of both time and cost. The major disorders that must be excluded are outlined in the box on page 304. The diagnosis is generally based on visualization of the colonic mucosa and biopsy of

Table 26-2 ***Clinical Manifestations of IBD***

Symptoms
Gastrointestinal
Abdominal pain
Weight loss
Nausea and vomiting
Extraintestinal
Nutritional abnormalities
Hypoalbuminemia, deficiencies (vitamins, calcium, zinc, magnesium, phosphate)
Hematologic abnormalities
Anemia, leukocytosis, thrombocytosis
Hepatic and biliary abnormalities
Fatty liver, percholangitis, gallstones, carcinoma of bile ducts
Renal abnormalities
Kidney stones, obstructive uropathy, fistulae to urinary tract
Signs
Gastrointestinal
Occult or overt stool blood, abdominal mass palpation, diarrhea
Extraintestinal
Skin and mucous membrane abnormalities
Arthritis: ankylosing spondylitis and sacroiliitis, large-bone involvement
Eye abnormalities: iritis, conjunctivitis, episcleritis
Psychological changes
Miscellaneous abnormalities: fever, increased thrombophlebitis

Data from reference numbers [3, 4, 5]

Disorders to be Considered in the Differential Diagnosis of IBD

Acute bacillary dysentery
Amebiasis
Pseudomembranous colitis
Ischemic colitis
Colonic neoplasms
Angiodysplasia
Acute appendicitis
Small intestine disease (lymphoma or tuberculosis)
Duodenal ulceration
General malabsorption
Infections
Radiation proctitis
Familial polyposis

Data from reference number[4]

affected areas, colon and ileum radiography, and microorganism culture or microscopy.[5] Unfortunately, laboratory studies are of no help in the differential diagnosis except in the exclusion of other disorders. However, because exclusion is the primary means of diagnosis at the present time, laboratory studies appropriate to the conditions outlined above remain very important.

There are, however, a number of laboratory tests that are being studied for their correlation to the presence or severity of IBD. Unfortunately, at this time none of these tests possesses the diagnostic specificity necessary for the diagnosis of IBD, since they can also be affected by many of the extraintestinal manifestations listed in Table 26-2. Presently, the most utilized of these tests, especially in determining the prognosis and monitoring the course of the diseases, are the erythrocyte

Table 26-3 ***Clinical Differences Between Ulcerative Colitis and Crohn's Disease***

	Ulcerative Colitis	Crohn's Disease
Bloody diarrhea	Common (>90%)	Less common (40%–60%)
Abdominal mass	Rare	Common (40%)
Perianal disease	Less common (20%)	Common (75%)
Signs of malabsorption	None	Common (small bowel disease)

Data from reference number [2]

sedimentation rate (ESR), tests of malabsorption, serum albumin, and hematologic tests. Recent studies have evaluated other tests that show promise in differentiating IBD from other disorders. Serum orosomucoid,[7, 8] C-reactive protein,[7, 8] and α_1-antitrypsin from blood[8] and fecal[9] samples have been found to correlate well with IBD activity, especially in Crohn's disease. These tests may yet prove useful in the diagnosis of IBD.

TREATMENT

The treatment of IBD is primarily medical, and is similar regardless of which form of the disease is present. The principal drugs used are anti-inflammatory agents. Return to normality of the indices of nutritional status and hematologic, renal, and hepatic function are at this time the only tools available from the laboratory to assist in the monitoring of patients being treated for IBD. The resolution of histologic and macroscopic abnormalities listed in Table 26-2 is also used in the assessment of successful treatment and recovery of the IBD patient. Further, there are indications that disease activity may be monitored by following the orosomucoid levels and the ESR with disease relapse as well as assessing activity by the level of C-reactive protein.[8] Finally, it is important for the nutritional status of the patient to be maintained. Indicators such as albumin[8] have been useful as to nutritional status.[4] Failure to respond to medical management, however, may result in surgical intervention.

CASE STUDY

A 20-year-old man was admitted for evaluation of an "eating disorder" and abdominal pain. The patient's recent history included reports of a chronic sore throat and dysphagia over the past 6 years. About 2 years after those began, the patient developed mild epigastric pain accompanied by vomiting after solid-food meals. At that time, the patient began a liquid only diet that relieved most of the symptoms. Diarrhea and abdominal pain were experienced intermittently over the course of the next 4 years. There was no history of smoking or drinking, and no fever, chills, or homosexual contacts.

The patient was a light-complected man who presented as thin for his size (weight 65 kg, height 190 cm). His temperature was 37.4° C, blood pressure was 140/70, pulse was 108, and respirations were 18. Bowel sounds were elevated, without hardness or palpable masses. Cardiac and pulmonary examinations were unremarkable. Rectal examination, however, presented with a maroon stool that gave a 4+ result in the test for occult blood; otherwise the examination was unremarkable. Upon questioning, both of the patient's parents were found to have experienced undiagnosed ulcerative colitis. This was deduced by histories of problems of chronic mild diarrhea, intermittent bloody stools, and cramping pain. His mother had had a 20-year history of diabetes mellitus.

Laboratory analysis revealed a hematocrit of 45%; white count of $9.5 \times 10^3/mm^3$, with 57% neutrophils, 25% lymphocytes, 9% monocytes, 7% eosinophils, and 2% basophils. The ESR was within reference limits at 2 mm/h. Other tests, such as liver and pancreatic function tests, were unremarkable. A biopsy via endoscopy was taken of the duodenum, with negative results upon microscopic examination, and a fiberoptic esophagogastroduodenoscopic examination was also negative. Stool examination was negative for parasites and ova. Upper gastrointestinal and small bowel radiographic studies showed an abnormal jejunum, with normal esophagus, stomach, duodenum, and ileum.

A diagnosis of Crohn's disease of the jejunum was made, based on results of a laparotomy that examined the small bowel and surrounding lymph nodes. Biopsy samples taken from the bowel and lymph were found, on microscopic examination, to include an acute inflammation, with noncaseous granulomas adjacent to the lesions.

The patient was treated with high-dose corticosteroids initially, with tapering of the dose over several months. Over this time the patient gained 7 kg. The daily stools only rarely presented with hematochezia. The patient continued to have occasional abdominal pain, and remained on a liquid diet.

Question

What assistance did the laboratory provide in making this diagnosis?

Discussion

The laboratory results, except for the occult blood test, were essentially within normal limits. These findings proved to exclude many disorders with symptoms similar to those of IBD. Because the diagnosis of IBD is primarily one of exclusion, the negative laboratory findings were important.

REFERENCES

1. Crohn BB, Ginsgurg L, Oppenheimer GD: Regional ileitis: A pathologic and clinical entity. JAMA 99: 1323–1329, 1932
2. Mowat NAG: Inflammatory bowel disease. Practitioner 228:803–810, 1984
3. Wright R: Crohn's disease: Diagnosis and management. Compr Ther 11:38–44, 1985
4. Andreoli TE, Carpenter CCJ, Plum F et al: Essentials of Medicine, pp 300–305. Philadelphia, WB Saunders, 1986
5. Shearman DJC, Finlayson NDC: Diseases of the Gastrointestinal Tract and Liver, pp 332–334, 863–903. Edinburgh, Churchill Livingstone, 1982
6. Steinhardt HJ, Loeschke K, Kasper H et al: European cooperative Crohn's disease study (ECCDS): Clinical features and natural history. Digestion 31:97–108, 1985
7. Shine B, Berghouse L, Jones JEL et al: C-reactive protein as an aid in the differentiation of functional and inflammatory bowel disorders. Clin Chim Acta 148: 105–109, 1985
8. Andre, Descos L, Andre F et al: Biological measurements of Crohn's activity—a reassessment. Hepatogastroenterology 32:135–137, 1985
9. Meyers S, Wolke A, Field SP et al: Fecal alpha$_1$-antitrypsin measurement: An indicator of Crohn's disease activity. Gastroenterology 89:13–18, 1985

Chapter 27

Gastrointestinal Malignancies

Dianne F. Johnson

Cancer may involve all areas of the gastrointestinal (GI) tract but most frequently occurs in the colon, where it is the second most common malignancy in adults in the United States. The most common type of cancer involving the GI tract is adenocarcinoma. Gastrointestinal adenocarcinoma is not common in persons under age 40, but its incidence increases steadily after that age.

In general, the clinical laboratory plays a limited role in the diagnosis of gastrointestinal malignancy. However, because this type of cancer may be relatively asymptomatic until late in its course, there is one valuable laboratory test that is used extensively to screen for early carcinoma of the gastrointestinal tract. This test, the examination of feces for occult blood, will be discussed below, as will other abnormal laboratory parameters associated with this type of cancer.

ESOPHAGEAL CARCINOMA

In the United States, carcinomas of the esophagus represent only about 10% of all the cancers of the gastrointestinal tract, but they cause a disproportionate number of cancer deaths. This type of carcinoma remains asymptomatic during much of its development, and so is often discovered too late to permit cure. Esophageal cancer occurs primarily in adults over the age of 50, and predominantly in males in a ratio of 4 : 1. For unknown reasons, blacks throughout the world are more vulnerable than whites. In the U.S., both black males and females have an approximately four-fold greater incidence than whites.[1]

The origin of this form of cancer is not well understood, but there are many strong suggestions that preexisting esophageal disease and environmental factors play important roles. The incidence of carcinoma is higher among those with esophagitis, achalasia (motor disorder of the esophagus), corrosive mucosal burns, esophageal diverticula, and esophageal webs (congenital annular narrowings of the esophagus). It seems reasonable that any esophageal disease that inappropriately exposes the mucosal surface to environmental influences might predispose to cancer. The environmental influences thought to contribute to causing this form of cancer are alcohol, smoking, and irritants such as excessively hot and spicy foods. Epidemiologic studies in the United States indicate a 25-fold increased risk among heavy drinkers, and a 6- to 7-fold increased risk among habitual smokers of cigarettes, cigars, or pipes.

About 60% to 70% of esophageal cancers are squamous cell carcinomas, 5% to 10% are adenocarcinomas, and the remainder are undifferentiated tumors. Approximately 25% of the squamous esophageal cancers are in the upper third, 50% in the middle, and 25% in the lower third of the organ. Lesions in the upper two-thirds are derived from squamous esophageal mucosa, the normal lining of the esophagus. In the distal esophagus, more than half of the cases prove to be adenocarcinomas, indicating that many cancers in this area originate from the stomach.

Clinical Presentation

Esophageal carcinoma is insidious in onset, producing symptoms gradually and late in the course of the disease. Difficulty in swallowing solid foods (*dysphagia*) is the patient's first and usually only complaint as the tumor encroaches on the lumen. Although initially intermittent, the dysphagia is progressive over a course of 6 months or less. Pain under the sternum, in the back, or in the neck is common; although it may be caused by associated spasm or esophagitis, it usually indicates spread of the tumor through the wall of the esophagus. In some cases, an early symptom may be substernal burning upon swallowing hot liquids. Extreme weight loss and debilitation result both from impaired nutrition and from effects of the tumor itself. Slow oozing of blood is a frequent complication, but brisk bleeding is rare. Occasionally, the first alarming symptom is the aspiration of food that enters the respiratory tree through a cancerous tracheo-esophageal fistula.[2, 3]

Physical examination is usually negative, and

even those patients with advanced disease may present with no more than signs of malnutrition. Although metastases to lymph nodes occur in three-fourths of the cases, only 5% have palpable lymph nodes that can be picked up on physical examinations. Because the liver and lung are each involved eventually in 20% to 25% of the cases, an enlarged liver (*hepatomegaly*) or pulmonary lesions may be evident. Other organs that may be involved with metastatic tumors of the esophagus are bone, kidneys, and adrenal glands. Sometimes direct invasion of contiguous structures leads to dramatic complications such as inflammation of the mediastinum and subsequent subcutaneous emphysema in the soft tissues of the neck, tracheoesophageal fistula with an apoplectic cough induced by swallowing liquids, or perforation of the aorta with precipitous exsanguination.

Diagnosis

An upper gastrointestinal radiographic series, the main method of diagnosis of esophageal cancer, has a diagnostic accuracy of 95% for advanced lesions. Esophagoscopy with a biopsy and cytology has a similar diagnostic yield.[2]

Therapy and Prognosis

The ideal therapy for cancer of the esophagus has not yet been determined. About 35% of patients when seen initially by the physician already will have clinical evidence of metastic disease. These patients are best treated with palliative irradiation, surgery, or insertion of indwelling tubes to circumvent the impending obstruction. Of the remaining 65% without clinically evident metastatic disease, only 20% will have truly localized disease. Therefore, a thorough workup to include a scalene lymph node biopsy (a particular lymph node in the neck that is frequently positive with this type of cancer), bronchoscopy, and liver scan should be performed before attempting curative therapy. The position of the cancer determines the mode of treatment: cervical and upper thoracic lesions are best treated with radiation, while lesions below the aortic arch are best treated surgically. The overall 5-year survival rate for all operable esophageal cancer is 15%.

GASTRIC CARCINOMA

Carcinoma of the stomach is the second most common gastrointestinal cancer in the United States, despite a continuous decrease in its incidence over the past 4 decades. The current U.S. death rate from this form of cancer is about seven to eight per 100,000 population; in 1930, it was 33 per 100,000. The reasons for this decrease are not known, but changing environmental influences are suspected. Nevertheless, gastric carcinoma remains a significant disease, responsible for approximately 8,000 deaths annually in the U.S. In Japan, the incidence of this type of carcinoma is greater: it causes approximately one-half of all cancer deaths, and is the leading cause of cancer mortality among adult males in that country. In the U.S., the incidence is higher in males and in blacks. Associated risk factors are gastric adenomatous polyps, chronic atrophic gastritis, and perhaps previous partial gastrectomy for benign peptic ulcer disease. In most patients, however, no obvious risk factors exist. Most of the cancers are adenocarcinomas.[1]

Clinical Presentation

Gastric carcinoma is an insidious disease that is generally asymptomatic until late in its course. In individuals with more advanced cancer, the frequency of symptoms is shown in Table 27-1. As noted, most of these symptoms are not very specific, rendering the diagnosis of this form of cancer quite difficult. The abdominal pain is usually referred to the epigastrium, but is often vague and intermittent. Occult bleeding is common, sometimes producing "coffee grounds" vomitus but more often associated only with guiaic-positive stools. Some patients (10%) experience massive hematemesis, sufficient to cause shock.

Table 27-1 *Advanced Gastric Carcinoma Symptomatology*

Symptom	% of Cases
Weight loss	80
Abdominal pain	72
Anorexia	57
Vomiting	44
Changed bowel habit	35
Anemic symptoms	12
Hemorrhage	10

Achlorhydria or hypochlorhydria is present in about half the patients.

All too often carcinoma of the stomach is discovered because of metastatic disease. Hepatomegaly due to metastases is already present at the time of first diagnosis in about 10% of cases. It may be accompanied by ascites and, less frequently, jaundice. Occasionally, spread to remote lymph nodes is the first sign of the gastric carcinoma. Metastases to the ovaries, referred to as *Kruckenberg tumors,* are sometimes discovered even before gastric symptoms appear.

Diagnosis

All upper gastrointestinal radiographic series, the primary method of diagnosis of gastric cancer, have a diagnostic accuracy of about 95% for advanced lesions. Gastroscopy with six to ten biopsies and cytology have a similarly high diagnostic yield.[2]

Therapy and Prognosis

The only successful treatment is surgical resection of the tumor. About 90% of patients undergo a laparotomy, with a resectability rate of about 50%. Regional lymph nodes are involved in about 70% of cases. For all patients, the 5-year survival rate is less than 10%.[1, 2, 3]

SMALL BOWEL MALIGNANCIES

Tumors of the small intestine are rare. Although the small bowel represents 75% of the length of the entire gastrointestinal tract, neoplasms in this location account for only 3% to 6% of all gastrointestinal tumors. Neoplasms of the small intestine are usually difficult to diagnose clinically because they are so uncommon and because the fluidity of the intestinal contents prevents obstructive symptoms.[1]

In contrast to other parts of the gastrointestinal tract, the most common type of malignancy in the small bowel is not carcinoma, but either an endocrine cell tumor (carcinoid) or lymphoma. Carcinomas are the third most frequently occurring type in this area.

Endocrine Cell Tumors (Argentaffinomas, Carcinoids)

Even though endocrine cell tumors have a benign histologic appearance, many invade and metastasize. Because it takes years for such cancerous behavior to be expressed, they have been called *malignant neoplasms in slow motion* or *carcinoma-like*—hence the name *carcinoids.* They arise from endocrine cells in the gut, known as *Kulchitsky cells* or *enterochromaffin cells* (because of an affinity for chrome salts). Most of these neoplasms are capable of elaborating a variety of amine and peptide products—histamine, serotonin, 5-hydroxytryptophan, ACTH, kallikrein, and sometimes prostaglandins. Some of these products may induce systemic manifestations known as *carcinoid syndrome.*

Endocrine cell tumors may appear at any age, and there is no sex predilection. These tumors are generally asymptomatic for some time, but eventually, they are likely to produce clinical manifestations in one of two ways: either by local invasion of the bowel and contiguous structures, or through their secretory products. The most common symptom is usually abdominal pain. Additional symptoms include weight loss, anorexia, nausea, weakness, rectal bleeding, and diarrhea. Occasionally, carcinoid tumors of the small bowel produce partial or complete intestinal obstruction. Less commonly, they present with metastatic nodular enlargement of the liver. Far more distinctive is the development of symptoms related to the elaboration of secretory products, listed in the box at the bottom of this page.

The major secretory product of carcinoid tumors is serotonin derived by the hydroxylation of tryptophan to 5-hydroxytryptophan, followed by its decarboxylation to serotonin. Most of this product is degraded to 5-hydroxyindoleacetic acid (5HIAA). The identification of 5HIAA in the urine provides an important diagnostic marker for this syndrome.

Carcinoid tumors may also occur in other locations in the gastrointestinal tract, such as the stomach, appendix, and rectum. Extra-gastrointestinal locations include the ovaries and lungs. The full-blown carcinoid syndrome tends to occur in carcinoid tumors located in ovaries and lungs, or in cases with extensive liver metastases. Only 5% to 10% of small bowel carcinoids produce the carcinoid syndrome.

Therapy and Prognosis

Surgical excision remains the only method of cure for this disease. Appendiceal carcinoids are usually discovered incidentally after the appendix has been removed, and are cured by the appendectomy except in the rare instances in which metastasis has occurred. In contrast, 5-year survival rates after surgical therapy range from 50% for carcinoids of the small bowel and appendix to 80% for those of the rectum. A major consideration in the management of patients with endocrine cell tumors is the associated increased incidence of other malignant neoplasms, some of which occur in extraintestinal sites. These are found in about 15% of patients with carcinoids of the rectum, and in about 30% of those with carcinoids of the small intestine. About half of these concurrent cancers occur in the gastrointestinal tract. It is therefore imperative that careful surgical exploration be done during excision of a gastrointestinal carcinoid, to rule out the possible presence of another malignancy.[1, 3]

Carcinoma of the Small Bowel

As stated above, adenocarcinomas are very uncommon in the small bowel. When they do occur, crampy pain, nausea, vomiting, and weight loss are the common presenting signs and symptoms, but such manifestations generally appear late in the course of these cancers. Thus, most have already penetrated the bowel wall, invaded the mesentery or other segments of the intestine, spread to regional lymph nodes, and sometimes metastasized to the liver. Despite these problems, wide "en bloc" excision of these cancers yields about a 70% 5-year survival rate.[1]

Secretion-Related Symptoms

1. Vasomotor disturbances—Episodic flushing of the skin and cyanosis (90%–100%)
2. Intestinal hypermotility—Diarrhea, cramps, nausea, and vomiting (90%–100%)
3. Bronchoconstrictive attacks—Cough, dyspnea, and wheezing resembling asthma (33%)
4. Right-sided cardiac involvement—Valvular thickening and stenosis (50%)
5. Hepatomegaly—Related to hepatic metastases (5%–10%)

COLORECTAL CARCINOMA

Colorectal cancer, 98% of which are carcinomas, is the second most common malignancy in adults in the United States. This type of cancer represents one of the prime challenges to the medical profession, because it produces subtle signals and symptoms relatively early, and at this stage is generally curable by resection. Too often these early symptoms are ignored by the patient and sometimes insufficiently investigated by the physician. Carcinoma of the large bowel has its peak incidence in the seventh decade of life. Fewer than 20% of cases are diagnosed in persons under the age of 50. When the neoplasm occurs in the rectum, there is a male-to-female ratio of approximately 2 : 1. In more proximal levels of the large bowel, there is no sex predominance.

Clinical Presentation

It is now appreciated that carcinoma of the large bowel is present for a considerable time before it produces clinical symptoms. Common symptoms and signs are abdominal pain, change in bowel habit, blood in or on the stools, anemia, and occasionally a palpable rectal or abdominal mass.[2, 3]

Diagnosis

The diagnosis of colorectal carcinoma relies on a great variety of techniques, including tests for occult blood in the stool, digital examination, proctoscopy, sigmoidoscopy, colonoscopy, contrast radiographic studies, and CT scans. Of all colorectal cancers, up to 10% to 15% may be detected by digital rectal examination, and up to 50% by proctosigmoidoscopy. It is essential to do a barium enema in all patients with colorectal symptoms, in order to detect lesions beyond the range of the sigmoidoscope and also to look for synchronous colonic neoplasms. A second cancer or benign polyp develops simultaneously in 20% of patients with one colonic cancer. Colonoscopy with biopsies is indicated if the barium enema is unsatisfactory.[2]

Therapy and Prognosis

Most patients require either curative or palliative resection of the tumor. The overall 5-year survival rate is about 40%. The prognosis depends on location, lymph node involvement, and cellular differentiation of the tumor. Chemotherapy and radiation therapy do not appreciably improve the survival rate. A regular program of followup visits should be established postoperatively because of the high incidence of recurrence.

LABORATORY ROLE IN DIAGNOSIS AND FOLLOWUP OF GASTROINTESTINAL MALIGNANCY

In general, laboratory tests are of limited value in diagnosing and evaluating patients with gastrointestinal carcinoma. Other diagnostic aids, such as x-ray examinations (upper GI series and barium enema) and directed visualization techniques (esophagogastro-duodenoscopy, proctoscopy, sigmoidoscopy, and colonoscopy), have proven to be much more sensitive. However, various laboratory tests are utilized in conjunction with the above methods to assist in the diagnosis and followup of patients with gastrointestinal malignancy.

Occult Blood

A very useful screening test is examination of the feces for blood. Usually this blood is occult, although sometimes it is grossly visible. Occult blood in the stool may be tested during the initial physical examination by using one of several commercial products available for this purpose. A single negative test, however, should not be interpreted as ruling out cancer. Multiple (at least three) examinations should be performed, and more than one area of the stool sample should be tested. Blood may also be found in gastric contents in patients with carcinoma of the stomach[4] (see also Chap. 23).

Carcinoembryonic Antigen (CEA)

When first described, CEA appeared to be a tumor-specific test for colon cancer that would enable early diagnosis in asymptomatic patients. This has not proved to be the case. Moreover, in screening large populations for colon cancer, CEA was found to have a false-positive rate of 15% and a false-negative rate of 40% to 60% in nonmetastatic disease. Thus, the test lacks both the specificity and the sensitivity to be useful for screening. Moreover, most asymptomatic patients with early stages of colon cancer have normal CEA values in their blood, and patients with elevated CEA tend to be those with more advanced cancer. More valuable is the use of CEA levels to assess the patient's condition following resection of the tumor. If total removal has been accomplished, the CEA levels disappear. Return of CEA positivity is a reliable indicator of recurrence of the tumor. Similarly, the CEA test can provide a rough estimation of the effectiveness of chemotherapy. However, caution must be used in interpreting this test because positive CEA levels may also be produced by cancers of the lung, breast, ovary, bladder, and prostate, as well as a number of nonneoplastic disorders, including alcoholic cirrhosis, pancreatitis, and ulcerative colitis.[1, 4]

Gastric Acidity

Varying degrees of hypochlorhydria and achlorhydria accompany atrophic gastritis and gastric cancer. However, a decrease in production of gastric acid occurs normally with the aging process, so that determination of gastric secretory function should not be used as a diagnostic tool for detecting gastric cancer. Some individuals believe that the absence of gastric acid after pentagastrin stimulation should raise suspicion of cancer in patients with gastric ulcers. In reality, about 50% of patients with gastric carcinoma have no gastric acid, even following stimulation, and 50% have normal or decreased gastric acid. Therefore, endoscopic evaluation with biopsy and cytology is a much more effective and direct approach to this diagnostic problem.

Serum Gastrin Levels

Some patients with hypochlorhydria associated with gastric cancer will also have an increased serum gastrin. Serum gastrin levels are quite high in patients who, in addition to their cancer, have chronic atrophic gastritis involving the proximal stomach with sparing of the antrum. However, when atrophic gastritis involves the entire stomach, including the antrum, serum gastrin levels are low or normal. Furthermore, patients with concomitant pernicious anemia and carcinoma may have very high serum gastrin levels. Because of this variability, serum gastrin levels are not useful as a screening test for gastric cancer.

Anemia

Between 35% and 45% of patients with gastrointestinal carcinoma are anemic at the time of presentation. This is usually due to chronic blood loss and iron deficiency. The anemia, therefore, is most often hypochromic and microcytic, except in those patients with underlying pernicious anemia or folate deficiency, in whom the anemia may be megaloblastic or mixed in type.

Liver Function Tests

Elevations of serum bilirubin levels, alkaline phosphatase, and 5-nucleotidase activities may indicate metastatic liver disease. If these are abnormal and hepatic metastases are suspected, radionuclide liver scan and ultrasonographic or computerized tomography of the liver should be performed. Hypoalbuminemia suggests malnutrition and advanced disease.

Serotonin and 5-hydroxyindoleacetic Acid (5-HIAA)

Patients with carcinoid syndrome will have increased levels of 5-HIAA in the urine. Blood and urine serotonin levels will also be elevated.[4] However, the ingestion of foods containing serotonin may complicate the biochemical diagnosis of carcinoid syndrome; both walnuts and bananas contain enough serotonin to produce abnormally elevated urinary excretion of 5-HIAA after their ingestion.[3]

Miscellaneous Laboratory Abnormalities

Elevated urea nitrogen or creatinine levels in the serum may be due to blockage of the ureters by expanding metastases. Decreased serum protein reflects protein loss in the stool or poor dietary intake. Leukocytosis and increased sedimentation rate occur with associated inflammation and necrosis of the tumor. Decreased serum potassium may occur as a result of potassium loss from a special histologic type of tumor of the rectum called a *villous adenoma.*

CASE STUDY

Mr. C., a 60 year-old man, presented to his physician with complaints of persistent, crampy abdominal pain, diarrhea, intermittent nausea and vomiting, anorexia, and a 20-lb weight loss over a 4-week period. He also related episodes of "flushing" of the face, at which time his heart seemed to beat "too fast." These episodes occurred more often following a meal. In addition, Mr. C. complained of an uncomfortable fullness in his right upper quadrant.

Physical examination revealed only an enlarged liver. Vital signs were within normal limits.

A liver-spleen scan showed the presence of several variably-sized mass lesions throughout both lobes of the liver, consistent with metastatic disease. An upper GI series with small bowel follow-through showed a small mass within the distal ileum. A short segment of small bowel that included this lesion was subsequently resected, and a representative biopsy of the liver mass was also taken during the surgical procedure. Histologic examination of both the small bowel and the liver masses had identical results.

Urine 5HIAA was measured, and found to be markedly increased.

Questions

1. What is the most likely diagnosis in this patient?
2. What laboratory test is needed to confirm the diagnosis of carcinoid syndrome?
3. Why is an appropriate diet necessary prior to collecting a specimen for 5-HIAA?

Discussion

1. Clinical symptomatology, metastatic lesions in the liver, and location of the tumor in the small bowel suggest that this patient is suffering from carcinoid syndrome.
2. The diagnostic hallmark of carcinoid syndrome is overproduction of 5-hydroxyindoleacetic acid. Normally, excretion of 5-HIAA does not exceed 9 mg daily. Elevations in the range of 9 to 25 mg may be seen with carcinoid syndrome, nontropical sprue, or acute intestinal obstruction. A urinary excretion of more than 25 mg 5-HIAA/24 hours is diagnostic of carcinoid syndrome.
3. Ingestion of foods containing serotonin may complicate the biochemical diagnosis of carcinoid syndrome; both walnuts and bananas contain enough serotonin to produce abnormally elevated urinary excretion of 5-HIAA after their ingestion.

REFERENCES

1. Robbins, Cotran, Kuman: Pathologic Basis of Disease, 3rd ed. Philadelphia, WB Saunders, 1984
2. Reller, Sahn, Schrier: Clinical Internal Medicine, Boston, Little, Brown Co, 1979
3. Isselbacher KJ: Harrison's Principles of Internal Medicine, 9th ed. New York City, McGraw-Hill, 1980
4. Henry: Clinical Diagnosis and Management by Laboratory Methods, 17th ed. Philadelphia, WB Saunders, 1984

Part VI

THE HEPATOBILIARY SYSTEM

Janet Duben-Von Laufen,
Associate Editor,
and Barbara Smith Michael

The liver is not only the largest organ in the body, it is also one of the most important and versatile. It is a complex organ responsible for a variety of functions, including production of bile, synthesis of serum proteins, regulation of blood glucose levels and fat metabolism, detoxification of drugs and other potentially harmful waste products, storage of several vitamins and other substances such as ferritin, and the excretion of substances such as bilirubin. The liver is also responsible for the phagocytosis of microorganisms and other foreign bodies, and the synthesis of various enzymes (*e.g.,* AST and ALT). Liver dysfunction can, therefore, result in a wide variety of clinical symptoms and effects.

The liver weighs about 1.5 kilograms in the average adult and is located in the upper right quadrant of the abdominal cavity, directly under the diaphragm. It consists of two externally distinguishable lobes and is supplied with an abundant amount of blood through the hepatic artery and portal vein. The illustration below shows a detailed diagram of the liver and biliary system. Internally, the basic structural and functional unit of the liver is the hepatic lobule (illustrated on page 320).

One important function of the liver is the production of bile. Drainage of bile from the liver occurs through a treelike network of excretory ducts (bile ducts or the biliary system) that ultimately empty into the duodenum through the common bile duct.

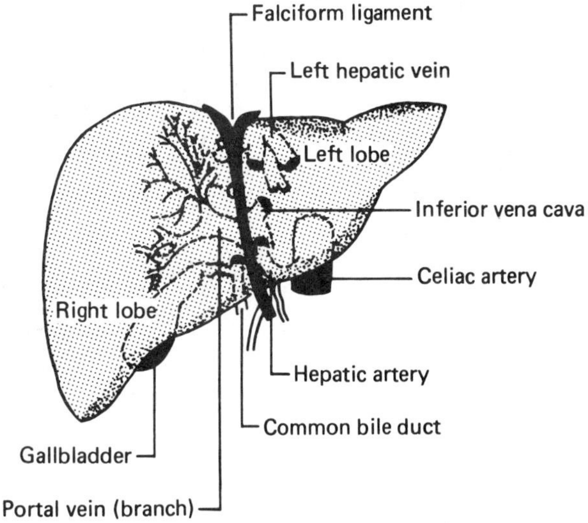

Gross anatomy of the liver showing major blood vessels and bile channels. (In Bishop ML, Duben-Von Laufen JL, Fody EP: Clinical Chemistry, p 438. Philadelphia, JB Lippincott, 1985. Adapted from Tietz NW: Fundamentals of Clinical Chemistry. Philadelphia, WB Saunders, 1976)

A second important function of the liver is the excretion of bilirubin, the principal pigment of bile. Bilirubin is derived from the breakdown of hemoglobin when aged red blood cells are phagocytized by the reticuloendothelial system (page 321).

The functional status of the hepatobiliary system may be evaluated through a range of diagnostic laboratory and radiologic tests; however, as will be shown in the chapters that follow, no one test is sufficient for diagnosis of a particular disorder, and a combination of different tests is needed to evaluate hepatobiliary function.

Laboratory tests are valuable for the diagnosis of hepatobiliary disorders as well as for differentiating specific dysfunctions and for monitoring patients with known hepatobiliary disease. Clinical laboratory tests typically used to diagnose liver disease are outlined on page 322.

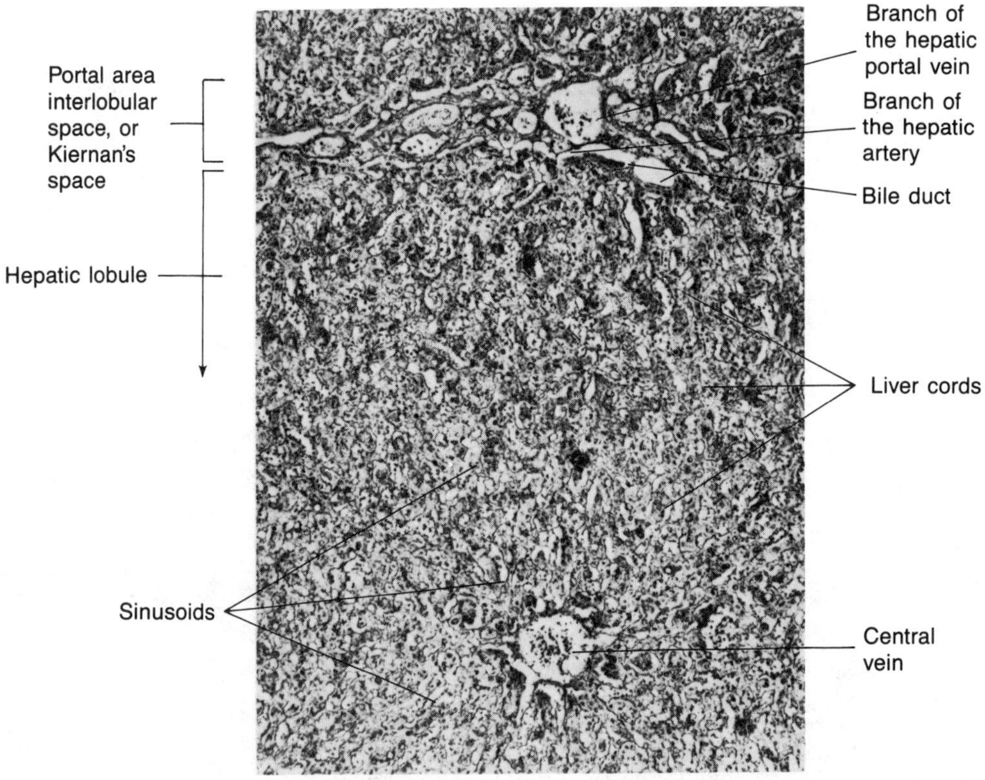

Liver lobule (panoramic view). (Photograph courtesy of James Furlong, MD)

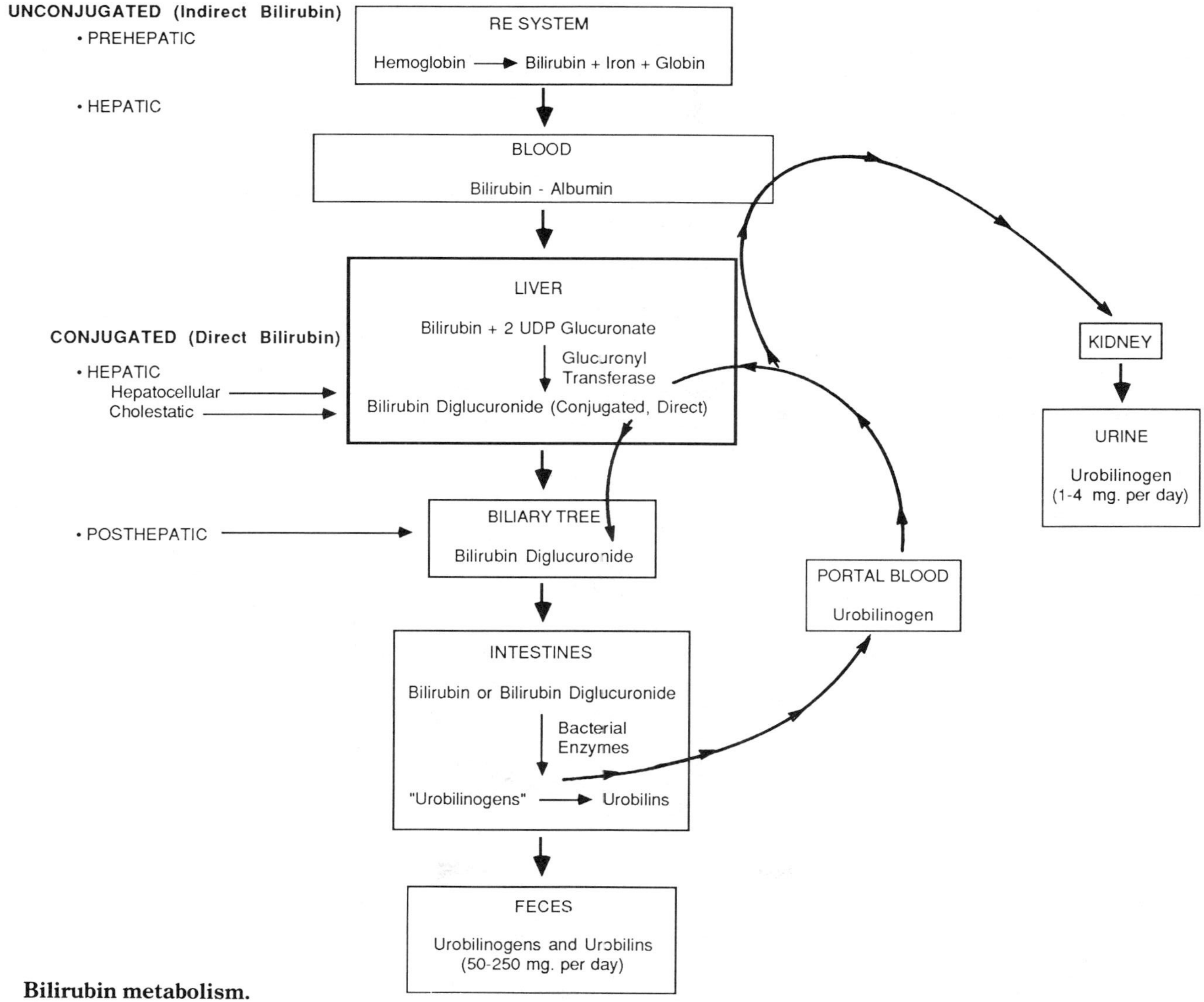

Bilirubin metabolism.

Laboratory Tests Commonly Used To Diagnose Hepatobiliary Disorders

Serum bilirubin (total and direct)
Urine bilirubin and urobilinogen
Total protein
Albumin
Aspartate aminotransferase (AST) (formerly SGOT)
Alanine aminotransferase (ALT) (formerly SGPT)
Alkaline phosphatase (ALP)
Prothrombin time

Because of the variety of clinical effects possible, classification of hepatobiliary disorders is not an easy task. Jaundice (hyperbilirubinemia) is the most obvious clinical sign, and often the most serious indication of hepatobiliary dysfunction. It is frequently used to classify the various types of disorders. The tabular material on page 323 presents a classification of jaundice, with the corresponding physiologic defect, and some examples of etiology.

Chapter 28 discusses jaundice as the major sign of hepatobiliary dysfunction. The remaining chapters of this section discuss the presenting symptoms, etiology, and diagnostic tests used in the diagnosis of specific hepatobiliary disorders.

Classification of Jaundice (Hyperbilirubinemia)

Classification	Physiologic Defect	Examples of Etiology
Unconjugated Bilirubin (Indirect)		
Prehepatic	Increased production of bilirubin	Hemolytic states Extensive hematoma
Hepatic	Defective transport of bilirubin from sinusoidal blood into hepatocyte	Gilbert syndrome Some toxins (*e.g.*, flavaspidic acid)
	Inability to conjugate	Crigler-Najjar syndrome Neonatal jaundice Some drugs (*e.g.*, Novobiocin)
Conjugated Bilirubin (Direct)		
Hepatic		
Hepatocellular	Hepatocyte injury	Viral or toxic hepatitis, cirrhosis, alcoholic hepatitis, other causes of hepatocyte injury
Cholestatic	Intrahepatic cholestasis owing to defective transport of bilirubin into the canaliculus	Some drugs (*e.g.*, anabolic steroids), viral hepatitis, primary biliary cirrhosis, some forms of familial jaundice
Posthepatic	Mechanical obstruction of biliary tree	Carcinoma of pancreas or common bile duct Choledocholithiasis (calculi) Other anatomic obstruction

Adapted from Henry JB: Clinical Diagnosis and Management by Laboratory Methods, p 223. Philadelphia: WB Saunders, 1984

Chapter 28

Jaundice

Robin Gaynor Krefetz

Jaundice is a yellow pigmentation of the skin and sclera of the eyes caused directly by an increase in the level of bilirubin in the serum. The first evidence of clinical jaundice may be seen in the sclera or whites of the eyes, because this tissue has a special affinity for bilirubin. Increasing levels of bilirubin subsequently cause the skin to take on a yellow color as well.

The clinical finding of jaundice can indicate several different types of disease. A careful medical history, including family history, as well as several important laboratory tests will help to identify the cause of the jaundice. Determining whether the increased bilirubin is primarily conjugated or unconjugated may also help to identify the cause of the jaundice.

Jaundice is a symptom and not a disease; however, it occurs because of one or more mechanisms that are related to specific disease processes. This chapter will discuss primarily these mechanisms. Other chapters in the text discuss specific disease entities in detail.

ETIOLOGY AND PATHOPHYSIOLOGY

The high levels of serum bilirubin that lead to jaundice can occur by means of mechanisms that can be classified as prehepatic, hepatic, and posthepatic, outlined as follows:

Prehepatic Jaundice

The term *prehepatic jaundice* refers to a type of jaundice resulting from an increased breakdown of hemoglobin. Usually there is no active liver disease, and the term "prehepatic" is used. The increased breakdown of hemoglobin to bilirubin occurs because of hemolysis of erythrocytes. A hemolytic state may develop, for many reasons. For example, hemolysis may occur because of an abnormality within the red blood cell, such as a vitamin B_{12} or folic acid deficiency, a defective cell membrane, an enzyme deficiency such as the lack of G-6-PD, or a hemoglobinopathy. Hemolysis may also occur due to chemical agents, disease states such as cancer, or antibodies or drugs coating the red blood cells. Hemolytic disease of the newborn is a hemolytic anemia caused by lysis of fetal red cells by maternal antibodies that coat them. Danger to the neonate occurs when bilirubin levels exceed 20 mg/dL (342 μmol/L), causing kernicteris or bilirubin encephalopathy and brain damage (see Chaps. 41 and 76).

Hepatic Jaundice

The second type of jaundice is *hepatic* or *hepatocellular jaundice.* Jaundice develops in this case because of a problem in the liver parenchyma. Hepatocellular jaundice can be further classified as diffuse hepatocellular jaundice, conjugation failure, and bilirubin transport problems. The latter two types refer respectively to the inability of bilirubin to be made water-soluble (conjugated) for excretion, and to a problem with transporting the conjugated bilirubin within the liver or outside the liver to the intestine.

The two primary *hepatocellular diseases* causing jaundice are hepatitis and cirrhosis. Both of these diseases are discussed in greater detail in Chapters 29 and 32.

Hepatitis, regardless of etiology, is characterized by necrosis and inflammation of hepatic cells. Because of impaired excretion by these cells, bilirubin reenters the systemic circulation, eventually causing jaundice. Unconjugated bilirubin may also increase, due to both impaired uptake and impaired conjugation of bilirubin.

Classification of Hepatocellular Disease

1. Diffuse Hepatocellular Diseases
   (a) Viral hepatitis
   (b) Toxic or drug-induced hepatitis
   (c) Cirrhosis
2. Conjugation Failure
   (a) Physiologic jaundice of the newborn
   (b) Criglar-Najjar disease—type I and type II
3. Bilirubin Transport Problems
   (a) Gilbert's disease
   (b) Dubin-Johnson syndrome
   (c) Rotor's syndrome

Liver cirrhosis is a chronic liver disease characterized by diffuse liver cell destruction with fibrosis and nodular regeneration of liver cells. Due to progressive loss of liver cells, there are elevated levels of both conjugated and unconjugated bilirubin, with conjugated bilirubin predominating.

Among the important functions of the liver is transforming bilirubin into a water-soluble substance, bilirubin diglucuronide. This form of bilirubin can then be excreted by the kidney. Presence of the enzyme UDP-glucuronyl transferase is required for this transformation to occur in the liver. Two liver conditions involve the absence or decreased level of this enzyme: physiologic jaundice of the newborn, and Criglar-Najjar syndrome—type I and type II.

Approximately 50% of full-term newborns become jaundiced in the first week of life. Bilirubin levels peak on the third day of life and diminish rapidly.[1] The jaundice in the neonate has been termed *physiologic jaundice of the newborn,* and occurs because the enzyme UDP-glucuronyl transferase is one of the last functions of the liver to develop. Full-term as well as premature infants can be born before the liver has developed sufficiently to produce this enzyme.[2] Any increased hemolysis of red cells also adds an additional bilirubin load for conjugation by an already immature liver.

The affected infants develop a rapid buildup of unconjugated bilirubin, which can pass into the brain and nerve cells and result in kernicterus if serum levels become sufficiently high. Most newborns' bilirubin levels return to a safe range within a few days because of the initiation of production of the required enzyme. Breast-fed infants tend to have increased bilirubin levels for longer time periods than do formula-fed infants.[3] Regular bilirubin levels performed on heelstick specimens are used to monitor the course of physiologic jaundice and to assure the clinician that normal bilirubin metabolism has been attained.

The *Crigler-Najjar syndrome* is a rare, inherited disorder affecting the enzyme UDP-glucuronyl transferase. Type I is the more severe form, involving the complete absence of the enzyme. This disease usually results in early death due to kernicterus. Type II is less severe, and involves reduced levels of the enzyme. Patients with this disease can live to adulthood yet remain moderately jaundiced.[4] Both forms of the disease involve an elevation of unconjugated bilirubin.

Several diseases involve jaundice caused by the inability of the liver to properly transport conjugated or unconjugated bilirubin within or from the liver. They are inherited chronic diseases, and include Gilbert's syndrome, the Dubin-Johnson syndrome, and Rotor's syndrome.

Gilbert's syndrome is a mild, chronic, unconjugated hyperbilirubinemia found in patients who do not have structural liver disease or overt hemolysis. It is an inherited disorder found in 5% of the population, and predominately in males.[5] It is usually detected in adolescence coincidentally with other diseases. It results from impaired ability of the liver to excrete an increased bilirubin load. It may also be due to a slight decrease in the enzyme UDP-glucuronyl transferase. A distinctive diagnostic feature is that bilirubin levels rise after prolonged fasting or calorie deprivation.[6]

The *Dubin-Johnson syndrome* is a benign hyperbilirubinemia characterized by dark pigmentation in the liver cells. There is a defect in the ability of the liver to transport conjugated bilirubin from the liver cells to the bile. The gallbladder or other parts of the biliary tract cannot be visualized with x-ray studies in this syndrome.

Rotor's syndrome is very similar to the Dubin-Johnson syndrome in that it is a chronic, conjugated hyperbilirubinemia without evidence of hemolysis. The major distinction between the two syndromes is that a liver biopsy from patients with Rotor's syndrome fails to have the dark pigment found in the Dubin-Johnson syndrome. Jaundice may increase when these patients develop an infection. Unlike in the Dubin-Johnson syndrome, the gallbladder can be visualized during x-ray studies in patients with Rotor's syndrome.[7]

Posthepatic Jaundice

Posthepatic jaundice does not result from a disease affecting liver function, but rather from an obstruction blocking the flow of bile from a normally functioning organ. The obstruction can be caused by gallstones in the common bile duct, a stricture severe enough to cause blockage, or an obstructing tumor.

The most common obstructive jaundice is from *gallstones* blocking the flow of bile in the common bile duct. Stones usually form in the gallbladder, but can cause blockage if they involve the common bile duct. Gallstones may be present for years without causing problems to the patient.

A *stricture* in the extrahepatic bile ducts can be caused by trauma during abdominal surgery or by a congenital defect. Jaundice may appear early, or may be delayed for several months or years. The stricture may cause a complete or a partial blockage.

Cancerous obstructions of the extrahepatic bile ducts are also causes of a posthepatic jaundice.

Other Causes of Jaundice

Jaundice that occurs during pregnancy is rare, with an incidence of approximately one case per 1500 pregnancies, and is rarely an indication to interrupt a pregnancy.[9] Jaundice during pregnancy can be caused by any of the processes described above, or by specific conditions seen only in pregnancy.

One such condition is *intrahepatic cholestasis of pregnancy.* Although very uncomfortable, it is generally not serious. This condition is also known as *jaundice of late pregnancy* (see also Chap. 31). The actual cause of this condition is not known, but may be related to an unusual response to estrogen.[8]

Acute fatty metamorphosis is the second type of jaundice of pregnancy. It is a much more serious disease, and most often occurs in a first pregnancy. It is often difficult to differentiate from acute viral hepatitis. About half of all patients develop renal failure. Mortality rates for the mother and the baby are high. Premature labor is common, with subsequent delivery of a stillborn child.

Other causes of jaundice of pregnancy have been documented in the literature. These include *megaloblastic anemia* (vitamin B_{12} deficiency), *hyperemesis gravidarum* (excessive vomiting during pregnancy), and *pregnancy-induced hypertension.* It is important to keep in mind when evaluating jaundiced women that the cause may not be related to the pregnancy.

Jaundice is a fairly common symptom during *postoperative* periods.

The use of anesthesia, especially halothane, is known to affect liver function in some patients; however, the majority of patients with no preexisting liver disease or shock during surgery will not demonstrate a significant increase in serum bilirubin levels.[8]

Patients who have undergone a cholecystectomy may become jaundiced because of a stone remaining in the common bile duct or a stricture in the duct. This leads to an obstructive jaundice that may require additional surgery. It is also possible for the surgeon to accidentally cut the common bile duct during abdominal surgery.

A number of drugs often given to postoperative patients are hepatotoxic. Certain antibiotics, phenothiazines, and anabolic steroids are among the drugs known to have caused jaundice.

Surgical patients who have received several units of blood may also become jaundiced. Stored blood can cause increased bilirubin loads on an already weak liver.

Postoperative jaundice may subside on its own as mysteriously as it developed.

CLINICAL MANIFESTATIONS

The clinical manifestations of diseases associated with prehepatic and hepatocellular jaundice are discussed in Chapters 29, 32, and 50. Clinical symptoms of conjugation failure and bilirubin transport are mild, perhaps no more than a slight malaise.

Posthepatic jaundice, however, particularly if due to gallstones, can be associated with acute attacks often involving nausea, vomiting, fever, right upper quadrant guarding, and severe pain. Symptoms may follow a heavy, fatty meal.[10] Bilirubinuria may also be present within 24 hours of acute pain. Patients often present with a markedly elevated bilirubin and rather yellow skin. They may have an enlarged liver and a palpable gallbladder. Their stools are usually pale. Chills and fever may accompany the jaundice.

Symptoms of intrahepatic cholestasis of pregnancy are mild, except for a severe pruritis. In acute fatty metamorphosis, however, patients are often overweight, have a bloated face, and often have pregnancy-induced hypertension. Symptoms occur after the thirtieth week of gestation, and include severe, persistent vomiting, abdominal pain, and headache. Tachycardia is present without fever, and jaundice develops within a few days.

LABORATORY ANALYSES AND DIAGNOSIS

The determination of the levels of conjugated and total serum bilirubin, urine urobilinogen and bilirubin, and the status of pigment in the feces are helpful in identifying the type of jaundice (see Table 28-1).

In addition, a routine blood smear can be a helpful tool in evaluating a hemolytic jaundice. Morphologic evidence for hemolysis includes the presence of spherocytes, target cells, schistocytes, and moderate anisocytosis. These abnormalities serve to identify the jaundice as hemolytic in nature. Special procedures such as the direct antiglobulin test, G-6PD assay, osmotic fragility test, and reticulocyte count can also be helpful. Serum bilirubin levels are usually lower than 10 mg/dL (172 μmol/L), with the indirect (unconjugated) fraction predominating.

In addition to bilirubin levels, other analyses help in evaluation of liver function. These include alkaline phosphatase (ALP), alanine aminotransferase (ALT), aspartate aminotransferase (AST), gamma-glutamyltransferase (GGT), albumin, and 5′-nucleotidase (5′-NT). Findings in these tests related to jaundiced disease states can be seen in Table 28-2.

With respect to Criglar-Najjar syndrome, patients with type I have no bilirubin in their urine, have normally-colored stools with a decrease in fecal urobilinogen, and show no evidence of hemo-

Table 28-1 ***Changes in Bilirubin in Normal and Jaundiced Patients***

	Serum		Urine		
Condition	*Total Bili*	*Direct Bili (Conjugated)*	*Bili*	*Urobilinogen*	*Feces Pigment*
Normal	0.5–2.0 mg/dL (8.5–37 μmol/L)	0.1–0.3 mg/dL (1.7–5 μmol/L)	Neg	0.5–4 mg/dL (8.5–68 μmol/L)	Brown
Prehepatic Jaundice	↑	N	Neg	↑	Brown
Hepatic Jaundice					
Hepatocellular disease	↑	↑	Pos	↓ or N	Light brown
Gilbert's disease	↑	N	Neg	↓ or N	Brown
Criglar-Najjar syndrome	↑	↓	Neg	↓	Light brown
Dubin-Johnson syndrome	↑	↑	Pos	↓ or N	Light brown
Posthepatic-obstructive Jaundice	↑	↑	Pos	↓	Light brown

Data from reference number [2]

Table 28-2 ***Disease States and Levels of Several Constituents***

	ALP	GGT	AST	ALT	Albumin	5′NT
Acute Hepatitis	↑	↑	↑↑↑	↑↑	N	↑
Alcoholic or Drug Hepatitis	N to SL ↑	↑↑↑	↑	↑	N to ↓	↑
Cirrhosis	N to SL ↑	N to SL ↑	N to SL ↑	N to SL ↑	↓	N to SL ↑
Cholestatic Disease	↑	↑↑	↑	↑	N	↑↑↑
Chronic Hepatocellular Disease	N to SL ↑	N to SL ↑	↑	↑	↓	N to SL ↑

Data from reference number [2]

lysis. Patients with type II have a few neurologic complications and a moderate decrease in fecal urobilinogen.

Children born with type I have unconjugated bilirubin levels of from 20 to 45 mg/dL (342–770 μmol/L), and usually die in their first year. Patients with type II may be free of jaundice until adolescence, when unconjugated bilirubin levels range from 6.0 to 18.0 mg/dL (103–308 μmol/L).

Patients with the Dubin-Johnson and Rotor's syndromes usually have a normal CBC, albumin, cholesterol, AST, ALT, alkaline phosphatase, and prothrombin time. Serum bilirubin levels are most often between 2.0 and 5.0 mg/dL (34–86 μmol/L), but occasionally are 20 to 25 mg/dL (342–428 μmol/L). Fifty percent or more of the bilirubin is conjugated, and bilirubin is also present in the urine.[11]

In posthepatic jaundice, serum bilirubin levels rise as high as 15 to 25 mg/dL (257–428 μmol/L), and may vary with the degree of blockage. Patients also have pale stools, no urobilinogen in their urine, a normal AST level, and an elevated alkaline phosphatase. Bilirubin elevations are predominantly direct or conjugated.[12]

Laboratory results must be interpreted carefully in the jaundiced pregnant patient (see also Chap. 40). The most valuable laboratory tests to use in monitoring the jaundiced pregnant patient are AST, ALT, prothrombin time, gamma-GT, and lactate dehydrogenase (LD) isoenzymes. These tests remain normal in uncomplicated pregnancies. Serum alkaline phosphatase levels are not very useful because they rise slowly in the first half of pregnancy and sharply during the seventh month, peaking at term. This elevation has been shown to be caused by the placental isoenzyme of alkaline phosphatase.[8] Laboratory features of acute fatty metamorphosis include WBC counts elevated to 26.0–30.0 × $10^3/mm^3$, and bilirubin levels usually below 10 mg/dL (171 μmol/L). AST and alkaline phosphatase levels are elevated, and the blood glucose is often decreased. Women who survive the disease show complete recovery of liver function.[8]

TREATMENT

There is no treatment for acute viral hepatitis, although supportive treatment and prophylaxis are discussed in Chapter 29. Treatment for cirrhosis is discussed in Chapter 32, and for cholestasis in Chapter 31.

Disorders associated with pregnancy usually subside when the pregnancy is terminated.

CASE STUDY #1

A two-year-old white child was admitted to the hospital having had vomiting and diarrhea for 3 days. She was jaundiced, and had light-colored stools and dark urine. Her symptoms were relieved with Tigan and Pedialyte. Her liver scan was normal, and no gallstones were seen by ultrasound studies.

Her admitting laboratory results were as follows:

LABORATORY FINDINGS

Na	139 mEq/L (139 mmol/L)
K	4.4 mEq/L (4.4 mmol/L)
Cl	103 mEq/L (103 mmol/L)
CO_2	24 mEq/L (24 mmol/L)
AST	203 IU/L
ALT	158 IU/L
LD	335 IU/L
ALP	1,296 IU/L
BUN	6 mg/dL (2.14 mmol/L)
Creatinine	0.4 mg/dL (35 μmol/L)
Total bilirubin	8.6 mg/dL (147 μmol/L)
Direct bilirubin	6.6 mg/dL (113 μmol/L)
Hgb	13.5 g (2 mmol/L)
Hct	40.9%
WBC	7.9 × $10^3/mm^3$
Differential (%)	
54 Segs	
3 Bands	
1 Eos	
36 Lymphs	
6 Monos	

Questions

1. What additional tests should be done to determine the patient's diagnosis?
2. What is/are the possible diagnosis(es)?
3. Which tests were the most diagnostic, and which were really unnecessary?
4. Explain the mechanism that caused the child's urine to darken and stools to become very light in color.

Discussion

1. An IV cholangiogram would be a useful procedure to visualize the common bile duct. If gallstones are not visualized, there might be other structural problems present that could be visualized with this test.
2. The patient has some sort of an obstructive or posthepatic jaundice. The liver is conjugating the bilirubin, and the hemoglobin of 13.5 g (2 mmol/L) does not indicate a hemolytic state.
3. The IV cholangiogram revealed a stricture in the common bile duct. The bilirubin levels, CBC, and enzyme levels helped to rule out other types of jaundice and were therefore necessary tests.
4. The stricture in the common bile duct did not allow conjugated bilirubin and urobilinogen to pass from the liver to the intestines. The stools became light because no urochrome was formed from urobilinogen in the intestines, and the urine became dark because bilirubin was excreted by the kidney.

Discharge Notes

The child had surgery to correct the stricture, and had an uneventful recovery. She was discharged with referrals for followup visits.

CASE STUDY #2

A four-day-old 8 lb, 13 oz full-term infant was admitted for jaundice. The baby was the second child of a 28-year-old mother, and had a 19-month-old sister. The infant was breast-fed, and was admitted after the bilirubin rose to 15.0 mg/dL (257 µmol/L). The baby was group O RH_0 D positive, and the mother was also group O Rh_0 D positive. The baby's temperature was 36.9° C, the heart rate was 148 beats/min, respirations were 70/min, and the current weight was 3.77 kg. Admitting laboratory results were as follows:

LABORATORY FINDINGS

Total bilirubin	16.6 mg/dL (284 µmol/L)		
Direct bilirubin	0.4 mg/dL (7 µmol/L)		
Hgb	18.4 g	*Urine*	Yellow, cloudy
WBC	$12.0 \times 10^3/mm^3$	*p*H	6.0
Retics	1.5%	Sp. gr.	1.005
Differential (%)		Protein	Negative
41 Segs		Sugar	Negative
42 Lymphs		Ketones	Negative
6 Atypical lymph's		Blood	Trace
9 Monos		*RBC*	0–1
2 Eos		*WBC*	HPF
297,000 Platelets		*Casts:*	0–6
		Epithelial	HPF
		cells:	none seen moderate

Questions

1. What is the most likely diagnosis, and why?
2. What is the best treatment?
3. Can you recommend other tests that should be performed?

Discussion

1. The most likely diagnosis is physiologic jaundice of the newborn. Both the mother and the child have the same blood type, and there is no evidence of hemolysis.
2. In this case the best treatment is phototherapy to lower the bilirubin level, forcing of fluids, and careful monitoring of the patient's bilirubin levels.
3. Serum liver enzyme tests—AST, ALT and LD—could be run on this patient. If the bilirubin

level drops with phototherapy, then the serum enzyme levels are probably not necessary.

REFERENCES

1. Kiviahan C, James E: The natural history of neonatal jaundice. Pediatrics 74(3):365–370, 1984
2. Kaplan L, Pesce A: Clinical Chemistry—Theory, Analysis, and Correlation, p 430. St Louis, CV Mosby, 1984
3. Kiviahan C, James E: The natural history of neonatal jaundice. Pediatrics 74(3):365–370, 1984
4. Warnes TW: Investigation of the Jaundiced Patient. Br J Hosp Med 28(4):385, 1982
5. June C, Benjamin S: Bright yellow—the extended spectrum of Gilbert's disease. Am J Gastroenterol 79(6):482–484, 1984
6. Petersdorf RG et al: Harrison's Principles of Internal Medicine, 10th ed, p 1785. New York City, McGraw-Hill, 1983
7. Workoff A: Inherited disorders manifested by conjugated hyperbilirubinemia. Semin Liver Dis 3(1):69, 1983
8. Schiff L, Schiff E: Diseases of the Liver, 5th ed, pp 1560–1583. Philadelphia, JB Lippincott, 1983
9. Hammeri UP: Jaundice during pregnancy with special emphasis on recurrent jaundice during pregnancy and differential diagnosis. Acta Med Scand (Suppl) 444(179):1–111, 1966
10. Roche: Handbook of Differential Diagnosis, p 12. Nutley, NJ, Hoffman LaRoche, 1976
11. Workoff A: Inherited disorders manifested by conjugated hyperbilirubinemia. Semin Liver Dis 3(1):66, 1983
12. Roche: Handbook of Differential Diagnosis, p 11. Nutley, NJ, Hoffman LaRoche, 1986

BIBLIOGRAPHY

Girarden MF, Saint Marc et al: Computer-aided selection of diagnostic tests in jaundiced patients. Gut 26:961–967, 1985

Henry JB: Clinical Diagnosis and Management by Laboratory Methods, 17th ed. Philadelphia, WB Saunders, 1984

Krejs G: Jaundice during pregnancy. Semin Liver Dis 3(1):73–81, 1983

Matzen P et al: Differential diagnosis of jaundice: A pocket diagnostic chart. Liver 4(6):360–371, 1984

Skornick YG et al: Cholelithiasis in Dubin-Johnson syndrome. Surg Gynecol Obstet 157(5):447–449, 1983

Sundberg W et al: Estimation of unconjugated, conjugated, and "delta" fractions in serum by use of a two-coated thin film. Clin Chem 30(8):1214–1317, 1984

Chapter 29

Hepatitis

Consuelo M. Kazen / Linda A. Smith

Hepatitis is the general term describing nonspecific inflammation of the liver, associated with a broad range of diseases and/or liver injury due to infectious and noninfectious agents. Types of hepatitis cannot be distinguished based on clinical symptoms alone, but require patient history, physical examination, and laboratory data.

In describing the type of hepatitis syndrome present, reference may be made to clinical presentation, persistence, or severity. The different terms used to describe hepatitis include anicteric, typical acute (icteric), chronic, and fulminant. *Anicteric hepatitis* is often subclinical because no jaundice is evident. It is usually a mild form of the disease. The patient often does not seek medical advice, and the only evidence of hepatitis is the presence of serological markers. *Icteric hepatitis* is the most readily recognized type of hepatitis, in that the patient exhibits the typical yellow color associated with jaundice.

Fulminant hepatitis results in acute liver failure due to massive hepatic necrosis. The disease is characterized by rapid onset and high mortality. Although this severe form of hepatitis occurs in <1% of patients with acute hepatitis caused by the hepatitis B virus, it occurs more frequently in those with non-A, non-B hepatitis.[1] It has also been known to occur rarely in hepatitis A, in toxic and alcoholic hepatitis, and in hepatitis of unknown origin.

Chronic hepatitis occurs in 5% to 10% of those patients with icteric hepatitis of viral origin (hepatitis B virus), and may develop in those with anicteric hepatitis.[2] Patients with chronic hepatitis, especially those with hepatitis B or non-A, non-B virus, may be clinically asymptomatic but serve as reservoirs of infection. Two types of chronic hepatitis may be identified: chronic persistent and chronic active. In *chronic persistent* hepatitis, the patient usually recovers clinically and has a favorable long-term prognosis. *Chronic active hepatitis,* on the other hand, is a progressive disease that often results in cirrhosis.

ETIOLOGY AND PATHOPHYSIOLOGY

Infectious Causes

Hepatitis may be caused by both infectious and noninfectious agents. The infectious causes are primarily viral; however, bacterial and parasitic organisms have been linked to individual cases of hepatitis. Table 29-1 shows the most common viral agents reported to cause hepatitis. The four hepatitis viruses—hepatitis A (HAV), hepatitis B (HBV), non-A, non-B (NANB), and hepatitis D (HDV)—are primary causes, while others such as cytomegalovirus and Epstein-Barr virus often produce hepatitis as a complication of the primary disease.

Table 29-1 ***Viral Agents Associated With Hepatitis***

Frequent/Primary Causes	Secondary Causes
Hepatitis A (HAV)	Cytomegalovirus (CMV)
Hepatitis B (HBV)	Epstein-Barr virus (EBV)
Non-A, non-B (NANB)	Herpes simplex virus
Hepatitis D (HDV)	Varicella-zoster virus

Hepatitis A virus (HAV) is transmitted primarily through the fecal-oral route from contaminated food and/or water, and causes the type of hepatitis known as *infectious hepatitis*. Exposure to the disease is linked to point sources as well as to poor sanitation and crowded living conditions. Parenteral transmission is rare, although there is a transient viremia of 7 to 10 days before clinical symptoms appear.[3] The virus is a nonenveloped RNA virus that replicates in the liver cells and is excreted in the stool. Stool specimens are infectious for 3 to 10 days before the onset of symptoms, and for up to 8 days after the onset of symptoms. The incubation period is approximately 30 days, with a range of 20 to 45 days. Symptoms, if present, have an abrupt onset. The disease, however, is usually mild, with 25% to 50% of the cases being subclinical. There are no documented cases of chronic hepatitis developing from infection with HAV.[4]

Hepatitis B virus (HBV), a member of the family *Hepadnaviridae,* is an antigenically complex virus that causes *serum hepatitis*. It is a DNA virus composed of an inner core of DNA and DNA polymerase and an outer protein layer. The entire molecule is referred to as the *Dane particle.* Core material is produced in the nucleus of the hepatocyte, and the protein in the cytoplasm. Coating of the core occurs before the molecule is excreted into the blood. Excess protein coat, known as the *Hepatitis B surface antigen (HBsAg),* is also excreted into the blood. There are four antigenic subtypes of the surface antigen—adw, adr, ayw, ayr; however, these are usually determined only for epidemiological studies.[5] The incubation period for HBV is 6 to 20 weeks, and clinical symptoms may last for 4 to 12 weeks. The most common route of infection is parenteral, although the virus may be transmitted through intimate contact.

The viral agent or agents responsible for *non-A, non-B hepatitis (NANB)* have yet to be identified; therefore, diagnosis is based on exclusion.[6] Negative tests for anti-HAV IgM, HBsAg, and anti-HBc IgM in the presence of clinical symptoms suggestive of hepatitis indicate NANB etiology. Transmission of NANB in the United States is primarily parenteral, with an incubation period of 2 to 20 weeks. Since the advent of routine HBsAg testing on donor units, NANB hepatitis has become the primary cause of transfusion-associated hepatitis.[7] Overall this virus causes a milder clinical form of hepatitis, with approximately 50% of the cases being anicteric.[8] However, NANB transfusion-associated hepatitis is more likely to cause persistent alanine aminotransferase (ALT) elevation and lead to chronic hepatitis.[9]

Hepatitis D virus (HDV), formerly known as the *Delta agent,* was described by Rizzetto in 1977 and is the most recently identified agent of hepatitis. The unique property of this virus is that it requires the presence of HBV, in particular the HBsAg, for replication.[10] Transmission, like that of HBV, is primarily parenteral in nonendemic areas. In areas where the virus is endemic, it may be spread through body fluids or intimate contact. There are typically three patterns of infection with HDV: (1) simultaneous infection of HBV and HDV, which causes an acute hepatitis (usually self-limited, but with a higher mortality rate than HBV infection[11, 12]; (2) acute HDV infection in a chronic HBV carrier; and (3) chronic HBV-HDV infection.

Bacterial agents of hepatitis are usually linked to cases of septicemia. Parasites that may cause hepatitis include *Toxoplasma gondii, Entamoeba histolytica, Echinococcus granulosus, Schistosoma* species, and hepatic flukes.

Noninfectious Causes

Noninfectious causes of hepatitis include chemicals, metabolic disorders, and idiopathic agents. The role of the liver in detoxification renders it especially susceptible to damage by *chemicals.* The mechanism for damage is not clearly understood, but it is believed that the enzymatic processes at the cellular level are involved.[13] The chemical most frequently cited as a cause of hepatitis is *ethanol,* and the resulting condition is typically referred to as *alcoholic hepatitis.* Many studies have been conducted to predict susceptibility to this condition, but they have not been conclusive. The mechanism for liver damage by ethanol has been proposed in three theories.[14] The most readily accepted theory states that the accumulation of acetaldehyde, a highly toxic chemical waste-product of ethanol metabolism, causes hepatocellular damage. A second theory holds that the presence of either ethanol or one of its metabolites causes antigenic components to be expressed in the hepatocytes, and these serve to stimulate lymphocyte activity, resulting in an autoimmune disorder. The third theory states that the presence of alcohol serves to sensitize the individual to hepatocyte damage by other viruses and chemicals. There is no specific test to diagnose alcoholic hepatitis.

Nitrofurantoin is commonly used to treat urinary tract infections, and has rarely been linked to hepatic damage. It has been known to result in chronic active hepatitis that is "lupoid" in nature.[15] *Halothane* hepatitis has also been well documented.[16] The use of halothane as an anesthetic is likely to continue for economic reasons, and it is important to recognize its potential role in liver disease. Other chemicals known to cause either chronic active hepatitis or cholestatic hepatitis are listed in Table 29-2.

Several *metabolic disorders* have also been known to result in hepatitis. Although the clinical symptoms may resemble viral hepatitis, treatment will be directed at the primary defect rather than being strictly supportive in nature. *Wilson's disease* is a hereditary disorder that may affect any age, and may present initially as fulminant hepatitis.[17] Other metabolic disorders that may present with a clinical picture of hepatitis include *galactosemia, fructosuria, tyrosinosis,* and *α_1-antitrypsin deficiency.* Ischemic hepatitis has been described in patients who suffer a fall in *cardiac output* with

Table 29-2 ***Chemicals Known to Result in Hepatitis***

Chemical Name	Common Name	Use
Chronic Active Hepatitis		
Allopurinol	Lopurin, Zyloprim	Antigout
Dantrolene sodium	Dantrium	Muscle relaxant
Halothane	Halothane	Anesthetic
Isoniazid	INH	TB therapy
Methyldopa	Aldomet	Antihypertensive
Methotrexate	Methotrexate	Chemotherapy
Nitrofurantoin	Furadantin	Urinary tract infection (UTI)
Cholestatic Hepatitis		
Chlordiazepoxide	Librium, Libritabs	Antianxiety
Imipramine	Tofranil	Antidepressant
Nitrofurantoin	Furadantin	UTI

noted left ventricular failure.[18] This condition can be differentiated from other types of hepatitis based on patient history and on the fact that the elevation of serum enzymes is not longlasting (1 to 2 days).

CLINICAL MANIFESTATIONS

When a patient presents with jaundice, complaints of nausea or vomiting, abdominal pain, and general malaise or fatigue, hepatitis should be suspected.

Infectious hepatitis, caused primarily by viral agents, exhibits four phases in a typical acute infection: incubation, prodromal (preicteric), icteric, and convalescent. During the incubation period in acute viral hepatitis, the patient rarely exhibits symptoms and the duration will vary depending on the etiologic agent. In the prodromal period, which may persist for 4 to 7 days before onset of jaundice, the patient exhibits generalized symptoms including malaise, anorexia, slight fever, weight loss, and upper right quadrant pain or tenderness. In addition, the patient may experience nausea and vomiting, headache, and myalgia. Ten to fifteen percent of patients exhibit a serum-sicknesslike syndrome.[4] Onset of jaundice marks the beginning of the icteric phase, which may last for 4 to 6 weeks in uncomplicated cases. The patient may also experience dark urine or pale stools. However, up to 50% of infections with HBV may be anicteric.[12] The disappearance of jaundice and other major symptoms marks the beginning of the convalescent period. *Noninfectious hepatitis* may present with these same phases, except that the incubation period is absent.

The clinical manifestations of *hepatitis syndromes* can vary greatly, from the mild gastrointestinal and systemic complaints of *anicteric hepatitis* to the fever, deep jaundice, coma, and seizures of *fulminant hepatitis.*

LABORATORY ANALYSES AND DIAGNOSIS

Chemistry

Chemical tests that are typically abnormal include the enzymes aspartate aminotransferase (AST) and alanine aminotransferase (ALT). Both are typically elevated during the final weeks of the incubation phase in viral hepatitis, and are usually the first abnormal biochemical tests regardless of the causative agent.[19] In viral hepatitis the values may be 10 to 100 times those of normal, while values of less than 10 times normal may suggest a nonviral etiology.[5] Alkaline phosphatase and the hepatic fraction of lactate dehydrogenase may also be elevated; however, these will not be elevated to the same degree as the transaminases. Urine bilirubin is usually detected before the appearance of jaundice. Serum bilirubin will begin to rise during the prodromal phase. As the disease progresses, the prothrombin time will become prolonged, and the erythrocyte sedimentation rate may be increased. Due to the longer half-life of albumin (21 days), hypoalbuminemia typically is present only in chronic hepatitis.

Serology

Identification of the causative agent is greatly dependent on the serology laboratory. Patients with suspected hepatitis should be tested for antibodies to hepatitis A virus and the antigens and antibodies of hepatitis B virus.

Diagnostic serologic markers for HAV are anti-HAV IgM and anti-HAV IgG. Anti-HAV IgM, which develops about 4 weeks after exposure and continues to rise for 4 to 6 weeks before dropping to nondetectable levels, is used to confirm acute HAV infection. The anti-HAV IgG develops after IgM, and may persist for years (see Fig. 29-1). The presence of anti-HAV (IgM and IgG) confirms previous HAV exposure, and usually indicates immunity to the virus.

Although hepatitis B viral particles have been isolated in saliva, semen, and other body fluids,[4] serologic methods are used to detect *infection.* Three *antigens* are *associated with HBV:* hepatitis B surface antigen (HBsAg), hepatitis B e antigen (HBeAg), and Hepatitis B core antigen (HBcAg). HBsAg and HBeAg serve as antigenic serological markers. HBcAg is not usually found free in the serum, but may be detected in hepatocyte nuclei.

HBsAg is the first detectable antigen, and is a useful marker for HBV infection. It usually appears 4 to 6 weeks after infection. It is not only present in patients with acute infections, but also persists in patients who are carriers. *HBeAg,* which is detected shortly after HBsAg, is a distinct component of the core, and its presence indicates infectivity.[19] Persistence of this antigen and lack of conversion to antibody directed against it (anti-HBe) indicate possible chronic HBV infection.

There are three *antibodies* that serve as serological markers for infection with HBV: anti-HBs, anti-HBe, and anti-HBc. *Anti-HBc* is the first antibody produced, usually 4 weeks after exposure or at the time clinical symptoms become evident. The anti-HBc IgM lasts about 60 days, but may persist for up to 6 months, and the anti-HBc IgG may persist for years. Presence of the anti-HBc IgM is indicative of acute HBV infection, and may be used to separate persons who are chronic HBsAg carriers from those with acute infections. *Anti-HBe* production usually begins during the first 10 weeks of the illness, and its presence indicates the beginning of the recovery period. *Anti-HBs* is the last antibody to be produced, usually 3 to 6 months after development of clinical symptoms. Production of this antibody indi-

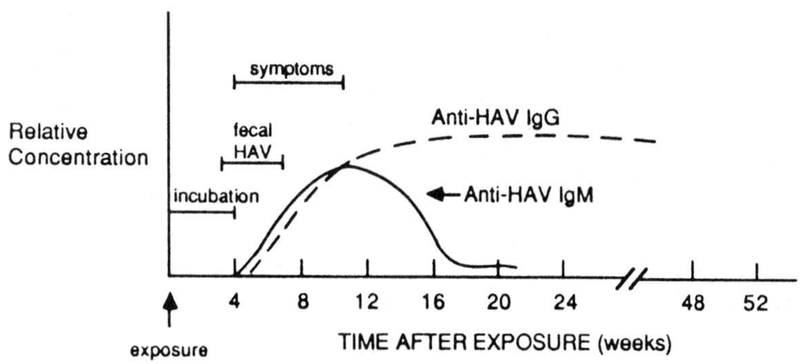

Figure 29-1 Serologic markers—hepatitis A virus.

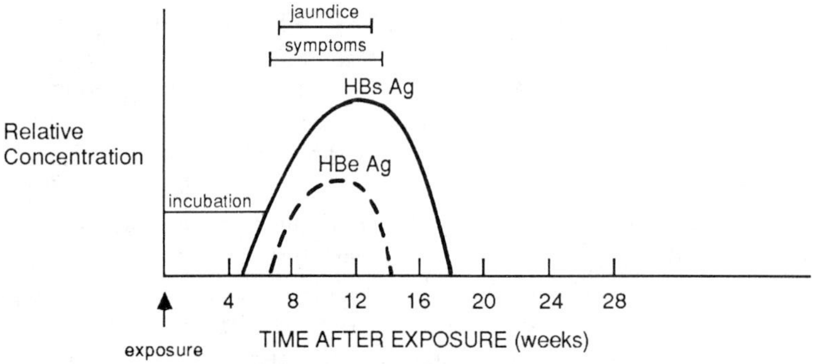

Figure 29-2 **Serologic markers—hepatitis B virus antigens.**

cates probable immunity to HBV. Thus the sequential order of serologic markers of HBV is usually HBsAg, HBeAg, anti-HBc, anti-HBe, and anti-HBs.[20] In acute HBV infection, there is a period of time, referred to as the *core window,* during which HBsAg is below detectable levels and only anti-HBc IgM is detectable to indicate recent infection. Anti-HBe may also be present. Recovery from HBV is indicated by presence of anti-HBc and anti-HBs in the patient's serum. Figures 29-2 and 29-3 indicate some of the usual patterns of serological markers in acute hepatitis infection.

Diagnosis of chronic hepatitis may be made by the persistence of HBsAg and HBeAg in the serum, presence of anti-HBc, and lack of production of anti-HBe. The presence of HBeAg indicates active viral replication, with conversion to anti-HBe indicating termination of active replication. HBsAg will, however, persist. In fulminant hepatitis due to HBV infection, HBsAg and HBeAg may be of lower concentration and cleared more rapidly than in an acute infection. In addition, there is an enhanced antibody response to these antigens.[21]

In *Hepatitis D infections,* where there is simultaneous HBV-HDV infection, tests for HBsAg, anti-HBc IgM, and anti-HDV will be positive. In acute hepatitis in a chronic HBV carrier, the presence of anti-HBc IgM will help to differentiate acute HBV infection from HDV superinfection, in which anti-HBc IgM is absent. In chronic HBV-HDV infection, the virus can be detected in hepatocyte nuclei by use of immunofluorescent techniques. Serological kits for detection of anti-HDV have recently become available. Anti-HDV IgM occurs in the early acute phase of the infection. Anti-HDV IgG may occur in the late acute phase, and persists for only a few months if the infection is self-limited.[22]

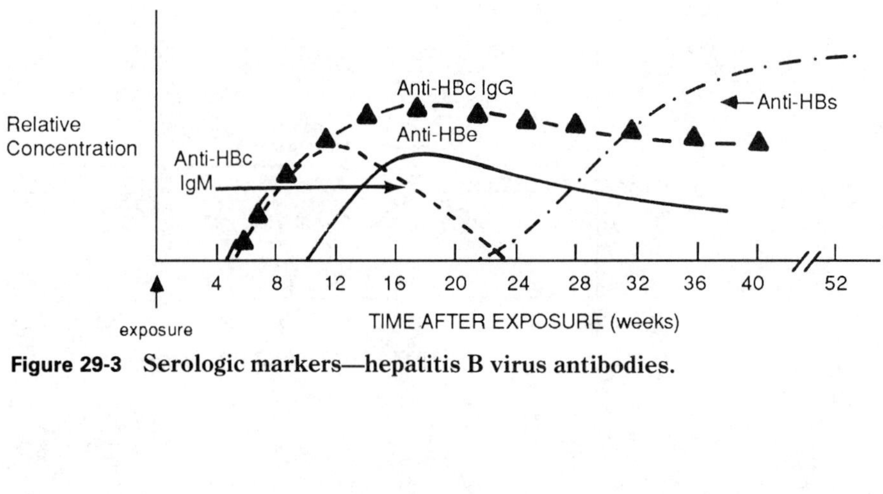

Figure 29-3 **Serologic markers—hepatitis B virus antibodies.**

Non-A–non-B hepatitis is characterized by negative tests for anti HAV IgM, HBsAg, and anti HBc IgM.

Table 29-3 lists some common patterns seen in testing for serologic markers of hepatitis, the possible diagnosis, and followup tests. The usual panel for diagnosing acute hepatitis consists of testing for anti-HAV (IgM), HBsAg, and anti-HBc IgM. Results of these tests may indicate the need for additional testing of serologic markers, including HBeAg, anti-HBe, and anti-HBs. Combinations of these tests may be used to monitor chronic hepatitis, followup infants who have been treated for perinatal exposure, or sexual contacts of persons with HBV infection.

Other

Biochemical tests are not specific for the different types of hepatitis, and will only indicate the presence of hepatocyte injury. *Alcoholic hepatitis* may be diagnosed based on patient history, liver biopsy, and failure to detect a viral cause.[23] *Drug-induced hepatitis* will follow the same protocol. *Nitrofurantoin hepatitis* may present with a positive antinuclear antibody and antismooth-muscle antibody. The LE prep may also be positive.

Due to the treatability or possible severity of *metabolic disorders,* it is important that these be ruled out in the differential diagnosis. In *Wilson's disease,* serum, urine, and liver levels of copper will be elevated, and serum ceruloplasmin levels will be decreased. Kayser-Fleischer rings may be present, and should be looked for. *α_1-antitrypsin deficiency* may be detected by serum protein electrophoresis, and is characterized by an absence or a greatly decreased level of the α_1 fraction. The phenotype may be identified by isoelectric focusing.[24] *Tyrosinosis* may be initially screened for by metabolic screening spot tests using urine. Definitive diagnosis may be made by specific enzyme assays. *Galactosemia* and *fructosuria* may also be screened for in urine, using nonspecific tests for reducing substances. Confirmation may be made by specific enzyme assays.

TREATMENT AND PROPHYLAXIS

There is no specific treatment for hepatitis, but supportive measures are usually instituted once the symptoms have begun.

Immune Globulin

The decision to use immune prophylaxis often depends on the type of hepatitis, type of exposure, and immune status of the patient.[25] In hepatitis A infections, the use of immune serum globulin may prevent or decrease the clinical symptoms if given within 2 weeks of exposure. However, because exposure to HAV is often not known until symptoms are evident, the immune serum globulin is not often used. Pregnant women rarely transmit HAV to the fetus because of the short viremic phase, but the infant may be given immune serum globulin at birth.[26] For HBV exposure, the current immune prophylaxis is hepatitis B immune globulin (HBIG), which is an immune globulin containing high levels of anti-HBs, usually $>1:100{,}000$.[2] HBIG should be given within 7 days after exposure to the virus to be effective in decreasing the attack rate.[5] The patient should be tested for immune status before HBIG is given. Tests used may include anti-HBc and anti-HBs as well as HBsAg. A positive result for any test contraindicates HBIG immunization. There is no current recommended prophylaxis against non-A, non-B hepatitis or hepatitis D virus infection. However, infants born to mothers with NANB hepatitis may also be given immune serum globulin at birth and at 28 days.[26]

Vaccine

Hepatitis B vaccine is recommended as preexposure prophylaxis in persons at high risk of infection by HBV. These include health care workers, intravenous drug users, male homosexuals, and hemodialysis patients. The vaccine contains purified HBsAg, and requires a three-dose regimen. Anti-HBs will develop in 90% to 95% of persons who receive the vaccine.[27] The age of the recipient

Table 29-3 ***Some Common Patterns of Acute Hepatitis Serologic Markers***

Results of Initial Diagnostic Profile				
Anti-HAV (IgM)	*HBsAg*	*Anti-HBc (IgM)*	**Most Likely Diagnosis**	**Some Suggested Followup Testing and Results**
=	=	=	? NANB, other causes	Test for other viral agents, toxins
+	=	=	Acute HAV infection	Usually none
=	=	+	Recent HBV infection	1. May want to test for anti-HBe to determine resolution, prognosis • If HBe Ag+ and anti-HBe=, indicates highly infectious • If HBe Ag= and anti-HBe+, indicates resolution of infection 2. Then test for anti-HBs. • If =, may be core window → retest in about a month • If +, indicates immunity/recovery
=	+	+	Acute HBV infection	1. Test for HBeAg and anti-HBe to determine infectivity. 2. Repeat HBsAg test approximately monthly. • When HBsAg=, HBeAg=, and anti-HBe+, indicates resolution • Then test for anti-HBs to determine immunity. 3. If HBeAg and HBsAg remain + over a period of several months, may indicate chronic carrier developing. Continue testing to determine if seroconversion to anti-HBe occurs, to indicate resolution
=	+	=	Early acute HBV or chronic carrier	Retest for HBsAg and anti-HBc IgM in approximately 2 weeks. 1. If both +, → acute HBV • Follow testing indicated above. 2. If HBsAg+ and anti-HBc IgM=, test for anti-HBc • Anti-HBc + indicates previous HBV infection and chronic carrier. Current acute infection most likely due to other causes (*e.g.*, NANB, HDV)

(=) Negative test result, (+) Positive test result

is a factor, with younger persons more likely to mount an immune response.[28] A second vaccine, developed by recombinant DNA methods using the S gene encoded into *Saccharomyces cerevisiae,* has been developed. This vaccine appears to stimulate an antibody similar in titer, affinity, and specificity to that produced by the plasma-based vaccine.[29] Prevaccination serologic screening using anti-HBs tests may be recommended, depending on prevalence of HBV serologic markers in the population, and cost.[25] Anti-HBs testing in one study detected 93% of the immune persons, while anti-HBc detected only 67% of those immune to HBV.[30] Anti-HBc can be used to identify anti-HBs-negative HBsAg carriers who do not need the vaccine.

Pregnant women who are HBV carriers present a problem in that they may transmit the virus to the infant, especially during birth. Approximately 90% of infected infants become chronic HBV carriers, with 25% of these dying due to HBV-related complications such as cirrhosis and primary hepatocellular carcinoma.[12] If prophylaxis is started at delivery, infections with HBV can be prevented in >90% of infants born to HBsAg-positive women.[31] A combination of active and passive immunization is used. The child is protected passively by HBIG during the time it takes to mount an immune response to the vaccine. HBIG is administered to the infant at birth, followed by doses of HBV vaccine within 24 hours, at one month, and at 6 months. The child should be tested for HBsAg and anti-HBs at 12 months to determine vaccine effectiveness. A positive test for HBsAg indicates immunization failure. If both anti-HBs and HBsAg are negative, another dose of vaccine may be given.

TREATMENT OF NONINFECTIOUS HEPATITIS

Alcoholic hepatitis has sometimes been treated with corticosteroids, but this has not proven very helpful in the majority of cases. Prophythiouracil has also been utilized, but has not been proven effective in all cases. Drug-induced hepatitis can usually be reversed by removing the precipitating drug before the hepatitis proceeds to liver failure.

Wilson's disease can be managed through lifelong administration of a chelating agent such as penicillamine, but must be treated early in its course.[32] α_1-antitrypsin deficiency, which results in liver disease, does not lend itself well to treatment. Experimental treatment using intravenous administration of concentrates of α_1-antitrypsin and oral use of androgen danazol to raise serum levels has been attempted.[33] Tyrosinosis, fructosuria, and galactosemia have been treated primarily by diet control. Foods that contain phenylalanine, tyrosine, and methionine are restricted for patients with tyrosinosis, while foods or medicines that contain fructose or sucrose must be withheld from patients diagnosed with fructosuria. Foods or medicines that contain galactose must be restricted for patients with a diagnosis of galactosemia.

CASE STUDY #1

A 32-year-old white woman was seen in the emergency room with jaundice, nausea, and malaise. She was afebrile. Several months earlier she had noticed darkening of her urine. She had no previous history of hepatitis or jaundice, and had never received a blood transfusion. She frequently suffered from urinary tract infections, and had been treated with nitrofurantoin for several years. She had no history of alcohol abuse.

LABORATORY FINDINGS

ADMISSION LABORATORY WORKUP	***PATIENT DATA***	***REFERENCE RANGE***
Aspartate aminotransferase	1000 U/L	(8–20 U/L)
Alkaline phosphatase	450 U/L	(20–70 U/L)

LABORATORY FINDINGS

ADMISSION

LABORATORY WORKUP	PATIENT DATA	REFERENCE RANGE
Total bilirubin	14 mg/dL (239.4 μmol/L)	0.2–1.0 mg/dL (3.42–17.1 μmol/L)
Prothrombin time	24 sec with a control of 12 sec	
IgG (serum)	360 mg/dL (36.0 g/L)	70–170 mg/dL (7–17 g/L)
HBsAg	Negative	Negative
IgM anti-HAV	Negative	Negative
Anti-HBc	Negative	Negative

FURTHER LABORATORY WORKUP

Antinuclear	Positive	Negative
Antinuclear Ab titer	1:320	Negative
Antismooth-muscle Ab	Positive	Negative
Antismooth-muscle Ab titer	1:10	Negative
LE prep	Positive	Negative

Questions

1. Based on the presenting features, the laboratory data, and the drug history, what is the presumptive diagnosis?
2. What is the most likely cause for this patient's illness?
3. For how long will the transaminase levels remain elevated after the primary cause of this patient's condition is removed?

Discussion

1. The patient appears to have active hepatitis that is lupoid in nature.
2. Nitrofurantoin has been known to cause an autoimmune chronic active hepatitis.
3. Transaminases may remain elevated for up to 2 to 6 weeks after withdrawal of nitrofurantoin.

CASE STUDY #2

A 37-year-old dentist consulted his physician when he experienced malaise, nausea, and vomiting over a 10-day period. Physical examination revealed slight tenderness in the upper right quadrant, but no enlargement of the liver. He had a fever of 100.8° F. The patient's history revealed that he was a nonsmoker and a moderate drinker. He denied taking any medications or drugs. He had visited Mexico and Central America about 4 weeks previously. Initial laboratory tests revealed a normal CBC and elevations of AST and ALT. Other routine chemistry tests were within normal limits.

Questions

1. What types of hepatitis are possible in this patient, given his history?
2. What initial tests for hepatitis serological markers should be performed? Why?
3. Given the following results, what is the most likely diagnosis for this patient?

   Anti-HAV IgM: negative
   HBsAg: negative
   Anti-HBc IgM: positive

   Do the results indicate administration of immune serum globulin?

Discussion

1. Hepatitis A and hepatitis B are both possible. The trip to Mexico and the patient's profession are indicators of possible exposure to either/both types of hepatitis.
2. Given the rise in liver enzymes and clinical symptoms, the routine screening panel for acute hepatitis should be performed. This consists of anti-HAV IgM, HBsAg, and anti-HBc IgM.
3. The results indicate acute hepatitis B infection. The anti-HBc IgM may indicate that the patient is in the "core window" period, when only this antibody is present and HBsAg, which would indicate active infection, is below detectable levels. The patient should be followed for devel-

opment of anti-HBe and anti-HBs to indicate recovery. Hepatitis B immune globulin (HBIG) is not indicated.

REFERENCES

1. Gerety RJ (ed): Hepatitis B, p 104. Orlando, Academic Press, 1985
2. Krugman S: Hepatitis B immunoprophylaxis. Lab Med 14(11):727–732, 1983
3. Hollinger FB, Melnick JL, Robinson WS: Viral Hepatitis. New York City, Raven Press, 1985
4. Hoofnagle JH: Type A and type B hepatitis. Lab Med 14(11):705–716, 1983
5. Sass MA, Cianflocco AJ: The diagnosis of acute viral hepatitis. Resident and Staff Physician 31(4): 17PC–34PC, 1985
6. Shorey J: Southwestern Internal Medicine Conference: The current status of non-A, non-B viral hepatitis. Am J Med Sci 289(6):251–261, 1985
7. Polesky HF, Hanson M: Transfusion-associated hepatitis: A dilemma. Lab Med 14(11):717–720, 1983
8. Gitnick G: Non-A, non-B hepatitis: Etiology and clinical course. Lab Med 14(11):721–726, 1983
9. Bradley DW: The agents of non-A, non-B viral hepatitis. J Virol Methods 10:307–319, 1985
10. Rizzeto M: The delta agent. Hepatology 3:729–737, 1983
11. Shiels MT, Cazja AJ, Taswell HF et al: Frequency significance of delta antibody in acute and chronic hepatitis B: A United States experience. Gastroenterology 89(6):1230–1234, 1985
12. Bredfeldt JE: Hepatitis B virus: Update on the spectrum of clinical infections and on prophylaxis. Postgrad Med 78(6):71–78, 81–83, 1985
13. Brunt PW, Losowsky MS, Read AE: The Liver and Biliary System, pp 48–69. London, William Heinemann, 1984
14. Saunders JB, Wodak AD, Williams R: What determines susceptibility to liver damage from alcohol?: Discussion paper. J R Soc Med 77:204–216, 1984
15. Young TL, Achkar E, Tuthill R et al: Chronic active hepatitis induced by nitrofurantoin. Cleve Clin Q 52(2):253–256, 1985
16. Stock JG, Strunin L: Unexplained hepatitis following halothane. Anesthesiology 63:424–439, 1984
17. Rakela J, Lange SM, Ludwig J et al: Fulminant hepatitis: Mayo Clinic experience with 34 cases. Mayo Clin Proc 60(5):289–292, 1985
18. Gibson PR, Dudley FJ: Ischemic Hepatitis: Clinical features, diagnosis, and prognosis. Aust NZ J Med 14:822–825, 1984
19. Keating LJ, Silvergleid AJ: Hepatitis: A Technical Workshop, p 18.10. Chicago, AABB, 1981
20. Mushahwar IK, Dienstag JL, Polesky HF et al: Interpretation of various serological profiles of hepatitis B virus infection. Am J Clin Pathol 76(6):773–777, 1981
21. Gimson AE, Tedder RS, White YS et al: Serological markers in fulminant hepatitis B. Gut 24(7): 615–617, 1983
22. Delta hepatitis: Identification, epidemiologic features, and prevention. Can Med Assoc J 134(4): 379–380, 1986
23. Frank D, Raicht RF: Alcohol-induced liver disease. Alcoholism 9(1):66–82, 1985
24. Kaplan LA, Pesce AJ: Clinical Chemistry—Theory, Analysis, and Correlation, p 433. St Louis, CV Mosby, 1984
25. Chang Y: Serological markers of viral hepatitis. Diagn Med 6:28–31, 1983
26. Snydham DR: Hepatitis in pregnancy. N Engl J Med 313(22):1398–1401, 1985
27. Coutinho RA: Hepatitis B vaccination. J Virol Methods 10:327–331, 1985
28. McLean AA: Hepatitis B vaccine: A review of the clinical data to date. J Am Dent Assoc 110(4):624–628, 1984
29. Brown SE, Stanley C, Howard CR et al: Antibody response to recombinant and plasma-derived hepatitis B vaccine. Br Med J (Clin Res) 292(6415): 159–161, 1986
30. Hanson M, Polesky HF: Prevalence of antiHBc in antiHbs-positive individuals: Implications for selecting vaccine candidates. Am J Clin Pathol 83(6): 716–719, 1984
31. Infectious Diseases and Immunization Committee, Canadian Paediatric Society: Hepatitis B: Update on perinatal management. Can Med Assoc J 134(8): 883–886, 1986
32. Rector WG, Uchida T, Kanel GC et al: Fulminant hepatic and renal failure complicating Wilson's disease. Liver 4:341–347, 1984
33. Maddray WC: Alpha-1-antitrypsin deficiency. In The Johns Hopkins Medical Grand Rounds, Vol 8, Program 9. May 1982

Chapter 30

Aminoaciduria

H. Jesse Guiles

ETIOLOGY AND PATHOPHYSIOLOGY

General Categories

Aminoaciduria (AAU) means high levels of amino acids in the urine. Generally, the cause of AAUs is either a malfunction in the manufacture of these compounds by the liver, or a malfunction in their transport or reabsorption by the kidney. AAUs can be grouped into four categories. The first three categories, known as *primary aminoacidurias,* are caused by a genetic defect that results in the nonmanufacture or faulty manufacture of an enzyme necessary for the synthesis, metabolism, or tubular reabsorption of a specific amino acid. These genetic defects are also known as *inborn errors of metabolism.* The categories follow:

1. *Overflow AAU*—caused by an enzyme defect that leads to an overproduction of one or more amino acid(s) by the liver. As a result, the amino acid(s) exceeds its renal threshold and spills into the urine. Both serum and urine amino acids will be increased in these diseases.
2. *Renal Transport AAU*—caused by a congenital defect in the reabsorption of an amino acid(s) by the kidney tubules. Serum levels for one or more amino acids are normal or decreased, whereas urine levels are high.
3. *No-Threshold AAU*—caused by a congenital enzyme block in the biochemical processing of an amino acid that leads to an accumulation in the urine of an intermediate amino acid not normally seen in the urine. It should be noted that these AAUs are due not to a congenital defect in the tubules but to a *normal* lack of a physiological mechanism for the reabsorption by the tubules of the intermediate metabolites.
4. *Secondary AAU*—caused by other diseases or toxins that result in liver necrosis or destruction of tubular function. Many or all amino acids are usually increased in these diseases.

A list of AAUs can be seen in Table 30-1. Although this table lists the major AAUs found today, more than 50 hereditary diseases of amino acid metabolism have been identified.[1] Fortunately, as can be seen from the table, the incidence of these diseases is low and identification of those AAUs with a relatively high frequency can easily be accomplished through screening tests.

Primary Overflow AAUs

PHENYLKETONURIA

Phenylketonuria (PKU) results from a block in the metabolism of phenylalanine (PHE) due to a congenital lack of the enzyme phenylalanine hydroxylase (PH), which causes a buildup of this amino acid in blood and urine (see Fig. 30-1). The enzymatic deficiency is inherited as an autosomal recessive, nonsex-linked trait. PKU is the prototype for overflow AAU and, as can be seen in Table 30-1, is the type that occurs most frequently. Variant forms exist, and are considered to be caused by partial deficiencies of the enzyme PH.

MATERNAL PKU

Because mass screening for PKU has been in existence for more than 18 years in some states and countries, a new problem has developed. Maternal hyperphenylalaninemia (mothers who were diagnosed and treated for PKU as infants but subsequently taken off treatment) has been steadily increasing in frequency. Among untreated pregnancies, the incidence of infant mental retardation, microcephaly, and congenital heart disease has greatly increased in the general population, and these increases correlate with blood levels of phenylalanine in mothers.[2] Several studies have indicated that harm to the fetus can accompany pregnancies compromised by any degree of hyperphenylalaninemia.[3] However, there is no consistent relationship between treatment during pregnancy and prevention of the abnormality in the offspring. It appears that, for treatment to be effective, dietary therapy may have to be initiated before and be in effect at conception.[2] Some centers, therefore, have started a registry of males

(*Text continues on page 348*)

Table 30-1 ***Aminoacidurias***

Disease	Prevalence	Deficient Enzyme	AA Increase	Clinical Features	Treatment
Primary Overflow AAUs (Autosomal Recessive)					
Phenylketonuria (PKU) with variants (I–V)	1:10,000	L-Phenylalanine hydroylase	Phenylalanine and metabolites	Mental retardation, seizures	Diet low in PHE
Tyrosinemia (variants) (neonatal)	1:100,000	Fumarylacetoacetate hydrolase, tyrosine aminotransferase (neonatal = liver immaturity)	Tyrosine, methionine, and metabolites (PHE in neonatal)	Hepatic cirrhosis, renal damage, tyrosine needles	Diet low in tyrosine, PHE, and methionine
Alkaptonuria	1:250,000	Homogentistic acid oxidase	Homogentisic acid	Degenerative arthritis	None known
Maple Syrup Urine Disease (MSUD) or Branched-Chain Ketoaciduria (BCKA)	1:200,000	Branched-chain ketoacid decarboxylase	Valine, leucine, isoleucine (ketoacids)	Spasticity, severe acidosis, convulsions, respiratory failure, mental retardation, leucine crystals, early death	Diet low in leucine, valine, and isoleucine
Histidinemia	1:20,000	Histidase	Histidine, alanine, and metabolites	Speech defects, motor deficiencies, mental retardation, to no symptoms	Diet low in histidine
Citrullinemia	Rare	Argininosuccinate synthetase	Citrulline, alanine (ammonia)	Seizures, vomiting, mental retardation	Low-protein diet

Primary No-Threshold AAUs (Autosomal Recessive)					
Homocystinuria (and variants)	1 : 200,000	Cystathionine beta synthase (and variants)	Homocystine, methionine (normal in variants)	Vascular thrombosis, ocular dislocation, skeletal deformity, mental retardation	Diet low in methionine, vitamins B_6 and B_{12} therapy
Cystathioninuria	1 : 70,000	Cystathionase	Cystathionine and metabolites	Benign to mild mental retardation	Vitamin B_{12} therapy
Primary Renal AAUs (Autosomal Recessive)					
Cystinuria (and variants)	1 : 7,000	Tubular dysfunction	Lysine, ornithine, arginine	Cystine crystals, renal calculi, renal damage	Hydration, alkaline urine, D-penicillamine
Hartnup's Disease	1 : 18,000	Tubular dysfunction	13 neutral amino acids	Normal to pellagra-like rash, retarded growth, mental retardation, and neurologic symptoms	Adequate protein diet, nicotinamide therapy
Iminoglycinuria	1 : 15,000	Tubular dysfunction	Glycine, proline, hydroxyproline	Renal tubular defect in reabsorption of iminoacids and glycine	None known
Causes of Secondary Aminoacidurias					
		Fulminant hepatic failure Acute massive necrosis of liver Acute yellow atrophy of liver Acute tubular necrosis Fanconi syndrome Galactosemia Wilson's disease Wasting/starvation Poisons (lead, mercury) Acetaminophen OD			

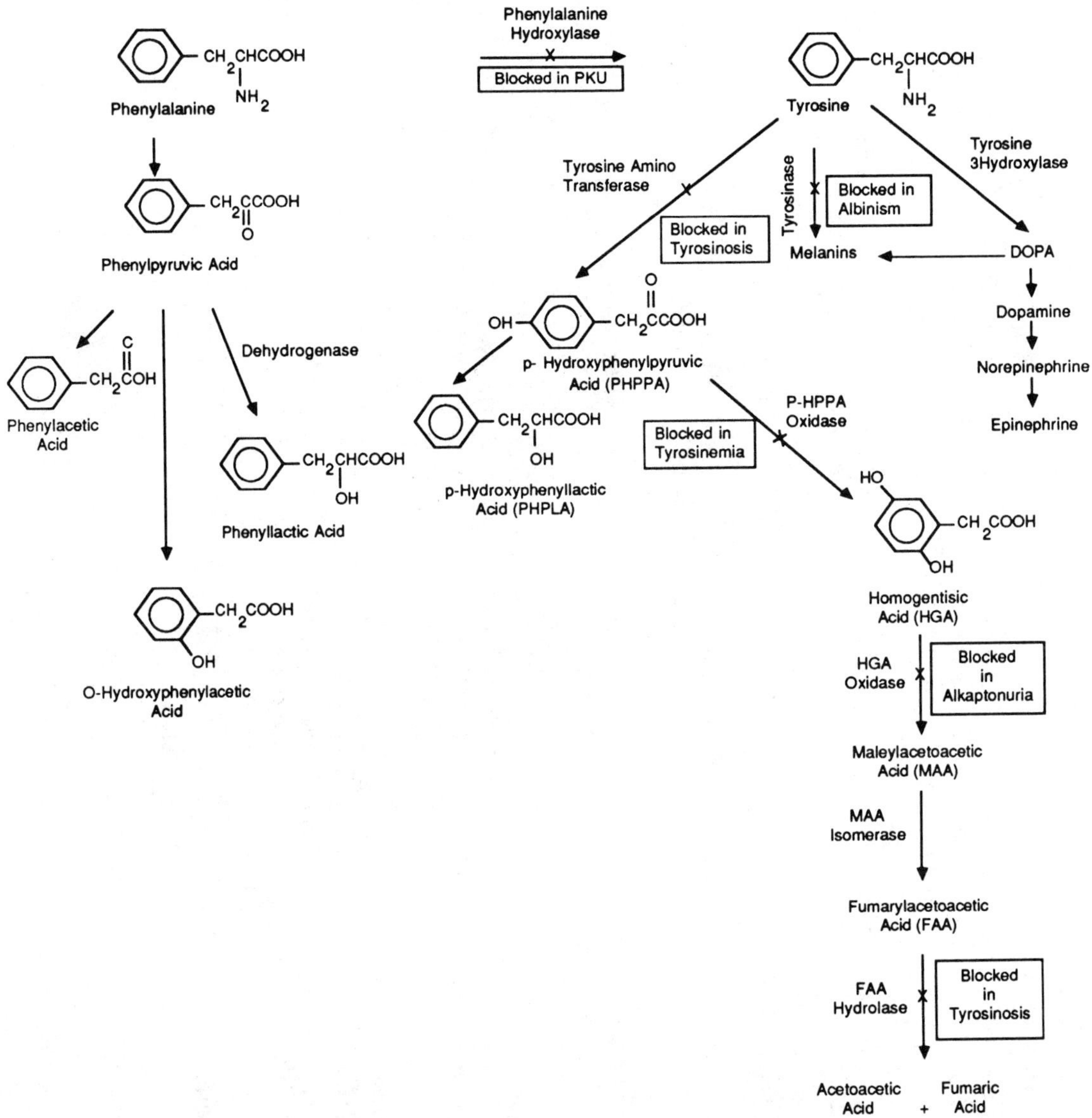

Figure 30-1 **Metabolism of phenylalanine and tyrosine.**

and females treated for PKU in order to provide counseling about the consequences of maternal PKU and the options to prevent it.[3]

TYROSINEMIA

The genetically-controlled lack of enzyme activity causing tyrosinosis/tyrosinemia is shown in Figure 30-1. Blockage leads to an alternate route for the metabolism of tyrosine, with a concurrent rise in the urine of tyrosine, DOPA, and other metabolites. Variant forms of the disease exist, depending on the specific enzyme affected and whether the genetic defect causes a partial or a total loss of enzyme activity. A milder, transient form of neonatal tyrosinemia is seen relatively frequently, caused by the decreased ability of the premature infant's liver to synthesize enzymes. This is a temporary condition that is self-correcting within 4 to 8 weeks. Although this is probably the most common form of tyrosinemia, it must be distinguished from the more severe forms in order to assure correct treatment. In transient neonatal tyrosinemia, phenylalanine will also accumulate because of an accompanying PH deficiency. The clinical laboratory scientist must be aware of this possibility when testing for PKU in order to avoid an erroneous diagnosis.

ALKAPTONURIA

Alkaptonuria results from an abnormality along the same metabolic pathway as PKU and tyrosinosis (see Fig. 30-1). Deficiency in the enzyme HGA oxidase leads to a buildup of homogentisic acid (HGA).

MAPLE SYRUP URINE DISEASE (MSUD) OR BRANCHED-CHAIN KETOACIDURIA (BCKA)

Maple Syrup Urine Disease (MSUD) is caused by an inborn error in the catabolism of branched-chain amino acids (BCAA)—leucine, isoleucine, and valine. The deficient enzyme appears to catalyze the decarboxylation of intermediate BCAA metabolites to alpha ketoacids (see Fig. 30-2). The enzyme is nonspecific, resulting in an increase in all three amino acids in serum and urine.

Variant forms of MSUD exist and have been identified by biochemical markers and clinical signs. In the intermittent form, enzymatic activity is sufficient during periods of relative health; however, in times of stress (*e.g.*, infections, surgery, vaccinations) children may show symptoms identical to classic MSUD. In milder forms, BCAA will be increased in urine but clinical symptoms will be less severe.

Renal Transport Aminoacidurias

Cystinuria is the classic example of renal transport aminoaciduria. It is caused by the defective reabsorption of cystine by the epithelial cells of the renal tubules, and is transmitted as an autosomal recessive trait (see Chap. 65).

No-Threshold Aminoacidurias

Examples of no-threshold AAUs are seen in Table 30-1. These are characterized by the presence in the serum and urine of an amino acid that is not normally detectable. No-threshold AAUs are caused by a blockage of an intermediate step in the metabolism of an amino acid, causing the metabolite to be filtered into the urine. Because there exists no physiological mechanism for tubular reabsorption of these intermediates, they are excreted by the kidneys.

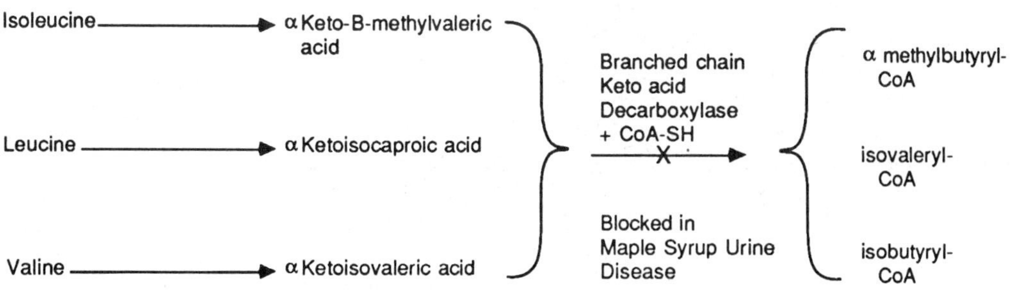

Figure 30-2 Catabolism of branched chain amino acids. (Adapted from Efron ML: Aminoaciduria. N Engl J Med 272:1058–1066, 1965)

Secondary Aminoacidurias

Causes of secondary AAUs are listed in Table 30-1. The AAU can be an overflow type (fulminant hepatic failure) or a renal type (Fanconi syndrome). Certain diseases, such as galactosuria, result in the accumulation of intermediate products of metabolism, which in turn can cause renal toxicity. Other causes of secondary AAUs include poisons, wasting from starvation, acute tubular necrosis, and acetaminophen overdose (see Table 30-1).

Secondary causes can result in an AAU involving a single amino acid or a generalized AAU. The latter is the usual case. Along with increases in amino acids, other substances such as glucose, protein, phosphate, and galactose can be, and usually are, increased in the urine.

CLINICAL MANIFESTATIONS

General

As can be seen in Table 30-1, clinical manifestations are similar in many of these diseases. They usually occur very early in life, beginning within a few days after birth and continuing through infancy into childhood and adulthood.

Clinical signs in infants and children that should alert the physician to the possibility of AAU include (1) mental retardation, (2) deterioration of motor skills or language, (3) profound developmental delay, (4) corneal clouding in the eye, (5) abnormalities in urine color or odor, (6) sparse, short, brittle hair, and (7) a family history of AAU or of siblings who died young.[4, 5] Very young infants who appear healthy at birth but begin manifesting signs of life-threatening illness (anorexia, vomiting, difficulty in breathing, coma) after the onset of feeding should be tested immediately for aminoacidopathy. The disease progression is very rapid once the first symptoms appear.

Phenylketonuria

Neonates with phenylketonuria appear normal at birth. After feeding begins, symptoms such as feeding difficulties, vomiting, and delayed development begin to appear. Brain injury occurs between the second and third weeks of life, and becomes maximal at 8 to 9 months. IQs of less than 60 occur in 98% of untreated patients.[6] Other symptoms include hypopigmentation, skin lesions and eczema, and urine with a characteristic "mousy" odor.

Tyrosinemia

Clinical symptoms of tyrosinemia include jaundice, failure to thrive, hepatosplenomegaly, ascites, edema, and bleeding. Symptoms usually begin in infancy and vary according to the severity of the disease (partial vs total enzyme depletion). Patients with partial enzymatic defects will develop cirrhosis. Death due to hepatocarcinoma and liver failure is the usual result in patients with a complete defect.[7]

Alkaptonuria

In infancy and childhood, the only symptom of alkaptonuria is darkening of the urine, which occurs when the urine stands in an alkaline *p*H or is exposed to air. The disease can be detected in neonates if dark stains in diapers are noticed and investigated. Clinical symptoms begin in adulthood, and include degenerative arthritis and dark pigmentation of cartilage. This is caused by the binding of HGA and its metabolites to collagen in cartilage and connective tissue.[8]

MSUD

The incidence of MSUD is rare (see Table 30-1). Although the neonate is normal at birth, symptoms such as listlessness, refusal to eat, and vomiting appear within the first 5 days of life. Symptoms rapidly progress to loss of reflexes, alternating hypotonicity and hypertonicity, lethargy, episodes of acute ketoacidosis (often triggered by recurring infections), irregular respiration, convulsions, and coma. Unless the disease is diagnosed promptly, the infant will die of respiratory insufficiency. Those who survive the acute neonatal period show severe retardation and cerebral palsy.[7]

No-Threshold AAUs

The clinical symptoms listed in Table 30-1 are the major reason for laboratory screening of suspected no-threshold AAUs. Symptoms may develop later in life or not at all. Both urine and serum samples should be sent to the laboratory, because a no-threshold AAU may show a positive result in the urine and a normal result in the serum.

Secondary AAUs

Clinical symptoms of secondary AAUs are consistent with the primary condition responsible for the liver or kidney malfunction that results in the AAU.

LABORATORY ANALYSES AND DIAGNOSIS

Screening Tests for AAU

Specimens for laboratory analysis come either from patients exhibiting symptoms mentioned above or from massive screening programs. Blood tests on infants for aminoaciduria, especially phenylketonuria, are mandatory in most states.

Screening tests are designed to call attention to suspicious cases; therefore, confirmation of a positive test is always necessary. Screening tests have a "high sensitivity," *i.e.*, patients with the disease will be positive for the test. In order to obtain this high sensitivity, some clinical specificity is sacrificed and there is a concurrent high rate of false positives. In most screening programs, only one of 15 infants with positive screens will have the disease.[9] This sacrifice of specificity for sensitivity is insignificant, in that treatment, consisting of a prescribed dietary regimen, can begin on all positive infants without any ill effects to the patients. However, prompt initiation of treatment is necessary to prevent permanent impairment of an affected infant.

The first, and still utilized, highly sensitive mass screening test is the Guthrie test system[10] (see Table 30-2), now available for several AAUs. Any positive result must be followed with confirmatory testing. It should be noted that there is a potential for false negatives using the Guthrie test. The laboratory scientist should be certain that the specimen was collected from an infant whose age is *at least* 48 hours, in order to assure that sufficient time has elapsed to allow for a rise in concentration of the amino acid in question to detectable levels.

Although state law may prescribe mandatory screening of neonates for one or more amino acids, infants up to several years of age may also present with symptoms of AAU. These individuals may have been missed in the screening program, or may have a defect not tested for in the initial screen. The next level of testing calls for urine and serum screening by qualitative chemical color-

Table 30-2 ***Guthrie Test Systems***

L-Amino Acid	Disease	Inhibitor	Reference Limits (mg/dL)
L-phenylalanine	PKU	B-2-Thienylalanine	4
L-tyrosine	Tyrosinemia	D-Tyrosine	8
L-leucine	MSUD	4-Azaleucine	4
L-methionine	Homocystinuria	Methionine sulfoximine	2

Data from reference number [8]

imetric methods, chromatography, or high voltage electrophoresis (HVE).

THIN LAYER CHROMATOGRAPHY SCREENS

One- and two-dimensional thin layer chromatography (TLC) is the preferred methodology for screening suspected AAU urine and blood samples (see Fig. 30-3). High voltage electrophoresis (HVE) can also be used, but it does not give the resolution of TLC and is more cumbersome. Principles of result interpretation are similar for both methods.

TLC will give a qualitative measure of the amino acids present. Interpretation of these screens requires great skill and experience. For this reason, many laboratories utilize reference laboratories experienced in interpretation of these tests. Generally, a positive result should be reported out with caution because this test is a screening test, and positive results can occur for a wide variety of reasons. Clinical laboratory scientists should be aware of the following limitations before making an interpretation of the chromatograph:

1. A *fresh* urine specimen is crucial for good results using this technique. Bacterial contamination can be an important source of false-positive and/or false-negative results. Bacteria utilize amino acids and produce metabolites that can cause interference. Laboratories must insist that the "clean catch random urine" protocol is strictly adhered to and that the specimen is brought to the laboratory for testing as expeditiously as possible.[11]
2. Administration of medication (especially penicillins) or dietary therapy can cause results resembling AAU.[12]
3. Oliguria with resulting concentration of metabolites can cause false positives. Suspected urines must be tested for specific gravity to rule out this possibility.
4. Inadequate metabolic development or enzymatic maturation in the infant can cause false negatives.

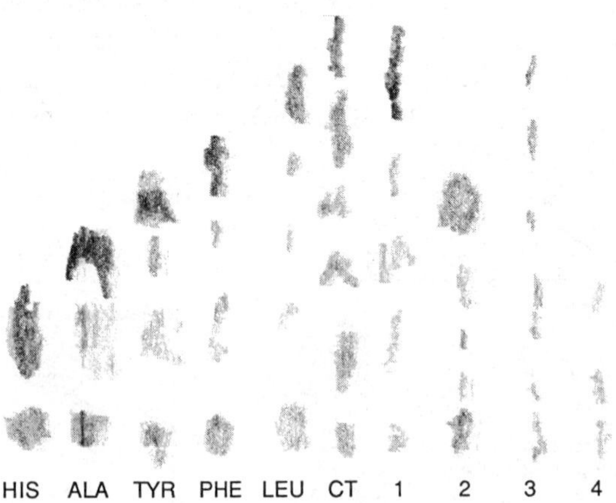

Figure 30-3 Thin layer chromatography (TLC) amino acid screen.

The TLC screen, like the Guthrie screen, is designed for high sensitivity, and there are limitations on specificity of the test. The laboratory will require patient information such as diagnosis, medication, and dietary regimen to help in the interpretation of the test.[12]

CHEMICAL SCREENING TESTS

Simple chemical screening tests are available and are easy to perform. They can be used *with* TLC, but should never be used alone as a screen. These tests are listed in Tables 30-3 and 30-4. They have drawbacks of being positive for a wide variety of metabolic disorders and drugs and negative in the presence of interfering substances, resulting in poor sensitivity and poor specificity.[13]

Quantitation of Amino Acids

If a screening test is positive, a quantitative determination is the next course of action. Quantitative results can be obtained by using High Pressure Liquid Chromatography (HPLC) with an ion exchange column and a fluorescent detection system. Interpretation of the test must be made with the precautions noted for the qualitative measurements.

A good separation technique to purify the sample and a good HPLC system designed for amino

Table 30-3 ***Some Diseases Detectable by Inborn Error Screening Tests***

	$FeCl_3$	Reducing Sub-stance	CTAB*	DNPH†	NaCN–Na Nitro-prus-side	Nitro-sonaph-thol	Nin-hydrin (4)	Amino Acid Chro-matog-raphy
Phenylketonuria	Green	±	–	+	–	–	±	+
Tyrosinuria	Quick-fading green	±	–	+	–	+	+	+
Galactosemia	–	+	–	–	–	±	+	+
Histidinemia	Olive	–	–	±	–	–	±	+
Maple Syrup Urine Disease	Greenish gray	–	–	+	–	–	+	+
Lowe's syndrome	–	±	–	+	–	–	+	+
Hartnup's disease	–	–	–	– ?	–	–	+	+
Wilson's disease	–	–	–	–	–	–	+	+
Arginosuccinicaciduria	–	–	–	– ?	–	–	±	+
Hyperglycinemia	Green	–	–	+	±	–	±	+
Citrullinuria	–	–	–	–	–	–	±	+
Homocystinuria	–	–	–	–	+	–	±	+
Cystinuria	–	–	–	–	+	–	+	+
Hyperlysinemia	–	–	–	+	–	–	±	+
Cystathionuria	–	–	–	–	–	–	±	+
Fructosuria	–	+	–	± ?	–	±	–	–
Alkaptonuria	Transient blue green	+	–	–	–	–	–	–
Hurler's syndrome	–	–	+	–	–	–	–	–
Morquio-Ullrich syndrome	–	–	+	–	–	–	–	–
Marfan's syndrome	–	–	±	–	–	–	–	–

* CTAB = Cetyltrimethylammonium bromide (for mucopolysaccharides)
† DNPH = Dinitrophenylhydrazine (for ketoacids)
Data from reference number [13]

acids are essential for reliable results. Should a delay occur in the reporting of the confirmatory (quantitative) results, it is advisable that a preliminary report indicating the probability of an AAU be issued so that appropriate therapy can be initiated promptly. Possible causes for false-positive results should be ruled out after a thorough review of the patient's status and the laboratory protocol as it relates to the specimen. An algorithm for handling specimens of suspected AAU is presented in Figure 30-4, and serum reference values for selected amino acids are shown in Table 30-5.

PREDICTING PKU

Suspected heterozygotes can be detected by a constant infusion of L-phenylalanine with concurrent measurement of PHE output. Detection is done by the usual laboratory methods, and a tolerance index is calculated.[14]

DNA sequencing analysis for suspected PKU is now possible, as is measurement of gene product catalytic protein and enzyme activity in cultured cells from amniocentesis.[4, 6] These techniques are currently available only in cytogenetic research laboratories.

Table 30-4 *Reactants in the Ferric Chloride Test*

Substance	Color Produced
Phenylpyruvic acid	Green or blue-green, eventually fading to yellow
p-Hydroxyphenylpyruvic acid	Green, fades in seconds
Homogentisic acid	Blue or green, fades slowly
Imidazolepyruvic acid	Green or blue-green
Xanthurenic acid	Deep green, later brown
Bilirubin	Blue-green
Maple Syrup Urine Disease	Gray with a green tinge
Melanin	Gray precipitate, turning black
3-Hydroxanthranilic acid	Immediate deep brown
Vanillic acid	Red-mauve, turns deep brown
Acetoacetic acid	Red or red-brown
Pyruvic acid	Deep gold yellow
α-Ketobutyric acid	Purple, fades to red-brown in 1–2 min
Salicylates	Stable purple
Phenothiazines	Purple
Phenol derivatives	Violet
p-Aminosalicylic acid	Red-brown
Antipyrines	Red
Acetophenetidines	Red
Cyanates	Red

Data from reference number [13]

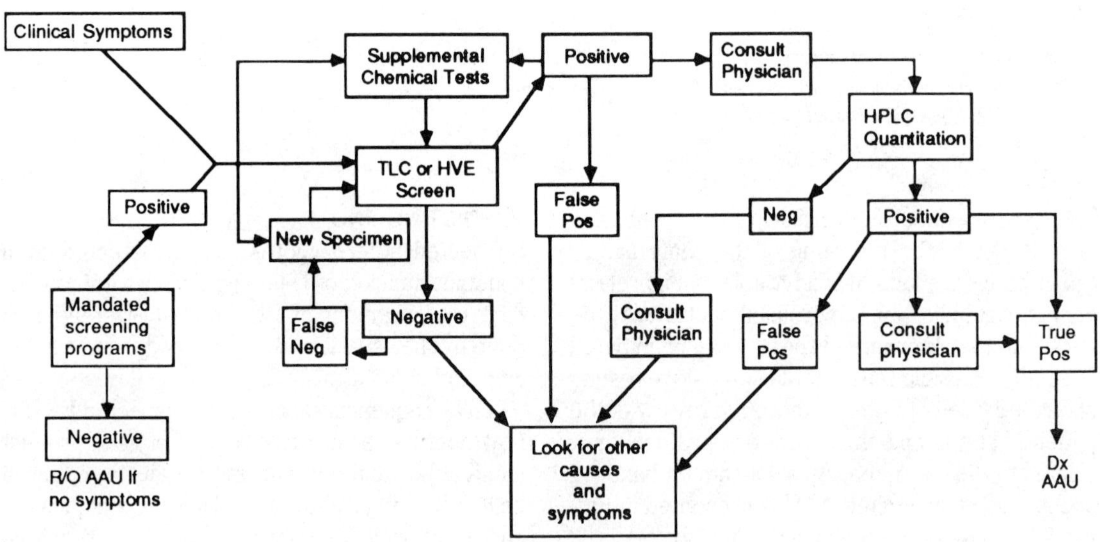

Figure 30-4 Use and interpretation of laboratory tests for aminoacidurias (AAU).

Table 30-5 ***Reference Values for Selected Amino Acids***

Serum Reference Values—Phenylalanine	
	mg/dL
Premature, 1 day	0.36–3.98
Newborn, 1 day	0.76–1.79
1–3 months	1.01–1.95
2–6 months	1.30–3.91
9 months–2 years	0.20–2.21
3–10 years	1.01–3.22
6–18 years	0.78–1.59
Adults	0.40–1.57
Urine Reference Values—Phenylalanine	
	mg/dL
Children	Low adult range
Adults	0.53–0.57
Reference Values—Tyrosine	
	mg/dL
Tyrosinemia I	4–10
Tyrosinemia II	
(0–7 yrs)	32.4–54.4
(8–55 yrs)	18–28
Reference Values—Branched-Chain Amino Acids	
	µmol/L
Leucine	180–700
Isoleucine	70–280
Valine	200–800

Tyrosinemia

A Guthrie system is available, but mass screening for tyrosinemia is usually not practical because of the low incidence of the disease. Urine samples can be used for qualitative screening, but serum must be used for final quantitation by chromatography. Urine contains interfering compounds in high enough concentration to give poor specificity. An enzymatic method is also available, which gives better sensitivity and specificity for tyrosine. *p*-Hydroxyphenylpyruvic acid (PHPPA) can also be detected by chromatography. This is considered one of the most reliable ways of diagnosing tyrosinemia, because urinary excretion of PHPPA can reach up to 25 times the normal amount.[8]

The nitrosonaphthol test (see Table 30-3) is considered more reliable than the ferric chloride test for tyrosine because the nitrosonaphthol test will be negative for other AAUs and will show a +/− reaction with galactose or fructose.

Hepatobiliary tests will be elevated with tyrosinemia, especially as the disease progresses. If a routine chemistry screen of a patient exhibiting characteristic symptoms indicates increased hepatic enzymes and bilirubin, a chromatographic screening is indicated.

Tyrosine crystals may be seen in the urine of patients with any form of tyrosinosis. The urine will also have a "cabbagelike" odor. The crystals must be distinguished from similar-looking crystals such as sulfonamides or x-ray dye crystals. Solubility tests will help to distinguish them. The discovery of tyrosine crystals in urine should always be considered a significant finding. The clinical laboratory scientist should check the age, symptoms, and suspected diagnosis of the patient to see if the patient fits the diagnostic profile of tyrosinosis. Tyrosine crystals can also be seen in patients with severe liver disease due to Oasthouse disease or to other etiologies.

Alkaptonuria

The darkening of urine over a 12- to 24-hour period when exposed to air or sunlight is a presumptive indication of alkaptonuria. A similar darkening of urine may be caused by other substances, however, such as phenols, melanin, and metabolites of salicylate and tryptophan. These substances must be ruled out by chemical testing. Furthermore, high levels of vitamin C, sometimes used to treat alkaptonuria, will reduce HGA and produce a false-negative result.

Homogentisic acid yields positive results with the ferric chloride test (see Table 30-4), but results should be interpreted with caution. Other tests that will give positive results for HGA are the silver nitrate test and Benedict's test, neither of which is specific for HGA.

A combination of positive screening tests and darkening of urine upon standing should lead to the performance of qualitative and quantitative chromatography procedures to confirm the presence of HGA. The chromatography results will correlate with symptoms in adults. Infants will be symptomless.

MSUD

The breath, skin, and *urine* of patients with MSUD have a characteristic burnt sugar or maple syrup odor, from which the disease gets its name. The odor is believed to be derived from the increase of isoleucine in the urine.[15] The urine will be positive in chemical tests but must be screened by TLC or HVE, which will show increases in all three amino acids.

Prompt diagnosis after appearance of the first symptoms is the single most important factor in determining the outcome of the disease. Morbidity is minimal if diagnosis is made and treatment initiated within 24 hours of the first symptoms. It is unpredictable if there is a delay of 3 to 14 days, and is inevitably grave, with severe mental retardation and cerebral palsy, if delayed longer than 14 days.[16, 17] Within 24 hours after birth, newborns with classic MSUD can have a diagnostically relevant plasma leucine concentration, regardless of feeding.[18] Because the infant may rapidly progress into episodes of acidosis, clinical symptoms and urine amino acid results should be correlated with other laboratory tests, particularly electrolyte studies and blood gas analysis.

Leucine crystals may be found in urine sediment of patients with MSUD. They are identified by their appearance and solubility characteristics. The finding of leucine crystals in urine is always abnormal, and should initiate a protocol similar to the one described when finding tyrosine crystals.

Because the incidence of the disease is so low, mass screening is impractical. MSUD can be diagnosed by characterization of the MSUD enzyme phenotype in cultured skin fibroblasts. This technique can be utilized when parents with MSUD-affected children propose to have another child and need prenatal diagnosis.[17]

No-Threshold AAUs

Chemical tests (see Table 30-3) can be useful for the detection of no-threshold AAUs but, again, they are not specific. Qualitative and quantitative assays are best performed by chromatography, in which the intermediate metabolites can be visualized.

Secondary AAUs

Clinical systems, laboratory data, and patient history should be utilized in the diagnosis of secondary AAU. Supporting laboratory data can include marked increase in liver enzymes, bilirubin, drug or toxin levels, electrophoretic abnormalities, and positive hepatitis profile.

TREATMENT

PKU

Treatment consists of a dietary regimen low in PHE. Overrestriction of PHE, however, can lead to impaired growth or brain damage. At the beginning of treatment, PHE measurements should be taken every 1 to 2 days until the level drops below 10 mg/dL (605 μmol/L); thereafter, weekly measurements for 1 or 2 months, followed by monthly measurements, are recommended.[6]

Infants are first placed on a PHE-free formula. These commercial formulas are hydrolysates of protein, and contain other amino acids and nutrients required for growth and development. Because PHE is also essential for growth, it is added to the diet in accordance with the patient's individual tolerance.

After infancy, conventional foods are added,

and slowly replace the PHE-free formula. High-protein foods such as meat, eggs, milk, and cheese are highly restricted or eliminated. Most other conventional foods, especially fruits and vegetables, are acceptable and are selected with consideration of the patient's needs in terms of age, weight, and development. The composition of conventional foods is readily found in standard tables of food composition,[19, 20] which are utilized by the physician and nutritionist to select foods that meet the patient's requirements and provide a varied and palatable diet.

Dietary control, along with PHE monitoring, should continue indefinitely. Physical examination, motor skills tests, neuropsychologic testing, hemoglobin levels, and bone age adequacy should also be monitored.[6] Data have shown that changes in cerebral function have occurred in children who, after several years of compliance, have discontinued their PHE-free diet.[21]

Tyrosinemia

Treatment of hereditary tyrosinemia includes restriction of tyrosine, phenylalanine, and methionine. Dietary treatment does not reverse liver damage nor prevent progression to hepatocarcinoma and liver failure. However, it can correct biochemical abnormalities, including renal tubular complications.[7] Liver transplant has been tried with some success.[22] Infants with transient neonatal tyrosinemia have been treated with high doses of ascorbic acid, which has been shown to help correct this disease.[23]

The treatment and laboratory protocol for monitoring tyrosinemia parallels that described for PKU. Hepatic tests will worsen as the disease progresses, and should be monitored for life. Renal complications can be demonstrated via routine urinalysis.

Alkaptonuria

There is no completely satisfactory treatment for alkaptonuria. If it is detected early, dietary restriction of tyrosine and phenylalanine may be beneficial. Vitamin C therapy has also been tried, since it has been shown that this vitamin is necessary for maximum activity of HGA oxidase.[8] Monitoring of HGA concentration should continue once a diagnosis is made, in order to monitor the progression of the disease and effectiveness of therapy.

MSUD

Treatment for MSUD, consisting of a diet low in BCAA, should be initiated within the first week of life but no later than the second week if permanent neurologic damage is to be prevented. It appears that leucine concentration is chiefly responsible for the neurologic symptoms of the patient;[15] therefore, valine or isoleucine supplements may be used safely to ensure normal growth and development.[7]

Commercial formula products that are devoid of one or more BCAA are available. The formulas contain other essential nutrients (*e.g.*, fat-soluble vitamins, minerals, and caloric sources) that provide a complete diet for infants with MSUD.[24] Older children can receive appropriately balanced mixtures of natural foods of known composition in accordance with the National Academy of Science report on recommended dietary allowances (RDA)[24] to meet nutritional requirements.

Two controversies concerning the dietary management of MSUD exist among the experts: (1) whether to regulate only leucine or all BCAA, and (2) whether to allow only those foods low in BCAA into the diet or, in order to provide a more varied diet, to allow any food as long as the portions are rigidly controlled.[25, 26] The philosophy of a given therapeutic team, therefore, may dictate the dietary regimen prescribed.

In the variant forms of MSUD, levels of BCAA can frequently be maintained within normal levels by limiting daily protein intake without need for special amino-acid mixtures, or by requiring a restricted diet only at times of acute stress. One variant form of MSUD is responsive to a regimen of thiamine ten times the normal daily requirement.

Measurement of serum concentrations of BCAA may be necessary on a daily basis early in life or whenever an acidotic crisis occurs. Daily analysis of urine for ketoacids should continue throughout life. This can be done at home, using dinitrophenylhydrazine strips. As long as urine is negative or contains only trace amounts of ketoacids, measuring serum amino acids at monthly intervals, accompanied by a simple chemistry screen, is usually sufficient.[7] Control ranges for serum concentration of leucine, isoleucine, and valine are included in Table 30-5.

No-Threshold AAUs

Treatment for no-threshold AAUs usually consists of diets low in intermediate metabolites supplemented with amino acids required for growth and development. Vitamin therapy is sometimes recommended.

Secondary AAUs

Treatment of secondary AAUs involves resolution of the underlying disease. Laboratory followup should continue during the course of the treatment.

CASE STUDY

A positive result on a Guthrie test screen for PKU is reported on a premature 5-day old infant. A ferric chloride screen on the same patient shows a green color that fades quickly. A diet low in phenylalanine is initiated, and serum and urine samples for TLC are ordered. In the interim the patient develops symptoms leading to a "failure to thrive" diagnosis, and additional testing is ordered. A sweat test is negative, and liver enzymes (AST and ALT) appear in the high normal range. Creatinine, BUN, and protein are normal as is glucose. The bilirubin has fallen from 15.6 mg/dL (267 μmol/L) on day 1 to 8.9 mg/dL (152 μmol/L) on day 5 (ref. range 1–12 mg/dL [17.1–205 μmol/L]). The TLC plate shows "an elevation in the reference areas of phenylalanine and tyrosine."

Questions

1. What is the most likely diagnosis?
2. What tests correlate with this diagnosis?
3. Why would a dietary regimen low in phenylalanine not improve the patient's condition?
4. What additional therapy is now indicated?
5. What additional tests are needed?
6. What are the advantages and limitations of the Guthrie test as it applies to this patient?

Discussion

1. Transient neonatal tyrosinemia is the most likely diagnosis.
2. The $FeCl_3$ test turns green, and phenylalanine *and* tyrosine are detected on TLC, along with normal chemistry test results (*e.g.,* ALT, bilirubin).
3. The problem was not PKU, but overall enzymatic deficiencies due to underdeveloped liver function.
4. Dietary restriction of tyrosine and phenylalanine and treatment with ascorbic acid are indicated.
5. HPLC quantitative testing for phenylalanine and tyrosine should be done, along with laboratory followup of the patient over the next few weeks.
6. The Guthrie test for PKU is sensitive but not specific. It is designed to bring a possible abnormality to the attention of the clinician, but it is not diagnostic. Further testing is always indicated with a positive Guthrie test. In this case it correctly identified an increase of phenylalanine in the blood, but this was not due to PKU.

REFERENCES

1. Woo J, Cannon DC: Metabolic intermediates and inorganic ions. In Henry JB et al (eds): Clinical Diagnosis and Management by Laboratory Methods, 17th ed, p 140. Philadelphia, WB Saunders, 1984
2. Lenke RR, Levy HL: Maternal phenylketonuria and hyperphenylalaninemia. N Engl J Med 303:1202–1208, 1980
3. Cartier L et al: Prevention of mental retardation in offspring of hyperphenylalaninemic mothers. Am J Public Health 72(12):1386–1389, 1982

4. Nyhan WL: Uncovering disorders of organic acid metabolism. Diagn Med 5(4): 45–57, 1982
5. Howel RR: Metabolic disease in children—crucial clues for the clinician. Consultant 23:133–140, 1983
6. Berry HK: Screening newborns for genetic disease: The PKU model. Diagn Med 7(1):50–59, 1984
7. Berry HK: The spectrum of metabolic disorders. Diagn Med 7(3):39–55, 1984
8. Silverman LM et al: Amino acids and proteins. In Tietz NW (ed): Textbook of Clinical Chemistry, pp 533–536, 545–554. Philadelphia, WB Saunders, 1986
9. McCabe ERB: Principles of newborn screening for metabolic disease. Perinat/Neonat 6:63–67, 1982
10. Guthrie R, Susi A: A simple phenylalanine method for detecting phenylketonuria in large populations of newborn infants. Pediatrics 32:338–343, 1963
11. Vidler J, Wilcken B: Prevalence of unsuspected urinary bacterial contamination: Effects of screening tests for detection of inborn errors of metabolism. Clin Chim Acta 82:173–178, 1978
12. Hill A, Casey R, Zaleski WA: Difficulties and pitfalls in the interpretation of screening tests for the detection of inborn errors of metabolism. Clin Chim Acta 72:1–15, 1976.
13. Graff L Sr: A Handbook of Routine Urinalysis, pp 241–259. Philadelphia, JB Lippincott, 1983.
14. Jagenburg R, Rodjer S: Detection of heterozygotes for phenylketonuria by constant intravenous infusion of L-phenylalanine. Clin Chem 23:1661–1665, 1977
15. Efron ML: Aminoaciduria. N Engl J Med 272(20): 1058–1066, 1965
16. Naughten ER et al: Outcome of maple syrup urine disease. Arch Dis Child 57:918–921, 1982
17. Clow CL et al: Outcome of early and long-term management of classical maple syrup urine disease. Pediatrics 68(6):856–861, 1981
18. Wendel U et al: Maple syrup urine disease (letter to the editor). N Engl J Med 308(18):1100–1101, 1983
19. Watt BK, Merrill AL (eds): Composition of Foods: Handbook No. 8. Washington, DC, Department of Agriculture, 1963
20. Bowes A, Church CF: Food Values and Portions Commonly Used, 11th ed. Philadelphia, JB Lippincott, 1972
21. Koch R et al: Preliminary report on the effects of diet discontinuation in PKU. Pediatr 100(4):870–875, 1982
22. Fisch PO et al: Homotransplantation of the liver in a patient with hepatoma and hereditary tyrosinemia. J Pediatr 93(4):592–596, 1978
23. Frimpter GW: Aminoacidurias due to inherited disorders of metabolism. N Engl J Med 289(16):837, 1973
24. American Academy of Pediatrics Committee on Nutrition: Special diets for infants with in-born errors of amino acid metabolism. Pediatrics 57(5):786–787, 1976
25. Noel MB et al: Dietary treatment of maple syrup urine disease (branched-chain ketoaciduria). J Am Diet Assoc. 69:62–68, 1976
26. Bell L et al: Dietary management of maple syrup urine disease: Extension of equivalency systems. J Am Diet Assoc 74:357–361, 1979

Chapter 31

Cholestasis

James Jackson

Cholestasis is not a disease, *per se,* but a clinical and biochemical syndrome that occurs whenever adequate amounts of both bile salts and bilirubin have failed to reach the intestinal tract and have accumulated instead in the blood. The impairment of bile flow or blockage may occur at any point from the liver cell canaliculus to the entrance of the common bile duct at the duodenum (ampulla of Vater) (see Fig. 31-1).

ETIOLOGY AND PATHOPHYSIOLOGY

In the outline on page 362, it can be seen that the etiology of cholestasis can be either intrahepatic or extrahepatic. Viral hepatitis and drug- or alcohol-induced liver disease are the more common causes of *intrahepatic* cholestasis, while a stone in the common bile duct and pancreatic cancer are the more common causes of the *extrahepatic* type. In addition, cholestasis with intense pruritus, jaundice, and dark urine may occur in the third trimester of pregnancy in certain patients who have an idiosyncratic response to estrogens that causes a slight disruption in bile transport. The condition disappears after delivery. When normal draining of bile into the intestine is substantially reduced or completely blocked, bile backs up into the liver and eventually into the blood as cholestasis progresses.

As the bile canaliculi become congested with bile, they tend to enlarge and eventually rupture.[1] This results in escape of bilirubin and bile salts directly into the blood (see outline on page 362). The initial influx of bilirubin is of the conjugated type. Eventually, as there is reduced uptake of bilirubin by the hepatic cells, unconjugated bil-

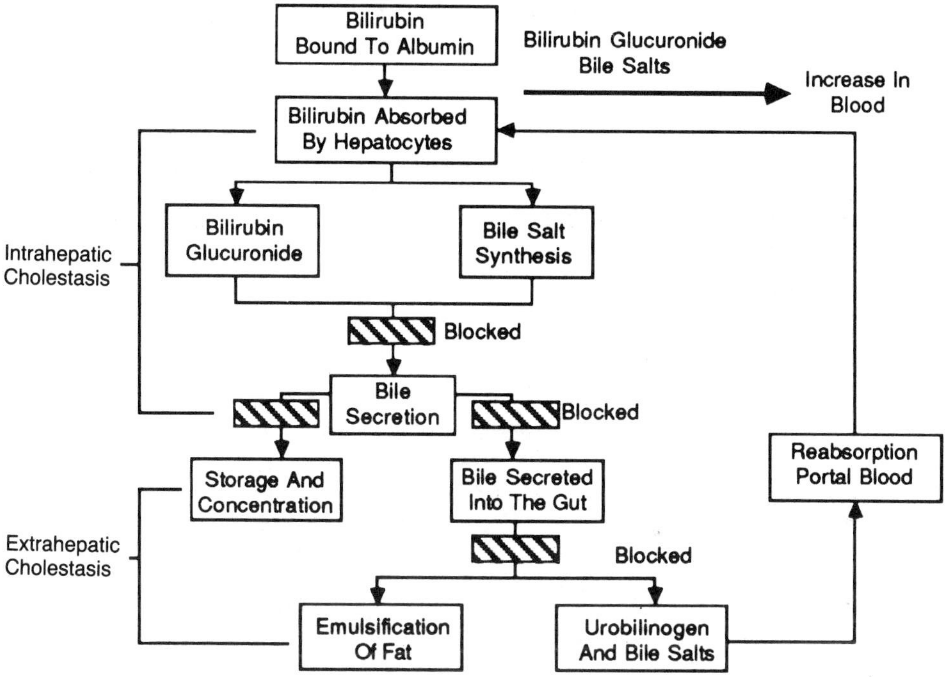

Figure 31-1 **Flow chart of intrahepatic and extrahepatic cholestasis.**

irubin also starts to increase in the blood, giving a mixed hyperbilirubinemia.[1] If the obstruction is complete, the feces will be gray-colored (the so-called "clay-colored stools"), which is the result of the lack of bile and of increased fat content in the feces.

Malabsorption of fat will occur due to the lack of the emulsifying action of bile in the intestine, and may result in several severe complications. Fat emulsification and fat absorption are diminished to about half of normal levels, resulting in *steatorrhea* (fat in the stools) and interference with fat-soluble vitamin and calcium absorption. Vitamin K is dependent on bile salts for its absorption, and is required for normal liver synthesis of various clotting factors. If cholestasis persists, there will be an increase in the prothrombin time, which may lead to bleeding tendencies. Malabsorption of vitamin D and calcium may lead to osteoporosis and bone pain.[1]

Exact causes of various hepatobiliary diseases that precipitate cholestasis are discussed elsewhere in this section and so will not be discussed to any great degree in this chapter.

CLINICAL MANIFESTATIONS

A patient with jaundice, pruritus, light-colored stools, and negative urobilinogen should be evaluated for cholestasis. The pruritus is a result of the movement of bile salts to the peripheral tissues.

LABORATORY ANALYSES AND DIAGNOSIS

Procedures for determining the etiology of cholestasis usually involve the nuclear medicine and radiology departments as well as the clinical laboratory. Some of the diagnostic procedures used are intravenous cholangiography, infusion tomography, ultrasound, and cholescintigraphy with technetium-99 iminodiacetic acid (^{99}Tc-IDA) or the analog of IDA, dimethyliminodiacetic acid (^{99}Tc-HIDA). ^{99}Tc-IDA and its analog are taken up by the

Etiology of Impaired Bilirubin and Bile Excretion

1. *Intrahepatic**—liver cell damage, or blockage of bile canaliculi
   (a) Hepatitis
   (b) Infiltrative tumors
   (c) Drugs or chemical toxins
   (d) Estrogens or pregnancy
   (e) Primary biliary cirrhosis
   (f) Intrahepatic biliary hypoplasia or atresia
   (g) Dubin-Johnson syndrome
2. *Extrahepatic**—obstruction of bile ducts
   (a) Extrahepatic biliary atresia
   (b) Intraluminal gallstones
   (c) Congenital choledochal cyst
   (d) Compression obstruction from tumor
   (e) Stenosis—postsurgical or inflammation

*In both conditions, hyperbilirubinemia results mainly from conjugated bilirubin, over 75% of the total.

hepatocytes and excreted unchanged into the bile. Functional and anatomical information can be obtained about the complete hepatobiliary system with these techniques.[2] The only contraindication to the technetium-99 tests is pregnancy. In cholestasis, ultrasound is probably the best initial diagnostic procedure for evaluating the jaundiced patient. It can pinpoint ductal dilation with a high degree of accuracy, and can often determine the level and cause of obstruction (See Fig. 31-2).

The characteristics of prolonged cholestasis are shown at the top of the opposite column.

The laboratory will be involved with tests associated with a "hepatic or liver panel" (see Table 31-1). The enzymes alkaline phosphatase (ALP) and gamma glutamyltransferase (GGT) are both helpful in identifying cholestasis because they are located on the surface of cell membranes bordering

Characteristics of Prolonged Cholestasis

1. Jaundice—75% conjugated bilirubin type
2. Pruritus—often severe
3. Malabsorption—due to lack of bile in intestine
4. Hypercholesterolemia—increased synthesis may result in fatty tumorlike masses in the skin called *xanthomas*

bile canaliculi and liver sinusoids (ALP),[3] and membranes of the canaliculi and epithelial cells of the bile ducts (GGT).[4]

Gamma glutamyltransferase is usually most significantly elevated by obstructive disease, has good specificity for the liver, and is not elevated in bone diseases or pregnancy (as is ALP) or in skeletal muscle disease (as is AST). GGT also can help to differentiate mechanical and viral from drug-induced cholestasis. In mechanical and viral cholestasis, GGT and ALP are about equally elevated,

Table 31-1 ***Diagnostic Hepatic Panel***

	Reference Range*
AST	8–20 U/L 30 C
ALT	8–20 U/L 30 C
Alkaline phosphatase (ALP)	25–90 U/L 30 C
Gamma glutamyl transferase (GGT)	9–50 U/L 37 C
Total bilirubin	0.2–1.0 mg/dL (3.4–17.1 μmol/L)
Conjugated (direct) bilirubin	0.0–0.2 mg/dL (0–3.4 μmol/L)
Prothrombin time	11–15 seconds
Total protein	6.4–8.3 g/dL (64–83 g/L)
Albumin	3.5–5.0 g/dL (35–50 g/L)
Urine bilirubin	Negative
Urobilinogen	0.2–1.0 E.U. (0.2–1.0 U)

*May vary depending on methodology used and patient population

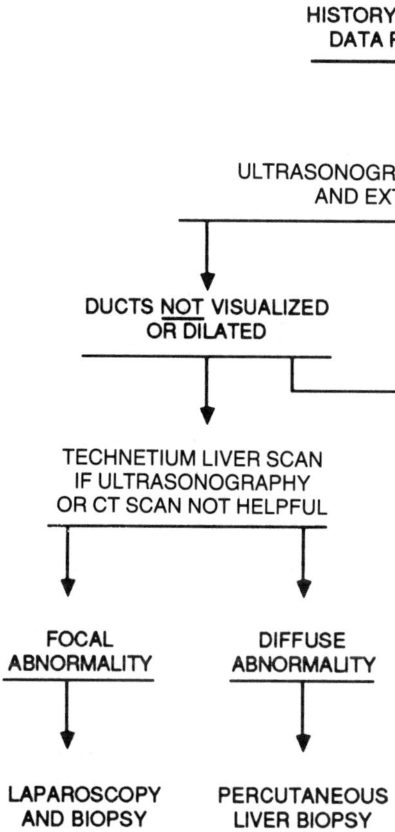

Figure 31-2 **Algorithm of work-up of patient with cholestasis.**

while in drug-induced cholestasis, GGT is increased more significantly than is ALP.[4] However, GGT is an inducible liver enzyme, and therefore elevated serum GGT levels may be found in patients who take such drugs as phenobarbital and phenytoin on a long-term basis (*e.g.*, treatment for epilepsy). These drugs induce the liver microsomes to increase protein synthesis and produce certain enzymes. Therefore, the patient's drug history must be considered in the evaluation of abnormal GGT levels.

Alkaline phosphatase, although increased in conditions other than cholestasis, is still one of the tests of choice for evaluating cholestasis and obstructive jaundice. ALP is only modestly increased in parenchymal damage—such as in hepatitis with cholestasis, in which ALP levels are rarely higher than twice the upper reference limits for adults. In disease or damage to the ducts with cholestasis, ALP levels may be two to four times the normal reference range for adults.[3]

Urine bilirubin should be positive due to the presence of conjugated bilirubin, while *urine urobilinogen* should be negative in obstructive diseases with cholestasis. It is important to remember that urine dipsticks do not have the ability to measure negative urobilinogen levels, and only detect normal or elevated amounts.[5] Only by using a quantitative test (2-hour or 24-hour) is it possible to detect an absence of urobilinogen.

Prothrombin times will be increased and the patient will exhibit bleeding tendencies if cholestasis is prolonged. As described above, this is due mainly to malabsorption of fats and vitamin K.

Marked *serum transaminase* elevations suggest an intrahepatic or hepatocellular cholestasis, but may also be seen in extrahepatic cholestasis with acute obstruction due to common bile duct stone. Elevated *serum amylase* levels usually indicate extrahepatic obstruction from the head of the pancreas. Liver biopsy may also help clarify the diagnosis.

TREATMENT

Treatment of cholestasis depends on the cause. A stone requires surgical intervention, which usually corrects the cholestasis. The practical problem of cholestasis is to determine at what level in the hepatobiliary system the block has occurred.[6] This, of course, will determine the type of treatment. If the block is in the hepatic ducts (usually distal to the bifurcation), surgical intervention may be necessary. If the block is at the level of the liver cell or the canaliculi, surgical intervention is not practical. If a patient presents with cholestasis and a normal-sized liver, a surgical lesion is very unlikely.[6]

Pruritus may respond to cholestyramine, a resinlike substance given orally that binds bile salts in the intestine. Calcium and fat-soluble vitamins A, D, and K supplements may be given as needed. Malabsorption and steatorrhea should disappear as bile flow to the intestine is restored. Urobilinogen should start to reappear in the urine, and bilirubin to disappear.

CASE STUDY #1

A white woman, 28 years of age and in the third trimester of her second pregnancy, complained to her physician of intense itching of her skin and of her urine turning "brownish green" in color. She also stated that her skin and eyes were turning yellow.

The physical examination was unremarkable except for small scratches on her arms and legs and a slightly jaundiced appearance. Laboratory data showed a negative HBsAg test and a slight anemia with mild leukocytosis. The total bilirubin was elevated, 5.0 mg/dL (86 μmol/L), with a conjugated bilirubin (direct reading) of 3.75 mg/dL (64 μmol/L). The serum alkaline phosphatase was about 1.5 times normal, and the GGT was 3 times normal. Serum transaminase levels were markedly increased, 5 times above normal range. The urine was dark brown in color, with 3+ bilirubin and "normal" urobilinogen using the Ames N-Multistix. Serum amylase was normal. There was a moderate increase in serum cholesterol and triglyceride levels. The patient history revealed that she had experienced some of the same symptoms with her first pregnancy, but that they had disappeared after delivery.

Questions

1. What is the probable diagnosis for this patient? Why?
2. Which laboratory tests ordered provided the most information and which tests provided the least? Why?

Discussion

1. Liver function, especially bile transport, is disrupted to a slight extent in pregnancy. Most liver function tests remain normal, with the exception of alkaline phosphatase, which may rise to 2 or 3 times normal due to placental production of ALP during the third trimester. However, for unknown reasons, a relatively common disorder may occur in patients who show an idiosyncratic response to certain steroid-type drugs—in this case, estrogens. Based on this patient's history, examination, and laboratory data, the diagnosis is that the patient is exhibiting cholestasis (pruritus) of pregnancy, a benign condition that occurs in the third trimester and is characterized by intense itching, dark urine, and jaundice. It disappears after delivery but tends to recur with each

pregnancy or if the same patient is given oral contraceptives. Treatment includes oral cholestyramine—8 to 12 grams daily in two or three doses—to relieve itching.

2. The transaminases are markedly increased in hepatocellular or intrahepatic cholestasis, more so than in the extrahepatic type. In this case the GGT is more significantly increased than the ALP, which suggests that the condition is a drug-induced cholestasis. Because of placental production, the ALP of a normal pregnant patient in her third trimester is usually elevated up to 2 to 3 times normal, and therefore the ALP level is of limited diagnostic value in this test. The positive urine bilirubin confirms the high direct-reading hyperbilirubinemia, because only conjugated bilirubin can appear in the urine. The urobilinogen results, in this case and in any case in which a negative reading is obtained, are useless, because none of the urine dipstick tests available can detect a negative urine urobilinogen.[6]

CASE STUDY #2

A 50-year old white woman was admitted to the hospital with jaundice, right upper quadrant tenderness, nausea, vomiting, and complaints of severe itching of skin. There was no history of alcohol abuse. Laboratory and radiology studies revealed the following data:

LABORATORY FINDINGS

CBC: "Within normal limits"
Total bilirubin: 3.5 mg/dL (60 μmol/L)
Direct (conjugated) bilirubin: 2.9 mg/dL (50 μmol/L)
ALP: 500 U/L 30 C
AST: 100 U/L 30 C
ALT: 175 U/L 30 C
Triglycerides: 280 mg/dL (3.2 mmol/L)
Cholesterol: 360 mg/dL (9.3 mmol/L)
Fasting blood sugar: 85 mg/dL (4.7 mmol/L)
Ultrasonography of liver: Ducts clearly visible and dilated
Urine bilirubin: Positive 2+
HBsAg: Negative
Serum amylase: Normal

Questions

1. The above findings are most consistent with what diagnosis?
2. Why did you select that diagnosis?
3. Which of the laboratory test results are abnormal? Which tests give the most information? The least information?

Discussion:

1. Cholecystitis is the most likely diagnosis.
2. The findings of right upper quadrant tenderness, jaundice, and severe itching (pruritus) suggest a liver problem. The lack of history of alcohol intake and negative HBsAg would rule out infectious hepatitis and alcoholic cirrhosis. The normal serum amylase rules out pancreatitis. These symptoms in a 50-year-old woman, especially the itching and the ultrasonography finding, indicate an intrahepatic cholestasis, most probably primary biliary cirrhosis (PBC). Nine out of ten patients with PBC are females between ages 40 and 60. Also, the markedly increased ALP and slightly increased AST and ALT would support a cholestatic problem rather than a necrotic or inflammatory one. The urine bilirubin and direct bilirubin would indicate an increase in conjugated bilirubin.
3. The ALP, total and direct bilirubin, AST, ALT, triglycerides, cholesterol, and urine bilirubin are all abnormal. Ultrasonography, total and direct bilirubin, ALP, AST, and ALT give the most information. The abnormal results point to a liver condition, and help to differentiate between a necroinflammatory and a cholestatic problem. The cholesterol and triglyceride levels do not provide much information, unless the patient has lipid deposits around the eyes (xanthelasma) or deposits elsewhere in the skin (xanthoma), which commonly appear in PBC. Other laboratory tests to use in this case are serum IgM levels (markedly increased), IgG and IgA levels (normal), and the presence of antimitochondrial antibodies, which are the hallmark of PBC.

REFERENCES

1. Emes JH, Nowak TJ: Introduction to Pathophysiology: Basic Principles of the Disease Process, pp 252–255. Baltimore, University Park Press, 1983
2. Weissman HM, Freeman LM: Evaluating hepatobiliary diseases with cholescintigraphy. Diagn Med 6(3): 32–46, 1983
3. Batsakis JG: Serum alkaline phosphatase: Refining an old test for the future. Diagn Med 5(3): 25–33: 1982
4. Shaw LM: Keeping pace with a popular enzyme. Diagn Med 5(3): 59–78, 1982
5. Jackson JA, Conrad ME: Technical aspects of urine dipstick reagent areas. Am Clin Prod Rev 12: 10–18, 1985
6. Iber FS, Latham PS: Normal and pathologic physiology of the liver. In Soderman WA, Soderman TM (eds): Pathologic Physiology: Mechanisms of Disease, 7th ed, pp 892–896. Philadelphia, WB Saunders, 1985.

Chapter 32

Cirrhosis

Bethany W. Hurtuk

ETIOLOGY AND PATHOPHYSIOLOGY

It is believed that diffuse liver cell death is the precursor of cirrhosis, a disease in which there is permanent structural damage to the liver, possibly in its entirety. Morphologically, cirrhosis presents with two features: increased fibrous tissue and nodular regeneration. The results are disorganization of the lobular structure and distortion of the vascular bed, which lead to disruption of normal liver function.[1]

Although there are several types of cirrhosis, in North America *alcoholic cirrhosis* is the most common. It is caused by the consumption of a pint or more of whiskey or its equivalent per day for at least 10 years. The effects on the liver are uniform liver cell loss, small islands of regenerating or preserved parenchyma, and diffuse fine scarring.[1]

Postnecrotic cirrhosis is the most common cirrhosis worldwide. The cause is unknown, but viral hepatitis has been a precursor in many cases. The pathology of the disease includes (1) irregular, large nodules of regenerating hepatocytes that vary from microscopic (<1 cm) to visible in size, (2) extensive liver cell loss, and (3) stromal collapse and fibrosis, which produce broad bands of connective tissue that contain the remains of many portal triads (hepatic vein, artery, and bile duct).

The cause is unknown for the third major kind of cirrhosis, *biliary cirrhosis*. Because 90% of the cases occur in middle-aged women, it is believed that the cause may have an endocrine origin. There is also evidence that viral destruction of the liver or drug hypersensitivity initiates the disease. Another aspect that may be related to the cause of the disease is the fact it often occurs in the presence of some specific or nonspecific immunologic abnormality. For example, about 80% of patients with biliary cirrhosis exhibit elevated IgM serum levels, and more than 95% of the patients exhibit a circulating IgG mitochondrial antibody. Hence, a disordered immune response may initiate or worsen the lesions of biliary cirrhosis.[1]

There is also a type of biliary cirrhosis that is secondary to an obstruction of the bile duct or its major branches. Gallstones, tumors or postoperative strictures may cause the obstruction. Whatever the cause of biliary cirrhosis, however, the disease is characterized by impaired bile excretion and progressive destruction of the intrahepatic bile ducts.[1]

CLINICAL MANIFESTATIONS

Most of the clinical manifestations of cirrhosis are common to all types. Jaundice, fluid accumulation in the peritoneal cavity (*ascites*), central nervous system dysfunction, and increased interstitial fluid volume (*edema*) are common. Additionally, the fibrosis results in distorted intrahepatic vasculature, which causes portal venous hypertension with splenomegaly and esophageal and gastric varices. The shape of the liver may also become distorted, and the intrahepatic venous and lymphatic radicals may become compressed, contributing to the ascites and portal hypertension.[1]

There are, however, some differentiating clinical features among the types of cirrhosis. After the symptoms of fluid retention, portal hypertension, and liver dysfunction, an individual with *alcoholic cirrhosis* may experience weakness, fatigue, anorexia, and weight loss. The liver may be firm and enlarged, and muscle wasting, gynecomastia, and testicular atrophy or amenorrhea may also be present. These features are generally secondary to the large intake of ethanol. The cause of death is usually hepatic coma or hemorrhage from ruptured esophageal varices.[1]

Postnecrotic cirrhosis presents somewhat differently than alcoholic cirrhosis. There may be more jaundice but fewer signs of wasting early in the disease process.[1]

Some of the clinical signs of *biliary cirrhosis* are different than the signs for alcoholic or postnecrotic cirrhosis. A patient (typically female) with biliary cirrhosis may complain of itching, pale stools, jaundice, and dark urine. Steatorrhea, diarrhea, osteomalacia, backache, bone pain, and yellowish plaques or nodules (xanthomas) in the subcutaneous tissues, resulting from lipid deposits, may also be present.[1]

LABORATORY ANALYSES AND DIAGNOSIS

The most nearly definitive means of diagnosing cirrhosis is a liver biopsy. Abnormalities in analytes that are useful in diagnosing *alcoholic cirrhosis* are summarized in Table 32-1. There may be some variations in the extent of increases of the analytes depending on the course and extent of the disease process, because analyte level is to some degree reflective of the degree of liver function impairment. For example, *cholestasis,* a lack of flow of bile from the liver cells into the common bile duct, is responsible for transient increases in bilirubin, GGT, and ALP. Increases in AST, ALT, and LD are transient with liver cell injury, and metabolic abnormalities are the reasons for changes in albumin, globulin, cholesterol, and prothrombin time.[2, 3] Anemia is usually caused by folic acid deficiency, gastrointestinal blood loss, or toxic effects of alcohol on bone marrow, and may be accompanied by thrombocytopenia and leukopenia.

The results of *postnecrotic cirrhosis* resemble those of alcoholic cirrhosis. However, the increase in bilirubin is usually higher, and increases in AST and ALT are usually more persistent.

In *biliary cirrhosis,* as with postnecrotic cirrhosis, the laboratory profile may differ somewhat from alcoholic cirrhosis. Serum ALP is the earliest abnormal result, with an elevation of two to five times the reference range. The bilirubin, AST, and ALT are only slightly elevated initially. Later in the disease the bilirubin increases further, but the AST and ALT remain only slightly elevated. A few other laboratory findings unique to biliary cirrhosis may aid in the diagnosis. These findings are antibodies that are present in the serum. They may be

Table 32-1 ***Changes in Analytes in Alcoholic Cirrhosis***

Analyte	Change
Bilirubin	Normal or increased
Gamma glutamyl transferase (GGT)	Normal or increased
Aspartate aminotransferase (AST)	Normal or increased
Alanine aminotransferase (ALT)	Normal or increased
Alkaline phosphatase (ALP)	Normal or increased
Lactate dehydrogenase (LD)	Normal or increased
Albumin	Decreased
Immunoglobulins	Increased
Cholesterol	Increased
Prothrombin time	Prolonged
Red blood cell count	Decreased
Hemoglobin	Decreased

antismooth-muscle antibodies, antimitochondrial antibodies, antinuclear antibodies, or antibodies directed against one or more liver antigens. These antibodies are present when the biliary cirrhosis is not secondary to an obstruction of the bile duct. Immunofluorescence is the technique most commonly used to assay them.[4]

In addition to the laboratory results already discussed, others may appear abnormal in certain types of cirrhosis. In *alcoholic cirrhosis,* respiratory alkalosis resulting from an increased depth of breathing may be noticed and, because of dietary deficiencies and urine loss, magnesium may be decreased. Ascites and edema may cause dilution, resulting in decreased sodium and potassium. Impaired liver function also results in elevated levels of ammonia in the blood.[1] Through successful treatment the physician may note improvement in these analyte levels, but there may still be permanent damage to the liver.

In *biliary cirrhosis* serum bile salts are increased and a unique low-density lipoprotein, called *lipoprotein X,* that contains 65% lecithin, 30% cholesterol, and 5% protein, is present. Another finding is increased levels of serum bile salts. For an unknown reason, liver copper levels are elevated in primary biliary cirrhosis[1] but may be reduced through appropriate treatment.

TREATMENT

As described above, the course of *alcoholic cirrhosis* is long and extensive. By the time the liver is damaged to the extent of cirrhosis, the prognosis is poor. If the patient abstains from alcohol and maintains good nutrition, and if liver damage is not severe, enzyme levels may return to normal, as may some of the other values. Liver damage resulting from cirrhosis, however, is advanced and irreversible.

Postnecrotic cirrhosis tends to progress even with supportive therapy. The majority of the cases terminate in death.[1] The laboratory values, therefore, cannot be used to monitor the success of treatment.

There is no known medical treatment to alter the course of primary *biliary cirrhosis.* Studies are under way to attempt to dissolve immune complexes in serum,[3] but it is too early to tell if this will be beneficial. Secondary biliary cirrhosis may be treated early by correcting the obstruction. Any abnormal laboratory results would subsequently return to normal.

CASE STUDY

A 63-year-old man, while helping his wife move some furniture, complained of not feeling well and vomited blood. Their physician admitted the patient to the hospital. Physical examination revealed edema and a hard, enlarged liver. Laboratory results revealed a decreased hemoglobin and hematocrit and increased bilirubin, GGT, AST, and ALT. The man had a history of alcohol abuse.

Questions

1. What is the probable diagnosis?
2. What is one aspect of treatment that should definitely be initiated as soon as possible?

3. What is the probable reason for the bleeding?
4. Is it possible that this patient's blood might not clot properly? Why?

Discussion

1. The most probable diagnosis is alcoholic cirrhosis.
2. Abstention from ingesting alcohol should begin immediately.
3. The bleeding is probably coming from a weakened vein in the esophagus that ruptured when the patient was moving the furniture.
4. This patient's blood might not clot properly because the clotting factors cannot be produced properly in a damaged liver.

REFERENCES

1. Petersdorf RG et al (eds): Harrison's Principles of Internal Medicine, 10th ed. New York City, McGraw-Hill, 1983
2. Tietz NW (ed): Textbook of Clinical Chemistry. Philadelphia, WB Saunders, 1986
3. Berkow R (ed): The Merck Manual of Diagnosis and Therapy, 14th ed. Rahway, NJ, Merck, Sharp & Dohme Research Laboratories, 1982
4. Henry JB: Clinical Diagnosis and Management by Laboratory Methods, 17th ed. Philadelphia, WB Saunders, 1984

Chapter 33

Hepatic Failure

Consuelo Kazen

Hepatic failure can be defined as the condition in which the liver fails to function adequately. Because the liver is responsible for such diverse functions as detoxification, carbohydrate metabolism, and protein synthesis, any or all of these functions will be affected should the liver fail. The degree and duration of the failure will determine the prognosis for survival.

ETIOLOGY AND PATHOPHYSIOLOGY

Hepatic failure may be the result of chronic liver disease or it may be of sudden onset caused by massive liver cell destruction.[1] Inadequate liver function is the immediate result of two processes: bypass shunting and necrosis. *Bypass shunting* is the process whereby blood flow through the lobules, blocked by fibrous or other tissue, may be rerouted to nearby vessels. Hepatocytes near the blockage site will be deprived of blood flow and will not receive the necessary substances for metabolic processing. *Tissue necrosis* will occur if cells are deprived of nutrients for a long enough period. Necrosis may also result from direct cell injury, such as occurs in drug toxicity. Failure thus occurs when liver cells cannot perform their functions because (1) they are not receiving the necessary substances for metabolism, or (2) they are undergoing necrosis.[2]

Due to the life-threatening nature of liver failure, it is imperative that its presence be detected as early in its course as possible.

Predisposing Conditions

Two of the most frequent conditions that may predispose an individual to hepatic failure are viral hepatitis and drug toxicity. Both may lead either to a rapid (acute) or an insidious (subacute) onset of liver failure. Drugs known to cause hepatotoxicity are listed below; ethanol is the most common cause.[3] Other conditions that may lead to liver failure are also listed. One of the first presenting features of Wilson's disease is frequently fulminant hepatitis.[4]

Certain susceptible individuals will develop some degree of hepatic failure as a result of stress or infection. Stress may be induced by surgical procedures such as shunting or by physical trauma.

Some Conditions That May Result in Hepatic Failure

- Viral hepatitis
- Drug toxicity
  - Ethanol
  - Paracetamol (acetaminophen)
  - Oral contraceptives
  - Halothane anesthesia
  - Methotrexate
  - α-Methyldopa
  - Chloroform
  - Industrial poisons
- Metabolic disorders
  - Wilson's disease
  - Galactosemia
  - α_1-antitrypsin deficiency
  - Fructosuria
  - Tyrosinemia
  - Reye's syndrome

Complications

Complications that accompany hepatic failure range from electrolyte imbalance to multiple organ failure (see listing below). Typically, hypoglycemia is present and must be monitored closely. Hyponatremia and hypokalemia also will often be observed. It is believed that the hyponatremia is a reflection of the fluid imbalance that occurs due to lowered oncotic pressure,[5] and that the hypokalemia results from intestinal loss of fluid. Edema and ascites are reflections of both fluid and electrolyte imbalances. The presence of ascites may predispose an individual to infection and septicemia. Neutrophil adherence is decreased in hepatic failure, and it has been suggested that this is a contributing factor to the high infection rate in these patients.[6]

Other complications include coagulopathy and hypertension. Bleeding may occur from any area, including the nose and venipuncture sites. Death is often caused by gastrointestinal hemorrhage as a complicating factor. Portal hypertension very often results from bypass shunting and lowered renal function.

For as yet unexplained reasons, a hepatorenal syndrome may develop in some individuals.[7] This is a condition in which renal failure will occur as a

Some Complications of Hepatic Failure

- Hypoglycemia
- Jaundice
- Infection
- Electrolyte imbalance
- Fluid imbalance
- Edema
- Ascites
- Coagulopathy
- Encephalopathy
- Cerebral edema
- Hepatorenal syndrome
- Pancreatitis

sequela to hepatic failure. The renal failure results in both oliguria and azotemia.

The accumulation of toxic substances in the presence or absence of renal failure may result in encephalopathy, which may progress to coma if the toxic substances are not removed at an effective rate. In some patients pancreatitis will be a further complication.

CLINICAL MANIFESTATIONS

Regardless of the cause of hepatic failure, one of the more typical clinical manifestations that may be seen is edema or fluid accumulation. Fluid may accumulate in the extremities or in the abdominal area as ascites. This is caused by the low oncotic pressure that results from the decrease in protein synthesis and transport (of albumin in particular) when liver cells fail to function. The fluid is typically a transudate.[2]

Jaundice is frequently a presenting feature, and should be looked for in the sclera as well as the skin (see Chap. 28). Bilirubin accumulation may arise from several causes but is due primarily to the liver's failure to conjugate it for elimination.

Because several important clotting factors are synthesized in the liver, bleeding diathesis is not uncommon. Typically, prolonged bleeding from puncture sites may occur, as may gastrointestinal hemorrhage.

As the severity of hepatic failure progresses, encephalopathy may occur. The symptoms associated with this condition will be dependent on the grade of encephalopathy that occurs, and may range from slight tremors, to drowsiness and forgetfulness, to coma, and finally to death (see listing above, right). Flapping tremor or asterixis is revealed through physical examination. A jerky motion of the hand is observed as the patient attempts to lift it while resting forearm and wrist on a flat surface. Hepatic fetor in the breath is attributed to the accumulation of certain toxic substances, and is typically associated with liver disease. Some individuals will begin to itch due to the accumulation of bile salts under the skin. Table 33-1 summarizes the presenting symptoms discussed, along with an explanation for their occurrence.

Encephalopathy Grades

Grade 1
- Slight flapping tremor
- Mild, temporary confusion
- Mood change
- Normal EEG

Grade 2
- Drowsiness
- Increased confusion
- Lost sphincter control
- Flapping tremor easily detected
- Abnormal EEG

Grade 3
- In stupor
- Can be roused
- Flapping tremor present
- EEG abnormal

Grade 4
- Comatose
- EEG abnormal

LABORATORY ANALYSES AND DIAGNOSIS

Diagnosis

Because of the severe and complex nature of hepatic failure, the laboratory usually plays a comprehensive and vital role in its diagnosis and treatment.

Although all individuals do not respond alike to similar disease processes, there are laboratory findings that have been observed to be representative of hepatic failure. They may vary among individuals. It should be noted that the degree of the laboratory abnormality will reflect the degree of liver failure.

Table 33-1 ***Symptoms and Their Causes***

Symptom	Cause
Jaundice	Unconjugated bilirubin accumulates.
Hepatic fetor in breath	α-Mercaptan accumulates, along with other toxic wastes.
Asterixis (flapping tremor)	Motor disturbance associated with encephalopathy is present.
Edema of extremities and/or ascites	Hypoalbuminemia causes low oncotic pressure that leads to fluid imbalance and the formation of a transudate.
Bleeding diatheses (petechiae, slowed clotting, hemorrhage)	Factors I, II, V, VII, IX, and X are not being synthesized at an effective rate by the liver. Platelets are being destroyed by the spleen or production is reduced due to BM suppression.
Encephalopathy	Toxic accumulation of NH_3, amines, bile salts, and other wastes leads to brain involvement.

Plasma and urine bilirubin levels are frequently elevated, and may be the first presenting features. Typically, the unconjugated fraction of bilirubin is elevated to a greater degree than is the conjugated fraction. Urine bilirubin often becomes detectable before the appearance of jaundice.[8] Urine urobilinogen may be decreased or normal initially because less conjugated bilirubin is available for conversion in the intestinal tract; as the disease progresses, however, the levels may become elevated. An elevated level of bilirubin is not in itself diagnostic of liver failure, but it is strong evidence that the hepatocyte is not functioning normally.

Several enzymes have been utilized as liver disease markers. These have been selected because they are normally present in the liver and their levels of activity can be affected by the presence of disease. Six enzymes normally present in liver include alkaline phosphatase (ALP), 5' nucleotidase (5'NT), aspartate aminotransferase (AST), alanine aminotransferase (ALT), lactate dehydrogenase (LD), and gamma glutamyltransferase (GGT). There are hundreds of other liver enzymes, but they have not been proven to be more effective in the study of liver disease than these six.

Typical liver profiles will usually include the measurement of ALP, AST, and ALT activity in serum. These are used in liver profiles because they are useful in distinguishing the type of liver disease that is present. ALP will show a greater degree of elevation in obstruction and liver metastasis, whereas the transaminases will show greater elevation in hepatocyte injury. In the presence of hepatic failure, all three will be elevated in serum during the early course of the disease, although ALP may be elevated only moderately. All three will eventually return to normal levels, either as the condition improves or as the liver cell injury becomes massive and virtually complete.

Other sources of ALP in the serum include bone, intestine, and placenta. The source of the elevated enzyme may be discovered by measurement of the isoenzymes or by measurement of the enzyme 5′NT, which is the hepatic fraction of alkaline phosphatase. The isoenzymes may be differentiated from each other by either heat or chemical stability testing. Chemicals such as L-phenylalanine or levamisole may be added to plasma in order to inhibit intestinal, placental, and Regan alkaline phosphatase isoenzymes.[9]

LD is present in many tissues in the body, including the myocardium, muscle, kidney, red cells, and liver. It is therefore more difficult to interpret an elevated level of total LD activity. It may be necessary to measure isoenzymes to determine the source of the elevated activity. Hepatocyte injury, as in hepatic failure, will result in an elevated activity of LD isoenzymes 4 and 5.

GGT is a very sensitive indicator of hepatocyte

toxicity, and is elevated in alcohol and drug abusers. It will also be elevated in liver failure.

Plasma levels of bile acids have been found elevated in hepatic failure, and it is believed that measuring the rate of clearance of free bile acids, such as cholic acid, can be helpful in predicting the likelihood of survival for individuals who have reached grade 4 encephalopathy.[10, 11] In one study, it was found that a higher survival rate was likely for persons who had a faster clearance rate of injected ^{14}C cholic acid from plasma than for those with a prolonged rate of clearance. Current methods for measuring bile acids include radioimmunoassays, enzyme-linked immunoassays, fluorometric assays, high performance liquid chromatography, and gas chromatography. Typically, an extraction process must be carried out before quantitation can be done.[12] Figure 33-1 is a representation of the typical approach to the assessment of encephalopathy.

Levels of albumin may be slow to fall because its half-life is 21 days; however, eventually low levels will be detected—usually in amounts below 4 g/dL (40g/L).[5] Cholesterol, which is synthesized in the liver, will also be found in decreased amounts in the plasma.

The single most important diagnostic hematologic test is the prothrombin time. Unlike enzyme and albumin levels, results of the prothrombin time test can be used to judge the progress of the hepatic failure. It is for this reason that serial measurements of prothrombin time are usually recommended. Also, unlike albumin, the half-life of the coagulation factors is relatively short (about seven days), and a decrease in synthesis will be manifested early in the course of the disease. The degree of liver failure parallels the degree of prolongation of the prothrombin time.[13] The prolonged prothrombin time can be attributed to two causes: (1) inadequate production of clotting factors, and (2) inadequate vitamin K absorption. The latter cause can be eliminated by administering vitamin K intravenously. The partial thromboplastin time will also result in a typically prolonged value.

Other diagnostic aids include the use of nuclear medicine technology. Colloid liver scans can aid in

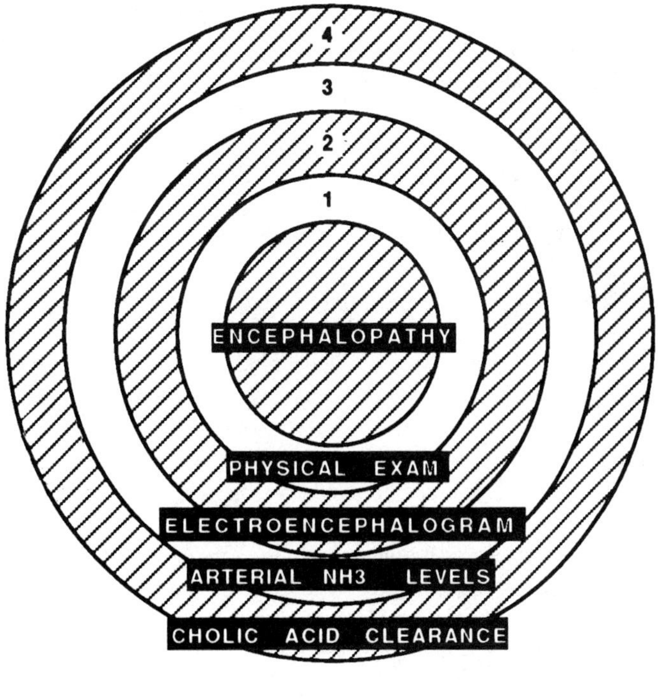

Figure 33-1 **Monitoring encephalopathy. Approaches to the assessment of encephalopathy normally proceed along the levels shown. Asterixis, degree of mental confusion, and neurological symptoms are looked for in a physical examination. Abnormal electroencephalogram (EEG) patterns are typically present in grades 2 through 4. Ammonia levels may be helpful in assessing levels of toxic accumulation. Cholic acid clearance is not routinely done but has been suggested as an aid in predicting recovery.**

the confirmation and detection of abnormal liver and spleen size, and can help locate abnormal growths or abscesses. Colloids that have been used include technetium and rose bengal. Ultrasound can serve a similar purpose, with the added benefit of not subjecting the patient to radiation. Because false interpretations of the results of these two procedures can easily be made, a more costly but perhaps more informative procedure is computerized tomography (CT scan). Liver biopsy may be necessary to ascertain the exact etiology, but must be approached with caution in a patient with severe bleeding problems.

Brain involvement may be assessed by the electroencephalogram (EEG), and serial measurements can aid in monitoring the progress of encephalopathy. See Figure 33-2 for an overview of the initial approach to a suspected case of hepatic failure.

Monitoring the Complications

Once the presence of hepatic failure has been established, it will be of utmost importance to monitor the life-threatening complications that may ensue. As described above, hypokalemia is frequently found in hepatic failure. It should be monitored closely and corrected as soon as possible. If allowed to reach very low levels, hypokalemia could be a precipitating factor for coma. If sodium is measured in plasma only, the results should be interpreted in light of the fact that the value attained may simply be a reflection of hemodilution. Urinary sodium should also be monitored in order to help determine whether the hepatorenal syndrome is occurring. In this condition, urinary sodium is typically decreased below normal levels, and a 24-hour collection is recommended. A decreased urinary output is also associated with hepatorenal syndrome, and urine volume should also be noted. Urea nitrogen and creatinine levels are elevated in this condition and may be measured as an added aid in its detection. Glucose and albumin levels should be monitored in order to determine replacement therapy.

Ascitic fluid may be withdrawn for its identification as a transudate or exudate; however, this procedure may compromise the patient's condition and should be done only if necessary.

Although ammonia levels are difficult to interpret due to problems with standardization and collection, they may be helpful as a measure of toxic waste accumulation. It has been suggested that an ammonia tolerance test can be helpful in predicting the chances of survival for individuals who undergo nonselective shunts that completely divert blood

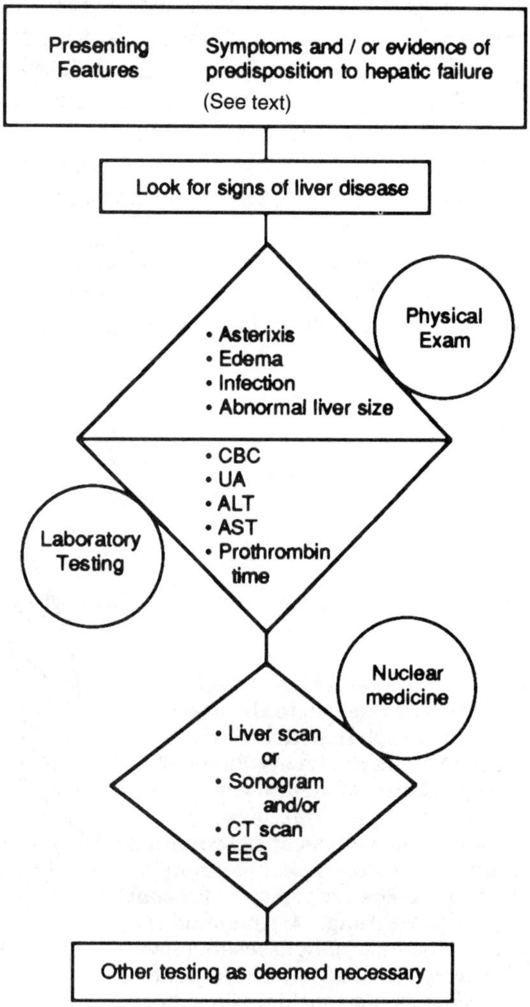

Figure 33-2 **Making the diagnosis in a patient suspected of having hepatic failure.**

flow to the liver.[14] These surgical procedures include end-to-side portacaval shunts, side-to-side portacaval shunts, and mesorenal shunts.

Blood gases are helpful in assessing the presence of alkalosis, which is a common finding and is believed to have several causes, including the presence of hypokalemia. Alkalosis has also been associated with reduced cerebral perfusion and lowered oxygen consumption.[1]

Because bleeding is a frequent complication, it may be necessary to monitor the hemoglobin and hematocrit to determine whether blood replacement therapy is needed and whether there may be a hemorrhagic protein overload, which can in turn contribute to hepatic encephalopathy.

TREATMENT

The ultimate goal of treatment is to cure hepatic failure and to return the individual to normal activity. It is commonly understood, however, that the mortality rate for this condition is extremely high. Acute hepatic failure has a mortality rate of 72% in the presence of severe hepatic necrosis,[15] and in persons who reach grade 3 or 4 encephalopathy the mortality rate increases to greater than 85%.[13] It is due to this high mortality rate that treatment plans usually follow three basic strategies.

The first strategy is to *correct or remove the primary cause* for the hepatic failure. Drugs or other toxic agents can be removed by the use of antidotes when they are available, by perfusion or, less commonly, by repeated plasmapheresis. To be successful, measures aimed at removing the toxic substances should be instigated shortly after their entry into the body.

Other primary causes of hepatic failure that may lend themselves to treatment include infections, α_1-antitrypsin deficiency, and Wilson's disease. Viral hepatitis is more easily prevented than treated. It is in situations such as this that the second strategy of treatment, *supportive care,* is important. The goal of supportive care is to gain time for liver regeneration or transplantation, the third strategy of treatment.

Because a common feature of hepatic failure is hypokalemia and fluid imbalance, potassium-sparing diuretics are often administered. Potassium supplements may also be given when laboratory data indicate that this is necessary. Sodium intake should be restricted in the presence of edema or ascites to avoid aggravating these conditions.

A diet low in protein and high in carbohydrate has been recommended as a further measure against precipitating encephalopathy.[16] Antibiotics should be used only when needed to treat an infection, and should not be used prophylactically. Neomycin may be given prophylactically, however, in order to reduce the urea-splitting bacteria of the gut. It is believed by some investigators that reducing the numbers of these bacteria aids in the prevention of coma, although this has not been proven.

Constipation may be treated by administering lactulose, a synthetic carbohydrate that is not absorbed. Lactulose is broken down to lactic acid by the enteric flora, further limiting the activity of the urea-splitting bacteria. Constipation that is not treated has been known to precipitate coma.

Gastrointestinal bleeding may be prevented by the prophylactic administration of cimetidine, which may be given orally or by intravenous infusion. Vitamin K administration has also proven useful. In the event that disseminated intravascular coagulation develops, subcutaneous heparin may be given, or plasmapheresis with replacement fresh-frozen plasma may be attempted.[17] Temporary relief can be attained by transfusing with platelet concentrates.

All of these supportive measures are utilized until *liver regeneration or transplantation* can occur. This is the purpose of the third strategy of treatment. In those persons with the potential for liver regeneration, several measures have been suggested. Infusions that have been suggested to support liver function include glucose, insulin, and glucagon.[18] A balanced amino acid infusion has also been attempted.[15] Plasmapheresis results in temporary relief for about 72 hours, while vitamin K and fresh-frozen plasma administration result in relief for only about 10 hours.[15]

Regeneration can be monitored by serial

α-fetoprotein levels and by other liver function tests such as the prothrombin time and the transaminases. In persons who fail to improve with time, liver transplantation may be the ultimate recourse.

CASE STUDY #1

A 20-year-old man was seen by his doctor for excessive nose bleeds. Physical examination revealed a flapping tremor and spider angiomas along the hands and forearms. He had no known history of exposure to viral hepatitis or drugs. He was admitted to the hospital for further evaluation. Cimetidine and vitamin K were administered intravenously.

Technetium scan revealed a liver slightly smaller than normal, with an enlarged spleen. A presumptive diagnosis of acute liver failure of unknown origin was made. On the third day of admission the patient became confused and openly hostile. He was able to respond to verbal commands.

LABORATORY FINDINGS

	(Reference Ranges)
	Day 1
Protime	16 s (control = 12 s)
APTT	43 s (control = 40 s)
ALT	400 U/L (8–20 U/L)
AST	900 U/L (8–20 U/L)
Bilirubin	0.9 mg/dL
Albumin	4.0 g/dL
Hepatitis screen	Neg
Stool occult blood	Neg
Bile acids (fasting)	3.0 μg/mL (0.3–2.3 μg/mL)
Platelet count	185 × 10^3/mm^3
NH_3	55 μg N/dL (15–45 μG N/dL)
	Day 3
Protime	19 s (control = 12 s)
APTT	48 s (control = 40 s)
ALT	1200 U/L
AST	1400 U/L
Bilirubin	1.6 mg/dL
Albumin	3.5 g/dL
Hepatitis screen	Neg
Stool occult blood	Neg
Bile acids (fasting)	3.3 μg/mL
Platelet count	180 × 10^3/mm^3
NH_3	70 μg N/dL

Conversion to SI units is as follows:
Bilirubin—mg/dL × 17.1 = μmol/L
Albumin—g/dL × 10 = g/L
Bile acids—μg/mL × 1.95 = μmol/L
NH_3—μg/dL × 0.714 = μmol/L

Questions

1. How is a flapping tremor detected, and what is its clinical significance?
2. What is the purpose of cimetidine administration?
3. What is the prognosis for this patient, based on the presumptive diagnosis?
4. Explain the significance of the abnormal laboratory data on days 1 and 3.

Discussion

1. Flapping tremor, also known as asterixis or liver flap, is detected by having the patient attempt to lift his hand while resting forearm and wrist on a flat surface. A flapping tremor will manifest itself as a jerky or flapping motion of the hand. Its presence is associated with liver disease and may be detected in grades 1 through 3 of encephalopathy.
2. Cimetidine, also known as tagamet, is used as a prophylactic agent to guard against intestinal bleeding, which could precipitate encephalopathy due to the protein overload that would result.
3. Acute hepatic failure has a mortality rate of 73% in the presence of massive necrosis, and the mortality increases to greater than 85% in patients who reach grade 3 or 4 encephalopathy.
4. The prothrombin time and activated partial thromboplastin time indicate either a reduced synthesis of coagulation factors or a vitamin K absorption problem. Administration of intra-

venous vitamin K did not correct the problem, so the former cause is indicated. The increased prothrombin time on the third day suggests further deterioration.

The elevation of both ALT and AST, along with the prolonged coagulation tests, further supports the idea that there is apparent hepatocyte damage. Bile acid quantitation is a very sensitive indicator of liver disease when elevated. Bilirubin elevation on the third day, along with low albumin levels, also indicates liver failure. Ammonia levels are helpful in assessing toxic waste accumulation in order to predict encephalopathy. The lowered levels of platelets may indicate increased spleen removal or a suppressed bone marrow.

CASE STUDY #2

A 65-year-old woman with a known history of alcohol abuse had been diagnosed as having cirrhosis with bleeding varices 6 years before her current hospital admission. She was admitted through the emergency room because of massive hemorrhaging. Her bleeding was controlled through an emergency side-to-side shunt. Twenty-four hours after surgery, the patient became disoriented as to time and exhibited all of the symptoms of grade 3 encephalopathy.

Questions

1. What chemistry and hematology results can reasonably be expected to be abnormal in this patient?
2. What are some measures that may be taken to assist this patient's recovery?
3. What tests may be used to monitor this patient's progress effectively and efficiently?

Discussion

1. The results expected to be abnormal include:
   Chemistries: ALT, AST, ALP, bilirubin, albumin, cholesterol, bile acids, ammonia, amino acids
   Hematology: Prothrombin time, APTT, platelet count, hemoglobin, hematocrit
2. Among the measures taken to assist in recovery are plasmapheresis, liver function support with glucose, insulin, glucagon, and balanced amino acid infusions.
3. Tests utilized to monitor progress include those for ALT, AST, prothrombin time, ammonia.

REFERENCES

1. Hetzel DJ: Fulminant hepatic failure. Anaesth Intensive Care 13: 272–282, 1985
2. Brunt, PW, Losowsky MS, Read AE: The Liver and Biliary System, pp 48–69. London, William Heinemann, 1984
3. Davis M, Tredger JM, Williams R: Drug Reactions and the Liver, pp 54–62. Great Britain, Pitman Medical, 1981
4. Rakela J: Fulminant hepatitis: Mayo Clinical experience with 34 cases. Mayo Clin Proc 60: 289–292, 1985
5. Reily CA: Acute hepatic failure in children. Yale J Biol Med 57: 161–184, 1984
6. Altin M, Rajkovic IA, Hughes RD et al: Neutrophil adherence in chronic liver disease and fulminant hepatic failure. Gut 24(8): 746–50, 1983
7. Kearns PJ, Polhemus RJ, Oakes D et al: Hepatorenal syndrome managed with hemodialysis and then reversed by peritoneovenous shunting. J Clin Gastroenterol 7(4): 341–343, 1985
8. Petersdorf RG, Adams RD, Braunwald E et al (eds): Harrison's Principles of Internal Medicine, 10th ed, pp 1771–1789. New York City, McGraw-Hill, 1983
9. Tietz NW (ed): Textbook of Clinical Chemistry, pp 713–717. Philadelphia, WB Saunders, 1986
10. Horak W, Waldram R, Murray-Lyon IM et al: Kinetics of [^{14}C] cholic acid in fulminant hepatic failure: A prognostic test. Gastroenterol 71: 809–813, 1976
11. Bremmelgaard A, Ranek L, Bahnsen M et al: Cholic acid conjugation test and quantitative liver function in acute liver failure. Scand J Gastroenterol 18(6): 797–802, 1983
12. Street JM, Trafford DJH, Makin HLJ: The quantitative estimation of bile acids and their conjugates in

human biological fluids. J Lipid Res 24: 491–511, 1983
13. Triger DR: Practical Management of Liver Disease, pp 187–201. London, Blackwell Scientific, 1981
14. Rikkers LF: Portal hemodynamics, intestinal absorption, and postshunt encephalopathy. Surgery 94(2): 126–133, 1983
15. Winikoff S, Glassman MS, Spivak W: Plasmapheresis in a patient with hepatic failure awaiting liver transplantation. J Pediatr 107(4): 547–549, 1985
16. Barber JR, Teasley KM: Nutritional support of patients with severe hepatic failure. Clin Pharm 3: 245–251, 1984
17. Chiba J, Asanuma Y, Matsubara S et al: A case of postoperative liver failure successfully treated with plasma exchange. Tohoku J Exp Med 146(3): 375–376, 1985
18. Jaspan JB, Landau RL, Schneider J: Insulin and glucagon infusion in the treatment of liver failure. Arch Intern Med 144(10): 2075–2078, 1984

Chapter 34

Liver Carcinoma

Alan H. B. Wu

Cancer affecting the liver cells is termed *hepatocellular carcinoma,* and accounts for the majority of all primary liver cancer cases (see Fig. 34-1). When the bile duct cells are malignant, the term *cholangiocellular* carcinoma is used. Both types can occur within the same individual, and their clinical courses are similar. The incidence of primary liver cancer in Western countries is very low. In the United States, this type is not among the top 20 causes of cancer death according to the National Cancer Institute.[1] Estimates of prevalence range from one to two cases per 100,000.

In contrast, primary liver cancer is one of the leading causes of cancer deaths in countries of Africa and Eastern Asia. The incidence among males living in Singapore, for example, is close to 30/100,000.[2] In China, some 100,000 persons die of it each year. It is clear that factors such as diet, environmental conditions, and preexisting disease play a role.

Secondary cancer results when a primary tumor invades surrounding tissues. Because the liver participates in many metabolic functions and is highly vascular, it is very vulnerable to meta-

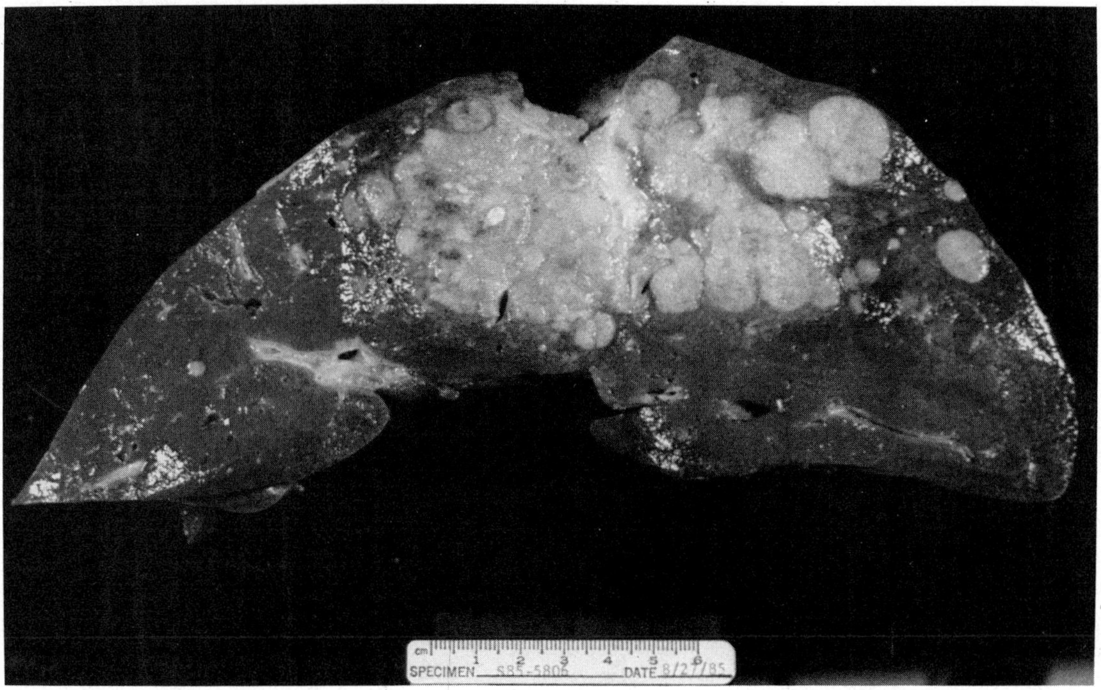

Figure 34-1 Hepatocellular carcinoma of the human liver.

stasis. Almost all types of cancer have the potential to metastasize to the liver, with the most common being cancers originating from the stomach, pancreas, colon, and lung.[3] As many as 50% of all cancer deaths in the United States show signs of hepatic malignancy at autopsy.

ETIOLOGY AND PATHOPHYSIOLOGY

Chemical Carcinogenesis

Numerous chemical agents are known to produce cancer in laboratory animals. For example, N-acetyl-2-aminofluorene will produce preneoplastic "nodules" in rats that will eventually culminate in a hepatoma.[4] Studying the cancer process in experimental models can provide fundamental information as to the etiology and progression of disease in humans. Aflatoxin B_1, which originates from the fungus *Aspergillus flavus,* is another potent carcinogen in rats. Because aflatoxin is found in high concentration in spoiled food, and because food storage conditions in undeveloped third-world countries are often conducive to this fungal growth, aflatoxin has been implicated as a major cause of the high incidence of primary liver cancer in these countries.[5]

Primary Liver Cancer With Hepatitis B and Cirrhosis

Several epidemiological studies have shown an association between the hepatitis B virus (HBV) and hepatocellular carcinoma.[6, 7] Some 80% to 90% of all patients with primary liver cancer are infected with hepatitis B virus. In some countries, 40% to 50% of patients who are carriers for hepatitis B surface antigen (HBsAg) will develop liver cancer sometime in their lifetimes. Other studies using immunofluorescence staining have shown a very high incidence of HBV-specific antigens, including HBsAg, in autopsy liver specimens from patients who died of liver cancer as compared with incidence in age- and geographically-matched controls.[7] Moreover, recent work has shown that DNA sequences originating from the B virus can incorporate into the tumor tissue of patients with positive HBsAg.[8]

Another related predisposing factor for primary liver carcinoma is chronic liver inflammation.[7, 9] In addition to the postnecrotic liver disease induced by hepatitis, other diseases such as alcoholic cirrhosis, biliary cirrhosis, and diseases caused by metabolic deficiencies, such as α_1-antitrypsin deficiency, have a high incidence of developing into liver cancer. Reports of a positive history of cirrhosis in cases of confirmed hepatocellular carcinoma range from 60% to 80%. In the U.S., most liver cancers are associated with a positive history of either hepatitis or alcoholic liver cirrhosis.

LABORATORY ANALYSES AND DIAGNOSIS

No single laboratory test is useful for early detection, diagnosis, and monitoring of cancer because this process is very diverse in humans. Consequently, markers of high clinical specificity must be coupled with markers of high clinical sensitivity for optimum use. Some markers such as gamma glutamyltransferase (GGT) are normally present in significant quantities in blood and are elevated in cancer. Although these markers can be highly sensitive, they lack specificity because many nonmalignant liver diseases can cause elevations. Other markers are normally absent in adult sera but are produced in association with cancer. Many of these markers, such as α-fetoprotein and carcinoembryonic antigen, are produced by the fetus. When found in association with cancer, they are termed *oncofetal antigens*. These markers often have high clinical sensitivity, but are not present in all tumors of the same type.

Oncofetal Tumor Markers

α-Fetoprotein (AFP) is an oncofetal antigen that is highly glycosylated and is produced *in utero* first by the yolk sac and later by the fetal liver. It is similar in molecular weight to albumin, and is thought to be the major protein in early prehepatic embryonic life. As the liver develops, it shifts from AFP to albumin production.

During normal fetal development, fetal blood levels of AFP peak in the first trimester, rising to 200 to 400 mg/dL (2–4 g/L) and slowly declining to about 5 mg/dL (0.05 g/L) at term. Maternal blood levels of AFP slowly increase from the first trimester due to increases in placental permeability. Maximum levels occur at the time of delivery, and are in the range of 5 to 35 μg/dL (50–350 μg/L). Amniotic fluid AFP levels roughly parallel fetal blood, but with a peak value of 2 to 4 mg/dL (20–40 mg/L). Elevation of AFP in amniotic fluid is associated with neural tube defects, anencephaly, intrauterine fetal death, spontaneous abortions, and congenital malformations. The reference range for AFP in the sera of nonpregnant adults is 0 to 3 μg/dL (0–30 μg/L).[10] (See also Chap. 41.)

Numerous studies have reported the diagnostic usefulness of AFP in hepatocellular carcinoma.[11, 12, 13] Because of differences in the sensitivity and specificity of the methods used, it is difficult to compare results directly. In general, however, moderate blood elevations of AFP, such as 4 to 100 μg/dL (40–1000 μg/L), are associated with (1) benign liver disease (*e.g.*, cirrhosis, acute hepatitis), due to the regeneration of hepatocytes, (2) early primary liver cancer, and (3) other tumors such as those of the gastrointestinal tract (*e.g.*, colon, pancreas, stomach), which may produce liver metastasis.[14] Differentiation among these groups can be made in two ways. Persistent AFP elevations of 6 to 12 months are associated with liver cancer, whereas transient elevations are associated with benign liver disease. In addition, the analysis of subfractions can help to distinguish these three groups from each other because the AFP have different glycosylations. Subfractions can be measured by concanavalin A crossed-line affinity immunoelectrophoresis.[15, 16] Large elevations of AFP (>100 μg/dL [>1000 μg/L]) are almost always associated with advanced hepatocellular carcinoma. Patients in this group are often beyond treatment.

The most effective use of AFP measurements is for screening populations who are at high risk for liver cancer.[2, 17, 18] Such a program was instituted in East China in 1971.[18] After examination of blood from some 5 million individuals using reverse hemagglutination, 1,000 cases of hepatocellular carcinoma were identified, of which 61% were in patients who did not present with any clinical signs of disease. This is significant because the success of treatment in such subclinical cases is dependent on early diagnosis.

Carcinoembryonic antigen (CEA) is a glycoprotein elevated in colon cancer, in liver diseases including primary and secondary cancer, and in alcoholic liver disease. It can be used in the assessment of patients in conjunction with AFP.[11] For example, a large elevation of AFP is suggestive of primary liver cancer, whereas a mild elevation of AFP coupled with elevation of CEA is suggestive of secondary liver carcinoma. Elevation of CEA without increased levels of AFP is suggestive of colonic cancer without hepatic malignancy.

Hepatic Enzyme Markers

Serum levels of *alkaline phosphatase (ALP)* are sensitive to obstructive liver disease and osteoblastic bone disease.[19] Thus it is not surprising that elevations in total serum ALP are observed in patients with liver metastasis, to the extent that the "space-occupying tumor" can cause hepatobiliary obstruction, and in cancer patients who have extensive bone metastasis. In these situations, total ALP elevations are indistinguishable from those in nonmalignant hepatic and osseous diseases. Total alkaline phosphatase activity is, therefore, only useful as a screen for malignant disease.

The measurement of *alkaline phosphatase isoenzymes* can demonstrate the presence of abnormal isoenzyme forms that are thought to originate from cancer cells. One such form, termed the *Regan isoenzyme,* has similar properties to placental alkaline phosphatase in terms of electrophoretic migration, heat stability, immunologic properties, and its ability to be inhibited by L-phenylalanine.[20] In clinical studies, this "placento-antigen" has only about a 25% sensitivity in cancer patients, with lower incidences in primary or secondary liver cancer. It is therefore not useful for diagnostic purposes.

In contrast to the Regan isoenzyme, a high-molecular-weight variant of alkaline phosphatase has been discovered that may have significant clinical utility. The α_1*-isoenzyme,* also termed the "fast liver" fraction because it migrates more anodic than does a normal liver fraction (see Fig. 34-2), is found with a high incidence in primary and secondary liver cancer.[21, 22] Reports comparing liver tumor markers show that the fast liver fraction may have the highest clinical sensitivity of all hepatic tumor markers. Although the exact nature of this isoenzyme is unknown, it appears to be released by the biliary obstruction caused by the neoplasm. In that respect, it is also elevated in nonmalignant liver diseases such as intra- and posthepatic biliary obstruction, which reduces its overall clinical efficiency.

Elevations of *enzymes* that show specificity towards liver disease have been proposed as potential markers of primary and secondary liver carcinoma. The more widely studied enzymes include *gamma glutamyltransferase* (GGT) and *5′-nucle-*

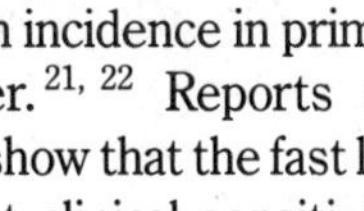

Figure 34-2 Electrophoretic migration of alkaline phosphatase isoenzymes on polyacrylamide gel at *p*H 9.5. FL = fast liver; L = liver; B = bone; I = intestinal fractions.

otidase (5′NT).[23, 24] Much of the interest in GGT in human liver cancer originates from work in experimental rat hepatocarcinogenesis, in which histochemical staining studies have shown that GGT is widely disseminated in tumor tissue.[25] Studies in human hepatocellular carcinoma have shown that GGT is elevated in the majority of cases and can be used in conjunction with AFP for diagnostic purposes.

Perhaps more significant is the potential of GGT and 5′NT as indicators of metastasis in extrahepatic tumors (*e.g.*, lung, breast, colon). These tumors are more common in the U.S. than is primary liver cancer, and usually carry a very poor prognosis. Thus, early indication of liver metastasis may alter the clinical management of these cancer patients. In general, studies have shown that both GGT and 5′NT are good markers of metastasis, with clinical sensitivities ranging from 75% to 85%.

A host of different markers have been examined for malignant neoplasms. Serum levels of *lactate dehydrogenase (LD)* are usually elevated in tumor patients; however, because LD is so nonspecific, it is not a useful marker for cancer. Atypical isoenzyme patterns of LD have been demonstrated by electrophoresis from the blood of patients with cancer, but the usefulness of this is uncertain. Atypical isoenzyme patterns of *creatine kinase (CK)* have also been observed in malignant diseases. A slow cathodic-migrating band, thought to be high-molecular-weight mitochondrial CK, has been shown to be an indicator of poor patient prognosis.[26, 27]

An area of active research is in the examination of liver tissues for biochemical markers of lesions that are preneoplastic. Studies in rat hepatocarcinogenesis and later in human hepatocellular carcinoma have shown that levels of GGT, for example, are elevated in the early stages of cancer.[4] Other enzymes such as *canalicular adenosine triphosphatase (ATPase)* and *glucose-6-phosphatase (G6Pase)* are negative markers, *i.e.*, they show reduced activity in preneoplastic lesions when compared to normal hepatocytes. These negative markers in early cancer cells may reflect the cells' reduced capacity for normal biochemical functions. Characterizing early changes in the liver is important in determining the mechanism of cancer.

Other Laboratory Determinations

An unfortunate consequence in many patients with primary cancers is the disruption of normal *hemostasis,* which is a delicate balance between proteins that produce coagulation and those that dissolve clots (fibrinolysis). Because the liver produces many of these factors, it is understandable that liver malignancies can disrupt this balance.[28, 29] For example, many cancer patients have increased levels of fibrinogen and are at greater risk for conditions of hypercoagulation such as disseminated intravascular coagulation (DIC). This condition, which is not uncommon in malignancy, is associated with extensive bleeding due to thrombocytopenia, decreased fibrinogen due to its consumption during the coagulation process, and increased levels of fibrin-split products due to fibrinolysis. Even non-DIC patients with primary or secondary liver cancer will usually have some abnormality in one or more of the clotting factors. In general, the effect on hemostastis is varied, and can be nonspecific and unpredictable.

The presence of primary or secondary liver cancer can affect the level of *therapeutic drugs* in many ways. For drugs that are highly protein-bound, *e.g.*, phenytoin, decreased levels of albumin can produce higher free drug levels for a given pharmacologic dose, which can lead to significant drug toxicity.[30] Cancer patients often have low levels of albumin because of either poor nutrition or the disruption of the hepatocytes responsible for producing albumin.

Liver cancer can also affect drugs that undergo hepatic metabolism. Unfortunately, the effect is generally unpredictable because the liver has significant reserve capacity for drug metabolism, and because cancer is a very heterogeneous process.[31] In addition, measuring various liver function enzymes (*e.g.*, AST, ALT) and metabolites (*e.g.*, bilirubin) does not aid in the determination of how therapeutic drugs will be affected by liver cancer. It is therefore necessary that drug levels be measured more frequently in cancer patients than in normal individuals.

TREATMENT

Surgical Resection

The success of treating primary liver cancer by surgically removing the tumor (*resection*) is dependent on the size and site of the neoplasm and the general health status and age of the patient. Small, encapsulated tumors that are limited to one lobe have the highest rate of success. Detection of these hepatomas requires early diagnosis, because most of these patients are subclinical. (Representative survival rates for resectable tumors in East China are shown in Table 34-1, below.[18]) In contrast to these, tumors in patients with concomitant liver cirrhosis are not resectable due to the diffuse nature of their tumors.

Hepatic Transplantation

Patients with primary liver cancers that cannot be surgically resected have 5-year survival rates of less than 5%. Because of this poor prognosis, many physicians have resorted to extreme treatment measures such as liver transplantation. Although this technique is not new, long-term success has only recently been possible with the development and use of the immunosuppressive drug cyclosporine A.[32] Today, more and more centers are performing liver transplantation for a variety of diseases. Survival times are increasing as technology and surgical techniques improve. Hepatic transplantations are not useful for treating secondary liver cancer, however, because remetastasis of the transplanted liver will occur if the primary site of the neoplasm is left untreated.

Table 34-1 ***Survival Rates in Treated and Untreated Liver Cancer Patients***

Patient Class	1-Year	2-Year	3-Year
Symptomatic	14.8%	7.4%	5.5%
Subclinical with conservative treatment	45.2%	16.4%	4.1%
Subclinical with surgical resection	79.1%	67.8%	61.6%

Data from reference number [18]

As with most systemic surgical procedures, basic supportive laboratory tests are necessary during liver transplantation. Rapid analysis and reporting of results are needed for arterial blood gases, electrolytes, glucose, hemoglobin, coagulation times, and blood counts.[33] Levels of *ionized* calcium are also important, because liver transplant patients can develop hypocalcemia.[34] Total calcium levels do not accurately reflect free calcium status because of its binding with the addition of citrated blood.

During the postoperative period, graft function can be monitored by various liver function tests. Large elevations of AST, ALT, ALP, and GGT are usually observed immediately after the operation. This is due to minor hepatocellular necrosis that occurs while the *ex-vivo* liver is being transported from the donor to the recipient. In successful operations, most of these enzymes return to normal within a few days.[35] GGT, however, can remain elevated in the absence of postoperative complications, and may not be as useful as ALP for detecting graft dysfunction. In addition to these, since liver transplant recipients must remain on life-long immunosuppressive therapy, regular monitoring of cyclosporine is necessary to minimize the possibility of graft rejection if values are low, or toxicity if values are high.

CASE STUDY #1

A 32-year-old white man presented with a 4-month history of lower back pain, intermittent chills and sweats, right upper quadrant pain, and weight loss of 7 to 8 pounds. Computed axial tomography (CT) and fine-needle biopsy presented evidence of primary hepatocellular carcinoma. The hepatoma was located between the lobes of the liver and was unresectable. The patient was given the options of being placed on chemotherapy or of undergoing hepatic transplantation. The patient chose the latter.

LABORATORY FINDINGS

Pretransplant	Patient Values (Reference Range)
AFP	< 25 ng/mL (< 25 ng/mL)
ALT	158 U/L (1–40)
LD	230 U/L (83–200)
PT	14 sec (9.5–13.5)
TT	50 sec (control 20 ± 2)
FSP	20 μg/mL (< 10)
ALP	723 U/L (34–108)
AST	92 U/L (7–40)
Ca	10.1 mg/dL (8.5–10.5)
PTT	53 sec (< 35)
Fibrinogen	212 mg/dL (170–410)

Conversion to SI units is as follows:
AFP—ng/mL × 1 = μg/L
FSP—μg/mL × 1 = mg/L
Ca—mg/dL × 0.25 = mmol/L
Fibrinogen—mg/dL × 0.01 = g/L

After a 10-hour orthotopic liver transplant, postoperative laboratory values appeared as follows:

ALP	126 U/L	ALT	690 U/L
AST	1100 U/L	LD	1270 U/L

Pathologic examination of the excised liver showed many firm masses, with diameters ranging from 1 to 1.5 cm. Immunoperoxidase staining for α-fetoprotein was negative. The tissue diagnosis of the tumor was "undifferentiated neoplasm," possibly of hepatocellular origin. The patient was discharged one month after the transplant and was placed on cyclosporine.

Questions

1. What is the cause of the normal serum α-fetoprotein?
2. What is the correct interpretation of the liver enzymes before and after transplantation?

Discussion

1. Although the clinical sensitivity of α-fetoprotein in primary liver cancer is high, no diagnostic test is 100% sensitive, and exceptions can always be found. In addition, Caucasians have a higher frequency of producing non-AFP-secreting liver tumors than do Orientals and African Blacks. One must also consider the possibility of laboratory error, as with any test that does not correlate with the clinical evidence. In this case, however, laboratory error is not likely because the test was repeated on two separate occasions with the same results, and because the AFP was not found in the tumor tissue itself.

   A second possible explanation is that the patient has secondary liver metastasis instead of primary hepatocellular carcinoma. It is not always possible to determine the primary site of a cancer even after post mortem examination. If the tumor in this case originated from an extrahepatic source, it is less likely to produce significant amounts of AFP.
2. Disproportionate elevations in ALP vs ALT and AST are typical in liver cancer, showing that the tumor causes obstruction of liver blood and bile flow without significant necrosis of normal hepatocytes. Elevations of ALP are not likely due to bone because calcium levels are normal. Marked elevations in GGT and 5'NT would also be expected, but may not add to the understanding of the clinical picture. After the transplant, ALP drops, shifting away from an obstructive picture toward one of cellular necrosis, as demonstrated by elevations in ALT and AST. As the new liver is revascularized, the liver enzymes are rapidly cleared and return to normal within a few days. Persistent elevations of any of these enzymes may represent liver dysfunction or graft rejection.

CASE STUDY #2

A 44-year-old white woman with colon cancer that was resected 18 months prior to admission was on chemotherapy, complained of poor appetite, weight loss, fatigue, dyspnea on exertion, and abdominal discomfort, and was admitted for fever. CT scan through her abdomen demonstrated marked metastatic disease to the liver with dystrophic calcification. Other medical problems included hemolytic anemia secondary to chemotherapy, infection, low-grade disseminated intravascular coagulation, and pulmonary edema. She died 4 weeks after admission due to these complications.

LABORATORY FINDINGS

Laboratory	Patient Values (Reference Range)
CEA	2385 ng/mL (< 3.0)
ALT	98 U/L (1–40)
LD	190 U/L (83–200)
PO_4	2.8 mg/dL (2.5–4.5)
PTT	25 sec (< 35)
RBC	3.4 × $10^3/mm^3$ (4.2–5.4)
Hematocrit	31% (37%–47%)
TT	23.5 sec (control 20 ± 2)
FSP	256 μg/mL (0–10)
ALP	800 U/L (34–108)
AST	198 U/L (7–40)
Ca	9.9 mg/dL (8.5–10.5)
PT	12.5 sec (9.5–13.5)
Hgb	10.8 g/dL (12–14)
WBC	26.5 × $10^3/mm^3$ (4.8–10.8)
Platelets	45 × $10^3/mm^3$ (13.3–33.3 × 10^3)
Fibrinogen	514 mg/dL (170–410)

Conversion to SI units is as follows:

CEA—ng/mL × 1 = μg/L
PO_4—mg/dL × 0.323 = mmol/L
FSP—μg/mL × 1 = mg/L
Ca—mg/dL × 0.25 = mmol/L
Hgb—g/dL × 0.155 = mmol/L
Fibrinogen—mg/dL × 0.01 = g/L

Arterial Blood Gas	Patient Values (Reference Range)
pH	7.25 (7.35–7.45)
PO_2	46 mm Hg (88–108)
PCO_2	39 mm Hg (35–45)
Bicarb	17.5 mEq/L [17.5 mmol/L] (22–26)

Questions

1. What is the clinical significance of the coagulation results?
2. What is the significance of liver metastasis for the death of the patient?

Discussion

1. Acute changes in plasma fibrinogen and elevations in fibrin-split products are often indicative of disseminated intravascular coagulation (DIC). The classic presentation of a patient in DIC is low levels of fibrinogen, Factors V and VIII, and platelet counts due to the consumption of these coagulation factors. A normal or high fibrinogen suggests that the synthesis rate has exceeded the catabolic rate, even if the latter is elevated. Patients may suffer shock and prolonged bleeding from venipuncture wounds.
2. Metastasis to the liver has been associated with the terminal stage of many cancers. In this case, it contributed to many of the metabolic imbalances observed. Because of the poor prognosis of liver cancer, much effort has been directed in making early diagnosis and treatment of cancer before metastasis occurs. The colon cancer in this case, for example, could have been surgically resected with early diagnosis. Many simple laboratory tests are now available, such as the fecal occult blood test, that can facilitate the initial diagnosis, which can be followed by appropriate treatment.

REFERENCES

1. Luna G, Florence L, Johansen K: Hepatocellular carcinoma: A 5-year institutional experience. Am J Surg 149: 591–594, 1985
2. Oon CJ, Yo SL, Chio LF et al: A pilot study on the screening of primary hepatocellular carcinoma in selected high-risk groups in the population using multiple tumour markers. Ann Acad Med Singapore 9: 240–244, 1980
3. Little JM: A comparison between primary and secondary liver cancer. Aust NZ J Surg 54: 341–343, 1984
4. Sell S, Leffert HL: An evaluation of cellular lineages in the pathogenesis of experimental hepatocellular carcinoma. Hepatology 2: 77–82, 1982
5. Stoloff L, Friedman L: Information bearing on the

evaluation of the hazard to man from aflatoxin ingestion. PAG Bull 6: 21–37, 1976
6. Munjal DD: Do asymptomatic, long-term carriers of hepatitis B virus develop liver cancer? Clin Biochem 14: 316–318, 1981
7. Nayak NC, Dhar A, Sachdeva R: Association of human hepatocellular carcinoma and cirrhosis with hepatitis B virus and core antigen in the liver. Int J Cancer 20: 643–654, 1977
8. Summers J, O'Connell A, Maupas P et al: Hepatitis B virus DNA in primary hepatocellular carcinoma tissue. J Med Virol 2: 207–214, 1978
9. Zaman SN, Melia WM, Johnson RD et al: Risk factors in development of hepatocellular carcinoma in cirrhosis: Prospective study of 613 patients. Lancet 1: 1357–1359, 1985
10. Tietz NW: Clinical Guide to Laboratory Tests, pp 194–196. Philadelphia, WB Saunders, 1983
11. Bell H: Alpha-fetoprotein and carcinoembryonic antigen in patients with primary liver carcinoma, metastatic liver disease, and alcoholic liver disease. Scand J Gastroenterol 17: 897–903, 1982
12. Alpert E: Serum alpha-fetoprotein (AFP) in benign and malignant gastrointestinal diseases: Evaluation of an immunoenzymatic assay. Clin Chim Acta 58: 77–83, 1975
13. McIntire KR, Waldmann TA, Moertel CG et al: Serum α-fetoprotein in patients with neoplasms of the gastrointestinal tract. Cancer Res 35: 991–996, 1975
14. Xu KL: Personal communication, 1986
15. Xu KL, Yu E, Lu L et al: Alpha-fetoprotein variants and their clinical significance. Chin Med J 97: 538–542, 1984
16. Ishguro T, Sugitachi I, Sakaguchi H et al: Serum alpha-fetoprotein subfractions in patients with primary hepatoma or hepatic metastasis of gastric cancer. Cancer 55: 156–159, 1985
17. Xu KL: Large-scale AFP screening for hepatocellular carcinoma in China. In Fishman WH (ed): Oncodevelopmental Markers: Biologic, Diagnostic, and Monitoring Aspects, pp 395–408. New York City, Academic Press, 1983
18. Tang ZY: Screening and early treatment of primary liver cancer—with special reference to the east part of China. Ann Acad Med Singapore 9: 203–205, 1980
19. Moss DW: Alkaline phosphatase isoenzymes. Clin Chem 28: 2007–2016, 1982
20. Stolbach LL, Krant MJ, Fishman WH: Ectopic production of an alkaline phosphatase isoenzyme in patients with cancer. N Engl J Med 281: 757–762, 1969
21. Burlina A, Plebani C, Dechecchi M et al: Occurrence of an atypical alkaline phosphatase fraction (biliary) in primary liver carcinoma. Clin Biochem 16: 346–349, 1983
22. Viot M, Thyss A, Viot G et al: Comparative study of GT and alkaline phosphatase and its isoenzyme as biological indicators of liver metastases. Clin Chim Acta 115: 348–358, 1981
23. Kim N, Yasmineh WG, Frier EF et al: Value of alkaline phosphatase, 5'-nucleotidase, α-glutamyltransferase, and glutamate dehydrogenase activity measurements (single and combined) in serum in diagnosis of metastasis to the liver. Clin Chem 23: 2034–2038, 1977
24. Tsou KC, Lo KW, Rosato EF et al: Evaluation of 5'-nucleotide phosphodiesterase isoenzyme-V as a predictor for liver metastasis in breast cancer patients. Cancer 50: 191–196, 1982
25. Gerber MA, Thung SN: Enzyme patterns in human hepatocellular carcinoma. Am J Pathol 98: 395–400, 1980
26. Wu AHB, Herson VC, Bowers GN: Macro creatine kinase types 1 and 2: Clinical significance in neonates and children as compared with adults. Clin Chem 29: 201–204, 1983
27. Kanemitsu F, Kawanishi I, Mizushima J et al: Mitochondrial creatine kinase as a tumor-associated marker. Clin Chim Acta 138: 175–183, 1984
28. Van der Walt JA, Gomperts ED, Kew MC: Hemostatic factors in primary hepatocellular cancer. Cancer 40: 1593–1603, 1977
29. Kies MS, Posch JJ, Giolma JP et al: Hemostatic function in cancer patients. Cancer 46: 831–837, 1980
30. Pippenger CE. Drug protein binding. In Moyer TP, Boeckx RL (eds): Applied Therapeutic Drug Monitoring, vol 1: Fundamentals, pp 55–61. Washington, DC, American Association for Clinical Chemistry, 1982
31. Hamilton CW, Evans WE. How neoplastic disease affects drug disposition. In Moyer TP, Boeckx RL (eds): Applied Therapeutic Drug Monitoring, vol 1: Fundamentals, pp 107–111. Washington, DC, American Association for Clinical Chemistry, 1982
32. Starzl TE, Iwatsuki S, Van Thiel DH et al: Evolution

of liver transplantation. Hepatology 2: 614–636, 1982

33. Bryan-Brown CW, Bracey AW, Lorimor KL: Intraoperative monitoring of the liver transplant patient. Acute Care 10: 207–212, 1983
34. Wu AHB, Bracey A, Bryan-Brown CW et al: Ionized calcium monitoring during liver transplantation. Arch Pathol Lab Med 11: 935–938, 1987
35. Simonsen R, Virji MA: Interpreting the profiles of liver-function tests in pediatric liver transplants. Clin Chem 30: 1607–1610, 1984

Part VII

ENDOCRINE DISORDERS

Virginia Sullivan Randolph, Associate Editor

Endocrine problems are among the most difficult to identify because they are often insidious, they mimic other diseases, and laboratory procedures are not specific in the identification of these disorders. Moreover, the various hormones have interrelationships that can confuse the patient's symptoms and the laboratory results. Some laboratory tests have cross-reactivity with other analytes, or measure the effect of the hormone rather than the hormone itself. In the chapters that follow an understanding of what each test measures and knowledge of the physiology of the endocrine system are both necessary to assist in the diagnosis of a disorder. It is important that the reader interested in the adrenal or thyroid disorders also read the chapter on pituitary disorders. The impact of the pituitary hormones on the adrenal and thyroid glands is direct. Pituitary disorders may also affect the male and female sex hormones, which in turn may alter reproductive capabilities as is discussed in Part VIII. Some disorders become multiendocrine in nature, particularly those due to autoimmune conditions; it is therefore suggested that, for any of the endocrine disorders, other gland deficiencies be investigated and monitored.

Chapter 35

Thyroid Disorders

Patricia Walsh

The adult thyroid gland is composed of two lobes of vascular tissue joined by an isthmus lying anterior to the cartilages of the larynx. The lumen of the gland contains colloid, and within the gland colloid is a protein unique to the thyroid, *thyroglobulin.*

The function of the thyroid gland is to secrete thyroxine (T_4) and triiodothyronine (T_3), the active, iodine-containing thyroid hormones important to a variety of metabolic activities. Disorders of the gland involve changes in hormone secretion, enlargement of the gland (*goiter*), or both.[1]

Thyroid hormone production is controlled by the level of circulating free hormone interacting with the hypothalamic-pituitary system in a negative feedback arrangement (see Fig. 35-1). Thyroid-releasing hormone (TRH) is a tripeptide produced in the hypothalamus that stimulates the production of pituitary thyroid-stimulating hormone (TSH). Like other pituitary hormones, TSH is a glycopeptide with two subunits. Specific tropic activity is associated with the beta subunit. Circulating TSH attaches to surface receptors on the thyroid follicular cells, initiating the cyclic AMP (cAMP) mechanism. TSH stimulates total thyroid gland activity, including cell proliferation, iodine trapping, organification, thyroglobulin synthesis, and the release of hormone from the colloid storage site. In primary disorders of the thyroid, which are the most common, TSH is increased in the hypothyroid patient and depressed in the hyperthyroid patient.[2]

The control mechanisms for the production of thyroxine (T_4) and triiodothyronine (T_3) in the thyroid are shown schematically in Figure 35-1. T_3 is

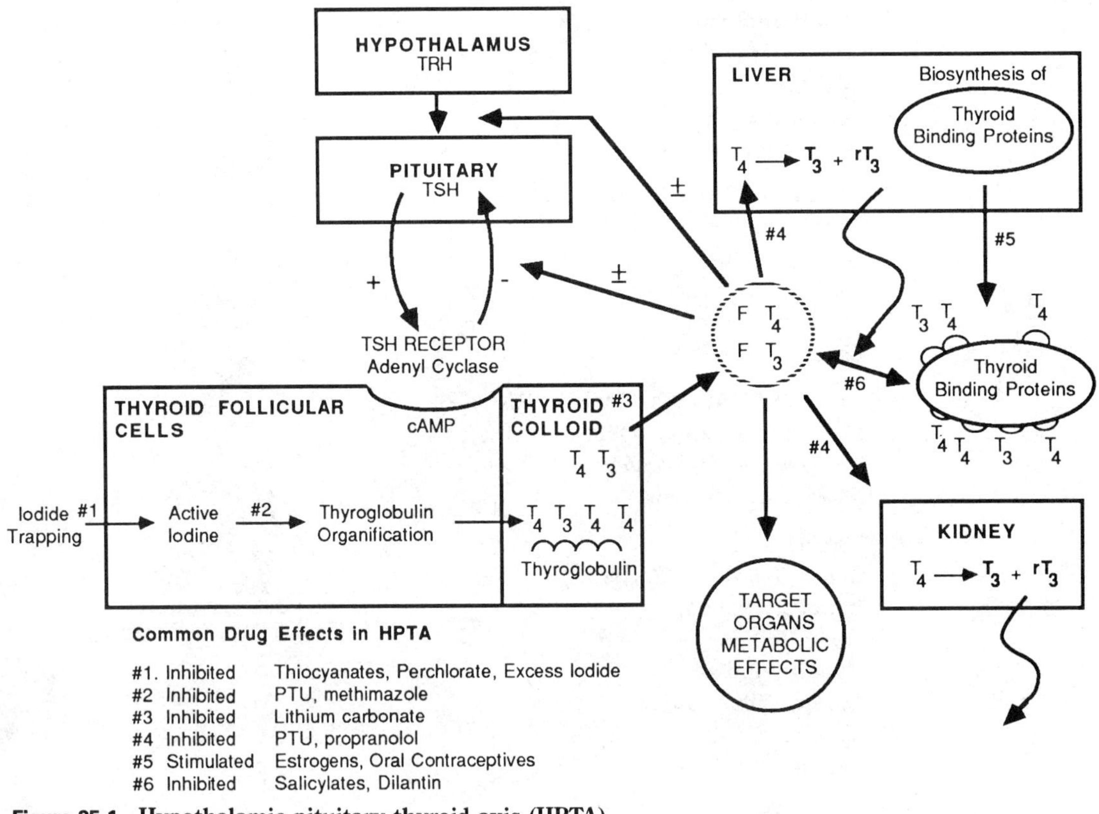

Figure 35-1 **Hypothalamic pituitary thyroid axis (HPTA).**

pharmacologically the most active thyroid hormone, but its concentration in the blood is approximately 1000 times less than T_4. Although the thyroid gland produces both T_3 and T_4, most T_3 (80%) is produced from T_4 in nonthyroidal tissues, such as the liver and kidney. These are the chief organs mediating the enzymatic deiodination of the *outer* phenol ring of T_4 to produce T_3. In severe illness and stress, this conversion is modified so that iodine is removed from the *inner* ring, producing reverse T_3 (rT_3), which is inactive. Some drugs (propranolol, propylthiouracil, glucocorticosteroids) also depress the T_4 to T_3 conversion.[3, 4, 5]

More than 99% of T_4 and T_3 circulates as protein-bound complexes; however, only free T_4 and T_3 (FT_4, FT_3) can function as hormones and modulators of the hypothalamic-pituitary-thyroid axis (HPTA). Thyroxine-binding globulin (TBG) specifically binds both hormones, although T_4 has a higher affinity for TBG than does T_3. T_4 also has a high affinity for thyroxine-binding prealbumin (TBPA), while T_3 binding is insignificant. Both hormones are bound by albumin as a nonspecific carrier. Variations in the amounts of binding proteins can result in depressed or elevated values for T_4 (or T_3) in some euthyroid patients.[2, 6]

ETIOLOGY AND PATHOPHYSIOLOGY

Simple Nontoxic Goiter—Diffuse or Nodular

The simple nontoxic goiter type of gland enlargement develops from chronic iodine deficiency or ingestion of goitrogens, as well as from genetic deficiencies in the iodine trapping mechanism, in organification enzymes, or in thyroglobulin production. Medications such as lithium can result in the formation of a euthyroid goiter. Thyroid hyperplasia suggests chronic overproduction of TSH in response to depressed thyroxine blood levels; however, TSH values in these patients are normal. It has been postulated that this occurs because an intrathyroidal hormone deficiency supersensitizes the gland to basal levels of TSH. In this event, total thyroxine production from the hyperplastic gland can satisfy metabolic demands. There is also the possibility that T_3 production in these patients is enhanced to the point that a euthyroid state is maintained.[7]

Hyperthyroidism (Thyrotoxicosis) (Toxic Goiter)

Graves's disease is the most common form of hyperthyroidism. Thyrotoxicosis can also result from a toxic nodular goiter, as well as from adenomas or carcinomas (follicular or papillary types). In some thyroid malignancies, thyroxine is produced not only by the primary lesion, but also in distant metastatic sites. In a small percentage of patients, thyrotoxicosis is due to overproduction of triiodothyronine rather than thyroxine (T_3 toxicosis).[7]

Factitious use of T_3 or T_4 is also a significant cause of hyperthyroidism. Factitious use can be iatrogenic (overmedication of a patient under a physician's care) or surreptitious (unprescribed abuse of thyroid hormone).[7, 8]

GRAVES'S DISEASE (EXOPHTHALMIC GOITER)

Despite extensive investigation into the origin of thyrotropin receptor antibodies (TRA), both stimulatory and blocking, the cause of Graves's disease remains unknown, although there is evidence that autoimmunity is a factor.[1] Considering the complexity of this disease and its multiple modes of progression, it might be more realistic to speak of "causes." Sometimes, symptoms of Graves's disease and Hashimoto's thyroiditis occur in the same patient—thus the clinical term "Hashitoxicosis."

A familial pattern has been detected in Graves's disease. Relatives of these patients often have the disease, thyroiditis, or some other thyroid problem. The disease occurs more frequently in women, ages 40 to 60 years.

A high percentage of patients produce thyroid stimulating immunoglobulins (TSI), which specifically stimulate the thyrotropin receptor sites on the thyroid membrane. Long-acting thyroid stimulator (LATS) is one such immunoglobulin. The presence of such stimulating factors is consistent with the symptoms of Graves's disease, but the role of immunoglobulins that *inhibit* the receptor sites is not clear. Unlike for Hashimoto's disease, there is no satisfactory animal model for Graves's disease, which is essential for establishing it as an organ-specific autoimmune process.[9]

Hyperplasia and increased vascularity are observed in the Graves's disease thyroid gland, accompanied by infiltration with both lymphocytes and plasma cells.[7]

Toxic Nodular Goiter

Although etiologic factors are not clear, some nontoxic goiters become toxic if untreated for a long period of time. X-irradiation of the neck or face early in life predisposes a significant number of individuals to nodular thyroid disorders, both benign and malignant, toxic and nontoxic.[7] Histopathology alone cannot differentiate between a toxic and a nontoxic nodule.

Hypothyroidism (Myxedema)

One of the most common causes of hypothyroidism is the ablation of goiterous tissue by surgery or radioisotopes that also destroy normal tissues. Other known causes are prolonged iodine deficiency, ingestion of goitrogens (which can include medications, such as propylthiouracil and methimazole), inherited defects in organification enzymes, and Hashimoto's chronic thyroiditis. The etiology in other cases is not known. Rarely is hypothyroidism due to deficient TRH or TSH secretion caused by necrosis or tumor growth.[7, 8] Autoantibodies to thyroglobulin have been observed in 75% of adult myxedemics. This similarity to Hashimoto's chronic thyroiditis is significant and may implicate undiagnosed chronic thyroiditis as a more common cause for hypothyroidism than was previously suspected.[7, 8]

Functional failure of thyroid tissue in newborns causes neonatal hypothyroidism in one of every 4000–5000 births. This is a serious condition that is treatable if detected early (see Chap. 73).

Chronic Thyroiditis

In chronic thyroiditis, the pathologic changes in the thyroid strongly indicate an antibody-dependent, cell-mediated autoimmune disorder involving lymphotoxicity. Hashimoto's disease (chronic lymphocytic thyroiditis) has been investigated extensively and found to meet the criteria established for autoimmune organ-specific diseases: (1) autoantibodies or cell-mediated immunity has been demonstrated; (2) thyroglobulin has been established as the antigen, and the autoantibodies produced are specific for this intrathyroid protein; (3) experimental animals sensitized with thyroglobulin will develop lesions similar to those observed in the human disease. Nonetheless, the pathogenesis of this condition has not been established.[7, 9] (See also Chap. 55.)

There is considerable speculation about the origin of the thyroid-specific autoantibodies, both antithyroglobulin and antimicrosomal. There is a familial pattern that may involve an inherited inability to recognize "self" or, more precisely, to control self-reactive lymphocytes. Different thyroid disorders, as well as autoimmune diseases, are found in relatives of these patients. Some of these are pernicious anemia associated with antiintrinsic-factor antibodies, atrophic gastritis with antibodies to cytoplasmic proteins of the gastric parietal cells, systemic lupus erythematosus, rheumatoid arthritis, and Sjogren's syndrome.[9]

SUBACUTE THYROIDITIS (GRANULOMATOUS, GIANT CELL, OR DEQUERVAIN'S THYROIDITIS)

Patients generally report a recent viral respiratory infection, but no autoimmune mechanism has been established for this disease. Histologically, it is distinct from Hashimoto's disease.

Adenomas

Statistically, most "hot" (hormone-producing) nodules are benign adenomas that do not invade surrounding tissue or metastasize. Patients are either euthyroid or hyperthyroid, depending on the size of the adenoma and the amount of T_4 or T_3 produced. Adenomas may be autonomous and synthesize a sufficient excess of T_4 to suppress TSH secretion. If TSH suppression is severe, adjacent normal thyroid tissue will not be visualized in scintiscanning unless TSH is administered to the patient prior to ingestion of radioiodide. Pathological examination of nodular cells is necessary for diagnosis.[10, 11]

Carcinomas

In scintiscanning, malignant tumors can appear as "hot" nodules or a solitary "cold" nodule.[10] The histopathology of a questionable nodule will reveal whether the lesion originates in the follicular epithelium (anaplastic, follicular, or papillary carcinomas) or in the parafollicular cells (calcitonin-secreting, medullary carcinoma).

The most common carcinomas are the well-differentiated follicular or papillary types that can concentrate I^{131}. Metastatic lesions, usually from a follicular carcinoma, can also concentrate I^{131} and produce "hot" nodules in the lungs or bone.

The anaplastic tumor with poor differentiation is highly malignant and produces a solitary "cold" nodule in scintiscanning. These patients are euthyroid, because the tumor does not produce thyroid hormone.

Patients diagnosed with adenomas and adenocarcinomas of the thyroid frequently have a medical history of radiation treatment to the face or neck during childhood.

Other Causes

Very rarely, ectopic thyroid tissue (*struma ovarii*) will cause thyrotoxicosis. Choriocarcinomas and hydatiform moles produce hCG, which is a mild thyroid stimulator; thyrotoxicosis is usually absent but T_4 values may be increased in these patients.[7]

CLINICAL MANIFESTATIONS

Simple Nontoxic Goiter

Symptoms of simple nontoxic goiter are related to the size and position of the mass in the throat area. Compression of the trachea or esophagus may result in difficulty in swallowing.

Hyperthyroidism

The symptoms of hyperthyroidism and thyrotoxicosis represent a general state of hypermetabolism. Goiter is frequently, but not always, present. The patient may experience any of the following symptoms: weight loss, intolerance to heat, irritability, excessive sweating, palpitations, and cardiac symptoms such as tachycardia and arrhythmias.

GRAVES'S DISEASE

In addition to the classic symptoms of hyperthyroidism, Graves's disease may be associated with either unilateral or bilateral exophthalmus and diffuse, nonnodular goiter. Exophthalmus occurs clinically in two forms: the milder type, which is best described as a staring expression, and severe infiltrative ophthalmopathy, which can result in blindness. The ophthalmic signs may be absent during the early stages of the disease. Also characteristic of Graves's disease is the development of pretibial myxedema, a hyperpigmented, raised, thickened skin lesion on the lower leg or ankle.[7, 8] *Pretibial myxedema* is a misleading descriptive term, since "myxedema" in all other contexts is associated with *hypo*thyroidism. Generally, full-blown cases of Graves's disease can be diagnosed on clinical observations alone.

Often elderly patients with Graves's disease

have a long-standing cardiac problem that deteriorates without obvious cause and is the reason why the patient seeks medical care. Thyromyopathy is frequently observed in the elderly; these patients may complain about unexpected difficulties in walking upstairs or performing simple tasks. Weight loss may be a factor, but more frequently it results from anorexia, a pattern not observed in younger patients.[7, 12]

Toxic Nodular Goiter

All of the clinical symptoms listed under "Hyperthyroidism" could be observed in patients with toxic nodular goiter. This form of thyrotoxicosis, however, is not as severe as that usually observed in Graves's disease. Because many patients with the disease are elderly, cardiac and muscle disorders may be most evident; however, exophthalmus is not observed.[7]

Hypothyroidism (Myxedema)

Myxedema is a dry, waxy, nonpitting type of edema caused by excessive accumulation of mucoprotein in the skin. It can affect any part of the body, and often produces swollen lips, nose, and eyelids.

Any or all of the following clinical signs are observed in myxedemic patients: lethargy, obesity despite poor appetite, poor muscle tone, delayed relaxation reflexes, intolerance to cold, dry coarse skin, constipation, and enlarged heart. Goiter may or may not be present. Myxedemic coma can occur and is an extreme event in which hypothermia ensues. Clinically, full-blown hypothyroidism can easily be recognized, and laboratory testing is ordered to quantitate the disorder and as a reference point for subsequent treatment.[7, 8]

Chronic Thyroiditis

Depending on the stage of the illness, the patient may be eu-, hypo-, or hyperthyroid. The metabolic picture can change during the course of the disease; however, the final outcome usually involves extensive destruction of thyroid tissue and permanent hypothyroidism.

Hashimoto's disease is the most common and best described disorder in this category. Patients present with a "rubbery" goiter with scalloped edges. Nodules are not found, and neck pain usually does not occur. The disease occurs more frequently in women (5 : 1), ages 30 to 60 years. It has, however, been reported as a cause for goiter in children and adolescents.[7, 8]

Table 35-1 ***Abbreviations***

HPTA	Hypothalamic-pituitary thyroid axis
TSH	Thyroid-stimulating hormone or thyrotropin
TRH	Thyroid-releasing hormone
T_4	Thyroxine (bound + free)
FT_4	Free thyroxine
FT_4I	Free Thyroxine Index*
T_3 or TT_3	Triiodothyronine (bound + free)
FT_3	Free triiodothyronine
FT_3I	Free Triiodothyronine Index*
rT_3	Reverse triiodothyronine (bound + free)
RT_3U or T_3U	T_3 resin uptake
RT_3U Ratio	T_3 resin uptake ratio**
TBG	Thyroxine-binding globulin
TBPA	Thyroxine-binding Prealbumin
Tg	Thyroglobulin
TRA	Thyroid receptor antibodies
TSI	Thyroid-stimulating immunoglobulins
LATS	Long-acting thyroid stimulator
PTU	Propylthiouracil
RAIU	Radioactive iodine uptake
FNA	Fine-needle aspiration
cAMP	3′5′ cyclic adenylate
hCG	Human chorionic gonadotropin

* Calculated: $FT_4I = T_4 \times RT_3U$ ratio
$FT_3I = T_3 \times RT_3U$ ratio
or
$FT_4I = T_4 \times RT_3U(\%) \div 100$
$FT_3I = T_3 \times RT_3U \div 100$

** Calculated: Patient RT_3U divided by RT_3U normal serum pool

SUBACUTE THYROIDITIS

The patient's history generally reveals a recent viral respiratory infection, and neck enlargement is observed in some cases. In many cases there may also be severe pain in the thyroid or on the face or lower jaw. If the gland is severely disrupted by the inflammatory process, hormone may pour into the circulation and cause symptoms of thyrotoxicosis. In this event, Graves's disease might be suspected.[7, 8]

LABORATORY ANALYSES AND DIAGNOSIS

Clinical Laboratory Assays (See Table 35-1.)

Highly specific and sensitive assays for T_4, T_3, and rT_3 are currently available that employ either radioimmunoassay (RIA) or one of the nonisotopic immunoassays. T_4 analysis is a cost-effective first choice in thyroid evaluation (see Fig. 35-2). Patients with borderline T_4 values are subjects for further testing. Patients with T_3 toxicosis and normal T_4 values would not be identified in this scheme; however, many of these patients have a history of thyroid disorders and/or clinical symptoms of hyperthyroidism.[7] Table 35-2 summarizes results of laboratory analyses in thyroid disease, and Table 35-3 provides information on reference ranges.[13] Various aspects of these analyses are discussed below.

Levels of FT_4 and FT_3 are most closely related to thyroid hormone activity. Generally, laboratories approximate this value by calculating the *Free Thyroxine Index* (FT_4I), using the data obtained from T_4 and T_3 Resin Uptake (T_3U). Calculation of the FT_4I frequently "normalizes" borderline or abnormal T_4 values by correcting for high or low levels of thyroid-binding proteins. Similar information can be generated using T_3 and T_3U in the calculations.[14]

FT_4 can be determined by *equilibrium dialysis* or by *ultrafiltration,* both of which are labor-intensive and unsuited for high-volume use. The most recent *RIA assays* for FT_4 involve either one or two steps, the one-step procedure using a labelled T_4 analog.[15] Currently there are serious technical

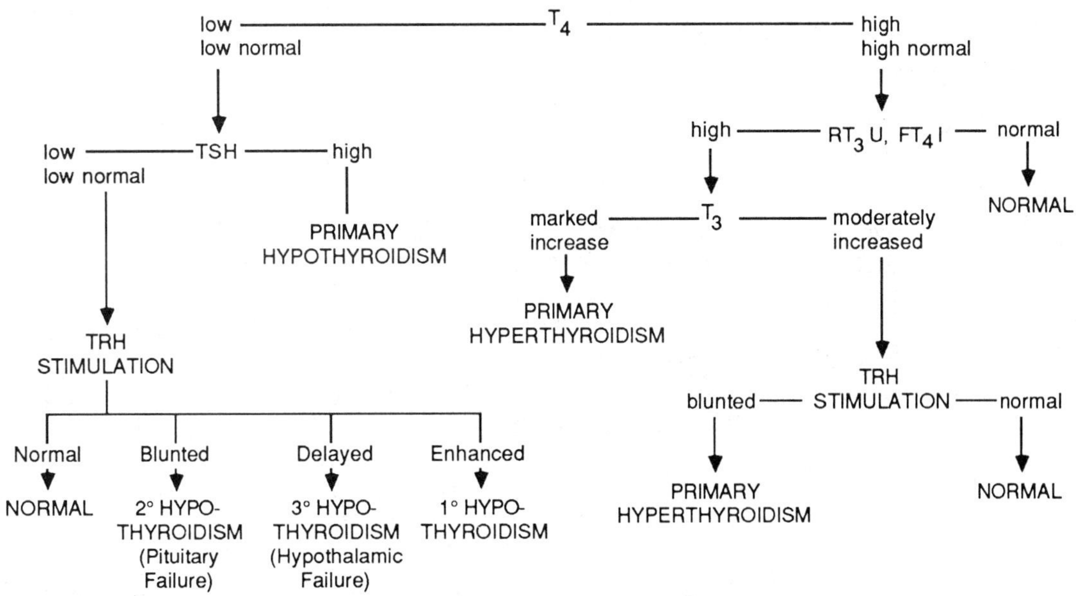

Figure 35-2 **Test-ordering strategies in patients suspected of having thyroid disorders.**

Table 35-2 ***Summary of Diagnostic Test Results in Thyroid Disease***

Clinical Disorder	T_4	T_3	RT_3U	FT_4I	TSH	TRH Stimulation	RAIU	Comments
Goiter, Simple	N	N	N	N	N	N	N	AntiTg Abs—absent
Hyperthyroidism								
Graves's disease	↑	↑	↑	↑	N↓	Blunted	↑	AntiTSI Abs—present, high titers
Toxic nodular goiter	N↑	N↑	↑	↑	N↓	Blunted	↑	Scintiscan—hot, warm, cold areas
T_4, T_3 abuse	↑	↑	↑	↑	N↓	Blunted	N	Tg normal
Hypothyroidism								Elevated cholesterol, CK, LD
Primary	↓	↓	↓	↓	↑	High	N↓	AntiTg Abs—often present
Secondary	↓	↓	↓	↓	N↓	Blunted	N↓	
Tertiary	↓	↓	↓	↓	N↓	Delayed	N↓	
Thyroiditis, chronic (Hashimoto's)	N↑ ↓	N↑ ↓	N↑ ↓	N↑ ↓	N↑ ↓		N↑	AntiTg Abs—often present; ↑ ↑ ESR
Adenomas/ Carcinomas	N↑	N↑	N↑	N↑	N↓	N/Blunted		Scintiscan—hot or cold nodules
Sick Euthyroid Syndrome (SES)	N	N↓	N↑	N↑	N			rT_3 increased
Euthyroid Graves's disease	N	N	N	N	N	Blunted/N	N	AntiTSI Abs—present

questions about serum protein binding of labelled analog in the one-step RIA procedures, which could invalidate results in patients with abnormal albumin values.[16, 17, 18]

TSH assays by RIA methodology are especially useful in corroborating clinical suspicion of hypothyroidism. In this condition, TSH values are higher than the reference range and remove speculation about the significance of a borderline low T_4 and FT_4I. The introduction of "ultrasensitive" TSH procedures has improved evaluation of the hyperthyroid patient without resorting to TRH stimulation. The ultrasensitive TSH assay accurately determines TSH in the low and low normal ranges, and permits accurate TSH monitoring of patients in whom TSH production is being suppressed using oral levothyroxine.[15, 19, 20, 21]

If TSH values are inconclusive, the *TRH Stimulation Test* may be helpful. After obtaining a baseline TSH value, TRH is administered to the patient and TSH blood levels are determined at 30 and 60 minutes. A "blunted" response is observed in primary hyperthyroidism, and an exaggerated response in primary hypothyroidism. Although most cases of hypothyroidism are not due to diseases of the hypothalamic-pituitary complex, the TRH Stimulation Test is used if there is a suspicion of secondary hypothyroidism. If TSH production is

Table 35-3 ***Reference Ranges for Thyroid Function Tests***

Total T_4	
Adult	4.5–13 μg/dL
Cord-blood	7.4–13.1 μg/dL
Newborn	7.0–17.0 μg/dL
RT_3U	25%–30%
RT_3U Ratio	0.8–1.35
FT_4I	4.5–12
FT_4	1.2–2.5 ng/dL
TSH	5–10 μU/mL
TRH stimulation (TSH)	>2 μU/mL after 20 min
TT_3	60–220 ng/dL
rT_3	27–62 ng/dL
FT_3I	85–205 ng/dL
FT_3	0.2–0.4 ng/dL
TBG	16–24 μg/mL
RAIU	10%–30%
Antithyroglobulin antibodies	<1 : 100
Antimicrosomal antibodies	<1 : 40

Data from reference number [13]

depressed because of pituitary disease, no response is observed with TRH stimulation; if the hypothalamic mechanism is impaired, the peak response is delayed.[7, 15]

Serum thyroglobulin (Tg) is assayed, using an RIA procedure. This glycoprotein is synthesized by the follicle cells of the thyroid, and it is the matrix for the formation of T_4 via iodotyrosine and iodothyronine biosynthetic intermediates. Except for very small amounts in the serum, Tg is normally confined to the interior of the gland; however, increased blood levels are observed in many thyroid diseases, including goiters and benign and malignant tumors.[15,22]

Caution should be used in interpreting abnormal thyroid test data obtained on patients with acute or severe chronic illness, some of whom may have coexisting thyroid disease. Frequently, T_3 will be depressed and rT_3 (an inactive form) will increase in such patients, and direct assay of rT_3 can clarify the diagnosis.[23, 24] In addition, hyperthyroidism in the elderly patient may be overlooked clinically because the presenting symptoms are atypical of thyroid disorders and, in some cases, resemble hypothyroidism. Laboratory tests are particularly useful in these cases.[12]

Radiological Techniques

NONIMAGING TECHNIQUES

Radioactive iodine uptake (RAIU) is a measurement of the ability of the thyroid gland to concentrate an oral dose of radioactive iodine. Approximately 5% to 33% of an ingested dose of I^{123} can be detected in the normal thyroid gland after 24 hours. Hyperthyroidism (high uptake) is more reliably assessed than is low or low normal uptake. Although the popularity of RAIU for diagnostic purposes is declining, it is still valuable as a monitor of radioiodine therapy.[25]

Autonomous function (independence from TSH control) is evaluated by the *T_3 Suppression Test.* If thyroid tissue is responding to TSH control, treatment of the patient with oral T_3 will suppress TSH production and RAIU. If no suppression is observed, functional autonomy is strongly suspected.[25]

IMAGING TECHNIQUES

Imaging or scintiscanning of the thyroid using an oral dose of I^{123} or sodium pertechnetate Tc 99m is done to identify the presence of abnormalities in the thyroid or ectopic thyroid tissue in metastatic lesions from a thyroid carcinoma. Pertechnetate, a man-made element, is trapped, but not organified by the thyroid gland.[10] The TSH stimulation test is occasionally used in conjunction with imaging techniques if it is necessary to visualize normal thyroid tissue that is being suppressed by an autonomous nodule. The terms "hot," "warm," and "cold" describe the relative uptake of radioisotopes by the thyroid gland or specific areas within the gland, and refer to degree of glandular activity.[10] Pathological examination of samples removed from the suspicious areas is always required for definitive diagnosis.

Aspiration Cytology (Fine Needle Aspiration)

Aspiration cytology or fine-needle aspiration is an increasingly popular technique that has reduced the costs of evaluating the goiterous patient, particularly in ruling out carcinomas. The cells obtained are stained with Giemsa, and evaluated by a pathologist while the patient waits. If necessary, additional needle aspirates can be drawn on the spot. This procedure eliminates costly diagnostic workups and exploratory surgery for the purpose of obtaining biopsy material.[11, 22]

TREATMENT

Simple Nontoxic Goiter

For simple nontoxic goiter, levothyroxine is prescribed in sufficiently high dosage to suppress TSH secretion and rest the hypertrophied gland. This treatment is reportedly very effective in reducing goiter size, particularly if the goiter is diffuse rather than nodular.

Surgery is not usually recommended, unless mechanical obstruction is extreme. The use of iodide to reduce gland size may present a problem, because iodide is known to induce thyrotoxicosis in both diffuse and multinodular nontoxic goiters (Jod-Basedow syndrome).

If the goiter remains untreated and colloid continues to accumulate, the structure of the thyroid gland changes so that nodules or focal areas of hyperplasia are interspersed throughout the gland. The transition from diffuse nontoxic goiter to nodular nontoxic goiter to toxic nodular goiter usually progresses slowly, the last of these being observed in elderly patients. If the goiter worsens, the thyroid can no longer compensate by producing more colloid, and hypothyroidism ensues.[7]

Hyperthyroidism (Thyrotoxicosis)

Because thyrotoxic symptoms are caused by an overproduction of thyroid hormone that can threaten the life of the patient, treatment focuses on the reduction of the level of circulating hormone. Two basic approaches can be used. One uses antithyroid drugs such as propylthiouracil or methimazole, and is a conservative approach that can continue indefinitely. Thyroid tissue is not destroyed, but suppressed. Patients can be removed from medication to observe whether remission has occurred, and if relapse occurs the treatment can be reinstituted. Some physicians prescribe levothyroxine along with antithyroid drugs to prevent hypothyroidism and suppress TSH activity. Other substances such as perchlorate and thiocyanate ions depress hormone production by inhibition of the iodine trapping system. Treatment with *excess* iodide can temporarily inhibit the thyroid through the same mechanism (Wolff-Chaikoff effect).[2]

Another approach uses ablation of hyperplastic thyroid tissue, through surgery or I^{131} "cocktail." These forms of treatment are more drastic because both are irreversible. Normal thyroid tissue is destroyed, resulting in permanent hypothyroidism and the need to maintain the patient on thyroid hormone for life. Laboratory monitoring of the treated patient using T_4 or TSH may extend over a period of years. It is critical, therefore, that both the accuracy and the precision of laboratory assays reflect subtle changes of organ function so that therapy can be promptly corrected.[7, 8]

Propranolol may be prescribed to alleviate the adrenergic symptoms of acute thyrotoxicosis; this drug also inhibits the peripheral conversion of T_4 to T_3.[7] Untreated Graves's disease progresses to a life-threatening situation. The so-called "storm" may be precipitated by stress from infection or surgery; thus thyrotoxic patients require careful preparation for surgery. Cardiac symptoms can be extreme and can result in death from heart failure.[7]

Toxic Nodular Goiter

In toxic nodular goiter, radioactive iodine "cocktail" is reportedly effective if the patient is first medicated with an antithyroid preparation until euthyroid status is achieved.[7]

Hypothyroidism

Several synthetic medications are available for treatment, including levothyroxine (T_4), liothyronine (T_3), and a combination of both (Liotrix). Unless an emergency exists (myxedemic coma), the metabolic status of the hypothyroid patient is gradually readjusted to normal with judicious use of these drugs. Although the physician will undoubtedly order laboratory assays to monitor recovery (T_4, TSH), the clinical state of the patient will be the overriding consideration. The laboratory should be informed at the time testing is ordered about any thyroid medication. If most of the thyroid gland is nonfunctional, the patient must be controlled by medication for life.

Chronic Thyroiditis

HASHIMOTO'S DISEASE

Patients are medicated with thyroxine during the active phase of Hashimoto's disease. Surgery is not recommended for chronic thyroiditis, nor is treatment with radioactive iodine, which may exacerbate the inflammation. Because permanent hypothyroidism often results, such patients are maintained in the euthyroid state, using hormone replacement as described above for hypothyroidism.[7, 8]

SUBACUTE THYROIDITIS

The painless or "silent" variety of subacute thyroiditis runs its course in a few months, usually with no sequelae. Salicylates reportedly control the symptoms in mild cases. Prednisone can be used in the more painful cases, and propranolol may be helpful to control the temporary symptoms of thyrotoxicosis if it occurs. Thyroid function usually returns to normal, although in a few cases thyroid tissue is extensively destroyed and the patient develops hypothyroidism.[7, 8]

Adenomas

Approaches to treatment include TSH suppression therapy using thyroxine or ablation of the nodule. Often, postoperative patients are maintained on suppressing doses of T_4, and are monitored using T_4 and TSH assays.[8]

Carcinomas

Surgical and I^{131} treatment of carcinomas are usual, and prognosis for the intrathyroidal papillary and follicular tumors is excellent.[8] Thyroglobulin assays are useful in detecting metastatic thyroid tissue that remains after treatment of the patient for thyroid adenocarcinoma.[15, 22] Thyroid suppression therapy is instituted and monitored as described above.[8]

CASE STUDY # 1

A 45-year-old woman complained of extreme fatigue for the past year, during which time her neck gradually enlarged. She had never experienced any neck pain. She complained of constipation and long menstrual periods. On physical examination, her physician found a diffuse goiter; the cervical lymph nodes were not enlarged.

LABORATORY AND RADIOLOGICAL FINDINGS (REFERENCE RANGES)

ESR	40 mm/hr (0–20 mm/hr)
T_4	3.0 μg/dL (4.5–13.0 μg/dL)
T_3U	23% (25%–30%)
T_3	120 ng/dL (60–220 ng/dL)
TSH	15 μU/mL (0.4–4.0 μU/mL)
RAIU	44% (10%–30%)
Antithyroglobulin antibodies	Titer: 1:1,000,000
Antimicrosomal antibodies	Titer: 1:128

Conversion to SI Units is as follows:

T_4—μg/dL × 12.9 = nmol/L
T_3—ng/dL × 0.0154 = nmol/L
TSH—μU/mL × 1 = mIU/L

Questions

1. What is the probable diagnosis indicated by the clinical and laboratory findings?
2. Can laboratory/radiological data that does not support this diagnosis be accounted for?

3. What additional procedure would confirm the diagnosis?

Discussion

1. The thyroid laboratory tests, particularly T_4 and TSH, strongly support the clinical diagnosis of hypothyroidism. Hashimoto's chronic lymphocytic thyroiditis is implicated as the cause of the hypothyroidism for the following reasons: a painless goiter with nodules is present, along with very high titers of antithyroglobulin antibodies, and elevated ESRs are often observed in these patients.
2. RAIU data indicating a moderately *elevated* uptake of radioactive iodine may be misleading at first glance. However, the earlier stages of this disease often produce contradictory data, as is the case here with RAIU. The autoimmune inflammatory process results in large amounts of iodoproteins (inactive as hormone) being discharged into the peripheral circulation. Thyroglobulin levels in the serum cannot be determined accurately because of the high titer of antithyroglobulin autoantibodies.
3. Pathological examination of a fine-needle aspirate of the thyroid gland would confirm the diagnosis.

CASE STUDY # 2

A 23-year-old woman visited her physician complaining of protruding eyes and serious vision problems. She had also experienced excessive sweating, extreme nervousness, and weight loss (20 lbs in 2 months). Pulse rate: 105; Blood pressure: 140/88; temperature: 98.4°F. No goiter was observed.

LABORATORY AND RADIOLOGICAL FINDINGS (REFERENCE RANGES)

T_4	10.5 μg/dL (4.5–13.0 μg/dL)
T_3	195 ng/dL (60–220 ng/dL)
T_3U	30% (25%–35%)
TSH	1.0 μU/mL (0.4–4.0 μU/mL)*
TRH Stimulation Test	blunted response
TSI (Thyroid-stimulating immunoglobulins)	strongly positive (none detected in normal serum)
RAIU	27% (10%–30%)

*Highly sensitive TSH procedure

Conversion to SI Units is as follows:

T_4—μg/dL × 12.9 = nmol/L
T_3—ng/dL × 0.0154 = nmol/L
TSH—μU/mL × 1 = mIU/L

Question

What is the probable diagnosis, based on laboratory and radiological findings?

Discussion

The laboratory thyroid tests, *i.e.*, T_4, T_3, T_3U, and TSH, indicate a euthyroid status for this patient. TRH stimulation resulted in a "blunted" response typical of hyperthyroidism. Clinically, the patient presents with some of the classic symptoms of Graves's disease (exophthalmus most prominently) and other physical signs of hyperthyroidism. A positive TSI further corroborates the diagnosis of euthyroid Graves's disease.

REFERENCES

1. Ingbar, SH, Walker, KA: Diseases of the thyroid. In Petersdorf, RG et al (eds): Harrison's Principles of Internal Medicine, pp 614–625. New York, McGraw Hill, 1983.
2. Fernandez-Viloa M, Maxon HR: Thyroid. In Kaplan LA, Pesce AJ (eds): Clinical Chemistry—Theory, Analysis, and Correlation, pp 748–772. St Louis, CV Mosby, 1984
3. Chopra IJ, Solomon DH, Chopra U et al: Pathways of metabolism of thyroid hormones. Recent Prog Horm Res 34:521–567, 1978
4. Braverman LE, Ingbar SH, Sterling K: Conversion of thyroxine to triiodothyronine in athyrotic subjects. J Clin Invest 49:855–864, 1970
5. Cavalieri RR, Rapoport B: Impaired peripheral conversion of thyroxine to triiodothyronine. Ann Rev Med 28:57–65, 1977
6. Oppenheimer JH: Role of plasma proteins in the binding, distribution and metabolism of the thyroid hormones. N Engl J Med 278:1153–1162, 1968
7. Ingbar SH. Diseases of the Thyroid. In Braunwald

E, Esselbacher KJ et al (eds): Harrison's Principles of Internal Medicine, 11th ed, pp 1732–1751. New York City, McGraw-Hill, 1987

8. Hershman JM: Management of Endocrine Disorders, pp 25–51. Philadelphia, Lea & Febiger, 1980
9. Rose NR, Lorenzi M, Lewis M. Endocrine Diseases. In Stites DP, Strobo JD et al (eds): Basic and Clinical Immunology, 5th ed, p 646. Los Altos, California, Lange Medical Publications, 1984
10. Okerlund MD, Hoffer PB, Matin P: Thyroid Imaging. In Matin P (ed): Nuclear Medicine Imaging, pp 226–242. New York City, Elsevier Science, 1985
11. Oertel YC. Fine-needle aspirations of thyroid, breast, and prostate. From Armed Forces Institute of Pathology, Exfoliative and Fine-Needle Aspiration Cytology course, 1986
12. Nystrom E, Lindstedt G, Lundberg PA et al: Recognizing hyperthyroidism in the elderly. Clin Chem 33:429, 1987
13. Burke MD: Thyroid function studies. Postgrad Med 68:169, 1980
14. Anderson SC: Thyroid Function. In Bishop ML, Duben-Von Laufen JL, Fody EP (eds): Clinical Chemistry—Principles, Procedures, Correlations, pp 470–481. Philadelphia, JB Lippincott, 1985
15. Chattoraj SC, Watts NB: Thyroid Function. In Tietz NW (ed): Textbook of Clinical Chemistry, 3rd ed, pp 1116–1136. Philadelphia, WB Saunders, 1986
16. Csako G, Zweig MH, Benson C et al: On the albumin dependence of measurements of free thyroxine. 1. Technical performance of seven methods. Clin Chem 32:108–115, 1986
17. Alexander NM: Free thyroxin in serum: Labelled thyroxin analog methods fall short of their mark. Clin Chem 32:417, 1986
18. Geiseler D, Chodha P, Ekins R: One-step immunoassays for free (unbound) hormones: The effect of tracer binding by serum proteins. Clin Chem 32:45–49, 1986
19. Clark PMS, Price CP: Enzyme-amplified immunoassays: A new ultrasensitive assay of thyrotropin evaluated. Clin Chem 32:88–92, 1986
20. Basset F, Eastman CJ, Ma G et al: Diagnostic value of thyrotropin concentrations in serum as measured by a sensitive immunoradiometric assay. Clin Chem 32:461–464, 1986
21. Musto JD, Pizzolante JM, Chesarome VP: A comment on thyrotropin measurement and evaluation. Clin Chem 30:329–330, 1984
22. Gruhn JG, Barsano CP, Kumar Y: The development of tests of thyroid function. Arch Pathol Lab Med 111:84–100, 1987
23. Chopra IJ, Solomon DH, Hepner GW et al: Misleading low free thyroxine index and usefulness of reverse triiodothyronine measurement in nonthyroidal illness. Ann Intern Med 90:905, 1979
24. Wartofsky L, Burman KD: Alterations in thyroid function in patients with systemic illness: The "euthyroid sick syndrome." Endocr Rev 3:164, 1982
25. Quaife MA, Nagel MV, Kotlyarov EV: The Endocrine System. In Bernier DR, Langan JK, Wells LD(eds): Nuclear Medicine Technology and Techniques, pp 241–255. St Louis, CV Mosby, 1981

BIBLIOGRAPHY

Tietz N (ed): Clinical Guide to Laboratory Tests, p 239. Philadelphia, WB Saunders, 1983

White GH, Walmsley RN: Plasma enzyme activities in primary hypothyroidism. Clin Chem 30:323, 1984

Chapter 36

Disorders of the Parathyroid

Sharon M. Miller

Abnormalities in parathyroid structure or function come to the attention of the physician when a patient presents with symptoms resulting from calcium "imbalance." Pathological consequences of this alteration in mineral metabolism range from minimal to profound.

Increased circulating levels of the calciotropic hormone *parathyrin* (PTH, parathyroid hormone) lead to clinical manifestations of hypercalcemia. If mild, this condition may warrant only continued observations by the physician and periodic laboratory monitoring of blood and urine to assure early detection of further changes. If progressive, differential diagnosis of the calcemia must be undertaken. When disruption is severe, immediate medical intervention to restore promptly and maintain normal calcium levels is mandatory for the preservation of life. In such an endocrine emergency, the laboratory's role often expands to include provision of data that will assist the medical team in localization and quantitation of parathyrin-secreting tissue for subsequent surgical removal.

Inadequate secretion of the parathyroids is reflected in lowered serum ionized calcium levels. Again, laboratory results are vital for early diagnosis and effective management. Preservation of calcium balance is achieved through numerous complex enzymatic and hormonal interactions. This chapter focuses on the role of the parathyroids in calcium homeostasis and the direct and indirect methods of laboratory assessment employed in the evaluation of gland function.

PARATHYROID STRUCTURE AND FUNCTION

Most individuals possess two pairs of parathyroid glands. The superior glands are generally located close to the upper posterior aspect of the thyroid. The location of the inferior glands is far more variable, ranging from the lower pole of the thyroid caudally to the thymus. The parathyroids are ellipsoidal and have a combined average weight of less than 150 mg.[1, 2] Knowledge of variation in gland number, position, and/or size is essential because surgery is the customary method of treatment for parathyroid lesions. Although 90% of individuals possess four parathyroids, as many as six or as few as two may be present. Therefore, the removal of even one gland may endanger the patient's ability to maintain calcium balance.

It is unusual to encounter a person with missing or rudimentary parathyroid glands. *DiGeorge's syndrome* is a rare congenital disorder in which neonatal parathyrin deficiency is caused by aplasia of the parathyroids and thymus. Patients die in early childhood of severe hypocalcemia and persistent infection.[3, 4] More common is the existence of an "above average" mass of PTH-secreting tissue. Up to 14% of adults are reported to have a fifth parathyroid, and six to eight glands are estimated to occur in as many as 5% of the population.[1, 2] Ectopic locations for the glands include the pericardium, anterior mediastinum in association with the thymus, and beneath the sheath of the carotid artery. Computer tomography (CT) scan, arteriography, ultrasound, and laboratory evaluation of parathyrin levels in blood samples from selective venous catheterizations are useful procedures in preoperative localization of abnormal parathyroid tissue.[3] If pathological enlargement of the parathyroid exists, one or more glands may be involved (see Table 36-1).[5] Roughly, the greater the increase in total parathyroid mass, the more severe the disease process and the more dramatic the clinical manifestations.[3]

Two types of cells are identified in the glandular parenchyma: chief cells and oxyphil cells. Oxyphil cells increase in number with age and may be mature, nonfunctional, or degenerative chief cells. It is the active chief cells that synthesize and secrete the polypeptide calciotropic hormone parathyrin.[2]

PTH synthesis begins with the formation of a 115 amino acid prohormone on rough endoplasmic reticulum (RER) of the chief cells. The precursor molecule, known as *PreProPTH,* is enzymatically cleaved twice before yielding the 84 amino acid hormone, parathyrin (see Fig. 36-1).[6] PTH may be stored intact within secretory granules of the chief cells or further degraded intracellularly to amino and mid-region/carboxy (C)-terminal fragments. In response to physiologic stimuli, principally the extracellular fluid (ECF) calcium ion concentration, polypeptide fragments and intact hormone are released into the circulation. A negative feedback regulation exists between ionized calcium levels and hormone release. Hypercalcemia reduces and hypocalcemia enhances the basal rate of parathyrin secretion. Among other factors observed to influence hormone synthesis and secretion are vitamin D metabolites, magnesium ions, catecholamines, and cortisol.[3]

Following entry into the peripheral circulation, intact PTH is metabolized in the liver and kidneys.

Table 36-1 ***Classification of Hyperparathyroid States***

Classification	Etiology	Lesion	Lesion Incidence (%)
Primary hyperparathyrodism	Idiopathic	Parathyroid adenoma	
		Single	80
		Multiple	3
		Parathyroid hyperplasia	16
		Parathyroid adenocarcinoma	<1
Secondary hyperparathyroidism	Compensatory response to chronic hypocalcemia, *e.g.*, vitamin D deficiency, renal failure	Parathyroid hyperplasia	
Tertiary hyperparathyroidism	Change in hyperplastic parathyroid of secondary hyperparathyroidism	Large functional parathyroid mass characterized by finite nonsuppressible PTH secretion	
Multiple endocrine neoplasia (MEN) syndromes	Congenital familial and sporadic disorder of cells derived from neural crest		
Type I (Werner's syndrome)	Inherited as autosomal dominant	Parathyroid hyperplasia or adenoma	80–90
		Pancreas adenoma	75
		Pituitary adenoma	60
Type IIa (Sipple's syndrome)		Parathyroid hyperplasia or adenoma	30–60
		Thyroid medullary carcinoma	95–100
		Pheochromocytoma	40–80
Ectopic hyperparathyroidism (pseudohyperparathyroidism)	Derepression of gene expression by malignant transformation of cells	Secretion of PTH or PTH-like peptides by malignant neoplasms in non-endocrine tissue	

Adapted from reference numbers [5, 14]

Impairment of renal function and clearance of mid-region polypeptide fragments are reflected in a significant increase in the relative proportion of these inert fragments in the circulation. Intact molecules and N-terminal fragments (amino acid residues 1–34) are biologically active. Thus they are removed from the circulation upon binding to the target tissues of the hormone, kidney and bone. *Immunoreactive parathyrin (iPTH)* consists of a mixture of intact molecules (1–84) and polypeptide sequences of varying lengths (see Fig. 36-2). Antisera employed in parathyrin immunoassays are classified on the basis of the location of their antigenic recognition sites. Intact and N-terminal procedures detect molecules and fragments containing the first 34 amino acid residues. Mid-molecule (35–55, 44–68) and C-terminal (53–84) assays react with the intact molecule as well as with their respective peptide sequences. Regardless of the absolute values used by a laboratory to establish an "expected normal range," the following relative percentages of PTH molecular forms are ob-

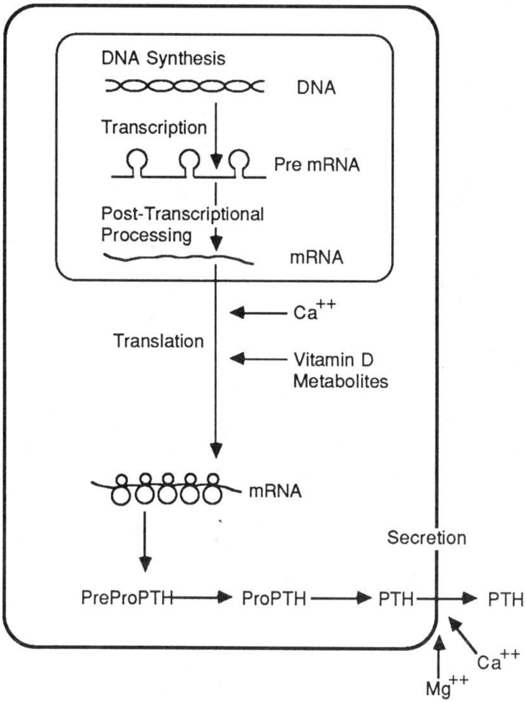

Figure 36-1 **Regulation of parathyrin formation and synthesis in chief cells of the parathyroid. (From Miller SM: Action and assessment of parathyrin, a calcium-regulating hormone. J Med Tech 3:335–341, 1986. Based on Habener JF, Rosenblatt M et al: Parathyroid hormone. Physiol Rev 64:985, 1984).**

served. Intact parathyrin and N-terminal fragments each account for approximately 10% of serum iPTH, and both are cleared from the blood in less than 6 minutes. Mid-region/carboxy-terminal fragments constitute 80% of total iPTH and have a longer circulating half-life, ranging from 20 to 40 minutes.[3, 7] It is this molecular heterogeneity and differential persistence of immunoreactive forms that makes laboratory evaluation of hormone secretion difficult.

HORMONE ACTION

PTH maintains serum levels of ionized calcium by (1) enhancing reabsorption of calcium in renal distal convoluted tubules; (2) acting in concert with the potent calciotropic steroid hormone 1,25-dihydroxyvitamin D (1,25-DHCC; 1,25-$[OH]_2D$; cholecalciferol) to mobilize calcium from bone; and (3) increasing activity of the renal enzyme 1α-hydroxylase, which promotes synthesis of 1,25-$[OH]_2D$ from 25-OHD (25-hydroxyvitamin D). It is the dihydroxyvitamin D metabolite that directly stimulates intestinal uptake of calcium. Cooperative action on bone and modulation of steroid hormone formation by parathyrin demonstrate the intimate relationship between the parathyroids and the vitamin D endocrine system in regulation of the body's calcium metabolism.

The polypeptide hormone calcitonin (CT), secreted predominantly by parafollicular or C cells of the thyroid, also affects calcium homeostasis by decreasing calcium release from bone mineral and increasing renal clearance of calcium. Calcium-liberating effects of parathyrin and 1,25-DHCC on skeletal tissue are opposed by calcitonin's inhibition of osteoclastic bone resorption.[1] The significance of the actions of calcitonin in calcium regulation under normal physiological conditions is still under review.

Serum phosphate concentration is also influenced by parathyrin. PTH promotes the osteoclastic release of phosphate from bone mineral. Simultaneously, phosphaturia occurs due to the hormone's inhibition of renal tubular reabsorption of phosphate. In addition to increasing urinary loss of phosphate, parathyrin acts in the kidney to enhance excretion of bicarbonate and sodium and to increase reabsorption of magnesium.[5, 8] Hyperchloremic acidosis is a common finding associated with increased secretion of parathyrin.[9]

Calcium in the serum circulates in three forms: free or ionized, protein-(mainly albumin) bound, and in diffusable but nonionized complexes. Only the free, ionized fraction, which accounts for approximately 50% of the total calcium, is physiologically active and parathyrin-regulated.[10] Plasma protein binding of calcium varies with the *p*H of the blood. By inhibiting both bicarbonate reabsorption and exchange of hydrogen ions for sodium ions in the proximal tubules, PTH gener-

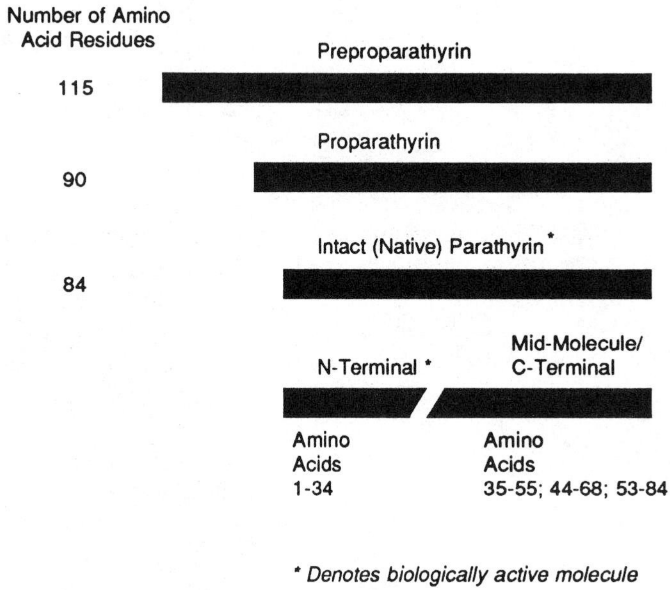

Figure 36-2 **Molecular precursors and metabolites of parathyrin. (From Miller SM: Action and assessment of parathyrin, a calcium-regulating hormone. J Med Tech 3:335–341, 1986)**

ates a metabolic acidosis. This condition favors displacement of calcium from the plasma proteins and bone, with a resulting increase in ECF ionized calcium. Parathyrin also increases activity of glucose-6-phosphate dehydrogenase in renal cells.

Direct PTH interaction with tissues of kidney and bone is by means of specific hormone-binding receptor proteins on the cell membranes (see Fig. 36-3). Because of the requirement for magnesium in this process, severe magnesium deficiency (< 0.8 mEq/L of serum [0.4 mmol/L]) leads to decreased parathyrin secretion and an impairment of hormone action on target tissues. Chronic alcoholics, the malnourished, and patients with malabsorption syndromes may be hypomagnesemic and, as a result, hypocalcemic. Before parathyroid function is assessed in these individuals, serum magnesium levels must be restored to normal. High concentrations of magnesium (> 4–5 mEq/L [2.0–2.5 mmol/L]) can also inhibit PTH secretion.[8] PTH stimulation of cAMP production and secretion, specifically by proximal tubule cells, forms the basis for an indirect laboratory method of assessing parathyroid function that is described later.[11]

ETIOLOGY AND PATHOPHYSIOLOGY

Hyperparathyroidism

Excessive production of parathyrin may be caused by increased total mass of secretory tissue, chief cell hyperfunctioning, or change in set point for calcium suppression of hormone release. Hyperparathyroid states have been classified as primary, secondary, tertiary, ectopic, and associated with congenital multiple endocrine neoplasia (MEN) syndromes (see Table 36-1).[5]

The most common parathyroid disorder, *primary hyperparathyroidism (HPT),* is characterized by an increased concentration of serum calcium and an inappropriately high level of parathyrin. On the basis of the frequency with which hypercalcemia is detected during routine blood analyses, it is estimated that one in every 900 adults in the United States has some degree of HPT.[12] This can be due to parathyroid hyperplasia, adenoma, and/or carcinoma. In more than 80% of cases, neoplastic transformation in the form of a single benign adenoma is the cause of hyperparathyroidism.

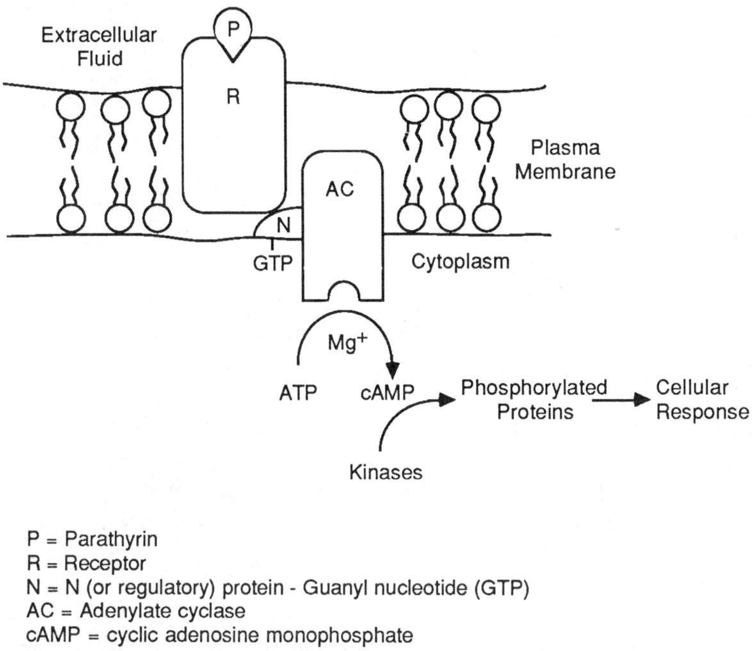

Figure 36-3 Hormone receptor-adenylate coupling. (From Miller SM: Action and assessment of parathyrin, a calcium-regulating hormone. J Med Tech 3:335–341, 1986. Based on Teitelbaum AP, Arnaud CD: Parathyroid hormone receptors. Diagn Med 5:69, 1982)

Multiple gland hyperplasia occurs in approximately 20% of patients, and carcinoma is seen in fewer than 1%.[1] Primary HPT occurs more frequently in the elderly, and is at least twice as common in females as in males. A disease incidence of 0.18% for females over 60 years of age has been reported.[3] Although an idiopathic etiology is not uncommon for primary HPT, the medical history of approximately one quarter of such patients reveals previous head and neck irradiation.[1] Dose-dependent, radiation-induced HPT may arise as long as 30 years after initial exposure.[13]

Elevated serum PTH levels also occur in 80% to 90% of patients with familial *multiple endocrine neoplasia syndromes (MENS),* Type I. These individuals exhibit parathyroid hyperplasia or adenoma as well as pituitary and pancreatic tumors (see Table 36-1).[14]

HPT may arise as a compensatory response to prolonged hypocalcemia. In long-standing impairment of kidney function there is an accompanying reduction in renal production of 1,25-dihydroxyvitamin D. Intestinal calcium absorption is sharply reduced, and hypocalcemia develops. Continual stimulation of PTH release through feedback regulation induces glandular hyperplasia and hypersecretion, which is thus secondary to chronic renal disease or vitamin D deficiency.[15] Classic chemical manifestations of *secondary HPT* due to chronic renal failure include hypocalcemia, hyperphosphatemia, and increased PTH. The mass of parathyroid tissue present in patients with secondary HPT is generally far greater than that found in patients with primary HPT.[5] Recent studies indicate a decreased sensitivity to the suppressive effects of ECF calcium on parathyrin release in both primary and secondary HPT.[16]

In *tertiary HPT,* hypercalcemia results when

parathyroids develop "autonomous" or nonsuppressible parathyrin secretion following an extended period of secondary HPT. Parathyroid hyperplasia may also occur when there is target-organ resistance to hormone action. In the condition of pseudohypoparathyroidism, low serum calcium triggers increased PTH secretion but effector organs (kidney and bone) are unresponsive presumably due to defective hormone receptor or an inherited deficiency in regulatory protein within the cell membrane.[17] Hypocalcemia persists despite increased parathyrin secretion.

The production of parathyrin by nonparathyroid neoplasms is rare. Solid tumors such as squamous cell carcinoma of the lung may produce PTH or PTHlike peptides, thereby creating the condition *pseudohyperparathyroidism*. Severe hypercalcemia accompanied by low or undetectable levels of parathyrin may indicate malignancy. Oncogenic hypercalcemia is attributable to development of osteolytic metastases, as in breast cancer, or the secretion of humoral, but nonPTH, bone-mobilizing factors such as osteoclast-activating factor (OAF) in multiple myeloma and other hematologic malignancies.[18] It is critical that the hypercalcemias of malignancy and primary HPT be differentiated as early as possible so that appropriate therapy may be initiated. It has been observed that, generally, primary HPT is associated with elevated serum calcium and normal to slightly elevated 1,25-$(OH)_2D$. In contrast, serum 1,25-$(OH)_2D$ levels are usually decreased in patients with tumor-associated malignancy. Unfortunately, clear separation of these conditions on the basis of laboratory findings is not always possible.

Hypoparathyroidism

Inadequacies in glandular secretion of parathyrin are often limited in duration and associated with a specific traumatic event. Acute PTH deficiency may be encountered among patients who have experienced a temporary disruption of blood flow to the neck, as in injury, surgery, or infarction. A period of hormone insufficiency, the so-called "hungry bone syndrome," may occur in patients with significant preoperative bone disease. Following removal of adenomatous or hyperplastic parathyroid tissue, hypocalcemia and recalcification tetany are often observed. The remaining glandular tissue, which is capable of normal functioning, temporarily remains suppressed in response to the preexisting, long-standing hypercalcemia. In addition, rapid remineralization of bone through increased osteoblastic activity quickly depletes circulating ionized calcium. Such a hypoparathyroid condition is usually transient.

Also of a temporary nature are the hypocalcemia, hypomagnesemia, and lowered circulating levels of parathyrin observed in patients with acute leukemia treated with adriamycin or cytarabine.[1] A number of drugs have been reported to alter parathyroid function. The organic thiophosphate compound WR-2721, employed to protect healthy tissue during radiation and chemotherapy, inhibits parathyrin secretion. Aminoglycosides and cisplatin may depress serum magnesium levels. Severe hypomagnesemia, in turn, causes hypocalcemia by suppression of parathyrin secretion and diminished end-organ responsiveness to the hormone.[1,3]

Permanent primary hypoparathyroidism may occur following removal of or damage to the glands, as a feature of DiGeorge's syndrome, or in association with autoimmune phenomena.[1, 3, 19] Surgery is the most common cause of hypoparathyroidism.[4] In the immediate postoperative period, a serum ionized calcium value of 8 mg/dL (2.0 mmol/L) has been interpreted as suggestive of partial hypoparathyroidism, and functional aparathyroidism by levels of 5–6 mg/dL (1.3–1.5 mmol/L).[3]

Functional hypoparathyroidism and hypocalcemia are often seen in pediatric patients, particularly preterm, low-birth-weight infants. This is attributed to a temporary "immaturity" or unresponsiveness of the glands to low circulating levels of calcium for several hours after birth.[10, 20] Fetal parathyrin secretion may be inhibited in utero in response to maternal hypercalcemia.[21] Serum calcium levels below 3 mg/dL (0.8 mmol/L) should be considered an emergency and treated aggressively. Plasma phosphate levels usually exceed 6 mg/dL (1.9 mmol/L) in children who are hypoparathyroid.

As suggested by its name, parathyroid function is normal, but hypocalcemia develops despite normal or increased parathyrin secretion in the rare X-linked disorder, pseudohypoparathyroidism. Abnormalities in sensitivity or numbers of membrane receptors or regulatory proteins in kidney and bone appear to be the basis for the decrease in end-organ response.[4, 5]

Idiopathic hypoparathyroidism refers to a broad category of disorders.[22] Onset of symptoms may occur in early childhood or late in life. While circulating glandular antibodies have been reported in some cases, the etiology of parathyroid destruction in these patients is unclear.

CLINICAL MANIFESTATIONS

Hyperparathyroidism

Clinical presentation of HPT ranges from asymptomatic to severe. Approximately 50% of HPT patients report no symptoms; the only evidence of the condition is laboratory-identified hypercalcemia, hypophosphatemia, and hypercalciuria during routine analysis.[23] Signs and symptoms associated with an HPT state are attributable mainly to hypercalcemia. Common nonspecific, mild complaints include malaise, general fatigue, anorexia, muscle weakness, aching, and excessive thirst and urination. (See Table 36-2). Constipation, caused by decreased smooth muscle activity in the gastrointestinal tract, is seen in approximately one-third of patients. Peptic ulcers and associated abdominal pain are also frequently reported in patients with confirmed HPT. Hypertension has been observed in up to 50% of primary HPT patients.[1, 3] Bone pain and arthralgia may occur without radiographic evidence of skeletal lesions. Chronic excessive secretion of PTH with resulting systemic manifestations of severe hypercalcemia produces a spectrum of dramatic, even life-threatening, alterations in nerve and muscle function (cardiac arrhythmias), central nervous system disruptions (paranoia or hallucinations), renal damage or failure due to alterations in calcium excretion (nephrolithiasis, nephrocalcinosis), metastatic calcifications (corneal calcification), and significant bone disease (osteitis fibrosa cystica) characterized by generalized patchy demineralization, cysts, brown tumors, and excessive bone resorption.[2]

Table 36-2 ***Clinical Manifestations of Primary Hyperparathyroidism***

Manifestation	Frequency (%)
Hypertension	53
Weakness	42
Fatigue	42
Renal colic	39
Weight loss	33
Mental disturbance	33
Constipation	32
Epigastric pain	32
Nausea/vomiting	23
Polyuria/polydipsia	19
Anorexia	18
Arthralgias	18
Peptic ulcer	17
Bone pain	16
Pruritus	9
Paresthesias	9
Headaches	9
Gout	9
Loose teeth	7
Spontaneous fractures	7
Pancreatitis	4

From reference number[3]

The clinical manifestations of primary HPT have been described classically as "the six moans": (1) stones (renal), (2) bones (pain, spontaneous fractures, skeletal deformities), (3) groans (abdominal pain), (4) ions (asymptomatic hypercalcemia), (5) neurons (neuromuscular and psychiatric disturbances), and (6) hormones (endocrine disorders as part of MENS).[2, 3]

Hypoparathyroidism

A lowered serum ionized calcium level is the chemical basis for the signs and symptoms associated with hypoparathyroidism (see Table 36-3).[5] It is the rapidity with which calcium deficiency develops, more than the absolute value of the serum ionized calcium, that determines the clinical manifestations of hypocalcemia.[4] Influenced by the extent and duration of calcium deficiency, a wide diversity of signs and symptoms are encountered.[22] For example, patients with chronic hypocalcemia may be asymptomatic, develop cataracts at an early age, or have such dermatologic diseases as moniliasis or psoriasis. Most often there is evidence of neuromuscular irritability and tetany, ranging from weakness and muscle cramps to seizures.[5] Indications of latent tetany include the ability to elicit contractions, in response to specific stimuli, of facial or wrist muscles. These spasmodic muscular contractions are known respectively as *Chvostek's* and *Trousseau's signs.* If respiratory muscles become involved, laryngospasm, bronchospasm, and respiratory arrest may follow.[3] Psychiatric manifestations range from anxiety and irritability to dementia. Cardiovascular difficulties include arrhythmias, digitalis insensitivity, hypotension, and congestive heart failure.[1, 3]

Table 36-3 ***Clinical Manifestations of Hypo- and Pseudohypoparathyroidism***

Manifestation	Frequency (%) in Parathyroidism: *Hypo-*	*Pseudohypo-*
Phenotypic abnormalities	10	60
Tetany	76	63
Convulsions	70	65
Cataracts	48	35
Muscle cramps, twitching	46	38
Laryngospasm	32	8
Ectopic ossifications	28	48
Paresthesia	24	12
Mental disturbances	24	10
Vomiting/constipation	20	2.5
Dental abnormalities	18	33
Moniliasis	16	0
Heart failure	8	0

Adapted from reference number [5]

In classical cases of pseudohypoparathyroidism (PHP), individuals are characterized by physical as well as biochemical abnormalities. They are short (< 5 feet), of stocky build or obese, and moon-faced. Most show some degree of mental impairment. Skeletal abnormalities include shortening of the phalanges as well as the fourth and fifth metacarpals and metatarsals. Ectopic ossifications are common. Most patients with PHP show signs of chronic hypocalcemia.[4, 5, 22]

LABORATORY ANALYSES AND DIAGNOSIS

Hyperparathyroidism

Assessment of parathyroid function is one of the ways in which the clinical laboratory scientist can assist the physician in the identification and management of diseases of bone and calcium metabolism. Evaluation of gland activity may be by means of either direct or indirect methodologies. Selection of a particular assay or group of tests is made with the goal of clearly distinguishing normoparathyroid from hypoparathyroid individuals, and differentiating patients with primary hyperparathyroidism (to be surgically proven) either from those with hyperparathyroidism secondary to chronic renal failure or from those with hypercalcemia of nonparathyroid origin (*e.g.,* malignancy). The clinical laboratory scientist's responsibility must be to provide recommendations to the clinician as to procedures most likely to provide data eliminating, or at least minimizing, overlap among patient populations. The most effective and efficient diagnostic protocols are most likely to be cost-effective as well.

Establishment and confirmation of hypercalcemia remains the pivotal event in the laboratory diagnosis of parathyroid dysfunction (see Table 36-4). While serum calcium level alone is an insufficient discriminator of parathyroid function, evaluation of this analyte offers a readily obtainable, inexpensive means of identifying individuals with possible gland pathologies.[10] Highly sophisticated algorithms have been developed for the most effective use of laboratory tests in the differential diagnosis of hypercalcemia.[24] At least three separate occurrences of hypercalcemia should be demonstrated. Either serum ionized (Ca^{+2}) or total calcium (Ca_T) can be measured. It is currently suggested that potentiometric measurements of ionized calcium give more meaningful clinical information than do total calcium results.[10] While improvements in ion-selective electrode (ISE) technology promise to make Ca^{+2} testing more routine in service laboratories, total calcium determinations are still preferred by most clinicians.

Table 36-4 ***Laboratory Results (Frequency) in Hyperparathyroidism***

Laboratory Test	Frequency (%)
Nonspecific	
Elevated ALP	25–30
Hypomagnesemia	10–15
Hyperuricemia	66
Anemia (Hct < 36)	21
Elevated ESR	48
Hypokalemia	5
Specific	
Hypercalcemia	100
Elevated parathyroid function	100
Elevated PTH	
Elevated nephrogenous cAMP	
% TRP < 80	Most
$Cl/PO_4 > 33$	Most
TmP/GFR decreased	Over 80%
Chloride	
>110 mEq/L	9
>107 mEq/L	39
>102 mEq/L	85
Hypophosphatemia	25–70
Hyperchloremic acidosis ($HCO_3 < 24$ mEq/L)	24

From reference number [3]

To evaluate total serum calcium results, correction must be applied for the serum protein status. For each change in serum albumin of 1.0 g/dL (10 g/L), total serum calcium changes in parallel by approximately 0.8 mg/dL (0.2 mmol/L). In hypercalcemia, serum calcium is often in the range of 10.2 to 11.0 mg/dL (2.6–2.8 mmol/L). Hypercalcemic crisis is reached when values exceed 14 to 15 mg/dL (3.5–3.8 mmol/L).[3] If the hypercalcemia remains untreated, muscular paralysis, ventricular arrhythmia, coma, and death follow.

Among hospital patients, the most common cause of hypercalcemia is malignancy with bone metastases.[25] Other conditions characterized by hypercalcemia include hyperthyroidism, renal disease, adrenal insufficiency, sarcoidosis, myeloma, milk-alkali syndrome, hypervitaminosis of A or D, chronic immobilization, and therapy with thiazide diuretics.[4] Persistent hypercalcemia in the absence of other identifiable causes is often the basis for a diagnosis of primary HPT. In secondary HPT, serum calcium levels are generally normal or decreased. Measurements by the clinical laboratory that have proved relevant, but not conclusive, in the diagnosis of disorders of the parathyroid include serum inorganic phosphate, chloride, chloride/phosphorus ratio, bicarbonate, alkaline phosphatase (ALP), 1,25-$(OH)_2D$, albumin, renal threshold phosphate concentration (TmP/GFR), tubular reabsorption of phosphate (TRP), and urinary calcium (see Table 36-4).

Two additional indices of parathyroid function are the urinary excretion ratios of cyclic adenosine monophosphate (cAMP) to creatinine or to glomerular filtration, and the ratio of the nephrogenous fraction of cAMP (NcAMP) to glomerular filtration. Under normal conditions total urinary cAMP originates equally from plasma (PcAMP) via glomerular filtration and from proximal tubular secretion in response to PTH (*i.e.*, UcAMP = PcAMP + NcAMP). When parathyrin secretion is increased, the rise in excreted urinary cAMP is due primarily to increased NcAMP. The renal contribution to urinary cAMP is elevated in more than 90% of patients with primary HPT.[23] However, although NcAMP distinguishes among individuals who have normo-, hyper-, and hypo-functioning parathyroids, alone it does not reliably differentiate among hypercalcemic disorders. NcAMP levels are also elevated in secondary HPT and oncogenic hypercalcemia. UcAMP and NcAMP measurements may be of use in the prompt evaluation of the success of parathyroidectomy. Values for both are elevated before surgery, and fall rapidly and significantly once the mass of PTH-secreting tissue is reduced.[1]

If urinary cAMP (nanomoles) is reported per dL of glomerular filtrate, the resultant expression provides information comparable to that obtained by calculation of nephrogenous cAMP.[26] This eliminates the need for the difficult and tedious determination of plasma cAMP.

Reference range for NcAMP is 0.34–2.7 nmol/dL of glomerular filtrate. For UcAMP, the reference range is 1.83–4.5 nmol/dL, with values greater than 3.5 nmol/dL suggestive of hyperparathyroidism.[3, 23]

Indirect tests measure the biological effect rather than absolute amount of hormone. Individually, such assays yield only limited diagnostic or predictive information. When results are evaluated in combination, however, particularly as they relate to PTH levels, the clinical usefulness of these procedures is increased. Diagnostic discrimination is significantly enhanced by the multivariate statistical treatment of multiple selected laboratory findings.[9, 23, 24, 27, 28] The HJMJ chloride index is a multivariate discriminant analysis that relates weighted serum chloride, albumin, and inorganic phosphate. A ratio of the HJMJ chloride index to parathyrin concentration reportedly gives a 100% diagnostic efficiency.[29] Various expressions of cAMP excretion, when combined with other indices of parathyroid function, also yield an extraordinary degree of precision in HPT disease classification.[27] When discriminant multivariate linear regression analysis is applied to the variables of plasma calcium, C-terminal PTH, and the ratio of the nephrogenous fraction of cAMP to glomerular filtrate, classification accuracy is 98%.[27]

In vitro bioassays are available for direct measuring of plasma parathyrin. Quantitation of minute amounts of parathyrin is best achieved through pretreatment of serum or heparinized plasma by immunoaffinity chromatography. Although bioassays are extremely sensitive, they are too time-consuming and costly for routine clinical use. These procedures are utilized currently as standards of reference against which other laboratory procedures are judged.[26]

At present, the method of choice for direct determination of circulating parathyrin species is radioimmunoassay. Reversed-phase high-performance liquid chromatography (HPLC) has been used on a limited basis for the analysis of hPTH in reference standards, parathyroid tissue, and biological fluids.[30] Quantification of PTH in the collected fractions has been accomplished by ultraviolet absorbance and, more commonly, with radioimmunoassay of the column effluents.

After the application in 1963 of RIA to the direct determination of serum parathyrin, it was anticipated that PTH levels alone would ultimately provide for definitive diagnoses.[31] However, the predictive value of an elevated hormone level, in isolation, has generally proven to be inadequate. A recent study reported the misclassification of 45% of patients with primary HPT when only parathyrin levels were assessed.[27, 29] When parathyrin levels are reported in relationship to serum total or ionized calcium, however, there is improved discrimination among patients with disorders of calcium homeostasis.[27, 32] A nomogram, in which the x axis is total serum calcium reported in mg/dL and the y axis is iPTH or a specific molecular subspecies of parathyrin (*e.g.*, mid-molecule PTH) expressed in pg/mL, is a common tool for evaluating parathyroid function (see Fig. 36-4). Various diagnostic areas are demarcated on the nomogram. These areas are established based on observed correlations of ion and hormone levels in confirmed diagnoses of calcium metabolism disorders. When plotted, the

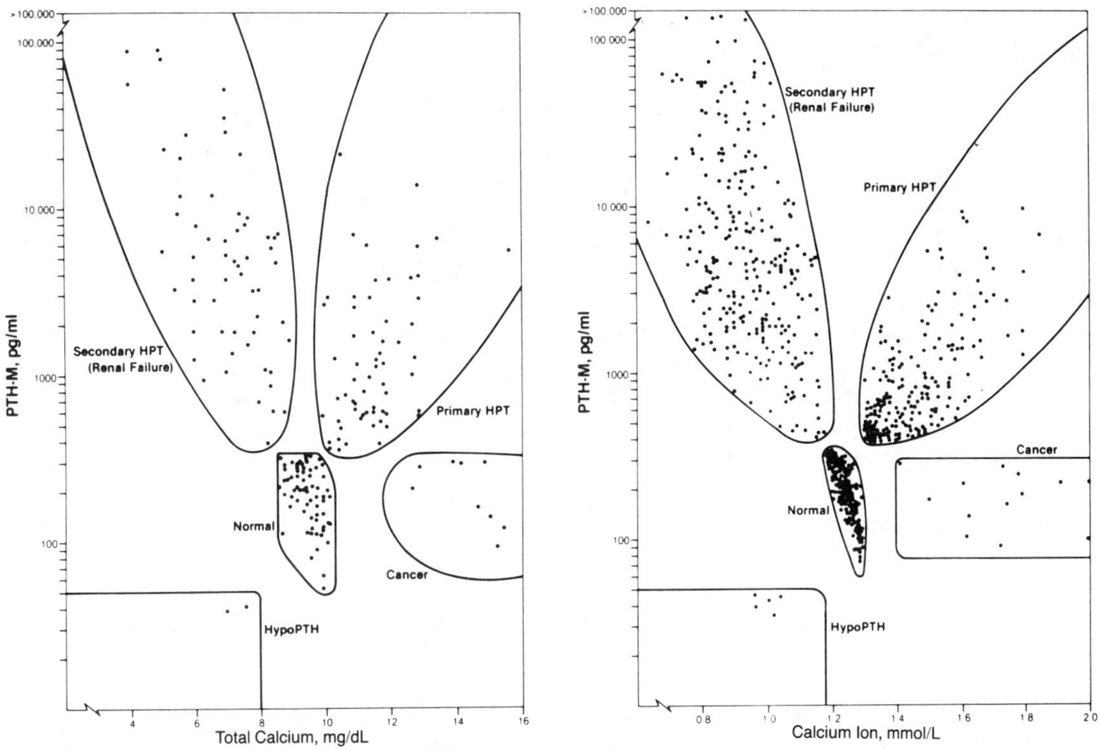

Figure 36-4 **Correlation of total and ionized calcium with midmolecule PTH in selected pathological conditions. (From Miller SM: Action and assessment of parathyrin, a calcium-regulating hormone. J Med Tech 3:335–341, 1986. Photo courtesy Endocrine Metabolic Center, Oakland, CA)**

coordinates of the patient's values define a point that, ideally, falls within the boundaries of a particular diagnostic region. Computer-generated probabilities for the association of specific calcium and PTH levels in various pathologies are available, accompanied by interpretive statements, through commercial laboratories, and increase the clinician's confidence in a particular diagnosis.

Technical difficulties associated with conducting and interpreting RIAs for iPTH and its molecular subspecies have, until recently, significantly limited the clinical usefulness of the direct method of assessing parathyroid function. Widely varying reference ranges for parathyrin are found in the literature. The early antisera used in this method exhibited highly variable affinity for and cross-reactivity with human PTH. With such limitations, it was particularly difficult to detect low concentrations of parathyrin or to measure directly the biologically active forms of the hormone.

Today, C-terminal parathyrin assays with virtually a 100% sensitivity for primary HPT are available. A mid-region PTH assay with sensitivity for primary HPT near 90% is available in kit form. Increased sensitivity and specificity of the new commercially-available parathyrin assays are possible because of the availability of homologous RIAs. Such assays employ synthetic hPTH for reference standards, in the radioligand (^{125}I-PTH), and to produce high-affinity antisera specific for particular peptide regions of the parathyrin molecule.[33] Turnaround time for the assay is relatively short. N-terminal assays may require two days or slightly less. Higher concentrations of mid-region/C-terminal fragments permit shorter incubation times, and such assays may be completed in less than a work day.[34, 35] One commercially-available RIA kit for measuring mid-region parathyrin has a four-hour turnaround time for results.[36] All procedures currently available detect picogram amounts of parathyrin; however, test sensitivities still vary with the particular antiserum employed.[37]

A two-site immunoradiometric assay (IRMA) for measurement of intact PTH has recently become commercially available. In RIA, it is the antigen that is radiolabeled, while in IRMA, it is the antibody that contains the radioisotope. The extreme sensitivity claimed for this immunoassay system should make it possible for the laboratory scientist to distinguish normal and reduced levels of PTH. Monoclonal antibodies are likely to replace polyclonal antisera for parathyrin assessment in the near future.[29]

DIAGNOSTIC PROTOCOLS

Parathyroid profiles routinely offered by laboratories include analyses for parathyrin (intact/N-terminal; mid-molecule; C-terminal), total and ionized serum calcium, inorganic phosphate, and creatinine. Serum 1,25-$(OH)_2D$, urine cAMP, and ALP measurements may also be provided. Initially, there must be establishment and verification of hypercalcemia. One schema for the sequencing of tests in the diagnosis and management of patients with hypercalcemia is shown in Figure 36-5. A fasting morning serum sample is preferable. Heparinized blood is often employed for parathyrin and vitamin D metabolite procedures. Intact PTH is extremely labile. Unless assessment is immediate, specimens should be maintained at -20° C.

If malignancy and drug-induced hypercalcemia can be excluded, diagnostic efforts will focus on the evaluation of parathyroid function, with a strong suspicion of primary hyperparathyroidism. Serum iPTH levels will then be determined. Most recent studies suggest the best discrimination between normal individuals and patients with primary HPT is consistently achieved by the use of mid-molecule/C-terminal PTH assays.[38] These assays are extremely sensitive to patient renal function.

If glomerular filtration rate (GFR) is reduced, as indicated by elevated plasma creatinine, it becomes advisable to utilize a PTH assay specific for intact/N-terminal parathyrin. Special problems exist in long-standing renal insufficiency because all forms of parathyrin remain in the circulation for an extended period of time. Intact and N-terminal fragments may persist for 30 minutes, while C-terminal fragments may have a half-life of 1 to 2 days.[39] Overabundance and accumulation of mid-molecule/C-terminal peptides, due to impaired renal clearance, mask subtle changes in levels of intact/N-terminal PTH. Under such circumstances, an assay specific to active hormone provides for a more direct assessment of parathyroid function. N-terminal assays available from commercial laboratories have sensitivities for primary HPT greater than 90%.

When intact PTH measurements are evaluated along with total serum calcium, overlap among reduced (*e.g.*, hypoparathyroidism, oncogenic hypercalcemia) and normal values, as well as above-normal values (*e.g.*, primary HPT) is largely eliminated.[37, 40] For maximum clinical usefulness, PTH levels should correlate with the severity of metabolic bone disease.[39] This is particularly important in monitoring patients receiving maintenance dialysis, in which early intervention will minimize renal osteodystrophy. Some studies indicate that results of N-terminal assays correlate better with histological changes seen in bone biopsies. N-terminal assays are specifically utilized in the localization of abnormal parathyroid tissue by means of selective venous catheterization. Suppression/stimulation tests, in which evaluation of rapid secretory response of the gland is desired, require use of intact/N-terminal assays.

Table 36-5 summaries the differential laboratory findings encountered most often in selected hypercalcemias of parathyroid and nonparathyroid origin.

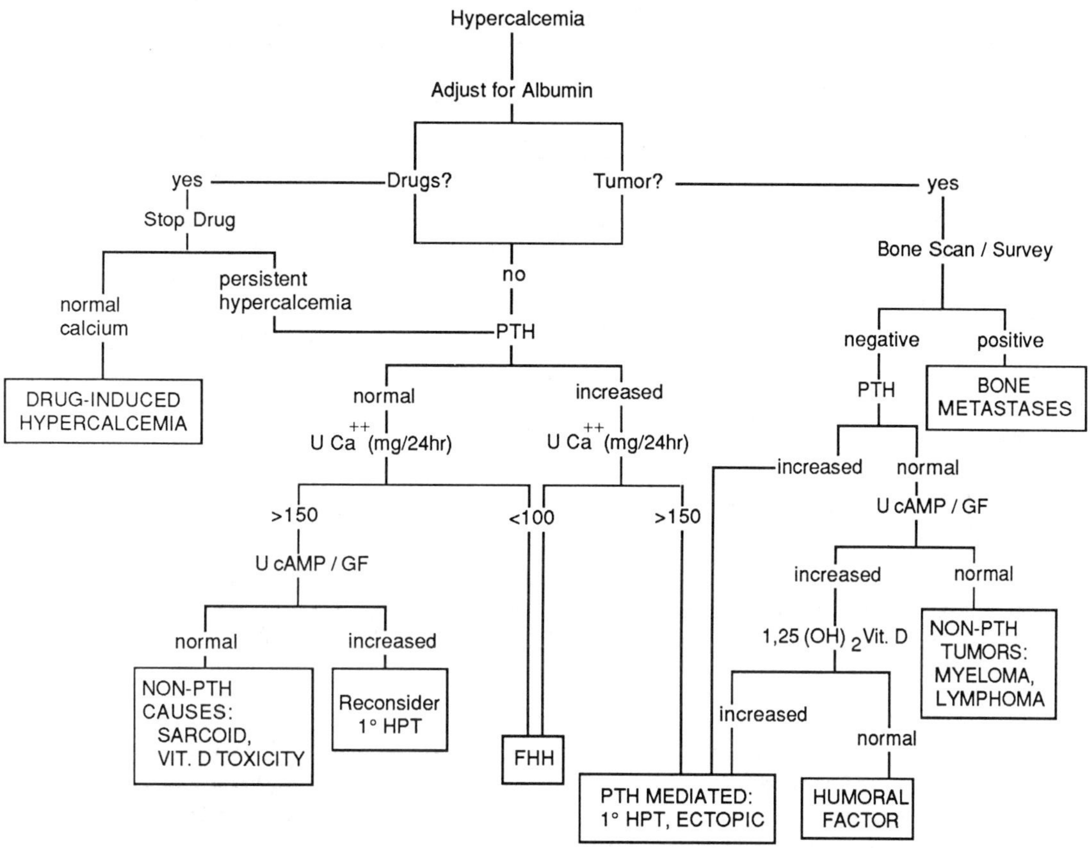

PTH = parathyroid hormone
cAMP = cyclic adenosine monophosphate
PHPT = primary hyperparathyroidism
FHH = familial hypocalciuric hypercalcemia

Figure 36-5 **Diagnostic protocol for hypercalcemia. (From Licata AA, Streck WF: Hypercalcemia. In Streck WF, Lockwood DH [eds]: Endocrine Diagnosis: Clinical and Laboratory Approach. Boston, Little, Brown & Co, 1983)**

Hypoparathyroidism

When total serum calcium is less than 8.5 mg/dL (2.1 mmol/L) and serum albumin levels are normal, hypocalcemia exists.[3] Differential diagnosis of hypocalcemia is routinely accomplished by assessing serum levels of total and ionized calcium, phosphorus, NcAMP, and iPTH. Additional assays found as part of a calcium metabolism testing profile may include calcitonin, osteocalcin, and vitamin D metabolites. Measurement of 25-OHD and 1,25-$(OH)_2D$ levels will permit identification of vitamin D deficiency. (See Figure 36-6). Hypoparathyroidism is associated with decreased activity of 1α-hydroxylase. If vitamin D nutrition is adequate, serum levels of 25-OHD are normal but

Table 36-5 ***Laboratory Findings in Hyperparathyroidism and Nonparathyroid Hypercalcemias***

	Serum										Urine	
Disorder	*Ca*	*iPTH*	*P*	*ALP*	*Cl*	HCO_3	*Mg*	*K*	*Uric Acid*	*BUN, Creatinine*	*Ca*	*cAMP*
Primary hyperparathyroidism	↑ ↑↑	↑ ↑↑	↓N	N↑	↑N	N↓	N↓	N(↓)	↑N	N	N↑	↑N
Secondary hyperparathyroidism												
Chronic renal disease	↓N	↑N	↑N	N↑	N	N↓	N↑	↑N	↑N	↑	N	↓
Osteomalacia	N↓	↑N	↓N	N↑	N	N	N	N	N	N	↓	N↑
Renal tubular acidosis	N↓	↑N	↓N	N↑	↑	↓	N↓	↓N	N(?)	N	↑	N
Oncogenic hypercalcemias	↑ ↑↑	↓N	N↑	N↑	N	N↓	N↓	N↓	N↑	N↑	↑ ↑↑	N↑

Symbols: ↑ = increased; ↑↑ = markedly increased; ↓ = decreased; N = normal. The first of a pair of symbols indicates the more usual finding. Symbol in parenthesis represents infrequent or rare findings.
Taken from Eliel LP: Disorders of calcium homeostasis. In Metz R, Larson EB (eds): Blue Book of Endocrinology, p 201. Philadelphia, WB Saunders, 1985

1,25-$(OH)_2D$ levels are decreased. If a deficiency of vitamin D exists in a normoparathyroid patient, parathyrin is increased but levels of vitamin D metabolites are reduced. In the absence of adequate gastrointestinal absorption of calcium due to hypovitaminosis D, and without the cooperative calcium-mobilizing action of parathyrin and 1,25-$(OH)_2D$ on bone, normal serum calcium levels cannot be maintained. Increased levels of parathyrin induce phosphaturia.

Primary hypoparathyroidism is characterized by low levels of parathyrin and calcium, hyperphosphatemia, and normal renal function. Nephrogenous cAMP levels are close to zero (see Table 36-6).

In pseudohypoparathyroidism, serum calcium is decreased despite elevated levels of parathyrin. If end-organ resistance to parathyrin is incomplete, there will be evidence of skeletal disorders and metabolic bone disease. PTH stimulation tests may be performed to assist in the diagnosis. Renal tubular resistance to PTH is demonstrated by minimal increase in UcAMP (rather than the usual four- to tenfold increase) and a blunted phosphaturic response when PTH is infused.[4]

DIAGNOSTIC PROTOCOL

Figure 36-6 details the routine sequence of laboratory procedures employed in the differential diagnosis of hypocalcemia. Measurement of serum iPTH is essential for a correct diagnosis. Assays employed must be sensitive enough to permit quantitation of the hormone at low normal or subnormal levels. The newer RIA and IRMA procedures appear to provide the required degrees of specificity and sensitivity.

TREATMENT

Hyperparathyroidism

Rapid correction of moderate to severe hypercalcemia involves restoration of intravascular volume with normal saline infusion and accelerated

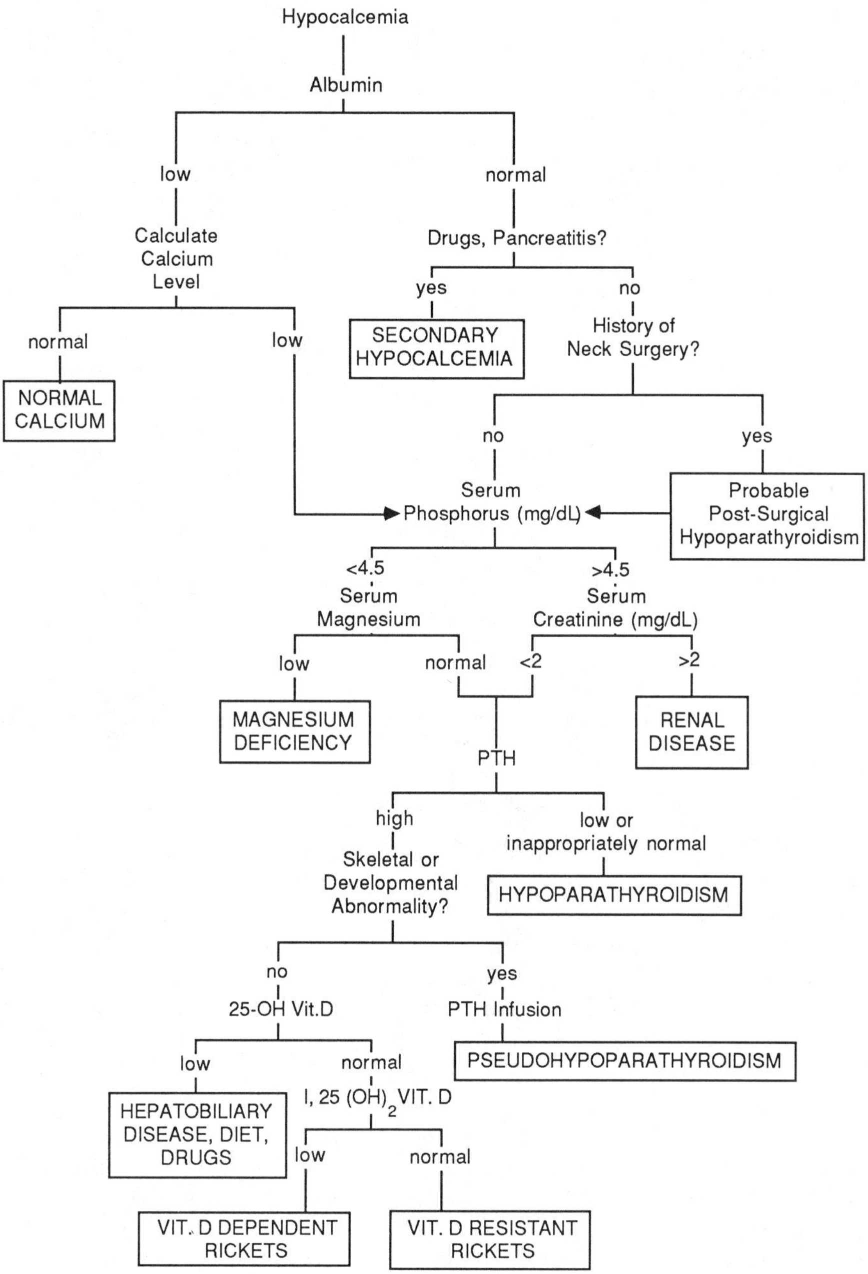

PTH = parathyroid hormone
25-OH Vit. D = 25-hydroxyvitamin D
1,25 $(OH)_2$ Vit. D= 1.25 dihydroxyvitamin D

Figure 36-6 **Diagnostic protocol for hypocalcemia. (From Licata AA, Streck WF: Hypocalcemia. In Streck WF, Lockwood DH [eds]: Endocrine Diagnosis: Clinical and Laboratory Approach. Boston, Little, Brown & Co, 1983)**

Table 36-6 ***Laboratory Findings in Hypocalcemic States***

Disorder	Serum						Urine	
	Ca	*P*	*ALP*	*iPTH*	*25(OH)D*	*1,25(OH)₂D*	*Ca*	*cAMP*
Hypoparathyroidism (congenital, genetic, or acquired)	↓	↑	N	↓	N	↓	↓	↓
Pseudohypoparathyroidism (PTH resistance)	↓	↑	N	↑	N	↓N	↓	↓ (Type I)
Deficient $1,25(OH)_2D$ synthesis; renal disease, inherited (vitamin D dependency)	↓ or N	↑, ↓*	↑ or N	↑	↑ or N	↓	↓ or N	↑, ↓*

Symbols: ↓ = low; ↑ = high; N = normal. The first of a pair of symbols indicates the more usual findings.
* High in renal disease, low in vitamin D dependency
Taken from Eliel LP: Disorders of calcium homeostasis. In Metz R, Larson EB (eds): Blue Book of Endocrinology, p 213. Philadelphia, WB Saunders, 1985

calcium excretion by forcing saline diuresis, using furosemide. Serum calcium levels will generally fall 3 to 4 mg/dL (0.8–1.0 mmol/L) in 24 hours if therapy is successful.[41] Careful monitoring of electrolytes is mandatory, because K^+ and Mg^{2+} depletion are likely to occur. Mithramycin, a cytotoxic antibiotic that inhibits osteoclast differentiation, can normalize serum calcium levels in 75% of hypercalcemic patients within 48 hours.[41] Toxic side-effects are rare if only one or two doses are administered. If, through further testing, primary HPT is identified as the cause of the hypercalcemic crisis, surgery is usually recommended. Postoperatively, serum calcium and phosphorus should be monitored every 6 to 12 hours until they stabilize.[3] Return to normal levels is usual within 24 hours.[1, 3] Monitoring of iPTH may also be conducted, but its usefulness in the immediate management of hypercalcemia is limited.[23] Calcium supplementation may become necessary to prevent development of transient hypocalcemia and tetany. Such an abrupt decline in ECF ionized calcium can occur due to rapid remineralization of skeletal tissue following prolonged bone disease, or because removal of adenomatous tissue leaves behind normal glandular tissue that has been suppressed in response to prolonged chronic hypercalcemia.

Hypoparathyroidism

The symptoms of severe hypocalcemia indicate impending neuromuscular and cardiovascular collapse. This is a medical emergency and requires the immediate administration of Ca^{2+} intravenously.[41] Chronic hypocalcemia is treated with calcium supplements and vitamin D analogs.[3]

CASE STUDY

During a routine preemployment physical examination conducted by her family physician, a 37-year-old woman was found to have a blood pressure of 148/95. The patient was of average height and weight. She stated that, although she had felt that she tired somewhat more easily over the past few months, she had no specific physical complaints. Both the patient and her physician considered her to be in good health. At the time of her last physical examination (18 months previously), her blood pressure had been 130/80 and all laboratory test results had been within reference range.

INITIAL LABORATORY FINDINGS

Serum

Analyte	***Result***	***Reference Range***
Calcium	11.8 mg/dL	8.5–10.5 mg/dL
Phosphate	1.6 mg/dL	2.5–4.5 mg/dL
Sodium	137 mEq/L	135–145 mEq/L
Potassium	4.2 mEq/L	3.5–4.5 mEq/L
Chloride	107 mEq/L	96–106 mEq/L
Bicarbonate	24 mEq/L	23–27 mEq/L

Conversion to SI units is as follows:
Calcium—mg/dL × 0.25 = mmol/L
Phosphate—mg/dL × 0.323 = mmol/L
Sodium—mEq/L × 1 = mmol/L
Potassium—mEq/L × 1 = mmol/L
Chloride—mEq/L × 1 = mmol/L
Bicarbonate—mEq/L × 1 = mmol/L

The complete blood count and urinalysis were normal. A chest x-ray taken at the time was unremarkable. The patient reported that the only medications she was taking were an over-the-counter multiple vitamin supplement once a day and a calcium supplement that she felt would minimize her risk of developing osteoporosis later in life.

The patient was instructed by her physician to return to the clinic later in the week for additional laboratory tests.

Questions

1. What element(s) of the physical examination and initial laboratory findings support a preliminary diagnosis of primary hyperparathyroidism?
2. In addition to a disorder of the parathyroids, what other etiologies of hypercalcemia would the physician be likely to consider?
3. What laboratory tests will the physician order to assess parathyroid function in followup testing of the patient?

Discussion

1. A diagnosis of primary hyperparathyroidism is suggested by the patient's hypertension, hypercalcemia, and hypophosphatemia, elevated serum chloride, and a chloride–phosphate ratio greater than 33.
2. In most clinical circumstances, hypercalcemia suggests either hyperparathyroidism or malignancy. Other causes of hypercalcemia that would need to be excluded are nonparathyroid endocrine disorders (*e.g.*, hyperthyroidism and MENS); drugs (*e.g.*, vitamins A or D intoxication, use of thiazide diuretics, chronic ingestion of calcium or alkali antacids); or the presence of granulomatous disease (*e.g.*, TB, sarcoidosis, histoplasmosis, coccidiomycosis).
3. The physician will require an additional serum calcium to verify the existence of hypercalcemia. Parathyroid profiles provided by most laboratories include serum calcium (ionized and total), phosphorus, creatinine, and a PTH assessment. An intact/N-terminal or mid-molecule PTH determination would be useful.

REFERENCES

1. Jubiz W: Endocrinology: A Logical Approach for Clinicians, 2nd ed. New York City, McGraw-Hill, 1985
2. Broadus AE: Mineral metabolism. In Felig P, Baxter JD, Broadus AE et al(eds): Endocrinology and Metabolism, pp 963–967. New York City, McGraw-Hill, 1981
3. Zaloga GP, Chernow B: Calcium Metabolism. In Geelhoed GW, Chernow B(eds): Endocrine Aspects of Acute Illness, pp 169–204. New York City, Churchill Livingstone, 1975
4. Licata AA, Streck WF: Hypocalcemia. In Streck WF, Lockwood DH(eds): Endocrine Diagnosis: Clinical and Laboratory Approach, pp 97–106. Boston, Little, Brown & Co, 1983
5. Rabin D, McKenna TJ(eds): Clinical Endocrinology and Metabolism: Principles and Practice. New York City, Grune & Stratton, 1982
6. Habener JF, Rosenblatt M, Potts JT Jr: Parathyroid hormone: Biochemical aspects of biosynthesis, secretion, action, and metabolism. Physiol Rev 64:985–1053, 1984
7. Scott DP, Teasdale PR, Swaminathan R: Value of measuring C-terminal parathyrin in differential diagnosis of hypercalcemia. Clin Chem 31:1838–1840, 1985
8. Balestrieri FJ: Magnesium metabolism in the critically ill patient. In Geelhoed GW, Chernow B(eds):

Endocrine Aspects of Acute Illness, pp 217–226. New York City, Churchill Livingstone, 1985

9. Lafferty FW: Primary hyperparathyroidism: Changing clinical spectrum, prevalence of hypertension, and discriminant analysis of laboratory tests. Arch Intern Med 141:1761–1766, 1981
10. Bowers GN Jr, Brassard C, Sena SF: Measurement of ionized calcium in serum with ion-selective electrodes: A mature technology that can meet the daily service needs. Clin Chem 32(8):1437–1447, 1986
11. Broadus AE, Mahaffey JE, Bartter FC et al: Nephrogenous cyclic adenosine monophosphate as a parathyroid function test. J Clin Invest 60:771–783, 1977
12. Boonstra CE, Jackson CE: Hyperparathyroidism detected by routine serum calcium analysis—prevalence in a clinical population. Ann Intern Med 6:468–474, 1965.
13. Rao SD et al: Hyperparathyroidism following head and neck irradiation. Arch Intern Med 140: 205–207, 1980
14. Williams TF, Streck WF: Multiple endocrine neoplasia (MEN) syndromes. In Streck WF, Lockwood DH(eds): Endocrine Diagnosis: Clinical and Laboratory Approach, pp 261–278. Boston, Little, Brown & Co, 1983
15. Aurbach GD, Marx SJ, Spiegel AM: Parathyroid hormone, calcitonin, and the calciferols. In Williams RH(ed): Textbook of Endocrinology, 6th ed, pp 922–1031. Philadelphia, WB Saunders, 1981
16. LeBoff MS, Shoback D, Brown EM et al: Regulation of parathyroid hormone release and cytosolic calcium by extracellular calcium in dispersed and cultured bovine and pathological human parathyroid cells. J Clin Invest 75(1):49–57, 1985
17. Teitelbaum AP, Arnaud CD: Parathyroid hormone receptors: An assay for circulating PTH? Diagn Med 5:69–74, 1982
18. Mundy GR, Ibbotson KJ, D'Souza SM: Tumor products and the hypercalcemia of malignancy. J Clin Invest 76:391–394, 1985
19. Fink JN, Beall GN: Immunologic aspects of endocrine disease. JAMA 248(20):2696–2700, 1982
20. Pena A: Hormonal and metabolic concerns in younger patients. In Geelhoed GW, Chernow B(eds): Endocrine Aspects of Acute Illness, pp 43–66. New York, Churchill Livingstone, 1985
21. Tsang RC, Steichen JJ, Chan GM: Neonatal hypocalcemia: Mechanisms of occurrence and management. Crit Care Med 5:56–61, 1977
22. Arnaud CD, Kolb FO: The calciotropic hormones and metabolic bone disease. In Greenspan FS, Forsham PH(eds): Basic and Clinical Endocrinology, pp 187–257. Los Altos, California, Lange Medical Publications, 1983
23. Licata AA, Streck WF: Hypercalcemia. In Streck WF, Lockwood DH(eds): Endocrine Diagnosis: Clinical and Laboratory Approach, pp 81–96. Boston, Little, Brown & Co, 1983
24. Wong ET, Freier EF: The differential diagnosis of hypercalcemia: An algorithm for more effective use of laboratory tests. JAMA 247(1):75–80, 1982
25. Fisken RA, Heath DA, Somers S et al: Hypercalcemia in hospital patients. Lancet 1:202–207, 1981
26. Heath H III: Tests of parathyroid function: Utility and limitations. AACC ENDO 2(8):1–10, 1984
27. Valsamis J, Van Peborgh J, Brauman H: Relative contribution of various expressions of cAMP excretion to other indices of parathyroid function, as tested by discriminant multivariate linear regression analysis. Clin Chem 32(7)1279–1284, 1986
28. Pribor HC, Fabisinski LF III: Artificial intelligence in laboratory medicine. III. The parathyroid hormone profile. Lab Man 21(6):21–24, 1983
29. Slatopolsky E, Martin K, Morrissey J et al: Current concepts of the metabolism and radioimmunoassay of parathyroid hormone. J Lab Clin Med 99(3):309–316, 1982
30. Zanelli JM, Kent JC, Rafferty B et al: High-performance liquid chromatographic methods for the analysis of human parathyroid hormone in reference standards, parathyroid tissue, and biological fluids. J Chromatogr 276:55–60, 1983
31. Berson SA, Yalow RS, Aurbach GD et al: Immunoassay of bovine and human parathyroid hormone. Proc Natl Acad Sci USA 49:613–617, 1963
32. DiBella FP, Hawker CD: Parathyrin (parathyroid hormone): Radioimmunoassay for intact and carboxyl-terminal moieties. Clin Chem 28(1):226–235, 1982
33. Reitz RE: Region-Specific Assays for Parathyroid Hormone. Oakland, California, Endocrine Metabolic Center, 1982
34. Hawker CD, Liebel MA, Clark SW et al: Parathyroid hormone measurement: Clinical utility of a

radioimmunoassay for the C-terminal and middle regions of PTH. Clin Confirm 5:1–7, 1984

35. Potts JT Jr, Segre GV, Endres DB: Assessment of parathyroid function with an N-terminal-specific radioimmunoassay for intact parathyroid hormone. Curr Clin Concepts, Nichols Inst 1–9, 1983
36. Haver VM, Rinker AD, Ko BM et al: Clinical and laboratory evaluation of a radioimmunoassay kit for measuring the mid-molecule fraction of parathyrin. Clin Chem 32(11):2056–2059, 1986
37. Armitage EK: Parathyrin (parathyroid hormone): Metabolism and methods for assay. Clin Chem 32(3): 418–424, 1986
38. Alexander LA, Famulare AJ, Worthy TE: Evaluation of a mid-region specific parathyroid hormone assay (abstr). Clin Chem 32(6);1153, 1986
39. Nebeker HG, Coburn JW: Parathyroid hormone and chronic renal failure. AACC ENDO 3(8), 1985
40. Alexander LA, Famulare AJ, Worthy TE: Evaluation of an assay for intact parathyroid hormone (abstr). Clin Chem 32(6):1152, 1986
41. Burch WM: Endocrinology for the House Doctor. Baltimore, Williams & Wilkins, 1984

BIBLIOGRAPHY

Goltzman D, Henderson B, Loveridge N: Cytochemical bioassay of parathyroid hormone: Characteristics of the assay and analysis of circulating hormonal forms. J Clin Invest 65:1309–1317, 1980

Johnson KR, Howarth AT, Hamilton M et al: Laboratory differentiation of hypercalcemic patients. Clin Chem 28:333–338, 1982

Nichols Institute Diagnostics: Allegro Intact PTH: Immunoassay for the Quantitative Determination of Intact Parathyroid Hormone in Human Serum. San Juan Capistrano, California, Nichols Institute, 1986

Schmidt-Gayk H, Schmitt-Fiebig M, Hitzler W et al: Two homologous radioimmunoassays for parathyrin compared and applied to disorders of calcium metabolism. Clin Chem 32(1):57–62, 1986

Chu Sy, Chu AK: Clinical assessment of an intact parathyroid hormone assay in the diagnosis of primary hyperparathyroidism. Lab Med 19(2):106–108, 1988

Zahradnik R, Brennan G, Nozawa UK: A two-site IRMA for intact N-terminal specific parathyroid hormone (INS-PTH) [abstr]. Clin Chem 32(6):1154, 1986

Chapter 37

Disorders of the Adrenal Cortex

Mary Ann McLane

The adrenal glands are located above the kidneys and are essential for life. Each gland consists of two histologically and developmentally distinct zones: the inner medulla, which produces the catecholamines epinephrine and norepinephrine, and the outer cortex, which is responsible for steroid hormone synthesis. The outer cortex is further divided functionally into the *zona glomerulosa* (outermost layer), *zona fasciculata,* and *zona reticularis* (innermost cortex layer). A review of the function and control of the corticosteroid hormones will provide a conceptual basis for correlating patient history and clinical data for the diagnosis of adrenocortical disorders.

STIMULATION OF THE ADRENAL CORTEX

Stimulation of the adrenal cortex is known to come from two sources, the anterior pituitary and the renin-angiotensin system. The anterior pituitary gives rise to the polypeptide adrenocorticotropic hormone (ACTH), which stimulates the *zona fasciculata* of the adrenal cortex to produce the glucocorticoid cortisol, and the *zona reticularis* to produce adrenal androgens. The renin-angiotensin system stimulates the *zona glomerulosa* to produce the mineralocorticoid aldosterone.

The anterior pituitary is itself stimulated by a tropic hypothalamic hormone, corticotrophin-releasing factor (CRF). CRF is considered to be a central nervous system hormone that responds to stress by causing an increase in ACTH and cortisol concentrations in direct proportion to the severity and duration of the stress.[1] "Stress" may take the form of anesthesia, trauma, hypoglycemia, anoxia, or anxiety.[2] The response of the adrenal cortex to such stress is limited, with a maximal possible output of 200 to 300 mg of cortisol per day. Elevation of plasma cortisol results in a decrease in pituitary ACTH levels by negative feedback. The lowered plasma ACTH concentration will then cause a decreased stimulation of the adrenal cortex, with an eventual lowering of cortisol levels in the plasma. In those instances in which severe stress causes a maximal elevation in both ACTH and cortisol, there seems to be an overriding of the normal negative feedback mechanism for the duration of the stress. In this event, the elevation in plasma cortisol does not immediately lead to diminished ACTH levels.

Causes of Altered Plasma CBG Levels

Increased CBG

Pregnancy
Estrogen administration

Decreased CBG

Androgen administration
Congenital deficiency
Liver disease
Nephrosis

Circulating cortisol can be bound reversibly to cortisol-binding globulin (CBG) (94%), can be loosely bound to albumin, or can be free (6%). Of these three forms, only free cortisol will be found in the urine; therefore, any condition that leads to a saturation of CBG will elevate the free cortisol level in the plasma as well as in the urine. While there are conditions unrelated to adrenal function that may alter the CBG concentration (see list above), thus elevating the bound cortisol level, the amount of free, biologically active cortisol in these conditions will not be altered.

Plasma cortisol concentrations exhibit a diurnal variation, with the highest levels found in the early morning.[3] The effect on tissues is varied, with both catabolic and anabolic characteristics as listed on page 430. Cortisol is well known for its anti-inflammatory properties, due to its interference in the synthesis of inflammatory prostaglandins. It is also noted as an immunosuppressive agent, since it will decrease the numbers of blood lymphocytes and eosinophils while stimulating erythropoiesis.

The adrenal glands also produce androgens under ACTH stimulation. Dehydroepiandrosterone and androstenedione are quantitatively the most significant. These are weakly androgenic, and are

Effects of Glucocorticoids on Tissues

Catabolic (skin, bone, muscle, lymphoid, adipose, connective tissue)
Protein synthesis ↓
Glucose, potassium, nucleoside, and amino acid transport ↓
Fatty acid release from adipose ↓
Serum potassium ↓
Serum sodium ↓
Serum calcium ↓

Anabolic (liver)
Glycogenesis ↑
Gluconeogenesis ↑
Triglyceride synthesis ↑

both prehormones of testosterone, being converted to the more active androgen by peripheral tissues. There is no known negative feedback mechanism between the adrenal androgens and ACTH production.

The synthesis of the mineralocorticoid aldosterone is not controlled specifically by ACTH. The renin-angiotensin system is the major control mechanism, responding to changes in blood volume, blood pressure, and/or serum sodium levels to initiate a compensatory cascade of enzymatic reactions. These culminate in elevated aldosterone secretion from the *zona glomerulosa,* in peripheral vasoconstriction, in sodium reabsorption, and in a return to normal blood volume and pressure (see Fig. 37-1).

Cortisol is a weak mineralocorticoid, and in normal individuals does not contribute significantly to the maintenance of normal blood pressure and sodium concentration. In severe stress, however, elevated cortisol exerts a profound effect on the maintenance of blood pressure, and is acknowledged to be essential in preventing acute vascular collapse.[1]

Disorders of the adrenal cortex will affect one or more of the steroid hormones synthesized by the gland. The direction of change (elevation, suppression) and consequent side-effects of overproduction/deficiency will determine the presenting signs and symptoms seen by the physician. These disorders may be classified as hyperadrenalism, hypoadrenalism, hyperaldosteronism, and congenital adrenal hyperplasia.

ETIOLOGY AND PATHOPHYSIOLOGY

Hyperadrenalism

The term *Cushing's syndrome* has become synonymous with *hyperadrenalism,* characterized by elevated plasma cortisol and loss of its diurnal variation.

By far the most common cause of hyperadrenalism today is iatrogenic. Corticosteroids are among the most frequently prescribed drugs in the United States.[1] Pharmacologic doses (1–3 grams) seem to aid in the treatment of overwhelming diseases such as gram-negative septicemia and septic shock.[1] Cortisone, a derivative of cortisol, has been used effectively since 1948 as therapy for patients with rheumatoid arthritis.[1] These patients are the easiest to diagnose, with a patient history confirming the cause of physical symptoms.

Differential diagnosis of the other types of hyperadrenalism centers on determining the cause of the elevated cortisol. Such causes may be considered "ACTH-dependent" or "ACTH-independent." *ACTH-dependent hyperadrenalism* constitutes 85% of all Cushing's syndrome cases.[4] It may result from increased ACTH production by an anterior pituitary adenoma (70%) or by an ectopic, extrapituitary source (15%). The latter source will most commonly be oat cell carcinoma of the lung, but may be epithelial thymoma, pancreatic islet-cell tumors, medullary cancer of the thyroid, or bronchial carcinoid tumor.[4] ACTH-dependent Cushing's syndrome will show bilateral hyperplasia of the adrenal glands and a loss of diurnal cortisol variation. Those with a pituitary adenoma (Cushing's *disease*) may present additionally with increased pigmentation of the skin. This is due to the

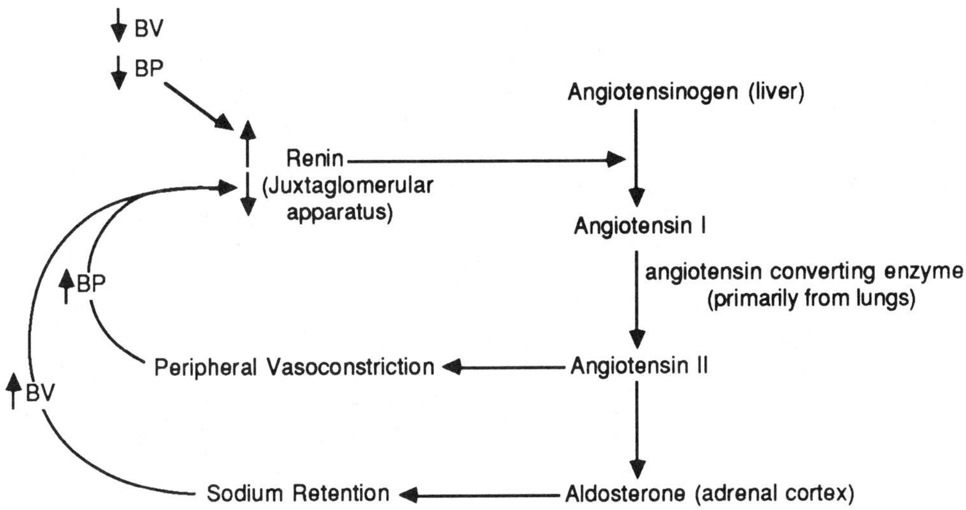

Figure 37-1 **Renin-angiotensin-aldosterone system in control of blood volume (BV) and blood pressure (BP). (Adapted from Bishop ML, Duben-Von Laufen JL, Fody EP [eds]: Clinical Chemistry. Philadelphia, JB Lippincott, 1985)**

structural similarities that exist between ACTH and α-melanocyte-stimulating hormone.[5, 6]

ACTH-independent hyperadrenalism (15% of all Cushing's syndrome cases) arises from adrenal gland tumors, with malignant carcinomas being slightly more common than are benign tumors. These patients will experience a suppression of their anterior pituitary ACTH production by negative feedback, which ultimately leads to atrophy of the adrenal cortex not involved by the tumor.[4] These tumors are more prevalent in women than in men (4 : 1 or 5 : 1), will usually be single and small, and may produce only cortisol or all of the adrenal hormones.[2] Weight loss may mask the classical Cushingoid appearance in these patients. As in ACTH-dependent Cushing's syndrome, diurnal variation in plasma cortisol levels is absent.

Hypoadrenalism

Addison's disease is the name associated with primary adrenal hypofunction. It is a rare, life-threatening condition, believed to be autoimmune in origin because adrenal antibodies are found in 60% of patients with the condition.[4] It is not unusual to find these patients concurrently showing signs and symptoms of other endocrine disorders, such as primary ovarian failure, diabetes mellitus, hypothyroidism, thyrotoxicosis, hypoparathyroidism, and pernicious anemia.[4, 7] In primary adrenal hypofunction, both cortisol and aldosterone synthesis are affected by the atrophy of the adrenal gland. Almost 95% of the adrenals must be destroyed, however, to produce the characteristic signs and symptoms of the disease.[2, 4, 7]

Secondary hypoadrenalism is commonly the result of prolonged therapeutic use of glucocorticoids such as cortisone and prednisone. Less commonly, it may be due to decreased ACTH formation caused by a pituitary tumor.[4] For these patients, there will usually not be the postural hypotension associated with Addison's disease because therapeutic regimens of corticosteroids will not affect aldosterone production. Hyperpigmentation will also be absent in secondary hypoadrenalism, because ACTH levels will be low.

For patients experiencing hypopituitarism, concurrent decreases in other pituitary hormones, such as growth hormone, thyroid-stimulating hormone, and gonadotropin-releasing hormone, may lead to symptoms associated with these deficiencies.

Secondary hypoadrenalism may also be caused by granulomatous diseases, such as tuberculosis, histoplasmosis, neoplasms, amyloidosis, or certain infections (especially fulminant meningococcal sepsis,[7] which may produce Waterhouse-Friderichsen syndrome, in which endotoxin release causes bilateral hemorrhagic destruction of the adrenals[2]). For all of these disorders, the adrenal dysfunction will result in decreased cortisol production, causing an elevation in ACTH from the removal of negative feedback.

Hyperaldosteronism

Hyperaldosteronism may be either primary or secondary. *Primary aldosteronism,* when caused by an adenoma of one adrenal gland (85% of all primary cases), is called *Conn's syndrome.* It may also be caused by an idiopathic hyperplasia of aldosterone-producing cells in both adrenals.[8] Rarely, a carcinoma of the adrenal cortex will produce sufficient mineralocorticoid to give symptoms of primary aldosteronism.

Secondary aldosteronism is more common than is primary. It will result from any condition that decreases blood volume, because lowered blood volume is a stimulus for activation of the renin-angiotensin system (see Fig. 37-1). Some conditions that lead to this event involve diuretic abuse, congestive heart failure, cirrhosis with ascites, and nephrotic syndrome.[4] It should be noted that the increased aldosterone is a response to the changes in the plasma volume, and may not result in hypertension.[9] There is an increase in aldosterone production unrelated to blood volume changes during normal pregnancy,[2] in toxemia of pregnancy, and in renal artery disease.[10]

Congenital Adrenal Hyperplasia (Adrenogenital Syndrome)

The term *adrenogenital syndrome* describes a group of diseases characterized by deficiencies in or blockage of one of the enzymes needed to synthesize cortisol. Figure 37-2 shows the interrelationships among the biosynthetic pathways in the adrenal cortex. Because the cortex is able to produce not only glucocorticoids but also mineralocorticoids and androgens, a defect in cortisol synthesis would be expected to affect the other two pathways, as well as the many intermediate metabolic pathways in the cortex, liver, and peripheral tissues.

Of the congenital defects known, 95% are caused by a deficiency in 21-hydroxylase and 2% by a lack of 11-β-hydroxylase. Both of these defects will result in lowered plasma cortisol levels, increased ACTH, and hyperplasia of the adrenal cortex. The steroid precursors synthesized *before* the block in the pathway will be elevated and will be found in plasma and urine.

CLINICAL MANIFESTATIONS

Cushing's Syndrome

The presenting signs and symptoms of a patient who is hyperadrenal, regardless of the cause, will reflect the elevation of hormones synthesized by the adrenal gland. Clinical features of Cushing's syndrome, listed in order of frequency of occurrence,[4] may include central truncal obesity, "moon face" and "buffalo hump," which reflect increased fat metabolism and redistribution of fat to the neck, shoulders, face, and abdomen; facial flushing (plethora); increased body hair (hirsuitism); menstrual disorders and acne, which reflect the elevation in adrenal androgens; hypertension, which reflects mineralocorticoid excess, although it will not be seen if the etiology is corticosteroid administration (iatrogenic Cushing's syndrome); muscular weakness, back pain, reddish-purple skin streaks (striae), thin skin, poor wound healing, and decreased bone and muscle mass, all of which reflect increased protein catabolism; osteoporosis, which reflects diminished bone formation and increased bone resorption and is seen especially in chronic glucocorticoid administration;[5] and emotional lability. A patient history will usually reveal a gradual onset of symptoms, with many present at least 1 year prior to diagnosis.[2]

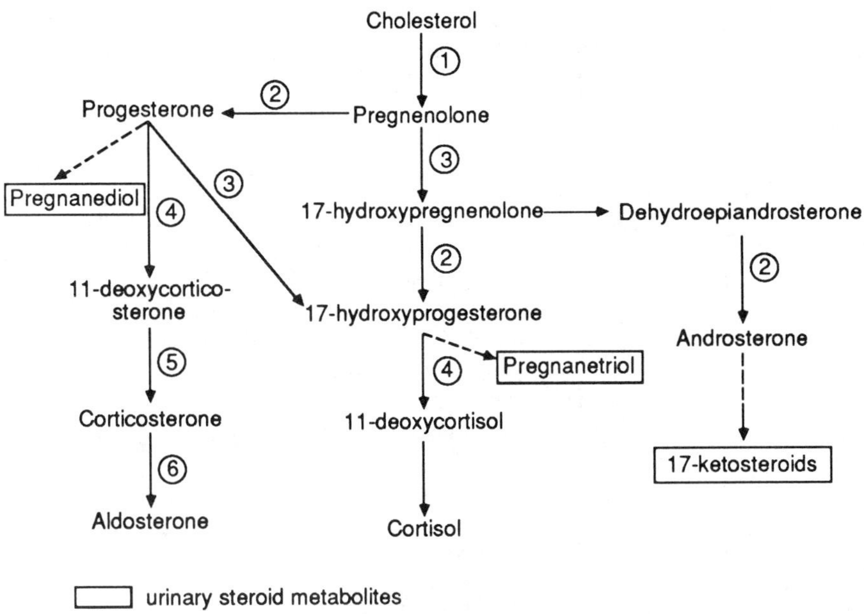

① Desmolase (rare): ↓ all adrenal hormones

② 3ß-OH dehydrogenase (rare): ↓ glucocorticoids, aldosterone

③ 17-hydroxylase (rare): ↓ glucocorticoids, androgens

④ 21-hydroxylase (95%): ↓ cortisol, aldosterone

⑤ 11ß-hydroxylase (2%): ↓ cortisol, aldosterone

⑥ 18-hydroxycorticosterone dehydrogenase (rare): ↓ aldosterone

Figure 37-2 Enzymatic defects in congenital adrenal hyperplasia.

Addison's Disease

The clinical manifestations of hypoadrenalism include weakness, fatigue (rejuvenated by rest), loss of appetite, weight loss, and gastrointestinal symptoms (nausea, vomiting, diarrhea), all of which reflect cortisol deficiency. Orthostatic hypotension reflects aldosterone deficiency, although some patients may be normotensive, with a fall in blood pressure occurring only in times of stress. There may be a decrease in axillary and pubic hair in females, which relflects decreased androgen synthesis. This will not be noticeable in males because adrenal androgens are a minor source of their total androgens.

There is often increased pigmentation of skin, which reflects an elevated ACTH level similar to the finding in ectopic Cushing's syndrome. The pigmentation will be noticeable, especially after sun exposure, and accentuated in body creases (palms of the hands), on extensor surfaces (knuckles, knees, elbows), at scars and pressure points, and along dental gingival margins. A variation of this sign is termed *vitiligo,* and presents as a patch of depigmentation, often with a hyperpigmented border, and often enlarging slowly. While hyperpigmentation may be helpful in the diagnosis, it may also be caused by many other conditions (see list on page 434), and must be differentiated from those.[2, 4, 7]

Conditions Characterized by Increased Pigmentation

Primary adrenal hypofunction
Hemochromatosis
Chronic nutritional insufficiency
Heavy metal poisoning
Peutz-Jeghers syndrome
Albright's syndrome
Estrogen therapy
Pregnancy
Wilson's disease
Pernicious anemia
Porphyrias
Gaucher's disease
Niemann-Pick disease
Pellagra
Sprue
Acanthosis nigricans
Whipple's syndrome

Hyperaldosteronism

Patients with primary or secondary hyperaldosteronism may present initially with headache, tetany, paresthesias (prickling sensations), and general muscle weakness. Hypertension will be the predominant symptom in most cases.[7]

Adrenogenital Syndrome

The initial presenting signs of adrenogenital syndrome vary widely, depending on the age and sex of the patient. In the 21-hydroxylase deficiency, infant females may present with abnormalities of the genitalia ranging from mild clitoral hypertrophy to a normal-appearing phallus. If the condition does not develop until later in life, the patient may present with hirsuitism, oligomenorrhea, and acne. The syndrome is unlikely to be diagnosed at birth in a male unless a salt-losing tendency is evident. Older males may show evidence of elevated androgens by rapid growth and maturation, early deepening of the voice, and acne.[2] Approximately 1/3 to 1/2 of all patients will have low blood pressure, dehydration, apathy, vomiting, and diarrhea. (See Fig. 37-3).

LABORATORY ANALYSES AND DIAGNOSIS

Cushing's Syndrome

Laboratory evaluation of the patient (see below) with suspected Cushing's syndrome should begin with the patient history to rule out steroid administration as a cause. Following this, a 24-hour urinary free cortisol may be used as a screening test. Normally only 1% of plasma cortisol is cleared by the kidneys as free, non protein-bound, cortisol. As described above, whenever the level of secreted cortisol saturates CBG, excess cortisol will be excreted and is a sensitive and specific index of plasma cortisol levels.

Radioimmunoassays (RIA) are available for this analysis, and are preferred to the less specific fluorometric, colorimetric, or competitive protein-

Laboratory Findings in Hyperadrenalism

Elevated white cell count
- ↑ Neutrophils
- ↓ Lymphocytes, eosinophils, monocytes

Polycythemia often present
Decreased serum potassium
Decreased glucose tolerance
Increased urine calcium (40% of patients)
Elevated plasma cortisol
Variable ACTH
Elevated HCO_3
Elevated blood *p*H
Ultrasound, computed tomography: localization and signs of pituitary/adrenal/ectopic tumor

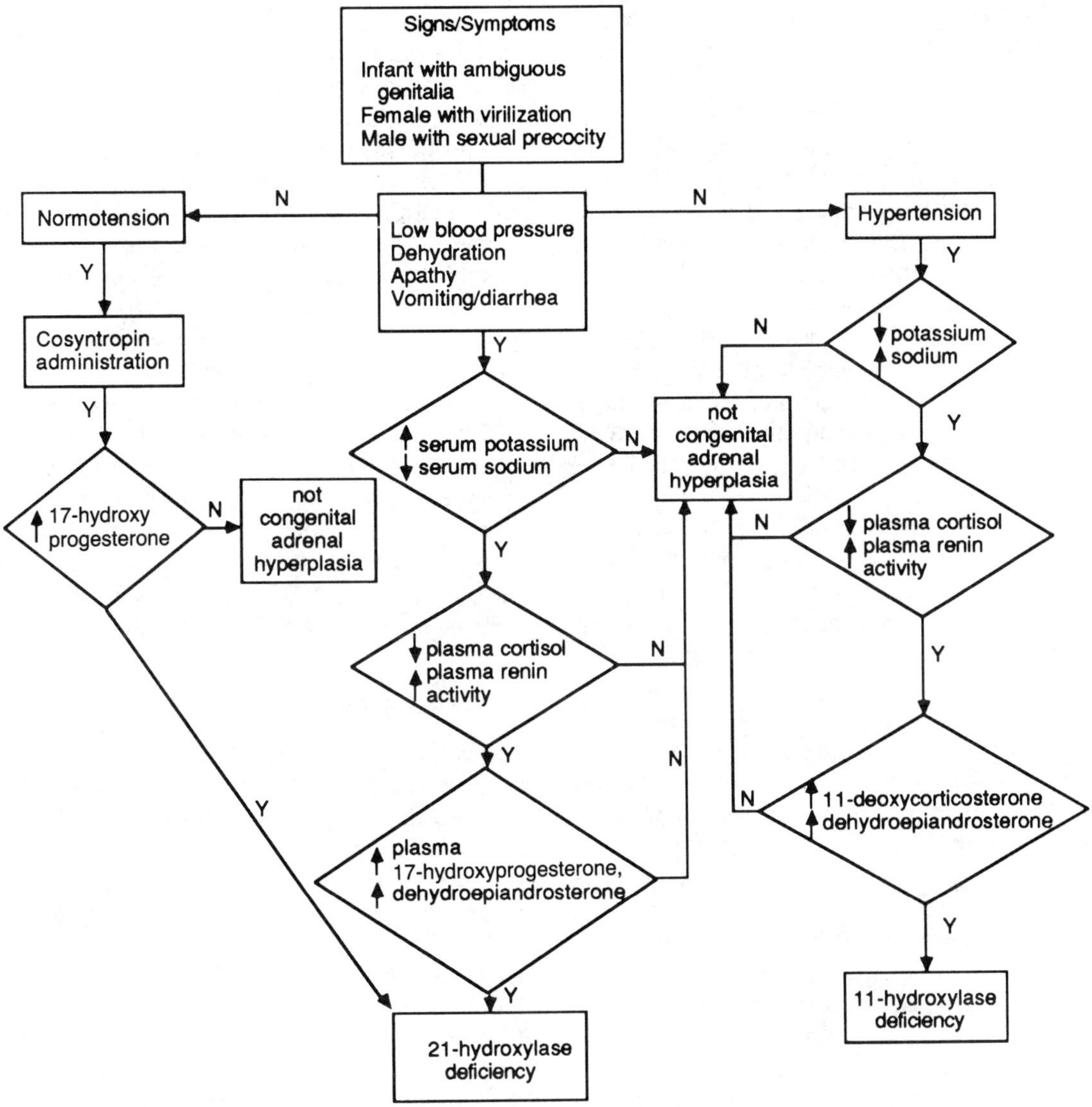

Figure 37-3 **Differential diagnosis of most common causes of congenital adrenal hyperplasia.**

binding assays. A normal value is strong evidence against Cushing's syndrome.[8] Values may be falsely increased with stress, and falsely decreased in renal disease.

Another screening test is the overnight dexamethasone suppression test. As a powerful synthetic glucocorticoid, dexamethasone, given at bedtime, will suppress the synthesis of ACTH and cause the morning plasma cortisol level to be low, rather than at its usual peak diurnal value. Cortisol values at 8 a.m. that are greater than 10 μg/dL (0.28 μmol/L) are suggestive of Cushing's syndrome. Testing interferences may be caused by stress, treatment with diphenylhydantoin or phenobarbital (which enhance dexamethasone metabolism), or endogenous depression.[8]

Stress as a cause of elevated cortisol may be ruled out by a low-dose dexamethasone test. This 4-day test involves assaying a 24-hour urine each day for free cortisol, 17-hydroxycorticosteroids (cortisol metabolites), and creatinine, with a low dose of dexamethasone given over days 3 and 4. Both the free cortisol and the 17-hydroxycorticosteroids should be decreased, even when the plasma cortisol has been elevated due to stress. A patient with Cushing's syndrome will not have the cortisol or metabolite production suppressed[8] (see Fig. 37.4).

17-hydroxycorticosteroids can be measured colorimetrically by the Porter-Silber method or by the 17-ketogenic steroid method. The former will not measure all major urinary metabolites of cortisol, and both procedures entail lengthy hydrolysis, extraction, and analysis times and are subject to considerable interference from nonsteroidal chromagens. False positives will be seen in patients who are obese or hyperthyroid. Low values may be seen in patients with severe depression, poor nutrition, liver disease, or hypothyroidism.[7] A plasma cortisol is therefore preferred to any of the urine assays, because it is easier to perform and is less subject to such interferences.

A high-dose dexamethasone suppression test may be used to rule out a pituitary adenoma as the cause of the hyperadrenalism. Because the pituitary-adrenal negative feedback mechanism is still functional in pituitary Cushing's syndrome, the higher-dose dexamethasone will be sufficient to suppress ACTH levels, thus lowering both urine free cortisol and 17-hydroxycorticosteroid excretion by more than 50% of baseline by the fourth day of the test. The plasma cortisol will continue to show a lack of diurnal variation, and will be elevated (>10 μg/dL [>0.28 μmol/L]) on day 5.[2]

Plasma ACTH levels will aid in the diagnosis of those patients whose cortisol production is not suppressed by dexamethasone. In ACTH-dependent, ectopic Cushing's syndrome, a very high ACTH level will be found, while the cortisol produced by an adrenal tumor will cause pituitary production of ACTH to be low or undetectable.[7] Ectopic Cushing's syndrome will, in fact, produce ACTH levels that exceed those of an ACTH-secreting pituitary tumor of Cushing's *disease.*[4] Radioimmunoassay is the method of choice for analysis of plasma ACTH. A number of technical considerations must be taken into account when assaying ACTH, including special requirements for collection and storage of samples.[8]

Two additional functional tests, metyrapone and ACTH stimulation tests, have been used as a means of differentiating the types of Cushing's syndrome. They do not add significantly to the diagnostic information achieved by using the tests already described, however.[7] Confirmation of a tumor source of ACTH or cortisol is made by ultrasound and computed tomography.

Hypoadrenalism

Diagnosis of hypoadrenalism begins by confirming a decrease in plasma cortisol with a loss of diurnal variation. Measurement of the plasma ACTH concentration will distinguish between Addison's disease (elevated ACTH) and secondary hypoadrenalism (normal to low ACTH).[4] Finding evidence of lowered aldosterone levels will also suggest Addison's disease. There will also be decreased serum sodium and elevated serum potassium, urea nitrogen, and creatinine. Dehydration will accompany the condition, and may make the sodium level appear normal. Other laboratory findings are listed on page 438.

Two functional tests are used to confirm a diagnosis of hypoadrenalism: The first is the *rapid ACTH test,* which uses a synthetic hormone, cosyntropin, to act as ACTH in stimulating the adrenal cortex. Patients with Addison's disease will not show a rise in their baseline cortisol level, while patients with secondary hypoadrenalism may give equivocal responses to the stimulation. Repeating the cosyntropin stimulation test over several days

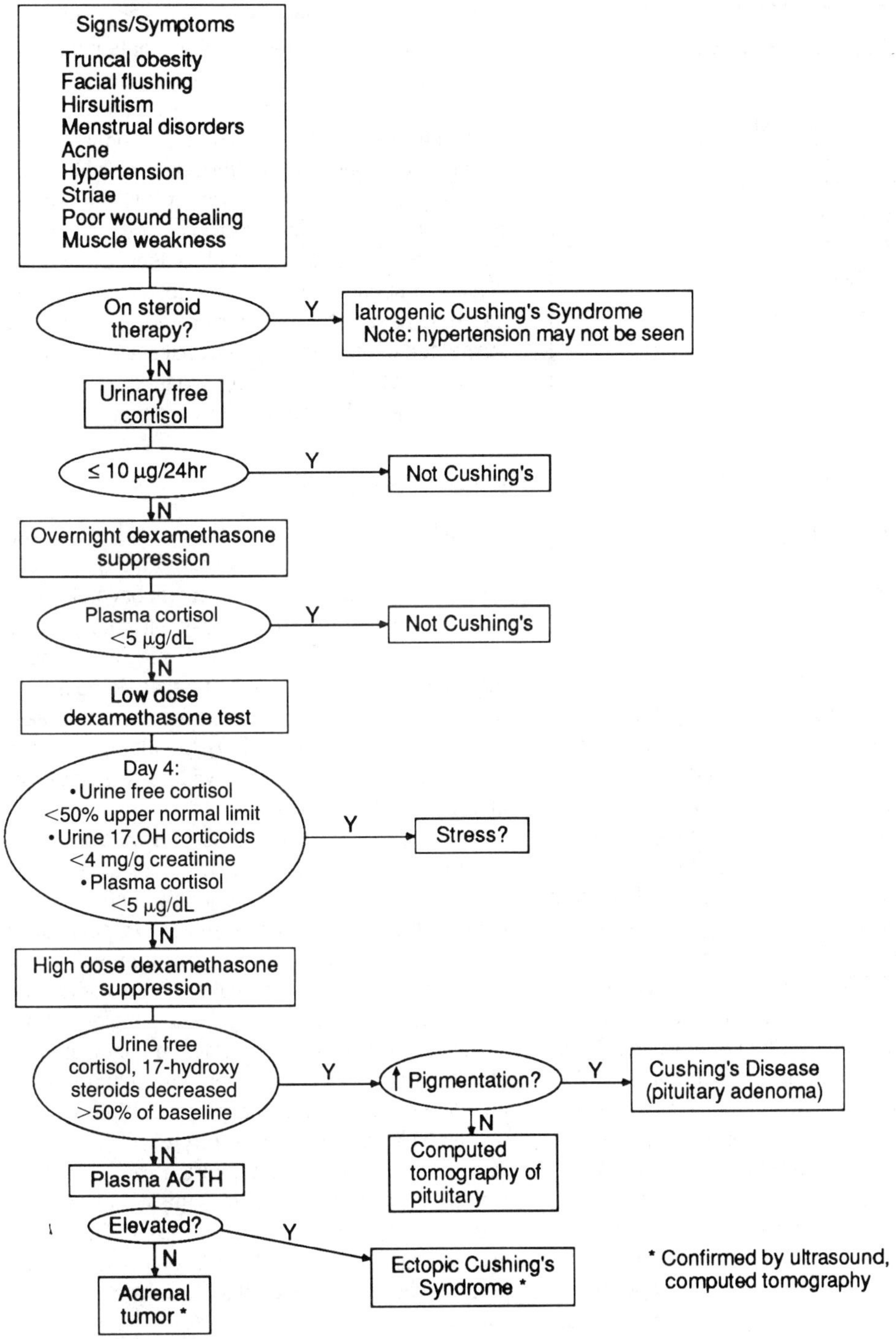

Figure 37-4 Differential diagnosis of hyperadrenalism.

Laboratory Findings in Hypoadrenalism

Addison's Disease Only
Low to normal serum sodium
Increased urine sodium
Increased serum potassium
Decreased urine potassium
Increased urea nitrogen
Increased creatinine
Adrenal antibodies
Increased ACTH

All Causes
Decreased plasma cortisol
Hypoglycemia
Normochromic, normocytic anemia
Decreased neutrophils
Increased lymphocytes, eosinophils
Increased serum calcium
Variable ACTH

will show no elevation in cortisol in patients with Addison's disease. Patients with secondary hypoadrenalism will respond in a delayed fashion, indicating the viability of their atrophied adrenals.[8] This response is also termed a "staircase" phenomenon because, observed over time, the cortisol levels will rise and plateau repeatedly during the course of the test.

The second confirmatory test is a *test for pituitary reserve of ACTH* that uses metyrapone, an inhibitor of 11-β-hydroxylase. This enzyme is the last one involved in the synthesis of cortisol. When it is inhibited, cortisol levels will fall and ACTH release should be stimulated. When given at night, metyrapone should cause increased synthesis of the cortisol immediate precursor, 11-deoxycortisol, the following morning. Patients with hypopituitarism will not show this characteristic rise.[2, 8] Plasma determinations of 11-deoxycortisol are performed by radioimmunoassay. A major disadvantage of this test lies in the many factors that may interfere with interpretation of negative results. Drugs that increase the liver's ability to metabolize drugs (phenobarbital, diphenylhydantoin) may lead to increased metyrapone metabolism. This will cause it to be cleared more rapidly from the blood, and have less effect on its target enzyme. Estrogens inhibit metyrapone's blockage of 11-hydroxylation of 11-deoxycortisol. Hypothyroidism, renal failure, cirrhosis of the liver, and malnutrition are also reported to decrease the adrenals' response to metyrapone.[2] It should be noted that this test, if performed on a patient suspected of primary hypoadrenalism, may create a life-threatening vascular collapse and shock through the fall in already low plasma cortisol.[10]

Hyperaldosteronism

Evaluation should begin with an analysis of the patient's electrolyte status (see Fig. 37-5). Patients with hyperaldosteronism will have elevated urine potassium (> 30 mEq/day). Eighty percent of patients will also have hypokalemia. The remaining 20% who are normokalemic may demonstrate decreased serum potassium after sodium intake. Elevated blood *p*H and pCO_2, resulting from the decreased serum potassium, will cause a metabolic alkalosis in these patients.[4]

Methods for assaying potassium will commonly use ion-selective electrode (ISE) or flame photometric technology. While both methods provide comparable data on most samples, a sample that is lipemic or contains elevated protein will show values that are falsely low in flame photometry and in ISE methods that incorporate a sample dilution. Because the plasma water fraction containing the electrolytes is decreased per unit volume of lipemic/hyperproteinemic sample, a routine dilution will actually cause the electrolytes to be diluted more than usual. Instrumentation cannot correct for this, and comparison of sample emission or activity to that of standards results in falsely decreased values. Such an "exclusion error" will not be found in ISE methods that do not use a diluted sample.[11]

Measurement of plasma aldosterone will also

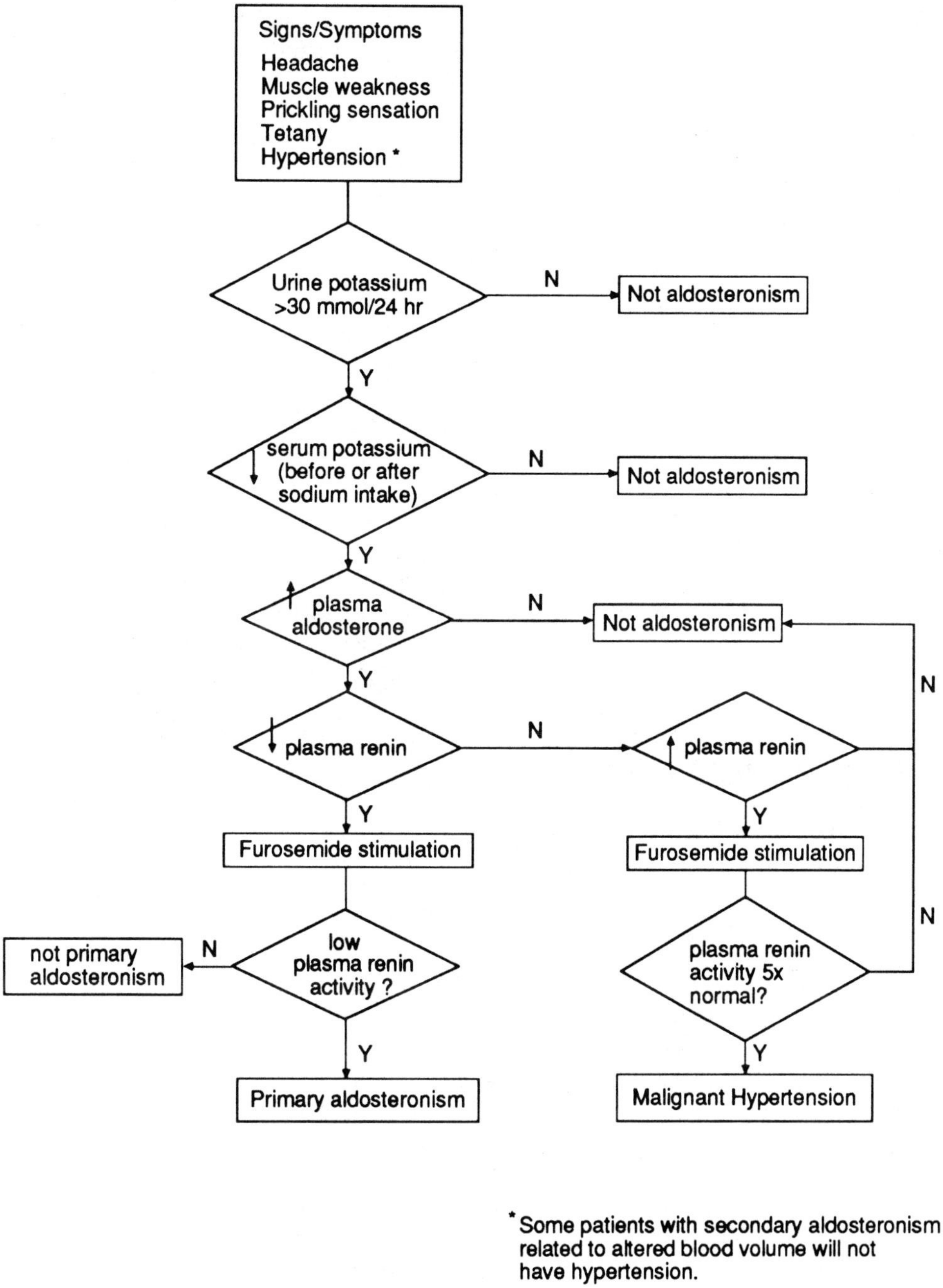

Figure 37-5 Differential diagnosis of aldosteronism.

confirm the diagnosis of hyperaldosteronism. A direct plasma RIA method may be used. Data from these assays must be interpreted in the light of sodium intake, posture, and diuretic administration history. Because hypokalemia has a suppressive effect on aldosterone production, serum potassium should be corrected and diuretic usage stopped 1 to 2 weeks prior to plasma aldosterone analysis. The sample itself should be taken while the patient is recumbent, because upright posture tends to increase blood pressure and suppress aldosterone secretion.

Plasma renin activity (PRA) levels, performed by RIA methodology, will differentiate between primary (decreased PRA) and secondary (increased PRA) aldosteronism. Plasma renin activity measures the conversion of angiotensinogen to angiotensin I per milliliter of plasma per hour. Samples should be collected in EDTA (which inhibits angiotensin-converting enzyme and angiotensinase), with plasma separated from cells quickly and frozen at -20°C until analysis. High values may be seen in patients taking diuretics or estrogen medications.[8]

A stimulation test that may be used to differentiate renovascular hypertension from Conn's syndrome involves administration of a potent diuretic, furosemide, with subsequent measurement of plasma renin activity. PRA will be five times normal in patients with renovascular hypertension. Patients with primary hyperaldosteronism will have PRA levels below assay sensitivity.

Two suppression tests may confirm the diagnosis of primary aldosteronism. Administration of a saline infusion will expand plasma volume and depress aldosterone secretion normally, but not in patients with primary hyperaldosteronism. Fluorocortisone, a potent mineralocorticoid, will suppress aldosterone synthesis normally, but not in patients with primary hyperaldosteronism. In both of these tests, any hypokalemia must be corrected before the test begins. The saline suppression test requires a plasma sample for aldosterone analysis, while the fluorocortisone test uses a 24-hour urine sample to measure aldosterone excretion.[4] If a tumor is suspected, computed tomography may be helpful in its localization.[7]

Adrenogenital Syndrome

Severe cases of adrenogenital syndrome, regardless of sex, will require prompt evaluation of fluid and electrolyte status. Elevated serum potassium and low serum sodium reflect the deficiency in mineralocorticoid synthesis, and will require immediate treatment to prevent vascular collapse.

All cases of 21-hydroxylase deficiency will show lowered plasma cortisol and increased plasma renin activity. The steroid elevated in direct response to the enzyme block is plasma 17-hydroxyprogesterone (17OHP). A radioimmunoassay method that includes a chromatographic step to remove progesterone has been described.[7] Caution in interpretation of a single result is necessary because this steroid shows diurnal variation. Assaying plasma for 17OHP is preferred to urinary analysis of pregnanetriol because of the decreased specificity of urinary steroid assays. It is also possible to detect a defect prenatally by assaying amniotic fluid for 17OHP. There is no evidence that the condition is hereditary.

Elevated androgens in these patients will be detected by testing for plasma dehydroepiandrosterone-sulfate (DHEA-S). Gas-liquid chromatography and competitive protein binding methods have been replaced by radioimmunoassay as the method of choice. This analysis is also preferred to assaying urinary 17-ketosteroids that are metabolites of testosterone and other androgens.[8]

Patients with 11-hydroxylase deficiency will experience hypertension and virilization due to an elevation in the aldosterone precursor 11-deoxycorticosterone (DOC), as well as in DHEA-S. The enzyme deficiency will also affect glucocorticoid synthesis in a manner similar to that in the metyrapone test discussed previously. Plasma elevations of 11-deoxycortisol may be assessed by RIA methods.

An adolescent or adult affected by the adrenogenital syndrome may not present with elevated plasma steroid levels as expected. A functional test, using cosyntropin stimulation as described above, will, however, result in such elevations.

TREATMENT

Cushing's Syndrome

Treatment for pituitary or adrenal Cushing's syndrome is usually surgical excision of the tumor. This effectively lowers the plasma cortisol levels in 80% of the pituitary cases, and in nearly 100% in patients with adrenal adenomas. There will be a concurrent return of laboratory data to normal levels as the blood cortisol concentration decreases. Surgery plus antisteroidogenesis drugs will alleviate some of the Cushingoid symptoms in cases of adrenal carcinoma, but prognosis is not good. In ectopic Cushing's syndrome, treatment is rarely successful.[10] It should be noted that adrenalectomy for Cushing's disease may result in higher plasma ACTH levels and hyperpigmentation postadrenalectomy (*Nelson's syndrome).*

Hypoadrenalism

Cortisol therapy is required for life in a hypoadrenal patient. An excellent prognosis follows, with most patients facing a crisis only during times of stress, such as respiratory or other infection, or gastrointestinal disturbances.[2] Patients with Addison's disease will also benefit from small doses of a mineralocorticoid. Glucose and electrolyte values will return to normal once therapy has been initiated.

Hyperaldosteronism

Conn's syndrome patients respond well to surgical excision of the causative adenoma. Patients with idiopathic adrenal hyperplasia will not respond to such treatment, but may respond to oral spironolactone. This substance blocks aldosterone's action, causing a lowering of blood pressure and return of potassium levels to normal. Renal artery hypertension will also respond to corrective surgery to remove any occlusion if treatment is done before irreversible kidney damage happens.[10]

Adrenogenital Syndrome

The severity of the disease and age of the patient will dictate the treatment required. Newborns will respond to intravenous fluids to correct electrolyte imbalance, glucocorticoids, and mineralocorticoids. Closely monitoring therapy, especially in children, will result in normal growth, sexual development, and fertility.[10] Abnormal blood and urine steroid levels will return to their respective age and sex reference intervals when the appropriate metabolic end-product is supplied. Those patients with treated hypocortisolism must be monitored during times of stress for the possibility of acute vascular collapse.

CASE STUDY

A 32-year-old white woman had been well until 8 months previous to her medical visit, when she had noticed herself bruising easily and gaining weight that seemed to be "localized" to her face, neck, and abdomen. She also had increased hair growth, acne, and generalized weakness. Physical examination revealed an anxious patient who was slightly hypertensive. The enlarged abdomen was characterized by reddish purple streaks. She denied the use of any drugs other than aspirin during the past year. Initial laboratory tests revealed the following data (reference intervals in parentheses):

LABORATORY FINDINGS

Analyte	Results	Reference Range
RBC	$7.3 \times 10^3/mm^3$	(4.2–5.4)
WBC	$16.2 \times 10^3/mm^3$	(4.5–11.0)
Neutrophils	86	(33–66)
Lymphocytes	11	(22–40)
Eosinophils	0	(1–4)
Monocytes	1	(4–8)
Basophils	0	(0–1)

LABORATORY FINDINGS

Analyte	Results	Reference Range
Plasma cortisol	(8 a.m.) 40 μg/dL	(5–23)
	(4 p.m.) 41 μg/dL	(3–15)
Serum potassium	2.9 mEq/L	(3.5–4.4)
Urine calcium	420 mg/24 hr	(100–300)
Total protein	7.4 g/dL	(6.4–8.3)
Glucose	(Fasting) 110 mg/dL	(70–105)
	(2-hr) 138 mg/dL	(< 120)
Plasma aldosterone	42 ng/dL	(5–30)

Conversion to SI units is as follows:
Cortisol—μg/dL × 0.028 = μmol/L
Potassium—mEq/L × 1 = mmol/L
Calcium—mg/24 hr × 0.025 = mmol/24 hr
Protein—g/dL × 10 = g/L
Glucose—mg/dL × 0.05555 = mmol/L
Aldosterone—ng/dL × 0.0277 = nmol/L

A urinary free cortisol was done and was elevated. This was followed by a low-dose dexamethasone test, which showed a continued elevation of urinary cortisol. A high-dose dexamethasone test did not suppress the cortisol production. Plasma ACTH taken at 8 a.m. and 4 p.m. both showed zero micrograms per deciliter.

Questions

1. What diagnosis should be suspected at this point?
2. What is the most likely source of the elevated cortisol, based on laboratory findings?
3. What treatments are available?

Discussion

1. Cushing's syndrome should be suspected.
2. Because the cortisol is not suppressed by dexamethasone, and ACTH levels are low, an adrenal tumor should be suspected.
3. Localization and excision of the adrenal tumor and antisteroidogenesis drugs will alleviate some of the Cushingoid symptoms, but prognosis is not good.

REFERENCES

1. Bethune JE: The Adrenal Cortex, p 33. Kalamazoo, MI, Upjohn, 1974
2. Nelson DH: The Adrenal Cortex: Physiologic Function and Disease, p 75. Philadelphia, WB Saunders, 1980
3. Sakiyama R, Ashcraft MW, Van Herle AJ: Cyclic Cushing's syndrome. Am J Med 77:945, 1984
4. Berner JJ: Effects of Diseases on Laboratory Tests, p 169. Philadelphia, JB Lippincott Company, 1983
5. Stuhlberg BU, Licata AA, Bauer TW et al: Hyperparathyroidism, Hyperthyroidism, and Cushing's Disease. Orthop Clin North Am 15(4):707, 1984
6. White A, Handler P, Smith E et al (eds): Principles of Biochemistry, 6th ed, p 1288. New York City, McGraw-Hill, 1978
7. Kaplan LA, Pesce AJ: Clinical Chemistry: Theory, Analysis, and Correlation, p 829. St Louis, CV Mosby, 1984
8. Teitz N (ed): Textbook of Clinical Chemistry, p 1066. Philadelphia, WB Saunders, 1986
9. Bishop ML, Duben-Von Laufen JL, Fody EP (eds): Clinical Chemistry, p 325. Philadelphia, JB Lippincott, 1985
10. Gornall AG: Applied Biochemistry of Clinical Disorders, p 260. Hagerstown, MD, Harper & Row, 1980
11. Flannery JM: Differences in electrolyte results as measured by direct potentiometry (ion-selective electrode) and flame photometry. Newton, MA, Nova Biomedical

Chapter 38

Impaired Glucose Metabolism

Bernhard Ludvigsen

Carbohydrates play a major role in the energy production necessary to sustain life. One carbohydrate in particular, glucose, is of particular importance in this respect. Aberration in glucose metabolism is a worldwide phenomenon, with as many as 200 million people suffering from just one group of such disorders, diabetes mellitus.[1] Although proper diagnostic measures and adequate therapy can now restore most of these patients to a quality of life that hardly can be distinguished from that of healthy persons, until the end of World War I, acquiring one of the forms of diabetes was tantamount to a sentence of death.

GLUCOSE METABOLISM AND REGULATION

Because glucose is the primary source of energy in animal life, knowledge of its normal metabolism is necessary to understand the events that occur when this metabolism is disturbed. Figure 38-1 gives a summary of metabolic events involving glucose directly or indirectly. Figures 38-2 and 38-3 indicate which of these reactions are preponderant in the healthy person, following a recent meal, and after a fast of many hours' duration. Intermediate steps are not shown—only branching and terminal points.

The demand for glucose necessary for various

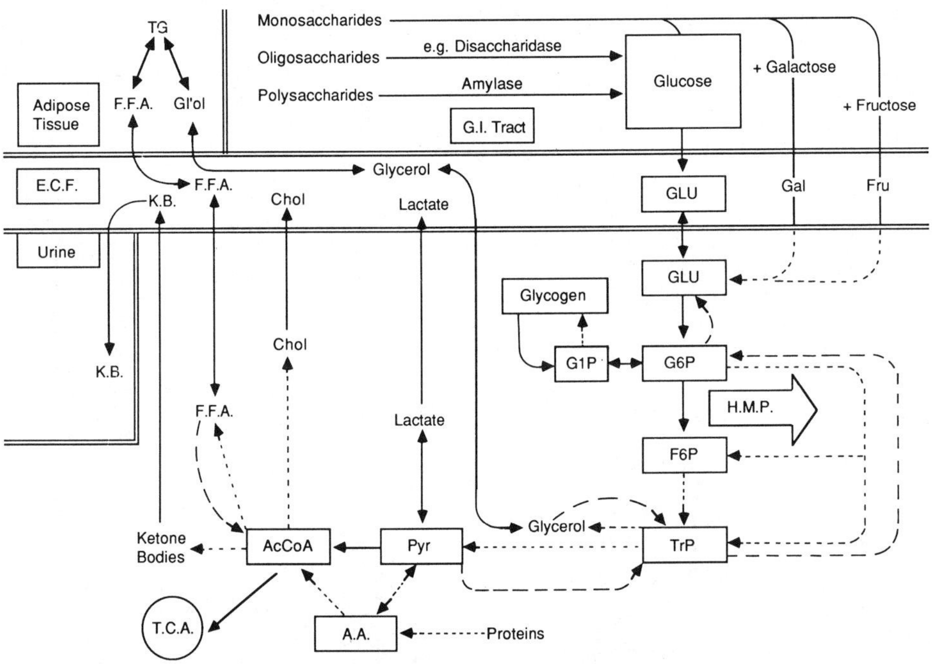

Figure 38-1 **Glucose metabolism: The stage.**

A.A. = Amino Acids; AcCoA = Acetyl CoA; ACTH = Adrenocorticotropic Hormone; Adr = Adrenaline; Chol = Cholesterol; Cort = Cortisol; E.C.F. = Extracellular Fluid; F.F.A. = Free Fatty Acids; Fru = Fructose; F6P = Fructose-6-Phosphate; Gal = Galactose; G'gon = Glucagon; G.I. Tract = Gastrointestinal Tract; Gl'ol = Glycerol; GLU = Glucose; G1P = Glucose-1-Phosphate; G6P = Glucose-6-Phosphate; HGH = Human Growth Hormone; Hi = High; H.M.P. = Hexose Monophosphate Pathway; HPL = Human Placental Lactogen; K.B. = Ketone Bodies; Lo = Low; Pyr = Pyruvate; S'st = Somatostatin; T.C.A. = Krebs Cycle; TG = Triglycerides; TrP = Triose Phosphates; T-4 = Thyroxine.

Symbols: ———————— = Single-Step Event
.... = Multi-Step Event, forward direction
- - - - - - - - - - - - = Multi-Step Event, reverse direction

\+ = Positive

Heavy lines indicate preferred direction under the given circumstances.

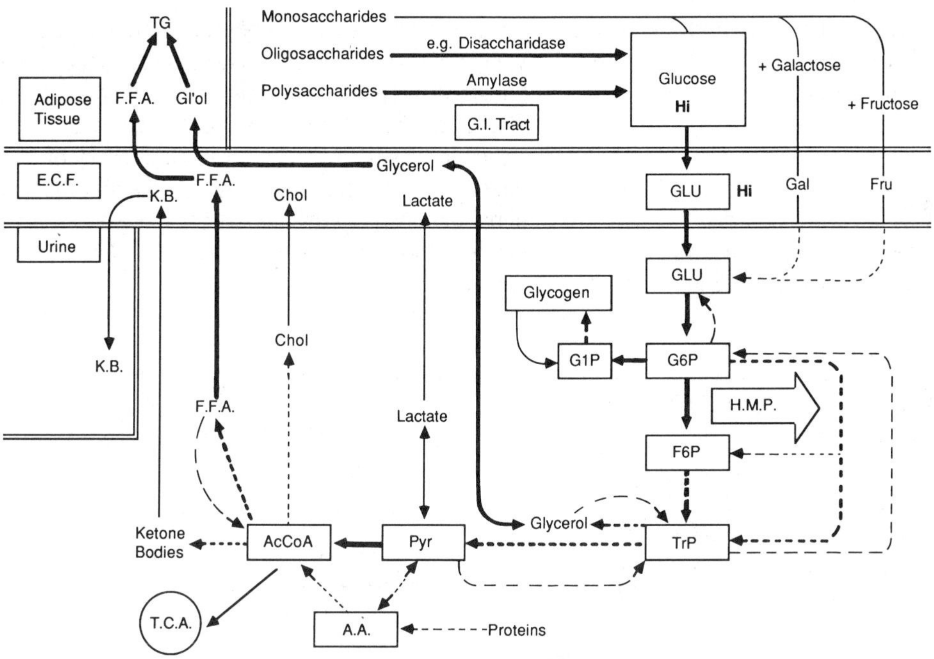

Figure 38-2 Glucose metabolism: Highlights of occurrences following a meal.

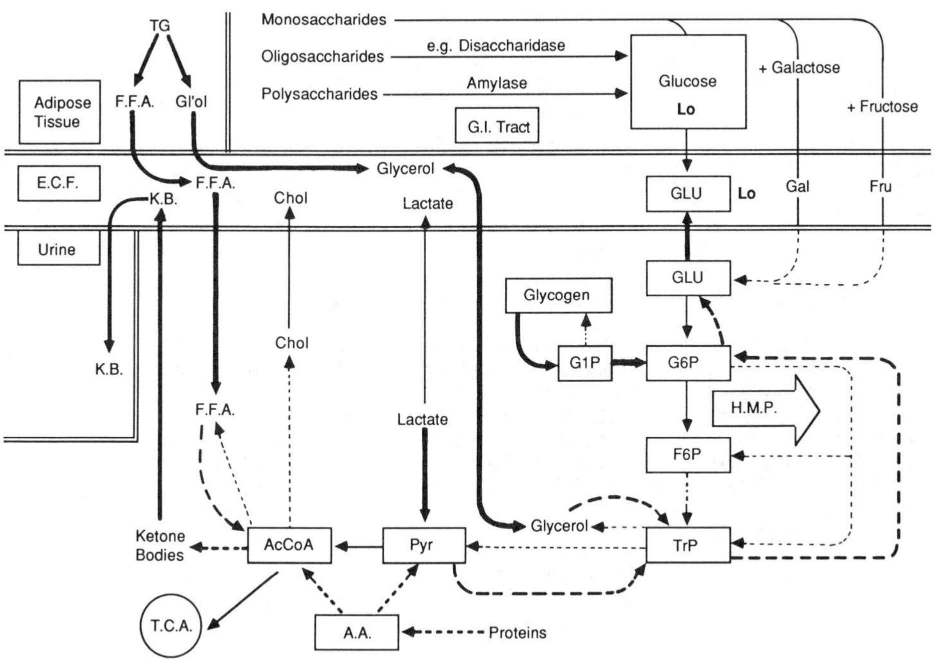

Figure 38-3 Glucose metabolism: Occurrences during a fast.

levels and forms of activities of the body is fulfilled through hormonal influence. Figures 38-4 and 38-5 show the sites of action of several of the glucose-regulating hormones.

Glucose Utilization

Only one hormone, *insulin,* is significantly involved in lowering the glucose level in the extracellular fluid. Insulin is a peptide with a molecular weight of about 6000 daltons and is produced in the pancreas by the B-cells of the islets of Langerhans. This hormone has two functions. It attaches itself to receptor sites on cells, facilitating entry of glucose for metabolic activities. Consequently and simultaneously, the glucose level in the extracellular fluid (plasma) is lowered. Insulin also inhibits lipolysis in adipose tissues.

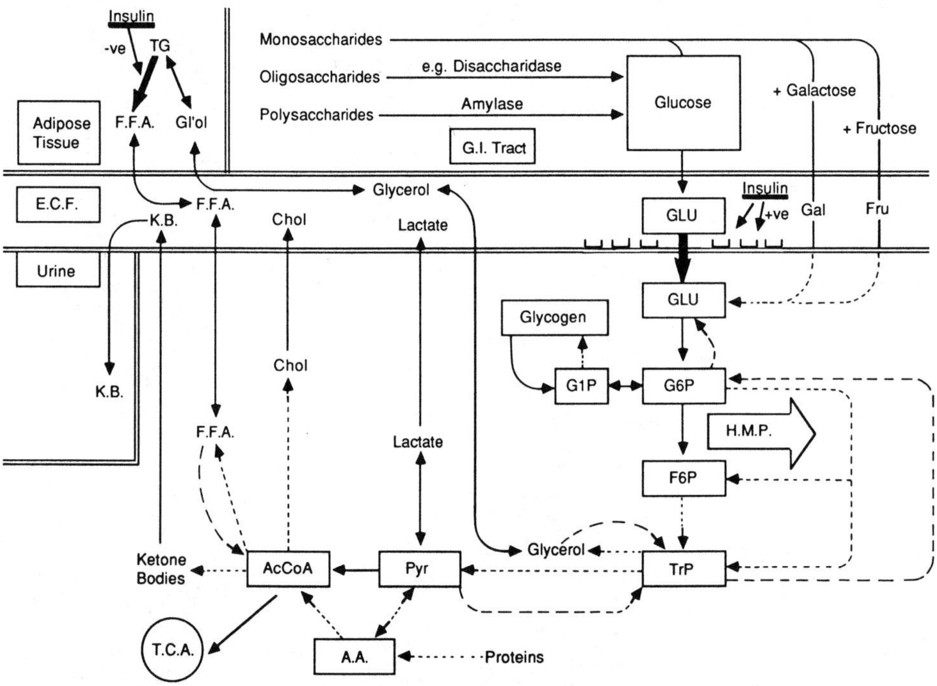

Figure 38-4 Hormonal influences on glucose metabolism. Effect of insulin.

A.A. = Amino Acids; AcCoA = Acetyl CoA; ACTH = Adrenocorticotropic Hormone; Adr = Adrenaline; Chol = Cholesterol; Cort. = Cortisol; E.C.F. = Extracellular Fluid; F.F.A. = Free Fatty Acids; Fru = Fructose; F6P = Fructose-6-Phosphate; Gal = Galactose; G'gon = Glucagon; G.I. Tract = Gastrointestinal Tract; Gl'ol = Glycerol; GLU = Glucose; G1P = Glucose-1-Phosphate; G6P = Glucose-6-Phosphate; HGH = Human Growth Hormone; Hi = High; H.M.P. = Hexose Monophosphate Pathway; HPL = Human Placental Lactogen; K.B. = Ketone Bodies; Lo = Low; Pyr = Pyruvate; S'st = Somatostatin; T.C.A. = Krebs Cycle; TG = Triglycerides; TrP = Triose Phosphates; T-4 = Thyroxine.

Symbols: ———————— = Single-Step Event
. . . . = Multi-Step Event, forward direction
- - - - - - - - - - - - - - - - = Multi-Step Event, reverse direction

⊔ = Receptors
+ or +ve = Promotion
− or −ve = Inhibition

Heavy lines indicate preferred direction under the given circumstances.

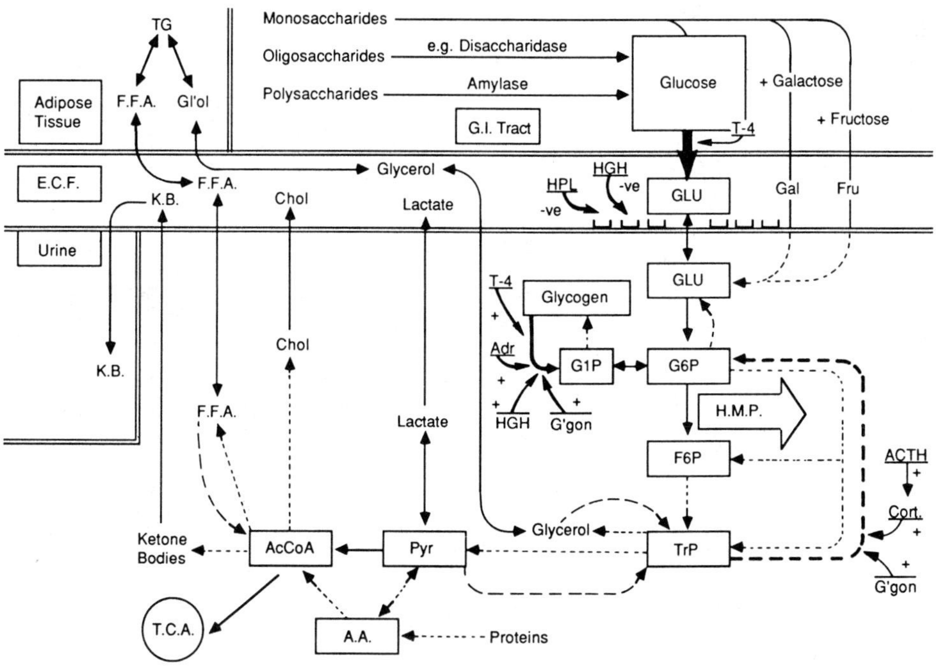

Figure 38-5 Hormonal influences on glucose metabolism. Effect of other hormones.

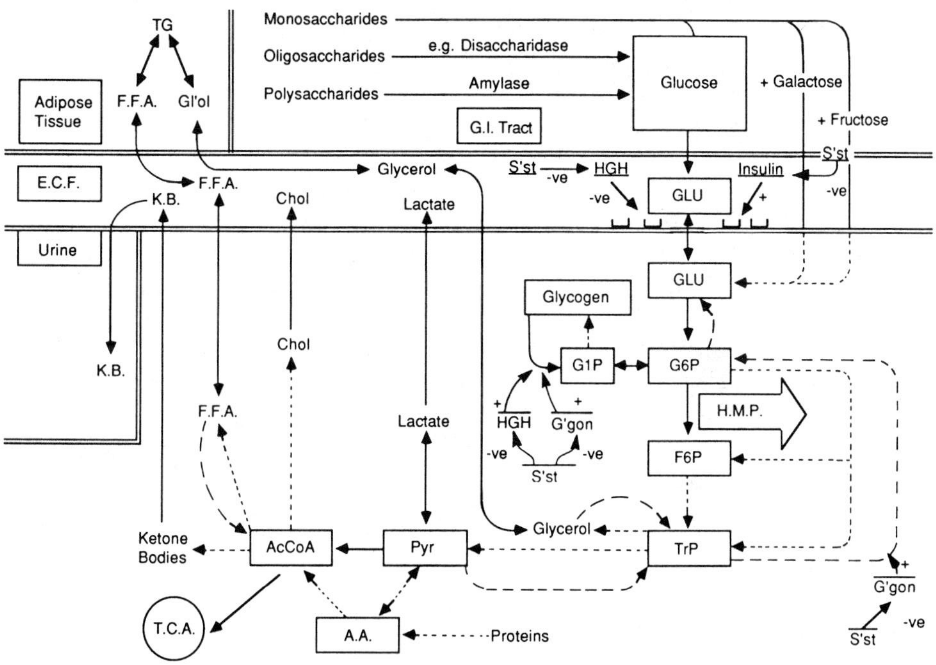

Figure 38-6 Hormonal influences on glucose metabolism. Effect of somatostatin.

Glucose Mobilization

In opposition to the action of insulin, several other hormones generate glucose by glycogenolysis or gluconeogenesis when demands are high and dietary glucose does not suffice. As a result, the levels of glucose in the extracellular fluids will be increased. *Glucagon,* like insulin, is a peptide hormone, and mobilizes glucose by inducing glycogenolysis in the liver. Glucagon is also produced in the pancreas, but, in contrast to insulin, by the A-cells of Langerhans's islets. *Cortisol* and *epinephrine* (*adrenaline*) are hormones generated during stressful situations, and both induce higher glucose levels. Cortisol promotes gluconeogenesis, and epinephrine induces glycogenolysis. Secretion of cortisol is stimulated by *ACTH,* which therefore has an effect similar to that of cortisol upon glucose metabolism. *Thyroxine* shows a twofold action when present in pathologically high amounts: it stimulates rapid uptake of dietary glucose, and it also causes glycogenolysis. *Growth Hormone (HGH)* also has a dual effect, in that it causes glycogenolysis in the liver and at the same time inhibits insulin in its promotion of cellular glucose uptake.

Glycogenolysis, stimulated through several pathways, is of limited capacity as a source of glucose. Liver glycogen stores will not last beyond 24 hours during a fast, and muscle glycogen is unavailable for glucose supply to the extracellular fluid. This is because muscle tissue does not contain glucose-6-phosphatase, an enzyme necessary for glycogenolysis to yield unphosphorylated glucose. *Human placental lactogen (HPL)* inhibits the insulin effect of promoting cellular uptake of glucose,[2] and may cause a diabetes like condition that develops late in pregnancy. The symptoms usually disappear following parturition. Another hormone produced in the pancreas, *somatostatin,* is a peptide, found in the D-cells of the pancreas. It also occurs in other parts of the body, especially in the hypothalamus. Somatostatin has an inhibitory effect on the release of three of the regulating hormones: insulin, glucagon, and growth hormone (see Fig. 38-6).[3, 4] It is of interest to note that the inhibition applies to hormones antagonistic to each other, and the effect is likely to be that of fine tuning the glucose supply.

ETIOLOGY AND PATHOPHYSIOLOGY

With such a multitude of interrelated balancing and counterbalancing reactions, it is understandable that many points in glucose metabolism may become unbalanced. A single disturbed reaction or effect, beyond normal variability, will almost always result in plasma glucose values beyond the reference range. If two points in the schema are affected, it is highly unlikely that the effects would negate each other, so plasma glucose would be abnormal and the laboratory diagnosis in such instances would be much more difficult. Based on laboratory findings only, it is thus reasonable to classify a substantial number of diseases, of widely varying etiology, as hyperglycemias and hypoglycemias; the terms refer only to the observed phenomena, and do not describe the underlying causes.

Hyperglycemias

Historically hyperglycemias, whatever their etiology, have been referred to as *diabetes mellitus.* The name, derived from the Greek, aptly describes the observable symptoms. The disease was named diabetes in the 2nd century A.D.,[5] but had been described in Egyptian papyri one-and-one-half millennia earlier.[6]

As can be seen in Figure 38-4, if either the receptor sites on the cell membranes are in short supply or nonfunctional, or the insulin is in short supply or nonfunctional, then glucose that has been derived from the diet will accumulate in the extracellular fluid (ECF) and must be disposed of via the kidney. Excretion of excess glucose will occur whenever the renal threshold is exceeded. Under these circumstances, cellular glucose uptake is compromised and the inhibitory effect on lipolysis by insulin is absent. Consequently, a condition will result that is similar to that observed during a prolonged fast, as shown in Figure 38-3. Whatever liver glycogen may be available will be converted to usable glucose. Fat stores will also be emptied, although at a slower rate, with the possibility of concomitant development of ketone bodies and acidosis. Due to the high production of acetyl-CoA from the lipolysis, there will often also be some excess production of cholesterol.

Two factors described above give similar, if not identical, symptoms: the lack of insulin, and the inadequacy of the receptor sites. Correspondingly, there are two major types of diabetes mellitus. *Insulin-dependent diabetes mellitus (IDDM),* formerly called juvenile or early-onset diabetes, is usually the result of pancreatic hypofunction. *Non-insulin-dependent diabetes mellitus (NIDDM),* on the other hand, seems frequently to be related to the quality and number of receptor sites. Although inadequate glucose utilization results, insulin production need not be impaired, and may actually be elevated.[7] The biochemical changes observed in these patients may not be as drastic as in IDDM, but tend to occur in the same direction.

Much less frequently occurring forms of hyperglycemia are those caused by the glucogenic factors, shown in Figure 38-5. The increased levels of glucose observed in these cases are milder. One instance is the so-called *gestational diabetes mellitus (GDM),* experienced by pregnant women and ascribed to the increased levels of HPL.[2] The condition subsides following delivery (see Chap. 40).

It should be noted that there is increasing evidence that diabetes mellitus is an autoimmune disorder, with the occurrence of antibody formation against the B-cells, against the receptor sites, or against insulin itself.[8, 9] Antibodies have been observed to be formed against insulin administered to diabetics, gradually causing insulin resistance.[10]

Although modern therapeutic measures can keep diabetics alive over decades, that victory comes, unfortunately, at a price. Even with the best of control of the glucose level, both IDDM and NIDDM patients suffer serious complications after some years.[11] The principal complications are vascular disease, primarily cardiovascular problems and arteriosclerosis, neuropathy, retinopathy and nephropathy.

Although these complications may be delayed in patients with long-standing diabetes, most diabetologists agree that they cannot be prevented, even when the patient's hyperglycemia has been well controlled. Fortunately, long-term studies, in this country as well as in Scandinavia, indicate that these secondary problems may be minimized with newer and more stable techniques for delivery of insulin, together with a closer watch for first symptoms.

Vascular disease has a much higher incidence among diabetics than in control groups. *Cardiovascular problems* are responsible for a substantial number of deaths among these patients, and cannot be correlated with the degree of hyperglycemia. *Arteriosclerosis* is also prominent in the lower extremities, with a concomitant decrease in blood flow. This, in conjunction with neuropathy (loss of sensory faculties) and a high concentration of food (glucose) for microorganisms, sets the stage for serious infections with possibility of gangrene and amputation. In this instance, micro- as well as macro-circulation is involved.

The diabetic *neuropathies* are the least well-researched major complication of diabetes. The effects become quite pervasive after some years, displaying loss of nerve function on the one hand and, at the same time, possibly causing pain elsewhere. Diabetic neuropathy is also apparently unrelated to the severity of the glucose abnormality. One effect, sensory loss, is described above. Bladder sensation may also be lost, causing backup of urine with subsequent pyelonephritis.

Ophthalmological involvement in the form of *retinopathies,* however, seems to be correlated with the severity and frequency of hyperglycemic episodes. The microvascular disease, the lipid disturbances, and the neuropathies seem to contribute to the destruction of the retinal tissue. Microaneurisms, lipid deposits, infarcts, and tissue proliferation may all lead gradually to total blindness after a few years.

Diabetic *nephropathy* is also correlated with the degree of hyperglycemia. Several years after the onset of diabetes, a slight albuminuria can be demonstrated, often in conjunction with an increased glomerular filtration rate. The latter can be normalized with control of the plasma glucose levels. With severe proteinuria and azotemia, the disease may progress to end-stage renal disease. Dialysis becomes necessary until a kidney can be found for transplantation. Interestingly, only a third of the patients who have kidney transplants re-develop nephropathy.

Hypoglycemias

The mechanisms opposing those that result in hyperglycemia will cause a disease state with diminished plasma glucose levels. *Lack of glucogenic activity* or *excessive consumption of glucose* may both lead to hypoglycemia, at least in theory. Fasting, even when prolonged, will not lead to hypoglycemia in normal individuals with functional glucogenic pathways. Only when sources of raw material for glucose production have been used up will starvation result in hypoglycemia.

Insulin-producing tumors, *insulinomas,* will cause hypoglycemia due to the constant output of insulin that is not triggered by increases above fasting level of plasma glucose.

Deficiency in the production of counter-regulatory hormones will cause normal insulin levels to have a proportionately stronger effect than would otherwise be the case. Adrenal insufficiency, whether medullar or cortical, is one example of disorders that may cause hypoglycemia.

Of the congenital defects of the regulatory system, *von Gierke's syndrome* probably occurs most frequently. A deficiency in the production of glucose-6-phosphatase will affect hepatic glycogenolysis in a negative manner, causing a buildup of glycogen in liver storage, and will prevent epinephrine from exerting its glucogenic effect.

As long as idiopathic hypoglycemia is kept under control, complications of the severity of hyperglycemia do not materialize. Because hypoglycemia often stems from a reaction to some other disorder, such as alcoholism, over-dosage of insulin, and adrenal insufficiency, complications may arise from the primary disease, in which case the hypoglycemia will have no causal relationship to such effects.

CLINICAL MANIFESTATIONS

Both hyper- and hypoglycemias are insidious and not readily detectable from the history only. Symptoms are nonspecific, and the disease may have been in progress for quite some time before being discovered, often unexpectedly. The exception to this is the frequently sudden onset of IDDM, which will manifest itself with heavy thirst and frequent urination. These symptoms are also seen in *diabetes insipidus,* a pituitary disorder, but the two conditions can be distinguished by the rapid weight loss that accompanies IDDM until it is brought under control. Tables 38-1 and 38-2 summarize complaints and clinical findings frequently observed in hyperglycemias and hypoglycemias.

An untreated case of IDDM will usually prove fatal within months, due to the wasting of the body's reserves and/or the hyperosmolality, ketoacidosis, and dehydration accompanying the metabolic disturbances.

The development of complications is not limited to untreated IDDM patients. Undiscovered NIDDM patients, and even known and controlled patients of both types, will often over the years develop secondary problems, as described above.

Patients presenting with symptoms of hypoglycemia should be considered possibly hypoglycemic, although in the majority of cases another diagnosis will eventually be established. Hypoglycemia has often been a convenient explanation for nonspecific complaints, when either low plasma glucose was surmised or laboratory data were interpreted beyond their level of clinical significance or predictive value.

Table 38-1 ***Clinical Observations in Untreated Hyperglycemia***

	IDDM	NIDDM	GDM
Acetone breath	Frequent	Occasional	Rare
Thirst	Frequent	Occasional	Rare
Polyuria	Frequent	Quite frequent	Occasional
Voracious appetite	Frequent	Occasional	Rare
Wasting	Yes	No	No
Obesity	No	Usual	Often
Circulatory problems	No	Yes	No
Age at onset	Before 30 yr	After 40 yr	N/A

IDDM = Insulin-dependent diabetes mellitus
NIDDM = Noninsulin-dependent diabetes mellitus
GDM = Gestational diabetes mellitus

LABORATORY ANALYSES AND DIAGNOSIS

Strategies for Diagnostic Workup

Because symptoms arising from impaired glucose metabolism are nonspecific and usually progressive in their manifestation, the disease may have progressed far before its detection. A diagnostic chain of events is often initiated by one of three occurrences:

Table 38-2 ***Clinical Observations in Untreated Hypoglycemia***

Plasma Glucose Dropping Fast (Adrenergic Symptoms):
Anxiety
Hunger
Shakiness
Sweating (cold)
Nausea
Dizziness
Plasma Glucose Dropping Slowly (Neuroglycopenic Symptoms):
Lethargy
Headache
Irritability
Unconsciousness
Coma

1. Response to complaints compatible with carbohydrate disturbances
2. Observation of an abnormality during mass screening (*e.g.*, at a health fair in a shopping mall)
3. Serendipitous detection during workup for other reasons (*e.g.*, an admission profile when patient is hospitalized for a broken leg)

When suspicion arises that a carbohydrate disorder is present, a strategy must be selected based on which disease is most likely involved, as indicated from the suspicion-triggering event. Most of these events would result in a blood sugar (plasma glucose) value outside normal range or a positive urine sugar. Suspicion would most frequently be directed toward a hyperglycemic condition.

HYPERGLYCEMIA

Suspicion of hyperglycemia should lead to determination of whether or not it is transient, considering the conditions during which it first manifested itself. If it is "nontransient," *i.e.*, fasting blood sugar (FBS) and/or 2-hour postprandial glucose are significantly elevated—>140 mg/dL (7.8 mmol/L)—on two consecutive occasions when determined with reliable methodology, then this is sufficient to establish a diagnosis of diabetes mellitus.[12] Problems arise when differentiation becomes necessary, and when severity is to be gauged. Usually *IDDM* can be presumed at this point, and confirmed with determination of immunoreactive insulin, which should be low or absent. The onset will normally have been abrupt and accompanied by ketoacidosis and rapid weight loss.

Early *NIDDM* is more difficult to establish, as FBS frequently is normal and postprandial values may be only marginally abnormal. In such instances, an oral glucose tolerance test is indicated. If two specimens, one of them drawn at 2 hours, postprandial, both exceed 200 mg/dL (11.1 mmol/L), a diagnosis of diabetes mellitus is considered confirmed,[12] and distinction between IDDM and NIDDM rests upon the accompanying clinical symptoms: weight loss vs maintenance or gain, ketones vs no ketones, excessive thirst vs little or no thirst (see Table 38-1).

Although a 2-hour GTT will often suffice to identify or confirm a case of NIDDM, a 3-hour GTT is preferred to diagnose *gestational diabetes.* When GDM is suspected, a 100-g glucose challenge is given to the patient, after no less than a 10-hour fast, and plasma glucose is determined before the glucose ingestion and hourly for 3 hours afterwards. Maximal allowable values follow:

Fasting: 105 mg/dL (5.8 mmol/L)
1 hour: 190 mg/dL (10.5 mmol/L)
2 hours: 165 mg/dL (9.2 mmol/L)
3 hours: 145 mg/dL (8.0 mmol/L)

If two of the observed values exceed these maxima, the diagnosis is considered confirmed.[12, 13] If there is no confirmed diagnosis early in the pregnancy, but the suspicion persists, the described GTT should be repeated in the third trimester.

HYPOGLYCEMIA

In suspected hypoglycemia, it must first be established whether or not the hypoglycemic episode occurs during a fast or in response to intake of food (*reactive hypoglycemia*). The *fasting hypoglycemia* is usually caused by factors not directly related to glucose metabolism, such as drug intake or endocrine disorders. If it can be established that during a fast the plasma glucose values remain low or gradually decrease toward dangerously low levels, then it is likely that the condition is self-induced (drugs, excess insulin use, alcohol) or is of an organic nature. A fast with periodic glucose testing may last up to 48 hours.

If, on the other hand, fasting values are not unreasonably low, but glucose levels seem to fall below fasting value some time after a meal, a 5-hour GTT is indicated. The subject should be kept under close scrutiny, specifically under observation for adrenergic symptoms, and these should be correlated with the lowest glucose value(s); levels below 50 mg/dL (2.8 mmol/L) are considered diagnostic.[14, 15] If no such correlation can be found, the concept of a reactive hypoglycemia may be discarded, and the search for another (organic or psychological) cause resumed.

Some patients, however, may display no symptoms at all and still have reactive hypoglycemia. An early hypoglycemic episode following glucose ingestion may be the result of rapid glucose uptake, with concomitant high plasma values and consequent forceful stimulus to produce insulin. A late hypoglycemic event may be seen with NIDDM patients who have a delayed but powerful insulin release following the challenge. In both instances, careful history-taking will aid in establishing the cause. *Insulinomas,* the most important cause of fasting hypoglycemias, are actively secreting tumors of pancreatic B-cells. Normally, fasting is associated with a progressive fall in serum insulin concentration; however, patients with insulinomas, even when hypoglycemic, usually do not exhibit this fall in insulin levels. Manifestation of inappropriate insulin release can be exaggerated by the response to insulin secretagogues such as tolbutamide. When given as a rapid intravenous infusion, tolbutamide causes an immediate release of insulin, resulting in hypoglycemia. The degree of hypoglycemia has been used to indicate the presence of an insulinoma. For confirmation of the diagnosis, insulin determination by RIA is essential.

Useful Laboratory Procedures

GLUCOSE DETERMINATION

Glucose determination in biological fluids has a long history, and few, if any, analytes have had more methodologies for them described over the years. Early methods involved the analysis of whole blood, while analysis currently takes place on serum or plasma as well as on whole blood. The specificity for glucose alone is very high, due to the glucose-specific enzymes utilized in almost all methods common today. Accuracy, however, is still very much dependent on the quality of sample used. A whole-blood specimen, whether anticoagulated or not, will consume significant amounts of the glucose content through action of the erythrocytes; to a lesser, but still significant, extent, glucose is metabolized in plasma or serum through glycolytic activity of enzymes. Bacterial contamination adds to the glycolytic activity, unless the specimen is drawn and maintained under sterile conditions.

Specimen collection should therefore aim at minimizing glycolysis between drawing and analysis. If glucose is to be determined as one analyte in a panel on a multichannel instrument, then serum is usually the sample provided. This is unfortunate in the sense that batch sample processing creates an opportunity for deterioration of glucose values. If serum must be used, blood should be drawn in a sterile container (containing a clotting activator if possible), allowed to clot at room temperature (but for no more than 30 minutes), and then centrifuged; the serum must be separated from the cells promptly and refrigerated until the time of analysis. If the specimen is drawn specifically for glucose determination, fluoridized plasma is much to be preferred.

Hexokinase Technique

At the present time, the hexokinase technique is the current reference method.[16] Because there is little to criticize in principle, technical requirements, skill required, or cost, the method is likely to remain state-of-the-art for a considerable time. NADH or NADPH is generated during the reaction, which is measured in the near UV. The reaction is supposed to go to completion; it is *not* kinetic.

Glucose Oxidase Method (Photometric, End-Point)

It should be noted that because the glucose oxidase method (GOD) is specific for β-glucose only, most commercial preparations of GOD-based analytical kits also contain mutarotase. As β-glucose is consumed, this enzyme will rapidly convert to β-glucose the 36% of α-glucose present in glucose solutions at equilibrium, so that all glucose eventually is used up.

Glucose Oxidase Method (Kinetic)

For the kinetic GOD method to be useful, it is essential that the reactions are carried out at constant temperature, that the reaction mixtures are saturated with atmospheric oxygen, and that the hydrogen peroxide formed is rendered inactive, or alternately used as the actual indicator of reaction rate.

Test Strip Technique

Reagent strips impregnated on the test pad with glucose-sensitive chemicals have improved considerably over the last decade; however, the visually-read strips *cannot* yet replace wet chemistry with respect to precision and reliability. The usefulness of the strips is in situations where a *rough* estimate of the glucose value will suffice.

Reflectance photometers have now been designed specifically for glucose reagent strips, and yield reasonable precision and accuracy. They are still not close to wet chemistry quality. Accuracy may be a more serious problem than is precision. Strips from the same container will compare in performance in the same analytical run, but sensitivity often changes during storage. Frequent calibration is necessary, and results will be inaccurate if instructions are not followed exactly. Application of the sample (usually whole blood), timing of each step, washing or wiping technique, and equipment maintenance are all critical components of the analysis. With good initial instruction, however, this methodology does serve a purpose in home testing, and to some degree in physicians' offices. Nonetheless, users should not rely too heavily on the data obtained, especially if the technique is applied in tolerance tests.

GLUCOSE TOLERANCE TESTS

When it is suspected that glucose metabolism is disturbed, a good test is to challenge the body with glucose and observe the response. Tolerance tests serve that purpose. They may take the form of a simple comparison between plasma glucose values before and 2 hours after a meal, or they may last several hours following intake of a measured amount of glucose, with restriction of the subject's activities for the duration of the test. Blood samples are drawn at specified intervals and analyzed for glucose. Urine samples may also be obtained hourly and semi-quantitated for glucose, although this aspect of tolerance testing is not quite as common as previously. Tolerance tests fell into some disfavor in the 1970s, but apparently are in the process of being restored to their former importance.

When performing an *oral glucose tolerance test (OGTT),* if the fasting blood sugar value by test strip methodology is above 160 mg/dL (8.9 mmol/L), the ordering physician should be notified and authorization secured before proceeding with the test. Alternatively, the fasting sample is analyzed by regular means for glucose and, if the value is above 140 mg/dL (7.8 mmol/L), a decision should be reached in consultation with the physician about whether or not to continue. If it is decided to proceed in such an instance, close watch must be kept on the patient.

All samples, properly stabilized to prevent glucose deterioration, should be analyzed in one series to minimize inter-run variation. Final specimens may also be sampled as whole blood on a test strip, as an indicator of a hypoglycemic condition before subjects are released to their own care.

In instances in which the subject suffers from malabsorption or is unable to keep down the ingested glucose, an *intravenous glucose tolerance test* can be performed. A test dose of glucose is given intravenously in a solution that is otherwise isotonic. Glucose does not contribute to the osmotic pressure, as it readily passes across membranes. The results of the test may be given as a chart of glucose value vs time, as for the OGTT. It is common to calculate the glucose disappearance constant from a plot of the $\log_{10}$ of the glucose value against time; this procedure theoretically will yield a straight line. From the slope, the disappearance of glucose per minute, expressed as a percentage of the 10-minute value, can be computed. One would expect the IV GTT to yield a better representation of the metabolic disposition of glucose, because variability in ingestion rate and absorption is circumvented. Practical experience has shown, however, that the predictive value of OGTT far exceeds that of IV GTT.[17]

An analysis for *reducing substances in urine* was used in the past as a tool in diagnosis and control of diabetes mellitus, presuming the *reduction of cupric ions* in the reagent was due to glucose. Sensitivity was adequate but specificity was lacking, mainly in cases of galactosuria and after intake of large amounts of ascorbic acid. The procedure has, by and large, been replaced with *glucose-specific test strips,* for which the test pad is impregnated with glucose oxidase and other reagents necessary for a reaction similar to the ones for plasma glucose described above.

Tests for total reducing substances are still used in pediatric care to detect the presence of other urinary sugars, most frequently galactose, which do not react on a strip. A positive reaction should be followed up with thin-layer chromatography.

Ketone bodies is the name commonly applied to a group of substances consisting of acetone, acetoacetic acid, and β-hydroxybutyric acid (which is not a ketone at all but a precursor). These substances are formed in large amounts when acetyl-CoA is produced in excess, and are a good source of energy for most tissues in an emergency, such as during prolonged fasting or inactive insulin production. The ketone bodies are a characteristic component of plasma, urine, and breath in ketoacidosis.

Detection of *plasma ketone bodies* may be useful in an emergency situation when rapid stabilization of a ketoacidotic patient is required but facilities for glucose assay are less than ideal. In such a situation, the administration of insulin and bicarbonate is followed closely by obtaining plasma samples and analyzing qualitatively for acetoacetic acid, using tablets, powder, or test strips containing nitroprusside and supporting chemicals. A purple color indicates the presence of acetoacetate and, by inference, the other ketone bodies. Glucose determination should be done later on the same specimens. With the advent of test strips for plasma glucose using uncentrifuged whole blood, data are rapidly available and the use of the nitroprusside tests has waned. Strip testing is also possible at the bedside, obviating the delays incurred when a laboratory is remote from the treatment area involved. *Urine ketone bodies* are determined with the same techniques as are used for plasma, and will determine if the subject has had a transient episode of ketosis since the last urine voiding; this is particularly useful if the plasma glucose is at a desirable level at the time of voiding.

Insulin was the first substance to be quantified with radioimmunoassay (RIA) methodology,[18] which is still the method of choice. The assay is particularly useful in evaluation of fasting hypoglycemia, but may eventually also prove useful as an adjunct to an OGTT. The rationale is to determine whether endogenous insulin is available at all in a patient with diabetes mellitus. If the result is affirmative, the disorder might then be controllable with diet alone (NIDDM).[19]

Insulin is generally stored as *proinsulin,* a protein of about 100 amino acid residues. When the need for increased peripheral insulin levels occurs, the proinsulin in the B-cells is cleaved to equimolar amounts of insulin and a connecting peptide called *C-peptide.* Both enter the circulation, but the former is quickly removed from the blood stream by the first passage through the liver, whereas the latter is excreted more slowly by the kidneys. The analysis for *C-peptide* in serum has diagnostic value as a measure of recent insulin production and release.[20, 21]

The *insulin tolerance test* is useful for determination of resistance to or intolerance of administered insulin. Due to its potential for triggering a severe episode of hypoglycemia, the test should be carried out only under controlled conditions, with a physician on standby for needed intervention. After 3 days' preparation as for an OGTT, fasting patients are given IV insulin, after which plasma glucose is determined at short intervals for 2 hours. A minimum glucose value of half the fasting level should be obtained after about 1/2 hour, and fasting value should be restored at 1 1/2 to 2 hours.

The *tolbutamide tolerance test* is based on the ability of the drug tolbutamide to stimulate the normal pancreas to secrete insulin.[22] Intravenous administration of tolbutamide after an overnight fast is followed by plasma glucose (and sometimes also plasma insulin) assays drawn in a pattern similar to that for the insulin tolerance test. In subjects with normal pancreatic function, the responses from the two tolerance tests will be similar.

The *epinephrine tolerance test* is a test to determine the presence in the liver of glucose-6-phosphatase. This enzyme is necessary for the final step in glycogenolysis. If it is missing, as is the case in von Gierke's glycogen storage disease, epinephrine, which stimulates mobilization of glucose from glycogen depots, is without effect. The injection of 1 mg of epinephrine in an adult should produce an increase in plasma glucose level of about 40 mg/dL (2.2 mmol/L) over fasting value in less than one hour.

Lactose tolerance tests are used to detect malabsorption secondary to lactose intolerance. This condition is the result of a defect in lactase production, of either congenital or acquired origin. Without disaccharidase (lactase) present in the digestive tract, lactose cannot be cleaved into glucose and galactose and lactose will remain in the lumen of the bowel, causing an osmotic diarrhea. Furthermore, subsequent bacterial degradation of the lactose will cause gas production, with further discomfort to the patient. (See also Chap. 67).

After the lactose is administered orally, plasma glucose is determined at 15-minute intervals for 90 minutes. A rise in glucose value over fasting level of 30 mg/dL (1.7 mmol/L) indicates adequate intestinal lactase production.[23, 24]

TREATMENT

Strategies in Emergencies

Patients presenting with symptoms indicating diabetic ketoacidosis and/or diabetic coma require instant symptomatic relief before a serious diagnostic workup can be initiated. Such indicators may include high plasma glucose values, plasma and urinary ketones, and metabolic acidosis with hyperventilation. Therapeutic measures, such as fluids to restore fluid balance, bicarbonate to offset the acidosis, and insulin to bring the glucose under control, are monitored for efficacy with frequent electrolyte and glucose assays.

Hyperglycemia

IDDM, as its name implies, requires insulin to normalize the blood sugar. NIDDM can usually be controlled by diet, although some patients do not respond and sulfonylureas or insulin must be given.

To normalize blood sugar throughout a 24-hour period, alternatives to the traditional therapy of one or two injections of insulin a day have been utilized. These include multiple subcutaneous insulin injection and continuous subcutaneous insulin infusion involving the use of a small battery-powered pump that delivers insulin throughout the day.[25]

Hypoglycemia

The treatment of serious hypoglycemia involves the immediate infusion of glucose, which continues until the patient is able to eat a meal. The meal is necessary to restore hepatic glycogen.

Surgery is required for insulinoma and for a number of the hormone-secreting tumors of the pancreas. Hormonal replacement is necessary for pituitary or adrenal insufficiency, but therapy for other forms of hypoglycemia is dietary.[26]

Laboratory Monitoring of Therapy

FASTING BLOOD SUGAR (FBS)

If the patient is hospitalized or in an outpatient clinic or physician's office, FBS may be of considerable value, particularly in cases of a history of limited or no compliance with treatment instructions. It should be recalled, however, that in many instances FBS is normal in diseased persons, such as in early cases of NIDDM, and in reactive hypoglycemia. For compliant patients FBS is of more value in detecting the worsening of existing disease that has been kept under control in the past.

GLYCOSYLATED HEMOGLOBINS

Analysis of glycosylated hemoglobins is especially useful in monitoring of patient compliance, but of little use in diagnostic work. Certain normally-occurring hemoglobin variants tend, slowly and irreversibly, to bind glucose at a rate proportional to the glucose concentration. A hemoglobin molecule therefore becomes a mirror of its past environment. Isolation and analysis of such hemoglobins and other similar proteins correlate well with the average glucose level during the previous several weeks to three months. Diabetic patients will have percentages of glycosylated hemoglobins higher than normal, but the actual values will reveal if the patient is in control or under- or over-medicated.

HOME TESTING

Not until recently has there been a significant number of laboratory tests suitable for use in the home by the patient. For some years, tests for diabetics could be purchased in pharmacies—nitroprusside papers and powders for urinary ketones, and tapes, strips, and tablets for urine sugars. Within the last decade, certain test strips have become reliable enough that patients can be trained in capillary blood collection from themselves and in determining glucose levels with strip-reading reflectance meters. Patients are also trained in algorithms used for adjusting their medication, without intervention from the health care team, and with only occasional control by the health care provider. Clinical laboratory scientists have a new, important, and logical role in patient education for home testing purposes.

CASE STUDY

A 32-year-old woman presented as an outpatient for a 5-hour oral glucose tolerance test (OGTT). Her past history, not known to the hospital laboratory personnel, included diminished appetite, an onset of shyness, general malaise, and fatigue; however, the initial physical examination revealed no diagnostic information, and it was the hope of her physician that the OGTT might be helpful. During the test, the patient did not collect urine samples, so these results are omitted below:

PLASMA GLUCOSE VALUES

Sample	***Results***
Fasting	97 mg/dL
30″	112 mg/dL
60″	108 mg/dL
120″	113 mg/dL
180″	102 mg/dL
240″	92 mg/dL
300″	95 mg/dL

SI units may be calculated as follows:
Glucose—mg/dL × 0.0555 = mmol/L

Questions

1. Was it a good decision to begin the laboratory workup of this patient with an OGTT? Why or why not?
2. With what diagnosis are these data most compatible?
3. Are the given glucose values significantly different from each other so that a "real" increase in glucose exists?

Discussion

1. An OGTT was not a good idea. With such nonspecific symptoms, a broader and better approach to detection or exclusion of a chemically-related disorder would be to order a biochemical profile.
2. A case could be made for malabsorption as the diagnosis. However, with so small a rise in glucose values, the condition would be severe. "Emaciated" is not mentioned in the physical findings. A hyperinsulinism also has a flat curve, but would show glucose values at a much lower level. These data must be characterized as nondiagnostic. Consideration should also be given to inadequate instruction to the patient about the test. If she vomited any of the glucose meal, as often happens, these glucose values would result.
3. From lowest to highest glucose value, the difference is 21 mg/dL (1.2 mmol/L). With these few samples, it is unlikely that one would be two S.Ds. above, and another two S.Ds. below the mean. Therefore, if the laboratory has established a C.V. of 5% or less for glucose, then these data are not representations of the same mean value, and the small rise *may* be real.

REFERENCES

1. WHO Expert Committee on diabetes mellitus: Second report. WHO Tech Rep Ser 646, 1980
2. Beck P, Doughaday WH: Human placental lactogen. Studies of its metabolic effects and disposition in normal man. J Clin Invest 46: 103, 1967
3. Gerich JE: Somatostatin and diabetes. Am J Med 70: 619, 1981
4. Vale W, Rivier C, Brown M: Regulatory peptides of the hypothalamus. Ann Rev Physiol 39: 473, 1977
5. Adams F: The Extant Works of Aretaeus the Cappadocian. London, Sydenham Society, 1856
6. Ebbell B (transl): The Papyrus Ebers. Copenhagen, Levin & Munksgaard, 1937

7. Olefsky JM: Insulin resistance and insulin action. Diabetes 30: 148, 1981
8. Del Prete GF, Betterle C et al: Incidence and significance of islet-cell autoantibodies in different types of diabetes mellitus. Diabetes 26: 909, 1977
9. Seino S et al: Characterization of circulating insulin in insulin autoimmune syndrome. J Clin Endocr Metab 62: 64, 1986
10. Kurtz AB, Nabarro JDN: Circulating insulin-binding antibodies. Diabetologia 19: 329, 1980
11. Santiago JV: Overview of the complications of diabetes. Clin Chem 32 (10B): B48, 1986
12. National Diabetes Data Group: Classification and diagnosis of diabetes mellitus and other categories of glucose intolerance. Diabetes 28: 1039, 1979
13. O'Sullivan JB, Mahan CM et al: Screening criteria for high-risk gestational diabetes patients. Am J Obstet Gynecol 116:895, 1973
14. Lev-Ran A, Anderson RW: The diagnosis of postprandial hypoglycemia. Diabetes 30: 996, 1981
15. Permutt MA: Postprandial hypoglycemia. Diabetes 25: 719, 1976
16. Neese JW, Duncan P, Bayse D et al: Development and evaluation of a hexokinase/glucose-6-phosphate dehydrogenase procedure for use as a national glucose reference method. HEW Publication No. (CDC)77-8330. Atlanta, Centers for Disease Control, 1976
17. Olefsky JM, Farquhar JW, Reaven GM: Do the oral and intravenous glucose tolerance tests provide similar diagnostic information in patients with chemical diabetes mellitus? Diabetes 22: 202, 1973
18. Yalow RS, Berson SA: Immunoassay of endogenous insulin in man. J Clin Invest 39: 1157, 1960
19. Turkington RW, Weindling HK: Insulin secretion in the diagnosis of adult-onset diabetes mellitus. JAMA 240: 833, 1978
20. Hoekstra JBL, van Rijn HJM, Erkelens DW et al: C-peptide. Diabetes Care 5: 438, 1982
21. Hoekstra JBL, van Rijn HJM, Thijsen JHH et al: C-peptide reactivity as a measure of insulin dependency in the obese diabetic patient treated with insulin. Diabetes Care 5: 585, 1982
22. Lebowitz HE, Feinglos MN: Sulfonylurea drugs: Mechanism of antidiabetic action and therapeutic usefulness. Diabetic Care 1: 189, 1978
23. Newcomer AD, McGill DB, Thomas PJ et al: Prospective comparison of indirect methods for detecting lactase deficiency. N Engl J Med 293: 1232, 1975
24. Gudmand-Hoyer E, Simony KO: Individual sensitivity of lactose in lactose malabsorption. Am J Dig Dis 22: 177, 1977
25. Foster DW: Diabetes mellitus. In Petersdorf RG et al (eds): Harrison's Principles of Internal Medicine, pp 664-666. New York City, McGraw-Hill, 1983
26. Foster DW, Rubenstein AH: Hypoglycemia, insulinoma, and other hormone-secreting tumors of the pancreas. In Petersdorf RG et al (eds): Harrison's Principles of Internal Medicine, pp 687-688. New York City, McGraw-Hill, 1983

Chapter 39

Pituitary Disorders

Mary Ann McLane

The pituitary, often called the "master gland," lies at the base of the skull in a bony depression called the *sella turcica.* Its two lobes differ in size, with the anterior larger than the posterior, and in function. The anterior lobe is concerned with hormone production and the posterior with hormone storage. Both lobes, however, have a similar innervation source, the neurons from the hypothalamus. Situated atop the pituitary, the hypothalamus neuroendocrine tissue is directly connected to both pituitary lobes by a pituitary stalk. Due to the intimate contact of the hypothalamus and glands, and the small concentrations of peptides secreted from them, it is often difficult to differentiate between these two glands as the primary source of a higher-level endocrine problem. The diagnosis of hypothalamic dysfunction usually depends on the exclusion of other probable causes.[1] Figure 39-1 depicts the structural relationship between the hypothalamus and pituitary and the controls involved in the production of anterior pituitary hormones. Because symptoms of pituitary dysfunction ulti-

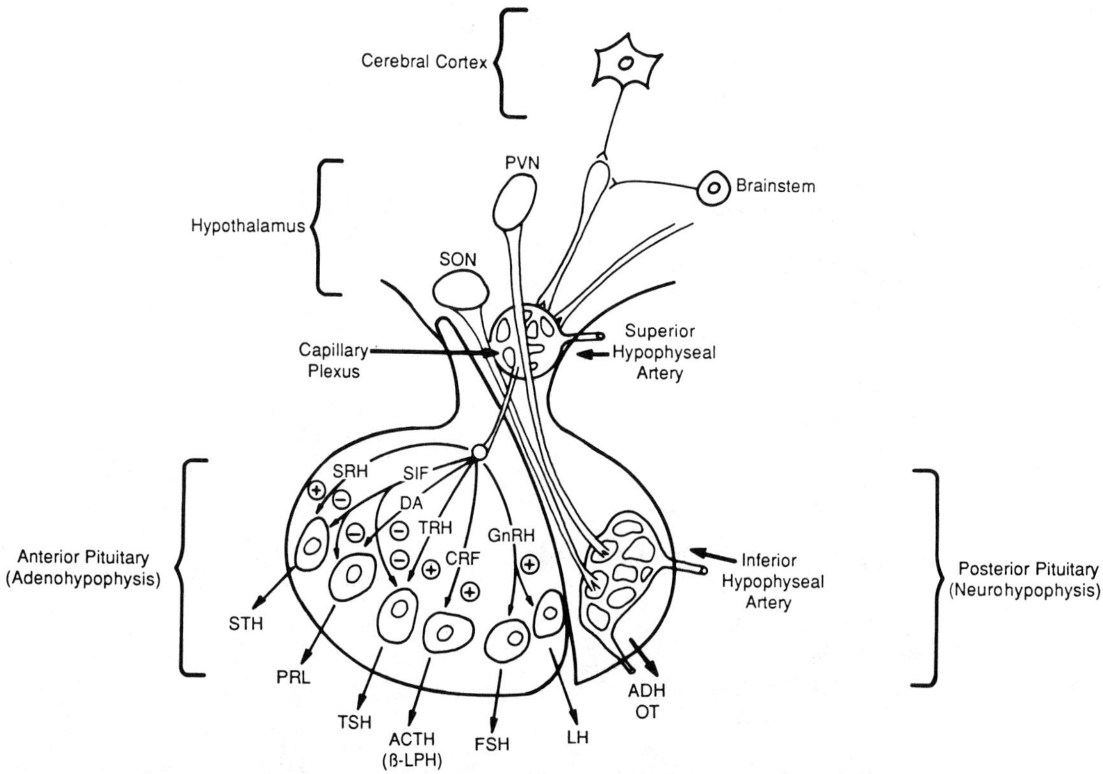

Figure 39-1 **Structure of the pituitary gland and control of the trophic cells of the anterior pituitary. ACTH = Adrenocorticotropic hormone; ADH = Antidiuretic hormone; CRF = Corticotropin-releasing factor; DA = Dopamine; FSH = Follicle-stimulating hormone; GnRH = Gonadotropin-releasing hormone; LH = Luteinizing hormone; β-LPH = β-lipotropin; OT = Oxytocin; PRL = Prolactin; PVN = Paraventricular nuclei; SIF = Somatotropin-inhibiting factor; SON = Supraoptic nuclei; SRH = Somatotropin-releasing hormone; STH = Somatotropin; TRH = Thyrotropin-releasing hormone; TSH = Thyroid-stimulating hormone.**
(Adapted from Gornall AG: Applied Biochemistry of Clinical Disorders, p 229. Hagerstown, Harper & Row, 1980)

mately reflect derangements of the final target hormone concentration, the reader is referred to the following chapters for dicussions of the hypothalamo-pituitary hormones: Chapter 37, adrenal cortex (CRF, ACTH), Chapter 35, thyroid (TRH, TSH), and Chapters 42 and 43, reproduction (GnRH, FSH, LH). This chapter will focus on the other four hormones produced or stored in the pituitary—growth hormone (GH), prolactin (PRL), oxytocin (OT), and antidiuretic hormone (ADH)—and those conditions that affect more than one pituitary hormone.

ETIOLOGY AND PATHOPHYSIOLOGY

Growth Hormone

Growth hormone (GH, somatotropin, STH) is the most abundant hormone produced in the anterior pituitary,[2] with roughly 50% of the endocrine cells in the gland being somatotrophs.[3] It resembles prolactin in its structure and action on tissues, acting directly on a wide spectrum of tissues rather than requiring an endocrine gland to produce a final target hormone.[4] Its effect on soft tissue, cartilage, and bone is to promote their increased uptake of amino acids, sodium, and potassium. It also promotes increased uptake of nonesterified fatty acids by muscle, and mobilization of fat by adipose.[2] It stimulates hepatic glycogenolysis and has an anti-insulin effect.[2] Most significant is its induction of hepatic synthesis of peptides known as *somatomedins.* These hormones mediate somatotropin's action on cartilage[5] and bone, and may act like GH on other tissues.[1]

HYPERSECRETION

The effect on patients with hypersecretion of growth hormone will depend on the age of the patient. If the prolonged exposure of skeleton and soft tissues to elevated GH occurs early in life, before long-bone growth is completed, the effect will be children of disproportionate size for their age. Sometimes these children exceed 8 feet in height, a condition referred to as *gigantism.*[5] If the hormone elevation occurs after puberty, the resulting condition is known as *acromegaly,* which is much more common than gigantism.[6] Acromegaly usually develops slowly. It is not uncommon for acromegaly to escape diagnosis until after the age of 30. Sixty-two percent of patients affected for fewer than 5 years and 26% of patients affected for fewer than 10 years will not be diagnosed as acromegalic[7] due to the subtlety of the clinical symptoms.[1, 4, 5, 6, 7]

Fifty percent of acromegalics will show abnormal x-rays or tomograms of the sella area, and 80% to 90% of the cases will reveal pituitary tumors on CT scan.[2] These benign somatotrope adenomas are the most frequent cause of elevated growth hormone. Less frequent causes can be carcinoma, ectopic growth hormone production,[6] dysfunction of the hypothalamus, or an intrinsic defect of the somatotrope cells themselves.[7]

HYPOFUNCTION

Patients experiencing an isolated deficiency of growth hormone will, as with hypersecretion, have symptoms that may vary according to age. Although in adults hyposecretion of somatotropin is the first chemical abnormality demonstrated in those patients with compressing pituitary adenomas or after pituitary radiation, it is rarely clinically significant.[2] For children, however, growth hormone deficiency may result in pituitary dwarfism, in which the child is small but proportionally built.[4] Diagnosis will usually not be made until after one year of age. Isolated growth hormone deficiencies will be either familial (rare) or sporadic, resulting from perinatal damage of the hypothalamus.[8] These may be difficult to differentiate from other causes of growth failure in children: a loss of tissue response to somatomedins,[2] or a deficiency in somatomedins themselves (Laron dwarfs).[1]

Prolactin

Prolactin (PRL) is the hormone responsible for initiation and maintenance of lactation. Its secreting cells, the *lactotrophs,* are known to experience transient hyperplasia during pregnancy and breast-feeding.[9] Prolactin has additional roles in fetal lung development, subcutaneous fat metabolism, carbohydrate, calcium, and vitamin D metabolism, and suppression of the normal preovulatory surge of LH and FSH.[10] Dopamine is a hypothalamic neurotransmitter that controls the synthesis of PRL through inhibition, hence its name *prolactin inhibition factor (PIF).* There is no known hypothalamic releasing factor for prolactin.

HYPERSECRETION

The hypersecreting lactotroph adenoma (*prolactinoma*) is the most frequently occurring cause of anterior pituitary dysfunction.[1] The tumors may be either micro- or macroadenomas, slow or rapid growers, and producers only of prolactin or of both prolactin and somatotropin.[3] Elevated PRL may also result from removal of dopamine's inhibition of the lactotrophs by a craniopharyngioma, by compression of the pituitary stalk by an adenoma, or by granuloma formation after pituitary stalk section.[11] All of these conditions cause problems with dopamine's movement from the hypothalamus down the pituitary stalk to the anterior pituitary. Drugs such as phenothiazines will block dopamine's action, and some, such as methyldopa, will prevent its synthesis.[2] Patients who are on estrogen therapy or who have primary hypothyroidism may experience hyperprolactinemia due to the stimulatory effect of estrogens and TRH. Other causes of increased prolactin are stress, chronic renal failure, pregnancy, breast stimulation, and chest wall trauma, as well as idiopathic etiology.[2]

HYPOPROLACTINEMIA

The only known clinical significance of low prolactin levels is in the inability of postpartum women to breast-feed. Testing for plasma PRL may provide additional information when panhypopituitarism is the suspected diagnosis.

Panhypopituitarism

Hypopituitarism will present with symptoms related to the cells affected. Such symptoms will not occur, however, until 75% of the cells have been destroyed.[4] Hyposecretion of more than one hormone may result from a pituitary tumor's destruction of the rest of the gland by compression. Both craniopharyngiomas in children and prolactinomas in adults are examples of such tumors. Any factor that destroys the pituitary gland and/or hypothalamus may lead to signs of hypopituitarism. Such factors are listed below. An acute occurrence of pituitary failure is known as *pituitary apoplexy,* and is a rare, often fatal condition. The more common form of hypopituitarism is chronic, with the loss of pituitary hormones following a predictable sequence: STH, LH, and FSH being lost first, with TSH next, and ACTH last.[5]

Antidiuretic Hormone (Vasopressin)

The posterior pituitary (*neurohypophysis*) is a storehouse of hormones produced by the neurons

Factors That May Lead to the Destruction of the Pituitary and/or Hypothalamus

Tumors

Craniopharyngiomas	Meningiomas
Oncocytomas	Trophic cell adenomas
Null cell adenomas	Mammosomatotroph adenomas
Gliomas	

Infections

Tuberculosis	Syphilis
Encephalitis	Meningitis

Granulomas

Vascular

Sheehan's syndrome (postpartum hemorrhage)
Diabetes mellitus
Hypertensive hemorrhage
Aneurysms

Surgery

Radiation

Trauma

of the hypothalamus. *Antidiuretic hormone (ADH, vasopressin, VP)* is a small peptide synthesized by the supraoptic nuclei of the hypothalamus. These neurons produce a carrier protein specific for ADH, and package the hormone and carrier in granules that travel down the axons to the posterior pituitary for storage and subsequent release upon appropriate stimulus (see Fig. 39-1).[1] ADH will be produced and secreted in response to the sensing by osmoreceptors in the hypothalamus of a 1% to 2% increase in plasma osmolality. Baroreceptors in the thorax, in response to a 5% to 10% drop in blood volume or blood pressure, will also stimulate the release of ADH. The baroreceptor response is thought to override the osmoreceptors in instances of significant blood loss, which leads to generalized vasoconstriction and elevated arterial blood pressure.[2] Such an overriding baroreceptor response will occur even in the face of decreased plasma osmolality.[12]

Vasopressin's primary function is to cause the distal tubules and collecting ducts in the kidney to reabsorb free water and thereby concentrate urine. It indirectly regulates electrolyte concentration in plasma, primarily that of sodium.

HYPOFUNCTIONING OF VASOPRESSIN (PRODUCTION/ACTION)

Numerous conditions will stimulate or depress ADH production and action. Each must be included in the differential diagnosis of pathologies associated with the hormone.

A physiological decrease in vasopressin production will be seen in response to hypoosmolality, after exposure to cold and after the ingestion of certain drugs, such as alcohol, dilantin, and glucocorticoids.[4] Pathological hyposecretion may result, most commonly after neurosurgery. If the destruction of the hypothalamus or posterior pituitary leaves enough axons intact, the hyposecretion may be transient. Less commonly, an infection, head trauma, or degenerative or infiltrative lesion of the pituitary or hypothalamus will lead to hyposecretion. Rarely, the cause may be idiopathic.[1] Such hyposecretion is termed *central (or hypothalamic) diabetes insipidus.* If the defect lies in a deficiency in the action of ADH on the kidney, it is termed *nephrogenic diabetes insipidus.* Factors affecting the kidney's response to ADH may be idiopathic, or may include amyloidosis, multiple myeloma, or association with drugs such as lithium, colchicine, demeclocycline, methoxyflurane, or propoxyphene.[2] A third condition may present with symptoms similar to both types of diabetes insipidus, and may be the most difficult to diagnose: *psychogenic polydipsia,* a psychiatric illness characterized by compulsive water-drinking.

HYPERSECRETION OF VASOPRESSIN

Physiological elevation of vasopressin may occur in response to nausea, pain, stress, exercise, sleep, and certain drugs such as nicotine, clofibrate, morphine, vincristine, and barbiturates.[4] Pathological increases may be relative or absolute. Relative increases reflect the normal baroreceptor response to a decrease in blood volume resulting from fluid or electrolyte loss. Paradoxically, this increase in ADH may cause fluid retention in spite of low plasma osmolality, evidence of the overriding effect that the thorax baroreceptors have on the hypothalamic osmoreceptors. Absolute hypersecretion of ADH will be associated with normal or increased blood volume. Forty percent of patients with oat-cell lung carcinoma will produce an ADH-like substance (*ectopic tumors*). Trauma to the central nervous system, some infections, pulmonary diseases, meningitis, or encephalitis may also result in this syndrome of inappropriate ADH production (*SIADH*).[12]

Oxytocin

Oxytocin is similar to vasopressin in structure and mode of synthesis, with the paraventricular nuclei in the hypothalamus being the site of production. Its function is in milk ejection from the breast and contraction of the uterus at parturition. Progestins and stress are believed to inhibit its action. Hyper- and hypooxytocin states are not characterized at present, nor are laboratory assays routinely performed.

CLINICAL MANIFESTATIONS

Acromegaly

Clinical signs and symptoms of acromegaly include history of changes in size of hat, shoes, gloves, or rings; deepened voice; arthralgia; coarsening of facial features (enlarged jaw, nose, tongue); oily, odorous, thickened skin; weight gain; and generalized visceromegaly (see Fig. 39-2). All of these findings reflect proliferation of cartilage, bone, and soft tissue. A concurrent elevation of prolactin, seen in 60% to 87% of females with acromegaly and 27% to 46% of males, results in menstrual disorders, galactorrhea (nipple discharge), and loss of libido and potency. Headache and visual complaints reflect sellar enlargement from tumor growth.[1, 4, 5, 6, 7]

Prolactinemia

Patients with elevated PRL may present with headache (50%) and visual complaints (females <25%; males 33% to 50%) that reflect the presence of adenoma and may be the only presenting signs. Galactorrhea (30% to 80%) reflects PRL stimulation of breast tissue, and amenorrhea (>50%), loss of libido, impotence (84%), obesity, female distribution of body fat in males, and decreased body and facial hair reflect PRL antigonadotropin effect.[11, 13]

Panhypopituitarism

Signs and symptoms of panhypopituitarism reflect the sequential loss of pituitary hormones. The presenting signs, therefore, in order of occurrence in chronic hypopituitarism may include slow growth (if a child) and thin, pale, finely wrinkled skin, which reflect decreased GH. Hypogonadism reflects decreased luteinizing hormone (LH) or follicle-stimulating hormone (FSH), and may be compounded if compression causes hyperprolactinemia. Disproportionate pallor, apathy, inertia, weakness, irritability, and hypothermia reflect decreased thyroid-stimulating hormone (TSH) and adrenocorticotropic hormone (ACTH). Headache and visual complaints are proportional to the tumor size.

Vasopressin Disorders

Regardless of the cause of the decrease of vasopressin, patients will present with polyuria (>2.5 L/24 hr) and insatiable thirst (polydipsia).

With hypersecretion of vasopressin, patients may initially present with complaints that reflect the extent of hyponatremia present: asymptomatic (Na >125 mEq/L [125 mmol/L]); anorexia, nausea, vomiting (Na = 115–125 mEq/L [115–125 mmol/L]); seizures, stupor, coma (Na <115 mEq/L [115 mmol/L]).

LABORATORY ANALYSES AND DIAGNOSIS

Acromegaly

Confirmation of acromegaly does not rely solely on the demonstration of a single elevated plasma GH level. This hormone is produced in short bursts throughout the day, and is best evaluated in a series of measurements over a 24-hour period, or as a part of provocative/suppression testing, using known stimuli or suppressors of GH secretion. The most widely-described tests are listed in Table 39-1. A normal response to a test involving the measurement of GH itself should show a post-stimulus elevation of more than 10 ng/mL (10 μg/L) above basal level. An elevation of 5–10 ng/mL (5–10 μg/L) is considered borderline, and an elevation of less than 5 ng/mL (5 μg/L) should be considered abnormal.[2] Because 20% to 30% of normal patients will be unable to show elevated GH with provocation, additional criteria require that at least two such stimuli be used at separate times, and that patients show no response to the stimulus in *both* tests before the results are considered abnormal.[2] Radioimmunoassay is the method of choice for assaying growth hormone in serum or

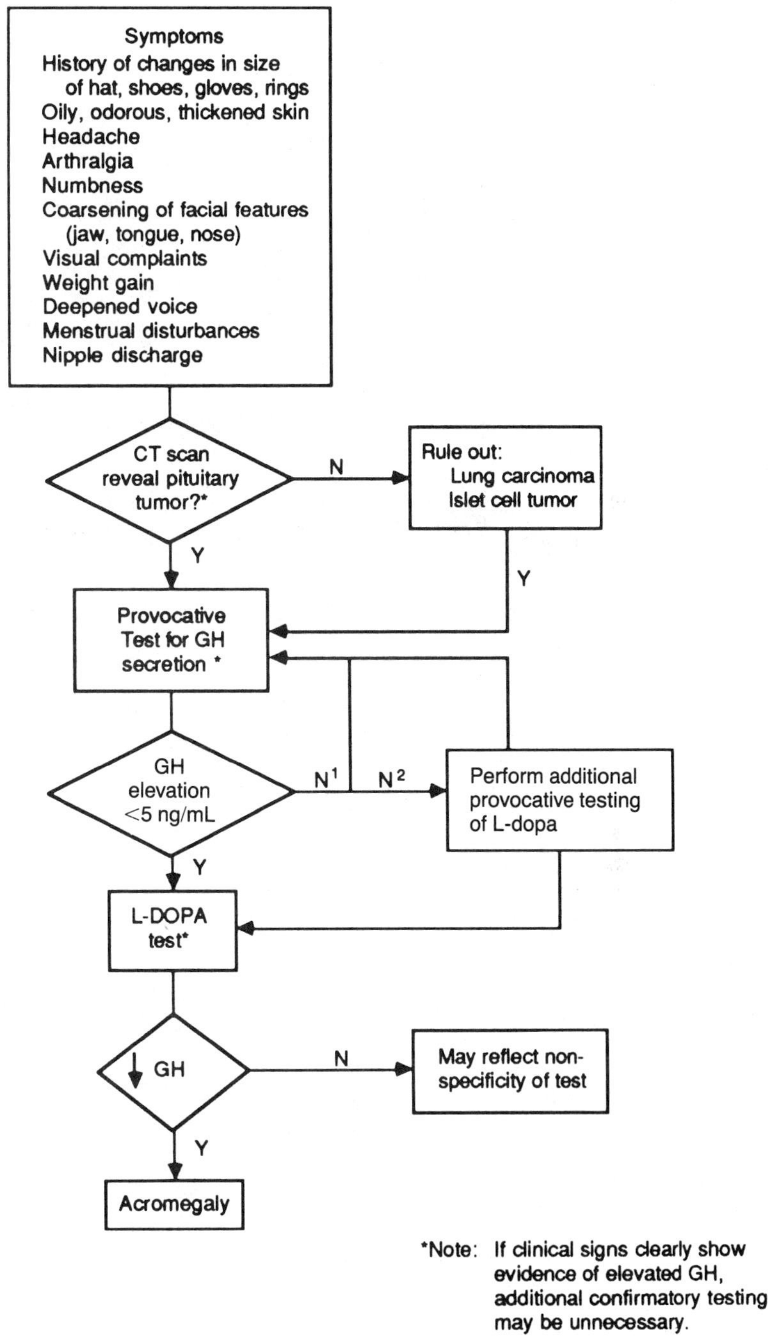

Figure 39-2 Diagnosis of acromegaly.

Table 39-1 ***Provocative Tests for Growth Hormone***

Stimulus	Patient Preparation	Normal Response	Acromegalic Response	Comments	Source*
Exercise		GH > 6 ng/mL	No response		Teitz, p 1022
Arginine (intravenous)	Overnight fast, bed rest	3-fold increase in GH	No response	Limited diagnostic value because response is variable even in health	Teitz, p 1025 Faglia, p 371
Insulin (intravenous)	Overnight fast, bed rest	Cortisol ↑ >7 μg/dL, GH > 20 ng/mL	No response	Valid only if glucose falls to <40 mg/dL or if symptoms develop (sweating, tremors); physician must be in attendance; limited diagnostic value (see arginine)	Teitz, p 1024
Oral Glucose Load	Overnight fast	GH < 5 ng/mL	No response; GH may ↑	Limited value if GH < 2 ng/mL or >10 ng/mL; may be useful postsurgery to reassess GH secretion; failure to show suppression may also be due to intermittent porphyria, metastatic breast carcinoma, chronic renal failure	Faglia, p 371 Gornall, p 137 Davis, p 164
L-dopa (oral)		↑ GH	↓ GH	Most widely used test; less powerful than insulin but also less dangerous	Faglia, p 371
Sulpiride (injection)		No effect	↑ GH	Response disappears postsurgery; therefore, good for diagnosis and followup	Faglia, p 373
TRH (intravenous)		No effect or ↓ GH	↑ GH	Response disappears after successful therapy; may see erratic GH response if patient has liver cirrhosis, chronic renal failure, mental depression, anorexia nervosa, primary hypothyroidism; normal patients may also show ↑ GH	Faglia, p 371

Conversion to SI units is as follows:
GH—ng/mL × 1 = μg/L
Glucose—mg/dL × 0.0555 = mmol/L

* See references.

plasma. Current methods that are sensitive may lack specificity due to the presence of growth hormone variants in patient samples.[14]

Unfortunately, there is not a strict correlation between a basal GH level and disease activity.[7] Somatomedin levels, however, do show good correlation with acromegalic signs before and after therapy. Levels greater than 2.5 U/mL (2500 IU/L) are suggestive of hypersecretion of GH.[7] Being fairly constant in production throughout the day, somatomedins need only be measured singly rather than in a series.[2] Current methods (radioreceptor and radioimmunoassay) for somatomedins will not react equally with all forms of the hormone, and therefore may lack precision.[2]

Other laboratory testing may reveal elevated insulin levels (in 80% of acromegalics), arterial hypertension (in 18% to 48%),[7] and elevated phosphate, alkaline phosphatase, serum/urine calcium, and serum/urine creatinine.[5]

Acromegalics may experience other endocrine difficulties in addition to an elevated GH. Thirty to forty percent of patients will show elevations of prolactin, with 3% to 9% showing thyroid hyperfunction. Adrenal function will usually be normal. Gonadal dysfunction may be an early presenting sign, usually as a reflection of the increased PRL.[7] Conversely, the pituitary adenoma causing the elevated GH may compress adjacent healthy pituitary cells, leading to deficiencies in the other pituitary hormones.[4, 5]

HYPOSECRETION OF GH

Although there are assays for somatomedins, there currently is no testing available for the isolated GH deficiency. Assays for growth hormone-releasing factor (GRF) seem promising.[8] Provocative testing with L-dopa or insulin may be used to observe the lack of GH response in these children. Insulin, although more dangerous, is considered by some to be a better choice of stimulant in those instances in which a panhypopituitarism is suspected, because it can provide information on overall pituitary status.[12]

Prolactinemia

Assessment of hyperprolactinemia should first note a patient history of stress or of dopamine antagonist ingestion. Evaluation of thyroid status for primary hypothyroidism should follow (see Chap. 35). Any history of irritation of the breast or intercostal nerves (thoracotomy, herpes zoster) or of head injury should also be ruled out. Posterior-anterior-lateral skull x-rays will reveal macroadenomas in most cases. Microadenomas, however, may escape attempts at visualization using x-ray, polytomography, or CT scan.[2] Basal levels of prolactin that exceed 200 μg/L (reference interval <20 ng/mL [20 μg/L]) are highly suggestive of an adenoma. Levels between 50 and 200 ng/mL (50 and 200 μg/L) are probably due to a microadenoma.[1] Performance of stimulation tests, using thyrotropin-releasing hormone (TRH) or insulin, are controversial.[14] RIA for the analysis of serum or plasma for prolactin is preferred to bioassay and radioreceptor techniques, because the latter techniques show cross-reactivity with growth hormone (see Fig. 39-3).

Panhypopituitarism

Because hyposecretion of pituitary hormones may be secondary to other endocrine disorders, it is important to exclude first any primary disease of the thyroid, adrenals, or gonads (see Fig. 39-4). Skull x-rays with tomography and CT scans may reveal masses in the sella, with the associated structural changes. A triple bolus hormone test may also be used. The test itself is costly, and interpretation may be difficult. Intravenous insulin, gonadotropin-releasing hormone (GnRH), and TRH are administered to the patient, and timed blood samples are taken for GH, cortisol, LH, FSH, TSH, PRL, and glucose. The test is valid only if glucose levels are suppressed below 40 mg/dL. A physician must be in attendance throughout the testing. Table 39-2 lists the normal and disease responses to the test.[1]

(*Text continues on page 470*)

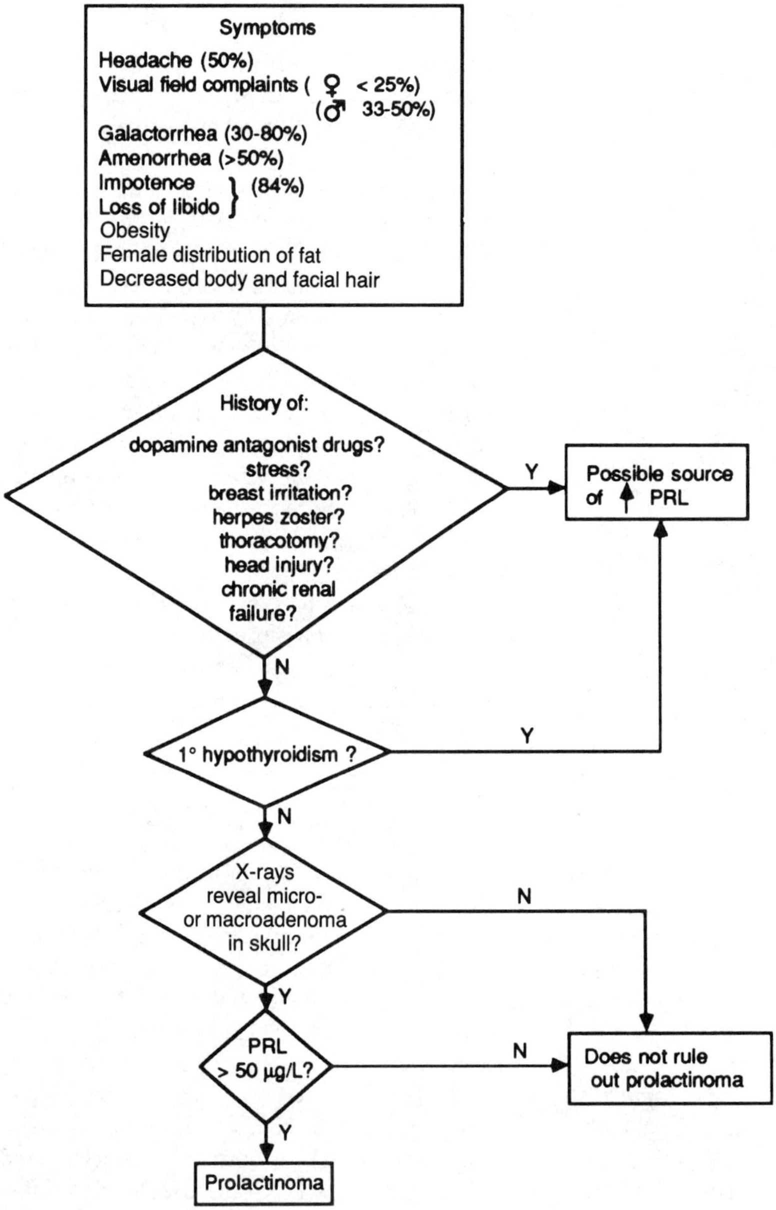

Figure 39-3 Diagnosis of hyperprolactinemia.

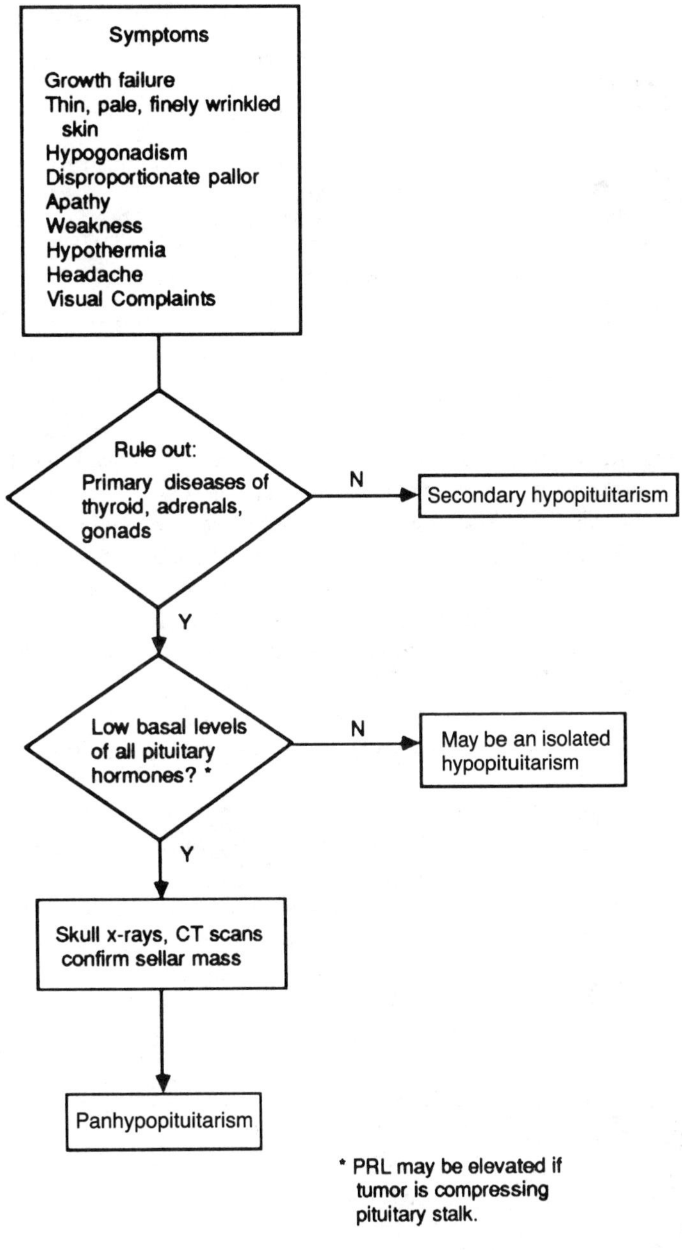

Figure 39-4 Diagnosis of panhypopituitarism.

Table 39-2 ***Responses to the Triple Bolus Hormone Test: Normal vs Hypopituitarism***

Assay	Normal Response	Hypopituitarism
Glucose	Decreased 50% of baseline	Decreased 50% of baseline
GH	Increased > 8 ng/mL (8 μg/L)	No response
Cortisol	Increased > 70 μg/dL (2.0 μmol/L)	No response
PRL	2-fold increase	No response
TSH	Increased > 5 μU/mL (5 mIU/L)	No response
FSH	Increased > 3 mU/mL (3 IU/L)	No response
LH	Increased > 3 mU/mL (3 IU/L)	No response

Vasopressin Disorders

HYPOVASOPRESSIN

Laboratory evaluation of hypovasopressin will rely on the demonstration of inability of the patient to concentrate urine. This is usually done with an overnight (8 hr) water deprivation test. The patient should avoid the use of nicotine, alcohol, and caffeine during this time because they inhibit vasopressin (ADH) action. Plasma and urine osmolalities are measured numerous times throughout the test. Table 39-3 gives expected results for each disorder.[2, 4, 5]

If serum ADH can be measured, a hypertonic saline infusion test may be performed. Normally, patients should experience a rise in ADH as the plasma osmolality rises, with a concurrent increase in urine osmolality and decrease in urine volume. Patients with central diabetes insipidus will have low or normal serum ADH levels that will not change in the presence of hyperosmolality. With nephrogenic diabetes insipidus, the basal ADH level will be elevated initially, and will not change after the infusion. The major disadvantage of this test is the unavailability of serum ADH assays due to method complexity and lack of sensitivity and specificity. The use of osmolality measurements seems to be sufficient, however, for a differential diagnosis. Specimens for osmolality may be serum, heparinized plasma, or unpreserved urine. Removal of all particulate matter must be accomplished. If analysis is delayed, the specimen should be refrigerated (serum, plasma, urine) or frozen (serum, plasma). Urine samples

Table 39-3 ***Response to Water Depletion Test***

Assay	Normal	Central Diabetes Insipidus	Neurogenic Diabetes Insipidus	Psychogenic Polydipsia
Prestimulation				
Plasma osmolality	<300 mOsm/kg	>300	>300	<300
Urine osmolality	>600 mOsm/kg	<270	<270	<270
Urine volume	~1 mL/min	>2 mL/min	>2 mL/min	>2 mL/min
Urine/plasma osmolality ratio	>1	<1	<1	<1
Poststimulation				
Urine osmolality	<5% increase	>5% increase	No change	<5% increase
Urine volume	<0.5 mL/min	<2 mL/min	No change	<0.5 mL/min

should be brought to room temperature before analysis.

Two analytical methods in common use for measurement of osmolality are freezing-point depression and vapor pressure (dew-point temperature) depression. Freezing point osmometers are preferred because they are reported to be more precise, are linear below 200 mOsm/kg H_2O, and will measure volatile solutes such as ethanol, ethylene glycol, methanol, and dissolved CO_2. Vapor pressure osmometers will not. Moreover, freezing-point osmometers will not be affected by lipemia as will vapor pressure osmometers.[2]

HYPERVASOPRESSIN SECRETIONS

Differential diagnosis of hypervasopressin states requires evidence of plasma hyponatremia and hypoosmolality. After any adrenal, thyroid, or renal disease is ruled out, a urine sodium will differentiate between total body sodium depletion (urine Na decreased) and dilutional hyponatremia (urine Na elevated). Comparison of the ratio of urine and plasma osmolalities will show a ratio value of less than one in hyponatremia from excessive fluid intake, while a ratio value of greater than one suggests SIADH. If needed, a water-loading test may be performed. A comparison is made of plasma and urine osmolalities before and after ingestion of a standard amount of water. A urine osmolality of greater than 100 mOsm/kg with less than 90% of the water load excreted confirms a diagnosis of SIADH. As with diabetes insipidus, plasma ADH (which should be high in SIADH) may be measured, but usually is not needed (see Fig. 39-5).

TREATMENT

Acromegaly

Transsphenoidal adenectomy and proton-beam radiation are current therapies for acromegaly.[1] Left untreated, acromegaly may cause severe disability, and death may result from cardiac or neurological complications.[2] As a temporary therapy, the dopamine antagonist bromocriptine will moderate GH levels.[1] Early treatment will reverse many of the abnormalities brought on by the excessive somatotropin; however, as described above, diagnosis will not occur for the majority of patients until the disease has progressed for five to ten years. Table 39-1 lists those tests that will show a reversal of results after successful therapy.

Prolactinemia

Therapeutic success in prolactinemia depends on the size of the adenoma causing the elevated PRL. Transsphenoidal adenectomy is usually successful for microadenomas, but not for large tumors. Dopaminergic antagonists, such as bromocriptine, will cause the disappearance or marked decrease in size of most tumors, and force PRL levels down. After removal of the drug therapy, PRL will rise again with a microadenoma but not with a macroadenoma.[11]

Panhypopituitarism

In panhypopituitarism, surgical excision of a causative tumor may actually result in the destruction of healthy pituitary tissue. Chronic anterior pituitary deficiency is usually irreversible, and requires long-term replacement of all target gland hormones. As in isolated pituitary dysfunction, stimulation or suppression testing of individual hormones may be required to evaluate the success of therapy. To the extent that target gland hormones are successfully replaced, laboratory results will return to normal and typical symptoms will disappear.

Vasopressin Disorders

HYPOVASOPRESSIN SECRETION

For hyposecretion of vasopressin, therapy is directed to reducing polyuria. Nasal sprays with an analog of arginine vasopressin, injectable ADH, or drugs that stimulate the release of or potentiate ADH will be effective for patients with central

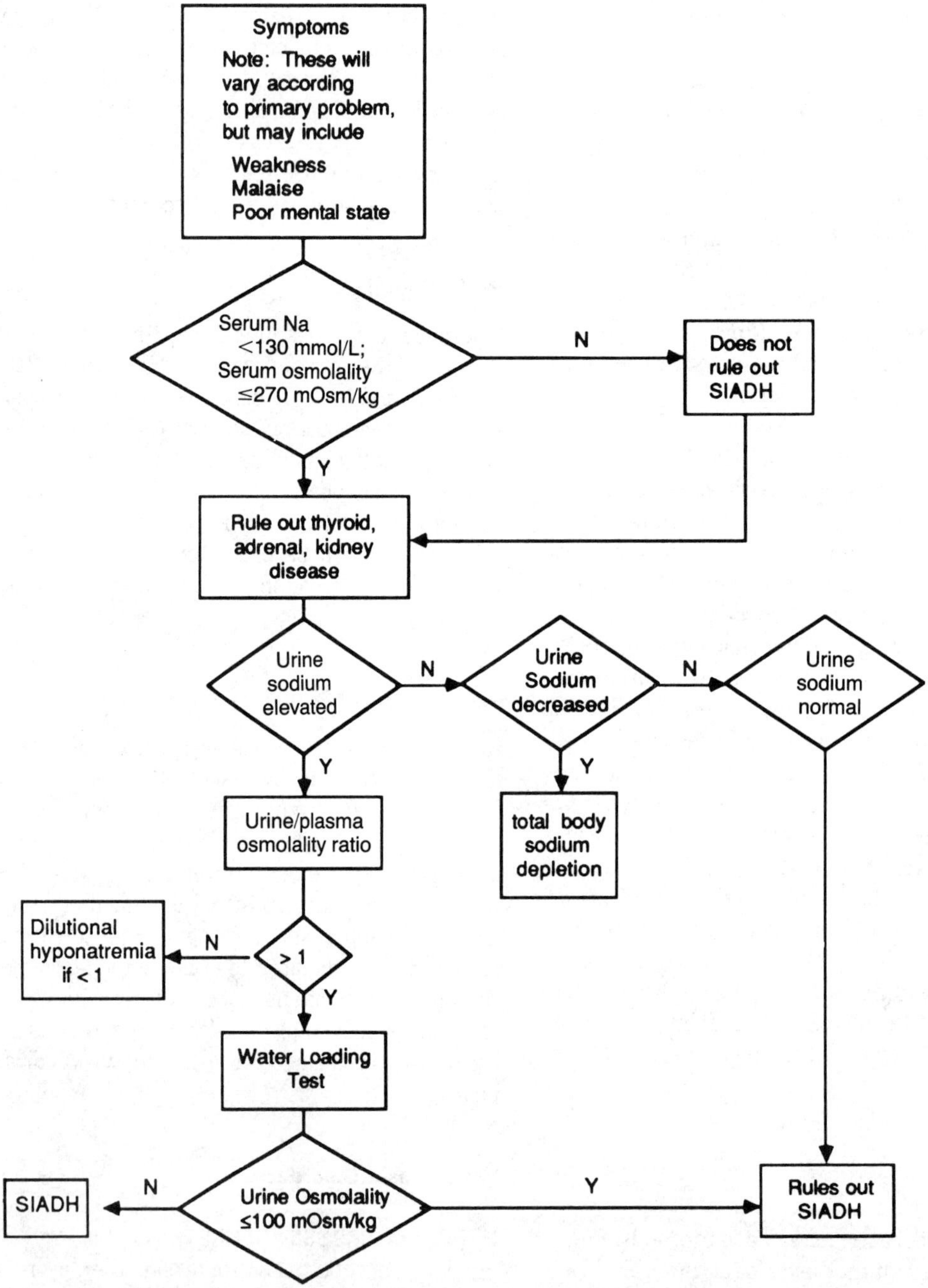

Figure 39-5 Diagnosis of syndrome of inappropriate ADH (antidiuretic hormone) production (SIADH).

diabetes insipidus. Nephrogenic patients respond to diuretics and dietary restrictions of protein and sodium to lower plasma osmolality. Patients with psychogenic polydipsia usually require psychiatric help.[1]

HYPERVASOPRESSIN SECRETION

For hypersecretion of vasopressin, therapy consists of removal of the stimulus of ADH secretion, as in tumor excision and correction of hypovolemia. In lieu of or in addition to this, water restriction or drug therapy may effectively lower ADH and return sodium to normal.

CASE STUDY

A 45-year-old man entered a fertility clinic for evaluation of decreased libido. He and his wife had tried to have a third child without success for the previous 3 years. Physical examination revealed a moderately obese patient with a history of frequent headaches and numerous problems with vision. He spoke of having to shave less frequently, and on further examination his pubic and axillary hair were found to be reduced. There were no other remarkable findings. He denied the use of any drugs except aspirin for his headaches.

Results of the laboratory studies performed follow (reference intervals in parentheses):

LABORATORY FINDINGS

Skull x-rays revealed mass in sella turcica

Analyte	*Result*	*Reference Range*
GH	Undetectable	(<2 ng/mL)
FSH	Undetectable	(4–18 U/d)
LH	Undetectable	(6–23 mU/mL)
TSH	8 μU/mL	(<10 μU/mL)
ACTH (0800 h)	83 pg/mL	(25–100 pg/mL)
PRL	376 ng/mL	(<20 ng/mL)
Testosterone	93 ng/dL	(437–707 ng/dL)

Conversion to SI units is as follows:

GH—ng/mL × 1 = μg/L
FSH—μU/d × 1 = μU/d
LH—mU/mL × 1 = IU/L
TSH—μU/mL × 1 = mIU/L
ACTH—pg/mL × 1 = ng/L
PRL—ng/mL × 1 = μg/L
Testosterone—ng/dL × 0.0347 = nmol/L

Questions

1. What is the probable diagnosis for this patient?
2. Which therapy will most effectively reduce the prolactin level?

Discussion

1. The probable diagnosis is macroprolactinoma, causing a hypopituitarism by compression, as evidenced by decreased GH and gonadotropins.
2. Use of a dopamine antagonist, such as bromocriptine, will decrease the size of the adenoma. There is a good chance that removal of the drug will *not* result in a return of the hyperprolactinemia.

REFERENCES

1. Gornall AG: Applied Biochemistry of Clinical Disorders, p 230. Hagerstown, MD, Harper & Row, 1980
2. Teitz N (ed): Textbook of Clinical Chemistry, p 1019. Philadelphia, WB Saunders, 1986
3. Kovacs K, Horvath E: Morphology of adenohypophyseal cells and pituitary adenomas. In Imura H (ed): The Pituitary Gland, p 27. New York City, Raven Press, 1985
4. Kaplan LA, Pesce AJ: Clinical Chemistry: Theory, Analysis, and Correlation, p 743. St Louis, CV Mosby, 1984
5. Berner JJ: Effects of Diseases on Laboratory Tests, p 161. Philadelphia, JB Lippincott, 1983
6. Wass JAH: Acromegaly. In Belchetz PE (ed): Management of Pituitary Disease, p 123. New York City, John Wiley & Sons, 1984
7. Faglia G, Arosio M, Ambrosi B: Recent advances in diagnosis and treatment of acromegaly. In Imura H (ed): The Pituitary Gland, p 364. New York City, Raven Press, 1985
8. Imura H: Hypopituitarism. In Imura H (ed): The Pituitary Gland, p 519. New York City, Raven Press, 1985
9. Saeger W: Anatomy of the pituitary gland. In

Belchetz PE (ed): Management of Pituitary Disorders, p 9, New York City, John Wiley & Sons, 1984
10. Belchetz PE: Hypopituitarism. In Belchetz PE (ed): Management of Pituitary Disorders, p 117. New York City, John Wiley & Sons, 1984
11. Von Werder K: Recent advances in the diagnosis and therapy of hyperprolactinemia. In Imura H (ed): The Pituitary Gland, p 405. New York City, Raven Press, 1985
12. Bennett BD, Wells DJ: Endocrinology. In Bishop ML, Duben-Von Laufen JL, Fody EP (eds): Clinical Chemistry, p 319. Philadelphia, JB Lippincott, 1985
13. Moult PJA: Hyperprolactinemia. In Belchetz PE (ed): Management of Pituitary Disorders, p 120. New York City, John Wiley & Sons, 1984
14. Davis JC, Hipkin LJ: Biochemical assessment of hormonal status. In Belchetz PE (ed): Management of Pituitary Disease, p 162. New York City, John Wiley & Sons, 1984

Part VIII

REPRODUCTION

Virginia Sullivan Randolph,
Associate Editor

The conditions discussed in the chapters that follow all have the pituitary gonadotropins in common with respect to normal homeostasis and response mechanisms. For some of the conditions, the gonadotropins are related to the etiology of the condition. Although infectious disease processes leading to reproductive dysfunction are not discussed in this section, it is important to consider them in determining the etiology of reproductive dysfunction in the previously normal patient. With respect to infertility, it is important to remember that both partners must be evaluated, and the chapters on both male and female reproductive disorders should be consulted. The chapters on pregnancy and fetal monitoring should be considered together, because the problem pregnancy often leads to the need to monitor the fetus. For this reason, a particular condition may be discussed in both these chapters but from different perspectives. For example, the chapter on pregnancy discusses the involvement and evaluation of the preeclamptic mother, and the chapter on fetal monitoring discusses the evaluation of fetal maturity in case this condition in the mother warrants early delivery of the child.

Chapter 40

Pregnancy

Sharon Jackson

Pregnancy is a special condition that induces many obvious and subtle changes in maternal metabolism and biochemistry. These changes are the natural responses of maternal organs to the increasing demands of the growing fetus and placenta. As a result, many pregestational reference intervals are of limited use during pregnancy. Knowledge of these naturally occurring changes is necessary for correct interpretation of analytical results and for differentiation of normal from pathological conditions.

DIAGNOSIS OF PREGNANCY

The diagnosis of pregnancy may be made based on information obtained from physical examination and results of laboratory tests. The signs and symptoms of pregnancy revealed during an examination are classified into three categories of evidence: presumptive, probable, and positive.

Laboratory assays for pregnancy typically measure *human chorionic gonadotropin (hCG)*, a glycoprotein hormone produced by the developing placenta. Production of hCG begins shortly after implantation, on the 21st to 23rd day of the cycle,[1] increases to a maximum level by 10 weeks of gestation, and then, by the 20th week, falls to a plateau that is maintained throughout the pregnancy (see Fig. 40-1).[2] It should be noted that the results of laboratory tests for hCG do not positively confirm or rule out the diagnosis of pregnancy. A positive test for hCG is not diagnostic of

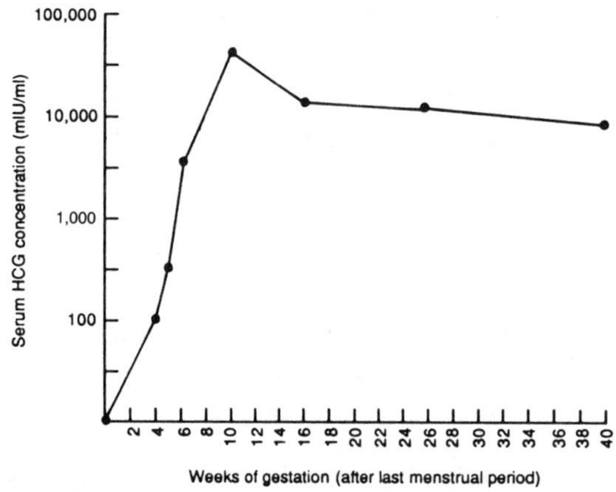

Figure 40-1 Serum human chorionic gonadotropin concentrations during pregnancy.

pregnancy because other conditions, *e.g.*, hCG-producing tumors, may result in hCG production. Likewise, negative results may be obtained if hCG levels are so low as to go undetected by the assay method. Low hCG levels may be found very early in pregnancy or in ectopic or abnormal intrauterine pregnancies.

Immunologic techniques are most often used in the assay of hCG in body fluids. The sensitivity and specificity of these methods are the determining factors in the predictive value of the test. The more sensitive the test, the lower the hCG levels detectable and, therefore, the earlier a pregnancy can be detected. Table 40-1 reviews the sensitivity of several methods for assay of hCG. Caution should be exercised when choosing tests based on sensitivity alone. A test that is very sensitive may not be sufficiently specific and could possibly react with nonhCG substances that may be present in the body fluid being tested.

The specificity of hCG methods is determined by the type of antibody used. Assay methods that use antibodies directed against the entire hCG molecule will cross-react with luteinizing hormone (LH), follicle-stimulating hormone (FSH), and thyroid-stimulating hormone (TSH) because all have similar alpha subunits. Assay methods employing this type of antibody usually adjust the sensitivity so that LH concentrations frequently encountered cannot react.

Because the beta subunits of hCG and LH differ, assay methods that employ antibodies directed against the β-hCG subunit are far more specific, do not cross-react with LH, and therefore discriminate between hCG and LH.

Slide and tube tests employing the technique of hemagglutination inhibition or latex particle agglutination inhibition are generally used as rapid-screening tests for pregnancy and are available in easy-to-use kits. Tube tests require more time and technical skill than do slide tests but, because they are generally more sensitive and yield fewer false negatives, they are used in many home pregnancy test kits.[3] The sensitivity of these tests is such that they become positive 8 to 14 days after the first missed menstrual cycle.[4] Generally, the kits are designed for urine testing. However, kits so formulated have been shown to give false-positive results in the presence of urine protein at a concentration of 0.06 g/dL (0.6 g/L), which is equivalent to a 1+ reading by urine dipstick.[5] Kits formulated to be used with either urine or serum are not similarly affected. It should be noted that the reliability of home pregnancy test kits depends, to a great extent, on strict compliance with written instructions. An increased rate of false negatives

Table 40-1 ***Comparison of the Sensitivities of Immunologic Methods for hCG Measurement***

Test Type	Sensitivity (mIU/mL)	Specimen
Agglutination-inhibition	1000–2000	Urine
β-hCG radioimmunoassay	1–10	Serum
Rapid β-hCG radioimmunoassay	25–150	Serum
Enzyme immunoassay (EIA)	5–25	Serum
Immunoradiometric monoclonal antibody	1.5–5.0	Serum

Reproduced with permission from Tietz NW (ed): Textbook of Clinical Chemistry, Philadelphia, WB Saunders, 1986

has been shown to occur when instructions are not followed exactly.[6]

By far the most sensitive tests for hCG are immunoassay procedures using serum and employing monoclonal antibodies to the beta subunit of the hCG molecule. These tests may become positive as soon as six to eight days after conception.[4] This sensitivity, although rarely necessary for diagnosing an uncomplicated pregnancy, does allow detection of the low hCG levels seen in patients with treated trophoblastic neoplasms and ectopic or abnormal intrauterine pregnancy. The sensitivity of these methods is also useful prior to surgery or administration of medication when pregnancy is a possibility.

UNCOMPLICATED PREGNANCY

Biochemical Changes

Biochemical changes associated with pregnancy may occur during the first, second, and third trimesters, often becoming more pronounced as the pregnancy progresses and returning to pregestational levels within weeks of parturition. Tables 40-2 and 40-3 summarize the biochemical changes that normally occur in uncomplicated pregnancies.

As is shown in Tables 40-2 and 40-3, hormones that appear in the maternal circulation may be derived from both placental and maternal endocrine glands. Generally, the concentration of placental hormones increases with placental mass. Human chorionic gonadotropin (hCG) is the excep-

Table 40-3 ***Biochemical Changes in Uncomplicated Pregnancy***

Analyte	Alteration from Nonpregnant Reference Range
Hormones	
Total T_4	Increased
Free T_4	Normal
Total T_3	Increased
Free T_3	Normal
Thyroxine-binding globulin	Increased
Total serum cortisol	Increased
Cortisol-binding globulin	Increased
Aldosterone	Increased two- to three-fold
Renin	Increased
Angiotensin II	Increased
Parathyroid hormone	Increased
Proteins	
Serum total protein	Decreased
Serum albumin	Decreased
Fibrinogen	Increased approximately 50%
α_1-antitrypsin	Increased
C-reactive protein	Increased
Enzymes	
Alkaline phosphatase	Increased two- to four-fold
Cholinesterase	Decreased
Leucine aminopeptidase	Increased

(Continued on next page)

Table 40-2 ***Hormonal Changes in Maternal Circulation of Placental Origin***

Hormone	Peak Concentration	Trimester
Human chorionic gonadotropin	50,000–100,000 mIU/mL (50,000–100,000 IU/L)	1st
Human placental lactogen	3.6–8.2 μg/mL (3.6–8.2 mg/L)	3rd
Progesterone	100–200 ng/mL (318–636 nmol/L)	3rd
Estrogens:		
Estradiol, total	127–281 pg/mL (466–1031 pmol/L)	3rd
Estriol, total	80–350 ng/mL (278–1214 nmol/L)	3rd
Estriol, free	10–34 μg/mL (35–118 nmol/L)	3rd

Table 40-3 ***Biochemical Changes in Uncomplicated Pregnancy—(Continued)***

Analyte	Alteration from Nonpregnant Reference Range
Lipids	
Total lipids	Increased 46%
Total cholesterol (free and esterified)	Increased 40%
Triglycerides	Increased
Phospholipids	Increased 37%
Free fatty acids	Increased 60%
Lipoproteins	Increased
Glucose	Normal (fasting levels sl ↓)
Electrolytes, Minerals	
Sodium	Normal to slightly decreased
Potassium	Normal to slightly decreased
Calcium, total	Decreased
Iron	Decreased if not supplemented
Renal Function Tests	
GFR (see creatinine clearance)	Increased
Serum urea nitrogen	Decreased
Creatinine	Decreased
Creatinine clearance	Increased (120–150 mL/min)
Blood Gas/Acid-base Parameters	
pCO_2	Decreased
HCO_3	Decreased

tion to the rule. The increases seen in some hormones of maternal origin (cortisol, T_4, T_3) may be explained by the estrogen-associated rise in serum concentration of their respective binding proteins. These hormonal increases are primarily in the bound, not the free, fraction.

The concentration of many plasma proteins is altered as a result of pregnancy. Rising estrogen levels may partly explain the increases seen in ceruloplasmin and thyroxine- and cortisol-binding globulins. With the exception of transferrin, which increases, the pattern of change in certain plasma proteins resembles the changes seen with the so-called "acute phase reactants." Albumin decreases, while α_1-antitrypsin, fibrinogen, several complement components, and C-reactive protein all increase.

The decrease in albumin coupled with a slight increase in globulins results in an albumin/globulin (A/G) ratio similar to that seen in certain hepatic disorders. Although the A/G ratio has been largely replaced by assays for individual protein fractions, the decreased ratio coupled with changes in enzyme activities discussed below points out the importance of careful evaluation of "liver profiles" when hepatic dysfunction is also suspected.

Serum alkaline phosphatase (ALP) activity may rise as much as two- to four-fold over prepregnancy levels during the third trimester. This increase is primarily due to the placental isoenzyme, although there is evidence to suggest that the bone isoenzyme may also contribute to total ALP increases.[7] ALP activity in leukocytes also increases during pregnancy, a response similar to the response frequently seen in inflammatory conditions.

Plasma cholinesterase (ChE) activity decreases during pregnancy, while leucine aminopeptidase (LAP) activity increases. The changes seen in ALP, ChE, and LAP may also be seen in certain hepatobiliary diseases.

A relative hyperlipidemia (as compared with values in nonpregnancy) exists during the latter half of pregnancy. Total lipids, total cholesterol (esterified and nonesterified), triglycerides, free fatty acids, phospholipids, and lipoproteins increase appreciably, ranging from a 37% increase in phospholipids to a 60% increase in free fatty acids.[8] This hyperlipidemia may be the result of increased lipid metabolism, storage, and utilization.

Even though pregnancy is potentially diabetogenic, fasting glucose levels in healthy women decline slightly. Random glucose levels are usually euglycemic. The finding of glycosuria, which is common during pregnancy, can be attributed to an increased glomerular filtration rate and a lowered renal threshold. However, the possibility of impaired carbohydrate metabolism should not be ignored when glycosuria is found.

In addition to increased fetal and placental demand, the changes seen in electrolyte and mineral concentration during pregnancy may result from hemodilution, lowered plasma protein concentration, or increased excretion. In fact, hemodilution may explain the slight decrease in sodium and potassium levels seen during pregnancy even though aldosterone levels are increased.

Changes in calcium levels during pregnancy do not appear to be significantly related to changes in either the concentration of circulating parathyroid hormone or calcitonin levels.[9] Thus the decreased total calcium concentration found during pregnancy is quite probably due to two factors: increased fetal and placental demand, and the decrease in albumin-bound calcium (45% to 50% of total calcium) caused by the decreased albumin concentration. Ionized calcium remains within nonpregnant levels.

During pregnancy, maternal need for iron increases secondary to increased fetal/placental demand and increased maternal erythropoiesis. Iron supplements are therefore needed during pregnancy.

Table 40-4 ***Hematologic Changes in Uncomplicated Pregnancy***

Analyte	Alteration from Nonpregnant Reference Range
Blood volume	Increased by 45%
RBC count	Decreased
Hemoglobin	Decreased
Hematocrit	Decreased
Reticulocytes	Increased
Platelets	Normal to slightly decreased
Erythrocyte sedimentation rate	Markedly increased
Coagulation parameters:	
Fibrinogen	Increased approximately 50%
Factor VII (proconvertin)	Increased
Factor VIII (antihemophiliac globulin)	Increased
Factor IX (Christmas factor)	Increased
Factor X (Stuart factor)	Increased
Partial thromboplastin time	Slightly decreased
Prothrombin time	Slightly decreased
Fibrin split products	Slightly increased
2,3 DPG	Increased

Hematologic Changes

Table 40-4 summarizes the hematologic changes that occur during uncomplicated pregnancies.

Although accelerated erythropoiesis increases the total red cell volume during pregnancy, typically the erythrocyte count as measured manually or by automated counter is slightly decreased over nonpregnant levels because plasma volume expands more rapidly than red cell volume (45% vs 33% respectively). The reticulocyte count and the mean cell volume (MCV) may be increased.

Because plasma volume expands more rapidly than does red cell mass, hemoglobin concentration and hematocrit are decreased. Hemoglobin on average may fall to a concentration of approximately 12.1 g/dL (1.9 mmol/L) from a nonpregnant level of 13.3 g/dL (2.1 mmol/L).[8] A hemoglobin of less than 11.0 g/dL (1.7 mmol/L) rarely occurs in a normal pregnancy, and therefore should be considered abnormal.

COAGULATION FACTORS

Several clotting factors are increased during pregnancy, including fibrinogen and factors VII, VIII, IX, and X. As a result of these increases, the activated PTT and the prothrombin time (PT) are both prolonged as the pregnancy progresses. Fibrinogen increases about 50% and may cause an increased sedimentation rate.

Fibrin/fibrinogen split products increase slightly during pregnancy, possibly as a result of increased fibrinogen and plasminogen and decreased antithrombin III.

COMPLICATIONS OF PREGNANCY

Etiology and Pathophysiology

Abruptio placentae (premature separation of a normally implanted placenta) is a relatively common complication of pregnancy that is especially dangerous to the mother and that can result in fetal or newborn mortality. Abruptio placentae has a frequency of about 1 in every 100 pregnancies, and accounts for approximately 30% of all cases of antepartal bleeding before fetal delivery.

The primary cause of abruptio placentae is unknown. However, certain predisposing factors have been suggested, including vascular injury or stasis, renal disease, pregnancy-induced or chronic hypertension, malnutrition, shortness of the umbilical cord, vasodilation, trauma, and smoking.

The sequence of events leading to the detachment of the placenta from the uterine wall begins with bleeding into the inner lining of the uterine mucosa, the decidua basalis. The hemorrhage may be concealed without an avenue of escape, as in retroplacental bleeding, or it may drain through the cervix, causing an external hemorrhage (see Fig. 40-2). The developing hematoma ultimately results in compression and destruction of the adjacent placental function. The severity of abruptio placentae is directly related to the extent of detachment that occurs.

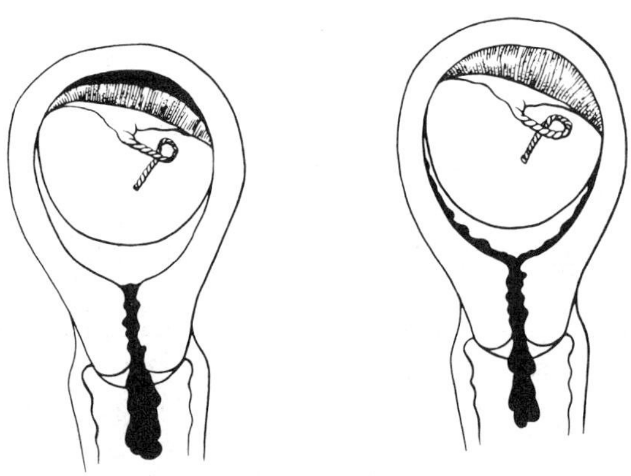

Figure 40-2 Placenta showing (*A*) retroplacental hemorrhage and (*B*) external hemorrhage.

Because the placenta is rich in thromboplastic agents, a consumptive coagulopathy (DIC) often results. The thromboplastic agents enter the maternal circulation and activate the coagulation cascade to fibrin formation. This results in the accelerated consumption and severe depletion of all coagulation factors (especially VIII and X), fibrinogen, and platelets. Fibrinolysis is also initiated with the conversion of plasminogen to plasmin, which exerts a lytic effect on the already depleted coagulation proteins. Fibrin/fibrinogen split products increase in concentration and inhibit fibrin formation. This series of events results in a greatly reduced capacity for coagulation and repair of the initial insult, and severe hemorrhage.

Pregnancy is potentially diabetogenic. This is evidenced by the development of gestational diabetes, the aggravation of diabetes mellitus, and the development of ketoacidotic states during pregnancy. Moreover, the induction and intensification of the condition may be reversible following delivery. In *gestational diabetes,* the condition may disappear following delivery.

While any approximation of the prevalence of *diabetes mellitus* must take into account diagnostic criteria used, generally diabetes mellitus presents as a complication in 1 out of every 300 pregnancies.[1] Diabetes mellitus results from deficient insulin secretion or a resistance to the peripheral action of insulin. While screening should be done on any pregnant woman around the 28th week of gestation, women who are at high risk, *i.e.,* who have a family history of diabetes mellitus, are overweight, or have a previous newborn that weighed more than 10 lb., should be screened early in the pregnancy.

The diabetogenic nature of pregnancy may be explained by the presence of increased levels of glucogenic hormones, namely human placental lactogen, estrogen, progesterone, cortisol, and thyroxine. Human placental lactogen causes a relative peripheral insulin resistance, while cortisol and thyroxine stimulate gluconeogenesis and glycogenolysis respectively. The glucogenic effects of estrogen may be indirectly related to the estrogen-associated rise in thyroxine- and cortisol-binding proteins, and therefore increased total T_4 and cortisol concentration. Additionally, placental insulinase may contribute to the overall diabetogenic state by accelerating insulin degradation.

Implantation of a fertilized ovum anywhere other than in the endometrial lining of the uterine cavity is referred to as an *ectopic pregnancy.* In order of decreasing frequency, the types include tubal (90%–95%), ovarian, cervical, abdominal, and combined (intra- and extrauterine). The frequency of ectopic gestation is approximately 1 in every 75–100 pregnancies. Because *tubal pregnancy* is by far the most common type of ectopic gestation, the remainder of this discussion will be limited to this type.

Factors or conditions that delay or prevent the passage of a fertilized ovum through the uterine tube and into the uterine cavity have been implicated as causes of ectopic pregnancy. Examples include pelvic inflammatory disease (PID), endometriosis, peritubal adhesions, and use of intrauterine contraceptive devices. Additionally, previous ectopic pregnancy has been associated with a high recurrence rate.[10]

The problem in ectopic pregnancy occurs because nonuterine organs cannot adapt to pregnancy. The trophoblast does not remain on the surface but rather penetrates the epithelium and rapidly invades the muscle. Maternal blood vessels are opened, with a resultant internal hemorrhage. As the trophoblast continues to grow, the tubal wall becomes distended and weakened and eventually ruptures.

Hypertensive disorders are among the most common medical complications of pregnancy. *Pregnancy-induced hypertension (PIH),** which for the purposes of this discussion will be limited to *preeclampsia,* is the most common hypertensive disorder of pregnancy. PIH develops in the latter half of pregnancy, usually after 24 to 28 weeks of gestation. Although PIH may occur prior to 20 weeks of gestation, as in association with a large and rapidly growing hydatidiform mole, generally hypertension that occurs prior to 20 weeks of gestation is considered to be preexisting or chronic hypertension. While there are admittedly wide variations in estimations of the incidence of PIH, due to such factors as method of diagnosis and proportion of primigravidas in the population, the incidence of PIH ranges from 6% to 8%.

Pregnancy-induced hypertension is an enigmatic disorder. There are any number of theories that have suggested possible causes of the disease.[11] The exact cause of PIH is still not known. Some suggested predisposing factors include diabetes mellitus, vascular and renal disease, malnutrition, nulliparity, pleural gestation, chronic hypertension, hydatidiform mole, fetal hydrops, hydramnios, and worms.

Currently, theories on the pathophysiology of PIH include increased vasoconstrictor tone (due to an increased responsiveness to the pressor effects of vasoactive agents such as angiotensin II), abnormal prostaglandin action (possibly due to reduced prostaglandin—especially prostacyclin—generation), and possible immunologic factors. Whatever the actual cause, PIH is characterized by intense vasospasm of peripheral arterioles that leads to ischemia, especially in renal, cerebral, and uteroplacental vascular beds. The degree of the vasospasm appears to be directly proportional to the severity of the disease.

*The terminology *toxemia of pregnancy* has been replaced with the more descriptive *pregnancy-induced hypertension,* which includes hypertension without proteinuria or edema, preeclampsia (hypertension with proteinuria and edema), and eclampsia (hypertension with proteinuria, edema, and convulsions).

Clinical Manifestations

The signs and symptoms of *abruptio placentae* may vary considerably (see Table 40-5). Women with milder, more common forms pose additional difficulties for diagnosis because symptoms may be subclinical. Physical symptoms in severe abruption include uterine pain, tenderness at the site of abruption, and petechiae of the uterus. External bleeding may or may not be present, and may not correlate with the amount of separation. Hypertonic, painful, and dysrhythmic uterine contractions, maternal anemia, fetal distress as evidenced by fetal heart sounds, shock, DIC, and coagulation defects may also be present.

The clinical symptoms of *gestational diabetes* are similar to the classical symptoms of *diabetes mellitus*. They include persistent hyperglycemia, glycosuria, polyuria, and polydipsia.

Unfortunately, there are no specific signs or symptoms that are diagnostic for *ectopic pregnancy* prior to rupture, and the clinical picture is at best variable. Women are frequently asymptomatic or mildly symptomatic prior to distention and rupture. Amenorrhea and vaginal spotting or bleeding may be present.

With distention and rupture, the symptoms include severe abdominal pain, abnormal uterine bleeding, and an adnexal mass. The percentage of cases that present with abdominal pain, abnormal uterine bleeding, and amenorrhea has been found to be 95% to 100%, 55% to 84%, and 68% to 86% respectively.[12]

Table 40-5 ***Signs and Symptoms Associated with Severe Abruptio Placentae***

Sign or Symptom	Frequency (%)
Vaginal bleeding	78
Uterine tenderness or back pain	66
Fetal distress	60
High-frequency contractions	34
Hypertonus	
Idiopathic premature labor	22
Dead fetus	15

Reprinted from reference number [8]

The classic triad of symptoms in *preeclampsia* includes hypertension, edema, and proteinuria. These symptoms present in varying intensity, leading to classification of the condition as mild or severe.

In addition to the symptoms of preeclampsia, *eclampsia* is characterized by convulsions. Physical symptoms may include headaches and visual disturbances, epigastric or right upper quadrant pain, nausea, vomiting, and oliguria.

Laboratory Analyses and Diagnosis

In *abruptio placentae,* thromboplastic agents released from the separated placenta may cause a consumptive coagulopathy; therefore, coagulation studies are critical. In suggested order, these include measurement of (1) PTT, PT, and fibrinogen, (2) platelet count, and (3) fibrin split products.

For both the PTT and the PT, sufficient amounts of Factors V and X as well as fibrinogen and thromboplastin must be present in order to have normal results. More specifically, the PTT enables evaluation of intrinsic clotting factors (VIII, IX, XI, and XII), whereas the PT enables evaluation of extrinsic clotting factors (VII). Both the PTT and the PT may be markedly prolonged in severe abruptio placentae.

Generally, when the PTT and PT are abnormal, other indices of coagulative abilities are usually abnormal. Fibrinogen levels are markedly decreased, with a concentration of less than 100 mg/dL (1 g/L) considered indicative of severe placental abruption. However, because the fibrinogen concentration may be elevated as a result of the pregnancy itself, "normal" concentrations of fibrinogen may be encountered in less severe cases of placental abruption. The thrombin time, which is unaffected by deficiencies in either the intrinsic or the extrinsic systems, may be more useful in extreme emergencies as an indication of relative fibrinogen concentration than will fibrinogen quantitation. Fibrinogen quantitation by precipitation or fibrin isolation is time-consuming. Immunochemical determinations of fibrinogen give quicker results, but their reliability depends on the purity of the antibody used and accurate standardization. Fibrin/fibrinogen split products are typically increased because plasmin acts on both fibrin formed from fibrinogen and the unconverted fibrinogen. Typically, a reduced platelet count and a normochromic, normocytic anemia may also be present.

It should be emphasized that all of the laboratory results mentioned occur more commonly in classic, severe placental abruption in which fetal death occurs, and are much less common in cases in which the fetus survives.

Diagnosis of *diabetes mellitus* depends on the results of laboratory tests of carbohydrate metabolism. These include a fasting blood glucose, two-hour postprandial (PP) glucose, and the glucose tolerance test (GTT), including both serum or plasma and urine. Figure 40-3 shows a scheme for screening diabetes in pregnancy during the first trimester. The procedure may be adapted for second-trimester screening by beginning with the two-hour PP test.

Because urine contains both carbohydrate- and noncarbohydrate-reducing substances, reduction tests for *glycosuria* are not recommended. Glycosuria is better evaluated by reagent dipsticks specific for glucose, i.e., those that incorporate glucose oxidase or other glucose specific enzymes in the reagent testing area. In any case, the finding of glycosuria alone is not diagnostic of diabetes mellitus in pregnancy because pregnant females often have a lowered renal threshold for glucose.

The reliability of the glucose tolerance test depends on correct patient preparation and proper specimen collection (*e.g.*, timing, preservation).

It should be emphasized that criteria for the interpretation of GTT results for diagnosis of *gestational diabetes* are different from the criteria used for classic diabetes mellitus (see Fig. 40-3).

The most important biochemical finding in an *ectopic pregnancy* is the presence of hCG at concentrations lower than that anticipated for a normal pregnancy of equal gestation. Additionally, repeat hCG testing may yield valuable information concerning the slope of the increase of β-hCG levels in suspected *tubal pregnancy*. Normally, β-hCG levels should approximately double every 2 to 3 days, up to a maximal level at 10 weeks. If this fails to occur, there is a strong possibility that the pregnancy is ectopic. This is not, however, diagnostic for ectopic pregnancy because the same phenomenon can be observed in cases of threatened abortion of an intrauterine pregnancy. However, failure of hCG doubling coupled with the symptoms previously mentioned provides a strong case for the diagnosis of ectopic pregnancy.

In order to detect the low hCG levels seen in ectopic pregnancy, very sensitive yet specific assay methods should be used. RIA assays to the beta subunit of the hCG molecule provide such sensitivity and specificity. RIA β-hCG assays have been developed with sensitivities in the range of 5–10 mIU/mL. Unfortunately, the more sensitive an hCG assay, the more time needed to perform the assay. Thus, the use of less sensitive, faster assay methods may be indicated in emergencies.

Hematologic parameters may support the diagnosis of ruptured ectopic pregnancy. Following an acute hemorrhage, possible findings include a normochromic, normocytic anemia, slightly reduced hemoglobin or hematocrit, normal to slightly increased leukocyte count, and slightly increased erythrocyte sedimentation rate. Both biochemical and hematologic alterations return to normal within two weeks of removal of the pregnancy.

There are several conditions with presenting symptoms similar to a ruptured ectopic pregnancy, including salpingitis, appendicitis, and abortion of an intrauterine pregnancy. Laboratory data can be useful in the differential diagnosis of these conditions. However, caution should be exercised when interpreting the results of laboratory tests. While hCG levels are absent in salpingitis and appendicitis, negative values may also be obtained with ectopic pregnancies, depending on the sensitivity

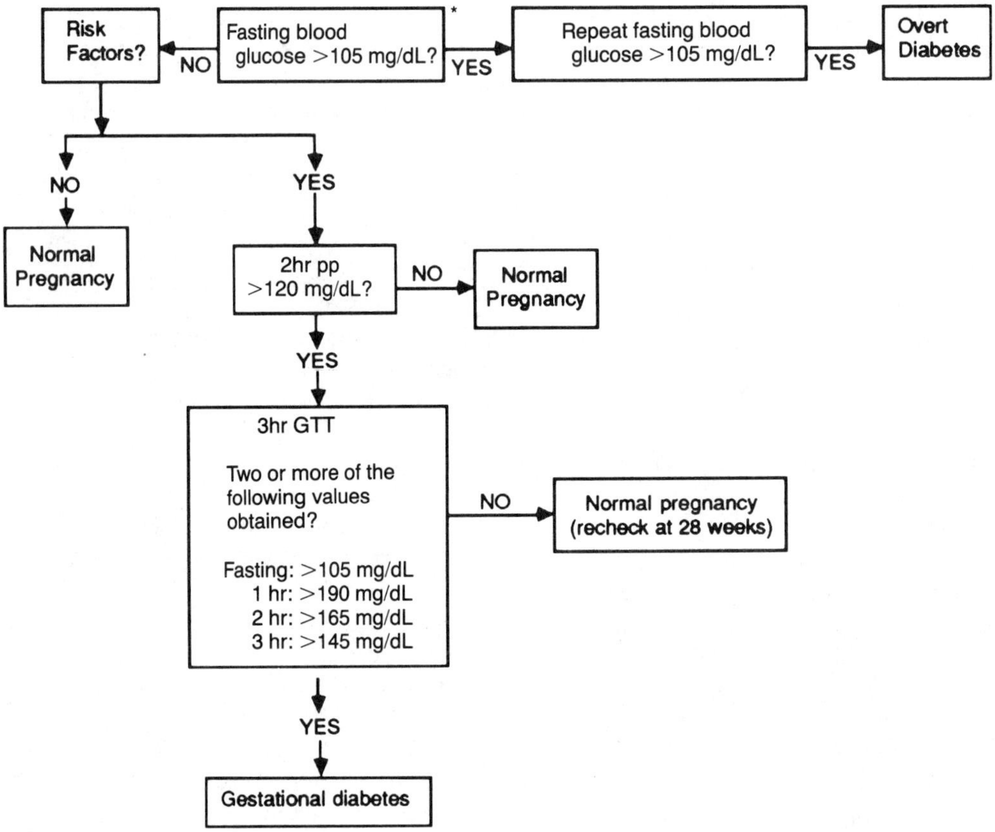

* Convert glucose values to SI units as follows:
mg/dL glucose × 0.0555 = mmol/L

Figure 40-3 **Schematic for screening of diabetes mellitus in first trimester.**

of the assay method. Detectable hCG levels are found in both ectopic pregnancy and abortion of an intrauterine pregnancy. Elevated amylase activity and leukocytosis, long hallmarks of acute appendicitis, may also be found in some cases of ruptured ectopic pregnancy. Thus, for differential diagnosis, laboratory tests must be augmented with other diagnostic aids such as laparoscopy, sonography, patient history, and physical symptoms.

Preeclampsia is a progressive disease in which the pathophysiology precedes the recognition and diagnosis by weeks to months. It is diagnosed when two out of three of the following conditions are present during the second half of pregnancy:

1. A blood pressure of >140/90 mm Hg on at least two occasions six or more hours apart, or a rise in systolic pressure of 30 mm Hg and/or diastolic pressure of 15 mm Hg
2. Edema of >1 kg/week
3. Proteinuria (≥1+ by dipstick or ≥300 mg/24 hours) on two occasions 6 or more hours apart

Although the concentrations of several laboratory analytes may be altered as a result of preeclampsia (see Table 40-6), there are inherent problems in using these alone either to establish or to rule out the diagnosis of preeclampsia. First, such results are not specific for preeclampsia. An elevated

Table 40-6 ***Biochemical Changes Associated With Preeclampsia-Eclampsia***

Analyte	Alteration
Albumin	Decreased
Uric acid	Increased
BUN	Increased
Creatinine	Increased
Sodium (plasma)	Increased
AST, ALT	Increased
GFR	Decreased
Urine protein	Increased

BUN, creatinine, and uric acid along with a decreased creatinine clearance may be caused by an underlying renal disease. When epigastric or right upper quandrant pain, nausea, vomiting, and abnormal liver function test results (*i.e.*, bilirubin, AST, ALT, ALP, LD) exist, preeclampsia may be confused with hepatobiliary dysfunction.

Second, these tests are not sufficiently sensitive to detect preeclampsia in its early stages. For example, proteinuria, described previously, is the most useful laboratory test in the diagnosis of the condition. However, proteinuria is usually a late sign. Cases have been documented in which convulsions have occurred without significant proteinuria. Additionally, proteinuria is a common finding in normal pregnancy.

Third, biochemical and hematologic changes that occur normally during pregnancy may mask the often subtle changes in concentration listed in Table 40-6. The glomerular filtration rate (GFR) normally rises in pregnancy. Thus the GFR, as measured by the creatinine clearance, may be misleading because the 25% to 50% decrease observed during preeclampsia may still result in a value above nonpregnant levels.

Hematologic changes such as seen with decreased to absent pregnancy hypervolemia, intravascular hemolysis, and coagulation abnormalities are frequently associated with preeclampsia. Hypofibrinogenemia, thrombocytopenia, and increased fibrin split products may or may not be present. These findings are more often seen in the more severe form of the disorder.

There is no one laboratory test or profile that is consistently accurate in the diagnosis of preeclampsia-eclampsia. However, laboratory tests commonly performed certainly may be used to help support the diagnosis of preeclampsia-eclampsia in the appropriate clinical setting.

Treatment

Treatment of *abruptio placentae* depends on the status of the mother and fetus. With severe abruption, fetal distress, and bleeding, prompt delivery is indicated. Fresh whole blood, cryoprecipitate, frozen plasma, platelet, and electrolyte solution transfusion may be indicated for severe maternal hemorrhage, anemia, and depleted coagulation factors. Following transfusion, coagulation studies may return to within reference ranges. Following delivery, coagulation factors return to within reference ranges spontaneously within 24 hours, with the exception of platelets, which take from 2 to 4 days to reach normal levels.[8]

In the treatment of *gestational diabetes,* usually by diet alone, measurement of the glycosylated hemoglobin level (Hgb A1C) is most useful for monitoring the effectiveness of glycemic control. When exposed to high plasma glucose concentrations, the beta chain of the hemoglobin molecule binds irreversibly with glucose. The glycosylated hemoglobin remains in the circulation for the life span of the erythrocyte, and therefore reflects inadequate control weeks to months preceding the test. Normal glycosylated hemoglobin (A1C) ranges from 3% to 6%, but may rise as high as 18% to 20% with prolonged hyperglycemia.

Treatment of *pregnancy-induced hypertension* varies according to the severity of the process. In mild cases, antihypertensives only may be used, while severe cases may require hospitalization and evacuation of the uterus if central nervous system involvement occurs. Proteinuria usually disappears within a few weeks after termination of pregnancy.[13]

CASE STUDY

A 33-year-old, gravida 1, para 1 white woman was brought to the antepartum unit of labor and delivery with a twin gestation of 36 weeks. Physical examination at her physician's office immediately prior to admission revealed a blood pressure of 154/92 (baseline blood pressure on first prenatal visit: 110/58), and notable pitting edema of the lower extremities. The remainder of the physical examination was normal. The patient's prenatal history was otherwise unremarkable. Initial laboratory data upon admission and data obtained 8 hours after admission are shown in the table below.

As the day progressed, the patient's antepartum course worsened, with the baseline blood pressure increasing to 180/110. The patient began to complain of headaches, dizziness, and seeing "spots" before her eyes. The patient was delivered by cesarean section. Laboratory data immediately following the C-section is shown below.

LABORATORY FINDINGS

Analyte	**Initial**	**8 hours**	**Post-C-Section**
Na, mmol/L	136	137	134
K, mmol/L	3.6	3.6	3.5
Glucose, mg/dL	88	85	86
BUN, mg/dL	20	21	23
Creatinine, serum, mg/dL	1.2	1.2	1.3
Uric acid, mg/dL	8.4	8.4	8.4
Total protein, g/dL	4.7	3.2	3.2
Albumin, g/dL	3.0	2.4	2.4
Bilirubin, mg/dL	1.3	1.3	1.3
AST, IU/L	19	20	20
ALT, IU/L	18	20	20
ALP, IU/L	419	–	–
LD, IU/L	254	–	–
24-hour urine protein, g/24 hours	2.08	–	–
Creatinine clearance, mL/min	88	–	–
PT, seconds (control: 12 s)	12	12	14
APTT, seconds (control: < 40 s)	41	42	50
Fibrinogen, mg/dL	500	450	90
Platelet count, cells/mm^3	150,000	90,000	25,000
Fibrin split products, μ/mL	normal		40

Convert to SI units as follows:
Glucose—mg/dL × 0.0555 = mmol/L
BUN—mg/dL × 0.357 = mmol/L
Creatinine—mg/dL × 88.4 = μmol/L
Uric acid—mg/dL × 0.059 = mmol/L
Protein—g/dL × 10 = g/L
Fibrinogen—mg/dL × 0.01 = g/L
Bilirubin—mg/dL × 17.1 = μmol/L

Questions

1. What was the most likely provisional diagnosis upon admission of the patient?
2. What is the significance of the elevations in serum creatinine, BUN, and uric acid?
3. Are the results of the creatinine clearance compatible with those for serum creatinine, BUN, and uric acid?
4. What is the significance of the change in coagulation studies?

Discussion

1. The presence of hypertension (154/92), proteinuria, and edema is strongly suggestive of preeclampsia (pregnancy-induced hypertension).
2. The elevations in BUN, serum creatinine, and uric acid suggest renal dysfunction, *i.e.*, decreased glomerular filtration secondary to preeclampsia.
3. The normal range for creatinine clearance in nonpregnant women is 88–128 mL/min. However, the creatinine clearance normally increases during pregnancy to 120–150 mL/min. Thus, this creatinine clearance of 88 mL/min is abnormal (decreased), and therefore compati-

ble with the other indices of decreasing renal function secondary to preeclampsia.

4. The decreasing platelet count and fibrinogen level, prolonged PT and APTT, and increased fibrin split products indicate that the preeclampsia is being further complicated by disseminated intravascular coagulation.

REFERENCES

1. Benson C: Handbook of Obstetrics and Gynecology, 8th ed, pp 62, 365. Los Altos, CA, Lange Medical Publ, 1983
2. Speroff L, Glass RH, Kase G: Clinical Gynecologic Endocrinology and Infertility, 3rd ed, p 286. Baltimore, Williams & Wilkins, 1983
3. Han JT et al: An evaluation of the sensitivity of five home pregnancy tests to known concentrations of human chorionic gonadotropin. Am J Obstet Gynecol 144(7): 778–782, 1982
4. Greene MF et al: Biochemical aspects of pregnancy. In Tietz NW (ed): Textbook of Clinical Chemistry. Philadelphia, WB Saunders, 1986
5. Cadoff E et al: Effect of urinary proteins on in vitro immunological tests for pregnancy. Am J Med Technol 49(3): 173–176, 1983
6. Valanis BG et al: Home pregnancy testing kits: Prevalence of use, false-negative rates, and compliance with instructions. Am J Public Health 72(9): 1034–1036, 1982
7. Adeniyi FA et al: Origins and significance of the increased plasma alkaline phosphatase during normal pregnancy and preeclampsia. Br J Obstet Gynaecol 91(9): 857–862, 1984
8. Pritchart JA, MacDonald PC, Gant NF: Williams Obstetrics, 17th ed, pp 190–192, 406. Norwalk, Connecticut, Appleton-Century-Crofts, 1985
9. Pedersen EB et al: Calcium, parathyroid hormone, and calcitonin in normal pregnancy and preeclampsia. Gynecol Obstet Invest 18(3): 156–164, 1984
10. DeCherney AH et al: Ectopic pregnancy. Clin Obstet Gynecol 28(2): 365–374, 1985
11. Worley RJ: Pathophysiology of pregnancy-induced hypertension. Clin Obstet Gynecol 27(4): 821–835, 1984
12. Quan MA et al: The diagnosis of pregnancy. Am Fam Physician 31(2): 201–207, 1985
13. Hollenberg NK: Vascular injury to the kidney. In Petersdorf RG et al (eds): Harrison's Principles of Internal Medicine, p 1665. New York City, McGraw-Hill, 1983

BIBLIOGRAPHY

Abdella TN et al: Relationship of hypertensive disease to abruptio placentae. Obstet Gynecol 63(3): 365–370, 1984

Bartl W et al: Evaluation and correlation of hormone levels in normal and pathologic pregnancies. Biol Res Pregnancy Perinatol 5(4): 143–148, 1984

Berg B et al: Reference values for serum components in pregnant women. Acta Obstet Gynecol Scand 63(7): 583–586, 1984

Chesley L: History and epidemiology of preeclampsia-eclampsia. Clin Obstet Gynecol 27(4): 801–820, 1984

Clemetson CA et al: Abruptio placentae. Int J Gynaecol Obstet 19(6): 453–460, 1981

Devoe SJ et al: Clinical manifestations and diagnosis of pregnancy-induced hypertension. Clin Obstet Gynecol 27(4): 836–853, 1984

Gilabert J et al: Abruptio placentae and disseminated intravascular coagulation. Acta Obstet Gynecol Scand 64(1): 35–39, 1985

Golan A et al: Human chorionic gonadotropin in the ectopic gestation. Int J Gynaecol Obstet 23(1): 65–69, 1985

Hayes PM et al: Plasma volume determination in normal and preeclamptic pregnancies. Am J Obstet Gynecol 151(7): 958–966, 1985

Javanovic L et al: Screening for gestational diabetes. Diabetes 34(Suppl 2): 21–23, 1985

Kletsky OA et al: Dynamics of human chorionic gonadotropin, prolactin, and growth hormone in serum and amniotic fluid throughout normal human pregnancy. Am J Obstet Gynecol 151(7): 878–884, 1985

Madsen H et al: Red cell 2,3-diphosphoglycerate and hemoglobin-oxygen affinity during normal pregnancy. Acta Obstet Gynecol Scand 63(5): 399–402, 1984

Marquette GP et al: Efficacy of screening for diabetes. Am J Perinatol 2(1): 7–9, 1985

McFarland CF et al: Clinical value of glycosylated serum protein and glycosylated hemoglobin in the diagnosis of gestational diabetes mellitus. Obstet Gynecol 64(4): 516–518, 1984

Moniz CF et al: Normal reference ranges for biochemical

substances relating to renal, hepatic, and bone function in fetal and maternal plasma throughout pregnancy. J Clin Pathol 38(4): 468–472, 1985

Moutquin JM et al: A prospective study of blood pressure in pregnancy: Prediction of preeclampsia. Am J Obstet Gynecol 151(2): 191–196, 1985

Pitkin RM: Calcium metabolism in pregnancy and the perinatal period: A review. Am J Obstet Gynecol 151(1): 99–109, 1985

Pittaway DE et al: Doubling times of human chorionic gonadotropin increase in early viable uterine pregnancies. Am J Obstet Gynecol 152(3): 299–302, 1985

Quan MA et al: The diagnosis of pregnancy. Am Fam Physician 31(2): 202, 1985

Rasor JL et al: An evaluation of 10 kits for the determination of hCG in serum. Clin Chem 29(10): 1828–1831, 1983

Romen Y et al: C-reactive protein in pregnancy and in the post partum period. Am J Obstet Gynecol 151(3): 380–383, 1985

Romero R et al: The effect of different human chorionic gonadotropin assay sensitivity on screening for ectopic pregnancy. Am J Obstet Gynecol 153(1): 72–76, 1985

Ryder KW et al: An evaluation of four serum tests for pregnancy. Am J Med Technol 49(3): 561–563, 1983

Senterfit LB et al: Early pregnancy testing: A comparison of hemagglutination inhibition and radioreceptor assay. Am J Med Technol 48(2): 145–147, 1982

Shaarawy M et al: A simple method for the early detection of pregnancy: (A) Comparative study with RIA beta-hCG; and (B), fallacies compared to other immunological pregnancy tests. Contraception 25(4): 375–386, 1982

Sill PR et al: Platelet values during normal pregnancy. Br J Obstet Gynaecol 92(5): 480–483, 1985

Tietz W (ed): Clinical Guide to Laboratory Tests. Philadelphia, WB Saunders, 1983

Tietz W (ed): Textbook of Clinical Chemistry. Philadelphia, WB Saunders, 1986

Weckstein LN et al: Accurate diagnosis of early ectopic pregnancy. Obstet Gynecol 65(3): 393–397, 1985

Widmann FK: Clinical Interpretation of Laboratory Tests, 9th ed. Philadelphia, FA Davis, 1983

Chapter 41

Fetal Monitoring

Kerry Upton

Fetal monitoring is required when any condition, whether of maternal or of fetal origin, may have a detrimental effect on the fetus. By careful monitoring, the effect may be determined and action taken at the appropriate time in the pregnancy.

DEVELOPMENT OF AMNIOTIC SAC

Around the 7th or 8th day of development of the normal ovum, the amnion develops into a small sac that covers the dorsal surface of the embryo. As the embryo grows, it gradually prolapses into the amniotic cavity. The amnion comes in contact with the internal surface of the chorion as the sac enlarges. These two membranes are slightly adherent, although unconnected. Thickness of the normal amnion ranges from 0.02 to 0.5 mm.[1] There are no blood vessels or nerves in the amnion, and no definite lymphatic channels have been found. Exchange of fluids and electrolytes across the membrane occurs passively.

BIOCHEMISTRY OF AMNIOTIC FLUID

The amniotic sac fills with fluid from a number of sources, primarily the placenta, fetal kidneys, and fetal skin and membranes. Biochemical changes in the amniotic fluid during pregnancy reflect the contributions from these sources. The fluid bathing the fetus prevents desiccation and serves as a cushion against physical shocks.

During the first half of pregnancy, amniotic fluid concentrations of sodium, chloride, and urea are closer to those in fetal serum than to those in maternal serum. At this stage of development, the fetal skin is permeable. Sodium and water can pass through the skin before keratinization occurs at about 20 weeks of gestation.[2] During this time, amniotic fluid is essentially an extension of the fetal extracellular fluid space. The sodium concentration in amniotic fluid is lower than that in fetal serum and the urea concentration is higher, suggesting that even this early in pregnancy small amounts of fetal urine influence the final composition.

During the second half of pregnancy, fetal skin is impermeable because of keratinization, and the composition of amniotic fluid is influenced predominantly by fetal urine. This is reflected by a decrease in osmolality and sodium concentrations and an increase in urea and creatinine as pregnancy progresses.[3] Phospholipids from the fetal lungs enter the amniotic fluid through respiratory movements made by the fetus.

The volume of amniotic fluid increases throughout pregnancy, reaching a maximum of about one L at 36 to 38 weeks of gestation. Fetal swallowing and urine production significantly influence fluid volume, and large individual variations are common. In cases in which fetal swallowing is impaired, such as anencephaly or esophageal atresia, an excess of amniotic fluid known as *polyhydramnios* develops. *Oligohydramnios,* a small amount of amniotic fluid, is seen in cases of fetal urinary tract obstruction.

AMNIOCENTESIS

Most fetal monitoring assays require a sample of amniotic fluid for testing. The fluid is usually obtained by transabdominal or vaginal amniocentesis. Transabdominal amniocentesis is the method most widely used and recommended. Generally, amniocentesis is not performed before the 16th week of gestation,[4] after which time it becomes easier to obtain a volume of fluid adequate for testing. Amniotic fluid obtained during the second trimester of pregnancy is used for genetic screening. Specimens obtained during the third trimester are most often used for monitoring the severity of Rh disease and assessing fetal pulmonary maturity.

Several risks are involved with the technique of amniocentesis: trauma to the fetus or placenta, infection, vaginal leakage of amniotic fluid, and premature labor or abortion. Damage to the placenta resulting in fetal–maternal transfusion and possible Rh sensitization of the mother is considered to be the major risk. This risk is lessened by the use of ultrasonography prior to amniocentesis to locate the placenta and the ideal site of puncture. Maternal sensitization may be reduced if all unsensitized Rh-negative women are given Rh-immune globulin after amniocentesis. After 20 weeks of gestation, the procedure of amniocentesis has less than a 1% risk of maternal or fetal morbidity or mortality.[5]

At any stage of pregnancy, the risks of amniocentesis must be weighed against the value of the information obtained by the technique and subsequent testing.

FETAL MATURITY

Except in cases in which immediate delivery is indicated for the survival of the mother or fetus, most complicated pregnancies are allowed to continue until the risk of neonatal death from immaturity is less than that of fetal death *in utero* from the complication. In general, the symptoms are treated and the fetus is allowed to remain *in utero* as long as the condition permits. Delivery of a functionally mature fetus as soon as possible is the major goal in fetal monitoring.

Fetal lung maturity, the major consideration, is dependent on the presence in the lungs of sufficient amounts of surfactant, which reduces surface tension by coating the alveolar walls. This provides the lungs with sufficient elasticity to prevent atelectasis and respiratory distress. Phospholipid-rich surfactant is produced by type II alveolar cells after 24 weeks of gestation, and is composed of lipid (80% to 90%) and protein (10% to 20%). The phospholipid dipalmitoyl phosphatidylcholine (more commonly known as lecithin) makes up approximately three-quarters of the lipid. The remaining one-quarter is composed of phosphatidylglycerol, phosphatidylserine, phosphatidylinositol, and sphingomyelin.

Lung maturation begins during the second half of pregnancy. As surfactant production increases in the lungs, surfactant flows into the amniotic fluid, which then may be tested in order to estimate surfactant concentration. In this way, fetal pulmonary maturity is estimated.

If an infant is born before the lungs are functionally mature, *respiratory distress syndrome (RDS)* results. RDS is caused by a deficiency in surfactant lining the alveolar surface. The diagnosis of *hyaline membrane disease (HMD)* as the cause of respiratory distress is made after death on the basis of autopsy findings. Lung sections of infants who have died from RDS show collapsed alveoli and the formation of hyaline membranes within them.

Immediately after birth, infants with RDS show increased respiratory effort with tachypnea, expiratory grunting, and cyanosis. Treatment consists of keeping the alveoli open by applying continuous positive airway pressure until surfactant production is adequate for unassisted respiration.

CONDITIONS REQUIRING MONITORING

Diabetes Mellitus

Diabetes complicates almost two percent of all pregnancies.[6] This figure includes women entering pregnancy with preexisting diabetes and those with gestational diabetes. *Gestational diabetes* refers to diabetes that develops during pregnancy but disappears post partum. The diagnosis of gestational diabetes (White's class A)[7] is made primarily on the basis of an abnormal glucose tolerance test (GTT) in pregnancy (see Chap. 40).

Diabetes exerts many adverse effects on pregnancy. Polyhydramnios occurs in approximately 10% of diabetic pregnancies, and excessively large infants are born in almost 30% of diabetic pregnancies.[6]

There is an increased incidence of perinatal mortality in diabetic pregnancies, especially if the pregnancy is not closely monitored, with mortality rates of 15% to 20% being reported.[8] As maternal age and weight increase, fetal risk also increases.[9] Fetal death occurring during the last month of gestation may remain unexplained in most cases. Neonatal deaths result primarily from respiratory distress syndrome or congenital anomalies. In an effort to minimize the risk of fetal death near the end of gestation, there is an increased number of cesarean sections performed in diabetic pregnancies. This contributes to the higher incidence of RDS.

Infants of diabetic mothers experience an incidence three times the expected rate of major congenital anomalies. This rate appears to increase with the severity of the maternal diabetes.[10]

Fetal macrosomia, a frequent complication in diabetic pregnancies, may be caused by overutilization of glucose *in utero*. Excessive amounts of glucose are delivered across the placenta in maternal hyperglycemia. There appears to be a positive correlation between the degree of macrosomia and the degree of hyperglycemia in the mother.[1] As a result of macrosomia, there is an increased incidence of birth trauma to both the mother and newborn if a caesarean section is not performed.

Insulin does not cross the placenta from the maternal circulation into the fetal blood. This causes the beta cells of the fetal pancreas to compensate for the large amounts of glucose present by producing excessive amounts of insulin. The pancreas continues to secrete large amounts of insulin after birth, even though the hyperglycemic environment is terminated. This may lead to hypoglycemia in the neonate and result in brain damage, neurologic disorders, or death, if not detected and treated promptly.[11]

Management of the diabetic pregnancy requires careful evaluation, beginning as early as possible and continuing throughout the pregnancy, labor, and delivery. Fetal maturity and fetoplacental function tests may be used to indicate optimal time for termination of the pregnancy in order to avoid fetal death *in utero*. Fetal lung maturity tests are widely used in diabetic patients to aid in the proper timing of delivery.

Intrauterine fetal death is rare in patients with gestational diabetes. In carefully managed pregnancies, perinatal mortality is no greater than that for the general population. These patients can be managed by dietary control alone, although the physician will probably request a greater number of office visits during the pregnancy. Approximately 10% to 15% of women with gestational diabetes will develop overt diabetes during pregnancy.[12] Because of this, the fasting blood glucose levels should be closely monitored throughout gestation. Fetal size may be monitored by ultrasonography. When macrosomia is detected, a cesarean section should be considered in order to decrease the risk of birth injury. In general, for women with gestational diabetes not requiring insulin, there is no need to terminate the pregnancy early.

In overt diabetes, more frequent visits to the physician are required, with hospitalization at the first indication of difficulties. Fasting plasma glucose levels should be maintained at 100–110 mg/dL (5.5–6.1 mmol/L), and postprandial levels at 140–150 mg/dL (7.8–8.3 mmol/L).[6] Insulin requirements may increase in pregnant patients, and frequent monitoring is necessary. After the twenty-eighth week of gestation, nonstressed monitoring of fetal reactivity may be used to assess fetal well-being. Serial measurements of maternal urinary estriol excretion may be used to assess fetal health and placental function; however, this test has not been used often in recent years.

Because of the increased risk of fetal death near term, amniocentesis should be performed at regular intervals beginning at about 35 weeks of gestation to evaluate fetal lung maturity. The lecithin/sphingomyelin ratio is the analysis most often used for this purpose. Through close monitoring, the delivery can be timed to occur at a point when the combined risks of fetal death and prematurity are at a minimum. The pregnancy is allowed to continue until the fetus is functionally mature unless maternal or fetal status begins to deteriorate.

Respiratory distress syndrome may still occur in infants of diabetic mothers in spite of a mature lecithin/sphingomyelin ratio. The cause of this is not known, although there are several hypotheses. It has been suggested that the fetal lungs synthesize and secrete a type of pulmonary surfactant that is adequate in lecithin but deficient in apoproteins, and that is not capable of preventing respiratory distress.[13] Increased incidence of respiratory distress may be caused by a delayed appearance of phosphatidylglycerol, which is necessary to stabilize the surfactant complex in the neonatal lung.[14] Phosphatidylglycerol first appears in the amniotic fluid about 1.5 weeks later in gestational diabetes than in normal pregnancies.[15] When phosphatidylglycerol is present, the incidence of

RDS is the same as that in the nondiabetic population.

Preeclampsia

Preeclampsia is the development of hypertension with proteinuria, edema, or both after the 20th week of gestation. The blood pressure rises solely because of pregnancy and then returns to normal after pregnancy. Eclamptic convulsions may develop if preeclampsia is allowed to progress untreated. The maternal mortality rate from eclampsia is 3% to 5%; the fetal mortality rate is 17% to 20%.[16] Incidence of preeclampsia and eclampsia is highest among indigent women who receive little or no prenatal care. They occur most often in the first pregnancy, and succeeding pregnancies are usually normal or mildly preeclamptic (see Chap. 40).

It is important to differentiate preeclampsia from chronic hypertension because of the increased perinatal mortality rate in the former. This may be difficult if the patient is first seen after 20 weeks of gestation. Patients with chronic hypertension are more likely to develop preeclampsia during pregnancy than those beginning pregnancy with normal blood pressure. In these patients, preeclampsia may occur earlier than 20 weeks of gestation and progress to eclampsia.

Vasospasm, characteristic of preeclampsia, increases resistance to blood flow and accounts for the development of hypertension and decreased circulation to the kidneys, brain, liver, and placenta. The decrease in placental perfusion described above may produce small placentas and lead to circulatory and nutritional deficits in the fetus.

In monitoring preeclamptic patients, the clinical severity of the maternal condition should be related to the maturity and condition of the fetus. Delivery of the fetus is the only treatment in severe cases. In milder cases, the pregnancy is allowed to progress as long as possible (see Chap. 40).

Proteinuria associated with hypertension carries a higher fetal mortality rate.[17] An increase in blood uric acid levels above 6 mg/dL (0.35 mmol/L) before 32 weeks of gestation in patients with hypertension has been shown to be associated with a perinatal mortality rate of 50%.[18]

Fetal evaluation should include amniocentesis for pulmonary maturity tests and ultrasonography. Failure of the fetus to grow, as observed by ultrasonography, is a sign that the fetus is in jeopardy and should be delivered as soon as it is functionally mature.

All treatment consists of management of symptoms until the fetus can be delivered. In almost all cases, the condition abates after delivery.

Fetal Hemolytic Disorders

Isoimmunization in the fetus occurs when a fetal antigen that is not present in the mother enters maternal circulation and stimulates antibody production. The antibodies then return to the fetus through the placenta, and fetal erythrocytes containing the specific antigen are destroyed, resulting in *erythroblastosis fetalis* or *hemolytic disease of the newborn.* Most fetuses and newborns who develop hemolytic disease are the product of an Rh-negative mother and an Rh-positive father. If the fetus is also Rh-positive, isoimmunization occurs. Usually, the first pregnancy is not affected unless the mother has previously been sensitized. In each succeeding pregnancy, the fetus is more likely to be severely affected.

There are many antigens that can cause hemolytic disease of the newborn, but the Rh antigen is most common and usually the most severe. ABO incompatibilities are usually associated with a much milder hemolytic disease than are Rh incompatibilities. Anti-Lewis antibodies, which are frequently encountered, are not associated with erythroblastosis fetalis because they are IgM antibodies and cannot cross the placenta. Anti-Kell, -Duffy, and -Kidd antibodies are rare, but they may be associated with erythroblastosis fetalis.

In order to detect a hemolytic disorder, the mother's ABO and Rh type should be determined as early as possible in the pregnancy. An antibody screen (indirect Coombs test) should also be performed to aid detection of any antibodies circulating in the blood. Repeat antibody screens at 28 and 34 weeks of gestation may also be helpful.

In previously unsensitized Rh-negative women, sensitization can be prevented by administering the appropriate doses of Rh immunoglobulin (RhIg) at certain times during the pregnancy. Immunoglobulin should also be administered to Rh-negative women who experience abortion, ectopic pregnancy, or amniocentesis. Typically, the Rh-negative woman receives RhIg routinely at 28 weeks of gestation, after any amniocentesis, and postpartum, to avoid isoimmunization from fetal–maternal bleeds that may occur before term. If a massive fetal–maternal hemorrhage is suspected, a larger dose of RhIg may be necessary. The general rule is to give RhIg when any doubt exists about the mother's Rh type or the occurrence of a fetal–maternal hemorrhage.

In hemolytic disease, maternal antibodies are absorbed on the fetal red cells and act as hemolysins, leading to an accelerated rate of red cell destruction. Severely affected infants may demonstrate *hydrops fetalis,* excessive subcutaneous edema, and effusion of fluid into the serous cavities. In cases in which the edema is severe enough to be detected by ultrasonography, the placenta is also markedly edematous. Prolonged hemolysis stimulates the bone marrow to produce red blood cells, and there is an outpouring of immature nucleated red cells into the fetal circulation. The liver and spleen become enlarged. Severely affected fetuses may die *in utero* from severe anemia and circulatory failure unless immediate action is taken to perform an intrauterine exchange transfusion or to deliver the baby.

The liveborn hydropic infant appears pale and edematous at birth, with severe anemia and enlarged liver and spleen. Exchange transfusions may be necessary to prevent death. Less severely affected infants may appear well at birth but develop jaundice after a few hours. Phototherapy to decrease bilirubin concentration may be adequate for these infants. (See also Chap. 76)

Neural Tube Defects

Neural tube defects are one of the most common groups of serious congenital malformations. *Anencephaly* and *spina bifida* are the two most common of this group. Together they account for approximately 95% of all neural tube defects.[19] It is important to distinguish between open and closed defects for the purpose of prenatal diagnosis. An *open defect* is one in which the fetal cerebrospinal fluid and amniotic fluid are continuous, and the neural tube is completely exposed or may be covered by a thin transparent membrane. A *closed defect* is completely covered by skin or a thick opaque membrane. Only an open defect can be detected by biochemical testing. Anencephaly is almost always an open lesion, and spina bifida lesions are open approximately 80% of the time.[19]

Infants surviving with spina bifida are often severely handicapped and require frequent surgical procedures and institutional care. Handicaps may consist of paralysis of the legs, hydrocephaly, and mental retardation. In one study, approximately one-third of the infants with open spina bifida lesions survived for five years. Of these, 84% were severely handicapped, 10% were moderately handicapped, and 6% had no handicap.[20] Anencephaly is fatal at or within hours after birth.

The prevalence of neural tube defects shows wide geographical variation. Incidence is highest in the United Kingdom, where the overall rate is four to five in 1000 births. Other parts of Europe and North America experience intermediate rates, with the lowest rates found in Africa, Asia, and South America.[21] The risk of occurrence increases by about 5% if the mother has had one previous child with a neural tube defect. This risk doubles if the mother has had two affected children.[22] Before α-fetoprotein (AFP) screening, recognition of pregnancies with an increased risk was based entirely on the mother's medical history. Nonetheless, about 95% of affected infants are born to women who have not previously had an affected child.[19]

Neural tube defects may sometimes be identified through ultrasound scanning of the fetus. Anencephaly is more readily detected by this method than is spina bifida. Ultrasonography is also used to estimate gestational age by measuring fetal biparietal diameter. Women who appear to have raised AFP levels may actually be normal if gestational age was initially underestimated. The use of ultrasound to estimate gestational age has been shown to increase the detection rate of spina bifida from 79% to 91%.[23]

The measurement of amniotic fluid AFP is the major diagnostic test for neural tube defects. Although some other fetal disorders are associated with elevated AFP levels, high AFP levels in both the maternal serum and the amniotic fluid strongly suggest the presence of a fetal neural tube defect. Using maternal serum AFP measurements as a screening test enables the physician to select cases in which amniocentesis is necessary. The overall rate of detection of anencephaly by amniotic fluid AFP determination is 94%, and of spina bifida is 75%.[24]

Genetic Disorders

Many inherited disorders and chromosome abnormalities can be identified successfully before birth. These include errors of metabolism, such as Tay-Sachs disease, and mucopolysaccharidoses and chromosome abnormalities, such as Down's syndrome and X-linked recessive diseases. Down's syndrome is the most common serious chromosome abnormality, and genetic screening is most often undertaken to detect this disorder.

Identification of families at risk for genetic disorders is the first step in genetic testing and counseling. This can be accomplished by screening on the basis of ethnic background, age, family history, and occupation. Many families will request genetic counseling if they have a child or close relative with a genetic disease and wish to know the recurrence rate of the disease. Genetic testing is usually recommended for pregnant women over the age of 35, in families in which a parent, child, or close relative has a chromosome abnormality, and in pregnancies at risk for a serious X-linked hereditary disorder.

Amniocentesis should be performed between the 15th and 18th weeks of gestation when there are likely to be sufficient fetal cells to obtain a successful culture. In many cases a cell culture can be completed before the 20th week of gestation. This is important if the parents are deciding whether or not to terminate the pregnancy.

Cultivated amniotic fluid cells are most often the material used for analysis. These cells may be used for studies in the diagnosis of chromosome abnormalities and metabolic defects. Metabolic defects are also identified by amniotic fluid enzymatic studies. Because extensive experience is required in tissue culture techniques, this type of testing is usually limited to health care facilities in large metropolitan areas.

A number of legal and ethical questions have been raised as a result of genetic testing and counseling. Physicians have an obligation to inform patients who are at risk for having a child with a genetic disorder, and to identify testing services available. Decisions made as a result of genetic counseling involve sensitive issues such as abortion and the reproductive future of a couple. After testing, extensive counseling plays a major role in the decisions made by a family.

LABORATORY ANALYSES AND DIAGNOSIS

Assays for Fetal Maturity

There are several tests for functionally mature lungs, a major consideration in the decision to terminate a pregnancy. These include the foam stability test, the L/S ratio, and several assays for phospholipids.

FOAM STABILITY TEST

The foam stability test is one type of the qualitative tests that measure the physical properties of fetal lung surfactant. Most of these tests are simpler, quicker, and less costly than chemical tests. The most common and widely used is the foam stability or shake test, which is based on the ability of pulmonary surfactant to produce stable foam in the presence of ethanol.[25]

Amniotic fluid is the specimen required. It should be removed directly from the amniotic sac to avoid contamination and, if possible, the test should be carried out immediately. Vaginal pool specimens are unacceptable. For same-day analysis, prompt refrigeration at 5° C is necessary. Freezing the fluid at −20° C is recommended if analysis cannot be carried out on the same day.

Although the foam stability test is inexpensive and quick, several problems are associated with it. The final concentration of reagents used is critical, and any remnants of soap or biological fluids on the glassware may cause foam, making the assay invalid. Movement of the tubes after shaking has stopped may break up the foam produced, making the test difficult to interpret. Most importantly, the test cannot be used if meconium or blood is found in the sample. Both produce stable foam even when present in low concentrations.

A clearly negative test has been found to be associated with a high risk of RDS, and a clearly positive test, with a low risk.[25] Tests giving intermediate results have been interpreted as showing a substantial possibility that the infant will have some degree of RDS. A high incidence of interlaboratory differences in interpretation and false-negative results has been reported. False-positive results have also been reported. One study found a false-positive rate of 18% and a false-negative rate of 7% when comparing the foam stability test to L/S ratios.[26] Another author concluded that the foam stability test gives too many false-negative results to be of value in routine clinical practice.[27]

The foam stability test may be used as a screening test for the detection of surfactant in amniotic fluid; however, in view of its lack of specificity, chemical assays should be used before the infant is delivered.

L/S RATIO

Among the tests for measuring the individual components of lung surfactant, the lecithin/sphingomyelin ratio (L/S), originally described in 1971,[28] is the most reliable and widely used.

The concentration of total lipid in amniotic fluid increases steadily throughout gestation; however, prior to 30 weeks of gestation, the sphingomyelin concentration is greater than that of lecithin. After this point, the lecithin concentration increases, rising sharply at approximately 35 weeks of gestation when maturation of the lung occurs (see Fig. 41-1). Throughout gestation, the sphingomyelin concentration remains relatively constant. This enables the use of a ratio, making the result independent of amniotic fluid volume.

An L/S ratio of 2.0 or greater signifies that the fetal lungs are mature and the risk of developing RDS is low. There is a high risk of developing RDS if the L/S ratio is less than 2.0. The severity of RDS has been found to be predicted by the L/S ratio—the lower the L/S ratio, the more clinically severe the RDS.[29]

In normal pregnancies, L/S ratios correlate closely with gestational age. High-risk pregnancies with certain maternal conditions may either accelerate or delay maturation of the fetal lung. Maternal conditions associated with accelerated production of phospholipids include hypertension resulting from severe toxemia, renal or cardiovascular disease, narcotic addiction, sickle cell disease, and prolonged rupture of membranes. Conditions that delay maturation are gestational diabetes mellitus, chronic nonhypertensive glomerulonephritis, and certain cases of hydrops fetalis.[30]

Amniotic fluid obtained by transabdominal amniocentesis is the specimen of choice. Vaginal samples may be used, but contamination with mucus and bacteria may alter results. Failure to refrigerate the sample will lower the L/S ratio.[31] The specimen should be frozen after centrifugation if analysis cannot be performed on the day of collection.

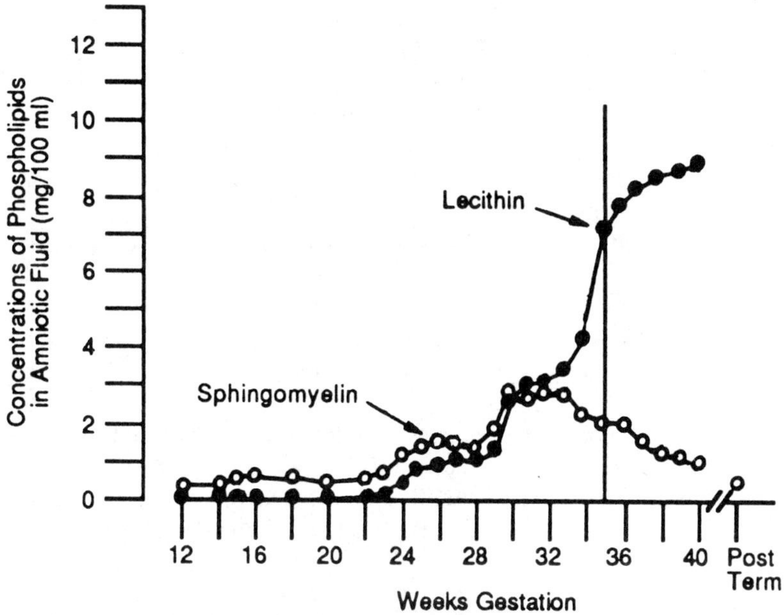

Figure 41-1 **Mean concentrations of lecithin and sphingomyelin in amniotic fluid during gestation in normal pregnancy.**

The presence of blood or meconium in the amniotic fluid will alter the results. Meconium has the effect of lowering the L/S ratio and, as the amount of meconium increases, so does its effect on the result.[32] Meconium also obscures the observation of lecithin and sphingomyelin during the analysis, making interpretation difficult. Blood has an L/S ratio of approximately 1.5; therefore the presence of blood in the sample may alter the L/S ratio.[32]

Minor variations in laboratory technique may result in major changes in the L/S ratio. High centrifugation speeds will decrease the L/S ratio if force is sufficient to spin out some of the phospholipids. Omitting the acetone precipitation step, a common modification of the Gluck technique, will result in an increased L/S ratio, and a new cutoff value must be set that indicates pulmonary maturity.[31]

In spite of the cost and time involved in performing L/S ratio measurement, it remains the most widely used test for predicting fetal lung maturity.

PHOSPHATIDYLGLYCEROL, PHOSPHATIDYLINOSITOL

Phosphatidylglycerol (PG), the second major phospholipid, makes up approximately 10% of surfactant phospholipids. Using PG measurements together with the L/S ratio increases the reliability of fetal lung maturity predictions. The presence of PG in the amniotic fluid sample, even in conjunction with a low L/S ratio, signifies fetal lung maturity. PG first appears in the amniotic fluid at 35 to 36 weeks of gestation, and continues to increase until term.

One study found that, once the PG concentration in amniotic fluid exceeded 3% of the total phospholipid concentration, no RDS occurred.[33] This was found to be true even in pregnancies complicated by diabetes mellitus, in which the L/S ratio alone has been shown to be unreliable in predicting the development of RDS. Pregnant women with any type of diabetes mellitus can be delivered safely when PG appears in the amniotic fluid.[15]

Another phospholipid occasionally monitored is *phosphatidylinositol (PI)*. Concentrations of PI increase after 30 weeks of gestation, peak at 35 to 36 weeks, and then decrease as fetal lung maturity occurs. Therefore, an absence of PI in the amniotic fluid signifies lung maturity in the fetus. PI is not a very useful test, however, because many problems in pregnancy occur prior to the 35th week of gestation.

PG is easily monitored along with the L/S ratio, and no extra amniotic fluid sample or extraction is required. Although one problem with the L/S ratio is the unreliability of results when blood or meconium is present in the sample, PG measurements are unaffected by the presence of blood and meconium if two-dimensional chromatography is utilized.[34]

The use of a lung profile consisting of L/S ratio, PG, and possibly PI measurements helps to form a clearer picture of fetal lung development. This is important in complicated pregnancies and in cases in which the L/S ratio is borderline.

OTHER PHOSPHOLIPID ASSAYS

In addition to the tests mentioned, there are numerous other tests used to predict fetal lung maturity. Assays dealing directly with the analysis of phospholipids are the most commonly used. Like the foam stability test, measurements of *surface tension of amniotic fluid* and *bubble clicking* take advantage of the physical properties of amniotic fluid. Although these tests are relatively inexpensive and quick, like the foam stability test they have a high incidence of false negatives and some false positives. If possible, they should be used only as screening tests before a chemical assay is performed.

Chemical tests such as measurements of *total phospholipid concentration, lecithin concentration,* and *palmitic acid concentration* in amniotic fluid are also in use. These tests show good correlation with L/S ratios, but in general offer few advantages over L/S ratio and PG measurements. Measurement of total lecithin concentration in amniotic fluid takes longer to perform than the L/S ratio, and results may be affected by amniotic fluid volume. As a result, the test has not been widely evaluated.[35]

Fluorescence polarization relates to the microviscosity and surface tension properties of amniotic fluid.[36] As surfactant increases in amniotic fluid, the result is lower surface tension and lower microviscosity, and therefore lower polarization values, indicating pulmonary maturity. Fluorescence polarization assay has not been widely utilized in the past because of the need for specialized, expensive equipment. In recent years, however, the test has been further evaluated and has been shown to be a promising assay for predicting fetal lung maturity. Moreover, techniques of measuring fluorescence polarization are being adapted to automated fluorescence instruments commonly used in the clinical laboratory for therapeutic drug monitoring.[37] This assay offers several advantages over the L/S ratio. A smaller amniotic fluid sample is required, and the time required for analysis is greatly reduced. Interlaboratory standardization, which is currently lacking in methods for L/S ratio determination, is possible with this technique.[38]

It is doubtful that any of these assays will replace the L/S ratio in the near future. The L/S ratio has been shown to be a reliable indicator of fetal pulmonary maturity, thereby making the prediction of respiratory distress syndrome possible.

AMNIOTIC FLUID CREATININE

Amniotic fluid creatinine measurements have been shown to have a positive correlation with gestational age. For many years, this test was widely used in estimation of fetal maturity. Because most clinical laboratories perform creatinine analysis on serum and urine, amniotic fluid analysis presents no problems. Amniotic fluid specimens usually have a creatinine concentration of 1–3 mg/dL, (88–265 μmol/L); therefore, the routine method for serum analysis may be followed without modification.

Creatinine concentration in amniotic fluid rises throughout pregnancy as a result of increased excretion by the maturing fetal kidneys. A concentration of 1.8–2.0 mg/dL (159–177 μmol/L) is reached at 36 to 38 weeks of gestation. Levels of 2.0 mg/dL or greater most often indicate fetal maturity.

Amniotic fluid creatinine is related primarily to kidney maturation and muscle mass of the fetus. Although the test correlates well with gestational maturity, its effectiveness in predicting fetal pulmonary maturity is small, because renal and pulmonary maturity may not occur simultaneously. Thus, fetal pulmonary maturity cannot be predicted on the basis of amniotic fluid creatinine alone. Factors that alter maternal serum creatinine concentration may also affect the amniotic fluid concentration. This could lead to a value greater than 2.0 mg/dL even though the fetus is not mature. Decreased fetal renal perfusion, which is seen in fetal hemolytic disease, will lower amniotic fluid creatinine levels.[39]

Assays for Fetal or Placental Abnormalities

ESTROGEN MONITORING

Urine and serum of pregnant women contain large amounts of estrogens that originate in the placenta. The placenta converts weak androgens made by the fetus to estrogens, primarily estriol, which are then excreted in the maternal urine. Maternal estriol measurements provide an index of placental function, because the fetus plays an important role in contributing precursors for estriol synthesis. Abnormal pregnancies may thus be identified by abnormal estriol levels.

Estriol monitoring usually begins early in the last trimester of pregnancy (32–34 weeks). For it to be useful, serial studies are needed. A progressive rise in estriol concentration is seen throughout normal pregnancies. Consistent declining concentrations indicate a pregnancy in trouble, possibly with imminent fetal death.

The method of analysis depends on whether urine or plasma is being monitored, with urinary procedures requiring a 24-hour sample. Methods used include colorimetric reactions, gas–liquid chromatography, radioimmunoassay (RIA), and enzyme immunoassay (EIA). The RIA and EIA methods offer the best precision and sensitivity. Plasma estriol measurements require a more sensitive assay than do urine measurements because of the lower concentrations present, and RIA is the method most often used.

Fetal congenital malformations of the central nervous system and certain drugs administered during pregnancy may cause abnormally low estrogen levels. Because of diurnal variations in blood estriol, samples should be obtained at approximately the same time every day. There is also a day-to-day variation in urinary excretion, which makes serial determinations necessary in order to see a trend. Unreliable 24-hour urine collections may also alter results. Plasma measurements have gained popularity because of the ease of sample collection. In general, estrogen assays are not useful in monitoring Rh-sensitized patients. Levels in these patients are usually increased because of the enlarged placenta.[40]

The level of estriol does not always accurately reflect the wellbeing of the fetus. One study suggests that the measurement of estriol has little clinical utility in efforts to reduce perinatal mortality or morbidity.[41] For these reasons, the use of this test has declined in recent years.

Rh ANTIBODY TITER

In Rh-sensitized patients, antibody titers should be performed on the mother's serum throughout the pregnancy. It is believed that, if the antibody titers remain less than 1:16 in an initial immunized gestation, the fetus is not in serious jeopardy.[42] Any titer is significant if the woman has had a previously affected baby. Titers are usually obtained every 2 weeks to monitor the severity of the disease. If the antibody titer rises above the critical level determined by the laboratory, the fetal condition should be investigated. This is done by spectrophotometric evaluation of the amniotic fluid at 450 nm, observing the increase in optical density above an expected baseline (Δ OD 450). The initial amniocentesis is usually performed between 22 and 24 weeks of gestation, with serial determinations every 1 to 3 weeks thereafter depending on the severity of the disease. Using this method, the fetal condition may be monitored closely.

BILIRUBIN IN AMNIOTIC FLUID

Spectrophotometric evaluation of amniotic fluid enables the physician to monitor the severity of fetal hemolytic disorders. In normal pregnancies, amniotic fluid bilirubin reaches a peak at 18 to 24 weeks of gestation and decreases steadily thereafter, approaching zero at 36 to 37 weeks. In hemolytic disorders, amniotic fluid bilirubin increases because of increased red cell destruction.

Bilirubin concentration is estimated by a spectrophotometric scan, and bilirubin typically absorbs with a peak at 450 nm. Liley found that the severity of hemolytic disease could be predicted by plotting the baseline corrected absorbance (Δ OD) at 450 nm against weeks of gestation on a three-zone graph (see Fig. 41-2).[43] Fetal condition is best determined by monitoring 1 to 3 weeks apart serial values of Δ OD at 450 nm. If the Δ OD remains in Liley zone I with a gradual decrease, either the fetus is unaffected or it is affected with mild hemolytic disease. These infants may be delivered close to term. If the Δ OD is in Liley zone II, the fetus is at moderate-to-severe risk. Readings in zone II may pass into zone I as pregnancy progresses, indicating mild disease, or enter zone III, indicating severe disease. If the Δ OD remains in zone III, the fetus is in severe jeopardy. Prompt delivery is indicated if this occurs after 32 weeks of gestation. If the values reach zone III prior to 32 weeks of gestation, intrauterine transfusion is usually performed.[42] Less risk is involved with early delivery and extrauterine transfusions if the fetus is mature enough to survive.

It is essential that the specimen for bilirubin analysis be protected from light at all times. Failure to do so will result in falsely decreased readings. In the original method, fluid containing blood or meconium rendered the sample worthless for evaluation.[44] Oxyhemoglobin contamination causes a large peak at 412 nm, which may overlap with the peak at 450. Meconium contamination increases absorbance from 350 to 400 nm, with decreasing absorbance up to 550 nm. These contaminants obscure the bilirubin peak, making it impossible to establish a satisfactory baseline.

A modification of the original method permits separation of bilirubin from interfering pigments.[45]

Intrauterine transfusions are usually performed after 23 weeks of gestation and before the 30th week.[46] After visualization of the fetus by ultrasound, a needle and catheter are inserted into the fetal peritoneal cavity, through which fresh group-O, Rh-negative red blood cells are infused. The transfused red cells are absorbed and enter the venous circulation, thereby improving the anemia. Gestational age and size of the fetus determine the volume of red cells infused. Transfusions are repeated every 2 weeks or until the fetus is mature enough for delivery. The procedure is most successful when the fetus is at 24 to 32 weeks of gestation. Before 24 weeks, the technical difficulty of a transfusion and the risk involved are greatly increased. At any stage of gestation, the procedure is not without risk to the fetus and requires considerable skill on the part of the physician.

α-FETOPROTEIN (AFP)

Several fetal conditions other than open neural tube defects are associated with increased AFP levels. These include congenital nephrosis, multiple pregnancy, intrauterine death, miscarriage, low birthweight, and exomphalos (congenital umbilical hernia).[19] However, AFP measurement is the primary screening technique for neural tube defects.

At 16 to 18 weeks of gestation, the optimal time for measurement of maternal serum AFP, the concentration of AFP in fetal serum is approximately 50,000 times greater than that in maternal serum. AFP levels in maternal serum normally rise throughout pregnancy due to the transfer of fetal

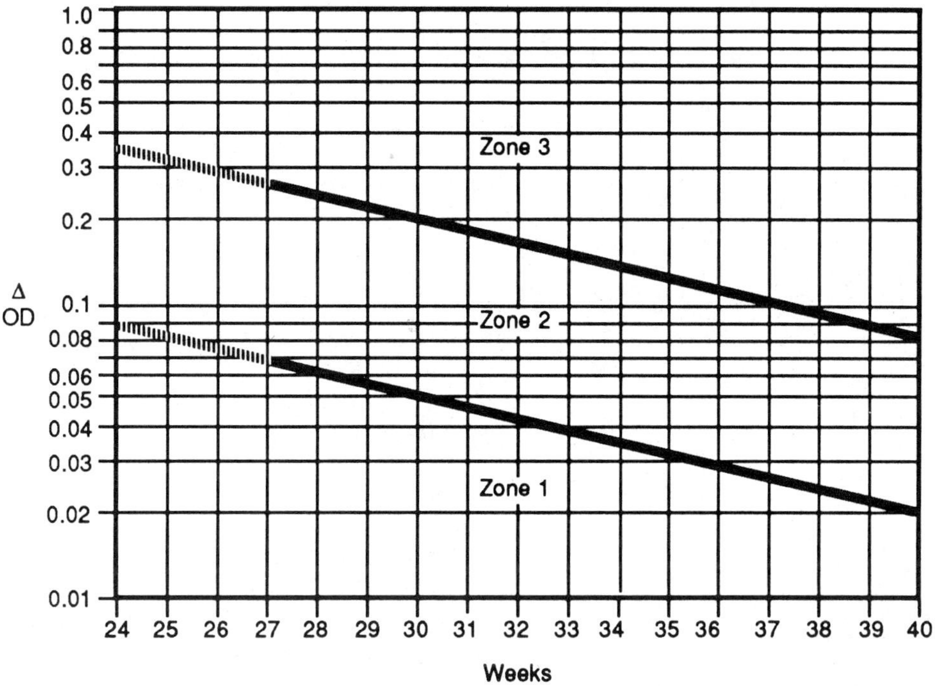

Figure 41-2 Modified Liley graph. The dotted lines represent linear extrapolations from the original Liley data (solid lines).

serum AFP across the placenta (see Fig. 41-3). In an open neural tube defect, amniotic fluid AFP levels are greatly increased because of leakage of fetal AFP through the lesion, and there is an increase in the maternal serum AFP levels. If the level of maternal serum AFP is significantly increased early in gestation, followup studies with ultrasonography and amniotic fluid AFP measurements are needed.

α-Fetoprotein measurements in maternal serum and amniotic fluid are most often performed by radioimmunoassay. This method offers more sensitivity and reproducibility than do other assays. A very sensitive assay is needed for detection of the low levels of AFP in maternal serum during early pregnancy. In recent years, enzyme-linked immunoassays have gained popularity in order to avoid the use of radioactive material. This method agrees well with RIA.

Contamination of amniotic fluid with fetal blood results in falsely increased AFP levels. If a sample is visibly contaminated with blood, the source (maternal or fetal) should be determined. Contamination by maternal blood will not have as great an effect on the AFP level, as long as the contamination does not dilute the sample.

Knowledge of a precise gestational age is essential to accurately evaluate AFP results. Underestimating gestational age may lead to a false-negative interpretation. If accurate dates are not available, ultrasonography should be used in estimating gestational age.

CASE STUDY

A 29-year-old white woman who had had diabetes mellitus since age 12 was followed throughout her pregnancy in an O.B. complications clinic. Two

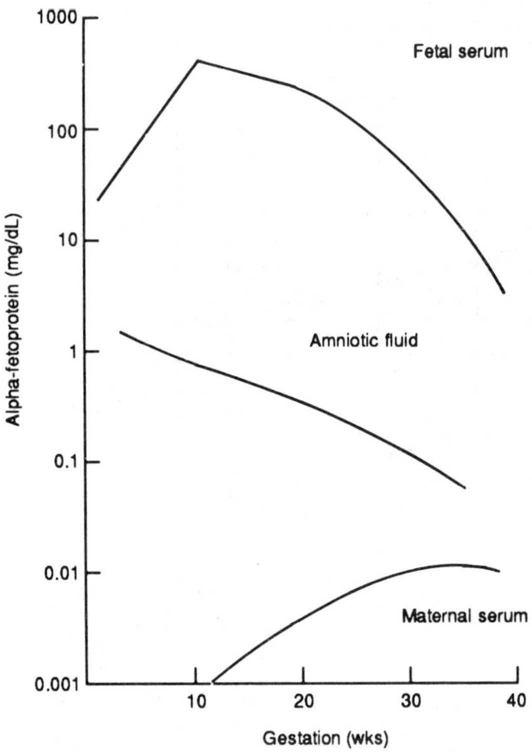

Figure 41-3 Normal concentrations of alpha-fetoprotein versus gestational age found in normal fetal serum, amniotic fluid, and maternal serum.

years earlier, she had delivered a stillborn baby at 24 weeks of gestation with severe intrauterine growth retardation.

The first clinic visit was at 5 weeks of gestation. The patient had routinely performed blood sugars on herself with a portable instrument, but admitted to poor control prior to this visit because of a broken instrument. She was receiving 77 units (50 NPH, 22 regular) of insulin in the morning and 20 units (10 NPH, 10 regular) in the evening. Initial laboratory results revealed elevated serum glucose levels but a negative urine glucose.

Throughout her pregnancy, the patient was seen weekly at the clinic. Her insulin requirement gradually increased. By hospital admission date, 7½ months later, she was receiving 204 units (102 NPH, 102 regular) of insulin in the morning and 32 units (10 NPH, 22 regular) in the evening. Blood pressure remained in control throughout pregnancy, with systolic fluctuating between 120 and 150 mm Hg and diastolic between 70 and 100 mm Hg. Urine glucose fluctuated, with several 4+ readings during the Christmas season, but generally remained negative or 1+.

Questions

1. What potential problems exist for the fetus?
2. What laboratory tests would be helpful for monitoring the mother?
3. What tests were most likely chosen to guide a decision for early delivery?

Discussion

1. Potential problems for the fetus/neonate include macrosomia with increased chances of congenital abnormality, and increased chances of neonatal mortality. Neonatal hypoglycemia and brain damage are also a possibility if the fetus was exposed to excessive amounts of glucose during gestation.
2. Tests useful in monitoring the mother during pregnancy would be serum and urine glucose analyses, urine protein determinations, and glycosylated hemoglobins.
3. Sonograms were performed periodically to monitor growth of the fetus. At 37 weeks of gestation, the sonogram suggested fetal macrosomia, with the weight of the fetus in the 90th percentile. Amniotic fluid was obtained for fetal pulmonary maturity testing. The lecithin/sphingomyelin ratio was 6.6, and phosphatidylglycerol was present. At 37 weeks and 2 days of gestation, the patient was admitted to the hospital because of suspicious results on a contraction stress test. An infant male was delivered by cesarean section that evening without complications. The baby weighed 3520 grams.

REFERENCES

1. Pritchard JA, Macdonald PC (eds): Williams Obstetrics, 16th ed. New York City, Appleton-Century-Crofts, 1980

2. Lind T, Kendall A, Hytten FE: The role of the fetus in the formation of amniotic fluid. Br J Obstet Gynaecol 79:289, 1972
3. Lind T: The biochemistry of amniotic fluid. In Sandler M (ed): Amniotic Fluid and Its Clinical Significance, p 1. New York City, Marcel Dekker, 1981
4. Bennett MJ: Amniocentesis. In Sandler M (ed): Amniotic Fluid and Its Clinical Significance, p 27. New York City, Marcel Dekker, 1981
5. Gerbie AB, Nadler HL, Gerbie MV: Amniocentesis in genetic counseling. Am J Obstet Gynecol 109:765, 1971
6. Rovinsky JJ: Diseases complicating pregnancy. In Romney SL, Gray MJ, Little AB et al (eds): Gynecology and Obstetrics: The Health Care of Women, p 697. New York City, McGraw-Hill, 1981
7. White P: Classification of obstetric diabetes. Am J Obstet Gynecol 130:228, 1978
8. Gabbe SG, Mestman JH, Freeman RD et al: Management and outcome of pregnancy in diabetes mellitus, Classes B to R. Am J Obstet Gynecol 129:723, 1977
9. Jarrett RJ: Diabetes Mellitus and gestational diabetes. In Wald NJ (ed): Antenatal and Neonatal Screening, p 382. Oxford, Oxford University Press, 1984
10. Pedersen LM, Tygstrup I, Pedersen J: Congenital malformations in newborn infants of diabetic women. Lancet 1:1124, 1964
11. McCann ML: Infants of diabetic mothers. Pediatrics 45:887, 1970
12. Gabbe SG, Mestman JH, Freeman RK et al: Management and outcome of class A diabetes mellitus. Am J Obstet Gynecol 127:465, 1977
13. Katyal SL, Amenta JS, Singh G et al: Deficient lung surfactant apoproteins in amniotic fluid with mature phospholipid profile from diabetic pregnancies. Am J Obstet Gynecol 148:51, 1984
14. Hallman M, Kulovich M, Kirkpatrick E et al: Phosphatidylinositol and phosphatidylglycerol in amniotic fluid: Indices of lung maturity. Am J Obstet Gynecol 125:613, 1976
15. Kulovich MV, Gluck L: The lung profile. II. Complicated pregnancy. Am J Obstet Gynecol 135:64, 1979
16. Hayashi T: Diseases specific to pregnancy. In Romney SL, Gray MJ, Little AB et al (eds): Gynecology and Obstetrics: The Health Care of Women, p 661, New York City, McGraw-Hill, 1981
17. MacGillivray I, Campbell DM: The effect of hypertension and oedema on birth-weight. In Bonnar J, MacGillivray I, Symonds M (eds): Pregnancy Hypertension, p 307. Baltimore, University Park Press, 1980
18. Redman CWG, Beilin LJ, Bonnar J et al: Plasma urate measurements in predicting fetal death in hypertensive pregnancy. Lancet 1:1370, 1976
19. Wald NJ, Cuckle HS: Open neural-tube defects. In Wald NJ (ed): Antenatal and Neonatal Screening, p 25. Oxford, Oxford University Press, 1984
20. Althouse R, Ward N: Survival and handicap of infants with spina bifida. Arch Dis Child 55:845, 1980
21. Brock DJH: Screening for neural tube defects. In Sandler M (ed): Amniotic Fluid and Its Clinical Significance, p 169. New York City, Marcel Dekker, 1981
22. Carter CO, Fraser-Roberts JA: The risk of recurrence after two children with central nervous system malformations. Lancet 1:306, 1967
23. Wald N, Cuckle H, Boreham J: Small biparietal diameter of fetuses with spina bifida: Implication for antenatal screening. Br J Obstet Gynaecol 87:219, 1980
24. Seppala M: Alpha-fetoprotein in the amniotic fluid in relation to neural tube defects and other congenital/genetic disorders of the fetus. In Fairweather DVI, Eskes TKAB (eds): Amniotic Fluid Research and Clinical Application, p 297. Amsterdam, Excerpta Medica, 1978
25. Clements JA, Platzker ACG, Tierney DF et al: Assessment of the risk of the respiratory-distress syndrome by a rapid test for surfactant in amniotic fluid. N Engl J Med 286:1077, 1972
26. Shephard B, Buhi W, Spellacy W: Critical analysis of the amniotic fluid shake test. Obstet Gynecol 43:558, 1974
27. Bhagwanani SG, Fahmy D, Turnbull AC: Bubble stability test compared with lecithin assay in prediction of respiratory distress syndrome. Br Med J 1:697, 1973
28. Gluck L, Kulovich MV, Borer RC et al: Diagnosis of the respiratory distress syndrome by amniocentesis. Am J Obstet Gynecol 109:440, 1971
29. Gluck L, Kulovich MV: Lecithin/sphingomyelin ratios in amniotic fluid in normal and abnormal pregnancy. Am J Obstet Gynecol 115:539,1973
30. Gluck L, Kulovich MV: Fetal lung development current concepts. Pediatr Clin North Am 20:367, 1973
31. Gluck L, Kulovich MV, Borer RC et al: The inter-

pretation and significance of the lecithin/sphingomyelin ratio in amniotic fluid. Am J Obstet Gynecol 120:142, 1974
32. Buhi WC, Spellacy WN: Effects of blood or meconium on the determination of the amniotic fluid lecithin/sphingomyelin ratio. Am J Obstet Gynecol 121:321, 1975
33. Kulovich MV, Hallman MB, Gluck L: The lung profile. I. Normal pregnancy. Am J Obstet Gynecol 135:57, 1979
34. Parkinson CE, Harvey D: Amniotic fluid and fetal pulmonary maturity. In Sandler M (ed): Amniotic Fluid and Its Clinical Significance, p 229. New York City, Marcel Dekker, 1981
35. Shinitzky M, Goldfisher A, Bruck A et al: A new method for the assessment of fetal lung maturity. Br J Obstet Gynaecol 83:834, 1976
36. Tait JF, Franklin RW, Simpson JB et al: Improved fluorescence polarization assay for use in evaluating fetal lung maturity. I. Development of the assay procedure. Clin Chem 32:248, 1986
37. Foerder CA, Tait JF, Franklin RW et al: Improved fluorescence polarization assay for use in evaluating fetal lung maturity. II. Analytical evaluation and comparison with the lecithin/sphingomyelin ratio. Clin Chem 32:255, 1986
38. Hinkley C, O'Neil L, Cassady G: Amniotic fluid creatinine in the Rh sensitized pregnancy. Am J Obstet Gynecol 117:544, 1973
39. Younger BJ: Estrogen monitoring in high risk obstetrical patients. In Current Practical Methods of Fetal Surveillance. Sponsored by Southern Perinatal Association, 1976
40. Duenhoelter JH, Whalley PJ, MacDonald PC: An analysis of the utility of plasma immunoreactive estrogen measurements in determining delivery time of gravidas with a fetus considered at high risk. Am J Obstet Gynecol 125:889, 1976
41. Liley AW: Liquor amnii analysis in the management of the pregnancy complicated by rhesus sensitization. Am J Obstet Gynecol 82:1359, 1961
42. American College of Obstetricians and Gynecologists: Management of Isoimmunization in Pregnancy. ACOG Technical Bulletin 90, 1986
43. Liley AW: Errors in the assessment of hemolytic disease from amniotic fluid. Am J Obstet Gynecol 86:485, 1963
44. Hochberg CJ, Witheiler AP, Cook H: Accurate amniotic fluid bilirubin analysis from the "bloody tap." Am J Obstet Gynecol 126:531, 1976
45. Freda VJ: The Antepartum Management of Rh Disease. In Garratty G (ed): Hemolytic Disease of the Newborn, p 33. Arlington, Virginia, American Association of Blood Banks, 1984

Chapter 42

Female Reproductive Disorders

Peggy Luebbert

A complex system involving neural stimuli, hypothalamus, pituitary, and ovaries regulates sexual maturation and reproduction in women. The system is modulated by several areas of the brain that contain neurons, the axons of which relay neurotransmitters to alter hypothalamus activity. Neurotransmitters involved include dopamine, epinephrine, norepinephrine, serotonin, acetylcholine, histamine, and γ-aminobenzoic acid.[1] In response, the neurons in the hypothalamus synthesize and secrete a decapeptide known as gonadotropin-releasing hormone (GnRH). This peptide, synonymous with luteinizing-hormone-releasing hormone (LHRH) and luteinizing-hormone-releasing factor (LRF), controls the production and release of the gonadotropins follicle-stimulating hormone (FSH) and luteinizing hormone (LH) from the anterior pituitary via the hypothalamic pituitary portal system.

In females FSH, as its name implies, is considered the gonadotropin responsible for ovarian follicular growth. LH stimulates ovarian production of the steroids estrogen, progesterone, and androgens. Three naturally occurring estrogens are involved in the menstrual cycle. 17-β-estradiol (E_2), the major secreted estrogen, is in equilibrium in the circulation with estrone. Estrone is further metabolized in the liver to estriol. Estradiol is the most potent estrogen, and estriol the least. Almost all of the estrogens during the menstrual cycle are derived from the ovary.

Progesterone, a C_{21} steroid, is secreted along with estrogens from the ovarian follicles. It is converted to pregnanediol in the liver, conjugated to glucuronic acid, and excreted in the urine. The androgens, testosterone and androstenedione, are also released by the ovarian follicles under the stimulus of LH and FSH.

A *negative feedback mechanism* is responsible for the interaction of these hormones. The primary stimulus for LH and FSH release is the concentration of estrogens in the peripheral circulation. That is, when the level of estradiol falls below a set point, the gonadotropins are released. Alternatively, when the level of estradiol is above a set point, release of the gonadotropins is reduced. Feedback actions of estrogen seem to occur at the hypothalamus where GnRH secretion is stimulated and at the pituitary where LH and FSH are released. Inhibin, a nonsteroid FSH inhibitor, has been demonstrated in ovarian follicles and may play a role in the regulation of FSH secretions.

PUBERTY AND THE MENSTRUAL PHASES

Puberty

The changes in the body that constitute puberty have been classified according to skeletal growth patterns, fat distribution, and the development of the gonads, reproductive organs, and secondary sex characteristics. In the female they include the development of the breast tissue, and the sprouting of pubic and axillary hair. The precise signal that initiates these events involves a complex set of neuromechanisms interacting with the hypothalamus, pituitary, gonads, and adrenal cortex.[2] Prior to puberty, this system is functional but inhibited by low levels of circulating steroid hormones, particularly estrogen. At puberty, for a reason yet unknown, the hypothalamic hormone receptor sites become less sensitive to the steroid hormones. Consequently, the hypothalamic release of GnRH prompts production by the pituitary of large amounts of the gonadotropins LH and FSH, which in turn stimulate gonadal production of estradiol and progesterone. Early in puberty episodic secretions of LH are associated with sleep. The FSH levels seem to plateau by midpuberty, while LH and estradiol levels continue to rise until late puberty. By midpuberty the ovary is ready to secrete estrogen in irregular cycles of 28 to 40 days. The estrogens promote the proliferation of the uterine endometrium. By mid- to late puberty the decrease in E_2 brings menarche. Approximately 6 to 12 months later the increase in circulating estrogens near midcycle induces a surge of LH and FSH, resulting in ovulation. The length of time involved in this evolution is usually 2 to 4 years.

Although the system follows an orderly progression, the age of onset of puberty is variable. Factors involved include genetic makeup, socioeconomic conditions, nutrition, and general health. There had been a progressive decrease in the mean age of menarche in the U.S. until the 1940s; since then it has remained constant. Now, puberty generally begins some time between 8 and 14 years of age, with menarche occurring between 9 and 18 years (mean 12.8).

Due to the wide variance in sexual maturation, abnormal conditions can be difficult to diagnose. In general, a young woman with menarche before the age of 9 or failure to menstruate after the age of 16 deserves evaluation.

Menstrual Phases

MENSTRUAL CYCLE

The complex changes in hormonal levels during the menstrual cycle are regulated by the estradiol gonadotropin feedback mechanism. The length of the cycle is variable, but averages around 28 days from the start of one menstrual period to the start of the next. The days of the cycle are often identified by number, starting with the first day of menstruation. The cycle can be divided into three primary stages: the follicular phase, ovulation, and the luteal phase.

The follicular phase is initiated by a rise in FSH that occurs in response to the decline in estradiol in the preceding cycle (see Fig. 42-1).[3] This initial phase lasts 10 to 14 days and results in one surviving mature follicle. Low levels of LH early in the cycle are thought to have no function other than to maintain low levels of steroids. During the late follicular phase, under FSH stimulation, the maturing follicle begins estrogen production. Estrogen levels, specifically estradiol, rise slowly at first and then rapidly reach a peak just before ovulation. The estradiol peak varies from 500 to 1000 pg/mL (1835–3670 pmol/L). It triggers a midcycle surge of LH and FSH. In order for the LH and FSH surge to occur, estradiol levels of more than 200 pg/mL (734 pmol/L) for a critical time period of 50 hours or more are required.[4] Ovulation of the mature follicle into the abdominal cavity occurs about 12 hours after the gonadotropin peak, or about day 14 to 16 of the menstrual cycle.[4] The ovum is picked up by the oviducts and transported to the uterus. Unless fertilization occurs, the ovum passes through the uterus and out the vagina.

In the majority of menstrual cycles, the system allows only one follicle to mature and reach the point of ovulation. However, multiple fraternal births may be due in part to the random maturation of more than one follicle per cycle. After the rupture of the follicle and release of the ovum, the follicle accumulates a yellow pigment, lutein, which lends its name to the third and final phase of the cycle, the luteal phase. The time period from ovulation to menses is consistently close to 14 days in length. The variability in cycle lengths among women is due to the varying number of days required for follicular growth.

The mature follicle, known as the corpus luteum, begins synthesizing estrogens, progestin, and androgen steroids. By day 8 or 9 after ovula-

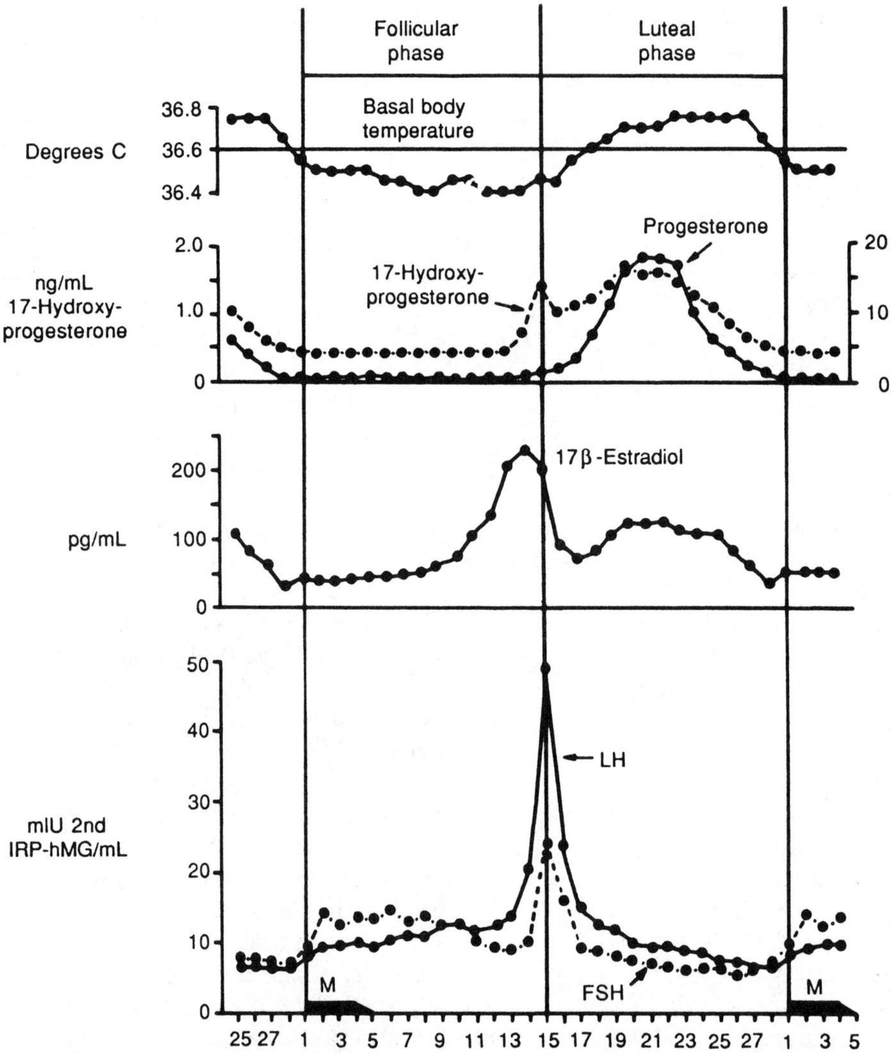

Figure 42-1 **Typical basal body temperature and plasma hormone concentrations during a normal 28-day human menstrual cycle. (From Midgley AR: Human Reproduction. Hagerstown, MD, Harper & Row, 1973)**

tion, peak levels of progesterone occur in the blood. Even though progesterone levels of 20 to 30 ng/mL (63.6–95.4 nmol/L) are not uncommon during the luteal phase, a level of 3 ng/mL (9.5 nmol/L) is considered a reliable indicator of ovulation and corpus luteum activity.[5] About 10% to 20% of the progesterone is excreted in the urine as the metabolite pregnanedione, which peaks at 3 to 6 mg/day (9.4–18.7 μmol/d) and is maintained until 2 days prior to menses. Due to the steroid negative feedback process, LH and FSH are now at their lowest levels in the cycle.

Ten to twelve days after ovulation, the corpus luteum enters a stage of regression in which progesterone and estradiol levels decrease, leading to menses and a new cycle. The corpus luteum is eventually replaced by fibrous tissue, forming a corpus albicans.

PREGNANCY

The menstrual cycle renewal is inevitable unless pregnancy occurs. With pregnancy the lifespan of the corpus luteum is prolonged by the emergence of a new stimulus, human chorionic gonadotropin (hCG). This gonadotropin appears at the peak of corpus luteum development (9 to 13 days after ovulation). It serves to maintain progesterone and estradiol levels until approximately the 9th to 10th week of gestation, by which time placental steroidogenesis is well established (see Chap. 40).

MENOPAUSE

At approximately 40 years of age, women enter a period known as the *climacteric*. This stage will last as long as 20 years and carries women through decreased fertility, menopause, and manifestations of progressive tissue atrophy and aging. Menopause, or the ceasing of cyclic menses, occurs in the U.S. between ages 48 and 55, with the median age being 51.4 years. Due to this age range, menopause may be presumed or misdiagnosed and the presence of other conditions may be missed. As a woman reaches menopause, residual follicles are least sensitive to gonadotropin stimulation and less likely to achieve complete maturation and estrogen production. Therefore, FSH and LH levels rise to their highest levels to stimulate the aging ovary. Levels of FSH greater than 40 mU/mL (40 IU/L) may be seen despite continued menstrual bleeding, while LH levels usually remain in the normal range. Eventually there is a ten- to twenty-fold increase in FSH and a three-fold increase in LH, reaching a maximum level 1 to 3 years after menopause, after which there is a gradual and slight decline. The circulating estradiol level after menopause is approximately 10 to 20 pg/mL (36.7–73.4 pmol/L), most of which is probably derived from peripheral conversion of testosterone and estrone. Interestingly, estrone levels are higher than estradiol levels at this point, with a mean level at approximately 30 pg/mL (111 pmol/L).

PRECOCIOUS PUBERTY

Etiology

In most cases of precocious puberty the clinical course is quite benign. In approximately 70% of affected girls, a specific etiology is not discovered. Frequently, familial disposition, congenital abnormalities, neonatal distress, or childhood infections or trauma may be involved. These children require long-term followup because cerebral abnormalities may not become apparent until adulthood. Other causes of true sexual precocity include intercranial diseases such as central nervous system (CNS) or pineal tumors, hamartoma or neurofibromas, McCune-Albright syndrome (polycystic fibrous dysplasia), or primary hypothyroidism.

In contrast, pseudoprecocious puberty usually indicates serious disease states such as ovarian cysts, ovarian or adrenal tumors, or adrenal hyperplasia. Both inadvertant ingestion of oral contraceptives and topical application of estrogens must be ruled out. In these conditions, development of secondary sex characteristics often progresses in an abnormal sequence or at an accelerated rate.

Clinical Manifestations

In precocious puberty, increased growth is often the first change noted, followed by breast development and pubic hair growth. If the child has cyclic ovarian activity resulting in menarche and ovulation, the syndrome is termed *true precocious puberty.* If a similar increase in steroid hormones occurs without gonadotropin stimulation and ovulation, a *pseudoprecocious puberty* exists. Although both are rare, true precocious puberty is seen five to six times more frequently than pseudoprecocious puberty.[6] Distinguishing the syndromes can be difficult and impractical. Both conditions can be due to serious disease; therefore, careful histories with dating of events, behavioral changes, and seizures along with thorough physical exams are crucial.

Laboratory Analyses and Diagnosis

Diagnostic radioimmunoassays (RIAs) of the gonadotropins LH and FSH, estradiol and progesterone, testosterone and androstenedione are readily available with established monoclonal double antibody technique and antibody-coated tube technology. These methods utilize a combination of tracer purified with monoclonal antibodies and human serum calibrators to provide sensitive and accurate assays. Because many hormone levels are affected by diurnal values, samples should be consistently collected in the morning. Values obtained on serum or urine will vary from technique to technique and even from run to run, so results should be compared cautiously. Simple kits for measurement of some of the peptide hormones (LH, hCG) are also entering the home (or self-) testing arena.

Blood estrogens and FSH : LH ratios compatible with those in sexually mature women are found in true precocious puberty. In contrast, low levels of LH and FSH with increased estrogens are often seen with tumors. Elevated hCGs may also indicate a teratoma or an ovarian dysgerminoma. High blood levels of 17-0H progesterone or 11-deoxycortisol that decline following oral administration of dexamethasone are useful in differentiating adrenal cortical hyperplasia from adrenal cortical adenomas, carcinomas, and ovarian tumors. An increase in testosterone suggests an ovarian cause of precocity. Increased dehydroisoandrosterone (DHA), the principal precursor of urinary 17-ketosteroids, is more consistent with adrenal sources of excess androgen.

Other tests useful in diagnosing sexual precocity include ultrasonic scanning of the adrenals and ovaries, CT scanning of the adrenals, and skull and bone age determinations.

Treatment

The treatment for precocious puberty is designed to suppress menstruation, ovulation, and fertility and to prevent excessively short stature. Administration of LHRH and/or appropriate replacement of thyroid hormone has been shown to cause regression in secondary sexual changes in precocious puberty. Treatment of choice for ovarian tumors causing pseudoprecocious puberty is surgical removal and, in some cases, chemotherapy. In cases of adrenocortical hyperplasia, glucocorticoid replacement therapy is indicated.

AMENORRHEA

Etiology

Amenorrhea is defined as follows:

1. No menses by the age of 14, with the absence of growth or development of secondary sex characteristics
2. No menses by the age of 16, despite the presence of normal growth and development and secondary sex characteristics
3. Absence of menses for 6 months or for the equivalent of three previous cycle intervals

As suggested by Speroff,[4] disorders producing amenorrhea can be classified into the following four compartments:

I. Outflow tract (uterus, cervix, vagina)
II. Ovary (follicular development and response)
III. Anterior pituitary (gonadotropin production and release)
IV. CNS and hypothalamus (gonadotropin-releasing hormones, production and release)

Once the compartment has been identified, the physician can usually identify a cause and formulate a treatment plan (see Fig. 42-2).

Because a minimal change in thyroid function can alter pituitary function, amenorrhea and infertility may be the first clinical symptoms of thyroid

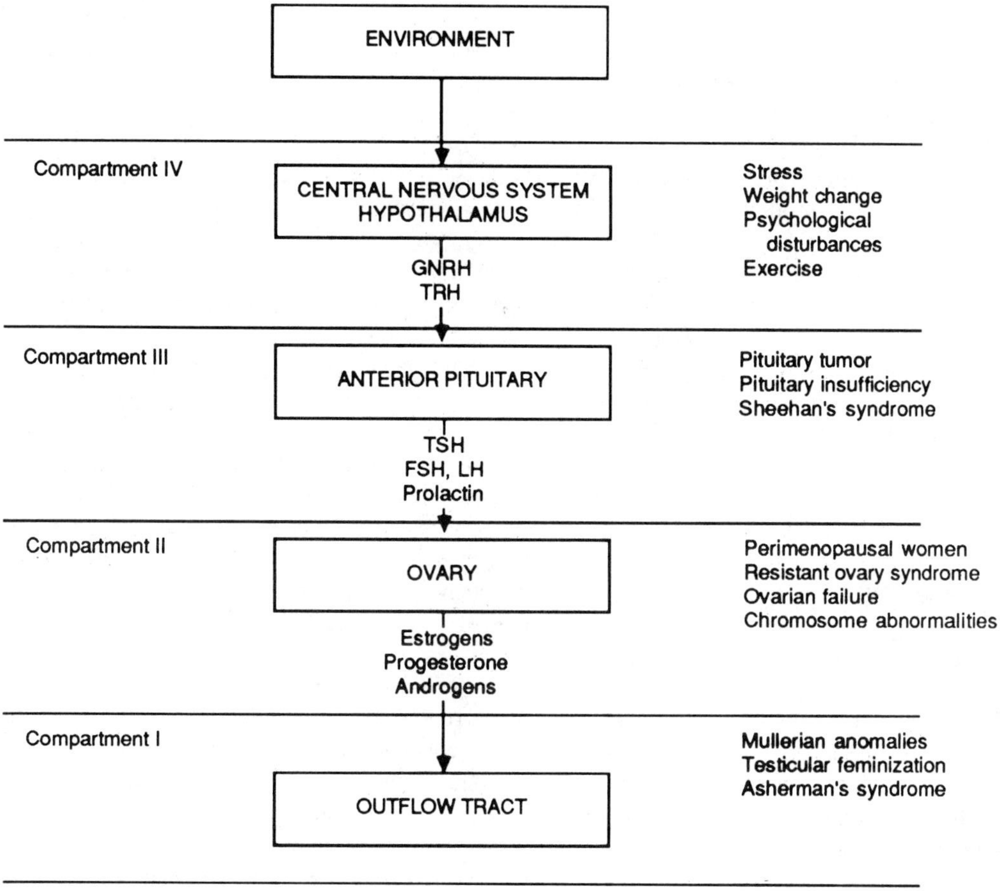

Figure 42-2 **Classification of common etiologies of amenorrhea by compartments and associated hormones.**

dysfunction. Increased TRH and TSH in primary hypothyroidism have been shown to induce hyperprolactinemia. Normal ovulatory function, however, usually returns after approximately 3 months of hormone replacement therapy.[7]

OUTFLOW TRACT ABNORMALITIES—COMPARTMENT I

Outflow tract defects can include congenital abnormalities such as mullerian agenesis or testicular feminization or can represent destruction of the endometrium as seen in Asherman's syndrome.

In the patient with a competent outflow tract who fails to bleed following progestational medication, inadequate levels of endogenous estrogen needed to stimulate endometrial growth are usually found. This fault may be due to ovarian unresponsiveness (Compartment II) or inadequate FSH gonadal stimulation (Compartment III or IV).

OVARIAN DYSFUNCTION—COMPARTMENT II

Ovarian dysfunction is almost always irreversible; however, cases do exist in which estrogen therapy triggered temporary return to ovarian activity.

The perimenopausal woman's gonadotropins may rise before bleeding actually ceases. Usually these women present with increased FSH and a normal LH value. It is likely that the elevated FSH levels are needed to stimulate the few remaining follicles that have diminished estrogen-producing ability. Once LH and FSH are elevated, total ovarian failure is likely.

Resistant ovarian syndrome is suggested in the amenorrhea patient with increased gonadotropins and functioning ovarian follicles. Large amounts of gonadotropins are needed to produce follicular growth in this rare syndrome. Achieving pregnancy is unlikely even with high doses of exogenous gonadotropins.

Premature ovarian failure is characterized by the cessation of ovarian function before the age of 40 years. It occurs secondary to increased atresia of the ovarian follicles. This may be a result of infection, radiation, chemotherapy, or autoantibody exposure. Sex chromosome abnormalities such as Turner's syndrome, silent Y chromosome, and a variety of other anomalies are also associated with premature ovarian failure.

Turner's syndrome, a gonadal dysgenesis in females, is the result of any of several defects of the X chromosome. About half of patients with this syndrome have a 45, X karyotype. The cytogenetic findings in the remainder vary. The 45, X defect may result from chromosome loss during gametogenesis in the parents or an error in mitosis during an early division of the zygote. This disorder must be distinguished clinically from Noonan's syndrome, which can occur in both males and females; however, patients with the latter disorder have a normal karyotype.[8]

The presence of a Y chromosome leading to mosaicism occurs, and testicular tissue may predispose the patient to malignancy or virilization. Approximately one-third of the patients carrying a Y chromosome do not exhibit signs of virilization. Thus a normal phenotypic female with amenorrhea and increased gonadotropins should be karyotyped, evaluated, and diagnosed accordingly. In the case of "testicular feminization" in which a genotypic male appears phenotypically female, a complete end organ resistance to androgens is present.

PITUITARY DISORDERS—COMPARTMENT III

With increased sensitivity of radiologic examinations along with increased utilization of prolactin assays, pituitary tumors are more frequently associated with amenorrhea. As many as one-third of patients with secondary amenorrhea will have a pituitary tumor.[6]

Pituitary insufficiency leading to amenorrhea may also be due to nearby lesions, carotid artery aneurysms, or an obstruction of the aqueduct of Sylvius or ischemia as seen in Sheehan's syndrome. This last disorder is caused by a postpartum vascular infarction of the pituitary. In these patients, the necrosis is due to extensive thrombosis of the pituitary circulation during or following delivery. It is usually associated with excessive blood loss and hypotension. Characteristically, patients with Sheehan's syndrome fail to lactate or menstruate. The association of these signs with low circulating levels of prolactin suggests this diagnosis. Some patients appear quite healthy, while others gradually lapse into severe anterior pituitary insufficiency involving gonadal, thyroid, and adrenal function. The pituitary gland has a large reserve, however, and substantial amounts of pituitary tissue must be damaged before significant hormone deficiency develops.

HYPOTHALAMIC AMENORRHEA—COMPARTMENT IV

Amenorrhea stems from an impaired release of GnRH with low levels of LH, FSH, and estrogens leading to anovulation.[9] It is postulated that the impaired release of GnRH is due to abnormal metabolism of dopamine and norepinephrine in the central nervous system; however, bromocriptine, a dopamine antagonist, has no effect on the abnormalities.[10]

Recently it has been shown that strenous physical activity as seen in avid marathon runners, ballet dancers, and swimmers has detrimental effects on reproductive functions, such as producing amenorrhea. It has been estimated that there are 4.4 million oligomenorrheic athletes.[11] In one study, more than 35% of the female runners of 60 miles per week experienced amenorrhea.[12] This chronic anovulation is influenced by a combination of physical, hormonal, and psychological effects. Changes in weight, percent of body fat, daily protein intake, and stress may all contribute to the problem.

Clinical Manifestations

OUTFLOW TRACT ABNORMALITIES—COMPARTMENT I

The clinical findings in these disorders depend on the nature of the anatomic or structural defect that precludes menstrual bleeding. Menstrual blood often accumulates behind the obstacle and these women may have cyclic episodes of abdominal pain. Surgery is the treatment.

OVARIAN DYSFUNCTION—COMPARTMENT II

A patient with amenorrhea due to ovarian dysfunction will have a variety of other symptoms depending on the cause of dysfunction. A thorough medical history will assist in ruling out some disorders. The patient with normal menses early in her history may be evaluated for previous treatments or development of an autoimmune disorder. Patients who have never achieved menses will have a variety of symptoms based on etiology. Turner's is one example.

Turner's syndrome (45,XO) is usually recognized in infancy by the classic physical characteristics of short stature, webbed neck, shield crest, and increased angle of the arms. The gonads are usually bilateral pale "streaks" of connective tissue; however, primary follicles have been described, with a rare occurrence of menarche and variable menses.[13]

PITUITARY DISORDERS—COMPARTMENT III

A patient with a disorder of the pituitary can have a variety of symptoms. In addition to amenorrhea, symptoms can include headaches, visual difficulties, acromegaly, cushionoid appearance, and lactation.

HYPOTHALAMIC DISORDERS—COMPARTMENT IV

Patients with hypothalamic disorders often have experienced physical or emotional stress, psychological disturbances, or drastic weight loss with a history of menstrual disorders. Many women on "crash diets" or suffering from anorexia nervosa initially have no complaints other than amenorrhea. Drastic weight loss as seen in anorexia is considered a psychiatric disorder associated with abnormalities of the feeding and endocrine functions normally controlled by the hypothalamus.

Laboratory Analyses and Diagnosis

INITIAL WORKUP

Before elaborate workups are undertaken, pregnancy in the sexually active patient should be ruled out. Today, pregnancy usually can be detected 1 to 2 weeks after conception when using monoclonal antibody pregnancy assays.

Following pregnancy testing, evaluation of an amenorrheic patient should include thyroid function tests (T_4, TSH), serum prolactin levels, and the progestogen challenge tests (Provera) used to assess the competency of the outflow tract (see Fig. 42-3). Normal results of these studies indicate a diagnosis of anovulation. Management of these patients depends on whether or not the patient would like to become pregnant. If pregnancy is desired, ovulation induction is indicated. If pregnancy is not desired, the patient can be placed on oral contraceptives or a barrier method of contraception because ovulation and fertility may return without warning.

OUTFLOW TRACT ABNORMALITIES—COMPARTMENT I

The lack of withdrawal flow within 2 weeks after a course of progestational medication can establish the diagnosis of a defect in compartment I.

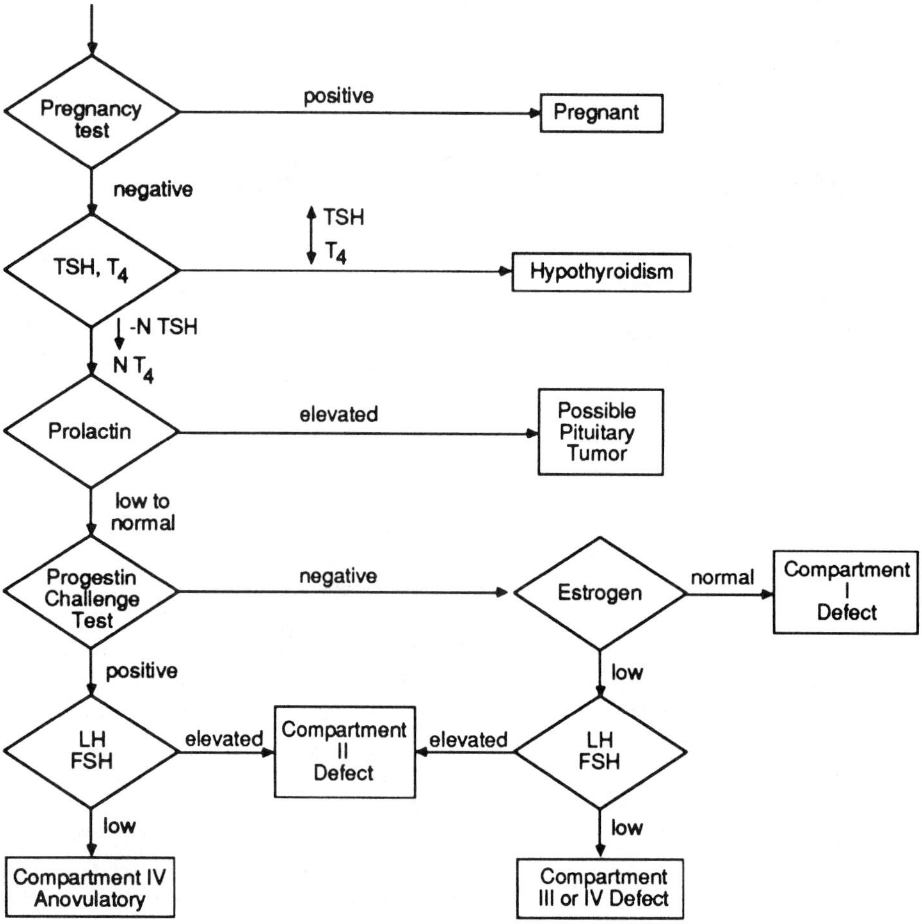

Figure 42-3 Evaluation of amenorrhea.

OVARIAN DYSFUNCTION—COMPARTMENT II

To rule out ovarian failure (compartment II), blood LH and FSH should be assayed. For accuracy, these hormones should be measured no earlier than 2 weeks after any hormonal medications are administered to the patient. Elevated gonadotropins indicate ovarian unresponsiveness (compartment II), whereas low or normal levels suggest hypopituitarism or pituitary dysfunction (compartment III).

An amenorrheic patient with FSH values over 20 mU/mL (20 IU/L) and low estrogen levels is considered to have ovarian failure.

Suspected Turner's syndrome patients can be screened by determination of the X chromosome pattern on a buccal smear, but should be diagnosed definitively by a blood lymphocyte karyotype analysis. Plasma gonadotropin levels, especially FSH, are useful in assessing the functional status of the gonads. Plasma FSH levels are usually elevated from birth to the age of 4 years, but decrease to high normal values between 5 and 10 years of age. After ten years, FSH levels reach their highest points. The pattern of change in LH is similar, but the concentrations are 1/3 to 1/10 those of FSH. GnRH-induced LH and FSH responses exhibit a pattern with age similar to that for basal levels. That is, patients under the age of 5 years and over the age of 10 years exhibit a rise in gonadotropins after GnRH, while between the ages of 5 and 10 years the response is less.

Before the age of 10 years, Turner's syndrome patients also show normal concentrations of adrenal androgens. However, after the age of 15, levels of dehydroepiandrosterone (DHEA), testosterone, and androstenedione are lower than normal due to the lack of gonadol production.[6]

Patients with silent Y syndrome (46,XY) have increased plasma LH and testosterone concentrations. Estradiol concentrations are higher than normally seen in men, and FSH levels are often normal or slightly increased.

PITUITARY DISORDERS—COMPARTMENT III

The association of pituitary tumors, amenorrhea, and elevated prolactin levels is high. Hyperprolactinemia has been reported in 15% to 40% of patients with secondary amenorrhea, and is the most common form of pituitary hyperfunction.[14] In addition to pituitary adenomas, factors leading to increased prolactin release can include the following:

1. Stress (trauma, exercise, surgery, psychological pressures)
2. Physiological (breast and nipple stimulation)
3. Pharmacologic (oral contraceptives, phenothiazines, tricyclic antidepressants, progestins, TRH)

Ideally a specimen for prolactin measurements should be obtained in midmorning in a relaxed patient who has not had a recent breast exam. Plasma prolactin levels in patients with prolactin-secreting tumors vary from 15 ng/mL (15 μg/L) to values greater than 10,000 ng/mL (10,000 μg/L).[15] In one study, all patients with levels in excess of 300 ng/mL (300 μg/L) had a demonstrable pituitary adenoma.[14] Phamacologic agents usually do not increase serum prolactin levels above 100 ng/mL (100 μg/L).[16]

A CT scan of the sella turcica is warranted for a positive diagnosis of a prolactinoma.

HYPOTHALAMIC AMENORRHEA—COMPARTMENT IV

A patient suffering from hypothalamic amenorrhea usually has a normal CT scan of the brain and normal prolactin levels. Patients may exhibit high growth hormone levels and plasma somatomedin activity, decreased T_4 and T_3, increased rT_3, and upper normal or elevated cortisol values. With the return of weight gain and normal hormone levels, menses usually return also.

Schwartz found that LH levels in amenorrheic runners were significantly higher than in their normal counterparts, whereas TSH levels were lower and basal steroids did not differ.[17] However, the ratio of estrone to estradiol was significantly higher in the runners. Increases in prolactin and beta endorphines, known LH and FSH inhibitors, have also been reported.[18]

Treatment

TURNER'S SYNDROME

Treatment is directed toward attempts to augment stature and correct somatic anomalies. Estrogen therapy, after 15 years of age, is also initiated to induce secondary sexual characteristics, to permit withdrawal bleeding, and to prevent osteoporosis. This therapy also reduces the risk of endometrial hyperplasia and possible endometrial adenocarcinoma later.[19]

SILENT Y SYNDROME

Therapy includes orchidectomy with estrogen replacement therapy, along with vaginal dilation and psychological reinforcement of female gender identity.

PITUITARY DISORDERS

Therapy for pituitary tumors is controversial at present. Neurosurgery (transphenoridal adenonectomy) is the preferred treatment for macroadenomas. For the patient with prolactin levels of less than 100 ng/mL (100 μg/L) and a normal CT scan, either bromocriptine therapy or surveillance can be chosen. If surveillance is chosen, annual CT scans and prolactin levels are advised to detect an emerging tumor.

HYPOTHALAMIC DISORDERS

Medical workup of the amenorrheic athlete depends upon her goals. Estrogen replacement for the hypoestrogenic female may be recommended to avoid osteoporosis. If pregnancy is desired, a reduction in exercise may be all that is necessary for ovulation to return. In severe cases, clomiphene gonadotropin therapy has been indicated.

INFERTILITY

Etiology

Infertility, which occurs in 15% of U.S. couples, is usually defined as 1 year of unprotected coitus without pregnancy. Women account for approximately 50% of fertility problems. Of these, 20% fail to ovulate, 4% have an inadequate luteal phase, 30% have abnormal tubal pathology, and 10% have cervical factors that complicate fertility. Although a specific cause for ovulation failure will not be found in the majority of women, anovulation or oligoovulation may result from abnormalities of the hypothalamic-pituitary axis or from ovary, thyroid, or adrenal dysfunctions.

LUTEAL PHASE DISORDER

The short or inadequate luteal phase is considered a possible cause of infertility in addition to anovulation discussed elsewhere in this chapter. This abnormality is characterized either by a short interval (less than 11 days) between ovulation and menstruation with a normal progesterone peak, or by a normal-length luteal phase with lower than normal progesterone levels. Both result in adequate stimulation of the endometrium, resulting in two or more unexplained short cycles or a history of habitual abortions. Decreased levels of FSH and estradiol during the follicular phase and a lower midcycle FSH peak suggest a subnormal stimulation prior to ovulation. Increased prolactin levels have also been associated with this abnormality.[20]

Clinical Manifestations

Clinical indicators of ovulation include mittelschmerz (abdominal pain midway between menstrual periods), ultrasound detection of preovulatory follicles and corpus luteum, or a serum progesterone level of 3 ng/mL (9.5 nmol/L) or more.[21] Progesterone at the midluteal phase should be 10 ng/mL (31.8 nmol/L) or more to indicate sufficient production by the corpus luteum. Biological effects of progesterone that may be used to evaluate ovulation indirectly include basal body temperature changes, a secretory endometrium, premenstrual molimina, thick cervical mucus, and a change in vaginal cytology.

Laboratory Analyses and Diagnosis

ANOVULATION

Many of the abnormalities resulting in anovulation are included under the discussions of amenorrhea and hirsuitism in this chapter. The history and physical examination of an anovulating woman should include laboratory quantitation of FSH, LH, prolactin, and progesterone. Thyroid studies and DHEA-sulfate and testosterone tests should be performed if symptoms suggest thyroid disease or hyperandrogenism.

LUTEAL PHASE DISORDER

The diagnosis of a luteal phase disorder can be approached in a variety of ways. A biphasic basal body temperature chart with a duration of the temperature rise of less than 11 days may indicate a shortened luteal phase. A serum progesterone level of 10 ng/mL (31.8 nmol/L) or more 5 to 10 days prior to the next menstrual period may rule out an inadequate luteal phase. The diagnosis of a shortened or inadequate luteal phase can be corroborated with an endometrial biopsy. A biopsy, taken 2 to 3 days prior to menstruation, found to be more than 2 days out of phase is diagnostic of this abnormality. Despite the discomfort and expense involved in this procedure, it remains the classical way to diagnose an inadequate luteal phase.

Treatment

When a specific etiology for infertility can be identified, therapy is directed toward the cause—for example, thyroid replacement therapy for hypothyroidism, or prolactin suppression with bromocriptine. For patients with no known identifiable cause, treatment is tailored to the goals of the woman. Ovulation therapy with clomiphene is warranted for the woman who desires pregnancy. Anovulatory women who do not desire to conceive require treatment with a course of oral progestin to correct cycle irregularities and to protect against abnormal bleeding episodes.

In luteal phase disorders, progesterone vaginal suppositories, hCG injections, and/or clomiphene have been used to lengthen the luteal phase and to achieve pregnancy.

HIRSUITISM

Etiology

Hirsuitism is usually defined as more hair growth than is considered cosmetically acceptable to a woman living in a certain culture. It is a symptom associated with abnormal androgen metabolism. The increase in hair growth will occur with increased androgen production, decreased hepatic clearance, or an increase in the sensitivity of the hair follicles to androgens.

The hormonal abnormalities leading to hirsuitism include elevations of the active androgens of testosterone (TST), dihydrotestosterone (DHT), dehydroepiandrosterone (DHEA), DHEA-sulfate, and androstenedione. Normally, 5% to 20% of circulating TST is secreted by the ovary, 0% to 30% by the adrenals, and 50% to 70% by peripheral conversion of precursors. 50% to 80% of androstenedione is produced by the ovaries, whereas DHEA is almost entirely of adrenal origin (80%).[22] In the hirsuit woman, the ovarian and adrenal components increase markedly and peripheral conversion decreases.

Metabolic clearance rate of TST is usually accelerated in women with hirsuitism. The steroid is taken up rapidly by the cells, where it is converted to DHT. DHT, the intracellular hormone most active in increasing hair growth, is converted from TST by 5-γ-reductase in areas such as the upper lip, chin, chest, and abdomen. Total testosterone levels may therefore not be elevated, but free TST concentration is always increased in hirsuits.

Polycystic ovary disease (PCO), first described in 1935 by Stein and Leventhal, is the most common cause of androgen stimulation in women. This condition includes bilaterally enlarged ovaries with multiple bluish follicular cysts, menstrual disturbances, infertility, and virilism.[23] Virilism, which consists of frontal balding, hirsuitism, deepening of the voice, acne, and clitoromegaly, is almost always associated with increased TST from an ovarian source such as PCO or the rare arrhenoblastoma. Obesity is also commonly seen in this disorder. Current hypotheses suggest this disorder to be a result of a hypothalamic neurotransmitter abnormality. The atypical ovaries in PCO produce TST and androstenedione, which are converted peripherally by the adipose tissue to estrone. Adrenal activity may also occur; however, controversy exists as to its predominance.

In congenital adrenal hyperplasia (CAH) and Cushing's syndrome, increased adrenal production of androstenedione and DHEA and their peripheral conversions to TST lead to hirsuitism. Evaluation of the corticosteroids will assist in identification of this cause of hirsuitism.

Clinical Manifestations

Most hirsuit women present initially to their physician with a cosmetic problem. Common findings include beard growth, sternal and areolar hair growth, irregular menses, and obesity. Patients usually have a normal menarche and only later develop menstrual disorders.

Laboratory Analyses and Diagnosis

Plasma TST levels may fluctuate with adrenal circadian rhythms, so it is often helpful to obtain three TST samples at different times and pool the samples for a single determination. It is difficult to distinguish ovarian and adrenal abnormalities; however, an increase in DHEA is highly suggestive of adrenal dysfunction. Suppression tests such as the dexamethasone or oral contraceptive suppression tests have also been useful.[23, 24]

In PCO, total TST levels and urinary 17-ketosteroids are usually normal or slightly elevated.[25] Serum prolactin levels also tend to be slightly elevated. Normal or low levels of FSH are seen, whereas LH levels may be elevated. A 1 : 5 ratio of LH to FSH is often characteristic of PCO.

Treatment

Treatment of hirsuitism is either by suppression of excess androgen production (oral contraceptives, medroxyprogesterone, or dexamethasone), by androgen blocking agents (cyproterone acetate), or by surgical removal of the ovarian or adrenal tumors.

GESTATIONAL TROPHOBLASTIC DISEASE

Etiology

Gestational trophoblastic disease involves a broad spectrum of interrelated neoplasms including hydatidiform mole, invasive mole, and choriocarcinoma. Hydatidiform moles are the most common trophoblastic neoplasm, and occur in approximately 1 out of 2000 pregnancies in the U.S. Two types of moles have been described.[26] The complete or classic mole has no evidence of fetal tissue and is androgenic in origin. That is, fertilization occurs by a haploid sperm, with duplication of its chromosomes without cell division resulting in the common karyotype 46,XX. In the partial mole, which occurs approximately 10% of the time, there is a fetal sac and/or fetus with associated degeneration of the villi.[27] The fetus usually shows trisomy on chromosome analysis. Only 4% lead to further neoplasms, whereas complete moles have neoplastic sequelae in 15% to 20% of cases.

Clinical Manifestations

Classic molar pregnancies present with early uterine bleeding, large uterus, excessive vomiting, and early preeclampsia toxemia. Hyperthyroidism and ovarian cysts may also develop. On the other hand, partial moles usually present with signs and symptoms of a spontaneous or missed abortion.

Laboratory Analyses and Diagnosis

Marked elevation of β-hCG levels and a characteristic "snowstorm" ultrasound pattern are valuable diagnostic tools in evaluating a molar pregnancy. β-hCG levels over 100,000 mU/mL (100,000 IU/L) after the twelfth week of gestation are common in molar patients. However, low or normal β-hCGs have been documented in these patients.[28]

Treatment

After diagnosis and stabilization of the patient, suction evacuation of the uterus is the treatment of choice. A hysterectomy may be performed on those who do not desire to preserve fertility. Prophylactic chemotherapy has also been recommended for those patients who are at high risk of developing further neoplastic sequelae. Pre-evacuation β-hCG levels of less than 50,000 mU/mL (50,000 IU/L) are considered indicative of high-risk trophoblastic disease.[29] In monitoring the patient, weekly serum β-hCG levels should be obtained one week after evacuation and continued weekly until the titer is normal. After normal values return, β-hCG measurements should be performed on a monthly basis for 6 months. A β-hCG regression curve should be plotted for each patient and compared with that of a normal molar β-hCG regression curve[30] (see Fig. 42-4). Any patient with a titer plateau (no decrease in a

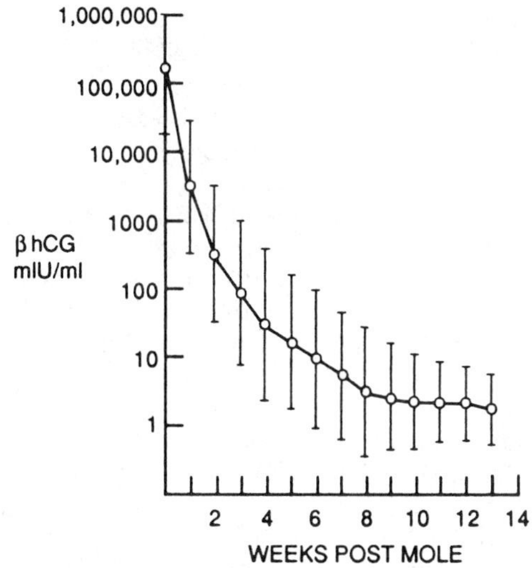

Figure 42-4 The mean value (0) and 95% confidence limits (vertical bars) describing the normal postmolar serum β = hCG regression curve. (From Schlaerth JB et al: Prognostic characteristics of serum hCG titer regression following molar pregnancy. Obstet Gynecol 58:478, 1981)

3-week period) or rise (two-fold increase in a 2-week period) should be evaluated for further trophoblastic tumors.[29]

TROPHOBLASTIC TUMORS

Etiology

Most trophoblastic tumors follow a molar pregnancy; however, they may develop after an ectopic pregnancy, abortion, or normal-term pregnancy. Local invasive tumors, limited to the uterus, develop in 15% of molar pregnancies. Metastatic disease occurs in 4% of patients and is usually associated with choriocarcinoma. Common sites of metastases also include lungs (80%), liver (19%), and brain (10%).[28] An anatomic staging system was adopted in 1979 along with a prognostic scoring system to help in objectively classifying and treating these patients.

Clinical Manifestations

Patients usually present to physicians with irregular vaginal bleeding, ovarian cysts, uterine subinvolution, and elevated β-hCG titers.

Treatment

Treatment for postmolar trophoblastic disease depends on the clinical situation, but the disease is virtually 100% curable. Treatment of choice for the women who prefer infertility is a hysterectomy. If β-hCG levels are less than 500 mU/mL (500 IU/L), treatment with a single agent such as actinomycin D is recommended until titers reach normal levels.[28] Higher β-hCG levels indicate the need for a more aggressive approach to testing and therapy, with brain and liver scans and a combination chemotherapy of methotrexate and actinomycin D. After normal β-hCG levels have been reached, patients should have levels repeated for a year and be analyzed every 5 years and/or for life after pregnancy.

CASE STUDY

A 16-year-old girl with a history of diabetes was admitted to the hospital with complaints of weakness and abdominal pain. Due to the patient's extreme obesity (277 lbs), abdominal probing by the physician was difficult. On examination, the physician noted a tall, well developed, sexually inactive teenager who had been amenorrheic for 8 months. She had slight hirsuitism of her face. The rest of the examination was unremarkable.

Results of initial laboratory hormone studies were as follows:

LABORATORY FINDINGS

Test	*Reference Values*	*Patient's Values*
T_4	5–12 μg/dL	10 μg/dL
TSH	2.0–6.0 μU/mL	4.0 μU/mL
LH	2–30 mU/mL	36 mU/mL
FSH	4–20 mU/mL	7 mU/mL
TST	0–90 ng/dL	114 ng/dL

Conversion to SI units is as follows:

T_4—μg/dL × 12.9 = nmol/L
TSH—μU/mL × 1 = mIU/L
LH—mU/mL × 1 = IU/L
FSH—mU/mL × 1 = IU/L
TST—ng/dL × 0.0347 = nmol/L

Questions

1. What condition is most often associated with these clinical findings?
2. What other procedure may be performed to confirm this abnormality?
3. What course of treatment might be prescribed?

Discussion

1. The obesity, amenorrhea, and abnormal androgens along with the 5:1 LH/FSH levels are most often seen in polycystic ovary disease.
2. In this case, a laparoscopy was performed. Small fallopian tubes with large ovaries of irregular dimensions were noted.
3. Typically, oral contraceptives to suppress TST levels and to induce menses are prescribed. In this situation the patient was dismissed on contraceptives with subsequent clinic visits scheduled. Her insulin was adjusted, and she was instructed to stay on a strict 1800-calorie diet.

REFERENCES

1. Yen S, Jaffe RB: Reproductive Endocrinology: Physiology, Pathophysiology, and Clinical Management, 2nd ed. Philadelphia, WB Saunders, 1986
2. Badawy S: Reproductive Endocrinology and Infertility. Chicago, Year Book Medical Publishers, 1980
3. Midgley AR: Human Reproduction, p 227. Hagerstown, Maryland, Harper & Row, 1973
4. Speroff L, Glass RH, Kase NG: Clinical Gynecologic Endocrinology and Infertility, 3rd ed. Baltimore, Williams & Wilkins, 1983
5. Gold JJ, Josimovich JB: Gynecologic Endocrinology, 3rd ed. Hagerstown, Maryland, Harper & Row, 1980
6. Wilson JD, Foster DW (eds): Williams Textbook of Endocrinology, 7th ed, p 344. Philadelphia, WB Saunders, 1985
7. Given JR: Endocrine Causes of Menstrual Disorders. Chicago, Year Book Medical Publishers, 1977
8. Wilson JD, Griffin JE: Disorders of Sexual Differentiation. In Petersdorf RG et al (eds): Harrison's Principles of Internal Medicine, p 728. New York City: McGraw-Hill, 1983
9. Schwabe AD, Lippe BM, Chang RJ: Anorexia nervosa. Ann Intern Med 94:371–381, 1981
10. Beaumont PJ, Abraham SI: Continuous IV fusion of luteinizing-Hormone-releasing hormone (LHRH) in patients with anorexia nervosa. Psychol Med 11:477–484, 1981
11. Bitner MR: Secondary amenorrhea in the female athlete. N Engl J Med 10:363, 1985
12. Feicht CB et al: Secondary amenorrhea in athletes. Lancet 2:1145, 1978
13. Kohn G, Yarkon S, Cohen MM: Two conceptions in a 45, X woman. Am J Med Genet 5:339–343, 1980
14. Quigley MM, Haney AI: Evaluation of hyperprolactinemia: Clinical Profiles. Clin Obstet Gynaecol 23 (2):337–348, 1980
15. Wyngaarden J, Smith L Jr: Textbook of Medicine, 17th ed, p 1263. Philadelphia, WB Saunders, 1985
16. Malo JW, Bezdicek BJ: Secondary amenorrhea: A protocol for pinpointing the underlying cause. Postgrad Med 79 (3):91, 1986
17. Schwartz B, Cumming DC: Exercise-associated amenorrhea: A distinct entry. Am J Obstet Gynecol 141:662–669, 1981
18. Colt EW, Wardlaw SJ, Frantz AG: The effect of running on plasma β-endorphin. Life Sci 28: 1637–1641, 1981
19. Gambrell RD Jr: The menopause: Benefits and risks of estrogen-progestogen replacement therapy. Fertil Steril 37 (4):457–474, 1982
20. Insler V, Lunenfeld B: Infertility: Male and Female, p 194. New York City, Churchill Livingstone, 1986
21. Keller DW, Strickler RC, Watten JC: Clinical Infertility, p 53. Norwalk, Connecticut, Appleton-Century-Crofts, 1984
22. Hare JW: Signs and Symptoms in Endocrine and Metabolic Disorders, p 73. Philadelphia, JB Lippincott, 1986
23. Hatch R, Rosenfield RL, Kim M: Hirsuitism: Implications, etiology, and management. Am J Obstet Gynecol 140:815, 1981
24. Givens JR, Anderson RN, Wiser WL: Dynamics of suppression and recovery of plasma FSH, LH, and

androstenedione and TST in PCO using oral contraceptives. J Clin Endocrinol Metab 38:727, 1974
25. Kaplan LA, Pesce AJ: Clinical Chemistry: Theory, Analysis, and Correlation, p 803. St. Louis, CV Mosby, 1984
26. Kohorn E: Molar pregnancy: Presentation and diagnosis. Clin Obstet Gynaecol 27 (1):181, 1984
27. Dodson MG: New concepts and questions in gestational trophoblastic disease. J Reprod Med 28 (11): 744, 1983
28. Kistner RW: Gynecology Principles and Practice. Chicago, Year Book Medical Publishers, 1986
29. Morrow CP: Post-molar trophoblastic disease: Diagnosis, management, and prognosis. Clin Obstet Gynaecol 27 (1):212, 1984
30. Schlaerth JB, Morrow CP, Kletzky OA et al: Prognostic characteristics of serum human chorionic gonadotropin titer regression following molar pregnancy. Obstet Gynecol 58:478, 1981

Chapter 43

Male Reproductive Disorders

Peggy L. Bottjen

The male reproductive system (see Fig. 43-1) consists of two testes that produce sperm and androgens, a penis, and a system of glands, the secretions of which produce most of the components of seminal fluid in which the sperm are conveyed. This gland system consists of two bulbourethral glands (Cowper's glands), the prostate, and two seminal vesicles. Ducts through which sperm pass outside the body include the epididymis, the vas deferens, and the ejaculatory duct.[1]

The mature testis is enclosed by a thick white capsule consisting of several layers. Eighty-five percent of the volume of the testis is composed of seminiferous tubules (see Fig. 43-2) that are separated by fibrous septa. The tubules are lined with Sertoli cells and spermatogenic cells. The interstitial tissue between the tubules contains Leydig cells, which are responsible for androgen production.[1]

The spermatogenic cells that line the seminiferous tubules mature progressively from spermatogonia to mature spermatozoa. Spermatogenesis in the human male takes about 72 days[2] and starts with the outer layer of dividing cells, called *spermatogonia*. Mitotic division provides a continuous source of new cells. Some of the spermatogonia move away from the lining of the

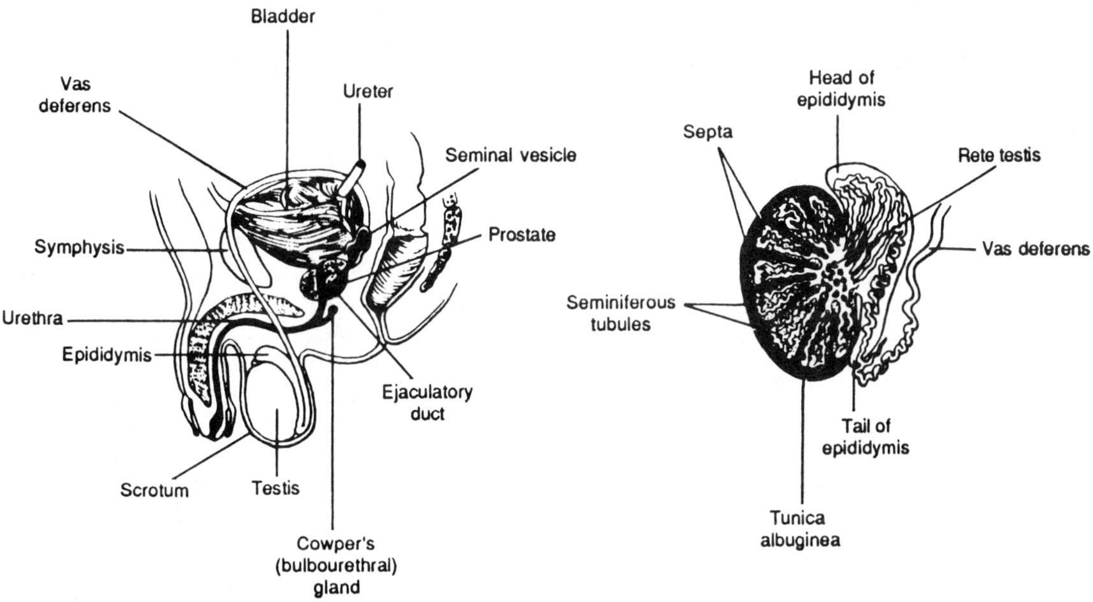

Figure 43-1 Male reproductive organs. (From Gonong WF: Review of Medical Physiology, 10th ed. Los Altos, Lange Medical Publications, 1981)

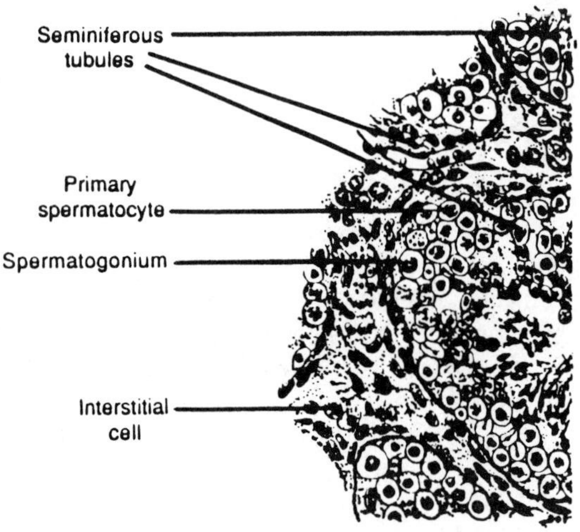

Figure 43-2 **Section of human testis. (From Gonong WF: Review of Medical Physiology, 10th ed. Los Altos, Lange Medical Publications, 1981)**

tubule and increase in size, becoming primary spermatocytes. Each spermatocyte then divides into two spermatids, which progress to mature spermatozoa (see Fig. 43-3)

The testes fulfill two functions, reproduction and hormonal control of secondary sex characteristics. Reproductive capacity is accomplished by the pituitary release of follicle-stimulating hormone (FSH), which acts on the seminiferous tubules to produce spermatozoa. Hormonal control of secondary sex characteristics is accomplished by pituitary release of luteinizing hormone (LH) (see Fig. 43-4). LH acts on the Leydig cells in the interstitial space of the testes to secrete testosterone, which is the primary androgen responsible for secondary sex characteristics. Testosterone is also important in maintenance of spermatogenesis in the seminiferous tubules.[3]

The pituitary release of LH and FSH is stimulated by gonadotropin-releasing hormone (GnRH or LHRH) from the hypothalamus (see Fig. 43-5). LH is believed to act primarily on the Leydig cells of the testes to control biosynthesis and secretion of testosterone, predominantly, and small amounts of dihydrotestosterone and estradiol. These steroids act in a negative feedback mechanism to shut off LH. FSH is believed to act primarily on the seminiferous tubules to initiate spermatogenesis. Sertoli cells within the seminiferous tubules are believed to produce inhibin, a hormone that acts to decrease FSH.[4]

This feedback mechanism is very important in understanding the clinical symptoms and laboratory results when evaluating a patient with hypogonadism or other male reproductive disorders.

SPERMATOGENESIS

SPERMATOGONIA
↓ mitosis and enlargement
°1 SPERMATOCYTE
↓ meiosis
°2 SPERMATOCYTE
↓ 2nd meiosis
SPERMATIDS
↓ spermiogenesis
MATURE SPERMATOZOA

Figure 43-3 Spermatogenesis.

HYPOGONADISM

Etiology and Pathophysiology

The etiology and characteristics of hypogonadism are outlined in the box on page 530.

Hyperprolactinemia can be caused by prolactin-secreting pituitary tumors, drugs, and functional secretion disorders.[5] The actual mechanism by which prolactin interferes with normal function is complex, and may involve the central nervous system, feedback control of gonadotropin secretion, Leydig cell sensitivity to LH, and enzymatic activity for steroidogenesis.[6]

Panhypopituitarism, which is generalized secretion deficiency of the anterior lobe of the pituitary gland, may be caused by adenomas, granu-

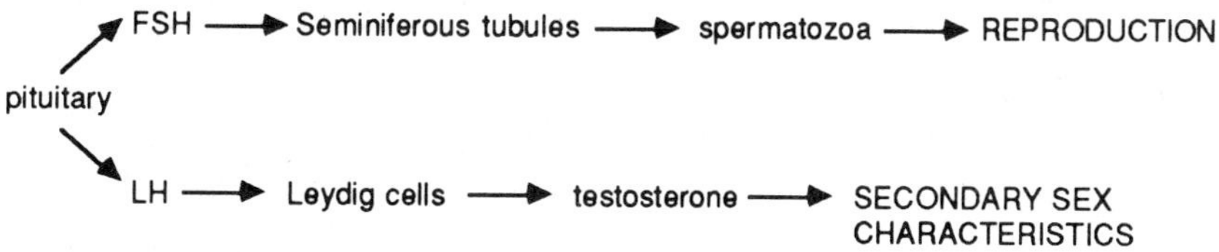

Figure 43-4 **Endocrine function of the testes and hormonal control. (From Jubiz W: Endocrinology—A Logical Approach for Clinicians, 2nd ed. New York, McGraw-Hill, 1985)**

lomas, sarcomas, aneurysms, carcinomas, hamartomas, or cysts. Hypogonadism is a secondary effect of these lesions.[5]

Kallmann's syndrome, also called hypogonadotropic hypogonadism and LH-FSH deficiency, is believed to be passed genetically in families.[7]

Other related syndromes that appear to be hypopituitary in etiology include *Prader-Willi syndrome,* with hypogonadism of hypothalamic origin; *Vasquez-Hurst-Sotos syndrome,* which resembles Prader-Willi; and the *Laurence-Moon-Biedl syndrome,* which is familial.[5]

Klinefelter's syndrome is the most common type of hypogonadism detected in males. It is caused by an extra X chromosome that results in an XXY chromosome pattern. More than one extra X chromosome has been reported, and the severity of clinical symptoms seems related to the number of

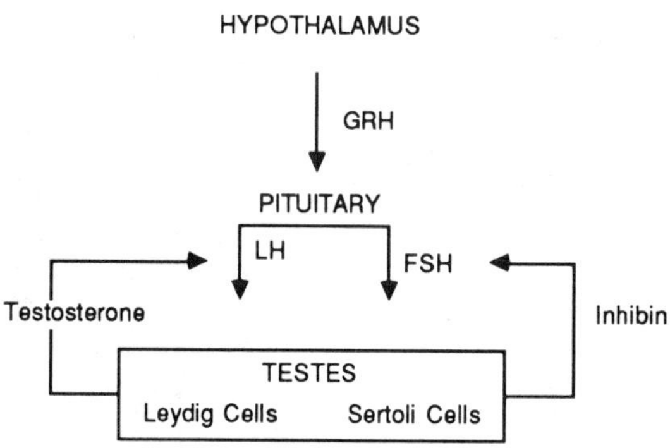

Figure 43-5 **Negative feedback mechanism. (Modified from Odell WD, Swerdloff RS: Abnormalities of gonadal function in men. Clin Endocrinol 8:149, 1978**

X chromosomes and whether some or all cell lines are involved.[5]

XX male syndrome closely resembles Klinefelter's, except that there is no evidence of a Y chromosome although testicular tissue is seen on biopsy. Several theories have been proposed to explain this: loss of a preexisting Y chromosome; an autosomal gene mutation; translocation of Y chromosome with X chromosome; deletion or inactivation of X chromosomal gene that affects testes determination.[8]

True hermaphroditism is characterized by the presence of both ovarian and testicular tissue. Classification is based on type and location of the gonads as follows: (1) *lateral*—30% of patients have a testis on one side and an ovary on the other; (2) *bilateral*—20% of patients have ovarian and testicular tissue on both sides, usually as ovotestes; (3) *unilateral*—50% of cases have testicular and ovarian tissue on one side and an ovary or testis on the other.[9]

Noonan's syndrome patients have normal XY chromosomes but exhibit primary gonadal failure. The disease is transmitted in an autosomal and dominant manner. Pubertal development and growth seem to vary widely in patients with Noonan's syndrome, but there is a general delay in maturation that affects growth and sexual development[10]

Low occurrence syndromes or diseases have in common low testosterone values, increased LH and FSH values, and abnormal XY karyotype with normal male genitalia. *Leydig cell hypoplasia* shows no Leydig cells on biopsy. *Myotonia dystrophica* is a slow atrophy of muscle along with gonadal atrophy.

Hypogonadism: Etiology and Characteristics

I. Hyperprolactinemia
II. Hypothalamic-pituitary function
   A. Panhypopituitarism
   B. Kallmann's syndrome
   C. Related syndromes
      1. Isolated FSH deficiency
      2. Isolated LH deficiency
      3. Prader-Willi syndrome
      4. Vasquez-Hurst-Sotos syndrome
      5. Laurence-Moon-Biedl syndrome
III. Primary gonadal abnormality
   A. Abnormal karyotype
      1. Male phenotype
         a. Klinefelter's syndrome
         b. XX male syndrome (sex reversal syndrome)
      2. Ambiguous phenotype
         a. XX male syndrome
         b. True hermaphroditism
   B. Normal karyotype
      1. Normal male genitalia
         a. Noonan's syndrome
         b. Acquired disorders
         c. Chemotherapy
         d. Low-occurrence syndromes
            i. Leydig cell hypoplasia
            ii. Myotonia dystrophica
            iii. Streak gonads
            iv. Testicular agenesis
      2. Ambiguous or female genitalia, enzyme deficiencies
         a. 20-α-hydroxylase deficiency
         b. 17,20-desmolase deficiency
         c. 3-β-hydroxysteroid dehydrogenase deficiency
         d. 17-hydroxylase deficiency
         e. 17-ketosteroid reductase deficiency
         f. 5-α-reductase deficiency
IV. Androgen insensitivity
   A. Normal FSH, normal or moderately elevated LH
      1. Complete androgen insensitivity
      2. Incomplete androgen sensitivity
   B. High LH, FSH
      1. 5-reductase deficiency

Streak gonads are pale streaks of connective tissue with an XY karyotype and no germ cells present. *Testicular agenesis* or vanishing testes syndrome occurs in phenotypic males, but no testes can be found in the scrotum or the inguinal canal as in cryptorchidism.[5, 9]

Six *enzyme deficiencies* of androgen synthesis have been described that cause decreased androgen production in males by blocking the conversion of cholesterol to testosterone.[5] (see Fig. 43-6).

Complete androgen insensitivity patients have normal XY chromosomes but, due to a defect of biochemical action of testosterone and dihydrotestosterone, show no response to androgens during embryogenesis or in adult life. Most of these patients consider themselves females, although there are usually palpable gonads (testes) in the inguinal area.[5]

Incomplete androgen sensitivity encompasses a variety of syndromes with a broad spectrum of hypogonadism. It may occur in males or females, and is passed in families.[5]

ACQUIRED DISORDERS

Orchitis is the most common acquired disorder of testicular failure. It is caused by the actual infection of the testes (unilateral or bilateral) by the mumps virus. It occurs in approximately 25% of all men who have mumps after puberty. In the acute phase, the testis may be swollen and inflamed. After recovery, atrophy of the testis occurs. Because the virus attacks the seminiferous tubules, testosterone production is low and increases in LH and FSH are seen. Gynecomastia may develop as testosterone becomes low in comparison to naturally occurring estrogens.[9]

Trauma is the second most frequently occurring acquired disorder of testicular failure. Radiation in very small amounts may cause damage to seminiferous tubules and thus affect spermatogenesis and testosterone production. Damage and long-term effects increase as the amount of radiation exposure increases.[9]

Clinical Manifestations

Hypogonadism is usually diagnosed secondary to some other clinical complaint of the patient. An alert clinician may find on physical examination (1) abnormal facial and body hair distribution; (2) decreased muscle mass with abnormal distribution; (3) abnormal fat distribution; (4) an increased ratio of arm span over height (average ratio of normal male is 0.96) or a decreased upper body to lower body ratio; (5) decreased testicular size; (6) decreased or absent sense of smell; and (7) gynecomastia.[4, 5]

A history should include questions about age of puberty and physical development, changes in libido, impotence, infertility, and marital difficulties related to sexual dysfunction.

In hypogonadism due to hyperprolactinemia, patients may present with galactorrhea, impotence, and decreased libido.[11]

Kallmann's syndrome is characterized by absent or decreased sense of smell, color blindness, renal agenesis, neurosensory deafness, cleft lip and palate, decreased or absent male secondary sex characteristics, and small testes.[7]

In related syndromes, the diagnosis is usually clinical. Prader-Willi syndrome patients are characterized by massive obesity, mental retardation, neonatal muscle hypotonia and, after puberty, hypogonadism that is hypothalamic in origin. Vasquez-Hurst-Sotos syndrome resembles the Prader-Willi syndrome but does not include hypotonia. Laurence-Moon-Biedl syndrome is a familial syndrome characterized by mental retardation, retinitis pigmentosa, webbed digits, and short fourth metacarpals.[5]

Typical clinical symptoms found in Kleinfelter's syndrome after puberty include eunochoid appearance, small firm testes, gynecomastia, azoospermia, and sometimes mental retardation.[5]

Clinically, the features of hermaphroditism are variable. There will be varying degrees of ambiguity in the genitalia; cryptorchidism, or undescended testes, is common; and usually a uterus is present.

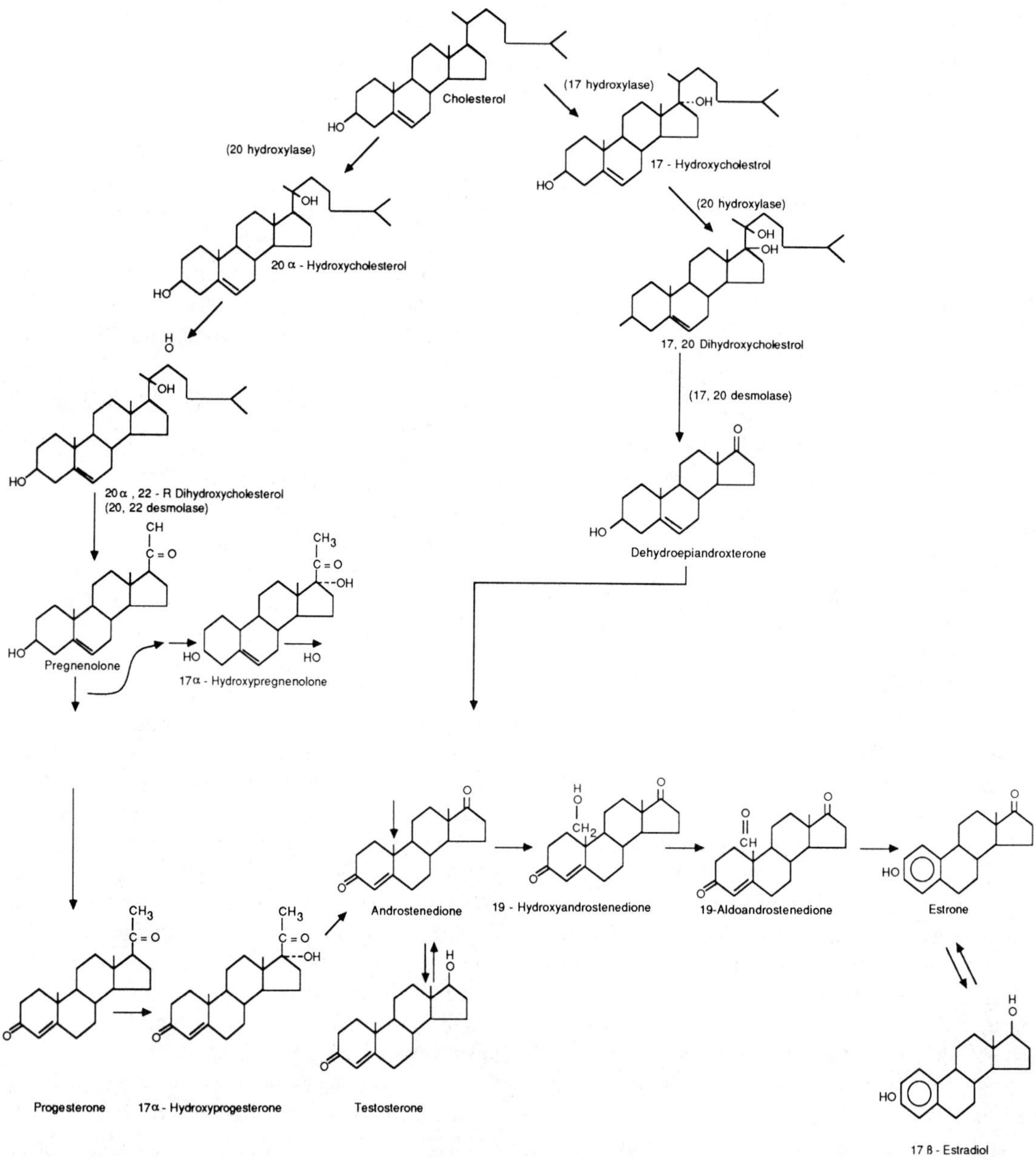

Figure 43-6 Pathways of biosynthesis of the sex steroids. (From Odell WD, Swerdloff RS: Abnormalities of gonadal function in men. Clin Endocrinol 8: 149, 1978)

Noonan's syndrome is characterized by short stature, shield-shaped chest, webbed neck, pectus excavation, cryptorchidism, and congenital heart disease. The diagnosis is usually made based on clinical findings.

Laboratory Analyses and Diagnosis

The diagnosis of hypogonadism can be supported well by the proper selection of laboratory tests. The most important of these is serum testosterone (TST). Secretion of testosterone by the testes is episodic; a pattern of maximal secretion in the early morning and minimal secretion about 13 hours later has been demonstrated.[1] Thus it is recommended that several blood specimens be collected approximately 30 minutes apart and pooled to obtain a more accurate testosterone measurement. Measurement of testosterone is best done by radioimmunoassay (RIA), using specific antisera. Most RIA assays require an extraction of the steroid into a solvent, although there are direct methods available. The latter probably are not as accurate, although there are claims of good correlation with extraction methods.[12]

To aid further in the diagnosis of hypogonadism, measurement of luteinizing hormone (LH), follicle-stimulating hormone (FSH), and prolactin (PRL) should be performed. PRL is believed to work with LH to stimulate androgen production and may be involved in sperm motility.[13] Hyperprolactinemia is also associated with decreased libido.

LH, FSH, and PRL are best measured by radioimmunoassay with specific antisera. Older RIA methods suffered from lack of specificity. Especially problematic was cross-reactivity with human chorionic gonadotropin (hCG) and thyroid-stimulating hormone (TSH). Current methods use highly purified human FSH and LH to produce specific antisera showing as little as 1% cross-reactivity to similar hormones.[12]

Measurements of LH, FSH, testosterone, and prolactin reveal the type of hypogonadism present[4, 5] (see Fig. 43-7 and Table 43-1). If the testosterone is low with an elevated prolactin, then a hyperprolactinemia may be the cause of disease. A low testosterone with an LH and FSH low or normal may indicate disorders of hypothalamic-pituitary function. A low testosterone with high LH and FSH is indicative of a primary gonadal abnormality. An abnormal karyotype with a male phenotype points to Kleinfelter's syndrome or XX male syndrome, while an ambiguous phenotype could be indicative of XX male syndrome or true hermaphroditism. A normal karyotype with normal male genitalia may demonstrate Noonan's syndrome, an acquired disorder, chemotherapy, or other low-occurring syndromes. A normal karyotype with ambiguous or female genitalia may be caused by enzyme defects in androgen synthesis. If the testosterone is normal or high, androgen insensitivity should be suspected. If FSH is normal and LH is normal to moderately elevated, then complete androgen insensitivity or incomplete androgen sensitivity may be present. High FSH and LH levels point to deficiency in 5-reductase, which is the enzyme responsible for conversion of testosterone to dihydrotestosterone in the cell.

In Kallman's syndrome laboratory tests will show below normal results for testosterone, LH, and FSH. Prolactin should be normal. If prolactin is elevated, then a tumor should be suspected. Semen analysis usually will demonstrate absence of sperm, although some cases have been reported in which limited spermatogenesis takes place.

The laboratory workup for a patient suspected of Klinefelter's syndrome will show testosterone to be low or low normal. LH may be normal or elevated, and FSH is consistently elevated. The buccal smear for chromatin is positive, and semen analysis shows lack of spermatozoa. One case study also reported toxic changes in neutrophils, including nuclear projections, which could represent an inactivated X chromatin when two or more X chromosomes are present in a cell.[14]

In patients with enzyme deficiencies, the testosterone level is low while LH and FSH are high. Further diagnostic testing that might differentiate which enzyme is deficient includes plasma and urinary cortisol, 17-ketosteroids in urine, preg-

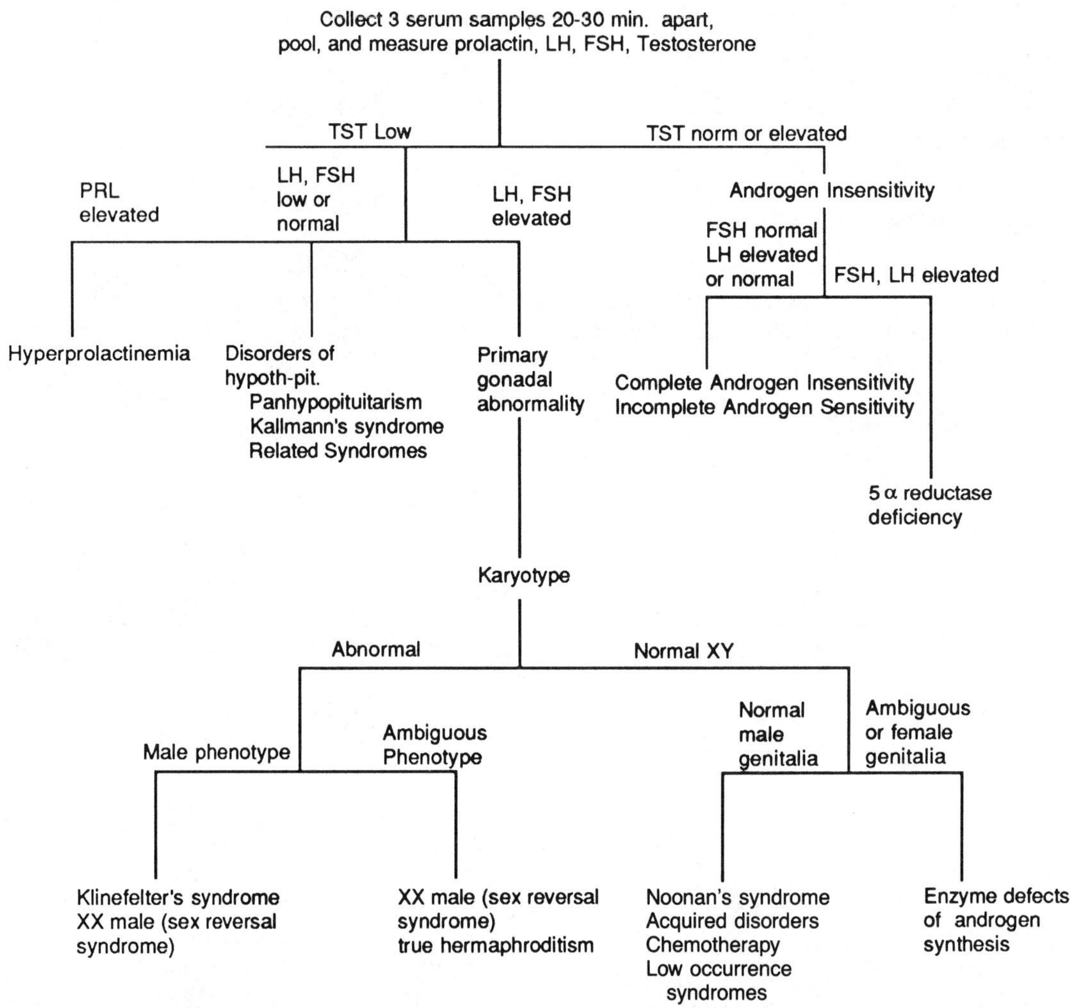

Figure 43-7 Flowsheet for laboratory and clinical diagnostic evaluation of male hypogonadism. (Modified from Odell WD, Swerdloff RS: Abnormalities of gonadal function in men. Clin Endocrinol 8: 149, 1978)

nanediol and pregnanetriol, and aldosterone (see Table 43-2).

Treatment

Treatment for pituitary tumors includes surgery, radiation, and medication, usually bromocriptine. Effectiveness of these treatments is closely related to the size and prolactin-secreting ability of the tumor.[15] Drug-related hyperprolactinemia may be helped by withdrawal from medications. Bromocriptine is used to lower prolactin levels in nontumoral hyperprolactinemia.[16]

The treatment for Kallmann's syndrome includes androgen therapy with testosterone esters. The aim of androgen therapy is to restore normal

Table 43-1 ***Laboratory Results in Hypogonadism***

Disease	TST	LH	FSH	Other
Hyperprolactinemia	↓	↓	↓	↑ PRL
Panhypopituitarism	↓	N or ↓	N or ↓	
Kallmann's Syndrome	↓	↓	↓	
Klinefelter's Syndrome	↓	N or ↑	↑	Karyotype XXY
XX Male Syndrome	↓	N or ↑	↑	Karyotype XX
True Hermaphroditism	↓	↑	↑	Biopsy shows testicular and ovarian tissue.
Noonan's Syndrome	↓	↑	↑	Clinical appearance
Acquired Disorders	N or ↓	N	↑	Testicular atrophy
Enzyme defects	↓	↑	↑	See Table 43-2
Androgen Insensitivity	N or ↓	N or ↑	N or ↑	

male secondary sex characteristics such as beard, body hair, and external genitalia. Therapy also increases muscle mass, hemoglobin, nitrogen balance, and closure of the epiphysia. Direct administration of testosterone, either orally or by parenteral injection, is not successful because testosterone is rapidly absorbed and degraded by the liver, and effective levels in the plasma are not achieved. Esterification of the 17-β-hydroxyl group of the steroid slows its release into the circulation and makes possible adequate plasma levels. Two agents found to be safe and effective, and the current treatment of choice, are testosterone cypionate and testosterone enanthate, which can be injected every 1 to 3 weeks.[17] Small initial doses of testosterone cypionate and testosterone enanthate followed by gradual increases are appropriate to bring plasma testosterone into the adult range slowly. When this therapy is started at the expected age of puberty, the normal events of male puberty take place. If therapy is delayed until later in life, results are more variable. As secondary male sex characteristics appear, serum testosterone, LH, and FSH should rise to normal adult levels. Other treatments, including administration of human chorionic gonadotropin, menopausal gonadotropin, and gonadotropin-releasing hormone to stimulate the pituitary, have been reported successful.[18]

Table 43-2 ***Laboratory Results in Androgen Enzyme Deficiencies***

Enzyme Deficiency	
20-α-hydroxylase	↓ Plasma & urinary cortisol ↓ Aldosterone
17,20-desmolase	↑ pregnanetriol excretion
3-β-hydroxysteroid dehydrogenase	↓ Cortisol ↓ Aldosterone N or ↑ pregnanetriol
17-hydroxylase	N Aldosterone ↓ Cortisol
17-ketosteroid reductase	↑ Ketosteroid excretion
5-α-reductase	Androgen resistance

Treatment for Klinefelter's syndrome is best accomplished by testosterone replacement therapy as described for Kallmann's syndrome. Treatment with testosterone esters should be followed by testosterone measurements in serum or plasma. The concentration should rise slowly to a normal level, depending on dosage and time of administration. LH and FSH concentrations should be suppressed to normal as the testosterone rises. Androgen therapy usually does not restore spermatogenesis, although there are reported cases of Klinefelter's patients fathering children.[5]

Treatment for hermaphroditism is dependent on the age at diagnosis. Most children are raised as males. In infants in whom gender has not been established, assignment of male or female gender can be made. Surgery is then used to remove structures contrary to that gender. Hormone replacement at puberty may be necessary.

Treatment for Noonan's syndrome includes stimulation with luteinizing-releasing hormone, which may or may not elicit a rise in LH or FSH. Treatment is usually androgen therapy beginning at puberty.[10]

INFERTILITY

Etiology

Infertility may occur in as many as 15% of all couples. In 30% to 40% of these couples, the male reproductive system is the major factor. Another 30% of infertile couples have a combination of male and female abnormalities, while the other 30% have female-related disorders. (A medical history for the infertile male should include questions about medications, alcohol consumption, smoking, toxic material exposure, radiation exposure, childhood diseases, and testicular trauma or disease.)

Clinical Manifestations

The physical examination should note any abnormalities in secondary sex characteristics and testicular size and consistency, and should include a careful check for a varicocele.

Laboratory Analyses and Diagnosis

The most important laboratory test in the early stages of diagnosis is a semen analysis. Care should be taken to instruct the patient to collect a complete specimen by masturbation into a sterile container. The semen analysis should include a check for coagulation, liquefaction within 30 minutes, semen fructose, and viscosity. The volume should be measured and the sperm count, motility, and viability evaluated under the microscope. Sperm morphology should also be evaluated. Special tests such as antisperm antibody, cervical mucus interaction, and sperm penetration tests are usually not available at all facilities, but reference labs are available to do them.[19] They should be used only after all other investigation is complete.

Laboratory results of the semen analysis should direct the clinician to the proper diagnosis (see Figs. 43-8 and 43-9). Natural variability in the semen quality may give an inaccurate picture. At least three specimens taken at weekly intervals should be evaluated. Normal semen should *coagulate* immediately. If it does not, then a fructose test should be done. A negative fructose test indicates a congenital absence of vas deferens and seminal vesicles. *Liquefaction* usually occurs within 30 minutes after collection of the ejaculate because of the presence of a prostatic enzyme. A prostatic enzyme deficiency may be suspected if it does not liquefy. *Viscosity* should be noted because an increase may affect fertility by trapping sperm, especially if both sperm count and motility are low. Normal *volume* for a semen specimen is 1.5 to 5 mL. High volume may dilute the sperm and decrease motility, while low volume could indicate retrograde ejaculation into the bladder, or an abnormality of the prostate or seminal vesicles.

The median *sperm count* of fertile patients is about 60 million sperm/mL, with a normal range of 40 million to 150 million sperm/mL. Less than 20 million sperm/mL is considered subfertile. Absence of any sperm (azoospermia) may be caused

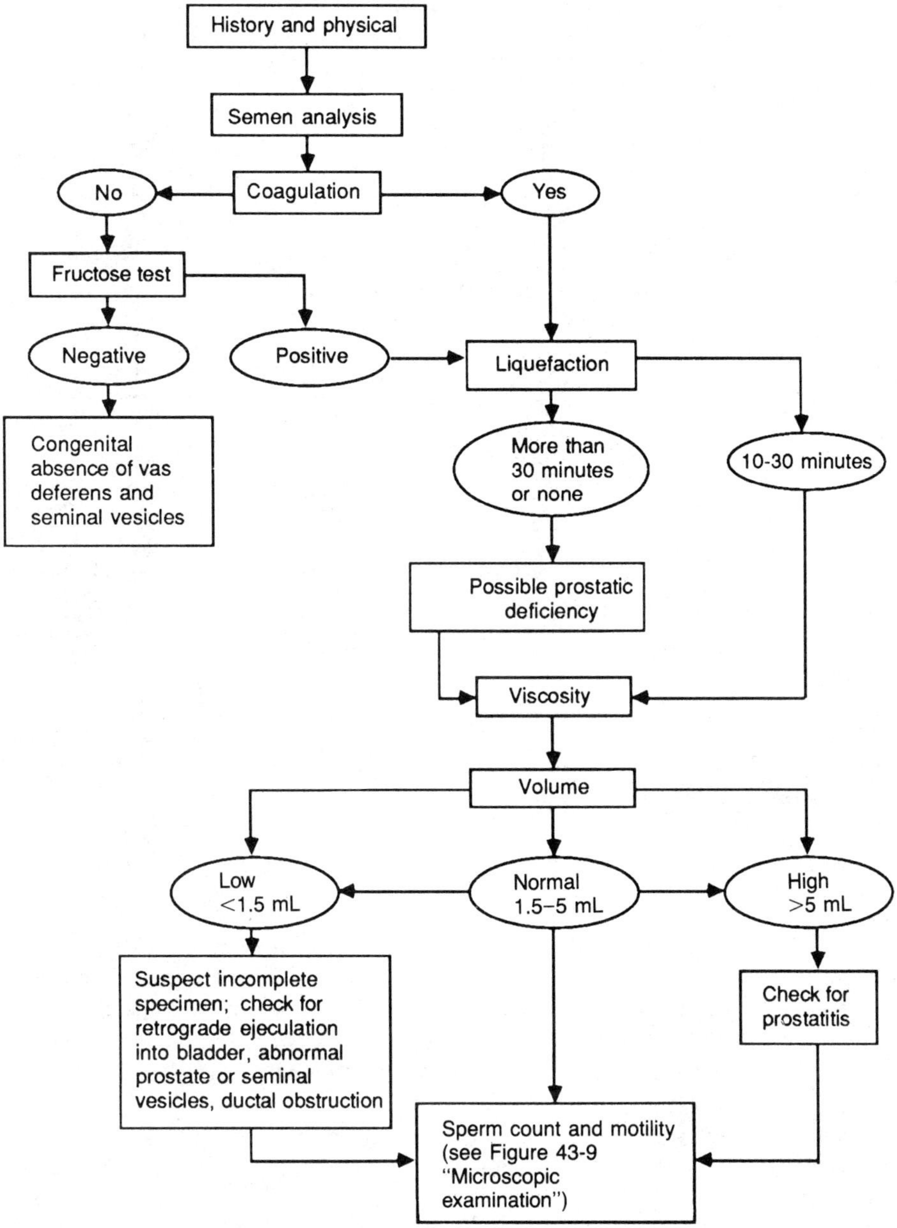

Figure 43-8 Male infertility: gross examination. (From Berger RE: Evaluating the infertile man. Diagnosis: July, 1983)

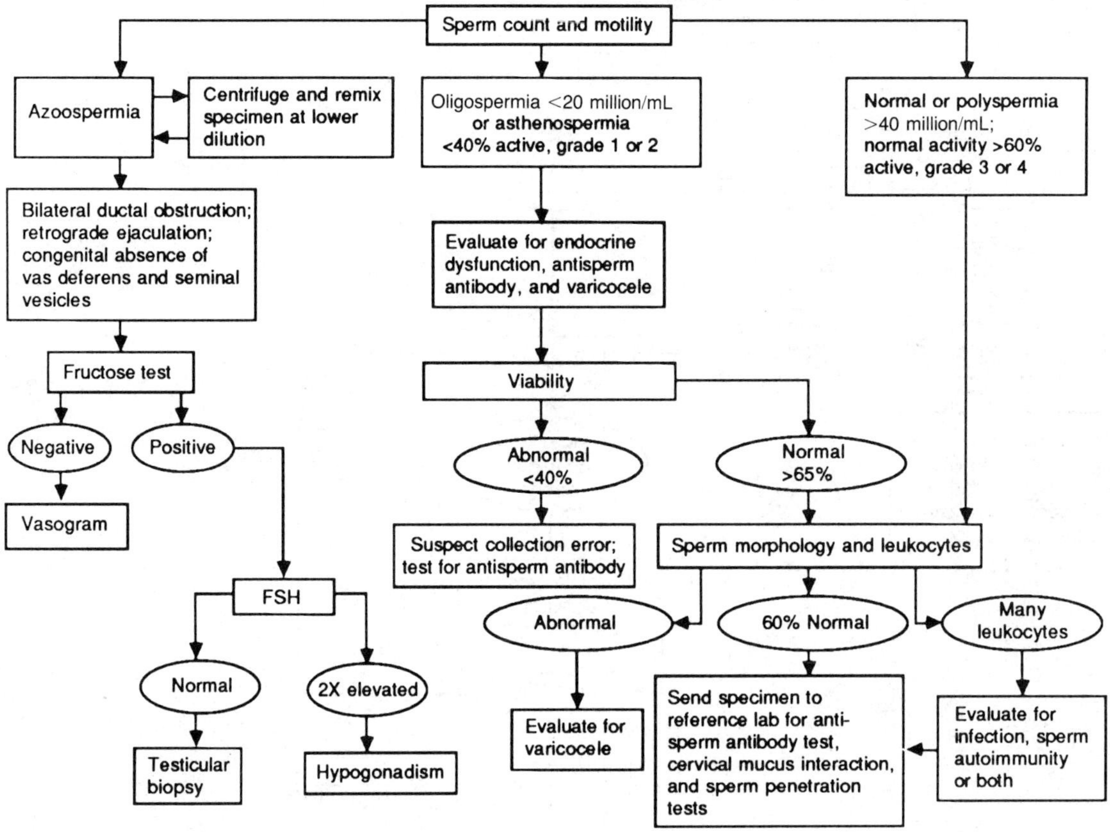

Figure 43-9 **Male infertility: microscopic examination. Diagnosis: July, 1983**

by bilateral ductal obstruction, retrograde ejaculation, or congenital absence of vas deferens or seminal vesicles. A negative *fructose* test and a *vasogram,* which gives a radiological picture of the vas deferens and seminal vesicles, will aid in the diagnosis. If the fructose is positive, a serum *FSH* should be performed. If it is elevated twice normal, the patient should be evaluated for hypogonadism. If a normal FSH is found, a testicular biopsy should be done.

Sperm motility should be studied on normal or high sperm counts as well as on low counts. At least 60% of the sperm should exhibit good motility. If it is low, then endocrine dysfunction, antisperm antibody reactions, and a varicocele should be considered. *Viability* of the sperm should be > 65% to be normal. Less than 40% is abnormal and may suggest poor collection of specimen or an antisperm antibody reaction. In *evaluation of morphology,* 60% of the sperm should appear normal. If morphology is abnormal, the patient should be further evaluated for a varicocele. The presence of *leukocytes* may indicate an infection or autoimmunity.

Normal morphology in patients with a low or normal sperm count indicates that further testing of sperm function is necessary. A *cervical mucus interaction* study measures the ability of the sperm to travel through cervical mucus to the site of fertilization. Results have been shown to correlate with fertility. *Sperm penetration* tests assess the sperm's ability to undergo physiological changes that make penetration of the human oocyte possible. There are reports of close association between male fertility and a positive result from this test.[2, 19]

Treatment

Treatment for infertility in the male is as varied as the causes of infertility. The clinician should look for and treat the most obvious symptoms first, such as drug and alcohol abuse, infection, exposure to toxins, and other disease processes that may cause infertility. If endocrine dysfunctions such as hyperprolactinemia, panhypopituitarism, or primary gonadal abnormalities are suspected, several options are available for treatment depending on the diagnosis. Androgen therapy, gonadotropin therapy, and drug therapy have been reported to restore fertility. A varicocele is the most common surgically correctable abnormality seen in infertile men. Ductal obstruction can be corrected surgically, but that is difficult. In patients with retrograde ejaculation, pregnancies have been reported after sperm recovered from the bladder were artificially inseminated in the female partner.[19]

IMPOTENCE

Etiology

Impotence is a complex problem involving psychological, neurological, pharmacological, hormonal, and vascular factors. Early reports that 90% of male sexual dysfunction was psychological are being discredited as better techniques for detecting organic disease are found.

Clinical Manifestations

The medical history of an impotent patient should include complete medical and surgical information, history of drug and alcohol use, and careful questioning concerning onset of symptoms, their duration, and related problems.[20, 21, 22]

Laboratory Analyses and Diagnosis

General laboratory testing for liver, renal, and thyroid disease as well as fasting glucose studies should be performed. A large number of diseases are known to be associated with impotence (see Table 43-3).[20] Endocrine evaluation should include blood sampling for testosterone, LH, FSH, and prolactin. Impotence is reported in men suffering from hypogonadism and hyperprolactinemia.

Treatment

Treatment for impotence is complex. In general, the clinician should look for and treat underlying disease first and then progress to treatment for specific dysfunctions.

TESTICULAR TUMORS

Etiology

Testicular tumors are the most common type of cancer in males aged 20 to 40 years. These tumors are divided into germinal (seminiferous tubules)

Table 43-3 ***Diseases Associated With Erectile Problems***

Diabetes mellitus	Spinal cord injury or compression
Renal failure	Temporal lobe lesions
Multiple sclerosis	Myocardial infarction
Aortoiliac disease	Hypertensive arterial disease
Hepatic failure	Pituitary adenomas
Thyroid disease	Hypogonadism
Alcoholic neuropathy	Adrenoleukodystrophy
Inflammatory neuropathy	Progressive systemic sclerosis
Peripheral nerve trauma (pelvic fracture)	Priapism
	Peyronie's disease
Tabes dorsalis	Adrenal disease (Cushing's, Addison's)
Nutritional neuropathies	Adrenocortical tumor

and nongerminal (interstitial cell) types. Germinal tumors include five types: seminoma, embryonal carcinoma, teratoma, teratocarcinoma, and choriocarcinoma. Nongerminal tumors originate in the Leydig cells.

Clinical Manifestations

Clinical presentation of a testicular tumor includes feminization, gynecomastia, decreased libido, and swollen or painful testes.

Laboratory Analyses and Diagnosis

The most helpful laboratory tests include serum testosterone, estrogen, and serum markers such as human chorionic gonadotropin (hCG), α-fetoprotein (AFP), and lactate dehydrogenase (LD). Normal results from these laboratory tests do not rule out the presence of a tumor, but elevated results are useful in the diagnosis. Researchers have found that 23% of seminomas had an elevated hCG and 75% to 80% of mixed germ cell tumors had an increased hCG, AFP, or both. LD is elevated in patients with a seminoma, and usually decreases with successful treatment. Choriocarcinomas are rare, and have the ability to secrete hCG and estrogens. Nongerminal tumors can secrete androgens and estrogens.[23, 24, 25, 26]

Treatment

Treatment for testicular cancer requires surgery for removal of the affected testis, followed by irradiation or chemotherapy. The choice of irradiation or chemotherapy is made according to the type of tumor present and its characteristic sensitivity to radiation or chemotherapy. Elevated testosterone, estrogen, AFP, hCG, and LD usually drop to normal after treatment and can be used to follow patients during recovery. However, these markers may not be sensitive enough to detect small metastases.[23]

CRYPTORCHIDISM

Etiology

Cryptorchidism, or undescended testes, is the most common disorder of sex differentiation and one of the most common congenital abnormalities in males.[27] Occurrence in more than one member of the same family is common. The etiology is essentially unknown, although investigators have studied breech births, hormones, and maternal estrogens as possible causes.[28] This condition is important because of strong associations with testicular malignancy and infertility. Its presence dictates a clinical workup for Kallmann's, Klinefelter's, and Noonan's syndromes as well as suspicion of testicular agenesis.

Laboratory Analyses and Diagnosis

Laboratory tests should include serum testosterone, LH, FSH, and prolactin to ascertain if hypogonadism is present.

Treatment

Treatment of underlying disease may cause descension of the testes. If no accompanying disease is found, treatment includes stimulation with hCG or administration of LHRH. Results of these two treatments are variable. Because fertility is depressed even after descent of the testes to the scrotum, treatment before age two is recommended to minimize damage. If drug therapy is unsuccessful, then surgery is recommended. If the testes are undescended in the adult male, careful evaluation for testicular tumors should be made as there is an increased risk in this group.

GYNECOMASTIA

Etiology

Gynecomastia, which is enlargement of the male breast, is most commonly found in adolescent boys or in older men secondary to another disease process or drug therapy.[29] Table 43-4 demonstrates the variety and number of causes for gynecomastia. One study of a hospitalized male population detected gynecomastia in 65% of all subjects examined in an age group of 27 to 92 years.[30]

Clinical Manifestations

When gynecomastia is present, a careful history should reveal the age at which symptoms were noticed as well as their duration. A drug history should be taken. An adolescent boy may need no further workup than a physical examination, since gynecomastia is so common during puberty. An adult with acute onset of symptoms, however, should be evaluated more carefully. The finding of gynecomastia on physical examination should trigger further investigation for underlying disease.

Laboratory Analyses and Diagnosis

General laboratory tests for liver, renal, and thyroid disease should be performed. Endocrine tests for hypogonadism include LH, FSH, testosterone, and prolactin. Gynecomastia is a common symptom in testicular cancer, and serum markers AFP, hCG, and LD should be performed as well as testosterone and estradiol.

Treatment

Treatment for gynecomastia is most often treatment for the underlying cause. Improvement in

Table 43-4 ***Causes of Gynecomastia***

Physiologic	Drugs	Endocrinopathies	Tumors	Chronic diseases

Neonatal
Pubertal
Senile
	Estrogens
	Testosterone
	hCG
	Spironolactone (aldactone)
	Digitalis
	Antihypertensive drugs
	  Thiazides
	  Methyldopa
	  Reserpine
	  Guanethidine
	Tricyclic antidepressants
	Phenothiazines
	Isoniazid (INH)
	Marijuana
	Cimetidine
	Diazepam
	Chemotherapeutic agents
		Klinefelter's syndrome
		Reifenstein's syndrome
		Hyperthyroidism
		Hypothyroidism
			Pituitary tumor
			Adrenal carcinoma
			Testicular tumors
			Choriocarcinoma
			Leydig cell tumors
			Hepatic carcinoma
			Carcinoma of the lung secreting gonadotropins and prolactin
			Breast cancer
				Cirrhosis of the liver
				Renal failure
				Malnutrition (followed by refeeding)

renal, liver, or thyroid function may decrease symptoms. If not, tamoxifen, danazol, and clomiphene have been used to reduce breast size.[29] Withdrawal from medications may clear up gynecomastia in those cases in which drugs are suspected. Surgical removal of tumors, especially those that secrete estrogens, is of benefit. Patients with hypogonadism are commonly started on androgen therapy, which may reduce breast size. Usually treatment for gynecomastia during puberty is unnecessary, unless the problem becomes psychological in nature due to teasing by peers or embarrassment. Treatment with danazol and tamoxifen have been reported to be successful.[29]

CASE STUDY

A 32-year-old man was seen at the infertility clinic along with his wife. They had been having regular intercourse for 2 years without a resulting pregnancy. Testing of the wife was not remarkable.

Physical examination of the husband showed slightly decreased testicular size, normal muscle mass and distribution, normal male hair amount and distribution, and absence of gynecomastia. Semen analysis showed normal coagulation, liquefaction, viscosity, and volume. No sperm were seen with microscopic examination. The fructose test was positive (normal).

Other laboratory tests showed normal liver, renal, and thyroid results. The testosterone was low, with an increased LH and FSH. Because an acquired disorder was suspected, the patient was questioned about childhood diseases, drugs, and environmental factors that had affected him. He reported having "mumps" at age 21. Diagnosis was infertility due to orchitis.

Questions

1. Which result(s) in semen analysis indicated the need for endocrine evaluation?
2. Why were liver, renal, and thyroid function tests ordered?
3. Which laboratory test(s) helped pinpoint or support the diagnosis?

Discussion

1. The fact that the semen analysis was essentially normal except for the absence of sperm indicated that the problem may be a seminiferous tubule problem. Because testosterone is required for spermatogenesis in the seminiferous tubules, evaluation of testosterone and its feedback mechanism should have been the next step in investigation.
2. Renal, hepatic, and thyroid function tests were ordered to rule out the presence of drug consumption, infection, tumors, and thyroid diseases that may result in infertility.
3. The high concentration of LH and FSH ruled out the hypothalamic-pituitary problems. The low TST concentration ruled out androgen insensitivity problems. The presence of normal male secondary sex characteristics and history of mumps ruled out probable abnormal karyotype and pointed to orchitis.

REFERENCES

1. Kicklighter EJ, Kulkarni B: The Gonads. In Kaplan LA, Pesce AJ (eds): Clinical Chemistry: Theory, Analysis, and Correlation, p 789. St Louis, CV Mosby, 1984
2. Swerdloff RS (moderator); Overstreet JW, Sokol RZ, Rajfer J (discussants): Infertility in the male. UCLA conference. Ann Intern Med 103: 906, 1985
3. Jubiz W: The Testes. In Jubiz W (ed): Endocrinology—A Logical Approach for Clinicians, p 387. New York City, McGraw-Hill, 1985
4. Odell WD, Swerdloff RS: Abnormalities of gonadal function in men. Clin Endocrinol 8:149, 1978
5. Odell WD, Larson JL: Reproduction: The New Frontier in Occupational and Environmental Health Research, p 293. New York City, AR Liss, 1984
6. Heshmatilt M, Turpin G, Nahal K et al: Testicular response to human chorionic gonadotropin in chronic hyperprolactinemia. Acta Endocrinol 108 (4):565, 1985
7. Lieblich JM, Rogol AD, White BJ et al: Syndrome of anosomia with hypogonadotrophic hypogonadism (Kallmann's syndrome). Am J Med 73:506, 1982
8. De la Chappelle A: The etiology of maleness in XX men. Hum Genet 58:105, 1981
9. Griffin JE, Wilson JD: Disorders of the testes and male reproductive tract. In Wilson JD, Foster DW

(eds): Williams Textbook of Endocrinology, 7th ed, p 259. Philadelphia, WB Saunders, 1985
10. Theintz G, Savage MO: Growth and pubertal development in five boys with Noonan's syndrome. Arch Dis Child 57: 13, 1982
11. Carter JN, Tyson JE, Tolis G et al: Prolactin-secreting tumors and hypogonadism in 22 men. N Engl J Med 299:847, 1978
12. Chattoraj SC, Watts NB: Endocrinology. In Tietz NW (ed): Textbook of Clinical Chemistry, p 1089. Philadelphia, WB Saunders, 1986
13. Pierrepoint CG, Jenkins BM, Wilson DW et al: An examination of blood steroid and gonadotropin concentrations in relation to fertility status and testicular function in men. Fertil Steril 38:465, 1982
14. Saumur JH: Case study: Klinefelter's syndrome. Am J Med Technol 49(10):715, 1983
15. Wollesen F, Bendson BB: Effect rates of different modalities for treatment of prolactin adenomas. Am J Med 78:114, 1985
16. March CM: Bromocriptine in the treatment of hypogonadism and male impotence. Drugs 17:349, 1979
17. Wilson JD, Griffin JE: The use and misuse of androgens. Metabolism 29:1278, 1980
18. Yoshimoto Y, Moridera K, Imura H: Restoration of normal pituitary gonadotropin reserve by administration of luteinizing hormone-releasing hormone in patients with hypogonadotropic hypogonadism. N Engl J Med 292:242, 1975
19. Berger RE: Evaluating the infertile man. Diagnosis July, 1983
20. Segraves RT, Schoenberg HW: Diagnosis and Treatment of Erectile Disturbances. New York City, Plenum Medical Book Company, 1985
21. Davis SS, Viosca SP, Guralnik M: Evaluation of impotence in older men. West J Med 142:499, 1985
22. Lue TF: Evaluation and treatment of impotence: Where are we going? West J Med 142:546, 1985
23. Catalona WJ: Tumor markers in testicular cancer. Urol Clin North Am 6:613, 1979
24. Montie JE: Testicular cancer: Diagnosis and staging. Semin Urol 2(4):194, 1984
25. Robertson AG, Read G: The value of lactate dehydrogenase as a nonspecific tumor marker for seminoma of the testes. Br J Cancer 46:994, 1982
26. Johnson DE: Testicular Tumors. New York City, Medical Examination Publishing Company, 1976
27. Swerdlow AJ, Wood KH, Smith PG: A case study of the aetiology of cryptorchidism. J Epidemiol Comm Health 37(3):238, 1983
28. Savion M, Nissenkorn I, Servadio C et al: Familial occurrence of undescended testes. Urology 23(4):355, 1984
29. Hooper PD: Puberty gynecomastia. J R Coll Gen Pract 35:142, 1985
30. Niewoehner CB, Nuhall F: Gynecomastia in a hospitalized male population. Am J Med 77:633, 1984

BIBLIOGRAPHY

Ford TF, Parkinson MC, Pryor JP: The undescended testes in adult life. Br J Urol 57:181, 1985

Hafez ESE, Ghaly IM, Ibrahim II et al: Endocrine profiles in pediatric andrology: human chorionic gonadotropin stimulation test in cryptorchid boys. Arch Androl 11:53, 1983

Karpe B, Eneroth P, Ritzen EM: LHRH treatment in unilateral cryptorchidism: Effect on testicular descent and hormonal response. J Pediatr 103:892, 1983

Part IX

NEUROLOGIC DISORDERS

Janet Duben-Von Laufen,
Associate Editor,
and Barbara Smith Michael

The nervous system forms a vital network for communication among the diverse parts of the body, and it is an important factor in the coordination and integration of body functions as a whole. Any disruption of the functioning of the nervous system, whether through genetic defect, injury, or disease, can, therefore, be catastrophic.

The nervous system can be divided into three parts, based on anatomical and physiological differences. The *central nervous system (CNS)* consists of the brain and spinal cord, as illustrated below. Because correlation and integration of information occurs in the CNS, the structures of the system must be well protected from trauma. Both the brain and the spinal cord are protected by bone and bathed in cerebrospinal fluid (CSF). The *peripheral nervous system (PNS)* consists of paired cranial and spinal nerves and ganglia that connect the CNS with all parts of the body. The *autonomic nervous system (ANS)* or visceral motor system innervates and regulates smooth muscle, cardiac muscle, and glands and generally controls the involuntary body processes.

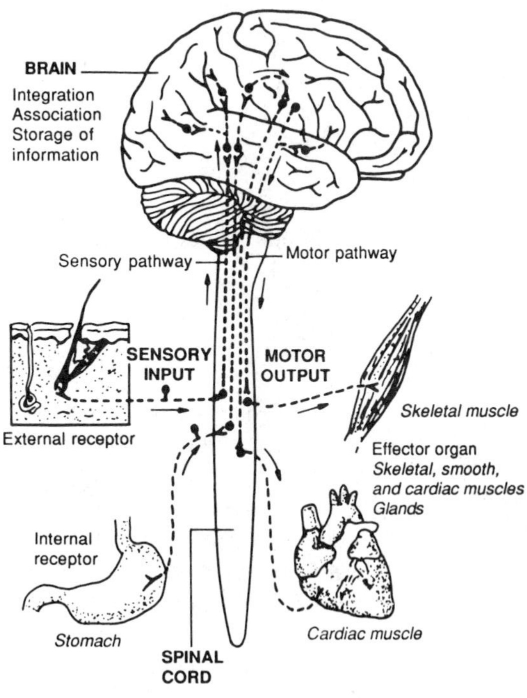

Brain and spinal cord.

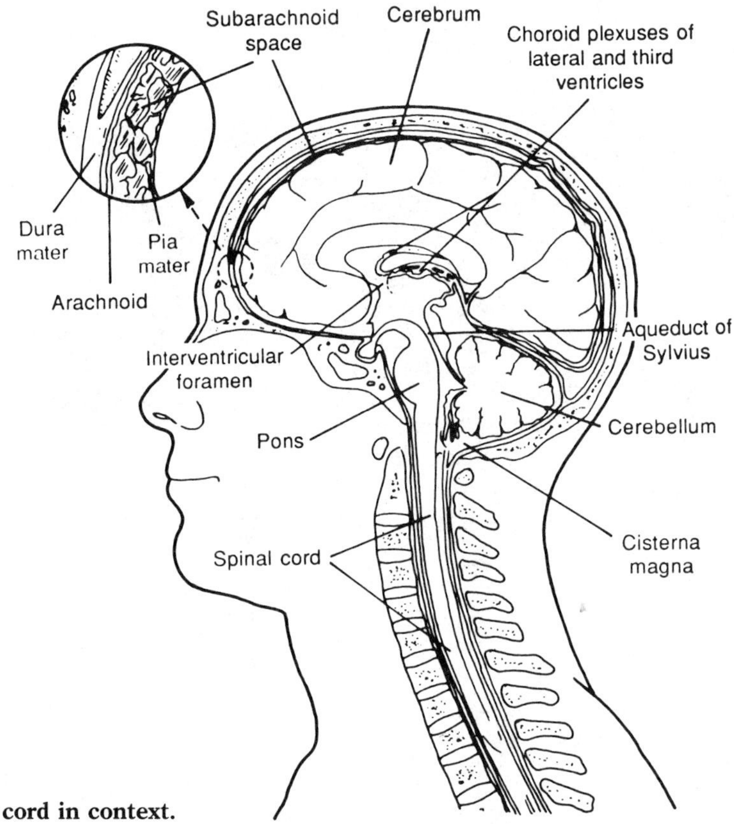

Brain and spinal cord in context.

The nervous system is the most highly organized and complex system in the body, in both structure and function. The brain and spinal cord may be seen in context (above). They are enveloped by three membranes collectively called the *meninges*. The membrane closest to the brain is the pia mater. The outermost membrane is the dura mater (or dura). Between the pia mater and dura mater lies the arachnoid. Together, the pia mater and the arachnoid are called the *leptomeninges,* and the space between these two is called the *subarachnoid space,* through which the CSF circulates. The relationships of the meninges are essentially the same for the spinal cord as for the brain.

The PNS conducts nerve impulses to and from the CNS. The afferent or sensory nerves carry impulses from the organs, skeletal muscles, tendons, joints, and skin to the CNS. The efferent motor nerves initiate voluntary or involuntary activities. The ANS or visceral motor system regulates the internal environment of the body in order to maintain homeostasis. The sympathetic ANS has a stimulating or accelerating effect on body function, and the parasympathetic ANS has an opposite but complementary function.

Diagnosis of neurologic disorders presents many problems, primarily because of the wide range of clinical symptoms that may be exhibited due to the complexity of the nervous system. Clinical manifestations range from headache, to loss of motor or sensory function, to changes in cognitive abilities and seizures. Examination of a patient presenting with one or more symptoms of a neurologic disorder includes many of the procedures outlined below.

Diagnostic Procedures Used in Neurology

Patient medical history
Neurologic examination of motor and sensory systems
Tests of cognitive functioning
Radiologic procedures (x-rays)
Electroencephalogram (EEG)
Computerized tomography (CT scan)
Laboratory analysis of CSF

The chapters in this section present a detailed discussion of the major neurologic and behavioral disorders. Each chapter covers the presenting symptoms, etiology, and diagnostic procedures used in differentiating specific dysfunctions of the nervous system.

Chapter 44

Degenerative Processes

Kozy M. Corsaut

Degenerative processes of the neurologic system are often difficult to diagnose. There is not a large menu of laboratory procedures available that are specific for many of these diseases. The physician must rely heavily on other data, such as on clinical features that may be typical, as in Parkinson's disease, or on family history, as in Huntington's disease.

The diseases presented in this section are often found classed with disorders in other chapters, (*e.g.*, Wilson's disease with hepatic disorders, Gaucher's disease with hematologic disorders, mucopolysaccharidosis with other genetic defects). However, these patients often present neurologic changes, such as mental retardation, loss of mental ability and muscle coordination, personality disturbances, or behavior disorders. In the majority of the following disease states, these symptoms are due to a progressive degeneration of the nervous system, and many of them are without cure.

DISEASES PRIMARILY AFFECTING ADULTS

Progressive Dementia

ALZHEIMER'S DISEASE

Alzheimer's disease, named for the German physician Alois Alzheimer, is a form of presenile dementia. The etiology is unknown, but theories have been advanced involving genetic, viral, and immunologic factors.[1, 2]

The disease can affect any age group, and has been reported in patients with Down's syndrome, but is mostly a disease of older patients, aged 50 to 60 years and older. Women are more likely to be afflicted than men. The disease may be more prevalent in some families, but is most often sporadic. It has been estimated that as many as 4% of the population over 65 are affected with Alzheimer's, and that 10% may have the disease but are still able to function in society.[3, 4]

The cerebral cortex of these patients appears atrophied, and the frontal and temporal lobes may be more seriously affected. On microscopic examination, the brain cortex shows neuronal loss, and demyelination may also be present. Senile plaques are characteristically present, and their numbers can be correlated with the loss of intellectual ability. In some patients, presynaptic defects with decreased levels in the brain of cholineacetyl transferase and acetylcholinesterase have been reported.[1]

Alzheimer's disease begins slowly. The initial complaints are of memory loss, difficulty in problem-solving, and depression. As the disease progresses, patients experience difficulty in walking, speech impairment, and the loss of bodily functions and mental ability. Eventually patients may require custodial care.[4]

In the clinical laboratory, blood findings are normal. Most often spinal fluid studies are also within normal limits, although a slight increase in total protein in cerebrospinal fluid (CSF) may be found. Tests on serum and CSF for syphilis, measles, and cryptococcus are also negative. It has recently been reported that patients with Alzheimer's are likely to display oligoclonal banding in CSF, though this is not a routine method for diagnosis at this time.[2]

Diagnosis is made by clinical symptoms and computerized tomography. The CT scan will show enlargement of the brain ventricles and cortical sulci.[4, 5] An exact diagnosis is obtained at autopsy with histologic studies of brain tissues.

The course of the disease is relentlessly progressive, often over a period of 8 to 10 years. There is no treatment and no cure for Alzheimer's disease at present; only custodial care can be given to these patients.[1]

Dementia and Other CNS Signs

JAKOB-CREUTZFELDT DISEASE

Jakob-Creutzfeldt disease is a rare dementia found in about 1/1,000,000 persons.[4] It is viral in origin, and affects the cortex, basal ganglia, and spinal cord. Inflammation is not apparent. At autopsy, cerebral atrophy and enlarged ventricles are seen, along with degeneration of the nerve cells.[4]

Jakob-Creutzfeldt disease generally occurs in late middle years. Patients complain of memory loss, personality changes, and behavioral disorders. The disease progression is rapid, and death occurs within an average of 15 months.[1, 4, 6]

Jakob-Creutzfeldt disease is caused by a transmissible spongiform encephalopathy agent. Transmission has been reported in corneal transplant patients and associated with inadequately sterilized sterostatic brain electrodes. No increased incidence has been seen in physicians and laboratory workers, however, which rules out the usual modes of transmission.[4] It can be considered a potential biohazard. The agent can be detected in most internal organs of the patients, but not in their body fluids and secretions (saliva, urine, feces, and blood). The disease has been transmitted to chimpanzees experimentally.[4]

The CSF total protein level may be slightly increased in these patients, but is most often normal.[4] Blood counts and routine chemistry tests are normal.[1] There are no signs of infection or inflammatory response. Later in the disease the EEG is abnormal.[1]

Central nervous system depressants such as bromide intoxication should be ruled out. Diseases such as subacute sclerosing panencephalitis, which will give an increased CSF IgG value, and neural syphilis, with a reactive VDRL on CSF, should also be considered.[6] There is no treatment for Jakob-Creutzfeldt disease, and death is inevitable.

HUNTINGTON'S DISEASE

Huntington's disease, also called Huntington's chorea, is an inherited autosomal dominant trait, affecting men and women equally, with an incidence of about 5/100,000. The symptoms of this disease do not begin before the age of 25, the time of life when many patients already have children. The children of these patients have a 50% chance of developing the disease.[4]

In patients affected with the disease there is death of the nerve cells that produce gamma-aminobutyric acid (GABA), accompanied by decreased levels of glutamic acid decarboxylase (GAD) and choline-acetyltransferase. The brain appears shrunken and atrophied, and on microscopic examination nerve loss is seen.

The disease begins slowly, at first with clumsiness, irritability, and forgetfulness. Speech ability deteriorates, along with intellectual ability. Uncontrolled movements (chorea) of arms, legs, head, and trunk worsen until the patient eventually degenerates to a state of helplessness and total disability.[6]

All laboratory findings for blood, CSF, and urine are essentially normal. The disease is usually diagnosed by clinical symptoms and family history. At the present time, research is being conducted to identify the defective gene to enable genetic counseling and prenatal testing. Two treatable diseases that should be ruled out before making a diagnosis of Huntington's are Wilson's disease and viral encephalitis.[5, 6]

There is no cure for Huntington's disease, and patients usually die within 15 to 20 years of diagnosis. Treatment with neuroleptic medications may alleviate some of the chorea, perhaps by blocking dopamine receptor sites. One hypothesis suggests that the chorea in these patients is due to a heightened receptor response to dopamine.[7]

Loss of Muscular Coordination and Control

AMYOTROPIC LATERAL SCLEROSIS

Amyotropic lateral sclerosis (ALS), also known as Lou Gehrig's disease,[5] is the most common of the motor neuron diseases. It is confined to the voluntary motor system of the skeletal muscles, and involves progressive deterioration of the alpha motor neurons.[4] The cause of the disease is unknown, but a chronic viral infection and immunologic factors have been suggested.

The disease usually begins in middle to late life and affects approximately 5/1,000,000 people.[4] Although ALS may appear to be inherited in some patients, most cases are sporadic. The symptoms generally begin with weakness in the arms and legs and a progressive atrophy of the muscles, sometimes affecting the facial muscles, tongue, and respiratory muscles. The patient's intellectual ability is not affected by this disease.[6] ALS has a rapid progression, and death occurs in 2 to 5 years due to the respiratory muscle involvement.[4]

Routine blood results are normal, except that some patients display an increased serum creatine kinase, as much as 50% above normal if rapid nerve loss is occurring.[4] In most patients the CSF total protein is within normal limits,[5] although in a few it may be increased 20 mg/dL (200 mg/L) above normal.[4]

Spinal cord compression due to tumors, chronic inflammatory disorders such as syphilitic meningomyelitis, metabolic disorders such as thyrotoxicosis and salt depletion, and lead toxicity are treatable diseases that should be ruled out.[5, 6]

There is no cure for amyotropic lateral sclerosis, and only supportive therapy can be offered to these patients.[4]

GUILLAIN-BARRÉ SYNDROME

Guillain-Barré syndrome affects the peripheral nervous system and is thought to be an acquired autoimmune disorder.[3] Throughout the cranial and spinal nerves there is infiltration of monocytic cells, accompanied by demyelination of the nerve cells. Guillain-Barré syndrome occurs in approximately 1/100,000 persons.[4] Often in these patients there is a preceding viral illness or vaccination, and a few cases have been associated with surgery.[3, 4] Although the syndrome can occur at any age, there is increasing incidence with increasing age of the patient.

Symptoms may be mild, or severe enough to cause respiratory failure. Weakness is the earliest symptom, along with loss of sensation in hands and feet and a slowing of the reflexes. There may be total paralysis of the limbs and/or total motor paralysis, including the muscles of respiration.[4]

There is no specific test for this disease. Electrophysiologic testing will show evidence of demyelination of the peripheral nerves. The CSF total protein is increased, often to very high levels, 100–400 mg/dL (1000–4000 mg/L), while the CSF cell count is most often within normal limits.[4] Some of these patients may also display oligoclonal bands in the CSF, along with an increased IgG synthesis rate. The IgG index is normal, while the albumin index is also increased, indicating increased blood–brain barrier permeability.[8] A preceding viral infection may be detected by demonstrating increased serum titers of antibody to the suspected viral antigen.

Most patients recover with remyelination of the nerves, and death is rare. Recovery is often slow and may take many months. Unfortunately, many patients will have some permanent disability even after the recovery period.[4]

MULTIPLE SCLEROSIS

Multiple sclerosis (MS) is one of the neurologic diseases most frequently seen, and is the most common of the demyelinating diseases. The term sclerosis refers to the hardened areas of scar tissue formed by the glial cells found throughout the central nervous system.[6]

The cause of multiple sclerosis remains unknown; however, immunologic processes or a virus of long incubation have been implicated.[4, 9, 10, 11]

Plaques (patches of demyelination) that are macroscopic (1–4 cm) are found on the cord, cerebellum, brain stem, cerebral hemispheres, and optic pathways. The plaques are infiltrated by macrophages, lymphocytes, and plasma cells. The macrophages may be implicated in the demyelination process. It appears that the peripheral nerves are not affected.[4, 6, 10]

Multiple sclerosis often begins in early adulthood, but can be found in children as well as in patients over 40. The disease is rare to nonexistent in the tropics, and increases in incidence north and south of the equator. Those that appear to be at most geographic risk are at latitudes of 45 to 65 degrees—Europe and North America. In these areas the disease has an incidence of 30–80/100,000, and even greater in certain populations. The risk factor seems to be determined by geographic location during adolescence. While MS is not inherited, it has a tendency to be familial, and siblings of MS patients are at greater risk than their own children. It is felt that there is a common link (perhaps exposure to virus) during childhood.[4, 11, 12]

Initial MS attacks seem to be precipitated by acute trauma, fatigue, pregnancy, emotional upsets, or vaccinations. Symptoms vary greatly with the area of CNS demyelination. Most frequently the eyes are involved (blurring of vision, loss of vision, double vision, loss of eye movement), and there is weakness, numbness and clumsiness in arms and legs, and urinary urgency and frequency. The symptoms may last for several weeks to months, interspersed with periods of complete or almost complete remission that last from months to years. As the disease progresses the periods of remission become shorter and less frequent, with only partial recovery of symptoms. The course is variable, ranging from an acute case of only a few months with unremitting symptoms, to the more common form of a remitting/relapsing course seen in most patients and lasting for 20 to 30 years. A few patients have symptoms on one occasion and are free of disease for the rest of their lives.[11, 12]

MS can be difficult to diagnose, as symptoms vary widely and are interspersed with remissions. The attempt to identify lesions in the CNS by computerized tomography (CT) may be helpful; lesions should be found on more than one occasion and at more than one site.[11]

More useful in diagnosis are studies of the CSF. About 30% of MS patients have a slightly increased CSF WBC count, rarely over 40/mm^3, with lymphs predominating. The CSF total protein is generally normal or slightly increased in about 40% of the patients.[4]

One of the most useful test results for the diagnosis of MS is the presence of oligoclonal bands, discrete bands of immunoglobulin found by specialized electrophoresis of the CSF. It should be noted that tests for oligoclonal bands generally must be ordered in addition to routine electrophoresis. At least one band is present in more than 90% of MS patients, and many patients have four or more bands present (see Fig. 44-1). A serum protein electrophoresis should be ordered at the same time to rule out paraproteinemia. If abnormal bands are seen in both serum and CSF, CSF oligoclonal bands are probably not present. If the bands are present in only the CSF and not in the serum, a diagnosis of MS is likely but not certain. Other diseases can also present oligoclonal bands, including Alzheimer's, neurosyphilis, both bacterial and viral encephalitis, Guillain-Barré, and polyneuropathy.[8, 11, 12, 13]

Patients with MS produce IgG in the CNS. Thus, it is necessary to prove that the presence of increased IgG in CSF is due to such *de novo* synthesis rather than to damage to the blood–brain

A

B

C

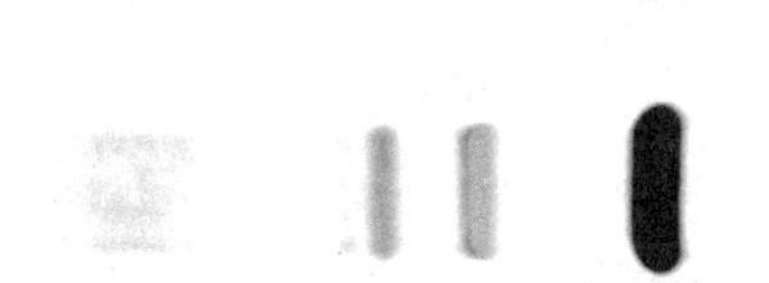

Figure 44-1 **(A) Normal cerebrospinal fluid (CSF) electrophoretogram. (B) SPE II CSF pattern positive MS patient with oligoclonal bands. (C) SPE II serum pattern from above patient negative for oligoclonal bands. (From reference numbers[8, 13])**

barrier (BBB). There are several calculations that attempt to correct for such interfering factors as traumatic taps:

1. Expressing the CSF IgG as a percentage of the total CSF protein or albumin
2. Calculation of the IgG index, in which the CSF IgG/blood IgG ratio is compared to the CSF albumin/blood albumin ratio
3. Calculation of the IgG synthesis rate in the CSF

These calculated values will vary from laboratory to laboratory, depending on methods of measurement of the proteins and on normal values and normal ratios.[14]

Another useful calculation in assessing the origin of CSF IgG, either *de novo* synthesis or blood–brain barrier damage, is calculation of the albumin index. This index is expressed as the ratio of CSF albumin to blood albumin. When the index is increased, damage to the BBB or traumatic tap is likely.[8, 11, 12, 13] (See Table 44-1.)

Levels of myelin basic protein (MBP) of greater than 8 ng/mL (8 μg/L) are present in almost all MS patients with recent exacerbations (less than 1 week) of the disease. Less recent attacks give lower values, 4–8 ng/mL (4–8 μg/L) (weakly positive), and fewer than 5% of patients in remission have a positive result—greater than 4 ng/mL (4 μg/L). The MBP test is useful for evaluating the severity of a recent demyelinating process, but it is not specific for MS and MBP levels can be found increased in other diseases in which primary or secondary demyelination is present.[8, 15]

Many laboratories offer a panel of tests for diagnosis of multiple sclerosis. These tests often include oligoclonal bands, MBP, CSF IgG and IgG synthesis rate, and IgG and albumin indices.[8]

When attempting to make a diagnosis of MS, diseases such as disseminated lupus erythematosus, polyarteritis nodosa, brain-stem gliomas, cord neoplasms, syringomyelia, and spondylosis should be ruled out.[4, 5]

Treatment for MS is generally supportive, although some physicians have some success with ACTH treatment.

Table 44-1 ***CNS IgG Synthesis Indices***

IgG Index	IgG Synthesis Rate/24 hrs	Albumin Index	Interpretation
Normal	Normal	Normal	Normal
Increased	Increased	Normal	CNS IgG synthesis likely
Sl increased	Increased	Increased	Equivocal results, BBB damage, or traumatic tap; cannot rule out CNS IgG synthesis.
Normal	Normal or increased	Increased	BBB damage likely
Increased	Normal or increased	Increased	CNS IgG synthesis likely

Date from reference number[8]

PARKINSON'S DISEASE

Parkinson's disease is a disease of the brain basal ganglia. Patients lack sufficient amounts of the neurotransmitter dopamine. The symptoms of the disease are due to an inhibitory influence on the ganglia. At autopsy the brain shows a loss of nerve cells and a loss of pigmentation of the substantia nigra.[4]

Parkinson's disease generally begins in middle to late life, and it is a leading cause of neurologic degeneration in patients over 60 years of age. It has been estimated that 1 in 1000 persons is affected by Parkinson's.[4]

The patient generally shows a characteristic tremor, stiffness in walking, and slowed movements. There may be a lack of facial mobility, loss of dexterity, and difficulty in speech, as well as other symptoms. Mental ability is not affected, however. The disease progresses slowly over a prolonged period, ending in a state of total invalidism. The etiology of this disease is still unclear.[4]

All routine blood tests and CSF tests are within normal limits. The clinical picture of Parkinson's disease is unique, but similar syndromes may occur with phenothiazine administration, carbon monoxide poisoning, heavy metal poisoning, head trauma, cerebral neoplasms, infectious encephalitis, and cerebral arteriosclerosis.[4]

Treatment with L-DOPA has been reported to relieve the symptoms in some patients, and a few have responded to surgery. However, the disease is progressive and there is no known cure.[4]

DISEASES PRIMARILY AFFECTING CHILDREN

Progressive Dementia and Other CNS Signs

WILSON'S DISEASE

Wilson's disease is characterized by a disturbance of the transport mechanism and storage of copper. The exact cause for the disturbance is as yet unknown, but is probably a genetic defect resulting in decreased ceruloplasmin synthesis. Wilson's disease is relatively rare, and is inherited as an autosomal recessive gene. Symptoms seen are a direct result of the copper deposition in body tissues, leading to lesions in the brain, liver, eye, and kidney.[4, 6]

Neurologic symptoms can be highly variable, but often tremors are present along with muscle spasms and rigidity. Often these patients move the upper extremities, especially hands and fingers, with a twisting or "flapping" type of movement,[16] and facial features show a fixed "smile." As mental deterioration progresses, psychological changes are noticed as the ganglion cells degenerate.[6] Later, liver cirrhosis is present and many patients display a rust-colored ring (Kayser-Fleischer) on the cornea due to copper deposits.[17]

Routine CSF tests are within normal limits; however, some patients will have an increased CSF copper level. Other laboratory tests may vary, but those that provide useful laboratory findings follow.[4, 6, 17]

Liver function tests may show changes: AST, increased; ALT, increased; bilirubin, increased; total protein and electrophoresis pattern similar to chronic active hepatitis; uric acid, decreased.[4, 6, 17] Liver function tests should be performed at frequent intervals, as these studies may be normal unless taken during periods of liver involvement.

There is a secondary aminoaciduria due to renal absorption defects. Plasma levels of amino acids are not increased. The presence of excess urinary amino acids may not occur until other clinical symptoms of the disease occur.

Of great diagnostic value is the ceruloplasmin level, which is usually decreased to less than 20 mg/dL (200 mg/L). It should be kept in mind that serum ceruloplasmin levels may be normal when liver involvement is advanced; thus normal values do not rule out Wilson's disease.

Measures of 24-hour urinary copper are also very useful. Early in the disease these levels may be normal or slightly increased. As the disease progresses, urine output of copper is markedly increased. Some physicians advocate measuring 24-hour urine copper levels before and after treatment with penicillamine. This chelating agent releases tissue-bound excess copper, resulting in dramatically increased urinary copper.

Liver biopsy will show increased deposits of copper, helping to make diagnosis certain.

Early diagnosis is important, so that patients can be treated before irreversible damage occurs to the brain and liver. Wilson's disease should be ruled out in any young patients complaining of symptoms similar to those of chronic hepatitis, accompanied by neurological changes.[17] Patients are advised to use low-copper diets and to take copper chelating agents such as penicillamine to minimize absorption of copper and facilitate its excretion. With treatment and early diagnosis, these patients have a good chance of survival with complete or almost complete remission of symptoms.[4]

Lipid Disorders with CNS Signs: Lysosomal Storage Diseases

Lysosomes are granules found in the cytoplasm of macrophages. Their function is to catabolize lipids ingested by those cells. Large molecular substances may require a number of hydrolase enzymes before the products are small enough to leave the cell. Any molecule incapable of being catabolized will accumulate in the macrophage.[17] A defect in the breakdown process of the lysosome will lead to the eventual buildup of these ingested materials.

Because macrophages are involved, the entire reticuloendothelial system will also be involved, due to the large number of phagocytes found in the spleen, liver, and bone marrow. Depending on the disease, the skeletal system and connective tissues may be involved as well as the central nervous system.[17]

The diseases discussed below are caused by inheritance of a defective autosomal recessive gene. The subsequent enzyme deficiency or defect results in lipid storage. These enzymes are necessary to degrade the lipid products of normal cell metabolism.

LEUKODYSTROPHY

The leukodystrophies can be considered dysmyelinating diseases, in which there is an enzymatic disturbance affecting the production and maintenance of the nerve myelin sheath. Lipids accumulate in tissues, primarily affecting the central nervous system and causing motor disturbances and mental retardation that can be severe.

Leukodystrophy has a high familial incidence and is inherited as an autosomal recessive gene. There are a number of diseases under this classification, two of which are Krabbe's disease and metachromatic leukodystrophy.

In *Krabbe's disease,* globoid cell leukodystrophy, there is widespread dysmyelination. Histologically, globoid cells are seen with multilobed nuclei in the white matter of the brain. Biochemically, deficiencies in two enzymes appear to be involved—betagalactase and sulfotransferase. These deficiencies may account for the increased deposits of cerebrosides found in the globoid cells.[4]

Krabbe's disease is rare. Generally it appears during infancy, although occasionally later in childhood. These children often display unexplained fever, light and noise sensitivity, and a halt in psychomotor development. Later, myoclonic jerks appear in the legs and arms, followed by blindness and mental deterioration.

The CSF will show an increased total protein, generally greater than 100 mg/dL (1000 mg/L). Determination of betagalactosidase deficiency by the substrate galactocerebroside, in serum or leukocytes, is highly indicative of Krabbe's disease. Parents can be tested for betagalactosidase activity to determine "carrier" status.[18]

There is no treatment or cure for this disease, and death usually occurs within 6 to 12 months.[4] Genetic counseling should be offered to those parents who already have an affected child. Prenatal diagnosis can be performed on amniotic fluid.[18]

In *metachromatic leukodystrophy,* sulfatide lipoidosis, there is a deficiency of arylsulfatase A. This deficiency leads to galactosyl sulfatide (lipid) accumulation in both the central and the peripheral nervous systems and in the renal tubules. The term metachromatic refers to the fact that the deposits of sulfatide change the color of certain tissue stains. Metachromatic granules can also be found in the urine sediment and WBCs. The excess galactosyl sulfatide is excreted in the urine of these patients.[17]

Metachromatic leukodystrophy is relatively rare, but more common than Krabbe's disease, with an onset in late infancy or early childhood.[17] These children display a loss of motor abilities and muscle weakness, thus losing the ability to walk. Mental functions show progressive degeneration.[1]

The CSF total protein is elevated, often to greater than 100 mg/dL (1000 mg/L).[1] A search for the metachromatic granules in the blood leukocytes or urine may be helpful. Determination of arylsulfatase A activity by the nitrocatecholsulfate test can be diagnostic. This test can be performed on urine, serum and cultures of WBCs and fibroblasts, thus making carrier status and prenatal testing available.[1, 18]

When clearcut laboratory results are not available, the following diseases should be ruled out: Neimann-Pick, Gaucher's, aminoacidurias, and subacute sclerosing panencephalitis.

There is no treatment for metachromatic leukodystrophy, and death usually occurs within 5 years. Parents should receive genetic counseling when heterozygotes can be identified by discovering decreased levels of arylsulfatase in cultured fibroblasts. Prenatal diagnosis can be made by cultures of amniotic cells and testing for decreased levels of arylsulfatase.[18]

MUCOPOLYSACCHARIDOSES

The mucopolysaccharidoses (MPS) are a group of inherited diseases with a defect in mucopolysaccharide metabolism due to an enzyme deficiency. Subsequently, there is an excess of dermatan sulfate, heparan sulfate, keratan sulfate, or chondroitin sulfate. These substances are stored in the body tissues and excreted in the urine. The severity of the symptoms varies with the type of mucopolysaccharidosis present.[4]

There are a number of different classifications for the MPS diseases. All are inherited as autosomal recessive genes except Hunter's disease, which is inherited as an X-linked gene.

Type I. Hurler's Disease

The deficient enzyme is α-L-iduronidase, and the excessive mucopolysaccharides are dermatan sulfate and heparan sulfate. This disease is characterized by skeletal deformities, dwarfism, mental retardation, and heart and liver involvement. Death usually occurs before the patient reaches 10 years of age.[19, 20]

Type II. Hunter's Disease

L-iduronide sulfatase is the deficient enzyme, with an increase in urinary dermatan sulfate and heparan sulfate. This disease is similar to Type I, but symptoms are milder and only males are affected. These patients may have a normal life expectancy.[19, 20]

Type III. Sanfilippo's Disease A and B

The enzyme deficiencies are respectively heparan N-sulfatase and N-acetyl-D-glucosaminidase, and the urine contains an excess of heparan sulfate. These patients have some skeletal deformities and severe mental retardation. Death usually occurs before the third decade.[19, 20]

Type IV. Morquio's Disease

The deficient enzyme is hexasamine-6-sulfatase, and an excess of urinary keratan sulfate is seen. Patients have severe skeletal deformities, corneal clouding, and respiratory problems. There is no mental retardation. Some patients live to age 60.[19, 20]

Type V. Scheie's Disease

α-L-iduronidase is deficient, causing an excess of dermatan sulfate and heparan sulfate. Symptoms may begin at age 10 with stiffness of hands and feet; corneal clouding and heart disease are also features. Little or no mental retardation is seen in these patients, who often have a normal life expectancy.[19, 20]

Type VI. Maroteaux-Lamy Syndrome

Arylsulfatase is deficient and there is excess dermatan sulfate. There is no mental retardation. Life expectancy is normal.[19, 20]

Type VII. Sly's Disease

The deficient enzyme is β-glucuronidase, with urinary excess of dermatan sulfate and heparan sulfate. These patients have a clinically variable picture.[19, 20]

All suspected mucopolysaccharidoses patients should have peripheral blood smears examined for the presence of Alder-Reilly bodies, which are significant evidence for the diagnosis.[6] The inclusions are seen as azurophilic and basophilic granules in neutrophils, eosinophils, and basophils, and sometimes in lymphocytes (Gasser's cells) and monocytes. The inclusions are more likely to be found in the bone marrow as Buhot's cells (large mononuclear cells). It can be easy to confuse the basophilic inclusions with toxic granulation.[6] In these patients and patients with other storage diseases, vacuolated lymphocytes can be seen (Mittwoch cells), and the smear may also show abnormally large platelets. It should be noted that these inclusions are most often seen in Hurler's, Hunter's, and Sanfilippo's diseases and are not seen in Morquio's disease.[21]

There are urine screening tests available for the detection of the mucopolysaccharidoses, such as the toluidine blue spot test which detects dermatan sulfate and heparan sulfate, and the acid albumin turbidity test. The acetylpyridium chloride test will also detect excess MPS in the urine. These screening tests may have false-positive as well as false-negative reactions, and will not detect keratan sulfate found in Morquio's disease. All positive reactions should be confirmed by either thin-layer chromatography or ion-exchange chromatography of the urine to determine the exact MPS present. Enzyme assays can also be performed on cultures of fibroblasts and leukocytes to identify the specific enzyme deficiency. The enzyme assays can be performed on cultured amniotic cells to make a prenatal diagnosis of MPS.[20]

The confirmatory tests are not routine in many laboratories, and usually must be performed by specialized reference labs.[14]

GAUCHER'S DISEASE

Gaucher's disease is the most common of the lysosomal storage diseases, and more frequent in those of Jewish descent than in other populations.[21]

The defect is in the lysosomal glucocerebrosidase and accumulation of the substrate glucocerebroside, a normal product of cellular breakdown. These lipids tend to build up in the reticuloendothelial system (RES) as the leukocytes are cleared from circulation.[17]

Patients with Gaucher's disease may be classed according to three types: adult onset, juvenile onset, and infantile onset. The earlier the clinical symptoms appear, the more severe the disease, with a shortened life span. The infantile form of the disease shows the most CNS involvement, and death before 2 years of age is usual. Adult onset is more common, with little or no retardation.[18]

Because of the RES involvement, patients will show an enlarged spleen and liver. There may also be bone destruction. Often there is a tendency to bruise and bleed easily after a small injury. Laboratory data will typically reveal a hypochromic normocytic anemia and a leukopenia—WBC $2.0–3.0 \times 10^3/mm^3$. There is thrombocytopenia (platelets $50–100 \times 10^3/mm^3$) and a marked increase in serum acid phosphatase with increased isoenzyme 5. Gaucher's cells are found occasionally in peripheral blood but more often in the bone marrow aspiration or liver and spleen biopsy. There is a deficiency in the specific enzyme β-glucosidase, in the peripheral leukocytes or, preferably, in cultured fibroblasts.[17]

Carrier status can be determined by identifying decreased enzyme activity in leukocytes or cultured fibroblasts. Usually carriers display approximately 50% of the enzyme activity of normal individuals; however, the "normal" varies considerably.[18]

Fetuses considered to be at risk can be monitored at 14 to 16 weeks by amniocentesis and testing the cultured fetal cells for enzyme activity.[18]

The clinical course of Gaucher's disease varies, from the severe form of infantile onset and early death to the relatively mild chronic form of adult onset with a normal life expectancy. There is little treatment available for Gaucher's disease at this time, although trials using enzyme replacement may prove successful in future.[18]

NIEMANN-PICK DISEASE

Niemann-Pick disease is also a lipid storage disease, caused by a deficiency of the enzyme sphingomyelinase. Niemann-Pick disease is inherited as an autosomal recessive gene, and is more common in persons of Jewish descent than in other population groups.[18, 21]

Occasionally the disease is not diagnosed until adulthood, but most commonly infants are affected and death occurs before the third birthday. Because of RES involvement (as in Gaucher's disease), patients display hepatomegaly and splenomegaly, accompanied by a mild jaundice due to liver damage. The nervous system is affected, leading to severe mental retardation. Approximately a third of these patients have a characteristic cherry red spot in the retina due to retinal degeneration.[18]

Routine laboratory tests are essentially normal. The anemia and thrombocytopenia seen in Gaucher's disease are not present or are very mild. Serum acid phosphatase is also normal, helping to differentiate this disease from Gaucher's.[21]

The diagnosis of Niemann-Pick disease can be made by finding Niemann-Pick cells in bone marrow aspirates. These are large macrophages filled with globules of sphingomyelin. Enzyme studies in leukocytes are useful in identifying the disease, using the substrate 2-hexadecanoylamino-4-nitrophenylphosphorylcholine, which closely resembles sphingomyelin. These tests can also be performed to identify carrier status of parents, to monitor the fetus, and to assist in genetic counseling.[18, 21]

At present there is no cure for Niemann-Pick disease, and most of the affected children die early. This makes recognition of heterozygotes important for purposes of family planning.

Other Etiologies

POSTINFECTIOUS AND POSTVACCINAL ENCEPHALOMYELITIS

Postinfectious encephalomyelitis can occur, although rarely, following certain childhood diseases such as measles, rubella, smallpox, and mumps. A similar disease can occur after vaccination for such diseases as rabies, smallpox, or measles. The exact etiology is unknown, but theories suggest that the virus or toxin associated with the virus causes neurological damage or that the patient's immune response (allergic reaction) is the cause (see Chap. 46).

SUBACUTE SCLEROSING PANENCEPHALITIS

Subacute sclerosing panencephalitis (SSPE) is considered a slow viral infection, caused by the measles virus. The pathology of this disease is not totally understood, but current theory suggests immune complex deposits in the brain as a factor (see Chap. 46).

CASE STUDY

A 24-year-old caucasian woman was seen by her physician. She complained of fatigue, weakness in arms and legs, difficulty in walking, and blurring of vision.

She reported weakness in her legs during the summer, when she found she was no longer able to water-ski. After the birth of her third child the weakness became progressively worse, to the point at which she had difficulty in walking and required assistance if there was no support to lean on. The weakness also appeared in her arms, making it difficult for her to set and comb her hair. When her vision began to blur, she sought medical help.

Up to this time the patient had been healthy. She had had only the usual childhood diseases. There was no history of recent illness or vaccinations. She had been raised in a rural area of Ohio and had not been out of the area recently.

LABORATORY FINDINGS

Blood	***Results***	***Interpretation***
Total protein	7.1 g/dL	Normal
Albumin	5.3 g/dL	Normal
IgG	998 mg/dL	Normal
Serum electrophoresis	Normal	Normal
WBC differential	Normal	Normal

Urine	***Results***	***Interpretation***
Routine urinalysis	Normal	
CSF		
Gross Examination	Clear and colorless	Normal
Cell count	26/mm^3	Increased
RBC	0/mm^3	Normal
WBC	26/mm^3	Increased
Lymph	26/mm^3	Increased
Granulocytes	0/mm^3	Normal
Glucose	52 mg/dL	Normal
VDRL	Nonreactive	Normal
Culture	No organisms	Normal
Total protein	55 mg/dL	Slight increase
Albumin	21 mg/DL	Normal
IgG	6.6 mg/dL	Increased
Oligoconal bands	4 seen	Abnormal
Myelin basic protein	wk pos (4–8 ng/mL)	Abnormal
IgG synthesis rate	5.7 mg/24 hr	Increased
Calculated Results		
IgG index	1.7	Increased
Albumin index	4.0	Normal

Conversion to SI units is as follows:
Protein—mg/dL × 10 = mg/L
—g/dL × 10 = g/L

Questions

1. What do the CSF oligoclonal bands and increased IgG index and IgG synthesis rate indicate?
2. What is a likely tentative diagnosis for this patient?
3. Does the patient's history correlate with the diagnosis?
4. Has the patient had a recent active episode?
5. What would be another diagnostic test to help confirm the diagnosis?

Discussion

1. These three test results point to de novo IgG synthesis in the CSF of the patient. Leakage in the blood–brain barrier is ruled out by the cell count (no RBCs) of the CSF, appearance of the CSF (no xanthrochromia), and a normal albumin index.

2. Multiple sclerosis may be likely.
3. The patient's history supports the diagnosis. She has been living in a geographic area where incidence of MS is high, and her symptoms worsened after the pregnancy. Her symptoms are common to MS: generalized fatigue, progressive weakness in both arms and legs, blurring of vision.
4. The weakly positive myelin basic protein indicates an active episode more than 1 week old, consistent with recovery from a flareup of MS or a slow demyelination.
5. A CT scan and finding lesions consistent with MS would be helpful in diagnosis.

REFERENCES

1. Baker AB, Baker LH (eds): Clinical Neurology. New York, Harper & Row, 1984
2. Williams A, Papadopoulos N, Chase T: Demonstration of CSF gammaglobulin banding in presenile dementia. Neurology 30:822–884, 1980
3. Kandel ER, Swartz JH: Principles of Neural Science, 2nd ed. New York City, Elsevier Science Publishing, 1985
4. Merritt HH: Textbook of Neurology, 6th ed. Philadelphia, Lea & Febiger, 1979
5. Collins DR: Illustrated Manual of Neurologic Diagnosis, 2nd ed. Philadelphia, JB Lippincott, 1982
6. Wintrobe M (ed): Harrison's Principles of Internal Medicine, 6th ed. New York City, McGraw-Hill, 1970
7. Price SA, Wilson LM: Pathophysiology: Clinical Concepts of Disease Processes, 3rd ed. New York City, McGraw-Hill, 1986
8. Specialty Laboratories: Laboratory Report Form and Update: Neuro-oncology and Neuroimmunology Come of Age. Los Angeles, Specialty Laboratories, 1987
9. Escourolle R, Poirier J, Rubinstein L (trans): Manual of Basic Neuropathology. Philadelphia, WB Saunders, 1971
10. Rowland L (ed): Merritt's Textbook of Neurology, 7th ed. Philadelphia, Lea & Febiger, 1984
11. Stahlheber PA, Peter JB: Multiple sclerosis: A clearer path to a complex diagnosis. Diagn Med 1:43–48, 1984
12. Johnson KP, Zobeeda H: Laboratory identification of multiple sclerosis. Lab Man 5:36–40, 1981
13. BioScience Laboratories: Assay Update: Oligoclonal Gammaglobulins in CSF by Agarose electrophoresis. Van Nuys, California, BioScience Laboratories, 1986
14. Jacobs D, Osten B, Demott W et al: Laboratory Test Handbook With DRG Index. St. Louis, Mosby/Lexicomp, 1984
15. BioScience Laboratories: Assay Update: Myelin Basic Protein. Van Nuys, California, BioScience Laboratories, 1986
16. Pansky B, Delamas JA: Review of Neuroscience. New York, Macmillan, 1980
17. Kaplan LA, Pesce AJ: Clinical Chemistry: Theory, Analysis, and Correlation. St Louis, CV Mosby, 1984
18. Brady RO, Kolodney EH: Sphingolipid storage disorders: Diagnosis and detection. Lab Man 7:27–37, 1982
19. Bennington JL (ed): Saunders Encyclopedia and Dictionary of Laboratory Medicine and Technology. Philadelphia, WB Saunders, 1984
20. Knight JA, Wu JY: Screening profile for detection of inherited metabolic disorders. Lab Med 13(11): 681–687, 1982
21. Miale J: Laboratory Medicine Hematology, 6th ed. St Louis, CV Mosby, 1982

BIBLIOGRAPHY

Bauer JD: Clinical Laboratory Methods, 9th ed. St. Louis, CV Mosby, 1982

Graff L: Handbook of Routine Urinalysis. Philadelphia, JB Lippincott, 1983

Henry JB (ed): Clinical Diagnosis and Management by Laboratory Methods, 17th ed. Philadelphia, WB Saunders, 1984

Robbins SH, Cotran RS: Pathologic Basis of Disease, 2nd ed. Philadelphia, WB Saunders, 1979

Wintrobe M: Clinical Hematology, 7th ed. Philadelphia, Lea & Febiger, 1974

Chapter 45

Meningitis

Paul G. Engelkirk

The term *meningitis* (pl. meningitides) refers to an inflammation either of the leptomeninges or within the subarachnoid space, or both. Meningitis is always cerebrospinal, meaning that the disease involves both the brain and the spinal cord.

The meningitides can be broadly divided into acute or chronic meningitis, the acute types having a short (symptoms of less than 24 hours' duration) and relatively severe course, and the chronic types persisting over a long period of time (at least 4 weeks). The term "subacute" meningitis refers to cases with symptoms of 1 to 7 days' duration.

ETIOLOGY AND PATHOPHYSIOLOGY

Acute Meningitis

Acute meningitis may be caused by a variety of infectious and noninfectious agents. When caused by bacteria, the disease is referred to as *bacterial meningitis.* The term *aseptic meningitis* (sometimes called acute nonbacterial meningitis) is used in conjunction with milder forms of meningitis, in which routine bacteriological culture techniques are unsuccessful. Most cases of aseptic meningitis are caused by viruses.

BACTERIAL MENINGITIS

Bacterial meningitis may be caused by a number of different pathogenic bacteria. The most common etiologic agents vary according to patient age group (see Table 45-1). In general, the bacteria causing acute bacterial meningitis are encapsulated, with the capsule serving to protect the organisms from phagocytosis by host leukocytes.

The three most common etiologic agents of acute bacterial meningitis are *Hemophilus influenzae* type b, *Neisseria meningitidis,* and *Streptococcus pneumoniae,* which collectively cause about 95% of the cases.[1] Neonatal meningitis, however, is most often due to other species of bacteria that were colonizing the maternal genital tract at the time of birth. This age group has the highest prevalence of meningitis and the highest mortality rate.[1]

Ninety-five percent of all cases of meningitis in

Table 45-1 ***Etiologic Agents of Acute Bacterial Meningitis***

Patient Age Group	Bacterium	CSF Gram-Stain Morphology	Comments
Newborn	Group B streptococci (*Streptococcus agalactiae*)	Gram-positive cocci	
	Enteric gram-negative bacilli (especially *Escherichia coli*)	Gram-negative bacilli	
	Listeria monocytogenes	Gram-positive coccobacilli ("diphtheroid" appearance)	Gram stains of CSF are often negative.
Infant and young child	*Hemophilus influenzae*	Gram-negative coccobacilli or short rods with rounded ends	May stain heavily at poles, resembling gram-negative cocci.
	Neisseria meningitidis	Gram-negative diplococci	Organisms within leukocytes may be indistinguishable from nuclear material.
	Streptococcus pneumoniae	"lancet-shaped" gram-positive cocci	Older pneumococci lose their capacity to stain gram-positive.
Young adult	*N. meningitidis*	As stated above	As stated above
Middle-aged and elderly	*S. pneumoniae*	As stated above	As stated above
Association with head trauma or surgery	*Staphylococcus aureus*	Gram-positive cocci	

the United States occur in children younger than 5 years of age.[1] Meningitis in this age group is most often due to *H. influenzae* type b, which tends to cause meningitis during the time period when maternal antibodies to this organism are no longer present, and before the child has produced antibodies to antigenically similar bacteria.[1]

The most common causes of bacterial meningitis in previously healthy adults are pneumococci and meningococci. In young adults, outbreaks of meningococcal meningitis are frequently associated with crowded conditions, such as military barracks and college dormitories, and occur among individuals lacking antibody to *N. meningitidis*. Serogroups A and C are most often associated with epidemics of meningococcal meningitis, whereas serogroup B is the principal cause of sporadic cases.[2] Conditions such as immunosuppression, alcoholism, splenectomy, diabetes mellitus, and intracranial shunts increase the risk of developing meningitis.

ASEPTIC MENINGITIS

The term *aseptic meningitis* was originally used to describe a disease characterized by an acute onset, meningeal symptoms, fever, increased leukocytes in the cerebrospinal fluid (CSF), and, most importantly, bacteriologically sterile CSF cultures. Today, it is known that aseptic meningitis is a condition of multiple etiologies, which include both infectious and noninfectious agents.

Infectious Agents

Although the vast majority of cases of aseptic meningitis are caused by viruses, this disease may also be caused by bacteria (*e.g., Mycobacterium tuberculosis, Treponema pallidum*), protozoa (*e.g., Naegleria fowleri*), and fungi (*e.g., Candida albicans, Cryptococcus neoformans, Coccidioides immitis*). The majority of these etiologic agents go undetected when routine CSF culture protocols are used.

The list of viruses that can produce aseptic meningitis is lengthy, and includes enteroviruses (echoviruses, coxsackieviruses), mumps virus, a number of arboviruses, herpesviruses (herpes simplex I and II, cytomegalovirus, Epstein-Barr virus), hepatitis virus, measles virus, adenoviruses, and lymphocytic choriomeningitis virus. Free-living amebic protozoa, such as *Naegleria fowleri* and *Acanthamoeba* species, can cause a disease known as primary amebic meningoencephalitis, which is an inflammation of both the brain and the meninges.

Microorganisms may gain access to the central nervous system (CNS) in any of several ways. The most common means is hematogenously, through the blood stream into the CNS by incompletely understood mechanisms. The microorganisms may also gain access via CNS shunts (see Chap. 46), or by direct inoculation following trauma to the head or a neurosurgical procedure. Some viruses are capable of entering the CNS along neural pathways (*e.g.,* herpes simplex) or via the olfactory tract (*e.g.,* adenoviruses). Free-living amebae may enter via the nasal mucosa and olfactory nerve following swimming or diving in contaminated (usually stagnant) freshwater ponds or lakes. Meningitis can also result from a ruptured or leaking brain abscess (see Chap. 46).

When local defense and clearance mechanisms are unable to eliminate the invading microorganisms, an infectious process develops with inflammation, tissue necrosis, and vasculitis. The resulting hypoxia, edema, and impaired flow of CSF can result in increased intracranial pressure and impaired neurologic function.

Noninfectious Agents

Noninfectious causes of aseptic meningitis include tumors, chemical agents (*e.g.,* contrast material, procaine, or disinfectants used during lumbar puncture), or material released into the subarachnoid space from cutaneous or noncutaneous cysts. Aseptic meningitis may also accompany such noninfectious disorders as sarcoidosis and systemic lupus erythematosus (SLE).

Chronic Meningitis

Chronic meningitides develop more slowly and tend to be less dramatic than the acute types. By definition, clinical and/or CSF abnormalities must have lasted at least 4 weeks before the diagnosis of chronic meningitis can be made.

Most cases of chronic meningitis are caused by slowly growing microorganisms such as *M. tuberculosis,* other mycobacteria, fungi (*e.g., C. neoformans, Histoplasma capsulatum*), *Nocardia* species, and *T. pallidum.* Other microorganisms that can cause chronic meningitis include *Leptospira, Toxoplasma, Brucella,* and *Taenia solium* (cysticercosis).

Patients most apt to develop chronic meningitis are those who are immunosuppressed, and those with diseases such as histoplasmosis, syphilis, tuberculosis, and brucellosis. Most of the etiologic agents of chronic meningitis gain access to the CNS by the same routes as the agents associated with acute meningitis. Exceptions are the leptospires, which apparently can penetrate tissues mechanically, and intracellular organisms that can be transported via the blood within phagocytic leukocytes.[3]

Humans acquire cysticercosis by ingesting *T. solium* eggs. After they hatch in the stomach and duodenum, oncospheres penetrate the intestinal epithelium, enter the lymphatic and vascular systems, and are carried to many different locations in the body. Approximately 60% of cysticercosis patients have cysticerci in their brains, and of these approximately 50% develop symptoms.[4]

CLINICAL MANIFESTATIONS

Acute Meningitis

The initial symptoms experienced by the patient with acute meningitis are chills, fever, lethargy, stiff neck, and a severe headache. Depending on the origin of the infection, the patient may also experience symptoms associated with pneumonia, sinusitis, or otitis media. With increased hypoxia and intracranial pressure, the headache may become increasingly severe, vomiting may occur, and there will be evidence of neurologic dysfunction (*e.g.,* photophobia, confusion, drowsiness, stupor, coma, occasionally convulsions). Attempts by the physician to flex the patient's stiff neck may cause meningeal irritation, resulting in neck and lower back pain.

Skin lesions (rash) occur in approximately 50% of cases of meningococcal meningitis,[5] a disease that can have a fulminant course and can cause death within a matter of hours. Rashes are also common in coxsackievirus and echovirus infections. A diagnosis of meningitis is somewhat difficult to establish in infants. Therefore, a tentative diagnosis of meningitis must be considered in any infant with temperature instability, respiratory difficulties, or feeding problems.[3]

Chronic Meningitis

In chronic meningitis, the disease progression is slow, and the patient experiences few, if any, symptoms that give an indication of the seriousness of the disease. Personality changes, altered levels of consciousness, and headaches may occur, although they tend to be much less severe than those associated with acute bacterial meningitis. Nausea and vomiting, together with the headaches and other symptoms resulting from increased intracranial pressure, may resemble the symptoms associated with the development of a tumor. Hydrocephalus and cerebral edema may cause a sudden deterioration of neurologic function. About half of patients with neurocysticercosis have meningeal cysts and the signs and symptoms of chronic meningitis, including intense inflammation, obstructive hydrocephalus, arterial thrombosis, and stroke.[4]

LABORATORY ANALYSES AND DIAGNOSIS

General

Should the physician suspect on the basis of the history and physical exam that the patient has bacterial meningitis, a CSF specimen will be required for a definitive diagnosis of the etiologic agent. However, when the CSF pressure is high (increased intracranial pressure, evidenced by headache and papilledema), lumbar puncture (spinal tap) is particularly hazardous, and can result in brain herniation. Thus, a computerized tomographic (CT) scan should first be performed to rule out a mass lesion such as a brain abscess (see Chap. 46).[6]

The seriousness of acute bacterial meningitis and other CNS infections cannot be overemphasized. Every effort to process the CSF specimen as quickly as possible must be made. Untreated bacterial meningitis is devastating and rapidly fatal. Ideally, it should never take longer than one hour to presumptively diagnose and begin treatment for this disease.

The traditional laboratory workup of a CSF specimen includes a gross examination, a total leukocyte count on the uncentrifuged specimen, a differential count on resuspended sediment following centrifugation of the specimen, culture and Gram stain of the sediment following centrifugation, as well as analyses of the protein and glucose concentrations. Additional tests may be helpful, as described below. In addition to a CSF specimen, blood should be sent to the laboratory for culture and for a complete blood count and differential.

Results of the various laboratory analyses useful in the diagnosis of CNS infections must be communicated to the physician as soon as they become available, even if it is necessary to provide this information in a piecemeal manner.

Acute Meningitis

MICROBIOLOGICAL PROCEDURES

Of the procedures listed in Table 45-2, culturing of CSF and blood and the microscopic examination of the Gram-stained sediment are the most useful in acute bacterial meningitis. The results of the latter procedure can be available shortly after collection of the specimen, but culture results will, of course, not be available until the following day, at the earliest. Because infected CSF usually contains only small numbers of microorganisms, some type of concentration procedure (*e.g.*, centrifugation or filtration) must be performed prior to culturing the specimen or preparation of a smear for staining. Failure to observe bacteria in the Gram-stained smear or failure to culture bacteria does *not* rule out bacterial etiology. The organisms may be too few in number to be observed microscopically, and prior antibiotic therapy may prevent the bacteria from being cultured from CSF or blood.

On the other hand, false-positive Gram stain results may be due to nonviable bacteria that were present either in the collection tubes or on the microscope slides, or to viable organisms present in the staining solutions or in the water used to rinse the smears. Thus, great care must be taken in interpretation of Gram-stained CSF, and the organism suspected should be one consistent with patient history and age and other lab findings. Whenever only a single specimen container is submitted to the laboratory, it must first be processed by the microbiology section to prevent contamination of the CSF specimen in other sections of the laboratory.

A drop of the CSF sediment may be stained using acridine orange stain, which permits a more rapid examination for bacteria, using the high-power microscope objective. Any suspicious smear can then be restained over the acridine orange stain using the Gram-staining procedure.[1]

Because they can be destroyed by centrifugation, motile amebae (*Naegleria* or *Acanthamoeba*) are best observed by examining a drop of fresh, uncentrifuged CSF by wet mount, using either a phase contrast or a brightfield microscope.[2] Whenever *C. neoformans* is suspected, a drop of CSF sediment should be examined in an India ink preparation. Because these organisms may be sparse in CSF specimens, appropriate culture media should also be inoculated. An acid-fast stain should be performed when mycobacteria are suspected, and, when deemed appropriate, CSF specimens should be cultured for anaerobes, fungi, and mycobacteria in addition to nonanaerobic bacteria.

Table 45-2 ***Results of Traditional CSF Laboratory Tests in Acute Meningitis***

Laboratory Test	Normal	Acute Bacterial (Septic) Meningitis	Aseptic Meningitis
Pressure (measured during lumbar puncture)	<140 mm H_2O (recumbent position)	Increased	Normal or increased
Gross examination	Clear	Usually turbid	Clear or slightly turbid (CSF may be clear, and yet contain as many as 300 to 400 cells/mm^3)
Gram stain of sediment	Sterile	Bacteria commonly observed; Gram stain reaction & morphology useful in tentative ID	
Culture	Negative	Positive in 70% to 80% of cases	Viral, fungal, or AFB cultures may be positive.
Blood culture	Negative	Positive in 40% to 60% of cases of meningococcal, pneumococcal, or *H. influenzae* meningitis	
Total leukocyte count	<5 cells/mm^3	Generally >1000 cells/mm^3 (av. = 5,000–20,000) (see text)	Generally <1000/mm^3 (usually 10–100), but can be 3000 or even higher (see text)
Predominant leukocyte type	All lymphocytes	>90% polymorphonuclear leukocytes (see text)	Usually >3/4 mononuclear (see text)
Glucose concentration	50–80 mg/dL (or >50% concomitant serum glucose level)	Decreased (<50% of serum level)	Normal (see text)
Protein concentration	15–45 mg/dL	Increased (>100 mg/dL); usually 150–500 mg/dL	Normal to increased

Conversion to SI units is as follows:
Glucose—mg/dL × 0.0555 = mmol/L
Protein—mg/dL × 10 = mg/L

Whenever viral meningitis is suspected, a variety of specimens (*e.g.*, stool, urine, saliva, throat washings, CSF) should be sent to the laboratory for culturing, and acute and convalescent sera should be sent for serologic studies. In most cases of viral meningitis, the agent will not be isolated from CSF (exceptions include mumps virus) or blood.[7] The CSF can be examined for viral antigen using either fluorescein-labeled antibody or immunoenzymatic methods.

OTHER TRADITIONAL LABORATORY TESTS

In acute aseptic meningitis, which is usually due to viral infection, the total CSF cell count is usually less than $1000/mm^3$, and mononuclear cells are the predominant cell type. However, during the first 24 to 48 hours of infection, the predominant cell type can be polymorphonuclear leukocytes, as in bacterial meningitis.[3] It is also important to remember that one-third of the cases of tuberculosis and viral meningitis will show a predominance of PMNs, and approximately 10% of the cases of bacterial meningitis will have greater than 80% lymphocytes.[2] Thus, the often quoted distinctions between bacterial and viral meningitis are not always clear-cut.

Blood leukocyte counts (WBC) are usually elevated in acute bacterial meningitis, with a shift to the left. Although the WBC count is usually normal in viral meningitis, leukopenia can be present in about one-third of patients.[7]

Although the CSF glucose concentration is usually normal in aseptic meningitis, certain viral meningitides (*e.g.*, those due to mumps virus, herpes simplex virus, CMV, and lymphocytic choriomeningitis virus) can be associated with decreased values, as found in bacterial meningitis.[3, 7]

ADDITIONAL PROCEDURES OF VALUE IN THE DIAGNOSIS OF ACUTE MENINGITIS

A number of additional laboratory procedures performed on CSF are available as adjuncts in the diagnosis of acute meningitis. These include capsular swelling (quellung) techniques, counterimmunoelectrophoresis (CIE) and agglutination procedures for the detection of bacterial and fungal antigens, lactic acid and lactate dehydrogenase (LD) determinations, and assays for the detection of endotoxin.

Although rarely used, antisera are commercially available for use in capsular swelling tests to identify tentatively certain of the encapsulated bacteria that could be present in CSF specimens; examples include *S. pneumoniae, H. influenzae* type b, and *N. meningitidis* groups A and C.

Latex agglutination, coagglutination, and/or CIE procedures are available for the detection of the same organisms (plus *S. agalactiae*) in CSF, urine, and serum specimens. These procedures are frequently of greater value in establishing a rapid presumptive diagnosis than is the Gram stain. A latex agglutination procedure is available for the detection of cryptococcal antigen, and enzyme-linked immunosorbent (ELISA) assays have been developed for the detection in CSF of antigens of *H. influenzae, S. pneumoniae, N. meningitidis,* and *M. tuberculosis.*

Reference values for CSF lactate are 10–22 mg/dL (1.1–2.4 mmol/L).[8] Levels of CSF lactic acid in excess of 35 mg/dL (3.9 mmol/L) have been reported to be associated with bacterial meningitis, including *M. tuberculosis,* although both false-negative and false-positive results occur.[5, 9] Levels lower than 35 mg/dL suggest nonbacterial (*e.g.*, viral) meningitis.[5]

Increased levels of LD isoenzymes have been reported to occur in the majority of cases of bacterial meningitis, with mean values of 113 units for isoenzymes 4 and 5 (normal range 2–7 units).[5] In viral meningitis, the average level is 23 units, and the isoenzymes consist mainly of fractions 1 and 2.[5]

The *Limulus* lysate test, which involves the use of amebocytes from the horseshoe crab, is capable of detecting endotoxin in CSF, thus indicating the involvement of either a gram-negative pathogen or *Listeria monocytogenes.*[1] Although both false-positive and false-negative results occur,[8] it is a sensitive adjunct in the diagnosis of meningitis caused by such agents as *E. coli, H. influenzae,* and *N. meningitidis.*[1]

Chronic Meningitis

As in acute meningitis, the physician will suspect chronic meningitis following careful consideration of the patient's history and complete physical examination. Whereas examination of CSF in acute meningitis can be diagnostic, such is usually not the case in chronic meningitis. However, an evaluation of CSF may be suggestive (see Table 45-3), and rapid processing of the specimen and expe-

Table 45-3 ***Results of Traditional CSF Laboratory Tests in Chronic Meningitis****

Laboratory Test	Result
Pressure (measured during lumbar puncture)	Normal to increased
Gross examination	Often clear; at least 200 leukocytes/mm^3 are required to cause slight turbidity
Gram stain of sediment	Rare spherules of *Coccidioides immitis* may be present
Acid-fast stain of sediment	Positive in 10% to 22% of cases of tuberculous meningitis
India ink preparation of sediment	Round, encapsulated, sometimes budding yeast in >50% of cases of cryptococcal meningitis
Culture	Positive in 33% to 50% of cases of coccidioidal meningitis; in >75% of cases of cryptococcal meningitis; in 38% to 88% of cases of tuberculous meningitis
Total leukocyte count	Generally 1000/mm^3
Predominant leukocyte type	Mononuclear
Glucose concentration	Usually decreased
Protein concentration	Increased (often markedly)

*Reference values are contained in Table 45–2.

ditious correlation, interpretation, and reporting of results are critical.

A history of diseases such as tuberculosis or syphilis can be helpful in establishing a diagnosis, and can serve to guide the clinical laboratory scientist in the selection of appropriate media, stains, and other laboratory procedures. The CSF should always be cultured and examined using appropriate staining techniques (e.g., Gram, acid-fast, and acridine orange stains). A cytologic examination of the sediment can help rule out the possibility of a tumor.

An India ink preparation can demonstrate the presence of *C. neoformans.* Serum and CSF should be tested for the presence of *Cryptococcus* and *Coccidioides* antigen and antitreponemal antibodies. Due to the blood–brain barrier, normal serum : CSF antibody ratios are greater than 200, meaning that the concentration (titer) of a given antibody in serum is usually 200 or more times greater than the concentration of that antibody in CSF.[3] Lower ratios usually indicate either that the blood–brain barrier has been injured or altered in some way, or that synthesis of antibody has occurred within the CNS. Thus, a serum : CSF ratio of less than 200 to a given etiologic agent may indicate CNS infection by that agent. As with infections not involving the CNS, identification of an etiologic agent may also be made by demonstrating a rise in specific antibody titers between acute and convalescent serum specimens.

The diagnosis of neurocysticercosis may be made by a combination of computerized tomography (CT) and radiography, antibody detection in CSF and/or serum, peripheral blood eosinophilia, and the presence of eosinophils in the CSF.

TREATMENT

Specific treatment of acute meningitis will, of course, depend upon its cause. Bacterial, fungal, and protozoal pathogens will be treated with appropriate antimicrobial agents; whenever possible, the selection of agent will be based on the results of antimicrobial susceptibility testing. Prior to the availability of susceptibility results, empirical treatment may be necessary, with the selection of agent being based on Gram-stain, India ink, or antigen detection results. The drug selected must be effective against the organism, must be capable of crossing the blood–brain barrier, and must be administered in an appropriate dose and by an appropriate route (usually intravenously).

Drugs that are used successfully to treat bacterial meningitis include penicillin (*S. pneumoniae* and *N. meningitidis*), ampicillin (*H. influenzae, L. monocytogenes, E. coli*), and chloramphenicol (*H. influenzae*). Because of possible infection with resistant strains of *H. influenzae,* children should be treated with both chloramphenicol and ampicillin until the results of culture and susceptibility tests are known.[10]

Intravenous amphotericin B is the most effective treatment for most systemic mycoses. However, because it penetrates poorly into CSF, intrathecal or intraventricular administration may also be necessary in cases of fungal meningitis (*e.g.*, coccidioidal meningitis).[11] Concurrent use of amphotericin B and flucytosine is sometimes used in the treatment of cryptococcal meningitis.[11] Amphotericin B and sulfadiazine are investigational drugs in the treatment of amebic meningoencephalitis due to *Naegleria* and *Acanthamoeba,* respectively.[12] In uncomplicated cases of viral meningitis, antiviral agents are usually not used.

Supportive therapy may include intracranial pressure monitoring, steroids, fluid replacement, and bed rest. Patients are usually monitored by direct observation, rather than by laboratory analysis of any convalescent specimens. Repeat lumbar punctures are usually not necessary, unless the patient's clinical response is atypical.

As with acute meningitis, antimicrobial therapy for chronic meningitis will of course depend on the specific etiologic agent involved. The same considerations with respect to effectiveness against the pathogen, ability to cross the blood–brain barrier, dosage, and route apply in the treatment of chronic meningitis. Although surgical intervention may be necessary, the investigational drug praziquantel is sometimes used successfully in the treatment of neurocysticercosis. Praziquantel will cross the blood–brain barrier and kill cysticerci, but apparently does not affect calcified cysts and thus will not always alleviate the patient's signs and symptoms.[4] In general, the prognosis for chronic meningitis will depend on the specific pathogen involved, the extent of the damage, and the susceptibility of the etiologic agent to the drugs used.

CASE STUDY

A 28-year-old woman gave birth to a 3,500-gram male infant at term, following an uneventful labor and delivery. Physical examinations of the neonate performed at birth and at 8 hours of age were essentially normal. At 18 hours of age, however, the infant began vomiting, refused to feed, and became irritable. By 30 hours of age the baby was lethargic (unconscious), and seizure activity was noted. Physical examination revealed a bulging of the anterior fontanelle (a membranous interval at the junction of several bones at the top of the infant's skull), a supple neck, clear lungs, a regular rhythmic heart, and a nonenlarged liver and spleen. A chest x-ray was negative. The infant's temperature was 37.8° C, blood pressure was 90/70 mm, pulse was 110/minute, and respiration rate was 36/minute. A lumbar puncture was performed, and blood and urine specimens were also submitted to the laboratory. Pertinent laboratory data are shown below.[13]

LABORATORY FINDINGS

Laboratory Test	***Result***
Hemoglobin	14.5 gm/dL
Blood WBC count	13.5 × 10^3/mm^3
Blood differential	60% neutrophils, 29% lymphocytes, 4% monocytes, 7% band forms
Urinalysis	Normal
Serum BUN, sugar, electrolytes	Normal
CSF appearance	Cloudy
CSF WBC count	2.8 × 10^3/mm^3
CSF differential	98% neutrophils
CSF glucose	30 mg/dL
Blood glucose	90 mg/dL
CSF protein	150 mg/dL

Laboratory Test	***Result***
CSF Gram stain	Many WBCs, gram-positive cocci in chains
CSF culture	Results pending
Blood culture	Results pending

Conversion to SI units is as follows:
Hemoglobin—gm/dL × 0.155 = mmol/L
Glucose—mg/dL × 0.0555 = mmol/L
Protein—mg/dL × 10 = mg/L

Questions

1. What prompted the physician to perform a lumbar puncture in this case?
2. Which etiologic agent(s) of meningitis would the physician be most apt to suspect in this case, prior to receipt of any laboratory results?
3. Based on your knowledge of the patient and the laboratory results, which etiologic agent do you suspect?
4. What additional laboratory procedures could have been performed to aid in the diagnosis of meningitis due to this particular pathogen?

Discussion

1. Because many of the usual signs of meningitis may be lacking in neonates, the diagnosis must be considered in any infant with temperature instability, respiratory difficulties, or feeding problems. In this case, the patient was also lethargic, was demonstrating seizure activity, and had a bulging fontanelle (indicating a late stage of infection in newborns). Because bacterial meningitis can be rapidly fatal, speed was essential in the processing of a CSF specimen and in the interpretation and reporting of laboratory results.
2. Although *N. meningitidis, S. pneumoniae,* and *H. influenzae* are common causes of bacterial meningitis in children and adults, the primary etiologic agents in neonates are Group B β-hemolytic streptococci (*S. agalactiae*), *L. monocytogenes,* and *E. coli,* any of which may be colonizing the birth canal at the time of delivery.
3. The appearance of the CSF specimen, its cellular contents, and the glucose and protein results are consistent with a diagnosis of bacterial meningitis. The Gram-stain results, gram-positive cocci in chains, are consistent with the appearance of streptococci. Therefore, because the patient is a newborn, *S. agalactiae* is the most likely cause of this patient's bacterial meningitis.
4. Latex agglutination and CIE procedures are commercially available, and permit rapid detection of bacterial antigens (to include *S. agalactiae* antigen) in CSF specimens. Such procedures are often positive in cases in which the Gram stains are negative.

REFERENCES

1. Finegold SM, Baron EJ: Bailey and Scott's Diagnostic Microbiology. St Louis, CV Mosby, 1986
2. McGee ZA, Kaiser AB: Acute Meningitis. In Mandell GL, Douglas RG, Bennett JE (eds): Principles and Practice of Infectious Diseases, p 560. New York City, John Wiley & Sons, 1985
3. Austin TW: Infections of the Central Nervous System. In Mandell LA, Ralph ED (eds): Essentials of Infectious Diseases, p 115. Boston, Blackwell Scientific, 1985
4. McGreevy PB, Nelson GS: Larval Cestode Infections. In Strickland GT (ed): Hunter's Tropical Medicine, p 771. Philadelphia, WB Saunders, 1984
5. Adams RD, Petersdorf RG: Pyogenic Infections of the Central Nervous System. In Petersdorf RG et al (eds): Harrison's Principles of Internal Medicine, p 2084. New York City, McGraw-Hill, 1983
6. Adams RD, Chiappa KH, Martin JB et al: Diagnostic Methods in Neurology. In Petersdorf RG et al (eds): Harrison's Principles of Internal Medicine, p 2010. New York City, McGraw-Hill, 1983
7. Harter DH, Petersdorf RG, Adams RD: Viral Diseases of the Central Nervous System—Aseptic Meningitis and Encephalitis. In Petersdorf RG et al (eds): Harrison's Principles of Internal Medicine, p 2091. New York City, McGraw-Hill, 1983
8. Kjeldsberg CR, Krieg AF: Cerebrospinal Fluid and Other Body Fluids. In Henry JB (ed): Todd-Sanford-Davidsohn Clinical Diagnosis and Management by Laboratory Methods, p 459. Philadelphia, WB Saunders, 1984

9. Ray CG, Wasilauskas BL, Zabransky R: Cumitech 14—Laboratory Diagnosis of Central Nervous System Infections. Washington, DC, American Society for Microbiology, 1982
10. The Medical Letter on Drugs and Therapeutics 28 (710): 34, March 28, 1986
11. The Medical Letter on Drugs and Therapeutics 28 (711): 41, April 11, 1986
12. The Medical Letter on Drugs and Therapeutics 28 (706): 10, January 31, 1986
13. Frothingham TE, Gutman LT, Idriss ZH et al: Pediatric Infectious Disease Case Studies. New York City, Medical Examination Publishing Company, 1978

BIBLIOGRAPHY

Ellner JJ: Chronic Meningitis. In Mandell GL, Douglas RG, Bennett JE (eds): Principles and Practice of Infectious Diseases, p 573. New York City, John Wiley & Sons, 1985

Chapter 46

Focal CNS Infections and Encephalitis

Paul G. Engelkirk

ETIOLOGY AND PATHOPHYSIOLOGY

Focal Suppurative Lesions

Brain abscesses, subdural empyema, and epidural abscesses are examples of focal suppurative lesions, *i.e.*, lesions confined to a specific location within the CNS, and associated with the production of pus. All are medical and surgical emergencies that can cause death or permanent neurological deficit. The key to successful treatment is early diagnosis.

The dura or dura mater is the outermost of the three membranes (meninges) covering the brain and spinal cord. It is the toughest and most fibrous of the three membranes. The term *epidural* refers to the area between the dura and the skull, whereas *subdural* refers to the potential space between the dura and the arachnoid (the membrane located between the dura mater and the pia mater). The only actual meningeal compartment within the skull under normal conditions is the subarachnoid space. Of the three types of focal suppurative lesions, brain abscesses (abscesses located within the brain parenchyma) are by far the most common (see Figs. 46-1 and 46-2).

BRAIN ABSCESS

Brain abscesses can be caused by bacteria, fungi, or parasites. Most cases of brain abscess are secondary to infection in some other area(s) of the body; thus, microorganisms involved in the abscess are those causing the underlying or initial infection. Such infections are frequently polymicrobial and often contain anaerobes in addition to other types of bacteria. Examples of the organisms frequently involved in brain abscesses are shown in Tables 46-1 and 46-2.

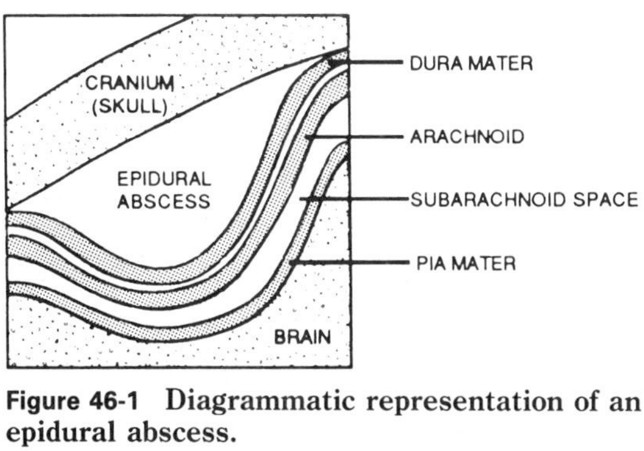

Figure 46-1 Diagrammatic representation of an epidural abscess.

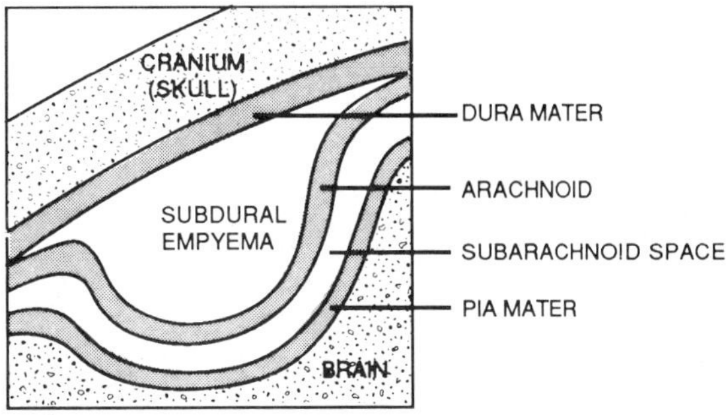

Figure 46-2 Diagrammatic representation of a subdural empyema.

The microorganisms listed in Tables 46-1 and 46-2 may gain access to the brain in any of several ways. They may travel from an original site of infection to the brain by direct extension of the infection (*e.g.*, from the sinuses or middle ear), or by the circulatory system from virtually any body site, most commonly from lung infections such as pneumonia, bronchiectasis, and abscesses, as well as heart infections such as endocarditis. Another method by which microorganisms gain access to the brain is by direct inoculation during or following some type of trauma (*e.g.*, neurosurgical procedure, automobile accident, gunshot wound).[1]

SUBDURAL EMPYEMA AND EPIDURAL ABSCESS

Subdural empyemas and epidural abscesses are focal collections of suppurative material that differ mainly in their anatomic location (see Figs. 46-1 and 46-2). A subdural empyema is located in the potential space between the dura mater and the arachnoid, whereas an epidural abscess is localized between the dura mater and the skull or in the epidural space of the spinal canal. The term *empyema* indicates suppuration in a preformed space.

Table 46-1 *Examples of Bacterial Etiologic Agents of Brain Abscesses*

Underlying Infection or Event	Microorganisms Likely to be Involved
Chronic sinusitis	Anaerobes (*e.g.*, *Bacteroides fragilis*, anaerobic gram-positive cocci) *Hemophilus influenzae* *Staphylococcus aureus* *Streptococcus pneumoniae* Other streptococci Enterobacteriaceae
Ear infection (otitis media)	Anaerobes (*e.g.*, *B. fragilis*, anaerobic gram-positive cocci) Enterobacteriaceae Streptococci
Dental sepsis	Polymicrobic, involving *Fusobacterium* and *Bacteroides* species, anaerobic gram-positive cocci
Lung infection	Streptococci *Fusobacterium* species *Bacteroides* species, occasionally *Nocardia* or *Actinomyces* species
Endocarditis	*S. aureus* Streptococci
Congenital heart problems	Streptococci (including the viridans group) Anaerobic gram-positive cocci *Hemophilus* species
Intraabdominal infection	Enterobacteriaceae Anaerobes
Trauma to head (*e.g.*, skull fracture, bullet wound, neurosurgery)	*S. aureus* Streptococci Enterobacteriaceae *Clostridium* species

Data from reference numbers[1, 4]

The two conditions frequently coexist in the same patient.

Subdural empyemas and epidural abscesses are essentially identical with respect to etiology, epidemiology, and pathophysiology. A variety of bacteria may be associated with these conditions, including streptococci (about 35% of cases of subdural empyema[2]), anaerobic gram-positive cocci, Enterobacteriaceae, *Bacteroides fragilis*, *Staphylococcus aureus* (17% of cases of subdural empyema;[2] 60%–90% of cases of epidural abscess[3]), *Streptococcus pneumoniae*, *Hemophilus influenzae*, and *Pseudomonas aeruginosa*. Anaerobes are isolated in 33% to 100% of cases of subdural em-

Table 46-2 ***Examples of Fungal and Parasitic Etiologic Agents of Brain Abscesses***

Fungi	Parasites
Aspergillus species	*Strongyloides stercoralis*
Mucor species	*Entamoeba histolytica*
Candida species	*Schistosoma japonicum*
Cryptococcus neoformans	*Paragonimus* species
Coccidioides immitis	*Toxoplasma gondii*
Cladosporium trichoides	*Taenia solium* (cysticercosis)
Curvularia species	
Blastomyces dermatitidis	
Histoplasma capsulatum (rarely)	

Data from reference number[1]

pyema.[2] *Mycobacterium tuberculosis* may be a cause of epidural abscess. Polymicrobial infections are quite common in subdural empyema, and occur in approximately 10% of cases of epidural abscess.[3]

As with brain abscesses, the etiologic agents gain access to the area by direct extension, hematogenous spread, or direct inoculation (*e.g.*, head trauma or surgery). Most cases of subdural empyema are secondary to infections involving the paranasal sinuses, middle ear, or mastoid. Epidural abscesses are frequently associated with osteomyelitis in an overlying area of the skull or vertebrae. Spinal epidural abscess may follow a penetrating injury, back surgery, lumbar puncture, or epidural anaesthesia.

Encephalitis

Encephalitis (pl. encephalitides) is defined as inflammation of the brain parenchyma, the cells that make up the functional elements of the brain. Unlike brain abscesses, encephalitis is not confined to a specific site within the brain, and in fact may be quite diffuse. *Meningoencephalitis* refers to inflammation of both the brain and the surrounding meninges; *encephalomyelitis* implies involvement of both the brain and the spinal cord; and *meningoencephalomyelitis* refers to inflammation of the meninges, brain, and spinal cord. Encephalitis may have a sudden onset (acute encephalitis) or there may be a slow, gradual progression of symptoms (chronic encephalitis).

Acute encephalitis may result from either infectious or noninfectious agents. The list of potential infectious agents is lengthy (see Table 46-3), and includes viruses, bacteria, fungi, protozoa, and helminths. Of these agents, arboviruses cause most cases of epidemic encephalitis.[4] Arboviral encephalitides of the United States include eastern and western equine encephalitis, St. Louis encephalitis, and California encephalitis. In each of these diseases, the viruses are transmitted to humans by mosquitoes. The most common sporadic form of fatal encephalitis in North America and Western Europe is that caused by herpes simplex virus type I.[4]

Noninfectious causes of acute encephalitis include vasculitis, neoplasms, toxins, metabolic diseases, and hypersensitivity reactions. Demyelinating processes (destruction of the myelin sheath of nerve cells), probably representing allergic reactions, have occurred following rabies and smallpox vaccinations.

Chronic encephalitides, also called "slow" virus infections, may result from "conventional" viral diseases or may be due to "unconventional" acellular infectious agents called *prions*. The conventional diseases include subacute sclerosing panencephalitis (SSPE; also called inclusion body encephalitis) due to measles virus, progressive multifocal leukoencephalopathy due to a papovavirus, and progressive rubella encephalitis due to a rubella virus. Prions, a name given to certain infectious agents that are smaller than traditional viruses, are thought by some authorities to cause two "slow" virus infections: kuru and Jakob-Creutzfeldt disease.[4]

Certain of the infectious agents gain direct access to the brain tissue via hematogenous spread or through peripheral nerves (*e.g.*, herpes simplex virus, rabies virus). Following their entry, these agents may cause focal or generalized infection.

Table 46-3 ***Potential Infectious Causes of Acute Encephalitis***

Category	Examples
Viruses	Herpes simplex virus, arboviruses, enteroviruses, mumps virus, measles virus, rubella virus, rabies virus, varicella zoster virus, adenoviruses, and many others
Bacteria	*Listeria, Brucella, Mycobacterium tuberculosis, Borrelia,* mycoplasmas, chlamydiae, rickettsiae (Rocky Mt. spotted fever; murine, epidemic, and scrub typhus), spirochetes (*Treponema pallidum, Leptospira*)
Fungi	*Candida, Aspergillus, Cryptococcus, Histoplasma*
Protozoa	*Toxoplasma, Plasmodium, Trypanosoma,* amebae (*Naegleria, Acanthamoeba*)
Helminths	*Taenia solium* (cysticercosis), *Trichinella spiralis,* schistosomes

Data from reference number[4]

Other infectious agents are capable of causing encephalitis without actually invading the brain. For example, demyelination of nerve cells near veins occurs during certain viral infections, such as measles, rubella, chickenpox, and smallpox. The demyelination process is thought to represent a hypersensitivity reaction, possibly being directed against myelin.[5]

The so-called "slow virus" diseases may result from ineffective host responses to the agents, or from protection of the viruses or viral genomes from host responses by their location within host cells. No host response seems to be elicited against the prion agents that cause kuru and Jakob-Creutzfeldt disease. In these latter two diseases, the CNS lesions tend to be spongiform (vacuolation of the brain tissue, resembling a sponge), rather than inflammatory or demyelinating. For this reason, these diseases are sometimes referred to as the subacute spongiform virus encephalopathies.

CLINICAL MANIFESTATIONS

Focal Suppurative Lesions

The signs and symptoms of *brain abscess* are the combined result of increased intracranial pressure and the particular site of brain tissue damage. Generalized or localized headaches occur, and are frequently severe. Other symptoms include nausea, vomiting, changes in mental status, and sometimes coma. Depending on the site of tissue destruction, other symptoms might include seizures and visual disorders. Additional symptoms will relate to the specific underlying infection (*e.g.*, sinusitis, ear infection, endocarditis). It is possible for a brain abscess to rupture into the subarachnoid space, producing a severe meningitis with a high mortality rate (see Chap. 45).

Symptoms of *subdural empyema* and cranial *epidural abscess* include fever and headaches, the latter being initially localized in the area of involvement. Increased intracranial pressure may cause vomiting, papilledema, seizures, focal neurologic dysfunction, and some decrease in mental status. Progression of the disease can lead to extensive neurologic damage, stupor, and coma. Additional symptomatology will relate to the underlying condition, if any, such as chronic sinusitis and mastoiditis. The conditions that need to be distinguished clinically from subdural empyema are cerebral thrombophlebitis, which is a common associated finding, brain abscess, acute hemorrhagic leukoencephalitis, and acute viral (inclusion body) encephalitis.

The most common symptoms of spinal epidural

abscesses are headache, fever, spinal pain and tenderness, progressive weakness of the legs, and urinary retention or incontinence. The differential diagnosis includes transverse myelitis, acute disk herniation, and compression of the spinal cord by tumor.

Encephalitis

The signs and symptoms of encephalitis vary widely, depending on a number of factors; these include the specific causative agent, the host response to the agent, and the area(s) of the brain that are affected. Illness can range from a mild headache and slight fever to an acute devastating disease with rapid progression to coma. Classical acute encephalitis involves sudden onset of fever, headache, stiff neck, and frequently changes in mental status.

Arbovirus infections are generally subclinical, but can develop to clinically overt disease that varies in severity. Herpes simplex infection may result in meningitis, focal encephalitis, mild diffuse encephalitis, or severe diffuse meningoencephalitis. Herpes simplex encephalitis tends to be a much more severe disease than herpes meningitis. Patients usually have headache, fever, and altered levels of consciousness. Seizures, the inability to smell (anosmia), speech defects, and hallucinations may also occur, depending on the area(s) of brain tissue involvement.

LABORATORY ANALYSES AND DIAGNOSIS

Focal Suppurative Lesions

Clinical laboratory techniques are of less value in the diagnosis of *brain abscess* than in meningitis. Routine blood and urine tests are seldom helpful. The collection of cerebrospinal fluid (CSF) is potentially dangerous in patients with brain abscess, increased intracranial pressure, and papilledema (edema of the optic disc). Therefore, lumbar puncture is not routinely done, both because it may precipitate brain herniation and death, and because normal CSF findings do not exclude the diagnosis.

Computer tomographic (CT) scans are of value, not only for diagnosis and providing information about the size and site of the mass, but also for followup of the patient. Radionuclide brain scan or CT scan with contrast enhancement are more than 90% effective in identifying and localizing brain abscesses.[1] Cerebral arteriography may also be required to define the exact location of the lesion.

Should CSF be obtained, it is processed rapidly, in the same manner as described in Chapter 45. The CSF results can be quite variable, ranging from essentially normal to quite abnormal. There may be a mild to moderate increase in pressure; some cells may be present (generally fewer than 200/mm^3; predominantly mononuclear, although polymorphonuclear leukocytes [PMNs] may also be present); protein may be mildly elevated; and glucose may be normal or reduced. Gram stains and CSF cultures are negative, unless the abscess is draining into the CSF in the subarachnoid space. Blood cultures are rarely positive. Hematologic findings may include leukocytosis with some shift to the left, and an elevated sedimentation rate, but such findings are certainly not specific for brain abscess. As in suspected cases of meningitis, the clinical laboratory scientist should correlate and integrate the CSF results, and communicate them to the requesting physician as rapidly as possible. Material obtained from the abscess during surgery should be cultured for organisms likely to be etiologic agents.

SUBDURAL AND EPIDURAL ABSCESS

As with brain abscess, a lumbar puncture is potentially dangerous due to the presence of increased intracranial pressure. A CT scan, carotid arteriography, or angiography can delineate the involved area, and routine skull x-rays may show evidence of sinusitis or mastoiditis when either of these conditions is the predisposing cause. Blood cultures should be performed, although subdural empyema is rarely associated with bacteremia.

When examined, the CSF of a patient with subdural empyema will show increased pressure; cloudiness; an elevated WBC count (50–1000/mm^3) that will include both PMNs and lymphocytes; an elevated protein concentration (75–300 mg/dL) (750–3000 g/L); and a normal glucose concentration.[6] The CSF cultures will be negative, unless the subdural space became infected as a result of extension of bacteria from the CSF or from a brain abscess. The CSF from a patient with an epidural abscess will be under normal pressure, will usually be clear, and may contain 20–100 lymphocytes and PMNs/mm^3, and the protein concentration may be slightly elevated.[6] Cultures of the CSF will be negative.

Encephalitis

Various radiologic and laboratory techniques are required to diagnose encephalitis definitively. Generally, laboratory tests are of less value than are procedures such as CT scans, electroencephalograms (EEGs), and radionuclide (technetium) imaging. Nevertheless, a lumbar puncture should be performed because examination of CSF is an essential diagnostic procedure in encephalitis.[5]

Pressure may be normal or slightly elevated, and the CSF is clear or only slightly turbid. There is usually an increased leukocyte count (<1000/mm^3), with a predominance of mononuclear cells (lymphocytes). In early stages of viral encephalitis, PMNs may be the predominant cell type. In severe cases of herpes simplex or *Naegleria* encephalitis, in which tissue necrosis occurs, red blood cells (>100/mm^3) may be seen in addition to PMNs. It should be noted that, in all other forms of CNS infection, fewer than 100 red blood cells/mm^3 will be observed, except in the event of "bloody" or traumatic spinal taps. Protein concentrations will be slightly to moderately elevated, and glucose concentrations may be normal or reduced (depending on the etiologic agent). CSF glucose concentrations are usually reduced in bacterial infections, and normal in viral infections. The glucose level can be reduced, however, in lymphocytic choriomeningitis virus and mumps virus infections. Glucose levels are also low in tuberculosis, fungal, *Listeria,* and amebic infections. Occasional viral encephalitides will show no CSF abnormalities, thus making the diagnosis more difficult.

Direct examination of the CSF by Gram stain, acid-fast stain, and India ink preparation may provide useful information, as may a wet preparation for amebae and a Giemsa stain for trypanosomes. CSF and biopsy specimens should be cultured for bacteria, mycobacteria, fungi, and viruses. Because the viremia is usually brief, and occurs prior to the onset of neurologic symptoms, viruses are rarely isolated from blood specimens.

Paired (acute and convalescent) serum samples and CSF specimens should be tested for rises in antibody titers. Most cases of epidemic viral encephalitis are diagnosed in this manner. Under normal conditions, the concentration of specific antibodies is about 200 times higher in serum than in CSF. The presence of antibodies to a particular pathogen (*e.g.*, mumps virus, herpes virus, rubella virus, *Treponema pallidum*) in CSF in a concentration as high as or higher than in serum, with CSF protein only moderately elevated, is indicative of CNS infection due to that pathogen.[5] Microbial antigen detection procedures, *e.g.*, for cryptococcal antigen, are often more sensitive than culture techniques.

TREATMENT

Focal Suppurative Lesions

BRAIN ABSCESS

Treatment for brain abscess consists of immediate appropriate antimicrobial therapy (intravenous, high-dose). Craniotomy may be performed to relieve the intracranial pressure and to drain as much infected material as possible.

Prior to receipt of the results of antimicrobial susceptibility testing, empirical therapy may be initiated, based on knowledge of the microorganisms most likely to be involved in the underlying infection and which drugs are capable of penetrating into the CNS. Because brain abscesses are frequently polymicrobic and commonly include anaerobes, a combination of penicillin G and chloramphenicol (or metronidazole) is often used.[1] Nafcillin or methicillin may be used when staphylococci are suspected, or vancomycin if the staphylococcus is known to be methicillin-resistant.[1] Following treatment, the lesion can be monitored by CT scan or radionuclide imaging. In spite of treatment, the mortality from brain abscess is about 15% to 20%.[1] Furthermore, survivors frequently have residual paralysis or other equally severe CNS sequelae.

SUBDURAL AND EPIDURAL ABSCESS
Treatment consists of surgical evacuation of the empyema (drainage of the pus), appropriate antimicrobial therapy, and steroids when intracranial pressure is elevated. *S. aureus* may be suspected in cases that occur following head trauma or surgery. These cases may be treated empirically until antimicrobial susceptibility tests are available. Samples taken at the time of surgery should, of course, be sent to the laboratory for aerobic and anaerobic culture and sensitivity testing.

The overall mortality rate for subdural empyema is approximately 14% to 18%,[2] and survivors have a high incidence of residual brain damage. If epidural abscesses are treated early, very few patients will die and many will have complete recovery. Delayed treatment in patients with spinal epidural abscesses may result in paraplegia.

Encephalitis

Specific antimicrobial therapy will obviously depend on the nature of the etiologic agent. Acyclovir or vidarabine may be used to treat herpes simplex encephalitis.[7] At the present time, there is no specific treatment available for the "slow" virus diseases. Supportive measures for the encephalitides are as described for the meningitides in Chapter 45.

INTRACRANIAL SHUNT INFECTIONS

Intracranial shunts are plastic tubes that are used to drain CSF from the brain for the relief of hydrocephalus (accumulation of CSF within the skull). These shunts are of two general types: ventriculoatrial and ventriculoperitoneal. The first type drains CSF from a cerebral ventricle (cavity) into a cardiac atrium (chamber), whereas the latter type drains the CSF into the peritoneal cavity.

Etiology and Pathophysiology

Infections associated with these shunts are usually due to bacterial skin flora such as coagulase-negative and coagulase-positive staphylococci. Other etiologic agents include Enterobacteriaceae and enterococci. In most cases of intracranial shunt infections, contamination probably occurred at the time of shunt insertion or replacement.

Clinical Manifestations

Approximately 10% to 30% of shunt patients develop meningitis (see Chap. 45).[8] In addition to exhibiting the usual signs and symptoms of meningitis, the patient may present with extracranial symptoms that will relate to the site of CSF drainage. If the lower end of the shunt lies in a cardiac atrium, for example, the patient may show signs of endocarditis. A patient whose CSF is being drained into the peritoneal cavity may develop peritonitis. Fever is a common finding, and, should the shunt be malfunctioning, the patient may show signs of increased intracranial pressure.

Laboratory Analyses and Diagnosis

The most useful diagnostic procedure is a complete examination of the CSF, which is collected either by lumbar puncture or percutaneously through the shunt reservoir. The CSF should be processed, and results reported, as described for meningitis (see Chap. 45). Both blood and CSF should be cultured.

Treatment

Treatment consists of removal of the contaminated shunt in most cases, surgical intervention when necessary, and appropriate antimicrobial therapy. When replaced, the shunt is inserted at a site as far removed as possible from the site of infection.

NEUROLOGIC COMPLICATIONS OF AIDS

Etiology and Pathophysiology

The etiology and general pathophysiology of acquired immunodeficiency syndrome (AIDS) are described in Chapter 53. The etiologic agent, human immunodeficiency virus (HIV), is capable of invading T-lymphocytes, resulting in adverse effects on the immunocompetence of the infected individual.

Computerized tomography (CT) scans of AIDS patients frequently show a shrunken brain, with larger than normal ventricles (the CSF-containing spaces within the brain).[9] Specimens obtained at autopsy reveal damage to both white matter (tracts of nerve fibers covered with sheaths of white myelin) and gray matter and vacuolar myelopathy (a vacuolization of the myelin tracts in the spinal cord).[9] Immunologic staining procedures have revealed the presence of HIV antigen in neurologic tissue, the vast majority (95%) of which is located within multinucleated giant cells derived from macrophages.[9]

Clinical Manifestations

Individuals infected with HIV may present with a variety of clinical manifestations, ranging from asymptomatic infection to severe immunodeficiency and life-threatening secondary infectious diseases or cancers. The Centers for Disease Control (CDC) have described a classification system[10] that places into Group IVB those AIDS patients with neurologic symptoms (*i.e.*, dementia, myelopathy, or peripheral neuropathy) and no concurrent illness or condition that would explain the findings. Dementia is a general mental deterioration, myelopathy is a disturbance or disease of the spinal cord, and peripheral neuropathy is a disorder affecting peripheral nerves.

Although the exact incidence of neurologic problems in AIDS patients is unknown, it has been estimated that as many as 60% will develop dementia.[9] In the early stages of disease, patients complain of forgetfulness, inability to concentrate, mild confusion, and being mentally slow. Later, symptoms may include leg weakness, an unsteady gait, poor coordination, and difficulty in writing, and the patient may become apathetic, withdrawn, agitated, or depressed.[9]

Laboratory Analyses and Diagnosis

Many persons infected with HIV have circulating antibodies to the virus, and serologic procedures for the detection of these anti-HIV antibodies are commercially available. HIV-specific antibodies have also been detected in CSF specimens of AIDS patients, and many of these patients have CSF titers higher than serum titers.[11]

HIV has been isolated from CSF and tissue specimens (*e.g.*, brain, spinal cord, peripheral nerve) of AIDS patients manifesting a variety of neurologic symptoms.[12] The virus has been recovered from patients with acute and chronic meningitis, dementia, subacute encephalitis, vacuolar myelopathy, and peripheral neuropathy.[12]

Taken together, these findings suggest intra-blood–brain-barrier production of HIV-specific antibody, infection by the virus within the blood–brain barrier, and HIV involvement in the neurologic diseases associated with AIDS.[11]

Treatment

Although the treatment of HIV infection remains experimental, some improvement in dementia and other neurologic symptoms has been noted in AIDS patients treated with azidothymidine (AZT).[13] Should quantitative analysis of HIV-specific IgG in CSF become a diagnostic test for HIV infection of neurologic tissue, then modulation of such antibody may become a quantifiable aspect in the evaluation of treatment for HIV-induced neurologic diseases.[11]

CASE STUDY

A 65-year-old man suffering from confusion was brought to the emergency room by his wife. Five days earlier he had complained of headache and malaise and had had a low-grade fever. These symptoms persisted, and the day before presentation his wife noted intermittent confusion. The patient had a long history of recurrent sinusitis, but had received no medicine during the previous month. Physical examination revealed the patient to be stuporous and disoriented, with slight nuchal rigidity. He had a temperature of 39° C, and a pulse rate of 110. Respiration rate and blood pressure were normal, as were the results of the remainder of the general physical examination. Neurologic examination revealed a slight drift of the left arm and leg, hemianopia (loss of vision for one half of the visual field) of the left eye, and a left Babinski sign (abnormal reflex of the toes following stimulation of the sole of the foot; indicative of neurologic impairment).[14]

Questions

1. At this point, what can be determined about the patient?
2. Is a lumbar puncture indicated at this time?
3. Would a laboratory examination of this patient's CSF be apt to be helpful in establishing a diagnosis?
4. What nonlaboratory procedure might be more helpful than CSF examination in establishing a diagnosis?
5. If this patient has a brain abscess, would you expect anaerobic bacteria to be involved? Would clindamycin be a suitable choice of antimicrobial agent?
6. What treatment is necessary in addition to appropriate antimicrobial therapy?

Discussion

1. The patient has presented with signs of a CNS infection as well as focal neurologic signs. The patient is more likely to have a brain abscess or encephalitis than bacterial meningitis.
2. A lumbar puncture would be very risky without additional information concerning this patient's intracranial dynamics. Cerebellar tonsillar herniation may result if cranial pressure is too high at the time of lumbar puncture.
3. CSF examination is not very helpful in cases of brain abscess or encephalitis. In brain abscesses, bacteria are usually localized to the brain substance, rarely gain access to the CSF, and thus are not apt to be isolated from CSF specimens.
4. A CT scan of this patient's brain is indicated, and the results should reveal whether it is safe to perform a lumbar puncture. In this case, a CT scan with contrast revealed a low-density right frontotemporal lesion surrounded by a ring of high density, suggestive of a brain abscess.
5. Anaerobic bacteria are involved in 80% to 85% of brain abscesses. While clindamycin is frequently effective in treating infections caused by anaerobes, it does not cross the blood–brain barrier well enough for treatment of CNS infections.
6. The most likely origin of infection in this patient is his recurrent sinusitis. Therefore, his paranasal sinuses should be drained.

REFERENCES

1. Scheld WM, Winn HR: Brain Abscess. In Mandell GL, Douglas RG, Bennett JE (eds): Principles and Practice of Infectious Diseases, p 585. New York City, John Wiley & Sons, 1985
2. Greenlee JE: Subdural Empyema. In Mandell GL, Douglas RG, Bennett JE (eds): Principles and Practice of Infectious Diseases, p 592. New York City, John Wiley & Sons, 1985
3. Greenlee JE: Epidural Abscess. In Mandell GL, Douglas RG, Bennett JE (eds): Principles and Practice of Infectious Diseases, p 594. New York City, John Wiley & Sons, 1985
4. Austin TW: Infections of the Central Nervous System. In Mandell LA, Ralph ED (eds): Essentials of Infectious Diseases, p 115. Boston, Blackwell Scientific, 1985
5. Griffin DE, Johnson RT: Encephalitis, Myelitis, and

Neuritis. In Mandell GL, Douglas RG, Bennett JE (eds): Principles and Practice of Infectious Diseases, p 579. New York City, John Wiley & Sons, 1985
6. Adams RD, Petersdorf RG: Pyogenic Infections of the Central Nervous System. In Petersdorf RG et al (eds): Harrison's Principles of Internal Medicine, p 2084. New York City, McGraw-Hill, 1983
7. Medical Letter on Drugs and Therapeutics 28:40, 1986
8. McGee ZA, Kaiser AB: Acute Meningitis. In Mandell GL, Douglas RG, Bennett JE (eds): Principles and Practice of Infectious Diseases, p 560. New York City, John Wiley & Sons, 1985
9. Barnes DM: AIDS-related brain damage unexplained. Science 232:1091, 1986
10. MMWR 35:334, 1986
11. Resnick L, DiMarzo-Veronese F, Schüpbach J et al: Intra-blood–brain-barrier synthesis of HTLV-III-specific IgG in patients with neurologic symptoms associated with AIDS and AIDS-related complex. N Engl J Med 313:1498, 1985
12. Ho DD, Rota TR, Schooley RT et al: Isolation of HTLV-III from cerebrospinal fluid and neural tissues of patients with neurologic symptoms related to the acquired immunodeficiency syndrome. N Engl J Med 313:1493, 1985
13. Medical Letter on Drugs and Therapeutics 28:107, 1986
14. Cobb CG, Griffin FM, Avent CK: Infectious Disease Case Studies. New York City, Medical Examination Publishing Company, 1986

Chapter 47

Cerebrovascular Accidents

Kathleen Becan-McBride

A cerebrovascular accident (CVA) is commonly referred to as a *stroke* and involves a disturbance or blockage in cerebral blood circulation. CVA is one of the major causes of death in the United States, and other Western countries have similar stroke incidence rates of approximately 150 to 250 per 100,000 population per year.[1] Because the vascular origin and sudden onset of a CVA are phenomena shared by other neurological disorders, it has been difficult to define stroke clearly. The National Survey of Stroke in the United States has devised the following definition:

Stroke is a clinical syndrome consisting of a constellation of neurological findings, sudden, or rapid in onset, that persists for more than 24 hours, and whose vascular origins are limited to: (a) thrombotic or embolic occlusion of a cerebral artery resulting in infarction, or (b) spontaneous rupture of a vessel resulting in intracerebral or subarachnoid hemorrhage. This definition excludes occlusion or rupture due to traumatic, neoplastic, or infectious processes that produce vascular pathology.[2]

ETIOLOGY

Specific Risk Factors

Risk factors have been identified that distinguish the stroke population from the rest of the community. These predisposing characteristics include hypertension, diabetes, heart disease, positive family history, hyperlipidemia, smoking, certain dietary factors, estrogen therapy, seasonal climate variations, daily variations of activity, obesity, and inactivity.

Hypertension is the most serious risk factor for a stroke.[3] Incidence of CVA increases approximately six-fold in hypertensive persons over incidence in persons of the same age group having normal blood pressure. Persons suffering from diabetes mellitus have been shown by the Framingham study to have a 2.5 (males) to a 3.7 (females) times greater risk of having a stroke.[4] The Framingham study also found that more than 75% of stroke victims have had some form of heart disease. Approximately 30% of stroke victims have coronary artery disease, and 15% have cardiac failure.

In addition, the Framingham study has shown a strong negative relationship between LDL-cholesterol and the risk of stroke in women. For HDL- cholesterol, a negative relationship to stroke incidence has been detected in both sexes. An elevated serum cholesterol level has been found to be a very important factor for myocardial infarction, but the association with stroke of the elevation of this blood lipid has been equivocal.[5]

The Framingham study has also shown that smoking is weakly linked to an increase in the risk of stroke in men. Other studies have agreed with this finding.[4]

A factor definitely associated with an increased risk of stroke is regular ingestion of estrogens. Women taking contraceptive pills are ten times more likely to suffer a stroke than women in the same age group who do not use this contraceptive method.[6] The risk is augmented in women who have coexisting hypertension, are over 35 years of age, suffer from diabetes mellitus, have hyperlipidemia, and/or who have taken contraceptives for a prolonged period of time.

The relationship of obesity to stroke incidence is still questionable; research studies are contradictory in findings. In Japan, one study found a positive correlation between obesity and stroke incidence.[7] In the Framingham study, however, stroke incidence was only moderately related to weight. It has been suggested that positive correlation between obesity and stroke may be the result of the close association between obesity, diabetes mellitus, and hypertension. Thus, the role of obesity alone as a risk factor for stroke has been difficult to ascertain.[5]

Seasonal variation has a definite association with the rate of stroke.[8] Declining temperatures and abundant snowfall have been positively correlated with increased mortality from CVAs. The relationship of daily variations and stroke incidence is not clearly defined at present.[4]

Familial susceptibility to stroke has been demonstrated in several studies. It appears that positive correlation between heredity and stroke incidence is the result of the close association between the family history and hypertension.

Major types of CVA are cerebral hemorrhage, cerebral infarction, and cerebral thrombosis.

Cerebral Hemorrhage

Cerebral hemorrhage into the subarachnoid space accounts for more than 50% of all spontaneous intracranial hemorrhages, and primarily affects individuals between the ages of 20 and 50 years. The most common cause is a ruptured berry (saccular) aneurysm, so called because of deficiencies in the muscle layer of the blood vessel wall (see Fig. 47-1). The reasons for development of saccular aneurysms have not been determined. When one ruptures, blood is spilled into the subarachnoid space. Most commonly, saccular aneurysms remain asymptomatic until they rupture. Three important factors contributing to rupture are ath-

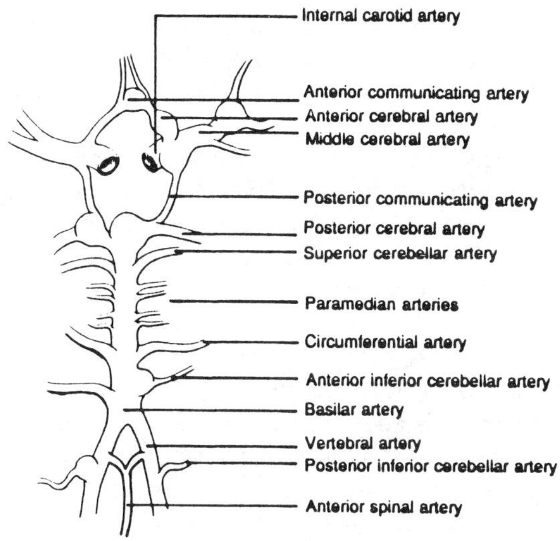

Figure 47-1 Cerebral arteries.

erosclerosis, hypertension, and emotional or physical stress.

Of the patients suffering from a subarachnoid hemorrhage, 70% to 75% die in 1 to 30 days from onset. The most common cause of death is rebleeding, which usually occurs within the first 2 weeks after the initial hemorrhage.

Cerebral Thrombosis

Thrombo-occlusive disease is usually associated with complications of hypertension and atherosclerosis.[9] Cerebral thrombosis is a disease of older persons. The usual age of occurrence is 60 to 69 years. With cerebral thrombosis, the patient may experience warning signs such as confusion, a speech defect, or blindness in one eye before the onset of the CVA. After onset, this type of stroke will lead to progressive damage over a period of several days as a result of extension of the thrombosis. The atherosclerotic lesions creating a blockage in the blood vessels can lead to infarction in older persons due to sudden hypotension or a cardiac arrhythmia that reduces the blood supply to the area.

Cerebral thrombosis, a solid aggregation of clotted blood that forms in circulating blood, can also occur as a result of certain primary blood disorders characterized by an excess of erythrocytes and platelets and/or an overproduction of fibrinogen. These disorders include polycythemia vera and Waldenstrom's macroglobulinemia. However, these are extremely rare causes of CVA.

Cerebral Embolism

Cerebral emboli are caused by clots and/or foreign material carried in the blood vessels and entering the cerebral arterial circulation, which becomes suddenly blocked when the emboli can no longer travel through the cerebral vessels. Many cerebral emboli originate from a thrombus in the heart, and the cerebral disorder is essentially a manifestation of cardiac disease. Other emboli may be derived from atherosclerotic plaques in the arterial system or from artificial heart valves, which are in increasing use. Victims of a cerebral embolism are usually younger than those with thrombosis.

Cerebral Infarction

Cerebral infarction (completed stroke) is a result of a thrombotic or embolic arterial occlusion. This type of stroke accounts for more than 60% of CVAs. It signifies blockage of a cerebral artery with the cessation of blood flow beyond the blockage (occlusion). Vascular occlusions result in death (infarction) of the segment of tissue supplied by that artery. The damaged brain tissue loses function within a short period of time and becomes necrotic within a few days.

Two disorders that frequently cause occlusion of cerebral blood vessels are cerebral thrombosis and cerebral emboli. The true incidence of thrombosis and embolus as the causes of cerebral infarction is not known; published figures are contradictory. It is estimated that one-half of all cerebral infarctions are to cerebral thrombosis and the other half to cerebral emboli.[2]

CLINICAL MANIFESTATIONS

Clinically, cerebral hemorrhage, thrombosis, infarction, and embolism are often indistinguishable, although sudden onset of an excruciating headache, followed by nausea, vomiting, a stiff neck, and then a coma are the typical symptoms of cerebral hemorrhage.

The size and site of the lesion affects the severity of a stroke. The manifestations may include dysphasia or aphasia (impaired language function), hemiplegia (weakness or loss of voluntary movement of the body opposite to the cerebral lesion), and loss of consciousness, which is quite frequent after cerebral hemorrhage and usually results in coma and death. Typical clinical features of stroke are summarized in Table 47-1.

The prognosis for a stroke victim depends on the extent of the damaged neurons and the etiology. Loss of consciousness is associated with an increased mortality.[10] Also, the mortality rates for stroke victims rise with increasing age.[11]

LABORATORY ANALYSES AND DIAGNOSIS

The clinical diagnosis of stroke is determined on the basis of the patient's history and physical examination. The two clinical features of utmost importance in the diagnosis are evidence of a disturbance of neurological function, and suddenness of onset (*e.g.*, between 5 minutes and 5 hours). However, the clinical features of a CVA, including loss of consciousness, confusion, and aphasia, may occur as a result of other disorders (see Table 47-2). For example, in hypoglycemia, the neurological manifestation of a rapid onset of impaired consciousness may occur. Because relatively small doses of oral hypoglycemic agents may produce this manifestation in the geriatric patient, as well as the more commonly encountered response to insulin, a blood glucose determination is essential in establishing the correct diagnosis.

Other disorders that clinical laboratory assays can assist in differentiating from stroke include severe hypothyroidism, drug intoxication, renal failure, hepatic failure, and meningitis. To distinguish possible hypothyroidism from CVA, thyroid function tests such as total T_4, resin T_3 uptake test and a serum TSH (thyroid-stimulating hormone) assay should be performed.[12] A laboratory drug screen is helpful to distinguish drug intoxication from a possible CVA. A complete urinalysis (*i.e.*, macroscopic and microscopic studies) plus blood electrolyte, serum urea, and creatinine determinations are important laboratory assays to differentiate uremia from a stroke. To distinguish hepatic encephalopathy from CVA, a liver panel is recommended that includes serum total bilirubin, serum conjugated bilirubin, serum alkaline phosphatase, aspartate aminotransferase (AST), alanine amino-

Table 47-1 ***Clinical Features of Different Types of Stroke***

	Onset	First Symptom	Outcome
Hemorrhage	Sudden	Headache most often	70%–75% die within a month
Thrombosis	Gradual and variable	Variable, often ill-defined	Ranges from minimal dysfunction to death within a week
Embolism	Sudden	Headache often	Recurrence in majority

Table 47-2 ***Differential Diagnosis for CVA***

Hypothermia	Hypoglycemia
Intracranial neoplasm	Uncontrolled diabetes mellitus
Cerebral abscess	Hypothyroidism
Head trauma	Hepatic failure
Subdural hematoma	Renal failure
Meningitis	
Drug intoxication	

transferase (ALT), albumin, and gamma globulin (see Chap. 33 on hepatic failure). Clinical microbiology culture studies can assist in differentiating between meningitis and a stroke (see Chap. 45 on meningitis).

In addition to these laboratory assays, other diagnostic procedures to diagnose and differentiate the type of CVA include: (a) computerized tomography (CT) scan, (b) arteriography and other investigations of the cerebral vascular system, (c) hematology and coagulation profile, and (d) electrocardiography (ECG) and other cardiac investigations.

Lumbar puncture is recommended only if meningitis or subarachnoid hemorrhage is suspected, due to the hazards and difficulties of performing this procedure on geriatric patients.

TREATMENT

Various factors have an effect on the prognosis of stroke, including the cause and severity of the stroke, the management of the acute phase, and the rehabilitation process. The method of treatment for a stroke varies with the type of CVA identified. If subarachnoid hemorrhaging has occurred or if an extracranial thrombus has formed, neurosurgery might be required. After the acute stage of a stroke, most patients are transferred to a rehabilitation center, where a team of health professionals assess and support the rehabilitation process. Various allied health professionals, including speech therapists, physical therapists, nurses, occupational therapists, and dietitians work with the patient to achieve the maximum possible rehabilitation. Unfortunately, of stroke survivors, one-half remain severely disabled by weakness or paralysis even after extensive rehabilitative therapy.

CASE STUDY

A 44-year-old white man was transported in an ambulance to the hospital by a paramedic team. The paramedics reported that the patient was unconscious upon their arrival at his home, and that the patient's wife had called their emergency number after the man had collapsed on the floor. Approximately an hour prior to his collapse, he had come into the house after mowing the lawn complaining of having an excruciating headache and had vomited.

In the emergency room, the attending physician requested a battery of laboratory tests and a CT scan. Upon review of the scan, an intracranial mass with increased density was identified. The patient was rushed to surgery.

Questions

1. What type of CVA had probably occurred?
2. What are the chances for survival from this type of CVA?
3. What type of clinical laboratory evaluation is helpful in distinguishing this type of CVA from other types?

Discussion

1. From the description of clinical features, the patient most likely suffered from a cerebral hemorrhage into the subarachnoid space.
2. The overall mortality rate for this type of intracerebral hemorrhage is 70% to 75%. However, many patients who survive the acute period may have a complete neurologic recovery.
3. Sometimes, if a subarachnoid hemorrhage is suspected but the CT scan fails to confirm the diagnosis, the presence of blood in an atraumatic lumbar puncture can confirm the presence of a hemorrhagic CVA.

REFERENCES

1. Aho K et al: Cerebrovascular disease in the community: Results of a WHO collaborative study. Bull WHO 58:113–130, 1980
2. Walker A, Robins M, Weinfeld F: Clinical findings in The National Survey of Stroke. Stroke 12 (Suppl 1):13–44, 1981
3. Wolf P, Kannel W: Controllable Risk Factors for Stroke: Preventive Implications of Trends in Stroke Mortality. In Meyer J, Shaw T (eds): Diagnosis and Management of Stroke and TIAs. Reading, Massachusetts, Addison-Wesley, 1982
4. Kannel W, Wolf P: Epidemiology of Cerebrovascular Disease. In Russell R (ed): Vascular Disease of the Central Nervous System. New York, Churchill Livingstone, 1983
5. Kannel W, Gordon T, Dawber T: Role of lipids in the development of brain infarctions: The Framingham Study. Stroke 5:679–685, 1974
6. Masi A, Dogdale M: Cerebrovascular diseases associated with the use of oral contraceptives: A review of the English language literature. Ann Intern Med 72:111–121, 1970
7. Rhoads G, Kagan A: The relation of coronary disease, stroke, and mortality to weight in youth and middle age. Lancet 1:492–495, 1983
8. Haberman S, Capildeo R, Rose F: The seasonal variation in mortality from cerebrovascular disease. J Neurol Sci 52:25–36, 1981
9. Taussig M: Processes in Pathology and Microbiology. London, Blackwell Scientific, 1984
10. Oxbury J, Greenhall R, Grainger K: Predicting the outcome of stroke: Acute stage after cerebral infarction. Brit Med J 3:125, 1975
11. Marguardson J: The natural history of acute cerebrovascular disease. Acta Neurol Scand 45 (Suppl):58, 192, 1969
12. Anderson S: Thyroid Function. In Bishop M, Duben-Von Laufen J, Fody E (eds): Clinical Chemistry: Principles, Procedures, Correlations. Philadelphia, JB Lippincott, 1985

Chapter 48

Seizures

Alexander Von Laufen

There is no single definition of epilepsy that is either universally accepted or completely adequate to describe all the different types of seizure disorders and their various manifestations. From a strict neurological perspective, seizure activity can be considered a sudden and identifiable dysfunction in the central nervous system in which there is an abnormal occurrence of highly synchronized electrical activity in the brain. Although this concept may serve the purposes of a neurological model, it is important to realize that abnormal electrical discharges are not always present in the electroencephalogram of an epileptic. More frequently, abnormal discharges can even be manifest on the exam in the absence of an observable behavioral disturbance.[1] Seizures and epilepsy, therefore, are not completely synonymous. Individuals with epilepsy continue to have recurring seizures throughout their lifetimes, and, most likely, maintain or control the frequency of their seizures with antiseizure medication. An individual seizure, on the other hand, can occur as a result of almost any physiological disease state, and does not necessarily indicate an epileptic disorder with repetitive seizure occurrence.

It is perhaps better to refer to epilepsy on the

basis of its presenting symptomatology rather than as a particular disease state. The current view is to regard the disorder as a potential symptom of almost any medical or psychopathological condition.[2] This alternative viewpoint takes into account not only the neurological process of the seizure itself, but also the psychological and social consequences of such a disorder. Furthermore, certain psychological mechanisms may well be viewed as maintenance factors that sustain or even precipitate an actual seizure.

A recent review suggested that approximately 1% of the U.S. population has been identified with some active form of epilepsy. Here epilepsy is defined as at least two seizures in the absence of an obvious precipitating factor, with at least one seizure occurring within the past 5 years.[3] This would place the estimate of prevalence somewhere between four and six cases per one thousand persons. In a similar survey, the estimate was placed slightly higher, at four million persons.[4] However, these figures are approximate at best, and the actual number of cases is probably one-third greater.[3]

ETIOLOGY AND PATHOPHYSIOLOGY

In order for the central nervous system to function efficiently, there must be highly coordinated activity among the billions of nerve cells in the brain. Nerve cells function by discharging small electrical waves. When neuronal activity becomes disorganized and these cells suddenly produce a burst of electrical activity that is greater than normal, a wave of electricity may be set up in the brain that causes an alteration in neurological function.

This physiological imbalance may cause problems associated with consciousness, sensation, strength, or coordination.[5] During a seizure or epileptic episode, normal brain functioning is upset

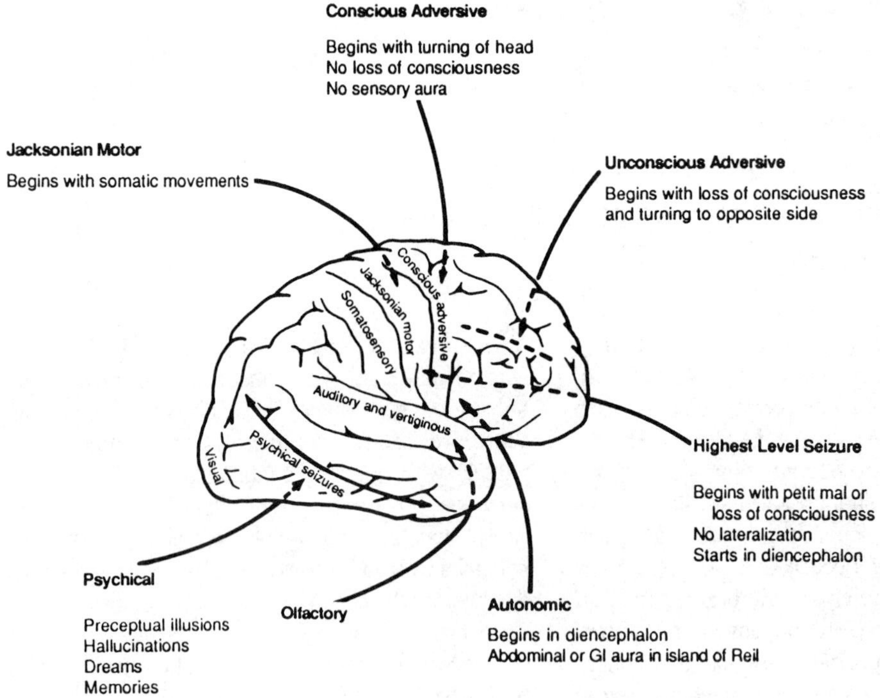

Figure 48-1 **Location and pattern of various nerve cell disturbances. (Reprinted from Review of Neuroscience by Pansky B, Allen DJ. Copyright © 1980 by Macmillan Publishing Co.)**

by focal or generalized disturbances in neuronal activity. The type of impairment that is actually manifested is determined by the location and severity of the nerve cell disturbances (see Fig. 48-1). This accounts for the many different varieties of seizure disorders.[5]

Symptomatic vs Idiopathic Epilepsy

Epilepsy has traditionally been divided into the two etiological categories of symptomatic epilepsy and idiopathic epilepsy,[1] based on the presumed origin of the disorder. "Symptomatic" epilepsy refers to those types of seizure disorders in which there is an identifiable cause associated with the disorder. For instance, certain types of cerebral trauma, brain tumors, encephalitis, or drug toxicity may be attributed as causal agents in the onset of epilepsy. In these conditions, seizures are simply seen as symptoms of another disease state. The term "idiopathic" epilepsy is used to refer to those seizure disorders either that do not have a prescribed cause or for which a cause has not yet been found.

The age of the patient when the seizures first occur can be a very important clue in determining actual etiology (see Fig. 48-2). For example, seizures that begin before the age of 6 months usually reflect some form of injury at birth, a congenital defect of the nervous system, a metabolic error, or an infectious disease process. Seizures that begin between the ages of 2 and 20 years are usually regarded as having a strong genetic component and are most likely idiopathic. Between the ages of 20 and 35, the onset of seizures is relatively rare. If they do occur, they are most likely due to an external cause, such as head trauma, drug abuse, or infection. When seizures begin after the age of 35, vascular diseases or brain tumors are common causes.[1] In general, it is probably accurate to conclude that seizures that have their onset before the age of 20 have primarily genetic origins, whereas seizures that are not manifest until after the age of 20 are probably a result of a more progressive condition. A thorough investigation into the family history of the patient will sometimes be the only reliable source of information available to the clinician.

Neurogenic vs Psychogenic Seizures

Perhaps even more important than the ability to attribute cause to a particular type of seizure is the responsibility of the diagnostician to determine differentially whether the presenting disorder is being precipitated by neurological or psychological factors. Although the presenting symptomatology may be quite similar, the two groups of disorders not only have different causes, but also respond in

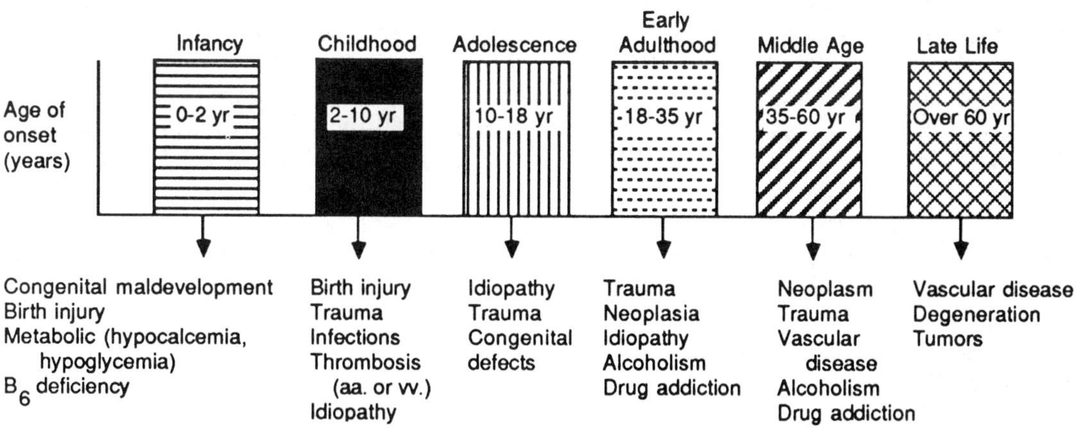

Figure 48-2 **Etiology of seizures at different age levels. (Reprinted from Review of Neuroscience by Pansky B, Allen DJ. Copyright © 1980 by Macmillan Publishing Co.)**

a different manner to various treatment modalities. It would be of little use, from a therapeutic standpoint, to treat a true psychogenic seizure with anticonvulsant medication, because the seizure disorder is not of neurological origin but is produced psychologically. In most instances, however, the clinician is not likely to be confronted with "pure" cases, but will encounter situations that display elements of both origins.

Functional Anatomy of Epilepsy (Seizure Elements)

The actual episode of a seizure can be broken down into various stages that follow a cyclical pattern. It may not be possible, however, to define these individual stages for every seizure.[6] During the buildup stage, if one should occur, certain areas in the brain begin to lose their efficient functioning as electrical disturbances begin to interfere with normal brain activities. There may be a very subtle change in the mood, the behavior, or the thinking of the individual, with nothing more than a subjective feeling of increased anxiety, depression, or simply inability to concentrate. If this brain activity is not brought under control, the electrical energy increases, becomes stronger, and spreads. The individual now begins to experience some disturbance of function or an identifiable aura of what is about to occur. If the discharge is localized to a certain area in the brain, the symptoms may be limited to a specific part of the body, such as the hand or the eye. This is called a *focal* or *partial seizure*. If the abnormal activity should begin to spread to other areas of the brain, more complex and dramatic symptoms become manifest. This is what is typically viewed as a *generalized seizure*. The obvious attack or seizure itself is referred to as the *ictus*. When the brain finally regains control over the abnormal discharging that has taken place, the nervous system is out of balance.[7] The brain, in an effort to maintain homeostasis, attempts to reestablish its previous balance. As it begins this task, there may be a period of time, called the *postictal phase*, in which there is a slowing of the usual brain functions, such as alertness, memory, concentration, or thinking. As the brain gains more control, normal functioning in the individual becomes more apparent and there is a gradual return to a normal state of alertness.

The distinction between partial and generalized seizures forms the basis of the International Classification of Epileptic Seizures, seen in Table 48-1.[8]

CLINICAL MANIFESTATIONS

Partial Seizures

Partial seizures are classified into three groups, depending upon the symptomatology presented: (1) simple partial seizure; (2) complex partial seizures; and (3) simple or complex seizures that evolve into generalized seizures (see Table 48-1).

Partial seizures with elementary symptomatology have a localized area of focus that results in specific characteristics. There is generally no impairment of consciousness. If the seizure begins in the frontal, parietal, or occipital lobes of the brain, the initial signs or symptoms will be focal ones of movement or sensation. This may involve an arm or leg jerking. If the seizure arises in the sensorimotor area adjacent to the central sulcus, symptoms of movement or sensation appear in one part of the body (usually the peripheral part) and generalize to larger areas. This type of seizure is called *Jacksonian* (after the man who first described them), and the symptoms can actually be observed as they begin in the fingers and progressively move up to involve the entire arm. Seizures that originate in the parietal area start with a sensation described as a breeze blowing on the skin or a light tingling or numbness. This is what is meant by an aura that precedes the actual attack. Seizures in the precentral region begin with a rhythmical twitching of the face, arm, or leg. Onset of seizures in the premotor area produces such contraversive movements as turning of the head or turning of the entire body. Seizures that originate in the occipital lobe begin with visual sensations, such as flashing colored lights (see Fig. 48-1).

Table 48-1 ***International Classification of Epileptic Seizures***

I. Partial seizures (seizures beginning locally)
   A. Partial seizures with elementary symptoms (without impairment of consciousness)
      1. Motor symptoms (includes Jacksonian seizures)
      2. Special sensory or somatosensory symptoms
      3. Autonomic symptoms (rare)
      4. Compound forms (elementary and/or complex symptoms)
   B. Partial seizures with complex symptoms (with impairment of consciousness) (temporal lobe or psychomotor seizures)
      1. Impairment of consciousness only
      2. Cognitive symptomatology
      3. Affective symptomatology
      4. "Psychosensory" symptomatology (hallucinations)
      5. "Psychomotor" symptomatology (automatisms)
      6. Compound forms
   C. Partial seizures secondarily realized: tonic–clonic seizures developing from a partial seizure
II. Generalized seizures (bilaterally symmetrical and without local onset)
   A. Absences (petit mal)
   B. Bilateral massive epileptic myoclonus
   C. Infantile spasms
   D. Clonic seizures
   E. Tonic seizures
   F. Tonic–clonic seizures (grand mal)
   G. Atonic seizures (loss of tone)
   H. Akinetic seizures (loss of movement)
III. Unilateral seizures (predominantly): seizures with clinical features restricted to one side of the body
IV. Unclassified epileptic seizures (due to lack of reliable information)

*Data based on reference number[8]

Partial seizures with complex symptomatology have their origin in the temporal lobe and involve more mixed symptomatology related to more complicated thoughts and actions, in contrast to the elementary movements and sensations of the focal seizures. The onset of a temporal lobe or psychomotor seizure can occur with or without an impairment in consciousness, and can involve any or all of the features described for simple partial seizures. In a more complicated fashion, temporal lobe seizures are usually characterized by changes in subjective experience. These can be very idiosyncratic types of sensations, such as a peculiar taste in the mouth, a visual hallucination of a person or scene, or an overwhelming feeling of familiarity with a place or an event (*déjà vu*). There may be the experience of strangeness, which involves the perception that objects are getting larger or smaller, or are approaching closer or receding into the background. There may also be the experience of overwhelming anxiety or fear, or perhaps the inability to comprehend what is being said or to express oneself.[9, 10]

One of the more interesting aspects of temporal lobe seizure activity is the automatic behavior that can occur. Automatisms may be preceded by a brief loss of consciousness or simply by a subjective sensation. The automatism begins with a brief arrest of activity, sometimes with increased chewing or swallowing present. There are frequently repetitive and stereotyped movements, like a continual scratching of the head or picking at one's clothes. Automatic types of behavior can vary from simple, uncoordinated movements all the way to complex activities. What is so unusual about this form of behavior, however, is that the individual is unaware of surroundings while performing the automatic behavior over and over again. Violent behavior during these episodes is very rare, but attempts at restraining the automatic behavior may be met with an aggressive reaction.[3, 11]

Partial seizures secondarily realized are seizures that begin in the simple phase and progress to generalized tonic–clonic seizures. They can also originate as complex seizures and evolve into a more generalized stage, or they can involve both processes, with an onset as a simple, partial seizure that evolves into a complex one and continues to develop into generalized tonic–clonic seizures.

Generalized Seizures

The second group of seizure disorders involves generalized seizures in which the electrical overactivity in the brain is no longer focused but is more diffuse. Several different types of generalized seizures have been identified.

Absence seizures or *petit mal epilepsy* is a disorder characterized by a brief loss of awareness during which there is no motor activity other than a blinking or a rolling up of the eyes. An attack of this nature may be very brief, usually lasting less than 10 seconds, but may proceed for several minutes. Patients do not fall to the ground, and there is a rapid return to full consciousness without retrograde amnesia or confusion, although there is no awareness of what took place during the attack. Petit mal epilepsy is typically found in children between the ages of 2 and 15 years, and is rarely seen in anyone over this age.[1, 3]

Myoclonic seizures are characterized by brief, repetitive jerking of the arms and trunk. Typically, the arms flex and the trunk jerks forward. The jerks are so quick that a lapse of consciousness is not evident; however, the jerks can become so rapid and repetitive that they begin to fuse into a generalized clonic seizure.[3] Myoclonic jerking sometimes occurs in nonepileptic individuals, and may be experienced just before falling asleep when in a relaxed state.

Tonic–clonic seizures or *grand mal epilepsy* is primarily generalized from the onset. There is a total loss of consciousness and stereotyped motor activity.[1] About 50% of grand mal patients have little or no warning that a tonic–clonic attack is imminent. In the initial tonic phase, the body suddenly becomes rigid, the extremities extend, and breathing stops. This is followed by a clonic phase characterized by a rhythmical jerking of the extremities and trunk. Gradually the jerking motions slow down, and they stop altogether after 2 to 10 minutes. The patient begins to regain consciousness, but may remain confused and drowsy for several minutes up to a day or two. This is the postictal depression or interictal phase referred to previously.

Akinetic seizures occur in children between the ages of 1 and 7 years, and are characterized by a sudden loss of their antigravity muscles.[1] The child simply falls to the ground without any warning. This kind of attack is usually very brief, and after a few seconds the child may get up without any postictal depression. Many authors believe that seizures of this type are not actually akinetic but rather are myoclonic, because they result from a severe flexion of the neck and hips. Although the onset is quick and the actual duration of the attack lasts only a few seconds, most of these cases are associated with brain damage, and children do not usually develop normal intellectual functioning.

Infantile spasms, which always begin before the age of 2 years, are actually massive myoclonic spasms in which there is a sudden flexion or extension of the body. Seizures of this type often go unrecognized in infancy because they are of such short duration, and are frequently mistaken for a startle reaction. Infantile spasms generally resolve as the child grows older, or they may evolve into other clinical seizures. Because this type of epilepsy results in a profound disruption of the central nervous system and occurs at such a young age, it can be expected to be associated with fairly severe forms of mental retardation.

DIAGNOSTIC EVALUATION

Although the epilepsies lend themselves to this method of classification, and their behavioral manifestations can be described on the basis of symptomatology, only about one out of four patients with an active form of epilepsy is diagnosed without any associated disabilities.[3] This suggests that the majority of patients who seek medical care for their seizures also have other disabilities, such as neurological deficits, cognitive impairment, or behavioral and adjustment problems. Patient evaluation is, therefore, of the utmost importance, not only to differentiate between a true and a pseudo- seizure disorder, but also to determine the etiology and nature of the disorder as a basis for treatment. Good diagnostic evaluation should include the following considerations: the tests that are required based on the clinical presentation of the patient, the meaning of their results, and what management might prove most useful.

The actual type of seizure itself frequently suggests the possible cause and consequently the most appropriate method of study. For instance, focal seizures are often caused by focal brain irritations.[7] Clinical studies are, therefore, more likely to include tests that will identify those structural changes in the areas of the brain under consideration, *e.g.*, electroencephalogram (EEG) or computed tomography (CT) scan of the brain. Because generalized seizures are more apt to be caused by problems affecting the entire brain, *e.g.*, chemical abnormalities, infections, or poisons, blood and chemical analyses as well as spinal fluid studies should be pursued.[7] The evaluation procedure typically advances along the lines of a decision tree much like the one presented in Figure 48-3.

Preliminary evaluation of a seizure disorder

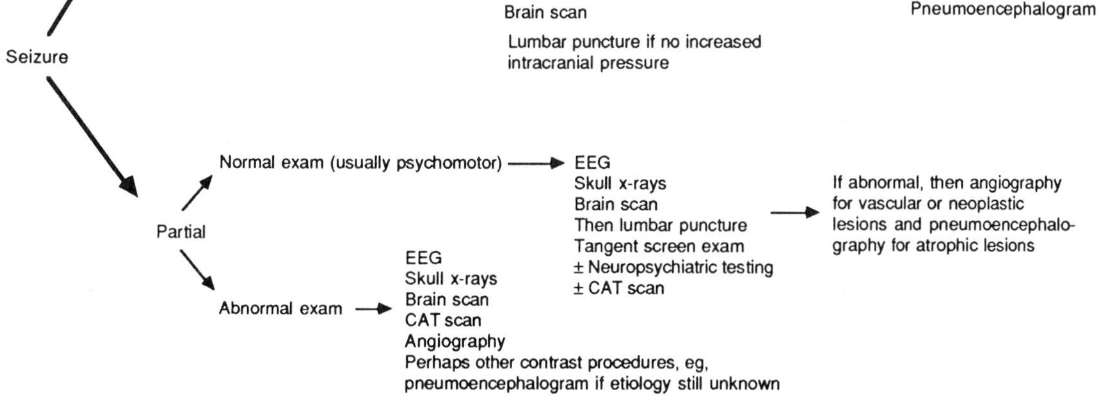

Figure 48-3 Diagnostic evaluation of seizures.

usually includes routine blood and urine tests, and sometimes an analysis of the cerebrospinal fluid, all performed by the clinical laboratory scientist. A neurological examination, electrophysiological studies, a CT scan of the brain, and comprehensive neuropsychological testing can also be beneficial, but these generally require the assistance of other health care professionals (see Table 48-2).

There are no clinical laboratory tests that specifically indicate a diagnosis of seizure or epilepsy. Laboratory analysis is generally limited to the monitoring of anticonvulsant drugs in the blood of the patient. The laboratory scientist does, however, perform a number of other analyses that aid the physician in ruling out a diagnosis of epilepsy, and in differentiating between seizures that are a result of a particular disease or illness and those resulting from a primary neurological disorder. A complete blood count (CBC), blood chemistries, and urinalysis are all generally within the expected normal range, unless associated with an underlying disease state. Analyses of the cerebrospinal fluid for glucose, total proteins, immunoglobulin G, and lactic acid all result in normal laboratory findings in epilepsy.[12]

TREATMENT OF ONGOING SEIZURE DISORDERS

Most of the many types of seizures can be managed effectively and treated successfully with anticonvulsant drugs. Alternative types of treatment, such as dietary manipulation, biofeedback, psychosurgery, or less conventional techniques should only be implemented when a drug regimen is clearly proved unbeneficial.[5] Anticonvulsant medication, however, should be kept as simple as possible. The goal is to reduce the frequency of ocurrence and eventually abolish the seizures themselves, with the least amount of and safest drugs possible.[13] Generally, one anticonvulsant is begun at a time, and the dosage gradually increased, with serum blood levels periodically checked, before a second medication is added. The particular medication that is first instituted depends on several contributing factors. The age of

Table 48-2 ***Diagnostic Tests in the Evaluation of a Seizure Disorder***

Basic Diagnostic Tests	
Hematologic studies	Complete blood count
Urine studies	Urinalysis
Biochemical studies	Serum calcium and phosphorus; fasting blood sugar
Serology	Studies to exclude TB, syphilis
Electrophysiological studies	EEG
Radiological studies	Skull x-ray, computed tomography (CT) scan of the brain
Psychological studies	Psychological, psychometric testing
Additional Studies in Select Cases	
Biochemical studies	5-hour glucose tolerance test, amino acid screen
Genetic studies	Chromosomal analysis
CSF examination	Infections of the nervous system
Electrophysiological studies	Special EEG activation procedures (sleep, telemetry, chemical)
Neuropsychological studies	Psycholinguistic evaluation for learning problems
Special Studies	
Electrophysiological studies	24-hour video and EEG monitoring, brain surface and depth EEGs
Radiological studies	Angiogram or air study

the patient, the particular type and severity of the seizure disorder, past medical history, and the patient's prior experience with anticonvulsant drugs all influence the physician's decision about what medication to use. If the first drug fails, other drugs should be tried one at a time until all reasonable choices have been selectively exhausted.[5] If one drug cannot control the occurrence of a seizure, then perhaps two or more anticonvulsant drugs in combination can prove beneficial.

Clinical research over the last several years has established certain medications as the drugs of choice for each presenting seizure type (see Table 48-3). The drug having the fewest adverse effects and the greatest efficacy is usually the one that is prescribed.[5] Most clinicians agree that phenytoin sodium (Dilantin) is still the most effective and safest drug available for treating generalized tonic–clonic seizures. Carbamazepine (Tegretol) is the first choice of many physicians for complex partial seizures. Primidone (Mysoline) can be considered a valuable alternative to carbamazepine if that drug fails to control this type of seizure activity.[5] Generalized absence seizures are probably best managed with ethosuximide and sodium valproate. Focal motor and focal sensory seizures respond best to phenytoin. An important advancement in the management of epilepsy was the introduction of certain techniques for measuring serum anticonvulsant levels. Evidence has now accumulated in the field demonstrating that the anticonvulsant properties and occurrence of potential neurotoxic side-effects of specific drugs are better correlated to the concentration of the drug in the serum, rather than to the dosage.[14] From research in this area, the concept of the therapeutic drug range has emerged—that is, the range of serum levels within which maximum seizure control can be expected with the minimum incidence of side-effects.[14]

Serum concentrations of all drugs used as anticonvulsants can be measured periodically by commonly available blood tests (see Table 48-4). The dosage required by a particular patient with seizures in order to maintain a therapeutic drug level in the serum can be measured precisely by periodic checking of the serum level. The frequency of how often the drug is checked depends on the rate at which the drug is metabolized in the body. The best time to check a serum drug level is usually at the end of the dose level, *i.e.*, just before the patient is about to take another dose of the drug.[5] (See also Chap. 71).

CASE STUDY

A 27-year-old woman came to the attention of a referring psychiatrist, who diagnosed her symptoms as "free-floating" anxiety and prescribed Librium. Her background had been extremely traumatic, with mentally-ill parents and institutionalization at an early age.

Psychodiagnostic assessment identified anxiety and depression, but also a marked perceptual confusion that required further differential diagnosis. Her past medical history was also significant, involving two head injuries, at ages 5 and 11. Both injuries had resulted in a loss of consciousness. She developed severe headaches that were described as frequent and becoming worse. She also experienced blackout spells, dizziness, nausea, blurring of vision, tingling in her fingers, an altered state of consciousness, and a prescient feeling that something terrible was going to happen to her. On one occasion, she suddenly and inexplicably struck out and hit a companion she was with.

The referring psychiatrist rejected the "psychological" findings and decided to obtain a neurological consultation. A second psychiatric opinion concluded that "the clinical picture is that of emotional instability that is probably secondary to her cerebral dysfunction and probably secondary to familial dysfunction."

Questions

1. Are the presenting symptoms "neurological" or "psychological" in nature? Is this diagnosis ac-

Table 48-3 ***Common Drugs Used In the Treatment and Management of Seizures***

Generic Name	Trade Name	Total Daily Dose (per kg body weight)	Partial (Elementary)	Partial (Complex)	Major Motor	Petit Mal	Myoclonic	Infantile Spasms
Diphenylhydantoin	Dilantin	4–7 mg	+	+	+			
Phenobarbital	Luminal	1–5 mg	As added to DPH	+	+			
Primidone	Mysoline	10–25 mg	+	+	+			
Carbamazepine	Tegretol	7–15 mg	+	+	+			
Ethosuximide	Zarontin	20–30 mg				+		
Trimethadione	Tridione	10–25 mg				+		
Paramethadione	Paradione	10–25 mg				+		
Mephenytoin	Mesantoin	7–12 mg	+	+	+			
Ethotion	Peganone	10–20 mg	+	+	+			
Metharbital	Gemonil	2.5–10 mg	+		+			
Mephobarbital	Mebaral	2.5–10 mg	+		+			
Methsuximide	Celontin	10–20 mg				+		
Phenacemide	Phenurone	25–45 mg		+				
Acetazolamide	Diamox	5–15 mg	+			+ and premenstrual		
ACTH		40–60 units total per day						+
Corticosteroids		5–60 mg total per day						+
Diazepam	Valium	0.15–2 mg				+ and status		
Chlordiazepoxide	Librium	1–4 mg			Alcohol withdrawl			
Paraldehyde		0.3–0.7 ml			Alcohol withdrawl			
Dextroamphetamine	Dexedrine	0.2–0.3 mg		Tonic seizures				
Methylphenidate	Ritalin	0.2–0.3 mg		Tonic seizures				
Clonazepam	Clonapin	0.1–0.2 mg				+	+	

Table 48-4 ***Therapeutic Serum Levels of Common Anticonvulsant Drugs***

Drug	Serum Levels (μg drug/mL serum)	Starting Dose (mg)	Daily Dose
Phenytoin	10–20	900	300–400
Carbamazepine	6–10	100–200	600–1,200
Valproic acid	50–100	250	1,000–3,000
Ethosuximide	50–100	250	750–2,000
Primidone	6–12	50–125	750–1,500
Phenobarbital	15–35	30–60	100–150
Clonazepam	0.013–0.072	0.5	1–2

curate, given the patient's medical and social history?

2. How might the psychiatrist treat the patient's various symptoms?

Discussion

1. Anxiety, depression, and emotional or behavioral disorders can frequently imitate (and often be mistaken for) an underlying neurological process. The course that actually occurs in an individual largely depends on the preexisting personality of the patient, the functional area of the brain in which the physiological imbalance occurs, and the speed at which the excitation spreads in the brain tissue. The actual diagnosis of this somewhat complicated case lies somewhere between a strictly neurological and a psychological explanation. Elements of both neurology and psychological reactions to that dysfunctioning come into play. It would be extremely difficult and nearly impossible to treat the "psychological" symptoms if the underlying neurological conditions were not first addressed. This "working" assumption is certainly a viable one, but it is also too obvious and, as a diagnosis, would also lend itself to very difficult treatment. An alternative diagnosis of post-traumatic seizures could explain some of the manifest symptomatology. However, the severity of the patient's developmental history should not be overlooked.

2. In this particular case, the patient was started on a therapeutic regime of anticonvulsant medication (Dilantin) and quickly responded with improvement in nearly all her symptoms.

   Not long afterwards, however, she returned to the clinic with continued complaints of increasing depression, irritability, restlessness, intellectual slowing, and relatively unstable mood swings. A blood sample was drawn as a routine procedure, and the serum level of Dilantin was subsequently checked. The anticonvulsant medication she was taking was found to be outside the therapeutic range of values and possibly causing toxic side-effects. Her medication was reduced, and her blood level was systematically monitored over the next several months. Her complaints gradually decreased, and her social worker reported greatly improved feelings with initial prospects for employment. The patient had to be maintained on the Dilantin with occasional returns to the clinic in order to monitor the drug's effectiveness, but she returned to a normal and active life.

   Although there is no conclusive proof that the patient's symptoms were directly related to seizure activity, her problems seemed to respond quickly to an appropriate level of anticonvulsant medication. The important thing to note is that the drug of choice has to be monitored periodically (usually every 2 to 3 months), and can easily cause negative side-effects if not properly adjusted.

REFERENCES

1. Pincus JH, Tucker GJ: Behavioral Neurology, 3rd ed, pp 3–69. New York City, Oxford University Press, 1985
2. Task Force on Nomenclature and Statistics of the American Psychiatric Association: Diagnostic and Statistical Manual of Mental Disorders (revised); 3rd ed. Washington, DC, American Psychiatric Association, 1987
3. Masland RL: The Nature of Epilepsy. In Sands H (ed): Epilepsy: A Handbook for the Mental Health Professional, pp 5–57. New York City, Bruner/Mazel, 1982
4. Strudler LA, Perlman LG (eds): Basic Statistics on the Epilepsies. Philadelphia, FA Davis, 1975
5. Lechtenberg R: The Diagnosis and Treatment of Epilepsy. New York City, Macmillan, 1985
6. Weisberg LA, Strub RL, Garcia CA: Essentials of Clinical Neurology, pp 167–194. Baltimore, University Park Press, 1983
7. Svoboda WB: Learning About Epilepsy. Baltimore, University Park Press, 1979
8. Gastaut H: Classification of the epilepsies: Proposal for an international classification. Epilepsia 10 (Suppl): 2–19, 1969
9. Blumer D: Temporal Lobe Epilepsy and its Psychiatric Significance. In Benson DF, Blumer D (eds): Psychiatric Aspects of Neurological Disease, Vol 1. pp 171–198. New York City, Grune & Stratton, 1975
10. Blumer D, Benson DF: Psychiatric Manifestations of Epilepsy. In Benson DF, Blumer D (eds): Psychiatric Aspects of Neurological Disease, Vol 2, pp 25–48. New York City, Grune & Stratton, 1982
11. Berman SA, Rosenfield DB: Neurobehavior and Temporal Lobe Epilepsy. In Fann WE et al (eds): Phenomenology and Treatment of Psychophysiological Disorders, pp 157–177. New York City, Spectrum Publications, 1982
12. Berner JJ: Effects of Diseases on Laboratory Tests, pp 207–208. Philadelphia, JB Lippincott, 1983
13. Wells CE, Duncan GW: Neurology for Psychiatrists, pp 115–132. Philadelphia, FA Davis, 1980
14. Grant I, Adams KM: Neuropsychological Assessment of Neuropsychiatric Disorders, pp 321–346. New York City, Oxford University Press, 1986

BIBLIOGRAPHY

Bannister R: Brain's Clinical Neurology, 6th ed, pp 186–211. London, Oxford University Press, 1985

Glaser GH: Epilepsy: Neuropsychological Aspects. In Reiser MF (ed): American Handbook of Psychiatry: Organic Disorders and Psychosomatic Medicine, 2nd ed, pp 314–355. New York City, Basic Books, 1975

Heilman KM, Watson RT, Greer M: Handbook for Differential Diagnosis of Neurologic Signs and Symptoms, pp 3–16. New York City, Appleton-Century-Crofts, 1977

Kaufman DM: Clinical Neurology for Psychiatrists, 2nd ed, pp 172–203. New York City, Grune & Stratton, 1985

Kirkpatrick B, Hall RCW: Seizure Disorders. In Hall RCW (ed): Psychiatric Presentations of Medical Illness: Somatopsychic Disorders, pp 243–258. New York City, Spectrum Publications, 1980

Lechtenberg R: The Psychiatrist's Guide to Diseases of the Nervous System, pp 76–105. New York City, John Wiley & Sons, 1982

Pansky B, Allen DJ: Review of Neuroscience, pp 488–495. New York City, Macmillan, 1980

Solomon G, Plum F: Clinical Management of Seizures. Philadelphia, WB Saunders, 1976

Strub RL, Black FW: Organic Brain Syndromes: An Introduction to Neurobehavioral Disorders, pp 335–368. Philadelphia, FA Davis, 1981

Wiederholt WC: Neurology for Non-Neurologists, pp 283–298. New York City, Academic Press, 1982

Williams DT: The Treatment of Seizures. In Sands H (ed): Epilepsy: A Handbook For The Mental Health Professional, pp 58–74. New York City, Bruner/Mazel, 1982

Chapter 49

Behavioral Disorders

Kathleen Becan-McBride

No precise definition of mental health exists. Thus, whether an individual is able to function normally in society is a matter of experienced evaluation. The severity of a behavior disorder is related to the extent to which the symptoms of the disorder interfere with the person's ability to function in society, and the degree to which the symptoms disturb others in society. Behavior disorders are usually distinct from diseases of the nervous system, in that most of them manifest themselves as behavioral changes rather than as neural motor (*e.g.*, paralysis) or sensory changes.[1]

ETIOLOGY

The origin of behavioral disorders may be either organic or functional, as is shown in Figure 49-1. These disorders are manifested by a wide array of symptoms, behavior changes, and subjective feelings, that generally are not specifically pathologic when considered in isolation. To differentiate between organic and functional behavior disorders, structural disease of the brain or metabolic disturbances (*e.g.*, hormonal imbalance) must be identified to attribute the illness to an organic cause. Because the symptoms are usually nonspecific and many behavior disorders are associated with physical illness as well as organic brain syndromes, clinical laboratory testing and a complete physical examination are necessary in the overall psychiatric evaluation.[2]

The classification of behavioral disorders is based on several parameters, including ability to correctly interpret reality, presence or absence of

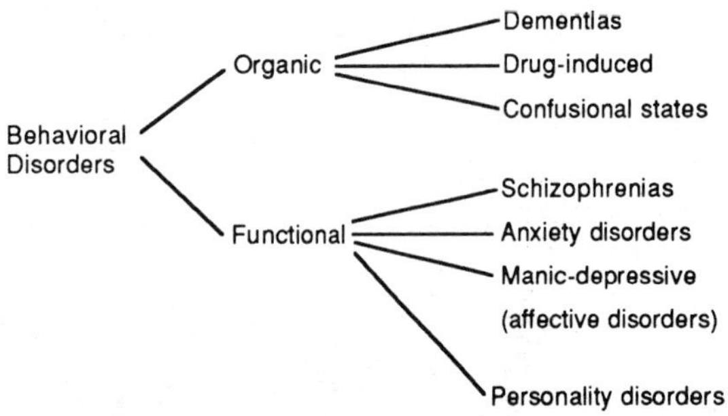

Figure 49-1 Major behavioral disorders.

Common Causes of Acute Organic Brain Syndrome

Intoxication—
- Drugs
- Chemicals
- Pollutants

Vitamin deficiency—Lack of
- B_1, B_6, B_{12}, niacin, folate

Metabolic disorder—
- Diabetes mellitus
- Renal failure
- Thyroid disease

Cardiovascular disorder—
- Occlusion
- Hemorrhage
- Hypertension

Drug withdrawal—
- Alcohol
- Barbiturates
- Narcotics

Neoplasm—Metastatic lesion of the central nervous system

Degenerative disease—Multiple sclerosis

Trauma—
- Concussion
- Contusion
- Hematoma

Postoperative complications—
- Anesthesia
- Blood loss
- Electrolyte imbalance

Infections

brain lesion, intelligence testing, personality assessment inventories, and duration of the condition.[3]

Organic Mental Disorders

Organic mental disorders involve mental disturbance due to a structural disease of the brain or metabolic alterations of the brain due to toxins, hormonal imbalance, or drugs.

ACUTE ORGANIC BRAIN SYNDROME

Acute organic brain syndrome is associated with a large number of acute biologic disorders that affect normal brain functioning. Some of the common causes are listed opposite. Acute organic mental disorders are usually manifested by delirium and intoxication. The treatment of choice for an acute organic mental illness is correction of the underlying medical or neurological condition. Clinical laboratory studies that are helpful in the diagnosis of an organic condition include a complete blood count (CBC), urinalysis, a chemistry profile, RPR, and a toxicology screen. Psychological testing is normally not of assistance in establishing the etiology of an acute organic mental illness, but can provide information regarding the form of illness.

CHRONIC ORGANIC BRAIN SYNDROME

Dementia, loss of recent memory, personality changes, and sometimes depression and hallucinations are the clinical, psychological, and behavioral manifestations associated with chronic organic brain syndrome. Chronic syndromes generally have a poorer prognosis than acute organic mental disorders. The most common type of chronic organic brain syndrome is senile dementia. In this condition, there is diffuse atrophy of the brain with loss of neurons.[4] Alzheimer's disease, Pick's disease, and Huntington's chorea are three conditions classified under chronic organic brain syndromes (see Chap. 44).

Functional Disorders

Functional mental illness is usually separable from organic mental disorders on the basis of a neurologic examination, clinical laboratory results, a mental status examination, and other special procedures.

SCHIZOPHRENIA

Schizophrenia is a functional disorder that is the most common form of psychosis. It affects approximately 1% of the adult population, and has no known biological etiology.[5] Most schizophrenic patients are under the age of 35 at the time of diagnosis. Schizophrenia is primarily manifested by bizarre or illogical thoughts, and is associated with other characteristics that include shyness, seclusiveness, oversensitivity, avoidance of close or competitive relationships, and perceptual distortions (illusions and hallucinations). The cause of schizophrenia is unknown, although genetic influences and environmental influences have been suggested as factors in the development of this behavioral disorder.[6]

There is no exact diagnostic scheme for the diagnosis of schizophrenia. The diagnosis is based on the clinical evaluation of the symptoms and duration of functional psychosis. Physical findings and clinical laboratory testing are of limited value. Although numerous biochemical abnormalities have been demonstrated in schizophrenic patients, none of them has been confirmed as the cause of the disorder.

Most patients with schizophrenia require long-term psychological treatment and maintenance on neuroleptic agents (tranquilizers).[7]

AFFECTIVE DISORDERS

One group of behavioral syndromes is called *affective disorders* because "alteration of mood" is the characteristic finding. *Mania* is a hyperactive, euphoric behavioral disorder that occurs in approximately 0.1% of the population.[8] It occurs more frequently in women than in men. Clinically, the manic syndrome includes motor hyperactivity, a euphoric, expansive, or irritable mood, rapid speech with flight of ideas, decreased need for sleep, and distractibility.[9] Lithium salts have antimanic properties. Lithium carbonate is presently the drug of choice in the treatment of acute manic episodes.[10]

Another affective syndrome is *depression*, which constitutes a sad or melancholy state with decreased activity. Depression is a constellation of interacting psychological, social, and biological symptoms and is the most prevalent of the psychiatric disorders. It is important to recognize this disorder because the rate of suicide among the depressed is 25 times the national average.[11] Some of the signs and symptoms of depression include tearfulness, helplessness, hopelessness, anxiety, hallucinations, insomnia, anorexia, and tension. The illness may be associated with alcoholism and/or drug abuse.

Many individuals with initial affective episodes of depression will have manic episodes some time later, and vice versa. These episodic moods are psychotic and can be classified as "bipolar" or "unipolar" affective illness. The bipolar behavioral disorder of manic–depressive psychosis is an inherited disorder manifested by periods of mania and periods of depression.[12]

Differential diagnosis for the affective disorders includes: (a) evaluation of the symptoms, (b) a complete longitudinal study and mental status examination, (c) a family history, (d) a physical examination, and (e) clinical laboratory procedures. Because many individuals with significant medical disorders are depressed, laboratory procedures should be performed to rule out illnesses that frequently lead to depression such as hypothyroidism, viral diseases (*e.g.*, infectious hepatitis, mononucleosis), carcinoma, and Cushing's syndrome. Also, some medications such as contraceptive hormones, antihypertensives, and corticosteroids can lead to depression. Thus, laboratory assays can play an essential part in differentiating organic disorders from this affective state.

ANXIETY DISORDERS (NEUROSES)

Neurotic illness consists of "acts that can be characterized as inappropriate, inadequate, unadaptive, and infantile, resulting in a subjective and objective discrepancy between psychological potential and actual performance."[13] Neuroses are similar to depression and schizophrenia in that they do not constitute a discrete disease entity. Neuroses are actually behavioral pathways resulting from interactions of biological, psychological, and social influences. A neurotic behavior pattern involves misjudgment of the inner world, whereas a psychotic pattern involves misjudgment of the outer as well as the inner world. Types of neurotic behavior include anxiety, hysteria, phobias, and obsessive–compulsive neuroses. The etiology of neuroses has been thought to be linked to unresolved conflicts that occurred in childhood. Treatment is generally long-term and occurs through psychotherapy to determine the underlying conflicts. For some types of neuroses such as anxiety neuroses or obsessive–compulsive disorders, clinical laboratory assays are needed to rule out clinical disorders such as pheochromocytoma or thyrotoxicosis.[14]

PERSONALITY DISORDERS

Lifelong patterns of behavior that cause inner distress or outer consternation can be classified as *personality disorders*. This group of disorders accounts for a high proportion of nonpsychotic psychiatric problems such as drug dependence, sexual deviation, and alcoholism. Some types of personality disorders develop into psychotic disorders (*e.g.*, manic–depressive disorders, schizophrenia).

Biochemical Bases of Behavioral Disorders

Brain function and behavior are directly linked to brain biochemistry. Some forms of dementia and delirium have been identified as biochemical abnormalities. The following chemical constituents have been associated with behavioral disorders.

Glucose. If blood glucose levels decrease below 70 mg/dL (3.89 mmol/L) for longer than an hour, the individual may become delirious.[15] If the hypoglycemia persists, the individual may experience severe brain damage with resultant dementia.

Electrolytes. Electrolyte and acid–base balance are essential in brain functioning. Delirium can result from imbalances such as acidosis, alkalosis, hypernatremia, hyponatremia, diminished blood zinc levels, hypercalcemia, and hypocalcemia.

ACTH and cortisol. Psychotic depression has been found to be related to increased cortisol secretion.[16] It has been suggested that this disorder is due to dysfunction in the hypothalamic–pituitary feedback mechanism involving adrenocorticotropic hormone (ACTH).

5-Hydroxyindoleacetic acid (5-HIAA). The major metabolite of serotonin, 5-HIAA, has been shown to be decreased in cerebrospinal fluid in depressed and manic patients, with persistent low levels even after recovery.[17]

Catecholamines. This group of chemical compounds includes dopamine, norepinephrine, and epinephrine. Research studies have indicated that major depression is linked to a deficiency of norepinephrine. The most effective treatment of depression, electroconvulsive therapy, has been found to increase the utilization of norepinephrine and dopamine in the brain. In addition, amphetamines, used in the treatment of major depression, have a stimulant effect that causes the release of norepinephrine and dopamine from neurons in the brain.[18]

Creatine Kinase (CK). Of the CK isoenzymes, the CK-MM(muscle type) isoenzyme has been found to be elevated in the blood of patients with schizophrenia and other psychiatric illnesses.[19]

LABORATORY ANALYSES AND DIAGNOSIS

In addition to the analyses described for acute organic brain disease and biochemical bases of behavioral disorders, other clinical laboratory procedures that have been helpful in distinguishing among behavioral disorders include the administration of oral lithium, with subsequent determination of the 36-hour urinary lithium concentration, to diagnose mania, because manics retain lithium more than do other individuals;[20] the penetration of lithium into, and efflux from, erythrocytes as a test for major affective disorders, because patients with these major affective disorders have a higher erythrocyte lithium index;[21] and the dexamethasone suppression test to evaluate endogenous depression, because endogenously depressed patients respond minimally to attempted suppression of the pituitary gland by dexamethasone.[22] Most of these laboratory tests are not used routinely because of a lack of absolute diagnostic specificity as well as a lack of familiarity of physicians with their utilization.

TREATMENT

Supportive care, psychotherapy, environmental manipulations, and psychopharmacology are some of the major treatments used for behavioral disorders. The treatment of choice for a behavioral disorder depends on the type of disorder and its severity. In the vast majority of cases, multiple approaches have been most desirable. For example, the use of major antipsychotic medications is essential to the treatment of schizophrenics, in addition to environmental and psychotherapeutic treatment.[23]

Four classes of psychotropic agents presently available for treatment of behavior disorders include neuroleptics, tricyclic antidepressants, lithium, and antianxiety agents. The neuroleptics are demonstrably effective in patients suffering from schizophrenia, mania, or organic brain disease. Pharmacologically, the neuroleptics block dopamine receptors.

The antidepressants include two groups of drugs: the tricyclics and the monoamine oxidase inhibitors. These compounds are used for major depressive disorders. The tricyclic antidepressants are ineffective if the dosage is too low, and may be even less effective if the dosage is too high. In fact, the patient's depression may actually become worse if the dosage level is too high. Because the rate of drug metabolism can vary significantly from one patient to another, plasma levels on patients treated with tricyclics must be monitored in the clinical laboratory in order to ascertain the proper dosage level.[24]

Lithium is indicated for the treatment of the manic episode of manic–depressive disorders. Serum lithium levels are needed on these patients to determine patient compliance and adequacy of drug dosage. Also, toxicity can result in certain circumstances such as salt or water retention or when antihypertensives are given to the patient.[25] Cardiac patients are quite susceptible to the toxic effects of lithium. Because the kidney is the main route for lithium excretion, normal renal function is a necessity for lithium therapy. Serum creatinine levels can be used to provide evidence of normal renal functioning.

Antianxiety agents are used to treat neurotic and anxiety disorders and have no established value in treating psychoses. Benzodiazepines are the most widely used antianxiety agents. Proper treatment of anxiety states with these drugs requires a careful assessment of the nature of the psychiatric illness. The assessment should include a physical examination, a medical history, and laboratory tests. The laboratory assays should include tests of plasma cortisol and ACTH for possible hyperadrenalism and a thyroid panel for possible hyperthyroidism, because both of these conditions can lead to anxiety symptoms.

CASE STUDY

A 21-year-old woman had recently dropped out of college and returned home. Psychiatric help was sought because for the past year she had had extreme variations in her behavior. She had been very vivacious and outgoing until that point, when she had started to become withdrawn and very shy, and had lost interest in everything, including her college courses. Her parents indicated that in all of her past school and college work she had been an outstanding student and had enjoyed her studies. Her parents had become alarmed because she had made bizarre comments from time to time and smiled inappropriately.

The physical examination was unremarkable. A toxicology screen revealed no evidence of drug abuse.

Questions

1. What psychotic behavior was probably being exhibited?
2. What type of medication was probably prescribed?
3. The medication prescribed for this behavioral disorder is also used for what other types of behavioral disorders?

Discussion

1. The psychotic behavior exhibited in this case study was probably schizophrenia.
2. The medication probably prescribed for this behavioral disorder was a neuroleptic agent such as phenothiazine.
3. The neuroleptics are demonstrably effective in patients suffering from schizophrenia, mania, or organic brain disease.

REFERENCES

1. Buros O: Mental Measurement Yearbook. Mt. Rainier, MD, Gryphon, 1979
2. Climent C, Burns B: Practical Psychiatry for the Health Professional. New York City: SP Medical and Scientific Books, 1984
3. Donlon P: Diagnosis and Treatment of Acute Psychotic Disorders. In Psychiatric Disorders: Diagnosis and Treatment. Bowie, Maryland, Robert Brady Company, 1982
4. Katzman R (ed): Congenital and Acquired Mental Disorders. New York City, Raven Press, 1979
5. Goldhamer H, Marshall A: Psychosis and Civilization: Two Studies in the Frequency of Mental Illness. New York City, Macmillan, 1953
6. Rosenthal D, Seymour K (eds): The Transmission of Schizophrenia. London, Pergamon Press, 1968
7. Davis J: Overview: Maintenance therapy in psychiatry: I. Schizophrenia. Am J Psychiatry 132: 1237–1245, 1975
8. Abrams R, Taylor M: A comparison of unipolar and bipolar depressive illness. Am J Psychiatry 137:1084–1087, 1980
9. Taylor M, Abrams R: The phenomenology of mania. Arch Gen Psychiatry 29:520–522, 1973
10. Schou M: Lithium Treatment of Manic-depressive Illness: A Practical Guide. New York City, Karger, 1986
11. Lester G, Lester D: Suicide—The Gamble With Death. Englewood Cliffs, New Jersey, Prentice-Hall, 1971
12. Kallman F: Genetics Principles in Manic–Depressive Psychosis. Hoch P, Zubin J (eds): Depression. Stratton, New York, Grune & Stratton, 1954
13. Redlich R, Freedman D: The Theory and Practice of Psychiatry, p 347. New York City, Basic Books, 1966
14. Taylor M: The Neuropsychiatric Mental Status Examination. New York City, Spectrum, 1981
15. Gilroy J, Meyer J: Medical Neurology. New York City, Macmillan, 1969
16. Jacher E et al: Disrupted 24-hour patterns of cortisol secretion in psychotic depression. Arch Gen Psychiatry 28:19–24, 1973
17. Coppen A, Noguera R: L-tryptophan in depression. Lancet 1: 1111, 1970
18. Schildkraut J: The Biochemistry of Affective Disorders. In Nicholi A (ed): The Harvard Guide to Modern Psychiatry, pp 81–91. Cambridge, Massachusetts, Harvard University Press, 1978
19. Meltzer H, Crayton J: Subterminal motor abnormalities in psychotic patients. Nature 249:373–375, 1974
20. Almy G, Taylor M: Lithium retention in mania. Arch Gen Psychiatry 29:232–234, 1973
21. Rybakowski J: Pharmacogenesis aspects of red blood cell lithium index in manic–depressive psychosis. Biol Psychiatry 12: 425–429, 1977
22. Feinberg M et al: A specific laboratory test for the diagnosis of melancholia. Arch Gen Psychiatry 38: 15–23, 1981
23. Tucker G, Ferrell R, Price R: The Hospital Treatment of Schizophrenia. In Bellack A (ed): Treatment and Care of Schizophrenia. Orlando, Florida, Grune & Stratton, 1984
24. Asberg M et al: Relationship between plasma levels and therapeutic effect of nortriptyline. Br Med J 3:331–334, 1971
25. Johnson F, Johnson S (eds): Lithium Medical Practice. Baltimore, University Park Press, 1978

Part X

HEMATOLOGIC DISORDERS

Karen Karni, Associate Editor

Disorders of the blood and lymphatic system generally are considered together because their components are interrelated and dependent on one another. These components include the blood, bone marrow, spleen, lymph nodes, and reticuloendothelial system. Anemias are among the more common hematologic disorders observed, while leukemias and coagulopathies are relatively rare. The clinical laboratory is key in the prompt, accurate diagnosis of these disorders and in many cases the monitoring of treatment as well.

Each chapter in this section addresses an important aspect of hematologic malfunction: anemia, leukocyte abnormalities and hematologic malignancies, and hemostatic disorders. In each, the author discusses salient etiologic considerations that form the basis for understanding the clinical and laboratory manifestations of these diseases and thus lead to a rational approach to the effective and appropriate utilization of the laboratory in diagnostic decision-making.

Chapter 50

The Anemias

Jacqueline Swoyer

ETIOLOGY AND PATHOPHYSIOLOGY

Anemia can be defined as a decreased oxygen-carrying capacity of the blood caused by diminished hemoglobin function or availability. It is often, but not always, associated with decreased erythrocyte numbers (red cell mass). Accurate interpretation of laboratory data is complicated by the necessity for separate reference ranges relative to sex, age, geographic location, and ethnic origins as well as the physiological needs of individuals at any one time. These needs may not remain constant, as with marked altitude changes or as in the newborn. Signs and symptoms of anemia will relate both to the degree of physiological need of the individual and to the degree of the reduced hemoglobin function.

The etiology of the anemia will determine the symptomatology. For example, early nutritional anemias may be characterized by pallor and fatigue, while massive blood loss may result in hypoxia and heart failure. Anemia *per se* is not a diagnosis, but rather a symptom of an underlying disease process.[1] Therefore, detection of the anemic state must be followed by a specific workup for the etiology. To simply improve the diminished oxygen-carrying capacity by providing increased oxygen availability or by replacing the decreased red cell numbers by transfusion will not resolve the underlying disease state.

Classification of Anemias

The pathophysiological classification of anemia is based on the mechanism of disease, *i.e.*, decreased bone marrow production of normally functioning erythrocytes or increased loss of red cells by hemorrhage or by hemolysis.[2] This seemingly simple differentiation is often complicated by overlapping or multiple etiologies. Moreover, the only relatively noninvasive laboratory procedure for differentiating these two mechanisms, the peripheral blood reticulocyte count, is unpopular because it is plagued both by imprecision and by labor intensity. When the reticulocyte count becomes automated, as is the platelet count, it may become more useful in the pathophysiological classification of anemia.

At the present time, the more clinically relevant or useful classification of anemia is that which more closely relates to the etiology and is based on readily available and sensitive laboratory measurements. It is a morphological classification derived from precise descriptions and measurements of erythrocyte size and hemoglobin content. Although in the past such description was available only from expert microscopic evaluation of blood smears, recent developments have provided numerical information derived from sophisticated automated instruments. When the laboratory detects and reports the anemic state and accompanying morphological classification, the physician correlates these data with information derived from a complete and pertinent patient history and physical examination.

Classification of anemias can be approached efficiently and cost-effectively based on red cell morphology derived from precise red cell indices and thorough microscopic examination of the well-made and stained blood smear. The morphological blood smear examination is one of the most informative laboratory tests performed in the evaluation of anemia. It and the red cell indices enable classification of the anemia into one of three major groups: microcytic, hypochromic anemia; macrocytic anemia; or normocytic, normochromic anemia. Etiologies associated with these three groups are outlined in Table 50-1.

Anemias Associated with Microcytic, Hypochromic Red Cells

The microcytic, hypochromic red cell is derived from normoblastic red cell maturation with decreased hemoglobination during the maturation process. This results in a small cell with a lower than normal amount of hemoglobin for the cell size and membrane content.

The most frequent etiology of this anemia is iron deficiency resulting either from decreased iron intake (especially in children) or from increased loss of iron stores due to chronic blood loss. The second most frequent etiology is the asynchrony of hemoglobin synthesis, as seen in thalassemia and lead poisoning, for example (see Table 50-1). The defective iron utilization anemias also may produce microcytic, hypochromic cell types, but these are usually mixed with more normally sized and hemoglobinated cells, resulting in the description of a "dimorphic" red cell population.

Iron deficiency states are often not so easily diagnosed, due to testing problems and etiologic overlaps.[3] It is important to remember that iron deficiency always has an underlying etiology, either not enough iron intake to supply the body with its metabolic needs for a variety of tissue cells, or excess iron loss. The most common and severe iron loss occurs in chronic blood loss, *e.g.*, GI-tract bleeding, excessive menstruation, and pregnancy, but extensive loss of other tissue such as skin, especially if over long periods of time, can eventually result in iron deficiency, especially if intake or absorption is decreased simultaneously.

If iron deficiency can be ruled out as the cause of microcytic, hypochromic anemia by findings of normal iron stores assessment, other less common causes are considered. Lead poisoning is relatively rare, and often is discovered by history and physical findings rather than by laboratory findings. The most common underlying cause of microcytic, hypochromic red cells in the presence of normal iron stores is a genetic disorder, thalassemia.[4, 5, 6] Defined as having quantitative reduction in one or more of the globin chains in the molecular formation of hemoglobin, the thalassemias are more fre-

Table 50-1 ***Classification of Anemias by Cell Size and Hemoglobin Content***

Microcytic, Hypochromic Anemias

1. Frequent cause—iron-deficiency anemia
   a. Insufficient iron intake
   b. Chronic blood loss
2. Less frequent causes
   a. Thalassemia—hereditary inability to make normal amounts of one of the polypeptide chains of globin
   b. Hypochromic, iron-utilization anemias—hemoglobin synthesis impaired because of an inability to synthesize heme (sideroblastic anemia)

Macrocytic Anemias

1. Macrocytic anemias with oval macrocytes and teardrop cells
   a. Megaloblastic anemias—also with hypersegmented neutrophils
   b. Myelofibrosis with extramedullary myeloid metaplasia (some nucleated RBCs, immature WBCs, and large platelets)
2. Macrocytic anemias with round macrocytes
   a. Hypothyroidism
   b. Chronic liver disease (target cells may be frequent)
   c. Hemolytic anemias with very marked reticulocytosis

Normocytic, Normochromic Anemias

1. Normocytic, normochromic anemias without abnormally shaped RBCs (poikilocytosis) and without polychromatophilic macrocytes (lack of polychromasia—no erythropoietic stimulation of the marrow; lack of poikilocytosis—no disordered erythroid maturation or hemolysis)
   a. Chronic infectious and inflammatory states (*e.g.*, rheumatoid arthritis, chronic tuberculosis)
   b. Malignancies (when there is anemia of chronic disease and/or bone marrow invasion)
   c. Chronic renal disease
   d. Endocrine hypofunction (hypothyroidism, hypopituitarism, hypogonadism, adrenal insufficiency)
   e. Marrow suppression by drugs or toxins
2. Normocytic, normochromic anemias with prominent poikilocytosis and occasional polychromatophilic macrocytes (disorders with markedly disturbed erythrocyte maturation or hemolysis)
   a. Uremia
   b. Leukemias
   c. Myelofibrosis with extramedullary myeloid metaplasia
   d. Carcinoma invading bone marrow
   e. Refractory normoblastic anemia
3. Normocytic, normochromic anemia with numerous polychromatophilic macrocytes
   a. Hemolytic anemias
   b. Acute blood loss

quently seen in certain ethnic groups of the world such as Mediterranean and Southeast Asian populations. The ethnic mix in the U.S. requires that the possibility of these abnormal hemoglobins be explored.

The presence of microcytic, hypochromic, red cells when iron stores are normal or increased suggests the "iron-loading" anemias. These are so named because (1) the red cells often show particulate iron inclusions (siderocytes), and (2) iron overload of tissue is seen, especially in reticuloendothelial organs such as the spleen, liver, and bone marrow. This disease process is also called sideroblastic anemia.

The sideroblastic anemias have one of three etiologies. Some are inherited; these are rare, and family history is important in identifying this cause. Some are drug-induced, as in alcoholism,[7] especially when complicated by poor diet, or in INH (isoniazid) treatment of tuberculosis.

In the drug-induced and/or severe dietary-depleted etiologies, the actual mechanism is pyridoxine (vitamin B_6) depletion. These drugs either cause destruction of vitamin B_6 or interfere with its absorption and/or function. Replacement by pyridoxine therapy may improve the anemia, but optimal response will usually occur only when the offending drug is discontinued.

The third and most common cause of sideroblastic anemia is the presence of a malignant clone of erythrocyte precursors that cannot properly metabolize iron to form hemoglobin. This condition demonstrates a variety of other blood cell abnormalities, and is commonly referred to as *dyserythropoietic* or *myelodysplastic anemia.* There may or may not be abnormal chromosome patterns in the precursors in the bone marrow. A common, although controversial, name for this disease state has been "preleukemic syndrome." The non-pyridoxine-responsive, nonfamilial sideroblastic anemias are included in this malignant myelodysplastic syndrome. Cure or remission with chemotherapy has not been successful. Supportive therapy such as transfusion and iron chelation are often necessary. Conversion to leukemia is common.

Anemias Associated with Macrocytic Red Cells

The origin of macrocytic red cells can be either megaloblastic or normoblastic maturation, with resulting differences in morphology. For this reason, in the past the logical approach was to use observation of red cell precursors in the bone marrow as the first step in diagnosis of these anemias. However, due to the availability of serum vitamin B_{12} and folic acid measurements in recent years, bone marrow biopsy and examination can usually be avoided.[8]

The morphological differences observed in macrocytic anemias can be explained by the different etiologies of these entirely different cell populations (see Table 50-1). Megaloblastic maturation is caused by unavailability of either vitamin B_{12} or folic acid (or both) at the site of blood cell formation, due to decreased intake or decreased absorption. Inability to utilize these necessary vitamins, even when available, as is seen in the malignant myeloproliferative disorders, also results in megaloblastic maturation. In the case of vitamin B_{12} and/or folic acid deficiency, similar nuclear maturation defects are seen in other cells as well, such as granulocytes and cervical cells.

Normoblastic maturation producing macrocytic cells is most frequently seen in liver disease and thyroid deficiency states. In thyroid deficiency, the resulting cell is often increased in size with normal hemoglobination. In liver disease, there is an increase in the cell membrane proportional to the hemoglobin content, which usually contributes to target cell formation.

Lowered levels of both vitamin B_{12} and folic acid, especially when combined with iron deficiency, are evidence of malabsorption, seen most frequently after surgical interventions of the GI tract or in the elderly. Decreased folic acid levels alone are most frequently seen in alcoholism or drug antagonism, as with some birth control medications, Dilantin, or antifolates such as methotrexate used in chemotherapy. Folic acid, although present in many foods, is not stored in the body for any length of time. This results in the development of deficiency states within a short time of dietary insufficiency or antagonism. Recent intake and absorption can mask deficiency, resulting in normal serum folate levels in the presence of a megaloblastic anemia.

Vitamin B_{12} is readily stored in a healthy liver, yielding months and perhaps years of available resources. Therefore, the lowered serum levels reflecting lowered stores available for red cell formation develop over a long period of time once absorption or intake is decreased or eliminated. The most common cause of B_{12} deficiency is pernicious anemia, due to intrinsic factor deficiency and subsequent failure to absorb dietary B_{12}. This is presumed to be an autoimmune process, and is a complex physiological condition usually accompanied by refractory gastric anacidity and significant levels of antiparietal cell antibodies. Distinction between B_{12} and folic acid deficiency in the etiology of megaloblastic anemias is necessary for two important reasons: (1) therapy using folic acid will not arrest the progression of the neurological deficit of B_{12} deficiency even if blood cell abnormalities improve, and (2) different causes of B_{12} or folic acid deficiencies may result in other symptoms or conditions as well as in anemia.

Anemias Associated with Normocytic, Normochromic Red Cells

Normocytic, normochromic anemia is the largest, the most frequently encountered, and the most varied of all the anemia classifications (see Table 50-1). The major pathogenetic division of this group is a distinction between marrow failure and increased red cell loss as the etiology of the anemia.

If acute blood loss can be ruled out, the differential diagnosis remaining is that of intracorpuscular (intrinsic) or extracorpuscular (extrinsic) hemolysis[9] (see Table 50-2). This etiologically variable group can present so mildly as to be almost undetectable, as in low-grade hereditary spherocytosis, or so acutely that the hemoglobin value drops precipitously.

If hemoglobinopathy, congenital spherocytosis, and disseminated intravascular coagulopathy are ruled out, autoimmune hemolytic anemia is assumed even if the direct antiglobulin test is negative. This condition is often secondary to lymphoproliferative and other malignancies (including metastatic solid tissue tumors), drugs such as penicillin, collagen vascular diseases (especially lupus erythematosus), and infectious diseases including mycoplasma pneumonia, infectious mononucleosis, and other viral illnesses (see Table 50-2).

Marrow failure anemias are suspected when there is no evidence of accelerated red cell replacement in response to the anemia, such as a peripheral blood polychromasia or reticulocytosis. The more severe the failure, the more evident are the changes seen in the peripheral blood, including pancytopenia (most severe in aplastic anemia)[10] and leukoerythroblastic reaction (LEBR), hallmark of the myelophthistic anemias. However, only bone marrow aspiration and examination will lead to the definitive diagnosis of marrow failure anemias. Table 50-3 describes various etiologies and findings in marrow failure anemias. Aplastic anemia has several etiologic possibilities, which are outlined on page 619.

CLINICAL MANIFESTATIONS

Anemia is an indicator of decreased oxygen-carrying capacity of the blood, and results in reduced oxygenation of body tissues. A range of symptomatology ensues, from minor fatigue to dyspnea, syncope, and angina pectoris. Reduction in circulating hemoglobin will produce pallor and eventually hypotension. Increased cardiac output results in symptoms such as minor palpitations, but may progress to actual heart failure as the hemoglobin capacity continues to decrease.

Because the etiologic possibilities are so broad, many factors must be assessed. The assessment should include information relative to age, sex, ethnic origin, diet, recent geographic habitation, toxic exposures including prescription and over-the-counter drugs, infection, neoplasm, bleeding tendencies, and family history of diseases and symptoms (see page 620).

Physical examination should include examination of skin for abnormal color changes, rashes, and ulcerations; appearance of tongue; nails; hair; lymph nodes; spleen; and liver. Secondary diagnostic tests may be needed for completion of neurologic, endocrine, and nutritional status of the patient.

LABORATORY ANALYSES AND DIAGNOSIS

The timeliness, accuracy, and precision of the laboratory's contribution to the diagnosis of anemia cannot be overestimated, and can eliminate the

Table 50-2 ***Classification of Hemolytic Anemias***

Intracorpuscular (intrinsic) Hemolytic Anemias

Hemolysis stems from a defect in the patient's red blood cells. Therefore, normal red blood cells are not destroyed rapidly when transfused into such a patient.

Most intrinsic anemias are hereditary.

1. Abnormal hemoglobins: S, C, H, unstable hemoglobins, *e.g.*, methemoglobin
2. Defective glycolysis
   a. Enzyme deficiency in main glycolytic pathway, *e.g.*, pyruvate-kinase deficiency
   b. Enzyme deficiency in hexose monophosphate shunt, *e.g.*, glucose-6-phosphate dehydrogenase (G6PD) deficiency
3. Membrane abnormalities
   a. Hereditary spherocytosis
   b. Paroxysmal nocturnal hemoglobinuria
   c. Hereditary elliptocytosis

Extracorpuscular (extrinsic) Hemolytic Anemias

The patient's red cells are normal but become damaged by an external factor. Transfused normal cells will be damaged as readily as the patient's own cells. Extrinsic anemias are acquired and often secondary to identifiable underlying disease.

1. Damage by antibodies
   a. Isohemagglutinins
      i. Transfusion of incompatible blood
      ii. Hemolytic disease of the newborn
   b. Autoantibodies
      i. Systemic lupus erythematosis
      ii. Lymphomas, lymphatic leukemias
      iii. Immunologic reactions, *e.g.*, infectious mononucleosis
   c. Drug-related antibodies
      i. Massive penicillin therapy
      ii. α-Methyldopa (Aldomet)
2. Mechanical damage
   a. Abnormally small and obstructed vessels (*i.e.*, with fibrin deposits)
      i. Thrombotic thrombocytopenic purpura
      ii. Hemolytic uremic syndrome
      iii. Disseminated intravascular coagulation (DIC)
   b. Prosthetic aortic heart valve, *i.e.*, with some regurgitant flow
3. Alterations in plasma lipids, leading to alteration of RBC membrane
   a. Complication of liver disease (Zieve's syndrome)
   b. Abetalipoproteinemia
4. Infectious agents and toxins
   a. Massive malarial infection
   b. Circulating *Clostridium* exotoxins
   c. Poisonous snake venom

Table 50-3 ***Bone Marrow Findings in Marrow Failure Anemias***

Aplastic anemia	Increased fat with markedly decreased to absent myeloid elements
Myelophthistic anemia	Marrow space occupied by invading malignant tissue such as leukemia, lymphoma, metastatic carcinoma, myelofibrosis
Chronic disease anemia (iron utilization deficiency)	Myeloid elements within normal limits and increased iron stores with decreased sideroblasts
Hypoplastic anemia	Myeloid elements within normal limits or decreased proportionally to the anemia present, suggesting suppression (or lack of stimulation) such as seen in renal disease (uremia or a combination of uremia and decreased erythropoietin stimulation) or other myelotoxic states
Red cell aplastic anemia	Marked decrease or absence only of erythroid precursors

Classification of Aplastic Anemia

1. Congenital or familial
   - Blackfan-Diamond type
   - Fanconi syndrome
   - Estrin-Dameshek type
2. Acquired
   - Idiopathic
   - Secondary
     - Exposure to chemicals and drugs
     - Exposure to radiant energy
3. Marrow exhaustion
4. Hemolytic disease in crisis
5. Aplasia in preleukemic states
6. Paroxysmal nocturnal hemoglobinuria
7. Infections
8. Pure red cell aplasia

ineffectiveness and complications of "trial and error" approaches to therapy.

Drugs or Chemicals Frequently Associated with Aplastic Anemia

Chemicals

Benzene and its derivatives, inorganic arsenic, DDT, parathion

Drugs

Cytostatic	6-Mercaptopurine, busulfan, melphalan, vincristine, methotrexate, and others
Antimicrobial	Chloramphenicol, penicillin, tetracycline, sulfonamides, sulfisoxazole
Analgesic	Phenylbutazone, aspirin
Anticonvulsant	Methylphenylethylhydantoin, trimethadione, diphenylhydantoin, primidone
Hypoglycemic	Tolbutamide, chlorpropamide
Tranquilizing	Chlorpromazine, chlordiazepoxide
Antithyroid	Carbimazole, tapazole
Others	Colchicine, acetazolamide

Initial Studies

The initial studies for detection, classification, and diagnosis of anemia include a complete blood count (hemoglobin, hematocrit, red cell count, red cell indices, white blood count, white cell differential) and an examination of the blood smear for shape,

Factors In the Evaluation of Anemia

History from a patient with suspected anemia should provide the following information:

1. Duration and onset of anemia symptoms
2. Severity of cerebral and circulatory symptoms relative to the severity of the anemia
3. The possibility of chronic blood loss
4. The possibility of episodes of hemolysis
5. The presence of neurologic symptoms
6. Prior therapy for anemia (vitamin B_{12}, folate, iron)
7. Use of other drugs and exposure to toxins
    - Megaloblastic anemia due to interference with folic acid metabolism
        - Diphenylhydantoin (Dilantin) and other anticonvulsants
        - Pyrimethamine ((Daraprin, antimalarials)
        - Chemotherapy for malignancies
    - Acute hemolysis in susceptible individuals induced by
        - Nitrofurantoin (Furadantin)
        - Sulfa drugs
        - Acetanilid
        - High doses of penicillin
        - α-Methyldopa (Aldomet)
    - Marked depression of red cell production
        - Chloramphenicol
        - Phenylbutazone (Butazolidine)
    - Interference in heme metabolism
        - Lead
    - Other (*e.g.*, benzene, insecticides)
8. Dietary history
    - Iron deficiency
    - Folic acid deficiency (alcoholics, patients on marginal diets)
9. Family history and racial background (*e.g.*, in black patients and ethnic groups from the Mediterranean basin or Near East)
    - Hemoglobinopathies
    - Thalassemia
    - Glucose-6-phosphate dehydrogenase (G6PD) deficiency
    - Hereditary spherocytosis
10. Underlying disease or surgical interference
    - Uremia
    - Chronic liver disease
    - Hypothyroidism
    - Gastrointestinal surgery
    - Splenectomy

Table 50-4 ***Laboratory Findings and Morphological Classification of Anemias***

	Microcytic, Hypochromic	Macrocytic	Normocytic, Normochromic
Red cell count	↓ N ↑	↓	N ↓
Hemoglobin	↓	↓	↓
Hematocrit	↓	↓	↓
MCV	↓	↑	N
MCH	↓	↑	N
MCHC	↓	N	N

size, and hemoglobin content of red cells (see Table 50-4). Other observations, *e.g.*, polychromatophilic erythrocytes and platelet count, are also made (see below). Currently available technology often allows the platelet count to be included in the automated part of these studies, at little extra cost. Further studies by the laboratory include analyses for iron, vitamin B_{12}, and folic acid as well as assessment of thyroid, liver, and kidney function.

Microcytic, Hypochromic Anemias

The most efficient approach to the diagnosis of microcytic, hypochromic anemias is to assess the iron stores. If they are below normal or frankly absent, the physician is alerted to the most common etiology in this group, iron deficiency anemia (see Fig. 50-1). This assessment must be followed by determining the cause of the iron deficiency—decreased iron intake or increased iron loss. This is often obvious from the patient's history, but may require testing for blood loss with occult blood studies and/or gastrointestinal examinations.

The assessment of iron stores, although controversial, has become technically sophisticated. Older methods were limited to serum iron and total iron binding capacity, yielding a calculated saturation percentage of approximately 40% when within normal limits. Many problems plagued this method as a precise indication of iron stores. First, the circadian variation[11, 12] of serum iron in healthy ambulatory subjects has a large but predictable amplitude, allowing some subjects to be within normal range at peak serum iron time but iron-deficient at the trough. The iron-binding capacity does not suffer from such variations but is affected by nutritional status, as is transferrin measurement. Free erythrocyte porphyrin (FEP) analysis can be used very economically as a screen for iron deficiency, but increases are also seen in lead poisoning. Although some interpretive value can be placed on various ranges of an FEP increase, there is tremendous overlap. The serum iron measurement is further complicated in the presence of inflammatory processes, usually resulting in low values that are not representative of the iron stores. The serum ferritin RIA methodology,

Initial Laboratory Evaluation

1. Complete blood count (CBC), preferably automated
   - RBC and WBC and platelet counts
   - Hemoglobin and hematocrit
   - Erythrocyte indices
2. Study of the peripheral blood smear
3. Reticulocyte count
4. Evaluation of plasma pigments
   - By observing the plasma at the top of the spun-down collection tube for bilirubin and/or hemolysis
   - By measuring the serum bilirubin and/or plasma hemoglobin levels

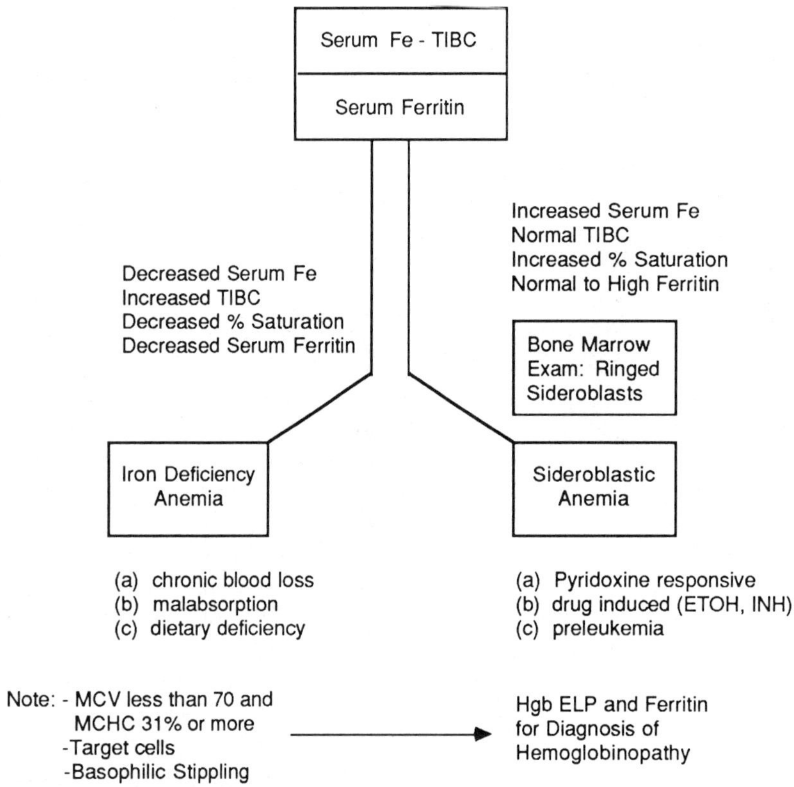

Figure 50-1 **Microcytic hypochromic red cells.**

which became available in the 1970s, is somewhat controversial but shows more predictable results in that it has a very flat circadian variation; it can be measured in very small amounts of serum, which is valuable in infant testing; and it is not spuriously low in inflammatory disease, although it may give falsely high results in severe systematic diseases such as renal failure or liver failure. The serum ferritin level is the preferred approach, therefore, especially in infants and children, because the finding of less than 10 ng/mL (10 μg/L) is essentially diagnostic of iron deficiency. Newborns and infants up to one year of age should have more than 50 ng/mL (50 μg/L) to represent adequate iron stores.[13] Although iron stores should not be assessed during times of acute illness or fever, this is often impractical in pediatric cases.

The bone marrow biopsy for assessment of decreased iron stores is used less commonly except in unusual circumstances such as evaluation of an iron-deficient subject who apparently does not respond to iron replacement therapy.

If iron stores are normal, defective iron utilization must be considered. If lead poisoning is suspected, actual lead levels must be measured to confirm this etiology and must be performed in laboratories proficient in this sophisticated methodology. Free erythrocyte protoporphyrin methods are very economical as well as readily available, and can be used effectively to rule out lead poisoning once iron stores are assessed to be within normal limits.

The laboratory method used in the diagnosis of thalassemia is the electrophoresis of hemoglobin. It should be noted that increases of hemoglobin A2 or F, the significant values seen in thalassemia, can only be detected in hemoglobin containing a normal amount of iron. Except in young children or in adults with increased blood loss, it is unusual to find an iron deficiency associated with thalassemia.

The most straightforward approach to the diagnosis of iron deficiency anemia or anemia with normal iron stores would seem to be one test at a time. However, this is often not practical or even cost-effective if diagnosis is delayed. For example, when a Southeast Asian child living in an old, lead-painted house in a lower socioeconomic area of the city is admitted to the hospital with microcytic, hypochromic anemia, the physician and laboratory must carefully plan an efficient testing profile that allows the diagnosis and subsequent treatment in a timely fashion on the smallest blood sample possible. In this instance, a test profile including a serum ferritin level, hemoglobin electrophoresis, and free erythrocyte porphyrin analysis meets these criteria. Adult anemias may require more elaborate followup studies because the underlying causes are often more complex.

Sideroblastic anemia is diagnosed by finding increased sideroblasts, abnormal sideroblasts (ringed sideroblasts), and increased intracellular iron in the aspirated and biopsied bone marrow specimen.

Macrocytic Anemias

Peripheral blood morphology is very helpful in determining the etiology of a macrocytic anemia (see Fig. 50-2). Macrocytic red cells derived from megaloblastic maturation are usually oval-shaped, with decreased central pallor and correspondingly increased MCV (always over 100 μm^3 [100 fL] and often over 120 μm^3 [120 fL]) as well as increased MCH. Those derived from normoblastic maturation are round, showing less anisocytosis and poikilocytosis, often with targeting, and with much

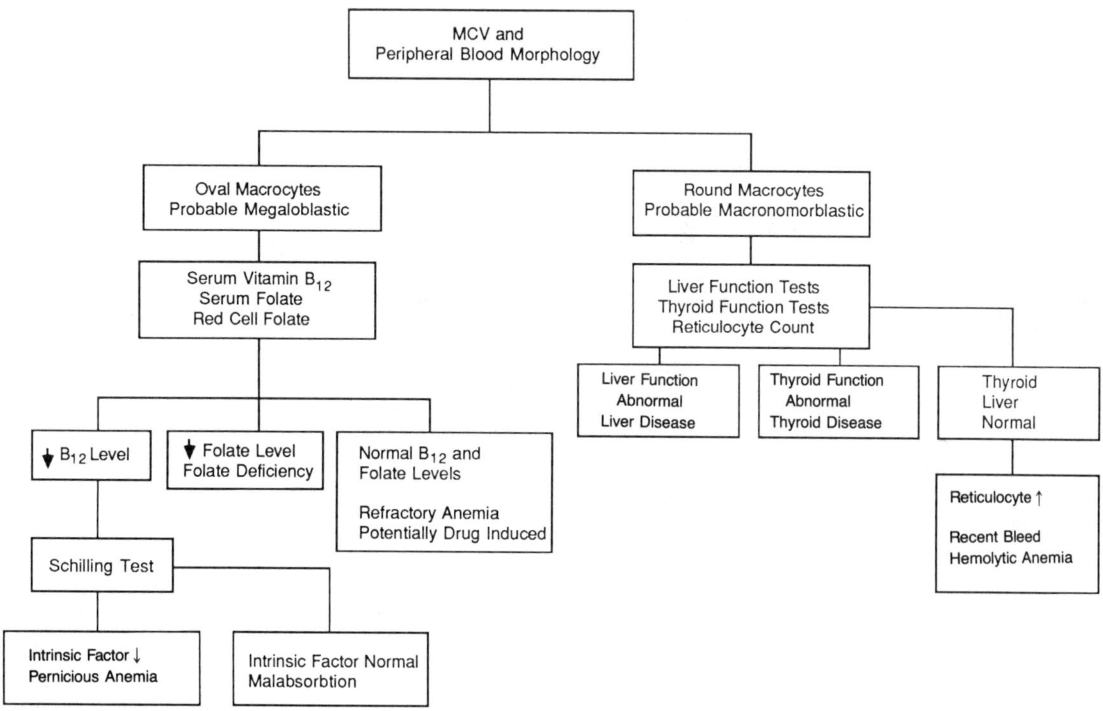

Figure 50-2 Macrocytic red cells.

less pronounced elevations of MCV and normal to decreased MCH.

After determination of the megaloblastic vs nonmegaloblastic (macro-normoblastic) maturation origin of the larger red cells, the next step is to assess thyroid vs liver disease if the origin is nonmegaloblastic, or vitamin B_{12} or folic acid deficiency states if the origin is megaloblastic.

Additional tests used to identify the etiology of B_{12} deficiencies include a complete Schilling test to distinguish malabsorption from intrinsic factor deficiency. This test is expensive, but does distinguish malabsorption, seen especially in older subjects or those with surgical intervention, from the true intrinsic factor deficiency that is the etiology of pernicious anemia. Although both are treated by intramuscular B_{12} therapy, pernicious anemia is frequently followed, accompanied, or preceded by other autoimmune disorders such as thyroiditis and even by gastric carcinomas. The typical patient with anemia of megaloblastic origin often presents with a hemoglobin of 5 g/dL (0.78 mmol/L) or less because of the slow progression of the anemia, which allows a physiological adaptation of the human body.

Normocytic, Normochromic Anemias

The peripheral blood smear examination for the presence and degree of polychromasia and the reticulocyte count, corrected for the degree of anemia, will usually yield the preliminary evidence to distinguish marrow failure from increased red cell loss (see Fig. 50-3). When no evidence of accelerated replacement is seen, a bone marrow examination must be performed to determine the reason for the failure of this organ (see also Table 50-3). Laboratory evaluation of red cell hemolysis is outlined on page 626.

TREATMENT

Unless an anemic state has resulted in cardiac manifestations or is due to marrow failure or acute blood loss, or there is a hemoglobin value of <9 g/dL (1.40 mmol/L), transfusion, even of packed red cells, is seldom indicated and may even be dangerous if volume overload occurs. Treatment is generally directed toward the etiology of the anemia, or, if it is incurable, to supportive therapies.

In the case of deficiency states, patients generally respond well to replacement therapy.[14] In iron-deficiency anemia, for example, iron replacement is simple and cost-effective. Iron therapy is not appropriate, however, when there is no evidence of deficiency. Although absorption is regulated by mechanisms found in the upper GI tract, iron overload can occur. This is especially true when the iron source is other than natural iron, and overload must be considered in the long-term therapy for the hemoglobinopathies. Iron therapy compliance is a particular problem in children because iron is not pleasant to take and is often given with liquids such as milk that interfere with absorption. Pediatricians occasionally order laboratory analysis of the iron prescription to determine therapy compliance when a child has not responded to therapy.

The administration of vitamin B_{12} or folic acid to deficient patients also results in dramatic improvement, with reticulocytosis observed four or five days after therapy is begun.[15]

Anemias secondary to other disorders or to exposure to drugs or other toxins improve if the underlying condition is corrected or the drug discontinued. Primary disorders of the bone marrow, however, are often irreversible, with only supportive therapy available. Bone marrow transplants have become an acceptable alternative in certain cases.[14] In this event, laboratory involvement is substantial.

Hemolytic anemias due to membrane abnormalities, especially hereditary spherocytic anemia, respond to splenectomy.[16] Immunohemolytic anemias often respond to corticosteroids, and splenectomy is not initially considered. Those patients with immunohemolytic disorders who need transfusions present particular crossmatch problems for the laboratory, and special procedures are undertaken to provide suitable blood products.[16]

Hemolytic anemias due to red cell enzyme de-

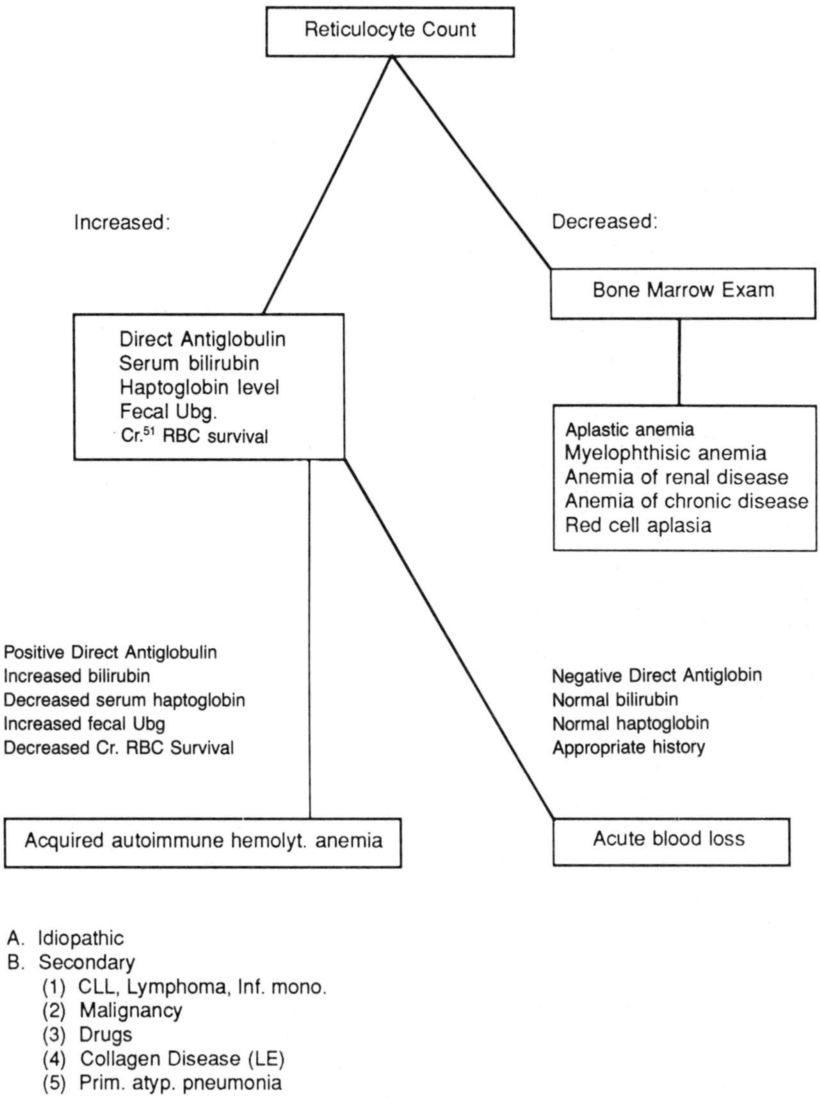

Figure 50-3 **Normocytic normochromic red cells.**

fects usually do not need treatment. In the case of G6PD deficiency, patients are advised to avoid oxidant drugs and fava beans. Hemolytic anemias due to hemoglobinopathies, such as sickle cell anemia and β-thalassemia, have no cure, but require supportive therapy, including folic acid administration.[17]

CASE STUDY

A 23-year-old female clinical laboratory scientist volunteered to have blood drawn to serve as a normal control for the laboratory in which she was employed. A complete blood count, a platelet count, and a reticulocyte count were performed to

Evaluation of RBC Destruction (Hemolysis)

Abnormal RBC morphology in peripheral smear

1. Spherocytes—an anomaly produced by several hemolytic mechanisms, *e.g.*, hereditary spherocytosis, acquired autoimmune hemolytic anemia, clostridial septicemia.
2. Fragmented RBCs — Mechanically damaged cells that occur
   a. In disorders with fibrin deposition
      i. Thrombotic thrombocytopenic purpura
      ii. Hemolytic–uremia syndrome
      iii. Disseminated intravascular coagulopathies
   b. In severe aortic valve disease and in patients with prosthetic heart valves (older valves more commonly implicated)
3. Agglutinated cells—hemolysis due to RBC antibody, *e.g.*, cold agglutinins
4. Ghost cells—broken cells that have lost their Hgb
5. Reticulocyte count—usually high
6. Cells containing aggregated Hgb crystals
   a. Sickle cell anemia
   b. Hb-C (homozygous and heterozygous)
7. Heinz bodies—clumps of oxidized Hgb visible with supravital stains
   a. Hemolysis due to G6PD deficiency
   b. Hemoglobinopathies

Plasma and Urine Pigments

Hemolysis produces serum and urinary pigment patterns that vary according to the hemolysis, being primarily extra- or intravascular.

1. Extravascular Hemolysis
   a. Removal of RBCs within reticuloendothelial system (RES)
   b. Exaggeration of normal pigment pattern
   c. Normally ± 0.6 g Hgb/day broken down

   Bilirubin released from RES cells binds to albumin and is removed by the liver (unconjugated bilirubin).
2. Intravascular Hemolysis—normally about 10% of daily breakdown (± 0.6 g Hgb/day)
   a. Hgb liberated binds to haptoglobin
   b. Hgb-haptoglobin complex removed by RES and converted to bilirubin

   Massive hemolysis overwhelms haptoglobin transport mechanism and decreases haptoglobin level.

confirm her "normal" status, with the following results:

LABORATORY FINDINGS

	Patient	*Reference Ranges*
Hgb	9.9 g/dL	(11.6–14.8)
Hct	28.5%	(34.2–43.7)
RBC	$2.34 \times 10^3/mm^3$	(3.79–4.91)
MCV	123 μm^3	(83–94)
MCH	42.2 pg/cell	(28.4–32.9)
MCHC	34.4%	(32.5–33.5)
WBC	$4.8 \times 10^3/mm^3$	(4.5–10.0)
Platelets	$98 \times 10^3/mm^3$	(150–350)
Reticulocytes	0.6%	(0.5–2.0)
Corrected	0.4%	(0.5–2.0)

Conversion to SI units is as follows:
Hgb—g/dL × 0.155 = mmol/L
MCV—μm^3 × 1 = fL
MCH—pg/cell × 0.0155 = fmol/cell

The stained blood smear demonstrated the presence of oval macrocytic erythrocytes and schistocytes. Hypersegmented neutrophils and eosinophils were also seen. The history and physical examination revealed an apparently healthy female with mild pallor of the conjunctiva and some complaint of fatigue of several months' duration. An adequate diet and no drug use or abuse were noted, and there was no history of pregnancy or excessive blood loss.

Questions

1. What is the most likely cause of this woman's anemia?
2. What laboratory tests will identify the primary etiology?
3. What secondary test is necessary to complete the diagnosis?
4. What other testing might follow the diagnostic secondary test?

Discussion

1. Megaloblastic anemia is most likely, given the presence of oval macrocytes.
2. Vitamin B_{12} and folic acid levels should indicate the primary etiology. Vitamin B_{12} deficiency is most likely in this case, considering the history and physical examinations.
3. The Schilling test with and without intrinsic factor yielded the definitive diagnosis of pernicious anemia and ruled out malabsorption.
4. Thyroid testing is recommended, because the pernicious anemia patient may have other autoimmune sequelae.

REFERENCES

1. Spaet TH: Editorial: Anemia is a symptom. Hosp Pract 15(2):17, 1980
2. Jacob HS: A pathogenic classification of the anemias. Med Clin North Am 50(6):1679, 1966
3. Herbert J: The nutritional anemias. Hosp Pract 15(3):65, 1980
4. England JM: Differentiation of iron deficiency from thalassemia trait by routine blood count. Lancet 1:449, 1973
5. Hoffman GC: Thalassemia minor—a common disorder. Lab Med 6(11):13, 1975
6. Milner DF: Laboratory detection of thalassemia. Am J Med Technol 44(5):431, 1978
7. Eichner ER: The hematologic disorders of alcoholism. Am J Med 54:621, 1973
8. Wallerstein RO: Role of the laboratory in the diagnosis of anemia. JAMA 236(5):490, 1976
9. Forget BG: Hemolytic anemias: Congenital and acquired. Hosp Pract 15(4):67, 1980
10. Goldstein M: The aplastic anemia. Hosp Pract 15(5):89, 1980
11. Haus E, Lakatua DL, Sackett-Lundeen L et al: Clinical Aspects of Chronobiology. In Reitveld WT (ed): Baarn:Bakker: 13–82, 1984
12. Haus E, Lakatua DL, Swoyer JK et al: Chronobiology in hematology and immunology. Am J Anat 168:467, 1983
13. Simmes MA, Addiego JE Jr, Dalman PR: Ferritin in serum: Diagnosis of iron deficiency and iron overload in infants and children. Blood 43(4):501, 1974
14. Bunn HF: Anemia. In Petersdorf RG et al (eds):

Harrison's Principles of Internal Medicine, p 291. New York City, McGraw-Hill, 1983
15. Babion BF, Bunn HF: Megaloblastic Anemias. In Petersdorf RG et al (eds): Harrison's Principles of Internal Medicine, p 1859. New York City, McGraw-Hill, 1983
16. Cooper RA, Bunn HF: Hemolytic Anemias. In Petersdorf RG et al (eds): Harrison's Principles of Internal Medicine, pp 1865–1875. New York City, McGraw-Hill, 1983
17. Bunn HF: Disorders of Hemoglobin Structure, Function, and Synthesis. In Petersdorf RG et al: Harrison's Principles of Internal Medicine, pp 1879–1885. New York City, McGraw-Hill, 1983

BIBLIOGRAPHY

Beck WS: Hematology, 4th ed. Cambridge, MA, Massachusetts Institute of Technology, 1985

Bessis MD: Blood Smears Reinterpreted. New York City, Springer International, 1977

Henry JB: Clinical Diagnosis and Management by Laboratory Methods, 17th ed. Philadelphia, WB Saunders, 1984

Hoffbrand AX, Pettit JE: Essential Hematology, 2nd ed. Boston, Blackwell Scientific, 1984

Hyun BH, Ashton JK, Dolan KD: Practical Hematology. Philadelphia, WB Saunders, 1975

Koepke JA: Laboratory Hematology. New York City, Churchill Livingstone, 1984

Miale JA: Laboratory Medicine: Hematology, 6th ed. St Louis, CV Mosby, 1982

Miller DR, Pearson HA: Smith's Blood Diseases of Infancy and Childhood, 5th ed. St Louis, CV Mosby, 1984

Nevalainen DE, Herbst GH, Sage BH: Hematology: Laboratory Evaluation of Blood Cells. North Chicago, Abbott Laboratories, 1978

Williams WJ: Hematology, 3rd ed. New York City, McGraw-Hill, 1983

Chapter 51

Leukocyte Abnormalities and Hematologic Malignancies

Jacqueline Swoyer

The malignant diseases of the hematologic system have in common the uncontrolled and seemingly purposeless proliferation of blood cells. There may be quantitative changes in cell numbers, qualitative or functional abnormalities, or both.

It is important to recognize that there are two major divisions in the origins of blood cells, lymphocytic and nonlymphocytic. Lymphocytes and their derivative cells, the plasmacytes, originate from bone marrow lymphoid precursors but do not continue to require this tissue for proliferation. Lymphocyte origins, lifespans, and proliferation are more complex than those of the nonlymphocytic or myeloid-derived cells. Lymphocytes are not "end" cells, as are the myeloid-derived cells. The latter, except for monocytes and histiocytes, have a development pattern that is well documented by microscopic and tissue culture studies of bone marrow and peripheral blood. Culture of bone marrow-derived myeloid elements has confirmed differentiation into erythropoietin-sensitive (dependent) cell lines, which end in mature red cells, and leukopoietin-sensitive (dependent) cell lines, which end in granulocytes, and has provided proof of a common precursor of these cells.[1]

In vitro lymphocyte cultures, on the other hand, can be initiated with peripheral blood lymphocytes that continue dividing indefinitely with the use of various mitotic stimulators. This technique demonstrates two major groups of lymphocytes, which are also demonstrated by various immunologic techniques: T lymphocytes (thymus-dependent) and B lymphocytes (bursa- or bone marrow-derived). Each of these has subclassifications, including killer and helper in the T-cell category, and specific immunoglobulin producers in the B-cell group (see Chap. 53).[1]

ETIOLOGY AND PATHOPHYSIOLOGY

Benign Leukocyte Abnormalities

Physiologic quantitative changes in specific leukocyte cell lines must be considered when comparing patient values to reference ranges. Quantitation of leukocyte cell lines should always be expressed in absolute numbers and related to age, *e.g.*, children have more lymphocytes than adults. Other factors affecting the numbers of specific leukocytes include sex, environment, and circadian variations.[2]

Benign pathologic changes in leukocytes reflect responses to abnormal environmental influences such as infection by bacteria, fungi, and viruses, or suppression of cell proliferation by toxic agents. These changes involve not only quantitative responses but also those that are functional in nature, *e.g.*, the toxic changes seen in neutrophils.

Familial leukocyte abnormalities are infrequent and are often overlooked in differential diagnoses. The Pelger-Huët (hyposegmentation) anomaly must be differentiated from the pseudo-Pelger-Huët characteristics seen in neutrophils in myeloproliferative and myelodysplastic disorders, including chronic myelogenous leukemia. Familial toxic granulation must be differentiated from the pathologic toxic granulation seen in inflammatory response. Chédiak-Higashi anomaly is a genetic defect with abnormal cell granulation that must be differentiated from toxic conditions. The May-Hegglin anomaly, demonstrating Döhlelike bodies in the cell cytoplasm, also has platelet abnormalities sometimes mistaken for the atypical platelets seen in the myeloproliferative and myelodysplastic disorders. Infrequently seen is familial vacuolization of lymphocytes, which must be differentiated from vacuolization seen in some storage diseases.

The leukopenias also pose difficulties in the differential diagnosis of benign and malignant conditions. Suppression, either from toxic substances or from immune processes, should be assumed until proven otherwise. Agranulocytosis is the most serious of the leukopenias, and is almost always drug-induced. Common agents implicated include the sulfonamides and chloramphenicol. This reactive suppression often presents with normal hemoglobin levels and normal platelet counts, and bone marrow studies are necessary to confirm and to determine the severity of the condition.

The neutropenias occur more frequently than agranulocytosis, and are more varied in etiology. Although many are toxic substance-induced, many are not. Of the latter, some have an immunologic etiology that is very difficult to establish, but they are commonly seen following viral illnesses. *Chronic neutropenia* is a term used when external causes have been ruled out and a long history of this condition has been observed. When a low degree of symptomless neutropenia is the case, individuals may be demonstrating their "normal" state. Cyclic neutropenia is very infrequent but can be dramatic in its presentation. Periodic infections bring this patient to the physician, and their occurrence can be traced to a predictable (21- to 28-day cycle) neutropenic pattern that includes eosinophilia and monocytosis.[2] Some patients succumb early in life to major infections, while others survive, retaining low but rhythmically flat neutrophil numbers.

Lymphopenia is usually caused either by toxic agents including drugs, *e.g.*, high-dose steroids and industrial poisons, or by viral infections, as seen in AIDS.[1] Caution must be used in evaluating mild lymphopenia because most reference ranges do not take into account circadian variations in cell numbers.[2]

The Leukemias

Leukemias, more than any of the hematologic neoplasms, display evidence in the peripheral blood of the increased proliferation and/or removal defect of hematopoietic elements. These are often represented by both an elevated white blood cell count and the appearance of abnormal, immature cells in the peripheral circulation.

The etiology of human leukemia is unknown; however, a number of factors are known to predispose individuals to the disease. These include (1) exposure to ionizing radiation (*e.g.*, atomic bomb survivors), radioactive phosphorus-treated polycythemia vera patients; (2) exposure to chemotoxins such as benzene, chloramphenicol, and malphalan; (3) hereditary aplastic anemias such as Fanconi's or Bloom's syndromes; (4) Down's syndrome; and (5) chronic hematologic malignancies such as polycythemia vera, some sideroblastic anemias, paroxysmal nocturnal hemoglobinuria (PNH), and myelodysplastic syndromes.[1, 3] Age is also a factor in the incidence of leukemia. The first peak occurrence is seen in children between the ages of 1 and 5 years; 90% or more are acute lymphoblastic leukemia. Adults over the age of 60 experience the second peak, with a variety of cell types affected. Acute leukemias are more common in children, although a second peak occurs in adults over 60 years of age. Chronic leukemias and myelodysplastic syndromes are more common in middle and older age groups.[1, 3]

Classification of the leukemias includes three major divisions, listed below in order of clinical significance.[4]

1. Pathogenic mechanism, implying course and prognosis
   - (a) Acute—clonal aberration occurring at the blast stage with endless uncontrolled mitoses and no maturation.
   - (b) Subacute—clonal aberration occurring at the blast stage but with less total proliferation than in the acute class. This may be the early onset of the acute phase.
   - (c) Chronic—clonal aberration allowing maturation but with aberrant adult cell function, abnormally increased cell survival, and increased proliferation.
2. Cell type, *i.e.*, lymphocytic vs nonlymphocytic origin
   - (a) Lymphocytic—histochemically myeloperoxidase- and Sudan Black B-negative
     - (1) Acute—L1, L2, L3 French-American-British (FAB) classification lymphoblastic leukemia, which is described below
     - (2) Chronic—chronic lymphocytic leukemia and variants
   - (b) Nonlymphocytic (myelogenous)—usually histochemically myeloperoxidase and Sudan Black B-positive
     - (1) Acute M1, M2, M3, M4, M5, M6 (FAB classification) myelogenous leukemia
     - (2) Chronic myelogenous leukemia
     - (3) Myelodysplastic and myeloproliferative syndromes

3. Tumor "load" or peripheral blood presence
   (a) Leukemic—leukocytosis with leukemic cells seen in peripheral circulation
   (b) Subleukemic—normal to slightly elevated leukocyte count and leukemic cells in peripheral circulation
   (c) Aleukemic—normal to diminished leukocyte count with no leukemic cells seen in circulation

In acute leukemia, the pathogenic mechanism is the principal determinant of prognosis and treatment. The acute mechanism, with rapid proliferation and little maturation of cells, results in a large tumor "load" and a corresponding decrease in normal cells (normal marrow failure). This results in the earliest demise (0–6 months) in untreated or unsuccessfully treated individuals. In acute lymphoblastic leukemia, the large number of immature cells may result in a more favorable response to therapy because cells in mitotic division are more vulnerable to destruction by chemotherapy and/or radiation; the chronic leukemias are less responsive to treatment.[1, 3, 5]

Clonal abnormalities can be demonstrated in hematologic malignancies by use of cytogenetic studies. These include quantitative defects such as hyperdiploidy as well as the presence of marker chromosomes. The first described chromosomal abnormality in a hematologic malignancy was the Ph′ defect t(9;22). Commonly called the *Philadelphia chromosome,* it is seen in chronic myelogenous leukemia. Such chromosomal findings are regarded as consistent with malignant clones unless they are found in phenotypically normal, healthy individuals.

Detection as well as differential diagnosis of the leukemias depends on certain findings in the peripheral blood and bone marrow that are characteristic for the various disorders. Detection of leukemia as early as possible is crucial to successful treatment, because increased numbers of malignant cells (tumor load) produce more symptoms and are more difficult to treat effectively.[1, 3, 5]

ACUTE NONLYMPHOCYTIC LEUKEMIAS (ANLL)

ANLL leukemias were previously referred to as acute myelogenous leukemias with variants, and have more recently been classified as acute nonlymphocytic leukemias by the FAB system, with the following subclassifications.[6]

M1 (acute myeloblastic leukemia)—this leukemia represents approximately 10% of the acute nonlymphocytic leukemias. It is common in adults but is very rarely seen in children. Even with aggressive chemotherapy, prognosis is poor, with survival from 6 months to 2 years.

M2 (myeloblastic leukemia with maturation or *subacute myelogenous leukemia)*—in this subclassification more maturation is observed in the granulocytic series of white cells than in M1. This form of leukemia is probably an early stage of M1.

M3 (acute promyelocytic leukemia)—M3 represents approximately 10% of the acute nonlymphocytic leukemias. DIC is a frequent complication, thought to be secondary to thromboplastin stimulation of excessive granulation in the increased numbers of promyelocytes found in this form. Patients who survive DIC have a prognosis similar to that for M1.

M4 (acute myelomonocytic leukemia)—M4 constitutes 20% of the acute nonlymphocytic leukemias. It demonstrates longer median survival times than M1, M2, or M3, although it is similarly resistant to chemotherapy. A chronic or "smoldering" form of this leukemia has been described and is often classified within the myelodysplastic syndromes.

M5 (acute monocytic leukemia)—this subclassification represents less than 10% of ANLL, and has a very poor prognosis (0–6 months). A variant of this leukemia demonstrates more maturation to promonocytes, has a longer median survival period (6–12 months), and is referred to as *M5b.*

M6 (erythroleukemia)—this leukemia represents less than 10% of ANLL. It has a prognosis similar to that of M1 and often progresses to M1, with steadily increasing proliferation of myeloblasts and corresponding decrease in abnormal erythroblasts.

An entity recently classified as *M7 (acute megakaryocytic leukemia)* was originally recognized as an M6 variant known as *erythromegakaryocytic leukemia.* Similar to M2–M6 leukemias, it is more likely a definable stage of an acute myelogenous clonal aberration.

ACUTE LYMPHOCYTIC LEUKEMIAS (ALL)

The large class of ALL leukemias is subclassified by both morphologic characteristics and immunologic markers. Incidence is more common in children 2 to 10 years of age. A second peak incidence is seen after middle age. The most frequent subclass observed is referred to as the *common-type ALL.* This form lacks B- or T-cell markers (nonT, nonB or null cell type), and is further defined immunologically by the presence of a distinct membrane antigen known as *common ALL antigen (cALLa),* consistent with preB-cell characteristics. Specific diagnosis of the latter subclass is essential because children have a remission rate of 80% to 90% with aggressive therapy.

The classification of ALL including immunologic markers is summarized in the box.[3, 6]

Characteristics of Lymphocytic Leukemia

B-Cell ALL

Detectable monoclonal immunoglobulin on cell surface
L3 morphology
Terminal deoxyribosidyl transferase (TdT)-negative
High incidence of associated abdominal lymphomas
2% of all ALL
Aggressive clinical course

T-Cell ALL

Spontaneous rosettes formed with sheep RBC
Reaction with T-cell monoclonal antibodies
Lymphoblasts have hyperchromatic and convoluted nuclei.
Terminal deoxyribosidyl transferase (TdT)-positive
Occurs more frequently in older (teenage) males
High incidence of mediastinal mass
Shorter initial remission than nonT-cell ALL with CNS relapse
10% to 15% of ALL

If the leukemic cells have neither T-cell nor B-cell characteristics, they are reacted with cALLa. If positive, the cells are classified as nonT, nonB. If negative with cALLa, they are classified as null cell. Approximately 60% to 70% of all ALLs are cALLa-positive (nonT, nonB), and 3% to 6% are null cell. Chromosomal abnormalities are observed in approximately 70% of ALL cases; however, the frequency varies with the different immunologic types.

The most widely accepted morphologic classification of the acute lymphocytic leukemias is that of the FAB study group.[6] In this typology there are three groups—L1, L2, and L3—which are differentiated primarily by cell size, quantity of cytoplasm, and presence and prominence of nucleoli. L1 is the most frequently occurring form of ALL (85%), in both children and adults. L2 occurs more frequently in adults. L3, circulating American Burkitt's lymphoma, is more often observed in children and young adults than in older persons, but overall is an infrequently occurring form of ALL.

CHRONIC LEUKEMIAS

The term "chronic" is used for those disorders in which the leukemic cell is sufficiently differentiated to be identifiable with respect to cell type.[7]

Chronic Myelogenous Leukemia (CML)

CML is commonly seen in patients between 25 and 50 years of age; however, it represents as many as 5% of childhood leukemias that convert to ALL-like leukemia before detection of CML occurs. Progression to one of the acute myelogenous leukemias is commonly seen, with addition of other chromosome markers. Progression to acute myelofibrosis is also seen.

Myeloproliferative variants with no Ph′ chromosome are even more resistant to chemotherapy. They are more commonly seen in childhood (juvenile CML) and in adults over 60 years of age.[1, 3]

Chronic Lymphocytic Leukemia (CLL)

CLL accounts for approximately 25% of all leukemias, and occurs primarily in the elderly. The median age of onset is 65 years, and there is a predominance in males.

Lymphocytes are well differentiated and, except for their homogeneity, are morphologically similar to normal lymphocytes. These cells show B-cell characteristics with monoclonal surface membrane immunoglobulins. Minimum diagnostic criteria are necessary, especially in the early stages of this disease, to differentiate CLL from benign lymphocytosis, as is discussed below.

In a small number of patients with common B-cell CLL, there will be a progression in the disease that is often referred to as *prolymphocytic transformation.* Characteristics of the transformation include increasing splenomegaly and lymphadenopathy, rising lymphocyte count, refractoriness to previously effective therapy, and a steady increase in the number of prolymphocytes seen. Prognosis becomes poorer when transformation occurs, with the expected survival period diminishing to less than 1 year.

Transformation of CLL may represent the onset of a secondary lymphoma, called *Richter's syndrome.* It is characterized by the presence in the lymphatic tissue and bone marrow of a large cell, pleomorphic, malignant lymphoma, containing multinucleate tumor cells and evidence of remaining residual proliferation of typical CLL lymphocytes. Two populations of abnormal lymphocytes are likewise seen in the peripheral blood.

Galton's prolymphocytic leukemia is another variant of chronic lymphocytic leukemia that also occurs primarily in older males.[5] Like Richter's syndrome, Galton's generally has a poor response to chemotherapy and a short survival period.

Chronic T-cell leukemia represents less than 5% of all CLL, and occurs in younger subjects more frequently than does common B-cell CLL. Other variants include *hairy-cell leukemia,* which is an infrequent disease primarily of 50- to 55-year old males, and Sezary syndrome. *Sezary syndrome* is usually included with the chronic lymphocytic leukemias, but, like hairy-cell leukemia, is probably a circulating lymphoma. Its characteristics include generalized exfoliative erythroderma with dermal and epidermal skin involvement (mycoses fungoides), with or without visceral organ involvement. Bone marrow infiltration may be minimal or absent, and the number of Sezary cells in the blood is extremely variable. These may be so infrequent as to require buffy coat smears to determine their presence. The malignant cell type in this case is a T helper lymphocyte.[1, 3]

Myeloproliferative Disorders Other Than CML

NonCML myeloproliferative disorders represent uncontrolled, purposeless proliferation of nonlymphocytic cells that demonstrate cell maturation. Some, such as myelofibrosis, have aplastic characteristics. Diagnosis is often determined by laboratory methods such as cytogenetic studies, tissue culture techniques, and histocytochemistry.

Although they are chronic in course, resulting in longer survival times, myeloproliferative disorders are markedly resistant to therapy and, except for bone marrow transplant, are often incurable.[1, 3, 5] Classification of these diseases remains the subject of debate and changes frequently.[1, 3, 8]

POLYCYTHEMIA VERA

Polycythemia vera is characterized by panmyelosis. It is specifically characterized by an increased red cell mass secondary to erythrocyte production not regulated by nor requiring erythropoietin stimulation. This characteristic differentiates polycythemia vera from secondary or relative polycythemia, in which hypoxia or decreased plasma volume is the underlying cause. Polycythemia vera may have a very prolonged course if successfully treated by chemotherapy and/or therapeutic phlebotomy; however, it commonly transforms to either acute myelogenous leukemia or bone marrow failure (myelofibrosis).

MYELOFIBROSIS

Myelofibrosis is characterized by patchy replacement of the bone marrow with fibrous tissue, often surrounding islands of bizarre megakaryocytes, and by extramedullary hematopoiesis in the liver and spleen (agnogenic myeloid metaplasia). This is distinct from the secondary myelofibrosis seen in nonmyeloid malignant diseases such as Hodgkin's lymphoma or metastatic carcinoma. The course of myelofibrosis is variable, with a median survival period of about five years, depending on the rate of proliferation of fibrous tissue or whether transformation to acute myelogenous leukemia occurs.

MYELODYSPLASIA (DYSMYELOPOIETIC SYNDROME)[6, 8, 9]

Myelodysplasia is characterized by evidence of malignant clonal aberration. It exhibits a presentation that is not classically leukemic (hyperproliferative); however, transformation to a rapidly proliferative process may occur. The terms *preleukemia* and *chronic myeloproliferative disorder* are often used for this syndrome. In most instances aberration of growth pattern and function in one to all myeloid cell lines occurs. Some attempts to further subclassify this group include distinction of refractory anemia with an excess of blasts (RAEB), and pyridoxine-resistant sideroblastic anemia.

Lymphoproliferative Disorders Other Than CLL

THE MALIGNANT LYMPHOMAS[1]

Although the cell type seen in malignant lymphomas is obviously related to the lymphatic leukemias, the malignant lymphomas more closely resemble solid tissue tumor disorders. Diagnosis must be made from biopsy of lymphoproliferative tissue such as lymph nodes, spleen, and liver, with secondary involvement of bone marrow and peripheral blood as important prognostic indicators.

Two major categories make up this large group—*Hodgkin's lymphoma,* characterized by the presence of Reed-Sternberg cells, and *non-Hodgkin's lymphoma (NHL).* Both categories demonstrate marked immunodeficiency, but Hodgkin's lymphoma appears to be a derangement of T cells, resulting in a decrease of numbers and/or function. The nonHodgkin's lymphomas are the more classic, malignant, uncontrolled proliferation of monoclonal B cells. The latter are often detected in peripheral blood smears during the leukemic phase of this disease.

Diagnosis, treatment, and prognosis of both types of lymphoma are determined using classifications that include cell type, histologic distribution of the malignant cells in the lymph nodes (nodular vs diffuse), and total amount of lymphoreticular tissue involved. While Hodgkin's lymphoma seems to have a unicentric origin and is spread contiguously, the nonHodgkin's lymphomas are more likely to have multicentric beginnings. Severity of both categories is in direct proportion to the amount of reticuloendothelial tissue involvement as determined by anatomic (clinical) staging and, in the nonHodgkin's lymphomas, to the immaturity or differentiation of the predominating cell type as well.

Even more evidence of environmental causes, such as viruses, is supported in the lymphomas than in the leukemias. In both Hodgkin's and Burkitt's lymphomas patients have circulating antibodies to the Epstein-Barr viruses, and in Burkitt's lymphoma viral particles have been detected by electron microscopy. A higher coincidence of Hodgkin's lymphoma in families, schools, and towns, revealed in epidemiologic studies, is more likely to be based on common environmental exposure than on genetics.

Terminology used for classification by both anatomic staging and cell type changes frequently in the lymphomas. The choice(s) for any given institution or locality is generally a matter of mutual discussion between pathologists and attending physicians who utilize such classifications in determining therapy and prognosis.

Hodgkin's lymphoma can be seen in any age group, but occurs more frequently in young to middle-aged adult males. NonHodgkin's lymphoma (NHL) also arises in lymphoid tissue, but the disease is not a single entity and its various forms can be found in all age groups. The majority are considered monoclonal B-cell neoplasms.

THE PLASMA CELL DYSCRASIAS[1, 3, 10]

The malignant states involving the proliferation of specific immunoglobulin-producing plasmacytes are also commonly called *dysproteinemias*. Extent of existing tumor is assessed by bone marrow examination and by radiologic bone studies.

Multiple myeloma is a typical and frequently occurring manifestation of plasma cell disease that occurs primarily in the middle-aged and elderly. It has a variable prognosis with respect to length of survival, 30 months being the median. Myeloma is characterized by an abnormal increase in monoclonal proteins, usually IgG, with a decrease in the other normal immunoglobulins. Because plasma cells play a key role in the development of the normal immune response, such abnormalities have serious potential for disruption of the normal immune state and subsequent infectious complications. Bone involvement due to plasma cell tumors in the bone marrow is also a prominent feature of the disease. Rarely, plasma cell leukemia develops in myeloma patients in which numerous plasma cells (more than 2,000/mm^3) are observed in the peripheral blood.

CLINICAL MANIFESTATIONS

The clinical effects of acute leukemia are due primarily to the effects of the replacement of normal blood cells with leukemic cells. Fever, weakness, and bleeding are, therefore, common symptoms. Onset may be rapid or more insidious, in which case recurrent infections are often observed. Enlargement of tonsils, lymph nodes, and spleen is common, and organs such as the kidney or liver may be enlarged if leukemic cells have infiltrated. There may also be central nervous system (CNS) involvement.[11] For example, in ALL, common clinical findings include pallor, lethargy, fever, malaise, weight loss, sore throat, spontaneous bruises, purpura, bleeding gums, ulcerative lesions in mouth and throat, tender bones, superficial lymphadenopathy, moderate splenomegaly and hepatomegaly, and meningeal syndrome due to infiltration by leukemia cells.[2, 6] In acute monocytic leukemia, infiltration of the gingivae is common.

In chronic leukemia, anemia, weight loss, and frequent infection are common symptoms, as is splenomegaly. One clinical distinction between CML and CLL is the usual lack of lymphadenopathy in the former and its characteristic prominence in the latter. Skin lesions are also a common finding in CLL.[7]

Similar findings are encountered in the myeloproliferative disorders. In polycythemia vera, clinical findings are variable although often striking. Increased blood viscosity and increased histamine from basophilia result in itching, especially after showering or bathing. There is a ruddy complexion, and splenomegaly is usually prominent.[1]

Clinical findings in the malignant lymphomas include non-tender, asymmetrical, firm, discrete, rubbery enlargement of the superficial lymph nodes. Cervical involvement is seen in 60% to 70% of cases. Clinical staging by means of radiologic techniques and surgical biopsy findings is important, and includes an indication of the presence or absence of symptoms such as fever, night sweats, and weight loss.[12] In multiple myeloma, symptoms are similar to the conditions described above, in which the normal function of the bone marrow is compromised by the replacement of normal with malignant cells. In addition, severe bone pain is a distinguishing feature of multiple myeloma.[10]

LABORATORY ANALYSES AND DIAGNOSIS[1, 3, 5]

Peripheral blood and bone marrow examinations are essential to the diagnosis of the majority of hematologic abnormalities. In addition to morphologic studies of blood, bone marrow, and lymph nodes, in the case of the lymphomas, immunologic and chemical studies are often useful as well. The results of useful histocytochemical studies are summarized in Table 51-1.

Acute Myelogenous Leukemia

M1

In M1, the bone marrow demonstrates markedly increased numbers of myeloblasts with very little maturation beyond the promyelocyte stage, combined with diminished numbers of erythroid and megakaryocyte precursors. The peripheral blood picture usually includes normocytic, normochromic anemia, thrombocytopenia, and variable numbers of myeloperoxidase-positive, immature cells (myeloblasts). In approximately 50% of patients, many myeloblasts are observed to contain Auer rods.

M2

In M2, the bone marrow demonstrates more maturation in the granulocytic series than in M1, with more than 10% promyelocytes and myelocytes and usually more than 30% myeloblasts. The myeloblasts are characteristically myeloperoxidase-positive, and many contain Auer rods. The peripheral blood often reveals abnormalities in nuclear and cytoplasmic maturation, including pseudo-Pelger-Huët. An anemia and thrombocytopenia exist that are directly proportional in severity to the number of myeloblasts in the bone marrow.

M3

M3 is characterized by demonstration in both the peripheral blood and the bone marrow of an increased number of myeloblasts and disproportionately increased numbers of hypergranular, intensely myeloperoxidase-positive promyelocytes, often with large numbers of delicate Auer rods in bundles (faggots). A variant form is seen, with the predominating promyelocyte demonstrating a monocytoid nucleus and microgranular to agranular cytoplasm. A chromosome abnormality t(15;17) is highly specific for but not always seen in promyelocytic leukemia.

M4

M4 is characterized by increased peripheral blood and bone marrow myeloblasts, many with Auer rods, and maturation forms that show monocytoid nuclei with neutrophilic cytoplasm. Adult monocytes are increased in both the peripheral blood and the bone marrow, with corresponding increases in serum lysozyme (muramidase) levels. Megaloblastic erythroid precursors and bizarre megakaryocytes are usually found in the bone marrow.

M5

Marked numbers of monoblasts (>80%) with very little differentiation are found in M5. The monoblasts contain plentiful delicate, azurophilic granulation in the abundant cytoplasm that is nonspecific esterase-positive with mild to absent myeloperoxidase positivity. Anemia and thrombocytopenia are commonly seen.

M6

Peripheral blood findings are extremely variable in M6, and include small to very large numbers of erythroid-looking blasts with mild to absent myeloperoxidase positivity. Anemia and thrombocytopenia are almost always seen. Bone marrow findings include a variable number of these abnormal erythroblasts, some of which contain Auer rods and/or periodic acid-Schiff (PAS)-positive

Table 51-1 ***Results of Histocytochemical Tests in Acute Leukemia***

	Peroxidase and Sudan Black B	Naphthol AS-D Choloroacetate (Specific Esterase)	Naphthol Butyrate (Nonspecific Esterase)	PAS	Oil Red O
ALL	Negative	Negative	Negative to weak	Positive, coarse; T-cell type may be negative	Positive; T-cell type may be negative
AML	Positive	Positive	Positive, fluoride-resistant	Negative to weak, diffuse	Negative
AMML	Positive	Granulocyte—positive Monocyte—negative	Positive, fluoride-sensitive and resistant	Negative to weak, diffuse or granular	Negative
AMoL	Positive	Negative to weak	Positive, fluoride-sensitive	Negative to weak, diffuse or granular	Negative

ALL = Acute lymphocytic leukemia
AML = Acute myelogenous leukemia
AMML = Acute myelomonocytic leukemia
AMoL = Acute monocytic leukemia

globules. The variable megaloblastic changes may create problems in distinguishing this leukemia from megaloblastic anemia due to B_{12} or folic acid deficiency.

Acute Lymphoblastic Leukemia

Hematologic findings in ALL commonly include normocytic, normochromic anemia, leukocyte counts that are quite variable, thrombocytopenia, and variable numbers of lymphoblasts. An aleukemic presentation is very common in children. The bone marrow is most often hypercellular, with a massive proliferation of leukemic blasts. The marrow may be difficult to aspirate (dry tap) because of marked hypercellularity and increased reticulum fibers.

The FAB differentiation of ALL is summarized in Table 51-2.

Note that the most useful cytologic features in differentiating L1 from L2 lymphoblastic leukemias are cell size, quantity of cytoplasm, and the presence and prominence of nucleoli. L3 is easily differentiated by the prominent cytoplasmic vacuoles. Cytochemically, 90% of all leukemic cells demonstrate terminal deoxyribosidyl transferase positivity, while most nonlymphocytic blasts are negative.

Chronic Myelogenous Leukemia

In chronic myelogenous leukemia, peripheral blood findings are variable but typically include normocytic, normochromic anemia, thrombocytosis with presence of large, atypical platelets and/or micromegakaryocytes, eosinophilia, and basophilia. Other findings include variably increased leukocyte counts with myeloblasts, promyelocytes, and

Table 51-2 ***FAB Classification of ALL***

Cytological Characteristics	L1	L2	L3
Cell size	Small, homogeneous	Large, heterogeneous	Large, homogeneous
Nucleus	Round, clefted, condensed chromatin	Round, indented, fine to coarse chromatin	Round to oval, fine chromatin
Nucleoli	Small, inconspicuous	One or more, prominent	One or more, large, prominent
Cytoplasm	Scanty, sl–mod basophilia	Moderate to abundant, variable basophilia	Mod, intense basophilia
Vacuoles	Variable	Variable	Sharply defined
Histochemistry			
PAS	+	+	–
Oil Red O	–	–	+
Myeloperoxidase	–	–	–
Sudan Black B	–	–	–

myelocytes. The last are sometimes disproportionately increased (myelocyte "hump"). There are also increased circulating normoblasts, decreased or absent leukocyte alkaline phosphatase scoring, and elevated serum uric acid, B_{12}, and LD levels. The bone marrow is markedly hypercellular and essentially depleted of fat, with aspiration difficult and smears indistinguishable from those of peripheral blood. Myelofibrosis is seen in approximately 40% of cases. The Ph′ chromosome t(9;22) can be seen in any myeloid cell in mitosis but not in lymphocytes.

Chronic Lymphocytic Leukemia

Laboratory findings in chronic lymphocytic leukemia include lymphocytosis with >70% of the white cells in the peripheral blood appearing as small, homogeneous lymphocytes with many damaged (smudge) cells. The same mechanical fragility allowing smudging of lymphocytes in the smear preparation may lead to spuriously lowered leukocyte counts performed by automated equipment. Normocytic, normochromic anemia and thrombocytopenia are more common in later stages of the disease. Bone marrow biopsy demonstrates variable amounts of focal or diffuse lymphocytic replacement of normal marrow elements. Reduced concentration of normal serum immunoglobulins is found in many patients, particularly in the advanced stages of disease, and hemolytic anemia with a positive direct antiglobulin test is sometimes seen.

In Galton's variant of this leukemia, laboratory findings include marked increases in peripheral and bone marrow lymphocytes that are large with moderately abundant, lightly basophilic cytoplasm. These cells have a round or oval nucleus with relatively condensed nuclear chromatin and a single large, centrally located, prominent nucleolus. The cells are morphologically indistinct from those found in the prolymphocytic transformation of CLL described above. Immunologic markers demonstrate approximately 70% with B-cell and 30% with T-cell characteristics. Surface immunoglobulin on these cells is usually more intense than that on the surface of the typical CLL B-lymphocytes.

Chronic T-cell leukemia is characterized by moderate increases in blood and marrow lymphocytes, with the predominant cell type having a large nucleus with condensed nuclear chromatin and abundant cytoplasm containing prominent azurophilic granulation. Marked neutropenia accompanies this distinct lymphocyte population.

Laboratory findings in hairy-cell leukemia include severe neutropenia. The proliferating cell type is slightly larger than most lymphocytes, with more delicate nuclear chromatin, nuclear folding or indentation, and cytoplasm that is moderate to abundant with a serrated cell border. The irregular and delicate cytoplasmic projections characteristic of these cells give this variant its name. This finding is more likely in smears made from blood without anticoagulants. Immunologically these cells demonstrate B-cell characteristics, and histochemically they demonstrate tartrate-resistant acid phosphatase activity. Bone marrow involvement is always present, and these lesions demonstrate extensive reticulum fibrosis with diffuse cellular infiltrates.

In Sezary syndrome, the lymphocytes demonstrate size variation but with consistently striking nuclear convolution, giving the nucleus a cerebriform appearance. The cytoplasm often contains PAS-positive vacuoles encircling the nucleus.

Laboratory findings, other than those mentioned above, are generally nonspecific and therefore not particularly useful in the diagnosis of leukemia. It should be noted that serum uric acid levels are increased in patients with large numbers of leukemic cells and in patients undergoing therapy with cytotoxic drugs. Phosphorus and potassium may also be increased for the same reason.[11]

CLL vs Benign Lymphocytosis

In some cases, CLL must be differentiated from benign conditions in which lymphocytes are greatly increased. The characteristics of CLL that serve to distinguish it from benign conditions include a persistent, peripheral blood absolute lymphocytosis of $>6.0 \times 10^3/mm^3$, with a median of $30.0–40.0 \times 10^3/mm^3$. Although bone marrow examination is not necessary for diagnosis, bone marrow findings would include increased lymphocytes in a hypercellular marrow, with a predominance of small lymphocytes. In CLL, not more than 30% of these cells would show prolymphocytic characteristics, and >20% would have irregular nuclei.

Myeloproliferative Disorders Other Than CML

POLYCYTHEMIA VERA

Peripheral blood findings in polycythemia vera are similar to those in CML, except for markedly elevated numbers of microcytic and often hypochromic erythrocytes. There is usually increased leukocyte alkaline phosphatase scoring. Characteristic bone marrow findings include increased myeloid elements and diminished to absent iron stores.

MYELOFIBROSIS

The peripheral blood picture is variable, but is generally characterized by the presence of atypical platelets, micromegakaryocytes, tear drop red cells, and coarse basophilic stippling. Mild basophilia and eosinophilia are sometimes seen. Normal to increased leukocyte alkaline phosphatase scoring is frequent.

MYELODYSPLASIA[6, 7, 8]

Myelodysplasia is characterized by erythrocytes showing megaloblastic changes that do not respond to B_{12} or folic acid therapy, and/or by increased ring-sideroblasts that are not responsive to pyridoxine. Granulocytes may show both nuclear hyposegmentation and cytoplasmic hypogranulation. Platelets often demonstrate both quantitative and qualitative defects.

Lymphoproliferative Disorders Other Than CLL[1, 12]

In Hodgkin's disease, peripheral blood findings are often unremarkable but, when abnormal, may include normocytic, normochromic anemia, eosinophilia, lymphopenia, and thrombocytopenia, especially in advanced disease. With marked marrow infiltration, bone marrow failure may occur, resulting in leukoerythroblastic reaction (LEBR), frequently seen in the peripheral blood. Diagnosis is made by histologic examination of involved lymph node(s), which must reveal Reed-Sternberg cells, a hallmark of this lymphoma category. A histologic classification scheme is employed based on tissue pattern and mix of lymphocytes and Reed-Sternberg cells.

NHL also involves a histopathologic diagnosis of lymphoid tissue. Abnormal cells infiltrate the peripheral blood more frequently than occurs in Hodgkin's, and these are often difficult to distinguish from those of certain leukemias.

In multiple myeloma, a severe normocytic, normochromic anemia is observed, often with neutropenia. Rouleaux of red blood cells are commonly observed on smears of peripheral blood, due to coating of the red blood cells with the monoclonal immunoglobulin produced in large amounts by the plasma cells. The abnormal amounts of protein also account for the blue background of smears stained with Wright's stain. If plasma cell leukemia has developed, the peripheral blood will contain very large numbers of plasma cells.

Serum immunoelectrophoresis reveals a characteristic monoclonal peak, usually IgG but sometimes IgA, IgD, etc., with decreased amounts of the other immunoglobulins. Urine electrophoresis often reveals the presence of Bence Jones protein (light chains) and is the procedure of choice for demonstrating this substance. Because Bence Jones protein is a globulin, it will not be detected by the usual urine dip stick methods that detect albumin. Other laboratory results of interest are those consistent with renal damage which often occurs in multiple myeloma. The bone marrow will contain large numbers of immature and atypical plasma cells having eccentric or multiple nuclei.[1, 3, 12]

TREATMENT

Untreated leukemias of any type are invariably fatal. The effectiveness of treatment is subject to many variables, including the age of the patient, the specific type of leukemia, and the individual patient's response to therapy. ALL is generally more responsive to treatment than are other types, with 90% of children and 85% of adults achieving complete remission.[11]

Treatment is aimed at the destruction of the entire abnormal clone of cells, with preservation of adequate normal stem cells and reticuloendothelial stroma to produce normal cells subsequent to treatment. All cells undergoing mitosis are vulnerable to destruction by mitotic poisons, including radiation and chemotherapeutic agents. Destruction of the abnormal cell population may also lead to destruction of the normal population of stem cells, particularly in the myelogenous leukemias. In this event, bone marrow transplant is the only alternative. Treatment of lymphocytic leukemias can be directed more specifically toward the lymphocytes and precursors, leaving the victim immunodeficient but with minimal destruction of myeloid elements.[1, 3, 5]

The selection of a treatment regimen is complicated because of the many variables involved and the lack, therefore, of standardized treatment protocols. Patients with acute leukemias require aggressive therapy because death can ensue within days of diagnosis. Most initial regimens in ALL include prednisone and vincristine. In ANLL, treatment is less effective than in ALL, particularly in older patients. Treatment usually includes an anthracycline and arabinosyl cytosine, and often a purine analogue. In all cases a major objective is to lower the cell count, and daily cell counts are necessary to follow treatment. Bone marrow transplants are being used more frequently following destruction of the leukemic cell population.

Good supportive care is necessary to control infection, bleeding, and anemia. Infusions of packed red cells, platelet concentrates, and fresh, histocompatible leukocytes (except in patients receiving amphotericin) may be helpful in this regard.[11]

CML is generally controlled by oral alkylating agents. Splenectomy is reserved for patients with repeated splenic infarcts or prolonged thrombocytopenia following treatment. Treatment in CLL is reserved for the point at which enlargement of nodes or spleen occurs or when normal hematopoiesis is disrupted. Corticosteroids and alkylating agents in combination are useful, but risk of infection is high. Splenectomy, except in the case of hairy-cell leukemia, is generally not effective in improving the hematologic picture.[7]

The treatment of the malignant lymphomas is in transition but has been effective nevertheless. Drugs and radiation therapy are used, and treatment of Hodgkin's and NHL requires great skill and experience on the part of the physician.[12]

Treatment of multiple myeloma is directed at eliminating the abnormal plasma cell population, and generally involves alkylating agents in combination with glucocorticoids. Plasma cell leukemia can occur as a result of treatment.[1, 10]

CASE STUDY #1

A 72-year-old woman presented to the emergency room with a burn from boiling water on her right leg and left ankle, now showing cellulitis.

LABORATORY FINDINGS

Peripheral Blood Findings	***Reference Range***
Hgb: 8.9 g/dL (1.38 mmol/L)	12–16 g/dL (1.86–2.48)
WBC: 136.0 × 10^3/mm^3	4.5–10.0 × 10^3/mm^3
Platelets: 680.0 × 10^3/mm^3	150.0–350.0 × 10^3/mm^3

Differential	*Relative (%)*	*Absolute (per mm^3)*
Blasts	2.5	0
Promyelocytes	2.5	0
Myelocytes and metamyelocytes	30.5	0
Neutrophil bands	27.0	150–1700
Neutrophil adults	25.5	1400–5000
Eosinophils	3.0	20–450
Basophils	3.5	0–150
Monocytes	2.0	70–700
Lymphocytes	3.5	1500–4200
Normoblasts	3/100 WBC	0

Peripheral Blood Findings	***Reference Range***
Leukocyte alkaline phosphate (LAP) score:	50-70
142 during burn infection	
10 after burn had healed	

Bone Marrow Findings

Aspirate—resembled peripheral blood

Trephine—marked hypercellularity with megakaryocyte hyperplasia

Cytogenetics—Ph′ chromosome present

Clinical Findings

Splenomegaly and hepatomegaly

Questions

1. Which findings distinguish this presentation as a malignant state rather than an inflammatory process?
2. Which leukemia does this patient have?
3. What is the prognosis in this case?

Discussion

1. Basophilia and eosinophilia are rarely seen in inflammatory reactions. Ph′ chromosome is seen only in malignant cell clones.
2. This patient has chronic myelogenous leukemia.
3. The prognosis is 3 to 5 years, with remission of proliferation after chemotherapy.

CASE STUDY #2

A 78-year-old man presented to the emergency room with swelling and pain in his left leg due to deep vein thrombosis and past diagnosis (2 years) of chronic lymphocytic leukemia.

LABORATORY FINDINGS

Peripheral Blood Findings	Reference Range
Hgb: 8.9 g/dL (1.38 mmol/L)	14–18 g/dL (2.17–2.79 mmol/L)
WBC: 220.0 × 10^3/mm^3	4.5–10.0 × 10^3/mm^3
Differential and morphology: monotonous mature lymphocytes, including some with clefts and nucleoli. Many smudge cells are seen.	
Platelets: 179.0 × 10^3/mm^3	150.0–350.0 × 10^3/mm^3
Reticulocytes: 3.6% (corrected 2.7%)	0.5–2.0%
Uric acid: 11.7 mg/dL (0.69 mmol/L)	3.5–7.2 mg/dL (0.21–0.42 mmol/L)

Bone Marrow Findings

Lymphocytes—98%

Mixed population of monotonous, mature cells with another population showing clefts and prominent nucleoli. Diffuse proliferation of both populations are seen in the trephine.

Questions

1. Is this picture significant of a conversion of chronic lymphocytic leukemia to acute lymphoblastic leukemia?
2. Name and describe this disease process.
3. What is the prognosis for this disease?

Discussion

1. Conversion to acute lymphoblastic leukemia occurs rarely, if ever, and mature cells are not consistent with an acute phase.
2. The disease process is Richter's syndrome, a combination of chronic lymphocytic leukemia and lymphoma.
3. The prognosis in this case is very poor (2–6 months).

REFERENCES

1. Williams WJ: Hematology, pp 560–996. New York City, McGraw-Hill, 1983
2. Haus E, Lakatua DL, Swoyer JK et al: Chronobiology in hematology and immunology. Am J Anat 168:467–517, 1983
3. Koepke JA: Laboratory Medicine, Vols I and II, pp 143–228. New York City, Churchill Livingstone, 1984
4. Linmann JW: Hematology: Physiologic, Pathophysiologic, and Clinical Principles, pp 539–822. New York City, Macmillan, 1975
5. Henry JB: Clinical Diagnosis and Management by Laboratory Methods, pp 704–748. Philadelphia, WB Saunders, 1984
6. Bennett JM et al: Proposals for the classification of acute leukemias. Br J Haematol 33:451–458, 1976
7. Canellos GP: The Chronic Leukemias. In Petersdorf RG et al (eds): Harrison's Principles of Internal Medicine, pp 808–810. New York City: McGraw-Hill, 1983
8. Bennett JM et al: Proposals for the classification of the myelodysplastic syndromes. Br J Haematol 51:189–199, 1982
9. Travis WD, Pierre RV: Preleukemia/Dysmyelopoietic Syndrome. Lab Med 16:157, 1985
10. Alexanian R: Plasma Cell Neoplasms and Related Disorders. In Petersdorf RG et al (eds): Harrison's Principles of Internal Medicine, pp 362–367. New York City, McGraw-Hill, 1983
11. Clarkson B: The Acute Leukemias. In Petersdorf RG et al (eds): Harrison's Principles of Internal Medicine, pp 798–807. New York City, McGraw-Hill, 1983
12. Ultmann JE, DeVita VT: Hodgkin's Disease and Other Lymphomas. In Petersdorf RG et al (eds): Harrison's Principles of Internal Medicine, pp 811–824. New York City, McGraw-Hill, 1983

Chapter 52

Hemostatic Disorders

Cheryl Swinehart

INTRODUCTION

Plasma Coagulation System

In most cases, the clotting proteins circulate as inactive precursors and become an active enzyme (serine protease) after proteolytic cleavage or conformational change. The clotting system has historically been divided into two pathways, the intrinsic and the extrinsic, both of which end in a final common pathway (see Figs. 52-1 and 52-2). The intrinsic pathway is initiated by surface-mediated reactions that are intrinsic to the vessel, while the

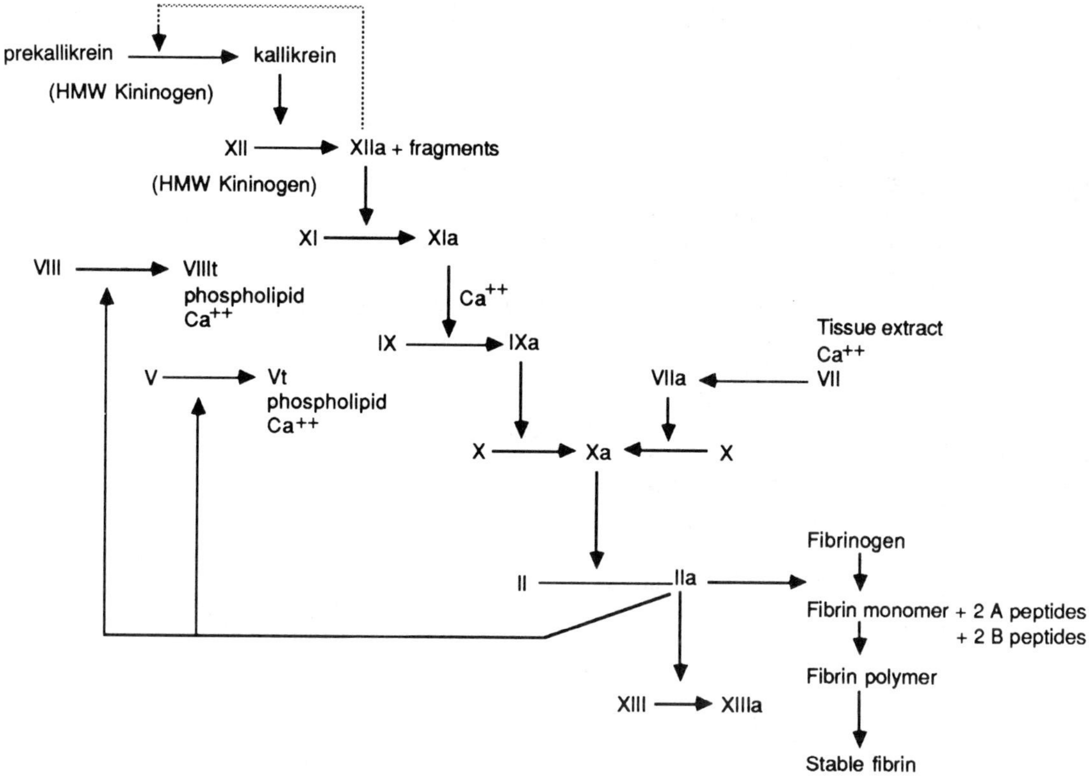

Figure 52-1 **Schematic of the plasma coagulation system.**

extrinsic pathway requires a tissue factor for activation. As more is learned, the distinction between these two pathways diminishes.[1]

The intrinsic pathway begins with the activation of factor XII. Although the initial process of activation of factor XII has been disputed, it now appears to involve two steps. The extrinsic pathway begins with the release of tissue factor from an injured vessel. Tissue factor that acts as a cofactor, Ca^{2+}, and factor VII activate factor X (see Fig. 52-2). After factor X is activated to Xa, the extrinsic pathway is the same as the intrinsic pathway activation of prothrombin and fibrinogen.

Platelets

When platelets are activated, a membrane phospholipid (platelet factor 3) is exposed. The phospholipid is involved in several steps in the coagulation pathway. These include the activation of factor II, factor X, and factor XI, and the activation of factor XII by kallikrein. Once the coagulation mechanism is activated and thrombin is formed, it reinforces the platelets with a fibrin mesh.

As platelets are activated they undergo many changes. These include shape change, adhesion, internal contraction, and aggregation. Platelets appear to undergo two types of adhesion. With minor breaks in the endothelium, platelets adhere to the endothelial cells and seal over the injury. No aggregation appears to take place with this type of injury. With more extensive injury, within seconds platelets adhere to the subendothelium and exposed collagen.

Adhesion requires platelet surface glycoprotein lb (GPlb), factor VIII/von Willebrand factor (VWF)

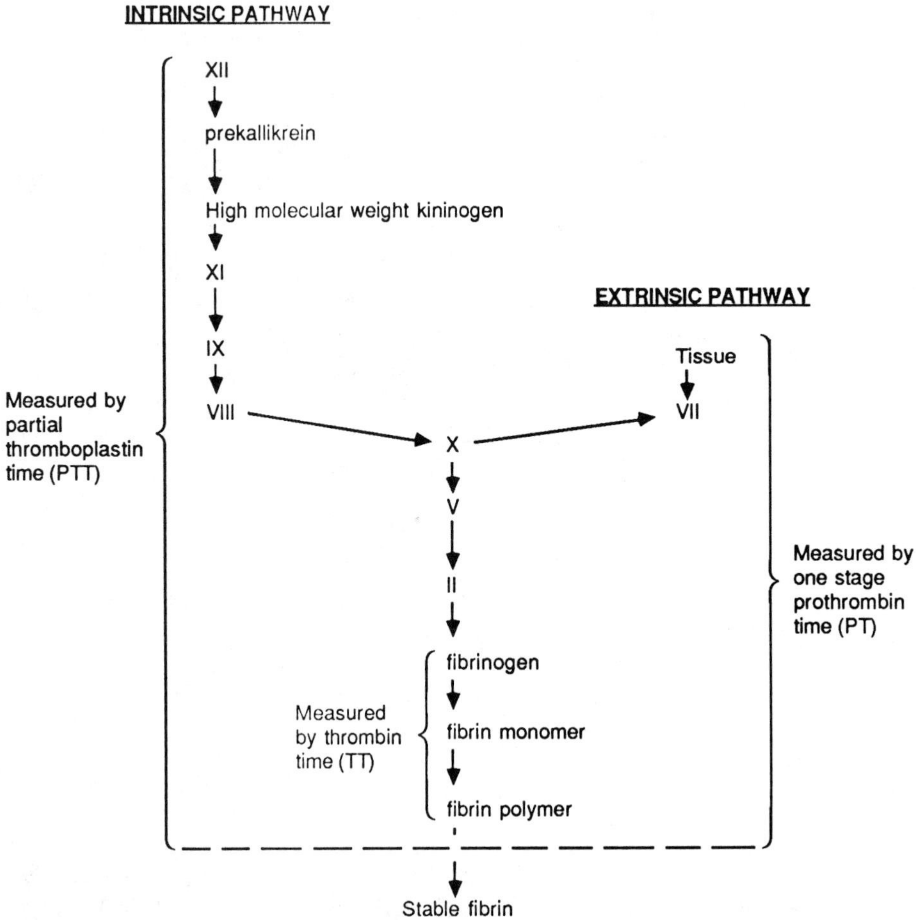

Figure 52-2 **Schematic of the extrinsic and intrinsic plasma coagulation system.**

as a cofactor, and exposed connective tissue elements of the subendothelium following vascular injury.[2] The platelet membrane GPIb appears to act as the surface receptor for VWF; therefore, absence of either GPIb or VWF results in defective platelet adhesion.

With more extensive injury, after the subendothelial tissue is exposed, it is rapidly covered by a layer of adhering platelets. This is usually followed very rapidly by the formation of platelet aggregates on top of the adhering platelets.[3] Platelet aggregometry is used to study this process *in vitro*. Platelet aggregation by adenosine diphosphate (ADP) requires platelet membrane GPIIb and GPIIIa, Ca^{2+}, and fibrinogen. Platelets will not aggregate if any of these components are missing.[2] Platelet aggregation occurs in two stages, primary and secondary. The shape change and primary aggregation are reversible reactions. Higher concentrations of agonists cause secondary aggregation, which is mostly irreversible.

During the aggregation process the platelets degranulate. Platelets contain both alpha granules and dense bodies. The alpha granules contain platelet factor 4, β-thromboglobulin, factor VIII/VWF, factor V, fibrinogen, fibronectin, mitogenic factor, and thrombospondin. The dense bodies contain ADP, serotonin, and Ca^{2+}. During secondary aggregation, ADP and many of these other substances are released from the platelet granules and secreted into the surrounding plasma. In the plasma, ADP may increase by as much as seven times. Secondary aggregation and secretion are mediated primarily by released ADP and thromboxane A2, and are mostly irreversible.

The aggregated platelets are loosely bound until a fibrin mesh, mediated through the clotting system and thrombin, stabilizes the clot. The platelets eventually retract into a dense thrombus. It is useful to think about platelet abnormalities in relation to the four steps described: adhesion, aggregation, release, and interaction of the clotting system.

Prostaglandins

Thromboxane A2 is a derivative of prostaglandins, which are synthesized after cleavage of arachidonic acid, found in membrane phospholipids. The prostaglandins that are formed are then acted upon by two different enzymes. If thromboxane synthetase acts on prostaglandin, the result is the production of thromboxane A2, which is a powerful platelet aggregant and vasoconstrictor. If prostacyclin synthetase is the enzyme, it leads to the production of prostacyclin, which is a powerful inhibitor of platelet aggregation and is a vasodilator. Anything that increases the synthesis of thromboxane A2 or decreases the production of prostacyclin will increase platelet aggregation. Aspirin affects the secondary aggregation of platelets by blocking the production of prostaglandins from arachidonic acid.

Vitamin K

The vitamin K-dependent factors (factors II, VII, IX, X, protein C, protein S) are produced by the liver, but require vitamin K for their complete synthesis. Vitamin K is required to carboxylate the glutamic portions of these molecules. Without carboxylation the protein cannot bind calcium ions, although the protein has the same antigenic determinants as a functional factor. The binding of calcium ions is important because the calcium forms bridges to phospholipid surfaces and allows the trace plasma proteins to be concentrated enough for activation and interaction with cofactors and substrates. Without vitamin K there is no calcium ion binding and the factors circulate with markedly impaired clotting activity. Factors made in the absence of vitamin K can be activated by nonphysiological activators such as the snake venom of Echis carinatus (saw-scaled viper), because this activation does not require adsorption to a phospholipid surface. Because vitamin K is only stored in the body for a few days, vitamin K deficiency can occur rapidly.

Fibrinolysis

The fibrinolytic mechanism is primarily an enzymatic process that removes fibrin deposits and reestablishes flow in vessels. The main component of fibrinolysis is the inactive precursor protein plasminogen. Plasminogen activators that are found in the blood stream and in tissues or the vessel wall activate plasminogen to the active enzyme plasmin. Plasmin then digests fibrin into X and Y fragments, and later into the smaller D and E fragments.[4] Fibrinogen, factors V and VIII, and other proteins also are substrates for plasmin. It appears that plasminogen is incorporated into the fibrin clot as it forms, and thus is readily available for lysis of the clot.

Inhibitors

The body must have a way of controlling clot formation if coagulation is initiated *in vivo*. Regulation usually occurs because of naturally occurring inhibitors, many of these being serine protease inhibitors. Two of the major inhibitors are antithrombin III and protein C. Antithrombin III primarily neutralizes thrombin (IIa); however, it can also neutralize factors Xa, IXa, XIIa, and kallikrein. After activation by thrombin, protein C inactivates activated factors V and VIII, which decreases the activity of the plasma coagulation system. Other naturally occurring inhibitors include α-2-macroglobulin, α-1-antitrypsin, C-1 esterase inhibitor, and α-2-antiplasmin. α-2-antiplasmin is a powerful inactivator of plasmin and helps control the lysis of clots. Deficiency of antithrombin III or protein C can lead to a thrombotic tendency, while deficiency of α-2-antiplasmin can lead to a bleeding tendency.

ETIOLOGY AND PATHOPHYSIOLOGY

Hereditary Coagulation Disorders

Identification has been made of deficiencies in all the coagulation proteins. Many proteins were discovered when a specific patient with an unexplained bleeding history or abnormal coagulation result was studied. The frequency of inheriting a plasma coagulation defect is about 1 in 10,000 persons. Von Willebrand's disease (Factor VIII/VWF deficiency) is the most common hereditary abnormality, followed by hemophilia A (Factor VIII deficiency) and hemophilia B (Factor IX deficiency). The other factor deficiencies are rare.

Clinical manifestations of these inherited abnormalities are variable, ranging from severe bleeding to normal clotting. The milder forms of the diseases occur with more frequency than do the severe forms. The diagnosis of severe forms is usually made clinically and is confirmed by laboratory tests. Mild forms may be recognized only when a patient is challenged hemostatically, and laboratory evaluation may be difficult.

Acquired Coagulation Disorders

LIVER DISEASE

In liver disease, a combination of coagulation abnormalities is common. This is due to the liver's involvement in many facets of hemostasis, including the synthesis of many clotting factors, the clearance of activated clotting factors from the circulation, and fibrinolysis. Approximately 85% of patients with liver disease have at least onc hemostatic abnormality, and 15% have clinical bleeding.[5] A low platelet count is often seen, which may be due to folate deficiency, increased splenic pooling, or decreased bone marrow production because of ethanol abuse. Higher than normal levels of fibrin(ogen) degradation products in the plasma, perhaps due to decreased clearance, may lead to platelet function abnormalities or an increased bleeding time. Disseminated intravascular coagulation (DIC) may accompany liver disease.

VITAMIN K DEFICIENCY

The usual sources of vitamin K in humans are dietary intake (green plants) and synthesis by gastrointestinal flora. Vitamin K is fat-soluble, and thus requires bile salts and pancreatic lipase for absorption in the GI tract. There are enough stores of vitamin K in the human body to last approximately 2 weeks. A common reason for a patient to become vitamin K-deficient in the hospital is removal of both sources of vitamin K by, for example, maintenance on I.V. fluids and broad-spectrum antibiotics or gastroenteritis. Dietary deficiency alone is rarely seen. Due to immaturity of the liver and low levels of the vitamin K factors, some babies may exhibit bleeding (hemorrhagic disease of the newborn). This is partly due to a lack of vitamin K in the diet (breast milk is a poor source of vitamin K) and a sterile gut. Bleeding usually occurs on the second or third day after birth. Although many babies do not bleed, vitamin K is now administered to most newborns at birth.[5]

PLATELET DEFECTS

Acquired qualitative platelet defects are fairly common and accompany a wide range of diseases and drugs. Drug effect causes the largest number of platelet dysfunctions, by a variety of mechanisms. Aspirin is probably the most common drug causing platelet dysfunction. Aspirin ingestion is characterized by a defective secondary wave of aggregation and often a mild increase in the bleeding time. While aspirin affects the function of the platelet for the life of the platelet, or about 8 days, many other drugs affect the function of the platelet only as long as the drug is in the circulation. Platelet function returns to normal when the drug is metabolized. Some drugs in each of the following categories have been reported to cause transient platelet dysfunction: nonsteroidal antiinflammatory agents, antihistamines, phenothiazines, sympathetic blocking agents, antibiotics, and diuretics.

Uremia also produces platelet dysfunction, which seems to intensify as the amounts of metabolic products increase in the blood. The treatment of choice is dialysis to remove the metabolic products.

Increased fibrin(ogen) degradation products (FDPs) can cause mild platelet dysfunction. Often this is difficult to evaluate because increased FDPs are often accompanied by many other hemostatic abnormalities, for example, in DIC.

Dysproteinemias or hyperfibrinogenemia (as seen in hemophiliac patients receiving large quantities of cryoprecipitate) can cause platelet dysfunction. The mechanism for this is not known, but may be due to interference by the protein at the reaction site on the platelet membrane surface.

Patients with myeloproliferative disorders (polycythemia vera, chronic myelogenous leukemia, agnogenic myeloid metaplasia, essential thrombocytosis) may exhibit platelet dysfunction. The abnormality demonstrated may vary from patient to patient. Abnormal platelet aggregation, especially with epinephrine, is common.

Von Willebrand's disease is sometimes classified as a platelet disorder, because the platelets do not adhere normally. The lack of adhesion is actually due, however, to a plasma cofactor deficiency, and the platelets are functionally normal.

DISSEMINATED INTRAVASCULAR COAGULATION (DIC)

DIC is a syndrome that has been given various names such as defibrination syndrome, consumption coagulopathy, and intravascular coagulation–fibrinolysis syndrome. It describes a condition in which platelets and fibrinogen are consumed. DIC is always a secondary phenomenon, the process being triggered by some underlying condition in the patient. There are several mechanisms that initiate DIC. One of these is extensive endothelial damage, with exposure of collagen. Collagen may activate the intrinsic pathway of coagulation or provide a surface for platelets to adhere to and thereby form a plug. Another means of initiating DIC is by the release of thromboplastic substances into the bloodstream, with the subsequent activation of the extrinsic pathway of coagulation. A third means of triggering DIC is by exposure to specific proteases such as snake venoms, trypsin, or some commercial factor IX concentrates. Thus, DIC can be initiated by activation of the intrinsic pathway, the extrinsic pathway, platelets, or any combination of these. There are many clinical conditions associated with DIC. Some of the most common are infections, obstetrical disorders, malignancy, surgery, and shock. It is important to remember that whenever the coagulation system is activated, the fibrinolytic system is also activated. This will lead to the degradation of fibrin(ogen) and factors V and VIII.

Either thrombosis, bleeding, or no abnormality may be associated with DIC, depending on the rate of production and the rate of consumption of the various components. In cases in which a small amount of thrombin is generated, levels of fibrinogen and platelets may actually increase and lead to thrombosis. An example of this is found in some cancers in which the slow destruction of cells releases a small amount of thromboplastin. The thromboplastin, in turn, causes small amounts of thrombin to be generated, which leads to increased risk of thrombosis for the patient.

Normal hemostasis will be observed in patients in whom the body is able to manufacture enough hemostatic components to compensate for the increased destruction. Platelets and fibrinogen are being consumed at greater than normal levels, but the body can compensate, and thus no bleeding occurs. Increased utilization in these patients can only be demonstrated with research tests such as survival studies of ^{51}Cr-platelets and ^{125}I-fibrinogen.[2]

Bleeding occurs because the components of coagulation are being consumed faster than they are being produced. In DIC patients, bleeding occurs by three main mechanisms or a combination of these mechanisms. One is the decreased levels of coagulation factors, including fibrinogen. Second, if enough platelets are consumed, thrombocytopenia occurs. Last, the increased lysis of fibrin(ogen) leads to degradation products that may interfere with normal platelet function.

MASSIVELY-TRANSFUSED PATIENT

Blood that is stored in the blood bank retains normal levels of most of the coagulation factors, except factors V and VIII. If a patient is transfused with large quantities (10–20 units) of stored bank blood, cryoprecipitate may also be required to increase the concentration of factor VIII and fibrinogen.[2] Thrombocytopenia is common in massively transfused patients; therefore, platelet concentrates may be needed. A platelet count near $100{,}000/mm^3$ is desirable.

INHIBITORS

Some inhibitors of clotting can be found in normal plasma. These include antithrombin III, α-1-antitrypsin, α-2-antiplasmin, C-1 esterase inhibitor, and α-2-macroglobulin. Circulating inhibitors may also be acquired. Certain inhibitors are acquired after blood or blood component transfusions, some are due to drugs, some occur frequently in certain diseases, and some arise spontaneously, especially in the elderly. Inhibitors may act upon one or several coagulation factors. Inhibitors may or may not be associated with a bleeding tendency.

The most common specific factor inhibitor is directed against factor VIII. Approximately 10% to 15% of hemophiliacs will develop antibodies directed against factor VIII.[4] Antibodies against factor VIII may also develop in postpartum women and spontaneously in the elderly. The clinical picture of these patients may resemble that of the hemophiliac, because the antibodies have destroyed their factor VIII. The bleeding diathesis that results may be mild to life-threatening.

Patients with lupus erythematosus can also have a number of problems with their hemostatic system, including thrombocytopenia, specific factor-VIII antibodies, a specific prothrombin deficiency, and a nonspecific inhibitor. While the first three of these may be associated with bleeding, the last is not. The nonspecific inhibitor has been found to react against phospholipid in some patients. In other patients the contact phase of coagulation is acted upon. Thus, there may be more than one type of antibody. When discovered before surgery, because the nonspecific inhibitor alone is not a cause for bleeding, it should be a concern only if any other coagulation abnormalities are present.

Some inhibitors are produced by drugs. One common drug-induced inhibitor is heparin, which enhances the inhibition of proteases by antithrombin III. Heparin is usually administered intravenously and is often used in the treatment of deep venous thrombosis or pulmonary embolism and during kidney dialysis or open-heart surgery. Another class of drugs that cause inhibition of the clotting mechanism are the coumarin drugs. Coumarin competes with vitamin K and prevents the carboxylation of the vitamin K-dependent factors. Without carboxylation, the factors circulate but have markedly impaired activity.

Thrombosis

While much is known about bleeding in patients, thromboembolic disease is less clearly understood. There are several physiological variables that can influence the formation of a thrombus, or blood clot, in a vessel or heart chamber. These include the flow rate of the vessel, alteration of the vessel wall, entry of large quantities of activators of coagulation into the blood stream, defects in the natural inhibitors of coagulation, and a decrease in the ability of the fibrinolytic system to lyse a clot.

The flow rate of arteries is usually undisturbed and rapid, and thus the clot formed is often a "white thrombus" consisting mostly of platelets and fibrin deposits. The flow rate of veins may be disturbed and slower, so activated coagulation factors become more important and a "red thrombus" consisting of trapped red blood cells and fibrin is more likely.[2] The thrombus that forms may adhere to the side of the vessel, allowing blood to flow, or it may be occlusive and block the vessel. If a white thrombus is occlusive, red thrombi may form behind it because the flow of blood is decreased behind the blockage.

Alterations in the vessel wall are important because exposure of the subendothelium uncovers collagen, which can activate platelets and the plasma coagulation system. The activated platelets not only adhere to the surface and aggregate together, but also provide a phospholipid surface on which the coagulation system can act. The endpoint of the coagulation system, thrombin, converts factor XIII to XIIIa, which stabilizes the clot. There are several mechanisms for altering vessel walls, including trauma (such as surgery or catheters) and immunologic or infectious agents.

Some situations do not require endothelial damage for thrombus formation. One example is the release of large quantities of activators of coagulation into the blood stream. During surgery, large quantities of tissue factor or thromboplastin may be released and activate the coagulation system, which can lead to thrombi in the circulation. Other conditions associated with activation of coagulation *in vivo* are malignancies, injection of snake venom, and bacteremia. These may lead to thrombosis or DIC, depending on both the rate of production and the rate of consumption of the hemostatic factors.

Defects in the natural inhibitors of coagulation, such as inherited deficiencies of antithrombin III or protein C, can lead to thrombosis. Antithrombin III (AT-III) deficiency has been recognized in several families with thrombotic tendencies. The disease is autosomal recessive, and the thrombotic events are primarily venous. AT-III deficiency can also be acquired, as is the case in patients with nephrotic syndrome. The decrease in AT-III does not have to be severe to cause thrombosis; half-normal levels appear to cause significant thrombosis. Patients with suspected AT-III deficiency should be tested for both functional and immunologic AT-III, because families with dysantithrombinemia also appear to have a thrombotic tendency. Patients who have decreased levels of AT-III cannot be treated with heparin because heparin requires AT-III as a cofactor. Long-term anticoagulation is usually the treatment of choice.

Other causes of thrombosis include protein C deficiency, which is inherited as an autosomal dominant trait. Patients with depleted levels of protein C appear to suffer recurrent thrombophlebitis and pulmonary embolism, probably because activated protein C is responsible for inactivation of factors Va and VIIIa. Patients with suspected protein C deficiency should be tested for both functional and immunologic protein C. Treatment for these patients is usually long-term oral anticoagulation.

Defects in the fibrinolytic system can also lead to thrombosis, because the body has less ability to lyse clots once they form. Some examples include hereditary excess of antiplasmin and dysfunctional plasminogen. Patients with suspected plasminogen deficiency should have tests for both immunologic and functional plasminogen performed, as genetically abnormal plasminogen has been reported. The mechanism for thrombosis in some dysfibrinogenemias may be a fibrinogen resistant to lysis. It is important to remember that, whatever the cause of thrombosis, stasis is a critical element. The more venous stasis that is present, the greater the risk of thrombosis.

CLINICAL MANIFESTATIONS

A useful way to approach clinical findings is to determine whether the hemostatic abnormality involves the primary or the secondary mechanism. Bleeding involving the primary or platelet system is often characterized by immediate bleeding that stops when direct pressure is applied. Hemorrhages into the skin and mucous membrane are common, as are petechiae and frequent bruises after minor trauma. Patients with an abnormal primary mechanism often have epistaxis, menorrhagia, and genitourinary and gastrointestinal hemorrhages.

Bleeding involving the secondary or clot-forming mechanism is often characterized by bleeding into deep tissue, especially into joints and muscles. Ecchymoses and hematomas are common findings. Delayed bleeding (which may be hours or even days later) may occur, and often cannot be controlled by direct pressure. Hemarthrosis and crippling due to injured joints may occur in more severe cases.

One of the more difficult diagnoses in hemostasis is the differentiation of hemophilia A (factor VIII deficiency) and von Willebrand's disease. The clinical pictures tend to be different in severe cases, but similar if the disease is mild. Severe hemophiliacs may have spontaneous bleeding into joint spaces and muscles. Mild hemophiliacs may have easy bruising and excessive bleeding after trauma. Von Willebrand's disease is characterized by mild mucous membrane bleeding, such as epistaxis, menorrhagia, and easy bruising; however, symptoms may vary from day to day in the same individual. Because patients with mild hemophilia and von Willebrand's disease may only bleed after a hemostatic challenge, they may have an inconclusive personal and family history.

The type of bleeding most often seen in vitamin K deficiency is oozing, easy bruisability and bleeding from venipuncture sites.

Bleeding is the complication most often seen in DIC, and can vary from bleeding from venipuncture sites and ecchymoses to severe gastrointestinal or central nervous system bleeds.

LABORATORY ANALYSES AND DIAGNOSIS

Whenever the competency of the hemostatic system is in question, a thorough history and physical examination must be performed. The history may be the most important screening test in the diagnosis of a bleeding disorder. Several questions should be asked during the taking of the history. These include

1. Age at onset of bleeding (whether the disorder is short-term or life-long)
2. Sites of bleeding (*e.g.*, nosebleeds, joints, G.I. tract)
3. Whether bleeding was spontaneous or induced
4. Duration of bleeding (with any blood replacement therapy or iron treatment)
5. Treatment for bleeding (*e.g.*, direct pressure, cauterization, blood products)
6. Prior challenges to the hemostatic system (especially tooth extractions, circumcision, fractures, sprains—including amount of swelling or disability)
7. Prior operations (including tonsillectomy)
8. Purpura (type and frequency)
9. Menstrual history
10. Drug history (including aspirin and anticoagulants)
11. Other local or systemic diseases (especially splenomegaly, lymphadenopathy, liver failure, or residual joint deformities)
12. Detailed family history (as much bleeding history as is possible for each family member. If the family history is positive, an effort should be made to establish an inheritance pattern.)

Laboratory Approach to Bleeding Disorders

PRIMARY VS SECONDARY COAGULATION SYSTEMS

When the information from the history and physical examination is combined with data from the screening tests listed on page 653, a decision can usually be made about whether the hemostatic problem is in the primary or secondary system. A schematic of the laboratory approach to a defect in the primary mechanism is shown in Figure 52-3.[5] The first consideration is whether the platelet count is normal or low. A low platelet count, thrombocytopenia, can be caused by decreased platelet production, increased platelet destruction, or changes in distribution. Because approximately one-third of the body's platelets are stored in the spleen, any condition that increases the size of the spleen will decrease the platelet count in the peripheral circulation. A bone marrow exam may help to decide the cause of the thrombocytopenia as well as determine the presence or absence of underlying marrow diseases. If the megakaryocyte number appears normal or increased in the bone marrow, the cause of the thrombocytopenia is probably accelerated destruction or a change in distribution. If the megakaryocyte count is reduced, the cause is probably decreased production. Some examples of disorders that involve thrombocytopenia are listed in Figure 52-3. Other laboratory tests that may be indicated if a patient is thrombocytopenic are an antiglobulin test for auto-

Laboratory Screening Tests for Hemostatic Abnormalities

Platelet count
Examination of the peripheral blood smear
Bleeding time
Prothrombin time
Activated partial thromboplastin time
Thrombin time
Fibrinogen

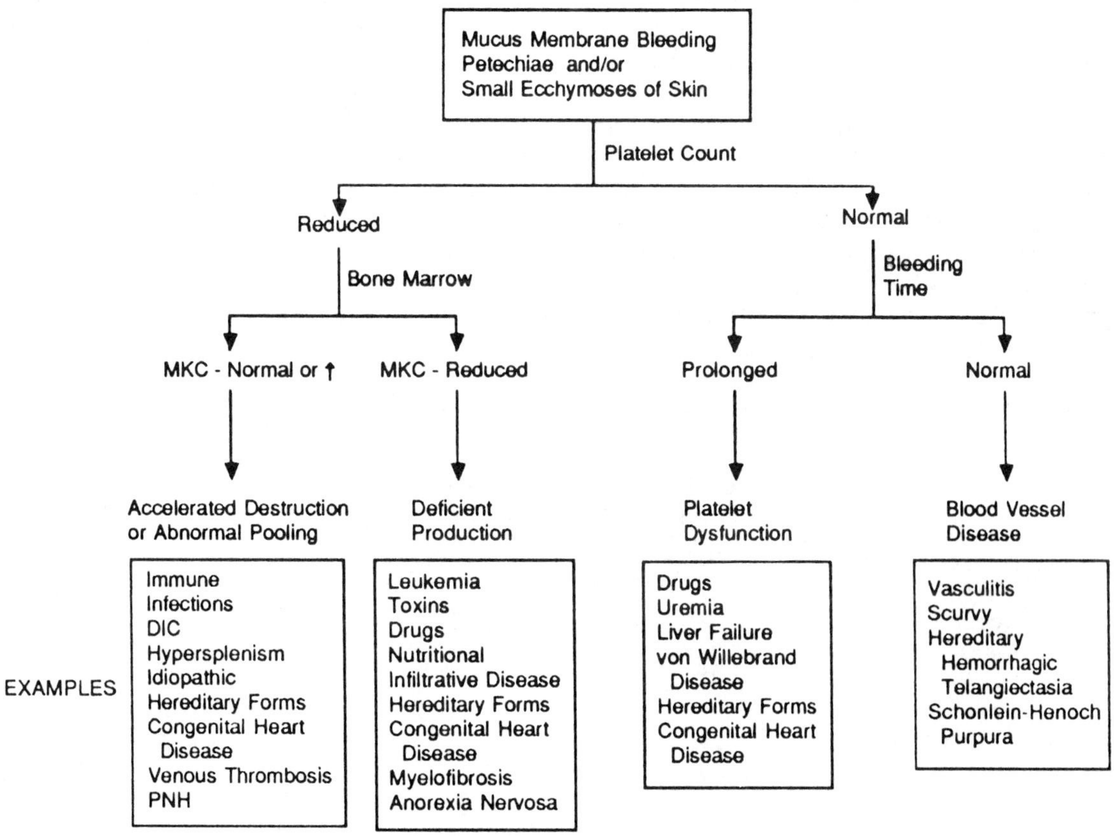

Figure 52-3 Work-up of patient with defect in the primary hemostatic mechanism. (From Corrigan JJ Jr. [ed]: Hemorrhagic and Thrombotic Diseases in Childhood and Adolescence. New York, Churchill Livingstone, 1985. Reprinted with permission)

antibodies, antinuclear antibody testing, or, on occasion, an ultrastructural examination or platelet antibody studies.

If the platelet count of the patient is normal and a bleeding history is positive, the next test usually performed is the bleeding time. If the bleeding time is also normal, a blood vessel disease should be suspected. Some examples are listed in Figure 52-3. If the platelet count is normal and the bleeding time is prolonged, a qualitative platelet disorder should be suspected. These platelet abnormalities may be inherited or acquired. Most are associated with a mild bleeding tendency, unless the hemostatic challenge is severe. Hereditary abnormalities are rare, so they will be discussed only briefly. The significant laboratory results for the major inherited disorders are given in Table 52-1.[6] The laboratory tests usually used to distinguish these diseases are platelet count, bleeding time, platelet adhesiveness test, and platelet aggregation studies. Storage pool deficiencies can be of either alpha granules or dense granules. The "gray platelet syndrome" has a nearly complete absence of alpha granules, while the Hermansky-Pudlak syndrome lacks dense granules and thus ADP. The type of abnormalities seen in the laboratory tests vary with the granule missing.

A schematic for laboratory evaluation of the secondary or plasma coagulation system is given in Figure 52-4.[5] The prothrombin time is used to test for factors X, V, II, and I, while the partial thromboplastin time tests for factors XII, XI, HMWK, IX, VIII, X, V, II, I, and prekallikrein (Fletcher factor), Figure 52-2. When using these two screening tests in a patient with a single factor deficiency, if the PT is long and the APTT is normal, the patient should have factor VII deficiency. If the APTT is long and the PT is normal, the patient should have a factor XII, XI, HMWK, IX, VIII, or prekallikrein (Fletcher factor) deficiency. Because of the higher frequency of occurrence of factor VIII and IX deficiency, it is probably one of these. If both the PT and APTT are prolonged, the patient should have a factor X, V, II, or I deficiency. Thrombin times are performed to check that enough fibrinogen is present to produce a clot and also to check for the presence of heparin. The above scheme works for single factor deficiencies, but does not work if multiple deficiencies are present. Many states such as liver disease, DIC, vita-

Table 52-1 ***Significant Laboratory Results for Inherited Platelet Disorders***

	Platelet Count	Bleeding Time	Platelet Adhesiveness	Platelet Aggregation		
				Epinephrine	ADP	Ristocetin
Glanzmann's thrombasthenia	N	P	D	A	A	D,N
Storage pool deficiency	N	P	D	A	A	V
Hermansky-Pudlak syndrome	N	P	D	A	A	N
Wiskott-Aldrich syndrome	D	P	D	A	A	N
Gray platelet syndrome	D	P	N	N	N	N
Bernard Soulier syndrome	D	P	D	N	N	D
Von Willebrand's disease	N	P	D	N	N	D

N = Normal
A = Abnormal
P = Prolonged
D = Decreased
V = Variable

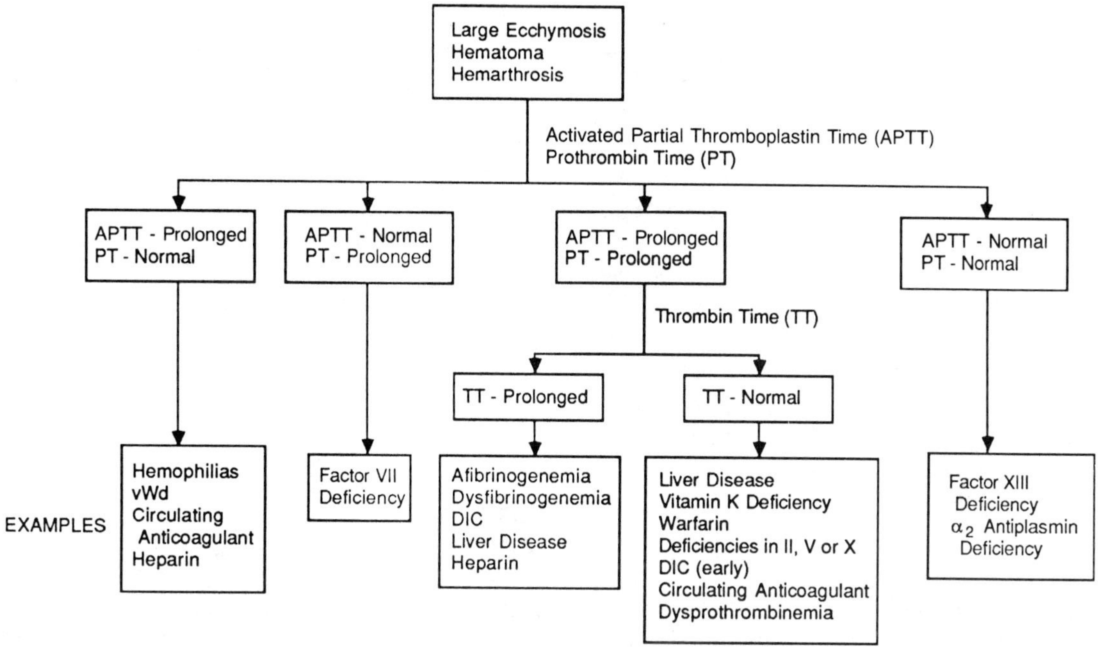

Figure 52-4 **Work-up of patient with defect in the secondary hemostatic mechanism. (From Corrigan JJ Jr. [ed]: Hemorrhagic and Thrombotic Diseases in Childhood and Adolescence. New York, Churchill Livingstone, 1985. Reprinted with permission)**

min K deficiency, and warfarin treatment do produce multiple deficiencies and a long PT and APTT. It is important to note that the screening tests do not measure for the presence of factor XIII or α-2-antiplasmin deficiency. These diseases must be picked up by history and subsequent special testing. An inhibitor may be suspected when a prolonged PT or APTT is not corrected by a 1:1 mixture of the patient's plasma and normal plasma.

SPECIFIC DISORDERS

For patients with a single factor deficiency, once the PT and APTT are performed and the factor deficiency has been narrowed down to one area of the plasma coagulation scheme (see Figs. 52-2 and 52-4), specific factor assays should be performed to arrive at a definitive diagnosis. Knowing which specific factor is deficient in the patient is important in the treatment of the patient with blood products. If inherited multiple factor deficiencies are suspected, specific factor assays should be run to determine which factors are deficient.

Hemophilia and Von Willebrand's Disease

The laboratory diagnosis of hemophilia can usually be made with a specific factor VIII assay. These patients should demonstrate a normal PT, long APTT, normal bleeding time, and normal platelet count. It is important to remember that several physiologic conditions such as stress, exercise, and pregnancy can increase the level of factor VIII, and that therefore in mild hemophiliacs these effects may mask slightly low factor VIII activity.

The diagnosis of von Willebrand's disease is often fairly difficult. Tests commonly performed to aid in the diagnosis include the platelet count, PT,

APTT, TT, bleeding time, factor VIII clotting activity, factor VIII antigen, ristocetin-induced platelet aggregation, and platelet adhesiveness. Table 52-2 compares the laboratory findings in hemophilia A and von Willebrand's disease. Several problems can arise when evaluating von Willebrand's disease. One problem is the variants that have been identified that may give normal results or even hyperreactive results for some of the tests usually used to diagnose von Willebrand's disease. Crossed immunoelectrophoresis and SDS-agarose gel electrophoresis can sometimes help to identify these patients.[4] Another problem is the variability in laboratory results in an individual from day to day. If a patient has a positive history suggestive of von Willebrand's disease but tests are normal, repeat studies should be performed.

Other Deficiencies

Factor IX deficiency is clinically indistinguishable from factor VIII deficiency. Definitive diagnosis must be made with specific factor assays. Diagnosis is very important because treatment is different for these two diseases.

The diagnosis of afibrinogenemia or dysfibrinogenemia should be made using a coagulation or immunologic assay for fibrinogen.

Other factor deficiencies should be diagnosed with specific factor assays to confirm the factor missing.

It is important to remember that factor XIII deficiency will not be detected in any coagulation screening tests. If factor XIII deficiency is suspected because of the patient history, a clot stability test using 5 M urea should be performed as a screening test. Specific assay of factor XIII will confirm the diagnosis.

Vitamin K Deficiency

The laboratory findings in vitamin K deficiency consist of a prolonged PT and an APTT that may be normal or abnormal, depending on the severity of the deficiency. Typically, the PT becomes prolonged before the APTT, because factor VII has the shortest *in vivo* half life and depletes most rapidly. The TT should be normal. When the PT and APTT are both moderately prolonged, the differentiation of vitamin K deficiency from DIC may be difficult. A factor V level may be helpful because factor V is not vitamin K-dependent;

Table 52-2 ***Laboratory Tests in Von Willebrand's Disease and Hemophilia***

Test	Hemophilia	Classical Von Willebrand's Disease
Bleeding time	N	I
Platelet adhesiveness	N	D
Platelet aggregation with ADP	N	N
Platelet aggregation with ristocetin	N	D
Von Willebrand antigen	N–I	D
Factor VIII coagulant activity	D	D
Crossed immunoelectrophoresis	N	N or A

N = Normal
D = Decreased
I = Increased
A = Abnormal

therefore the factor V activity should be normal in vitamin K deficiency but low in DIC because it is consumed.

Liver Disease

The PT and APTT are often prolonged in liver disease due to decreased production of the factors or to decreased carboxylation of the vitamin K-dependent factors that leads to decreased function. An increased TT may be seen if the fibrin(ogen) degradation products are greatly increased. DIC may accompany liver disease and confuse the diagnosis and treatment.

DIC

The diagnosis of DIC is based on the clinical condition of the patient and on laboratory tests. If the patient has a disease that is often associated with DIC and is bleeding or has signs of thrombosis, screening tests should be performed. The screening tests should include a platelet count, PT, APTT, TT, and fibrinogen test. A diagnosis of DIC can be made if the values are very low, or if the levels are falling in a successive series of tests. The examination of a blood smear for fragmented red blood cells is sometimes suggested as a screening test for DIC, but this seldom proves useful. Fibrin(ogen) degradation products are usually positive in DIC, but are not diagnostic of DIC. A factor V assay may be helpful in the differential diagnosis of DIC from vitamin K deficiency, as described above. In vitamin K deficiency, the platelet count and fibrinogen are also often normal. The differential diagnosis of DIC from liver disease can also be difficult. A factor VIII level may be helpful because factor VIII is often elevated in mild liver disease. If the liver disease is more advanced, the factor VIII level may be low in both conditions.

Massive Transfusion

Most coagulation screening tests will be affected in massively transfused patients given stored bank blood. The PT, APTT, TT, and bleeding time may all be long. The fibrinogen and platelet count may be low. Because the screening tests are similar in massively transfused patients and in patients with DIC or liver disease, massive transfusion should always be considered as part of the differential diagnosis.

Inhibitors

Deficient inhibitors of fibrinolysis can cause a bleeding tendency. Some deficient α-2-antiplasmin patients have been reported to bleed excessively. Screening tests for this condition would be whole blood clot lysis or euglobulin clot lysis. Specific α-2-antiplasmin assays may be run to confirm the diagnosis.

Laboratory Approach to Thrombosis

Laboratory tests to identify patients with increased thrombotic risk are not very useful at the present time. The exception occurs in those families with a history of recurrent thrombotic events, especially if the events occur in young adults. These individuals should have tests run for antithrombin III, protein C, plasminogen, and fibrinogen.[2]

Specific Laboratory Analyses

PLATELET COUNT

Platelet counts are now usually performed on electronic counters, although very low counts should be determined manually by phase microscopy. It is often important to review the peripheral smear before releasing a platelet count because there are clinical situations that can cause false results. Some of these include a clotting specimen, EDTA-associated platelet satellitism, cold agglutinins, and the undergoing of chemotherapy (because white cells may fragment and the fragments may be counted as platelets).

EXAMINATION OF THE PERIPHERAL SMEAR

The examination of the peripheral smear should include an estimate of the number of platelets, the size of the platelets, the variation in the size and granularity of the platelet, how the granules are distributed, and whether there are any pseudopods on the platelet. The peripheral smear may also suggest other diseases that affect hemostatic status.

BLEEDING TIME

The template Ivy bleeding time approach is the recommended method for performing bleeding time tests. Commercially-made bleeding time apparatus is now available. It is important to remember that the bleeding time is inversely related to the circulating platelet count when it falls below $100,000/mm^3$. It is a good practice to obtain the platelet count before beginning the bleeding time test so that the test may be avoided in patients with low platelet counts.

A patient with a long bleeding time but a platelet count greater than $100,000/mm^3$ is said to have platelet dysfunction. More specific tests of platelet function such as platelet adhesiveness and aggregation are usually needed to establish a specific diagnosis.

PROTHROMBIN TIME (PT)

The prothrombin time test measures the extrinsic pathway of coagulation (factors I, II, V, X, VII) (see Fig. 52-2). When the test is performed, thromboplastin is added as a source of tissue extract and phospholipid. Thromboplastin is combined with calcium ions and platelet-poor plasma, and the formation of a fibrin clot is observed. The final result is dependent on the concentration of thromboplastin and calcium used as well as on the method used to detect the clot. Because of this, results may vary a great deal from laboratory to laboratory.

ACTIVATED PARTIAL THROMBOPLASTIN TIME (APTT)

The activated partial thromboplastin time test measures the intrinsic pathway of coagulation (factors I, II, V, X, VIII, IX, XI, XII, prekallikrein, high-molecular-weight kininogen) (see Fig. 52-2). The term "activated" refers to the fact that an inert substance (such as kaolin, celite, ellagic acid, micronized silica) is added to the test to maximally activate the contact factors. The other reagents in the test are a source of phospholipid and calcium ions. The endpoint is the formation of a fibrin clot, which is dependent on the concentrations of activator, phospholipid, and calcium as well as on the method used for fibrin detection.

As can be seen in Figure 52-2, factors I, II, V, and X are measured by both the prothrombin time and the partial thromboplastin time. Deficiencies in any of these factors may result in the prolongation of both of these tests, depending on the severity of the defect. In most laboratories the APTT test is more sensitive to factor deficiencies than is the PT test.

THROMBIN TIME (TT)

The thrombin time test measures the time it takes for fibrinogen to be converted to a fibrin clot. It does not measure any other coagulation factors (see Fig. 52-2). The reagent used in the test is a dilute thrombin. Because calcium is added, the formation of the fibrin clot is dependent on the thrombin–fibrinogen reaction. This test is commonly used to monitor heparin therapy. Some conditions for prolongation of the TT, in addition to heparin therapy, are dysfibrinogenemia, severe hypofibrinogenemia, and increased fibrin(ogen) degradation products.

FIBRINOGEN

There are many methods available for the measurement of fibrinogen, including the modified thrombin time test and various clottable protein methods and immunologic methods. High levels of fibrin(ogen) degradation products or heparin may influence the modified thrombin times. Fibrinogen is an important consideration in all clotting assays because the conversion of fibrinogen to fibrin is the endpoint for all these tests. In general, a fibrinogen level below 100 mg/dL (1 g/L) will influence the PT, APTT, and TT.

OTHER HEMOSTATIC STUDIES

To establish a definite diagnosis, coagulation studies other than the screening tests may be indicated. Many of these tests are difficult to perform and should only be done in a reference laboratory that does them on a regular basis where proficiency can be maintained.

SPECIFIC FACTOR ASSAYS

Specific factor assays for clotting activity can be performed using either the prothrombin time or APTT assay plus a substrate deficient in a specific factor and dilutions of the patient plasma. The clotting results for the patient are compared to a control with a known amount of factor, and the answer is expressed as a percentage of the normal. Commercial chromogenic assays are also becoming available for many of the specific factors. Factor XIII is analyzed by a clot stability test using 5 M urea. Immunologic tests can also be performed for most coagulation factors, but indicate only if the molecule is present, not if it is functional.

FIBRIN(OGEN) DEGRADATION PRODUCTS (FDP)

Tests for fibrin(ogen) degradation products are usually semiquantitative methods performed by slide agglutination. Any substance that causes fibrinogen or fibrin to be digested will cause the FDP level to increase.

PLATELET ADHESION

Two tests of platelet function are often performed in hemostatic workups. These are tests for platelet adhesion and aggregation. Platelet adhesion tests measure the platelets' ability to stick to a surface, often glass beads. Blood is passed over a glass bead column and a platelet count is performed on the blood before and after it is passed over the beads. The difference between these two values is the number of platelets that adhere to the beads.

PLATELET AGGREGATION

The ability of platelets to aggregate is usually tested using a nephelometer or platelet aggregometer. A platelet agonist is added to stirred platelet-rich plasma. As the platelets aggregate, the increase in light transmission is recorded. The three main characteristics that can be detected on the tracing are shape change of the platelets, primary aggregation due to the addition of the agonist, and secondary aggregation due to the release of the platelets' own internal constituents. The platelet shape change and primary aggregation are reversible, while secondary aggregation is usually irreversible. Agonists often used are adenosine diphosphate (ADP), epinephrine, collagen, thrombin, arachidonic acid, and ristocetin. Using a special aggregometer that measures luminescence, the release of ATP by platelets can be detected. This instrument allows measurement of the time relationship between platelet aggregation and secretion of ATP.

INHIBITORS

Some patients develop circulating anticoagulants that may be directed against a specific coagulation factor or, as in the case of lupus erythematosus, may be less specific. These can be assayed in two ways. One is to make serial dilutions of patient plasma in normal plasma and test this, using either a PT or an APTT assay, at 0 time and 2 hours later. Some antibodies are time-dependent and require the incubation time to react. Other anticoagulants, such as the one found in lupus, act immediately. The other assay method for antibodies is to run specific factor assays to see the effect of the inhibitor on the coagulation factor. An example of this type of assay is the Bethesda assay, done for factor VIII inhibitors.

TREATMENT

Hemophilia A is treated with cryoprecipitate, factor VIII concentrate, or DDAVP which triggers release of endothelial factor VII reserves. Von Willebrand's disease is treated with fresh frozen plasma, cryoprecipitate, or DDAVP. Factor VIII concentrates do not contain the portion of the von Willebrand factor molecule needed, so should not be used. Hemophilia B (factor IX deficiency) is treated with fresh frozen plasma or commercial factor IX concentrates. It should be remembered that concentrates may contain the virus of hepatitis and may contain the HIV virus. Factor IX concentrate also seems to increase the patient's risk of thrombotic episodes.

Treatment of hemophiliacs who have antibodies can be very difficult. Treatment of nonhemophiliac patients with factor VIII antibodies may be accomplished with high-dose steroids, massive doses of factor VIII, or plasmaphoresis to remove the antibody. Specific inhibitors to other factors have been described, but are less common than factor VIII antibodies.

Other factor deficiencies are usually treated with fresh frozen plasma. Deficiencies in fibrinogen or factor XIII are usually treated with cryoprecipitate because it contains high concentrations of these two substances.

Treatment of bleeding disorders due to liver disease must take into account the multiple causes for hemostatic abnormalities. Giving fresh frozen plasma may correct the PT and APTT but not affect platelet function, and the patient may still bleed. All possible causes of bleeding must be treated with the correct blood product. Treatment is often only supportive.

Treatment for vitamin K deficiency depends on the severity of the bleeding. If the patient is bleeding massively or in an operative setting, fresh frozen plasma or whole blood should be given to replace the vitamin K-deficient factors. For most patients, slow intravenous administration of water-soluble vitamin K or oral administration is preferred.[2] A water-soluble preparation should be used in patients with a fat malabsorption problem if the vitamin K is given orally. If a patient has severe liver problems, the vitamin K factors may not correct the bleeding problem because precursors may not be synthesized. Prothrombin complex should not be used in patients with severe vitamin K deficiency, even if they are bleeding severely, because of the large risk of hepatitis from the concentrates.

The primary treatment for DIC is to remove the underlying cause, if possible, and to take supportive measures. If the patient is not bleeding, removing the cause is enough. If the patient is bleeding, but not severely, replacement with fresh frozen plasma often will replace enough of the clotting factors to stop the bleeding. In addition, platelet concentrates may be required. If the fibrinogen is very low, cryoprecipitate should also be given.

Whether or not heparin should be administered to a patient with DIC remains controversial. Some physicians administer heparin to block the ongoing consumptive process; however, heparinization may exacerbate the bleeding tendency. Heparin, if used, should be monitored carefully. Along with coagulation parameters, the platelet count should be monitored because heparin can induce thrombocytopenia in some patients.

Treatment for acute thromboembolic disease is directed at control of the thrombotic process and usually involves the administration of heparin. In some patients whose thrombotic disease is not associated with surgery or trauma, fibrinolysis is attempted using streptokinase. When a major artery is occluded due to a thromboembolitic event, surgery may be required. The treatment of pulmonary thromboembolism is discussed in Chapter 9.

Prophylaxis in patients who are at risk for thromboembolic disease usually involves heparin therapy.[7]

Various tests have been used to monitor heparin therapy, including the APTT, TT, and recalcification time. Heparin must be monitored carefully to prevent bleeding. Protamine sulfate can be administered to neutralize the effects of heparin.

Treatment for platelet disorders involving thrombocytopenia not due to an autoantibody includes platelet transfusion. Disorders of platelet function due to drugs or other underlying causes improve when the underlying condition is corrected. Inherited disorders of platelet function are also treated with periodic platelet transfusions. Because platelets are quite immunogenic, the development of platelet antibodies is not unusual and greatly complicates the use of platelet therapy.[8]

CASE STUDY #1

Fifteen months previous to his present hospital admission, a 28-month-old boy had ingested lye, which damaged his esophagus. Presently, he was admitted for surgery for the repair of the esophagus. The following coagulation results were obtained preoperatively. Reference ranges are in parentheses.

LABORATORY FINDINGS

PT = 12.5 seconds (11.5–15.0)
APTT = 35.7 second (35.0–45.0)
TT = 14.5 seconds (13.0–20.0)

One month later, after IV feedings during his convalescence, the following coagulation results were obtained.

LABORATORY FINDINGS

PT = 27.1 seconds (11.5–15.0)
APTT = 116.8 seconds (35.0–45.0)
TT = 19.0 seconds (13.0–20.0)
Factor V = 85.0% (70%–130%)
Platelets = Normal

Questions

1. What is the most likely cause of this patient's problem?
2. Why was a factor V performed?

Discussion

1. Because of the repair to his esophagus, the patient had been on IV feedings with little or no oral intake for 1 month, which caused him to become vitamin K-deficient. Vitamin K was administered and his coagulation parameters soon returned to normal.
2. Factor V will help to differentiate between vitamin K deficiency and DIC. Because factor V is not vitamin K-dependent, it will be normal in vitamin K deficiency and low in severe DIC.

CASE STUDY #2

A 28-year-old white man presented with a history of nosebleeds as a child, once or twice weekly with occasional cauterization required. The nosebleeds had stopped as he matured. He was circumcised as a neonate and had a tonsillectomy at age 5, both with no abnormal bleeding. At 16 years of age he injured his left knee, and considerable fluid was removed. He had a history of bruising easily and bleeding from the gums. The patient's paternal grandfather and father both had histories of nosebleeds. At the time of presentation, the patient had strained his chest attempting the "strong man" feat at a fair. In the emergency room, his APTT was 38.4 seconds (R.R. 35.0–45.0) and his factor VIII was 63% (R.R. 70%–120%). He was treated with cryoprecipitate, and 2 L of blood were evacuated from his chest.

The following laboratory data were obtained several weeks later, once the current problem had resolved. The reference range is in parentheses.

LABORATORY FINDINGS

PT = 11.9 seconds (11.5–15.0)
APTT = 44.5 seconds (35.0–45.0)
TT = 15.5 seconds (13.0–20.0)
Clauss fibrinogen = 0.33 g/dL (0.17–0.35 g/dL)
Factor VIII = 34% (70%–130%)
Factor IX = 140% (70%–130%)
Factor XI = 134% (70%–130%)
Factor XII = 119% (60%–200%)
Platelet count = 315 × 10^3/mm^3 (200–400 × 10^3/mm^3)
Bleeding time = 11.5, 14 minutes (up to 9.5)
Platelet adhesiveness = 10% (>80%)
Platelet aggregation with epinephrine, ADP, collagen = Normal
Platelet aggregation with ristocetin = Abnormal
Platelet morphology = Normal
Ristocetin cofactor = Not detectable (60%–144%)
VIII antigen = Not detectable (60%–164%)
VIII crossed immunoelectrophoresis = Not done

Questions

1. What is the most likely diagnosis for this patient?

2. If this patient has a bleeding episodc, what should be used to treat the bleed?

Discussion

1. This patient has classical von Willebrand's disease. His APTT is prolonged, factor VIII is low, bleeding time is prolonged, aggregation with all reagents is normal except ristocetin, platelet adhesiveness is low, ristocetin cofactor is low, and VIII antigen is not detectable so a crossed immunoelectrophoresis was not performed.

2. If this patient bleeds, he should be treated with cryoprecipitate.

REFERENCES

1. Koepke JA: Laboratory Hematology. New York City, Churchill Livingstone, 1984
2. Thompson AR, Harker LA: Manual of Hemostasis and Thrombosis, 3rd ed. Philadelphia, FA Davis, 1984
3. Schumacher HR, Garvin DF, Triplett DA: Introduction to Laboratory Hematology and Hematopathology. New York City, Alan R Liss, 1984
4. Pittiglio DH, Sacher R: Clinical Hematology and Fundamentals of Hemostasis. Philadelphia, FA Davis, 1987
5. Corrigan JJ Jr: Hemorrhagic and Thrombotic Diseases in Childhood and Adolescence. New York City, Churchill Livingstone, 1985
6. Ratnoff OD, Forbes CD: Disorders of Hemostasis. Orlando, Florida, Grune & Stratton, 1984
7. Standness DE: Vascular Disease of Extremities. In Petersdorf RG et al (eds): Harrison's Principles of Internal Medicine, pp 1492–1497. New York City, McGraw-Hill, 1983
8. Nossel HL: Platelet Disorders. In Petersdorf RG et al (eds): Harrison's Principles of Internal Medicine, pp 1896–1898. New York City, McGraw-Hill, 1983

Part XI

IMMUNOLOGIC DISORDERS

Sharon L. Zablotney, Associate Editor

The immune system is a collection of cells, tissues, and organs that mediate the body's immune response. This response in a state of health provides protection from potentially harmful agents or substances that gain entrance to the body. Pathological states may arise, however, when a cell, tissue, or organ is not present, does not interact appropriately, or malfunctions. The result is harm to the organism rather than protection. This section has been organized around the three major areas of pathological disorders that befall the immune system.

The first chapter, Immunodeficiencies, describes the range of conditions that may result when the immune system does not respond to potentially harmful agents or substances. These patients may have deficiencies that range from reduction in the ability to produce adequate amounts of the third component of the complement system to a total lack of stem cells, which serve as the progenitors for the critical B and T cells of the lymphocytic cell series. The resulting pathology may exhibit a similar breadth of expression, from recurrence of mild infections to a total inability to respond to the simplest and least pathogenic of the opportunistic organisms, a life-threatening state.

The second chapter, Allergies, addresses an immunologic state exhibited daily by millions of people. Although the allergic state may be a common phenomenon, the underlying mechanisms responsible for the conditions are complex and diverse. The immunologic mediators in these conditions range from the production of immunoglobulins, such as IgE, to the release of lymphokines from sensitized lymphocytes. In these instances the immune system mounts a response to substances that frequent our environment or that we encounter in other ways. The resulting reaction precipitates an "allergic response," which may range from watery eyes or a skin rash to the destruction of essential tissue.

The third chapter, Autoimmune Diseases, focuses on a conglomerate of disorders in which every conceivable malfunction of the immune system can be expressed. The pathological immunologic reaction may be mediated by the production of immunoglobulins and/or sensitized lymphocytes. These reactions may follow the hyper- or hypo-reactive T or B cells or the production of an immunoglobulin that crossreacts with a cellular antigen associated with normal tissue. These reactions lead to the immunologic destruction of normal tissue as the body appears to mount an immune response against itself.

The following chapters provide an introduction to the variety of immunologic disorders associated with each of these categories. Each chapter will review the underlying pathophysiology of each disorder and the associated clinical symptoms. The laboratory provides significant data upon which the clinical diagnosis may be based. Through careful selection of appropriate laboratory tests and interpretation of the results, the abnormality within the immune response may be identified and treatment selected. These chapters were designed to guide in this decision-making process.

Chapter 53

Immunodeficiencies

Scot C. Buessow/
Shirley MacManigal/Hal S. Larsen

In the past few years, knowledge of the immune system has expanded more rapidly than almost any other area in clinical laboratory science. The crucial role of cell-mediated immunity (CMI) in host defense, the role of the mononuclear phagocyte in the generation of an immune response, and the role of the major histocompatibility complex (MHC) in health and disease are but a few examples of the tremendous variety of immunologic information that has direct impact on the clinical laboratory.

The most primitive cellular response is phagocytosis, mediated by granulocytes and monocyte-derived cells. Humoral and cellular immunity is provided by the lymphoid cells. The activity of these cellular systems is augmented by the biological amplification systems, primarily complement and the acute-phase proteins.

Within the marrow, lymphoid stem cells are stimulated to differentiate by poorly understood hormonal influences, collectively termed the *lymphopoietic inductive microenvironment.* The resulting prelymphocytes migrate into the peripheral blood and thence to the primary lymphoid organs.

The primary lymphoid organs, the thymus and the bone marrow, are responsible for immunologic programming. Prelymphocytes within the thymus are referred to as *thymocytes.* These cells are programmed under the influence of thymopoietins and interactions with class I and II MHC antigens on thymic stromal cells, resulting in the deletion of autoreactive clones. The mature cell is released into the peripheral blood as a thymus-derived, or T, cell. The lymphocytes mediating humoral immunity are presumably processed in a similar fashion in the bone marrow, hence the term B cells.

Following differentiation and programming, these immunocompetent T and B cells migrate into the peripheral lymphoid organs. The major secondary lymphoid organs are the spleen, lymph nodes, tonsils, and gut-associated lymphoid tissue (GALT), which provide a systemic network of antigen-responsive cells. Within secondary lymphoid tissue, T and B cells occur in relatively discrete

Table 53-1 ***Lymphokines Secreted by Antigen-Stimulated T Lymphocytes***

Lymphokine	Other Names	Biologic Activities
Interleukin-2	IL-2 T-cell growth factor	Stimulates division of T cells to enhance immune response
Gamma interferon	Macrophage-activating factor (MAF)	Stimulates macrophage phagocytosis and NK cell-killing; antineoplastic; regulates antibody production
B-cell growth factor	–	Stimulates B-cell growth and plasma cell differentiation
Lymphotoxin	–	Cytotoxic
Chemotactic factor	–	Attracts macrophages to site of antigen
Migration inhibition factor	–	Enhances macrophage adherence at site of antigen

regions, with macrophages dispersed throughout. This sequence of maturation is depicted in Figure 53-1.

The primary stimulus for the generation of an immune response is the interaction of immunogen and the mononuclear phagocyte system (MPS). The MPS is a body-wide collection of specialized fixed macrophages. Immunogens are phagocytized by these cells and partially degraded. The processed antigen is then displayed on the cell membrane. These antigen-presenting cells (APC) interact with lymphocytes through MHC membrane proteins. Simultaneously, the APC begins secreting the immunoregulatory monokine interleukin-1 (IL-1), a potent lymphocyte-activating factor triggering the clonal expansion of both T and B cells.

The interaction of the APC with the T cell triggers dedifferentiation into a T lymphoblast, followed by intense proliferation of the stimulated

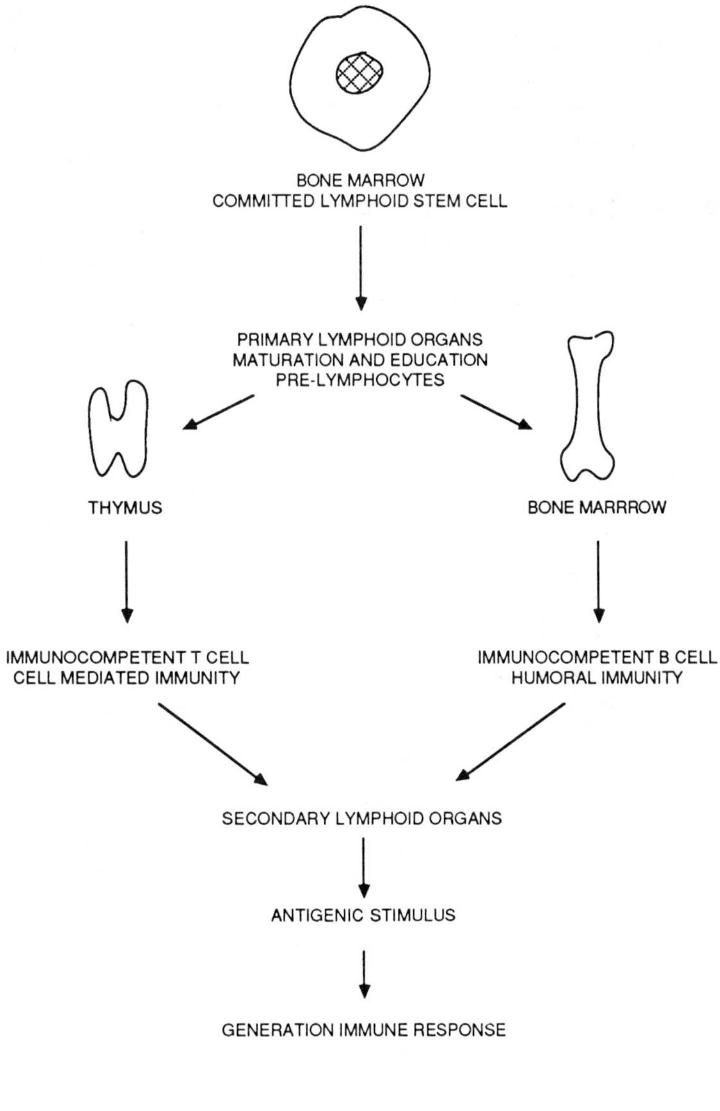

Figure 53-1 Maturation of the immune system.

clone. This clonal expansion results in a number of T-cell subpopulations (see Fig. 53-2), which are classed as effector, memory, or regulatory. Effector T cells promote cell-mediated cytotoxicity (CMC) and delayed type hypersensitivity (DTH). Memory T cells are responsible for anamnesis. The regulatory T cells are the helper/inducer and suppressor cells. The relative proportion of these two populations of cells regulates the strength and duration of both cellular and humoral immune responses, often directly mediated by the elaboration of a heterogeneous group of glycoproteins classed as lymphokines (see Table 53-1).

A humoral immune response is produced by the interaction of APC, T cells, and B cells, which stimulates the production of long-lived memory cells and short-lived, antibody-secreting plasma cells. Primary immune responses produce predominantly IgM; however, prolonged exposure or reexposure to immunogen will produce an Ig class switch, promoted by the helper T cell. The plasma cells will now secrete predominantly IgG or IgA. Antibody production is regulated by the suppressor T cell, which acts by inhibiting the helper T cell or the B cell itself (see Fig. 53-3). Table 53-2 lists the five major Ig classes and their biological activities.

ETIOLOGY AND PATHOPHYSIOLOGY

All immunodeficiencies (ID) can be classed as either primary (congenital) or secondary (acquired). Within these broad groups, the abnormality might be the result of either an embryologic abnormality or a defective or absent enzyme, or idiopathic. The presenting symptoms and clinical course of each deficiency state are a reflection of which defense mechanism has been affected.

B-Cell Deficiency States

The B-cell deficiency states range from a virtual absence of all Ig classes to selective defects in one class.[1, 2] Therefore, the clinical symptomatology and therapy depend predominantly on the Ig class affected and the totality of that defect. Because of

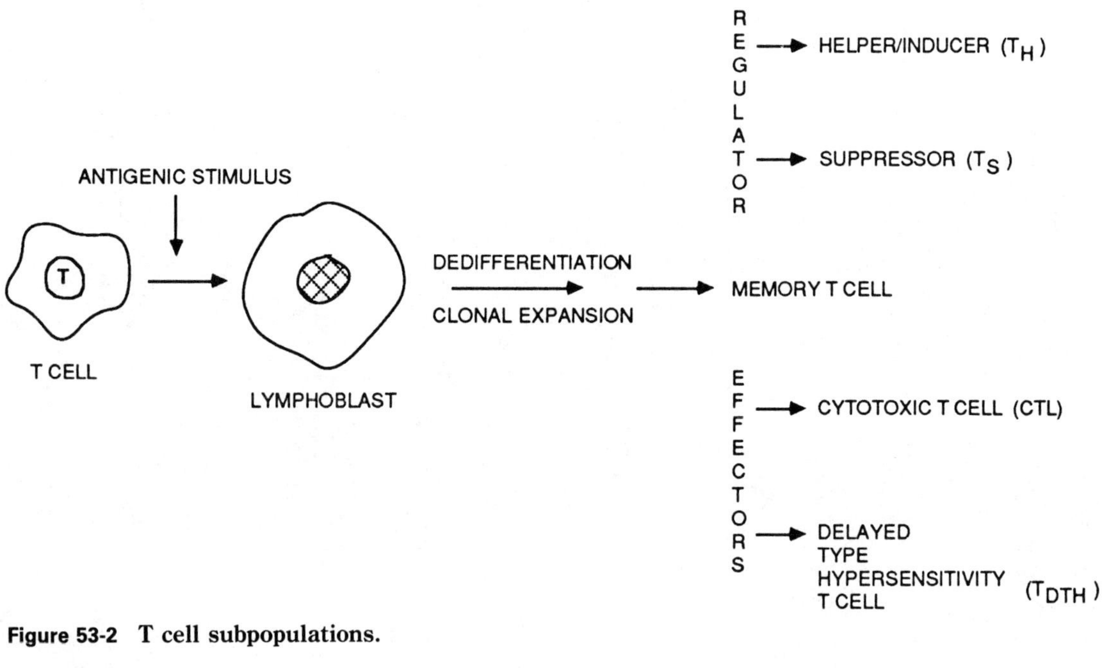

Figure 53-2 T cell subpopulations.

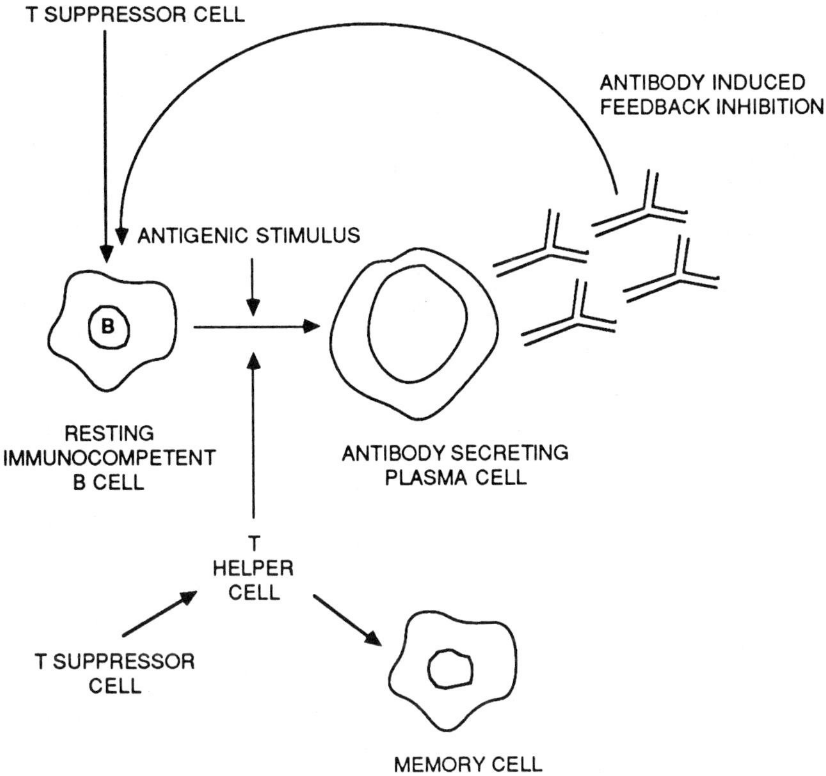

Figure 53-3 **Regulation of the antibody response.**

the relative ease of detecting a hypogammaglobulinemic condition, patients are usually diagnosed promptly, with rapid therapeutic intervention.

BRUTON'S AGAMMAGLOBULINEMIA

Bruton's agammaglobulinemia, an immunodeficiency state also termed *X-linked infantile hypogammaglobulinemia,* was described by Bruton in a male child in 1952 (considered the first description of a primary immunodeficiency). Estimates indicate that 1/100,000 males may be affected. Although there is an absence of mature B cells in the peripheral blood, recent investigations have detected preB-cell populations in the bone marrow. These cells fail to mature and do not secrete Ig, probably as a result of an as yet undetermined maturation block or absence of helper T-cell interactions.[3]

TRANSIENT NEONATAL HYPOGAMMAGLOBULINEMIA

Transient neonatal hypogammaglobulinemia mimics Bruton's in some ways; at present, the etiology is unknown.[4] In isolated cases, maternal antibodies to IgG allotypic markers have been found that could produce a transient suppression of IgG-secreting cells. Alternatively, a selective defect in T helper cells has been proposed.[5]

ACQUIRED HYPOGAMMAGLOBULINEMIA

Although the etiology of acquired hypogammaglobulinemia, also called variable unclassifiable immunodeficiency, is not known, these patients do

Table 53-2 ***Immunoglobulin Class and Biologic Activities***

Class	Subclass	M.W.	Biologic Activity
IgG	IgG1–IgG4	150,000	Antiviral Antibacterial Antifungal Opsonizing
IgM	IgM1 and IgM2	900,000	Antiviral Antibacterial Antifungal
IgA	IgA1 and IgA2	160,000 or 400,000	Mucosal immunity
IgE	–	190,000	Allergy Antiparasitic
IgD	–	180,000	B-lymphocyte differentiation

have normal levels of circulating B cells. This has led to an hypothesis that implicates either an increase in suppressor T cells or a decrease in helper T cells.

SELECTIVE IGA DEFICIENCY

A selective lack of IgA is the most common immunodeficiency state to be identified, with reported incidences ranging from 1/600 to 1/800. It appears that IgA deficiency, like other ID states, predisposes the affected individual to a number of other diseases. As in most immunodeficiency states, the pathogenesis of selective IgA deficiency is not definitively known. Studies have demonstrated normal levels of circulating IgA-bearing B cells. A subpopulation of patients have suppressor T cells that inhibit IgA production from B cells of normal individuals. Drug-induced IgA deficiencies have been described in patients taking penicillamine or phenytoin; the deficiency often resolves upon removal of the drug.

Cell-Mediated Immunodeficiencies

Because of the interactions between T and B cells, a pure T-cell immunodeficiency state is rare. Generally speaking, any defect in T-cell number or function will result in some aberration in Ig synthesis. Patients with CMI deficiencies are prone to develop acute or chronic infections with numerous viral, fungal, or protozoal pathogens.

DIGEORGE'S SYNDROME

Also known as *congenital thymic aplasia,*[6] DiGeorge's syndrome is a result of an embryologic malformation producing physical abnormalities as well as immunodeficiency. Between the sixth and eighth weeks of gestation, an unknown embryologic insult perturbs the normal development of the thymus and parotid glands; they are either totally absent or partially developed in an abnormal anatomic location. It has also been suggested that some cases may be the result of failure of thymopoietin production and faulty T-cell maturation.

Combined Humoral and Cell-Mediated Immunodeficiency

Several different etiologies have been proposed for the different classifications of the severe combined immunodeficiency diseases (SCID), which range from partially-depressed immunity to a complete lack of responsiveness. Genetically, SCID may be inherited as an X-linked recessive (X-linked lymphopenic agammaglobulinemia) or as an autosomal recessive (Swiss-type lymphopenic agammaglobulinemia). Because many of the affected children die before a diagnosis can be made, the exact incidence of SCID is unknown. There are two theories about the origin of SCID and its variants. The first assumes a failure of the lymphoid stem cell to differentiate into mature lymphocytes; the second, that normal stem cells exist but the primary lymphoid organs are nonfunctional.[7] *Nezelhof's syndrome* is a loose grouping of variable immunologic deficiencies with no known etiology, characterized by marked cell-mediated defects and variable humoral abnormalities. *Ataxia–telangectasia* involves not only the immune system, but also the nervous, endocrine, and vascular systems. *Wiskott-Aldrich syndrome* is an X-linked immunodeficiency characterized by hypercatabolism of immunoglobulins. No satisfactory etiology has been advanced for ataxia–telangectasia or Wiskott-Aldrich syndromes.

ADENOSINE DEAMINASE/NUCLEOSIDE PHOSPHORYLASE DEFICIENCY

Adenosine deaminase (ADA) and nucleoside phosphorylase (NP) are both involved in the normal catabolism of purines (see Fig. 53-4). Deficiencies in either of these enzymes results in a gradual buildup of biochemically-toxic intermediates.[8]

Deficiencies of Phagocytic Cells

The primary deficiencies of phagocytic function are usually related to an inability to complete the bactericidal pathway, often due to an enzyme deficiency.[9, 10, 11] There is generally little difficulty in responding to viral infection. A list of all major phagocytic deficiencies appears on page 674.

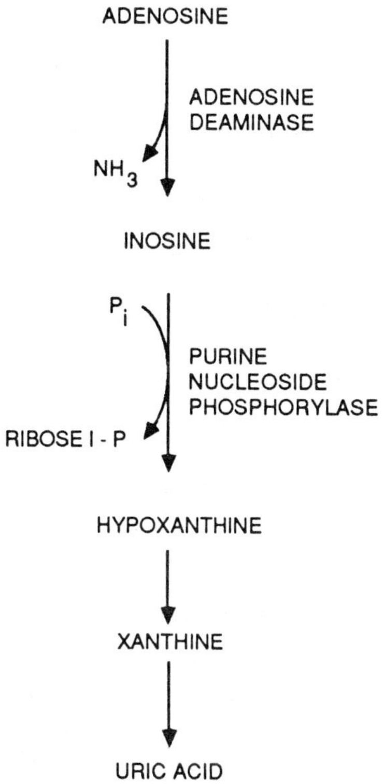

Figure 53-4 Enzyme-induced immunodeficiencies.

CHRONIC GRANULOMATOUS DISEASE (CGD)

There are numerous biochemical defects described that produce CGD,[12] but the most common is defective or absent NADH/NADPH. This results in decreased oxygen metabolism and consequently ineffective bactericidal activity. Inheritance is predominantly as an X-linked disorder, although a female variant has been described.

CHÉDIAK-HIGASHI SYNDROME

Chédiak-Higashi syndrome is an autosomal recessive multisystem disorder.[13] The bactericidal de-

Immunodeficiency Disorders Affecting Phagocytic Cells

Defective Bactericidal Enzyme Systems

NADH/NADPH oxidase, NADH reductase (CGD)
Lysosomal proteases (Chédiak-Higashi)
Glucose-6-phosphate dehydrogenase
Myeloperoxidase
Alkaline phosphatase

Defective Chemotactic Responses

Tuftsin deficiency
Lazy leukocyte syndrome
HyperIgE syndrome
Glycogen storage diseases

fect is seen as an increased killing time, likely due to abnormal lysosomal enzymes. Natural killer cell activity is also reduced.[14]

Complement Deficiencies

Activated components of the complement cascade are necessary for optimal bactericidal activity, neutrophil chemotaxis, and immune adherence. The etiology of complement component deficiency is most often a result of either a decreased synthesis or an increased catabolism.[15, 16, 17]

Secondary Immunodeficiency States

Secondary immunodeficiency states (see Table 53-3) are the result of some exogenous influence. These may be disease-related, as with tumors or infectious agents, drug-induced, or even dietary.[18] Depending on the etiology, secondary immunodeficiencies may be transient or permanent.

ACQUIRED IMMUNODEFICIENCY SYNDROME (AIDS)

There are few diseases in recent history that have attracted such intense scientific scrutiny as has acquired immunodeficiency disease.[19, 20] Thus, the etiology and pathophysiology of AIDS are much more clearly understood than those of almost any other immunodeficiency. AIDS is a result of infection by human T-lymphocytotropic virus-III (HTLV-III), now referred to as *human immunodeficiency virus* (HIV). This virus has also been known as *lymphadenopathy virus* (LAV), and *AIDS-related virus* (ARV).[21, 22, 23, 24] Following infection of the T helper cell, HIV produces a lytic effect.[25, 26, 27] From an immunologic standpoint, this results in decreased or absent responses to immunogenic challenge, due in part to the loss of helper cell function but also due to decreased clonal expansion mediated by helper cell-produced interleukin-2.[28] At one time, it was felt that HIV had an absolute tropism for helper T cells, but viral infection has recently been demonstrated in macrophages.[29]

CLINICAL MANIFESTATIONS

Very often the presenting symptoms (see below) provide the first indication as to which part of the immune system is abnormal. For example, abnormalities in humoral immunity often result in chronic or recurrent infections with pyogenic bacteria. Patients with defects in cell-mediated immunity are subject to disseminated viral and fungal infections (see the box on page 676).

B-Cell Immunodeficiencies

BRUTON'S AGAMMAGLOBULINEMIA

The majority of individuals affected by Bruton's agammaglobulinemia do not encounter any clinical problems for the first 4 to 6 months of life, due to the protective influence of maternal IgG. However, past this age the affected child will begin to suffer from chronic, recurrent bacterial infections. Diagnosis may be delayed at this point because of good response to antibiotic therapy. The most common presenting symptoms are otitis media, bronchitis, pneumonia, meningitis, dermatitis, and rarely, arthritis and malabsorption. Generally, the

Table 53-3 ***Secondary Immunodeficiency Disorders***

Etiologic Agent	Affected Immune Parameters
Pathogens	
Rubella	Decreased T-cell function Decreased antibody response Immunoglobulin deficiency
Leprosy/Tuberculosis	Decreased DTH response HyperIg in leprosy
Coccidioidomycosis	Decreased T-cell function
Cytomegalovirus	CMI anergy to CMV HyperIgM and -IgA
Human immunodeficiency virus	T-cell lysis; depressed IL-2
Malignant/Autoimmune Disease	
Leukemias/lymphomas	Variable T- or B-cell defects
Myelomas	Abnormal antibody response
Nonhematopoietic tumors	Increasing T- and B-cell anergy with tumor burden
Connective tissue disease	Decreased T-cell levels Abnormal T-cell function Hypergammaglobulinemia Variable complement defects
Chronic hepatitis	Decreased T-cell numbers Decreased T-cell function Hypergammaglobulinemia
Miscellaneous Clinical Conditions With Variable Deficiencies	
Diabetes Alcoholism Malnutrition Burns Sarcoidosis Splenectomy Sickle cell disease Uremia Down's syndrome	
Immunosuppressive Regimens	
Steroids	Short-term decrease in T- and B-cell numbers Reduced Ig synthesis Reduced phagocytosis
Antimetabolites Alkylating agents Radiation	Generalized suppression
Antithymocyte globulin	Variable effects on T-cell numbers and function, some T-dependent antibodies depressed
Cyclosporin A	Depressed synthesis of IL-2

Presenting Symptoms in Immunodeficiency Disorders

Often Found

1. Chronic or recurrent infections
2. Opportunistic or unusual pathogens
3. Incomplete response to therapy
4. Failure to thrive

Occasionally Found

1. Skin rash/eczema
2. Chronic diarrhea/malabsorption
3. Hepatosplenomegaly
4. Growth retardation
5. Abscesses
6. Autoimmune disease

infections are of a pyogenic nature, with *Streptococcus pneumoniae* and *Hemophilus influenzae* implicated most often. Gram-negative infections are also common. One indication that hypogammaglobulinemia may be present is an incomplete response to antimicrobials, or failure to clear infections completely.

For the most part, patients with defective antibody synthesis have an intact cell-mediated response and are not usually at risk for viral or fungal infections.

TRANSIENT NEONATAL HYPOGAMMAGLOBULINEMIA

Transient, or physiologic, hypogammaglobulinemia mimics Bruton's in many of the clinical manifestations, and a differential diagnosis must be made with care.

ACQUIRED HYPOGAMMAGLOBULINEMIA

Patients with variable unclassifiable immunodeficiency will present with the classic symptoms of X-linked immunoglobulin deficiency. Recurrent upper respiratory infections with pyogenic bacteria are common. A small percentage will progress to a protein-losing malabsorption syndrome. The two major differences are that the acquired condition does not appear until later in life, typically 15 to 30 years, and that both sexes are affected. This group of immunodeficient patients may also present with cell-mediated abnormalities, and seems to be more prone to a variety of autoimmune diseases and tumors.[30]

SELECTIVE IGA DEFICIENCY

As might be expected, the most common presenting symptom in patients with selective IgA deficiency is recurrent infections, chiefly viral or bacterial sino-pulmonary events.[31] There is a strong linkage between selective IgA deficiency and atopy. Of clinical importance is the subgroup of IgA-deficient individuals who produce high titers of IgG antiIgA, which places them at risk for anaphylactic reactions to plasma proteins.

Because of the role of IgA in mucosal immunity, it is not surprising that these patients suffer from a variety of gastrointestinal disorders. Celiac disease, ulcerative colitis, and regional enteritis are all associated with IgA deficiency. IgA-deficient individuals are also at increased risk for pernicious anemia, with autoantibodies to both intrinsic factor and gastric parietal cells. IgA deficiency also predisposes the individual to other autoimmune disorders, particularly systemic lupus erythematosus and rheumatoid arthritis. Other autoimmune disease associations described are thyroiditis, Coombs's positive hemolytic anemia, and chronic hepatitis.

Cell-Mediated Immunodeficiencies

DIGEORGE'S SYNDROME

The congenital physical abnormalities of DiGeorge's syndrome are usually the means of early diagnosis. The embryologic trauma results in a newborn with structural defects in the eyes, ears, and mouth, hypoparathyroidism, and congenital heart disease. The most common symptomatology in a DiGeorge's patient is early-onset refractory hypocalcemia. Should the newborn survive the gross anatomic abnormalities, the immunologic defects will become manifest. Chronic infections with numerous pathogens may produce pneumonia, diarrhea, mucosal candidiasis, and failure to thrive.[32]

SEVERE COMBINED IMMUNODEFICIENCY DISEASE (SCID)

SCID patients are prone to infection with any potential pathogen; in fact, they rarely survive longer than 1 year after birth. Maternal IgG offers only limited protection. Presenting symptoms of individuals with SCID include pneumonia, sepsis, oral candidiasis, otitis media, and a generalized failure to thrive.[33] These patients are particularly susceptible to the opportunistic pathogens, notably *Candida,* cytomegalovirus, and *Pneumocystis carinii.*

Symptomatology of the SCID variants is similar, with some exceptions. Nezelhof's syndrome often presents with lymphadenopathy and hepatosplenomegaly.

Ataxia–telangectasia can be identified by neurologic and endocrine disorders. Selective IgA deficiency is a common finding,[34] as well as consistently elevated levels of α-fetoprotein.

Wiskott-Aldrich syndrome patients develop recurrent bacterial infections, beginning at the age of about 6 months; viral infections will occur as the patient ages.[35] Nonimmunologic manifestations include thrombocytopenia present from birth, with bleeding tendencies during infectious episodes. Eczema is found at the age of about 1 year.

Phagocytic Deficiencies

CHRONIC GRANULOMATOUS DISEASE (CGD)

Patients with CGD often present in early childhood with recurrent infections caused by a variety of nonpathogenic or opportunistic organisms.[36] Draining nodes, lymphadenopathy, and hepatosplenomegaly are also seen.

CHÉDIAK-HIGASHI SYNDROME

The major symptomatology in Chédiak-Higashi syndrome includes recurrent bacterial infections, hepatosplenomegaly, CNS defects, natural killer (NK) cell dysfunction,[37] and increased risk of lymphoreticular neoplasms.

Complement Deficiencies

Depending on which specific component of complement is defective or absent, there may be no clinical symptoms, chronic bacterial infections, or an increased incidence of autoimmune disease.

C1 deficiency has been described in individuals with other immunodeficiencies and some autoimmune disorders. The degree of increased risk of bacterial infection will vary sharply.

C2 deficiency has been strongly linked to systemic lupuslike disorders with renal disease and positive antinuclear antibodies (ANAs).[38] These patients are at risk for bacterial infections.

C3 deficiencies have been described in several patients, with increased risk of infection and nephritis.[39]

C4 abnormalities have been found in a range of patients, from those who are asymptomatic to those with lupuslike syndromes. HLA associations have been noted in some cases. These patients exhibit decreased chemotactic responses and diminished immune adherence.

C5 deficiency has only been seen in a single case, that of a patient with SLE. C5 dysfunction has been documented as a familial defect.[40] It presents as a failure to thrive coupled with recurrent bacterial infections, diarrhea, and dermatitis. Chemotaxis will be ineffective; leukocytosis and hypergammaglobulinemia are often concomitant phenomena.

C6, C7, and C8 deficiencies have been seen in numerous cases, predisposing the affected individual to repeated meningococcal or gonococcal infections. C7 deficiencies are strongly linked to connective tissue disease.

C9 deficiency has been described, but affected individuals remain in good health.

Secondary Immunodeficiencies

In general, the clinical manifestations of secondary immunodeficiencies are extremely variable, and largely dependent on the agent producing the deficiency. Any or all combinations of humoral and cellular, phagocytic, or complement defects have been described.

ACQUIRED IMMUNODEFICIENCY SYNDROME (AIDS)

The clinical manifestations of AIDS will most often be centered around opportunistic infections, due to the severe depression of both T- and B-cell responses, a direct result of the lysis of helper T cells. With the recent description of macrophage infection by HIV, mononuclear phagocyte dysfunction may also be found. The most common opportunistic pathogens identified to date are *Candida albicans* and *Pneumocystis carinii.* Symptomatology will often present as thrush, pneumonia, or nonspecific fatigue, weight loss, and gastrointestinal distress. AIDS patients are also at increased risk of neoplasia, in particular Kaposi's sarcoma, a tumor relatively rare in the general population.[41] AIDS-related encephalitis and dementia have also been reported with increasing frequency, due to HIV infection of glial cells in the brain.[42]

LABORATORY ANALYSES AND DIAGNOSIS

The appropriate laboratory tests for the evaluation of ID states are shown on page 679.

B-Cell Deficiency States

BRUTON'S AGAMMAGLOBULINEMIA

Diagnosis of a hypogammaglobulinemic state can be made easily, based on serum electrophoretograms and serum Ig class quantitation. In most cases, total serum Ig levels will be in the range of 200 to 250 mg/dL (2000–2500 mg/L), with IgG constituting about 80% of the total Ig. Levels of the other four classes of antibody will be extremely low or even undetectable. Peripheral blood will show a variable loss of B cells, depending on the severity of the Ig deficiency. Tests for cell-mediated immunity, such as DTH skin testing or mitogenic stimulation, will most often prove normal in individuals over 1 year of age.

TRANSIENT NEONATAL HYPOGAMMAGLOBULINEMIA

Laboratory evaluation is essential in a differential diagnosis of transient neonatal hypogammaglobulinemia and Bruton's. This is done by determining the levels of individual Ig classes. While the levels of IgM and IgA will be abnormal in Bruton's, patients with transient hypogammaglobulinemia will have normal age-matched levels of these two Ig classes.[43] Serial Ig level determinations will indicate increasing levels of IgM and IgA, further supporting the diagnosis of a temporary physiologic aberration in Ig production.

ACQUIRED HYPOGAMMAGLOBULINEMIA

Patients with acquired hypogammaglobulinemia do have normal levels of circulating B cells, but lymph node biopsies will reveal an absence of plasma cells. Ig levels are usually in the region of 300 mg/dL (3000 mg/L), and IgG is usually less than 250 mg/dL (2500 mg/L). Both IgA and IgM levels will vary. Cell-mediated immune abnormalities include absent DTH skin tests, depressed mitogen stimulation, and low levels of circulating T cells.

SELECTIVE IGA DEFICIENCY

By convention, IgA deficiency occurs when an individual presents with a serum level of IgA of less than 5 mg/dL (50 mg/L), with normal or increased levels of the other Ig classes. The number of circulating peripheral B cells will be in the normal range. Generally, all tests of cell-mediated immunity will be normal. Those patients who have cell-mediated

Laboratory Tests in the Evaluation of Immunodeficiency Disorders

Cell-Mediated Immunity

1. Absolute lymphocyte count
2. Monoclonal analysis of T-cell subpopulations
3. Mitogen- and antigen-induced proliferation (blastogenesis)
4. Delayed type hypersensitivity skin testing

Humoral Immunity

1. Absolute lymphocyte count
2. Monoclonal analysis of total B cells, SIg subpopulations
3. Quantitation of immunoglobulin levels
4. *In vitro* antibody production to mitogen or antigen challenge

Phagocytic Function

1. Phagocytosis, with and without antibody-coated particles
2. Chemotaxis
3. NBT reduction and chemiluminescence
4. Myeloperoxidase levels

Complement

1. Total hemolytic complement
2. Quantitation of individual components
3. Chemotactic activity of serum

defects must be carefully monitored for the possible development of ataxia–telangectasia.

Cell-Mediated Immunodeficiencies

DIGEORGE'S SYNDROME

Because of the immaturity of the cell-mediated immune response in a normal neonate, the functional immunologic testing required to determine a T-cell defect must be interpreted with caution. Nevertheless, the total T-cell count is usually depressed (<1200/mm^3). Determination of T-cell numbers with monoclonal antibodies will reveal a striking decrease in T-cell populations. Functional studies of the immune system, such as delayed type hypersensitivity or lymphocyte mitogen stimulation, will usually result in negative responses.

Other nonimmunologic laboratory tests that will help to establish a diagnosis of DiGeorge's syndrome are x-rays to determine the absence of a thymic shadow. When coupled with the demonstration of elevated serum phosphorus, low serum calcium, and absent parathyroid hormone, these findings are strongly supportive of DiGeorge's.

SEVERE COMBINED IMMUNODEFICIENCY DISEASE (SCID)

Humoral immune responses in suspected SCID patients should be evaluated by serial determinations of IgM and IgA, which normally increase with time. Serum IgG is more difficult to assess because of the presence of maternal IgG; however, a continually declining IgG level combined with a failure of IgM and IgA to increase is an important finding, especially in infants with repeated infections. Most SCID patients will have severely depressed or totally absent peripheral B-cell levels.

Likewise, tests for cell-mediated immunity will be abnormal. Peripheral T-cell levels will be significantly depressed. Functional studies such as mitogen stimulation or mixed lymphocyte culture generally show no response. DTH testing will not provide meaningful data. Because of the possibility of SCID resulting from a deficiency in enzymes of the purine metabolic pathway, differential diagnosis must include a determination of ADA and NP levels, both of which should be in the normal range.[44, 45]

NEZELHOF'S SYNDROME

All laboratory tests of immune function are variable in patients with Nezelhof's. Although the levels of circulating B cells are usually within normal limits, the levels of each Ig class will vary. There is no specific antibody response following immunization. A differential diagnosis based on these findings can be difficult. It is often necessary to do further nonimmunologic testing to rule out ataxia–telangectasia or Wiskott-Aldrich.

ATAXIA–TELANGECTASIA

The immunologic defects seen in ataxia–telangectasia are similar to those seen in Nezelhof's in that most cell-mediated and humoral immune parameters are affected to a variable degree in each patient.[35] Selective IgA deficiency is a common finding. The presence of neurologic and endocrine disorders is important in establishing a differential diagnosis. Consistently elevated levels of α-fetoprotein are a common finding.

WISKOTT-ALDRICH SYNDROME

Early in the Wiskott-Aldrich syndrome, cell-mediated immunity is within normal limits, but it may decline progressively with age. Normal levels of circulating B cells will be present, but serum Ig analysis will reveal decreased IgM and increased IgA and IgE. This pattern may not appear until 1 year of age. Paraproteinemia may also be present.

Phagocytic Deficiency States

CHRONIC GRANULOMATOUS DISEASE (CGD)

The peripheral white cell count is often elevated in CGD, even when no active infection is present. Ig and complement levels may be elevated, with normal function. Cell-mediated immunity is normal. The best diagnostic test indication for CGD is the failure to reduce nitro-blue tetrazolium. The ability to reduce this substance is an indication of effective bactericidal capacity. Chemotactic assays will be normal.[46] There is also a correlation between CGD and the Mcleod phenotype on red cells.

CHÉDIAK-HIGASHI SYNDROME

On routine peripheral blood smears, giant cytoplasmic granular inclusion bodies can be found in both white cells and platelets in cases of Chédiak-Higashi syndrome. The bactericidal defect of the phagocytic cells is seen as an increased killing time due to abnormal lysosomal enzymes.

Complement Deficiencies

Very often an abnormal hemolytic complement level is the first indication of a complement deficiency. Quantitative analyses of the individual components will be necessary to establish a firm diagnosis.

Secondary Immunodeficiencies

Because of the diverse etiologies and the transient nature of the secondary immunodeficiencies, diagnosis can be difficult at best. A close examination of the medical history can often give a clue. A "screening panel" of Ig and complement levels, absolute lymphocyte count, and phagocytosis should provide further information.

ACQUIRED IMMUNODEFICIENCY SYNDROME (AIDS)

With the increasing incidence of HIV in the general population, test methodology readily adaptable to screening large numbers of samples has been developed. As in other infectious diseases, a serological approach has been chosen and is in use today. The basis for these tests is the detection in the serum of antibody that is produced following the host's exposure to virus. The preliminary screening test now in use for detecting HIV is an ELISA procedure that uses antigen derived from HIV and bound to a solid phase. While the sensitivity of the test is deliberately quite high, generally both the sensitivity and specificity vary among manufacturers of reagents for the test. Moreover, due to the crudeness of the antigen preparation used in the initial screening test, a seropositive result is only reported and followed up if two of three determinations on the sample are positive.

A more specific evaluation is available with the Western Blot technique, which is used to confirm an ELISA-positive result. In this technique, the crude viral antigen is subjected to electrophoresis to separate its viral components. The serum (antibody) sample is applied and, if HIV antibody is present, it will react with that specific component. This methodology identifies specific antibody against HIV and confirms its presence in the patient's serum.

Because of the grave prognosis for and current level of concern about AIDS, it is important to remember that both types of serologic methods in use evaluate *only the antibody content* of patient serum, and are currently considered supplemental tests by the Federal Drug Administration. Antibody is developed following exposure to viral antigen, with or without manifestations of the disease state. Although the presence of antibody is indicative of *exposure* to HIV, it by no means confirms that the disease itself is present, and the significance of the presence of the antibody in relation to the development of the disease is presently unknown. As yet, no laboratory method is available to evaluate directly the presence of the HIV antigen, although research has been underway for some time to develop testing that will do so. Further laboratory investigation of the patient's lymphocyte population and consideration of the nature of any symptoms that may exist are necessary to determine disease status.

A recent scheme for the staging of AIDS patients has somewhat simplified laboratory diagnosis. The presence of lymphadenopathy, opportunistic infections (particularly *Candida* and *Pneumocystis*), or Kaposi's sarcoma, combined with an absolute helper T-cell count below 400/mm^3, is considered presumptive evidence of AIDS.

TREATMENT

B-Cell Immunodeficiencies

BRUTON'S AGAMMAGLOBULINEMIA

The treatment of choice for hypogammaglobulinemic patients is intramuscular preparations of gamma globulins supported by broad-spectrum antibiotics.[47] The dose and timing of the gamma globulin should be tailored to the patient's clinical course. Antibiotics should be continued even when no infection is evident, as this appears to decrease the incidence of irreversible tissue damage. It has been suggested that fresh plasma infusions be given occasionally to replace the IgA that is virtually absent in commercial gamma globulin preparations. The major adverse reaction seen in these patients is anaphylaxis, most likely a result of intravenous delivery of aggregated IgG.

With better understanding of the disease and advances in therapy, many hypogammaglobulinemic patients have lived into their late 20s or early 30s. Chronic low-grade infections often result in progressive tissue damage, especially respiratory or neurologic. There also appears to be an increased risk of developing leukemias or lymphomas.

Serial determinations of IgG and IgM levels should be performed after each dose of gamma globulin to monitor effective serum levels and to determine when additional doses are required.

TRANSIENT NEONATAL HYPOGAMMAGLOBULINEMIA

If therapy for transient, physiologic neonatal hypogammaglobulinemia is required, it is identical to that for the X-linked condition. In some cases transient hypogammaglobulinemia has lasted for 18 to 24 months before spontaneously normalizing.

SELECTIVE IGA DEFICIENCY

At the present time, there is no effective immunologic replacement therapy for selective IgA deficiency. Patients should not be transfused with plasma or Ig fractions because of the increased risk of immunization against IgA and subsequent anaphylactic reactions. Broad-spectrum antibiotic therapy is the treatment of choice for this immunodeficiency state.

Although some patients with selective IgA deficiency have had normal life spans, the majority of affected individuals present with clinical problems within the first ten years of life. Careful monitoring and aggressive antibiotic intervention are necessary to keep morbidity at a minimum.

Cell-Mediated Immunodeficiencies

DIGEORGE'S SYNDROME

Once a diagnosis of congenital thymic aplasia has been made, a fetal thymic transplant should be performed as soon as feasible. To avoid potential graft-vs-host reactions, the thymus should be obtained from a fetus of less than 14 weeks of gestation. Alternatively, treatment with thymosins or other thymic hormones has been attempted, with mixed success. The prognosis for the individual with DiGeorge's syndrome is guarded at best. While there are some reports of good short-term survival, the numbers of patients who have received thymic grafts is insufficient to draw any firm conclusions. Those with successful grafts have displayed a variable reconstitution of their immune functions. An added problem is that patients who have been successfully engrafted still may suffer morbidity and mortality from their other congenital anomalies.

SEVERE COMBINED IMMUNODEFICIENCY DISEASE

Unless heroic measures are taken, the overwhelming majority of SCID individuals do not survive the first year. The major goal is to prevent systemic infections and the ensuing complications. Supportive therapy consists of aggressive antibiotic treatment and gamma globulin infusions as often as required. The only definitive therapy for SCID is bone marrow transplantation. Limited success has been reported with fetal liver or thymus transplants. As with DiGeorge's, a successful transplant will result in the appearance of some immune functions, but there are too few patients to permit a general conclusion. The major drawback to marrow transplantation is the present inability to adequately control graft-vs-host disease.

NEZELHOF'S SYNDROME

Therapy consists of aggressive antibiotic support and gamma globulin infusions. Experimental therapies have included bone marrow and thymic transplants, but neither have proven beneficial. Patients rarely survive beyond the age of 18 years.

ATAXIA–TELANGIECTASIA

Prophylactic antibiotics and gamma globulin will lessen the severity of the recurrent infections in ataxia–telangiectasia, but no curative therapy is available. Although some patients have survived into their fifth decade, the majority will succumb earlier to infection or neoplasm.[48]

WISKOTT-ALDRICH SYNDROME

Intravenous gamma globulin and antibiotic therapy are the best treatment available for Wiskott-Aldrich syndrome, although bone marrow transplantation is an experimental therapy.[49] Therapy is complicated by the concurrent thrombocytopenia. Although the prognosis has improved somewhat, patients who survive infectious complications often develop lymphoreticular or hematopoietic neoplasms.

ADA/NP DEFICIENCY

ADA-deficient individuals have been treated with red cells as a temporary source of the enzyme, but the definitive treatment for either enzyme deficiency remains bone marrow transplantation. Successful engraftment will result in normalization of enzyme levels. ADA deficiency may be treated with experimental gene therapy in the near future. The prognosis is variable, depending on the severity of the defect.[50]

Phagocytic Deficiency States

CHRONIC GRANULOMATOUS DISEASE

In the absence of a definitive cure, aggressive broad-spectrum antibiotic therapy is the treatment of choice to prevent or reduce the severity of the inevitable bacterial infection. Although improved diagnosis and therapy have produced survival into the second decade, chronic infection and organ dysfunction remain the major causes of morbidity and mortality.

CHÉDIAK-HIGASHI SYNDROME

The only treatment for Chédiak-Higashi syndrome is specific antibiotic therapy for each infection. Prognosis is poor, due to the increase with age in incidence of severe infections, coupled with increasing neurologic deficits. Death usually occurs in childhood.

Complement Deficiencies

C1—No specific therapy other than antibiotics has been accepted.

C2—Complement-replacement therapy is unwise due to the increased risk of immune complex-mediated tissue damage. The basic therapy involves treating the autoimmune disease and giving antibiotics when infection occurs.

C5–8—Therapy is limited to specific antibiotics during infectious episodes, although there have been some reports of successful reconstitutive therapy.

Secondary Immunodeficiencies

Because of the diversity of exogenous agents that can produce immunodeficiency states, the best therapy remains identification and removal (if possible) or replacement of the causative agent. Laboratory testing should be directed to identifying the specific immunologic defect and determining when these parameters have normalized. If the defect is found to be permanent, then selective support or replacement therapy is indicated.

ACQUIRED IMMUNODEFICIENCY SYNDROME (AIDS)

The current therapies for AIDS are all designed around immunomodulation or potentiation. Numerous clinical trials have been reported with antiviral agents, antiparasitic agents, interleukins, and interferons, to name but a few.[51, 52] At best, these regimens have produced prolongation of life span. At present, more than 50% of individuals with clinical AIDS have died.[53] There is no definitive cure, but work on a vaccine is progressing.[54]

CASE STUDY

A 17-week-old-male, weighing 9 lbs, 2 oz, was seen for chronic diarrhea and sinus infection. *Staphylococcus aureus* was isolated and antibiotics were prescribed; response was rapid and complete. At 6, 10, and 14 months the child was seen for respiratory infections, which responded partially to antibiotics. At 23 months the child was hospitalized for *Hemophilus influenzae* pneumonia; both height and weight were significantly below normal. Laboratory analyses at this time revealed normal levels of lymphocytes in the peripheral blood; further analysis by flow cytometry detected normal levels of T cells but less than 1% B cells (normal 5%–15%). Serum immunoglobulin levels were quantitated, and IgG, IgM, and IgA were all found to be significantly depressed (<10% normal). No other family members were found to have problems.

Questions

1. During the first year of life, what two immunodeficiencies must be considered, given this patient's history?
2. Given the patient's history over the first 2 years of life and the laboratory findings at the time of hospitalization, what is the most likely diagnosis?
3. What therapy is appropriate with this diagnosis, and what is the role of the laboratory in monitoring its effectiveness?

Discussion

1. Bruton's agammaglobulinemia and transitory neonatal hypogammaglobulinemia should be considered.
2. Bruton's agammaglobulinemia is the most likely diagnosis. Recurrent infections in a male infant with only partial response to antibiotics is typical of Bruton's. In addition, the decreased number of B cells, normal level of T cells, and decrease in immunoglobulins of all classes are consistent with this diagnosis. Only gamma globulin would be decreased in transient neonatal hypogammaglobulinemia.
3. Intramuscular injection of immunoglobulin on a periodic basis is the appropriate treatment in this case, with laboratory monitoring of the immunoglobulin levels.

REFERENCES

1. Cooper MD, Lawton AR, Prud'homme JL: Primary antibody deficiencies. Springer Semin Immunopathol 1:265, 1978
2. Schur, PH: Selective gamma-G globulin deficiencies in patients with recurrent pyogenic infections. N Engl J Med 283:631, 1970
3. De la Concha EG, Garcia-Rodriquez MC, Zabay JM et al: Functional assessment of T and B lymphocytes in patients with selective IgM deficiency. Clin Exp Immunol 49:670, 1982
4. Tiller TL, Buckley RH: Transient hypogammaglobulinemia of infancy: Review of the literature, clinical and immunologic features of 11 new cases, and long-term followup. J Pediatr 92:347, 1978
5. Siegel RL, Isseekutz T, Schwaber J et al: Deficiency of T helper cells in transient hypogammaglobulinemia of infancy. N Engl J Med 305:1307, 1981
6. Barrett DJ, Ammann AJ, Wara DW: Clinical and immunological spectrum of the DiGeorge syndrome. J Clin Lab Immunol 6:1, 1981
7. Pahwa SG, Pahwa RN, Good RA: Heterogeneity of B lymphocyte differentiation in patients with recurrent pyogenic infections. J Clin Invest 66:543, 1980
8. Hirschorn R, Martin DW: Enzyme defects in immunodeficiency diseases. Semin Immunopathol 1:299, 1978
9. Arnaout MA, Pitt J, Cohen HJ: Deficiency of a granulocyte membrane glycoprotein (gp150) in a boy with recurrent bacterial infections. N Engl J Med 306:693, 1982
10. Lehrer RI, Cline MJ: Leukocyte myeloperoxidase deficiency and disseminated candidiasis: The role of myeloperoxidase and resistance to Candida infections. J Clin Invest 48:1478, 1978
11. Quie PG, Root RK, Metcalf JA: Phagocytic defects. Springer Semin Immunopathol 1:323, 1978
12. Johnston RB, Baehner RL: Chronic granulomatous disease: Correlation between pathogenesis and clinical findings. Pediatrics 48:730, 1971
13. Blume RS, Wolff SM: The Chédiak-Higashi syndrome: Studies in four patients and a review of the literature. Medicine 51:246, 1972
14. Haliotis T: Chédiak-Higashi gene in humans: 1. Impairment of natural killer function. J Exp Med 151:1039, 1980
15. Agnello V: Complement deficiency states. Medicine 57:1, 1978
16. Frank MM: Hereditary angioedema: The clinical syndrome and its management. Ann Intern Med 84:580, 1976
17. Muller-Eberhard HJ: Complement abnormalities in human disease. Hosp Pract 13:65, 1978
18. Miller CL: Secondary immunodeficiency in burns

and surgical trauma. Clin Immunol Allerg 1:641, 1981
19. Gottleib MS, Groopman JE, Weinstein WM: The acquired immunodeficiency syndrome. Ann Intern Med 99:208, 1983
20. Reinherz EL, Geha RS, Wohl, ME et al: Immunodeficiency associated with loss of T4$^+$-inducer T-cell function. N Engl J Med 304:811, 1981
21. Clavel F, Gu'etard D, Brun-V'ezinet F et al: Isolation of a new human retrovirus from West African patients with AIDS. Science 233:343, 1986
22. Hahn BH, Shaw GM, Taylor ME et al: Genetic variation in HTLV-III over time in patients with AIDS or at risk for AIDS. Science 232:1548, 1986
23. Brown F: Human immunodeficiency virus. Science 232:1486, 1986
24. Kanki PJ, Barin F, M'Boup S et al: New human T-lymphotropic retrovirus related to simian T-lymphotropic virus type III (STLV-IIIAGM). Science 232:238, 1986
25. Folks T, Powell DM, Lightfoote MM et al: Induction of HTLV-III/LAV from a nonvirus-producing T-cell line: Implications for latency. Science 231:600, 1986
26. Marx JL: The slow, insidious nature of the HTLVs. Science 231:450, 1986
27. McDougal JS, Kennedy MS, Sligh JM et al: Binding of HTLV-III/LAV to T4$^+$ T cells by a complex of the 110K viral protein and the T_4 molecule. Science 231:382, 1986
28. Lifson JD, Reyes GR, McGrath MS et al: AIDS retrovirus-induced cytopathology: Giant cell formation and involvement of CD4 antigen. Science 232:1123, 1986
29. Gartner S, Markovits P, Markovits DM et al: The role of mononuclear phagocytes in HTLV-III/LAV infection. Science 233:215, 1986
30. Hermans PE, Diaz-Buxo JA, Stobo JD: Idiopathic late onset immunoglobulin deficiency: Clinical observations in 50 patients. Am J Med 61:221, 1976
31. Chipps BE, Talamo RC, Winklestein JA: IgA deficiency, recurrent pneumonias, and bronchiectasis. Chest 73:519, 1978
32. Schlegel RJ, Bernier GM, Bellanti JA: Severe candidiasis associated with thymic dysplasia, IgA deficiency, and plasma antilymphocyte effects. Pediatrics 45:926, 1970
33. Hitzig WH, Martin DW: Severe combined immunodeficiency diseases. Springer Semin Immunopathol 1:238, 1978
34. Rivat-Peran L, Buriot D, Salier J: Immunoglobulins in ataxia–telangiectasia: Evidence for IgG4 and IgA2 subclass deficiencies. Clin Immunol Immunopathol 20:99, 1981
35. Ochs HD, Sclichter SJ, Harker LA: The Wiskott-Aldrich syndrome: Studies of lymphocytes, granulocytes, and platelets. Blood 55:243, 1980
36. Parry MD, Root RK, Metcalf JA: Myeloperoxidase deficiency: Prevalence and clinical significance. Ann Intern Med 95:263, 1981
37. Sirriani MC, Fiorilli M, Pandolfi F: Natural killer activity and lymphocyte subpopulations in patients with primary humoral and cellular immunodeficiencies. Clin Immunol Immunopathol 21:12, 1981
38. Day NK: C2 deficiency: Development of lupus erythematosus. J Clin Invest 52:1601, 1973
39. Apel CH, Bloch RG, Rosen LS: Increased susceptibility to infection in a patient with type II essential hypercatabolism of C3. N Engl J Med 288:601, 1973
40. Miller NE, Nilsson UR: A familial deficiency of the phagocytosis-enhancing activity of serum related to a dysfunction of the fifth component of complement (C5). N Engl J Med 282:354, 1970
41. Curran JW, Morgan WM, Hardy AM et al: The epidemiology of AIDS: Current status and future trends. Science 229:1352, 1985
42. Barnes DM: Brain endothelial cells infected by AIDS virus. Science 233:418, 1986
43. Schur PH, Rosen F, Norman ME: Immunoglobulin subclasses in normal children. Pediatr Res 63:301, 1979
44. Giblett ER, Anderson JE, Cohen F: Adenosine deaminase deficiency in two patients with severely impaired cellular immunity. Lancet 2:1067, 1972
45. Webster AD: Metabolic defects in immunodeficiency diseases (Review). Clin Exp Immunol 49:1, 1982
46. Gallin JL: Disorders of phagocyte chemotaxis. Ann Intern 92:520, 1980
47. Amman AJ, Ashman RF, Buckley RH: Use of intravenous gammaglobulin in antibody deficiency: Results of a multicenter-controlled trial. Clin Immunol Immunopathol 22:60, 1982
48. Kersey JH, Spector BD, Good RA: Cancer in children with primary immunodeficiency diseases. J Pediatr 84:263, 1974
49. Parkman R: Complete correction of the Wiskott-Aldrich syndrome by allogeneic bone marrow transplantation. N Engl J Med 298:921, 1978

50. Mitchell BS, Kelley WN: Purinogenic immunodeficiency disease: Clinical features and molecular mechanisms. Ann Intern Med 92:826, 1980
51. Barnes DM: In search of the best drugs against AIDS. Science 233:419, 1986
52. Barnes DM: Measuring antibodies may predict disease. Science 233:419, 1986
53. Norman C: AIDS trends: Projections from limited data. Science 230:1018, 1985
54. Sarin PS, Sun DK, Thornton AH et al: Neutralization of HTLV-III/LAV replication by antiserum to thymosin alpha 1. Science 232:1135, 1986

Chapter 54

Allergies

Hal S. Larsen /
Shirley MacManigal /
Scot C. Buessow

The immune system is an essential part of our defenses against pathogenic microorganisms and environmental exposures. In the majority of cases the immune response is beneficial, although in certain situations a state of hypersensitivity can result in immune-mediated disease.

ETIOLOGY AND PATHOPHYSIOLOGY

Immunologic hypersensitivities have been classified into four general categories. These are based on the kinetics of the response and the mechanisms for tissue injury. The four types of hypersensitivity reactions (Types I, II, III, and IV) are summarized in Table 54-1.[1] Although this classification is useful, it is important to keep in mind that, except for anaphylactic reactions, human disease processes involving hypersensitivity usually involve mechanisms from more than one type.

Type I hypersensitivity is characterized by an immune response within minutes following contact with the antigen. The allergic response can be either generalized or cutaneous. Both types of reaction are dependent on specific triggering of immunoglobulin E-sensitized mast cells by the antigen, followed by release of powerful pharmacologic mediators of inflammation.

The IgE molecule shows the four-chain basic antibody structure: two identical H or heavy chains and two L or light chains (see Fig. 54-1).

Although IgE has many similarities to the other classes of immunoglobulin, there are distinct differences. Some characteristics of the human immunoglobulins and a comparison with IgE are found in Table 54-2.

The mast cell and basophil are important sources of substances that mediate the clinical effects of immediate hypersensitivity. Mast cells are widely distributed in the connective tissues and are especially prevalent along small blood vessels. Their cytoplasm is filled with granules that are the source of the mediators of inflammation. Basophils are found in very low numbers in the circulation and are rarely seen in the tissue of normal individuals. They resemble mast cells in that they contain deep violet blue granules, pharmacologic mediators, and bind IgE, but they differ in a number of other characteristics.

The role of eosinophils in allergy is unclear. They are capable of phagocytizing and killing microorganisms, and can be degranulated by appropriate stimuli. These cells appear at the site of hypersensitivity reactions and produce substances that inhibit the release or action of some of the mast cell mediators.[2, 3, 4]

The common allergic respiratory diseases affect an estimated 40 million persons in the United States. Inhalant allergens are most frequently involved, and are usually derived from natural organic sources such as house dust, mold spores, insect products, pollens, and animal epithelial products. Seasonal allergic disease is usually due to pollens such as ragweed, molds, and insects. Inhalant allergens are most often responsible for rhinitis, conjunctivitis, and asthma, and occasionally cause urticaria or systemic anaphylaxis. Year-round allergies are due to exposure to nonseasonal allergens such as dust, animal danders, some plant products, and molds. In addition, occupational exposure to certain chemicals has been

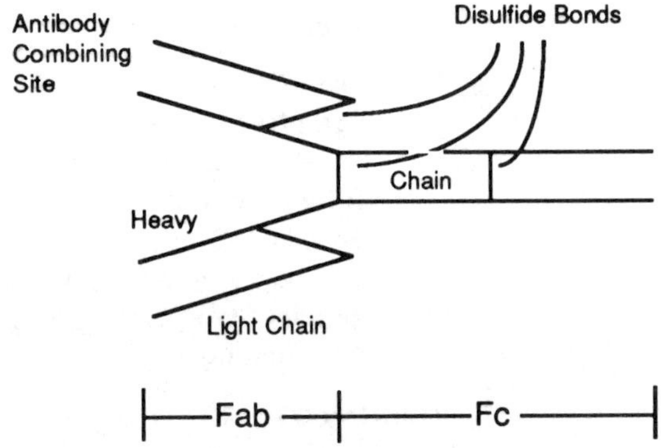

Figure 54-1 **The IgE molecule is comprised of two heavy and two light chains connected by disulfide bonds. The portion designated Fc has a constant amino acid sequence when different IgE antibodies are compared. The antibody combining site or Fab portion has a variable amino acid sequence that reflects the response to different antigens.**

Table 54-1 ***Comparison of the Four Types of Hypersensitivity Reactions***

	I Immediate	II Cytotoxic	III Immune Complexes	IV Delayed
Mechanisms	Mediator release from sensitized mast cells following antigenic challenge	Antibody-mediated damage to host cells or tissue	Immune complexes deposited in tissue	Sensitized T cells release lymphokines following secondary contact with antigen
Antigens	Usually exogenous small proteins or drugs	Cell surface antigens, *e.g.*, tissue, blood group antigens, viral particles or compounds attaching to cell surface	Extracellular, *e.g.*, serum proteins, DNA, viruses, drugs	Cell surface or extracellular, *e.g.*, tuberculin, poison ivy, nickel
Reactions following intradermal injection of antigen				
Time for maximum response	30 min	–	3–8 hr	24–48 hr
Macroscopic appearance	Wheal and flare	–	Erythema and edema	Erythema and induration
Histologic appearance	Eosinophils; degranulated mast cells	–	Acute inflammatory reaction; polymorphonuclear leukocytes	Mononuclear cells
Passive Sensitization	Serum	Serum	Serum	Lymphocytes
Disorders	Allergic rhinitis Asthma	Transfusion reactions Drug reactions	Serum sickness SLE	Contact dermatitis Allograft rejection

shown to be an increasing cause of allergic rhinitis, asthma, or both.

Symptoms of *allergic rhinitis* can occur when the sensitized individual inhales allergen. This initiates a rapid release of various mediators from mast cells. These mediators cause vasodilation and edema (nasal congestion), increased mucus secretion and cellular recruitment (rhinorrhea), and increased capillary and mucosal permeability. The mediators probably also disturb the balanced nervous control of nasal function, which leads to direct and reflex vascular dilation and hypersecretion and also reduces the sneezing threshold. *Allergic asthma* is an IgE-mediated problem in which pa-

Table 54-2 ***Characteristics of Human Immunoglobulins***

	IgG	IgA	IgM	IgD	IgE
Normal serum concentration (mg/dL)	1000	200	120	3	0.05
Serum half-life (days)	23	6	5	2–8	1–5
Synthetic rate (g/day/70 kg)	2.3	1.7	0.1	0.03	2×10^{-4}
% carbohydrate	3	7	12	13	12
Molecular weight	150,000	155,000	900,000	180,000	190,000
Complement fixation (classic)	+	–	+	–	–
Placental transfer	+	–	–	–	–
Reaginic activity	–	–	–	–	+

Conversion to SI units is as follows:
Proteins—mg/dL × 10 = mg/L

tients have a specific sensitivity to common inhaled substances such as house dust, mold spores, and plant pollens. It is not uncommon for patients to demonstrate allergic rhinitis along with the asthma symptoms[3, 5, 6] (see Chap. 8).

Hypersensitivity pneumonitis is a general term that identifies a variety of clinical conditions, all with more fanciful descriptions. Names such as "pituitary snufftaker's lung," "doghouse disease," "farmer's lung," "wheat weevil disease," and "bird fancier's lung" are a few of the clinical descriptions. The list of recognized causes of hypersensitivity pneumonitis continues to grow. All of these illnesses have in common the inhalation of organic material that leads to airway and lung parenchymal hypersensitivity reactions in susceptible persons.[7, 8]

Allergic bronchopulmonary aspergillosis (ABPA) is an inflammatory bronchial and interstitial lung disease occurring in patients with preexisting asthma. The disease is caused by the host response to the fungal organism.

There is evidence of defects in the cell-mediated immune response in patients with *atopic dermatitis (AD)* These patients have an increased susceptibility to infections with viruses such as herpes simplex and vaccinia. The results of skin testing for delayed-type hypersensitivity reactions with antigens such as *Candida* and poison ivy extract are delayed or less than normal. A number of cell-mediated immune parameters such as response to mitogens are decreased. In addition, a variety of leukocyte dysfunctions have been reported in AD, including defective neutrophil chemotaxis.

Patients with AD also show a number of physiologic and pharmacologic abnormalities, such as abnormal vascular reactions, increased skin histamine in affected areas, and a host of other features.[6, 7, 9]

Urticaria–angioedema can be classified into six groups: reactions that are idiopathic, and those mediated by IgE, physical stimuli, complement, direct mast cell-releasing agents, and arachidonic acid metabolism abnormalities.

The majority of cases of chronic urticaria and angioedema are *idiopathic*. Proof of hormonal abnormalities, malignant conditions, foods, medications, or emotional factors as causes is lacking. Specific antigens such as foods, drugs, pollens, and bee stings can induce severe reactions that are *IgE-mediated. Physical urticaria* occurs after a variety of stimuli such as pressure, cold, sunlight, heat, and exercise. *Complement-mediated* urticaria–angioedema is associated with the absence of the serum inhibitor of the activated first component of complement. This hereditary condition, known as hereditary angioedema, may involve the upper respiratory and gastrointestinal tracts and may cause severe manifestations. Mediators may be released directly from *mast cells* following the administration of opiates, polymyxin B, curare, and radiocontrast media.[6, 9, 10, 11]

Anaphylaxis is an acute life-threatening event resulting from antigen-induced, IgE-mediated release or formation of chemical mediators that affect smooth muscle and vascular permeability.[12]

Mast Cell Activation and Release of Mediators

Type I hypersensitivity occurs when IgE antibodies, produced in response to an otherwise innocuous antigen, bind to the surface of mast cells and basophils. Mast cells and basophils have high-affinity binding sites for the Fc portion of IgE. When the appropriate antigen is encountered again, the antigen cross-links or connects the cell-bound IgE molecules with one another, which triggers degranulation of the cell (see Fig. 54-2). Breakdown products of complement (C3a, C5a) serve to degranulate mast cells, as do calcium ionophore, mellitin, synthetic ACTH, codeine, and morphine. This causes an exocytosis of preformed mediators such as histamine, and the induction of prostaglandins and leukotrienes, as outlined on this page, at the top of the opposite column.

Mediators of Immediate Hypersensitivity

Preformed Mediators
Histamine
Eosinophil chemotactic factor-A (ECF-A)
Heparin
Serotonin
Enzymes

Newly-Generated Mediators
Platelet aggregating factor (PAF)
Arachidonic acid metabolites
- Leukotrienes (LTB_4, LTC_4, LTD_4, LTE_4)
- SRS-A (LTC_4 + LTD_4)
- Prostaglandins (PG)
- Thromboxanes

The physiological effects of degranulation are summarized in Figures 54-3 and 54-4. Among the effects of histamine are bronchial and intestinal smooth-muscle contraction; an increase in vascular permeability; pulmonary vasoconstriction; stimulation of nasal mucus production; and enhancement or inhibition of granulocyte chemotaxis.[4, 13]

CLINICAL MANIFESTATIONS

An estimated 17% of all Americans have at least one common allergic disease. Practically any organ or tissue may become the target of immu-

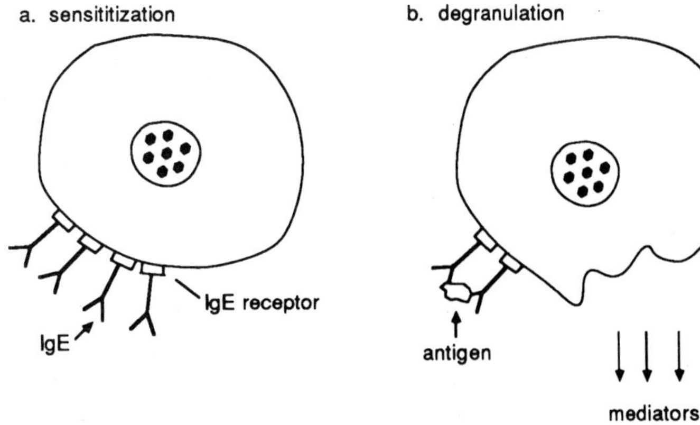

Figure 54-2 **Mast cells bind IgE via their Fc receptors and are sensitized. When antigen is encountered, crosslinking occurs with subsequent degranulation and release of mediators.**

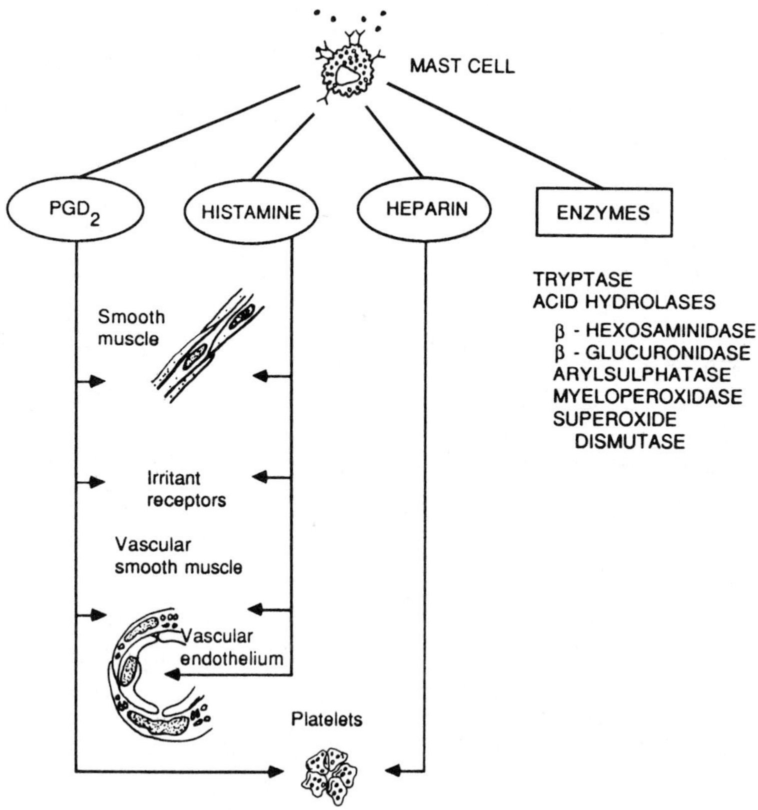

Figure 54-3 Products of mucosal mast cell activation. The effects of heparin and prostaglandin D_2 (PGD_2) on platelets are inhibitory, whereas the effects of histamine and PGD_2 on other target cells are stimulatory. Enzymes are released during activation and may generate mediators from precursors in plasma. (From Lessof MH [ed]: Allergy, Immunological and Clinical Aspects. New York, John Wiley & Sons, 1984)

nologically-mediated disease. Allergic disease may be grouped into the following categories, according to the site of antigen contact and the severity of the disease: respiratory, cutaneous, digestive, and anaphylaxis (see Table 54-3). These categories are not mutually exclusive, because antigen exposure at any site may lead to symptoms at a distant site or to anaphylaxis.

Allergic Rhinitis

A variety of types of rhinitis and other nasal conditions must be considered in the differential diagnosis of allergic rhinitis. These include eosinophilic nonallergic rhinitis, vasomotor rhinitis of pregnancy, vasomotor rhinitis, rhinitis medicamentosa, and disturbed nasal function associated with a number of clinical conditions (tumors, ciliary dyskinesia, hypothyroidism, aspirin intolerance, and others). As many as 60% to 70% of patients with chronic rhinitis are assigned to one of these poorly understood categories.

Allergic rhinitis is associated with symptoms of nasal discharge or obstruction, sneezing, itching of the nose, eyes, palate, pharynx, and conjunctivae, and mucous discharge.

Patients may show irritability, fatigue, depression, and anorexia. Maxillofrontal headache, postnasal discharge, and persistent nasal stuffiness may indicate complicating inflammatory sinusitus. Symptoms related to accompanying serous otitis and eustachian tube dysfunction may also be present, particularly in children.[5, 8]

Asthma

Asthma involves the large and small bronchi and is characterized by wheezing and breathlessness, of-

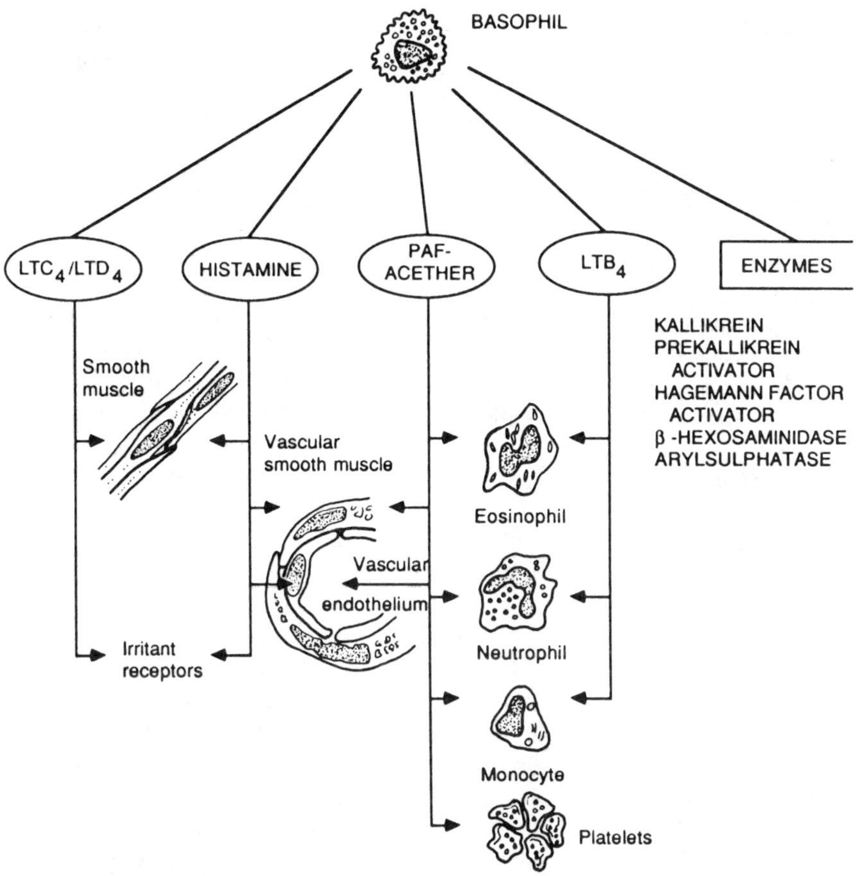

Figure 54-4 **Products of basophil activation. Histamine and products of phospholipid metabolism (leukotrienes B_4, C_4, and D_4 [LTB_4 LTC_4, and LTD_4] activate smooth muscle and inflammatory cells. Enzymes may generate mediators from precursors in plasma. (From Lessof MH [ed]: Allergy, Immunological and Clinical Aspects. New York, John Wiley & Sons, 1984)**

ten with cough and sputum production. There is reduction in the airway diameter due to construction of smooth muscle, edema of the mucous membranes and bronchial wall tissues, accumulation of thick tenacious secretions, and inflammatory changes in the bronchial mucosa. This obstruction of the air flow can be reversed with medication or with time, and the term "reversible obstructive airways disease" is often used in place of "asthma" (see Chap. 8).

Some patients with intrinsic asthma have a clinical intolerance to aspirin that manifests as rhinitis, nasal polyps, or exacerbations of asthma. The mechanism of aspirin-induced asthma is thought to be mediated through alteration of arachidonic acid metabolism.[8, 11]

Hypersensitivity Pneumonitis

The reaction that occurs in patients susceptible to hypersensitivity pneumonitis is different from that seen in asthma, in that the allergic reaction does

Table 54-3 ***Clinical Manifestations of Allergic Disease***

Site of Antigen Exposure	Diseases
Respiratory	Allergic rhinitis Asthma Hypersensitivity pneumonitis
Cutaneous	Atopic dermatitis Urticaria Angioedema (anaphylaxis)
Digestive	Food allergy (Urticaria) (Angioedema) (Anaphylaxis)
Anaphylaxis	Anaphylaxis due to Allergenic extracts Drugs Insect stings Food

not occur immediately following inhalation of the allergen. The onset of signs and symptoms occurs from 4 to 6 hours after exposure, with cough, fever, and dyspnea commonly seen.[8]

Aspergillosis

Allergic bronchopulmonary aspergillosis is characterized by eosinophilia, pulmonary infiltrates, and bronchial plugging by secretions that contain eosinophils and *Aspergillus*.[6]

Cutaneous

Allergic skin diseases are common problems that occur in both adults and children. Conditions to be discussed include atopic dermatitis, allergic contact dermatitis, and urticaria and angioedema.[11]

Atopic Dermatitis

Atopic dermatitis (AD) is a difficult disease to characterize and define. It is a common dermatitis characterized by severe pruritus, frequent onset in infancy, a strong familial propensity, and a tendency to chronicity.

The dermatitis usually begins on cheeks in the first few months after birth. The face, scalp, neck, diaper area, and extensor surface of the extremities are the areas most commonly affected in an infant. The patches are erythematous and edematous and may have weeping or crusted surfaces. During childhood, the face is involved less often, while the sides of the neck show lesions. The teenager or adult tends to have localized plaques of dry, thickened skin with varying degrees of redness and scaling.

Patients with atopic dermatitis often have increased levels of serum IgE, family histories of allergic disease, and development of allergic rhinitis or asthma.[3, 6, 9, 14]

Urticaria–Angioedema

Urticaria–angioedema is a common problem that has its highest incidence in young adults. Urticaria, or *hives,* appears as pruritic, circumscribed, and elevated erythematous areas of cutaneous edema that involve the superficial portions of the dermis. When the edema extends deeper into the skin or mucous membranes, it is referred to as *angioedema.*

A common response to aspirin ingestion is development of urticaria–angioedema. Aspirin and related compounds inhibit the biosynthesis of prostaglandin E_2 from arachidonic acid. This favors the synthesis of prostaglandin F_2, which is a bronchoconstrictor, and leukotrienes (SRS-A).[11]

Digestive

Immediate hypersensitivity reactions to foods begin within minutes to hours following ingestion. Symptoms may be confined to the digestive tract or may involve other target sites, particularly the skin. Allergic reactions to foods may begin at the initial site of exposure with itching, burning, and swelling of the lips or oral cavity. Gastrointestinal symptoms may occur as the antigen travels through the intestinal tract. Intestinal symptoms include nausea, vomiting, cramping, abdominal distention, and diarrhea. The most profound reaction to foods is systemic anaphylaxis.[10, 15]

Anaphylaxis

Symptoms of anaphylaxis can begin within seconds or take up to an hour to develop. Onset is usually within 5 to 10 minutes. The cardiovascular system, respiratory tract, gastrointestinal tract, and skin are the major organs affected. The most common manifestations of anaphylaxis are urticaria, flushing, and angioedema, although symptoms involving multiple organ systems may be seen. Reactions involving the cardiovascular and respiratory systems are the most serious, and deaths have occurred as the result of laryngeal edema and shock.[12]

LABORATORY ANALYSES AND DIAGNOSIS

Laboratory findings are of little value in anaphylaxis because the diagnosis must be made and treatment begun in a very short time-frame. On the other hand, the diagnosis of the less acute allergic diseases can be aided by the proper *in vitro* and *in vivo* studies.

Determining the diagnosis of chronic allergic rhinitis is difficult because there is no objective test that is pathognomonic. Consequently, diagnosis must be made on the basis of medical history and interview, examination, and laboratory data, including a nasal smear and skin tests. Seasonal allergic rhinitis due to pollens seldom presents a problem in diagnosis except in efforts to differentiate it from the common cold.[6, 14, 16]

Complete Blood Count

A complete blood count (CBC) should be done on all patients suspected of having allergic disease. Eosinophilia is not an uncommon finding and, when consistent with the patient's allergic signs and symptoms, often requires no further investigation. Unexplained numbers of eosinophils, particularly in the absence of allergic disease, may indicate parasitic infestation, collagen vascular diseases, malignancy, or drug reactions. Allergic bronchopulmonary aspergillosis is characterized by a significant eosinophilia. In general, allergic diseases are associated with eosinophilia, although the occurrence of eosinophilia is not a consistent finding. Diagnosis, in most cases, is made on the basis of physical findings and history, with the CBC playing a minor role. Patients with food allergy, however, may demonstrate anemia due to occult gastrointestinal bleeding. In this case a CBC, with or without eosinophilia, will be of diagnostic importance.

Although eosinophilia is usually determined by relative means, by the use of the peripheral blood differential, absolute eosinophil counts may be more useful in some cases.

Nasal Cytology

Nasal cytology can be used to evaluate patients with chronic rhinitis. When correlated with historical data and physical findings, these results aid in the determination of the type of rhinitis present. Nasal cytologic examination can be performed on expelled mucus, but a more satisfactory specimen is obtained by scraping the nasal turbinates and mucosal surfaces with a flexible nasal probe. Nasal smears are usually limited to questionable cases and to determinations of chronic allergic rhinitis.

Total Serum IgE

Total serum IgE levels are elevated in many, but not all, patients with allergic (IgE-mediated) disease. There are also nonallergic diseases that are associated with an increase in serum IgE. These include parasitic, infectious, immunologic, and cutaneous diseases. The total serum IgE level, therefore, does not precisely correlate with the presence or absence of allergy in a patient. Measurement of serum IgE is helpful in following patients with allergic bronchopulmonary aspergillosis, because a rise in IgE may indicate a relapse. The most frequently used assay for the measurement of total IgE levels is the PRIST (paper radioimmunosorbent test) assay. This technique enables measurement of picogram quantities of IgE, which are reported as units or nanograms per mL (one unit is equivalent to 2.4 ng).

Specific IgE

Measurement of specific IgE can be accomplished by the radioallergosorbent test (RAST). The RAST is similar to the PRIST except that specific antigens, rather than IgE molecules, are the objects of analysis. The RAST is a sensitive test that measures picogram quantities of IgE and correlates well with other classic techniques such as the Prausnitz-Küstner test and skin tests. Advantages of RAST testing include that there is no risk of anaphylaxis or of sensitization, it is unaffected by skin diseases, there is no need to interrupt antihistamines, and it is especially useful in infants. Problems include the expense, use of radioactivity, interference by non-IgE antibody, and lack of quantification. There is some controversy about the use of the RAST instead of skin testing. Skin testing, properly performed, is the method of choice for assessment of antigen-specific IgE in most patients.

Leukocyte Histamine Release

Basophils will release histamine when challenged by the antigen to which they have been sensitized. An *in vitro* test (leukocyte histamine release) is available for measurement of this release. Leukocyte histamine release is a time-consuming, difficult test to perform and is not practical as a routine diagnostic procedure.

Arterial Blood Gases

The determination of arterial blood gases is an important method of laboratory evaluation of the asthmatic patient, especially in an acute episode. Arterial blood gas determinations are indicated if the patient is steroid-dependent, fails to respond to therapy rapidly, or has a history of frequent hospitalizations for asthma. Blood should be obtained when the patient is breathing room air and not receiving supplemental oxygen. Abnormalities are usually respiratory alkalosis and hypocarbia, followed by hypoxia.

Skin Testing

Direct skin tests are the most commonly used of all tests in clinical allergy. Testing may be performed by intradermal or prick-puncture methods, with the latter being preferred in most cases. Testing sites (back or forearm) are cleansed, and a drop of antigen solution is placed on the skin. A needle or prick-puncture device is inserted into the skin through the antigen. Only superficial penetration is made, and no bleeding should occur. The antigen is removed by blotting one minute after puncture, and the site is observed for a wheal-and-flare reaction 15 minutes later. Skin testing is inexpensive, rapid, precise, and sensitive. In addition, a multitude of antigens are available.

Considerations in skin testing include the potential for anaphylaxis, skin disease, the potential for sensitizing the patient, and the age of the patient (infants and elderly individuals can be difficult). In general, skin testing is a reproducible, accurate (particularly with food antigens), sensitive, and patient-accepted method of allergy testing, and has been found to be very helpful in a number of allergic conditions.

TREATMENT

The treatment of an allergic disease may be as simple as removing the offending antigen from the patient's environment or as complex as the individualized treatment protocols used in asthma. For some conditions, such as seasonal allergic rhinitis, the use of an antihistamine may be adequate for relief. For others, more aggressive therapy, such as antigen desensitization, is attempted. Treatment of sensitized individuals focuses on either preventing the antigen from reaching the sensitized mast cell or preventing or lessening the effects of the mediators that are released if antigen makes contact with the cell-bound IgE.

Antigen desensitization (hyposensitization) therapy involves the injection of increasing doses of allergen over time. Many patients benefit from such treatment, although the exact mechanism by which it works is unknown. Following treatment there is an increase in antigen-specific IgG and a fall in antigen-specific IgE. This fall is thought to be due to an increase in suppressor T-cell activity, which in turn leads to a suppression of the IgE response. In the case of individuals allergic to bee venom, the IgG produced by the hyposensitization protects by neutralizing the injected antigen. There is also evidence that there are nonspecific suppressor factors affecting IgE synthesis and subsequently allergy. Much work remains to be done, however, to determine the mechanisms involved in hyposensitization and how to apply these mechanisms to treatment.[5, 6, 7, 14]

DELAYED HYPERSENSITIVITY

In most instances the term allergy is synonymous with immediate hypersensitivity. However, the classification of hypersensitivity is not clearly separated, in that patients may demonstrate allergic disease based on a complex mechanism involving elements of more than one of the four hypersensitivity types.

Type IV, or delayed-type hypersensitivity (DTH), is characterized by a reaction consisting mainly of erythema and induration. The cellular interactions and mediators involved in DTH are very complex. Unlike other forms of hypersensitivity, DTH is dependent not upon antibodies, but rather upon sensitized T lymphocytes. Also, the reaction that occurs following intradermal injection of antigen into a sensitized individual peaks within 24 to 48 hours.

A common dermatologic problem is *allergic contact dermatitis,* which is characterized by a 48-hour delayed eczematous response to the antigen. The most common contact-sensitizing antigens encountered in clinical practice are plants (poison ivy, oak, or sumac), paraphenylenediamine, nickel compounds, rubber compounds, and the dichromates. The diagnosis is based on the distribution of the lesions, medical history, and examination for environmental exposures. The diagnosis can be confirmed by patch testing, which consists of applying the suspected antigen to the patient's skin and covering it with a dressing for 48 hours. An eczematous reaction at the site of the patch test constitutes a positive response. The patch test is of importance because an eczematous reaction is not otherwise pathognomonic of allergic contact dermatitis. Treatment involves avoidance of the offending antigen or application of hydrocortisone cream if dermatitis is present.

Tuberculin-type hypersensitivity is characterized by local induration and swelling, with or without a fever. There is an intense infiltration by mononuclear cells, of which about 50% are lymphoctyes and the remainder monocytes. As the lesion develops it may become a granulomatous reaction. This type is often associated with the presence of an infectious agent such as *Mycobacterium tuberculosis, Mycobacterium leprae,* and *Leishmania tropica.* However, nonmicrobial antigens may also induce this type of reaction, and it may be seen in individuals treated with BCG.

Granulomatous hypersensitivity is clinically the most important form of delayed hypersensitivity. This type, which causes many of the pathological effects in diseases that involve T cell-mediated immunity, results from the presence of a persistent agent within macrophages. This agent is usually a microorganism that the macrophage is unable to destroy. It may also be caused by the continued presence of immune complexes (*e.g.,* allergic alveolitis). The result is an epithelioid cell granuloma formation that, histologically, is quite different from the tuberculin-type reaction.[1, 17]

CASE STUDY #1

A seven-year-old girl demonstrated conjunctivitis and rhinitis during August and September. The child had sunken, dark-appearing infraorbital areas and constantly rubbed the tip of her nose upward with the palm of her hand. The tympanic membranes were well visualized and appeared normal in appearance and in mobility. Hearing was normal. The nasal mucosa was boggy, glistening, and bluish-grey, with swelling over the inferior turbinates.

LABORATORY FINDINGS

Hematocrit	38%
Hemoglobin	13.5 g/dL (2.09 mmol/L)
WBC	$8.5 \times 10^3/mm^3$
PMNs	56%
Lymph	29%
Mono	4%
Eosin	11%
Serum immunoglobulins	
IgA, M, G	Normal range
IgE	Markedly elevated
Nasal smear	Many eosinophils
Urinalysis	Normal

Questions

1. A presentation such as this could have an infectious etiology. Which tests distinguish between infectious and allergic processes?
2. Are any other tests indicated?

Discussion

1. This case demonstrates the laboratory findings seen in allergic rhinitis: eosinophilia, positive nasal smear, and elevated serum immunoglobulin E levels.
2. Nasal cultures could be done; however, on the basis of cost, treatment for an allergic condition should be attempted first.

CASE STUDY #2

A 26-year-old male with an eight-year history of asthma was admitted to the hospital for acute shortness of breath.

LABORATORY FINDINGS

CBC	Normal except for 7% eosinophils
Urinalysis	Normal
Nasal smear	No eosinophils seen
Sputum smear	No eosinophils seen
Arterial blood gases	
*p*H	7.50
PCO_2	37 mm Hg
PO_2	70 mm Hg
Bicarbonate	25 mEq/L (25 mmol/L)
Skin tests	4+ reaction to all grasses tested

Questions

1. Does lack of nasal or sputum eosinophils cast doubt on the allergic basis for the patient's condition?
2. Evaluate the arterial blood gas results. How can they be explained in this patient?

Discussion

1. Although peripheral blood eosinophilia is demonstrated, no eosinophils were seen in the sputum or nasal smear. The presence of eosinophils is not essential for the diagnosis, although both specimens will often contain eosinophils.
2. The arterial blood gases are compatible with a diagnosis of respiratory alkalemia with hypoxemia. There is often an early decrease in arterial Po_2, with a greater decrease as severity of the condition increases. Compensatory hyperventilation results in an early decrease in Pco_2, which increases toward normal as compensation fails. The *p*H increases early and then decreases as the condition worsens (respiratory alkalosis→respiratory acidosis).

CASE STUDY #3

A 53-year-old woman was hospitalized for congestive heart failure. It was noticed on regular CBCs that the percentage of eosinophils, which had been normal upon admission, had risen to 9%. Two days later a severe pruritic rash appeared all over the body and the eosinophils rose to 24%. Therapy included Atarax and Benadryl, and in 10 days the rash had cleared. The peripheral blood cell differential showed 1% eosinophils.

Question

Are any other laboratory tests indicated?

Discussion

Because treatment with antihistamines was successful, no further tests are necessary. If further problems occur, however, a more complete workup would be indicated.

REFERENCES

1. Coombs RRA, Gell PGH: Classification of Allergic Reactions Responsible for Clinical Hypersensitivity and Disease. In Gell PGH, Coombs RRA, Lachmann PJ (eds): Clinical Aspects of Immunology, p 761. Oxford, Blackwell Scientific, 1975
2. Bennich H, Johannsson SGO: Structure and function of human immunoglobulin E. Adv Immunol 13:1, 1971
3. Geall GN (ed): Allergy and Clinical Immunology. New York City, John Wiley & Sons, 1983
4. Roitt IM, Brostoff J, Male DK: Immunology. St Louis, CV Mosby, 1985
5. Kaplan AP (ed): Allergy. New York City, Churchill Livingstone, 1985
6. Patterson R (ed): Allergic Diseases: Diagnosis and Management, 3rd ed. Philadelphia, JB Lippincott, 1985
7. Lessof MH (ed): Allergy: Immunological and Clinical Aspects. New York City, John Wiley & Sons, 1984
8. Mathews DP: Respiratory atopic disease. JAMA 248:2587, 1982
9. Buckley RH, Mathews KP: Common "allergic" skin diseases. JAMA 248:2611, 1982
10. Atkins FM: The basis of immediate hypersensitivity reactions to foods. Nutr Rev 41:29, 1983
11. Mathews KP: Urticaria and angioedema. J Allergy Clin Immunol 72:1, 1983
12. Patterson R, Valentine M: Anaphylaxis and related allergic emergencies including reactions due to insect stings. JAMA 248:2632, 1982
13. Wasserman SI: Mediators of immediate hypersensitivity. J Allergy Clin Immunol 72:101, 1983
14. Middleton E, Reed CE, Ellis EF (eds): Allergy: Principles and Practice. St Louis, CV Mosby, 1983
15. Buckley RH, Metcalfe D: Food allergy. JAMA 248:2627, 1982
16. Grieco MH, Meriney DK (eds): Immunodiagnosis for Clinicians: Interpretation of Immunoassays. Chicago, Year Book Medical Publishers, 1983
17. Patterson R, Anderson J: Allergic reactions to drugs and biologic agents. JAMA 248:2637, 1982

Chapter 55

Autoimmune Diseases

Barbara J. Minard

Autoimmune diseases appear to be disorders of immunoregulation with increased autoantibody production or cellular proliferation, resulting in immune complex formation, cell death, or altered function. The autoantibody specificity may be a ubiquitous self-antigen and therefore naturally occurring, or a neoantigen, cross-reactive antigen, or chemical or viral antigen. The subsequent antibody production or overproduction may be due to genetic predisposition, polyclonal activation of B lymphocytes, alteration of T-suppressor to T-helper cells, alteration of idiotypic–antiidiotypic network (antibodies produced by one individual), or impaired C4 activation–macrophage phagocytosis. The immune injury caused may result in *vasculitis, arthralgias,* or *glomerulonephritis* due to circulating immune complexes; *innocent bystander syndrome* due to cross-reactivity of tissue antigen and an organism or virus; *cell death* due to an autoantibody to a specific tissue antigen; or *altered function* of a specific tissue due to the autoantibody to a receptor or specific antigen. Drug-induced disorders may result from impaired clearance of immune complexes because the drug impairs C4 activation and consequently impairs macrophage phagocytosis. The clinical manifestations and laboratory findings are related to the specificity of the autoantibody and the resultant immune injury mechanism.

The term *autoimmune disease* specifically refers to an immunopathological condition caused by autoimmunization to "self" components. Although there are autoimmune responses to self components that occur naturally and are nonpathological, the immune response seems to exhibit either a controlled or a noncontrolled loss of tolerance to self in autosensitization. The effects are quite variable. An autoimmune disease may be organ/tissue-specific or nonorgan/tissue-specific in scope. It may destroy, mimic, or enhance the target. It can range in severity from being only an irritation to being fatal to the individual. Aside from the immunopathology associated with the development of autoimmune response or autoimmune disease, it is important to understand the etiologic factors that permit autoimmunization to self components.

ETIOLOGY AND PATHOPHYSIOLOGY

A normal, immunocompetent individual has an intact autorecognition system that distinguishes self from nonself. The causes of the phenotypic change in autorecognition are unknown. Etiologic factors that have been implicated include viral and/or chemical modifications of self, defective immune regulation, hyperimmunization, and immunogenetic alteration. In assessing the implications of each of these broad-based etiologic factors, certain etiologies are more attributable to specific autoimmune disease than others.[1]

Viral or Chemical Modifications

The autoimmune diseases with suspected chemical or viral etiologies are more often organ/tissue-specific disorders. Diabetes, Type I, is apparently the result of a previous infection with coxsackievirus, the antibody of which is cross-reactive with the islet cells of the pancreas. The resultant autoantibody disrupts normal production of insulin, thereby causing an insulin-dependent diabetes (IDD). A percentage of patients with systemic lupus erythematosus (SLE) have been shown to have IgM antibodies that react with HIV. Chemical modification of lung basement membrane by gasoline fumes has been implicated in the development of Goodpasture's syndrome. It is believed that the virus stimulation produces an immune response (antibody or lymphokine) either with cross-reactivity to a self antigen or with the ability to expose a hidden antigen that is new, rather than self.[1, 2, 3]

Defective Immune Regulation

Defective immune regulation is a potential cause of the development of autoimmune disease, both organ/tissue-specific and nonorgan/tissue-specific. Mouse models for SLE demonstrate both hyperactivity of B lymphocytes to T-helper cell-produced lymphokines and hyperreactivity of T-helper cells in lymphokine production. Of the various strains of mice that develop lupuslike conditions, the New Zealand black/white strain (NZB/NZW) appears to have a population of B lymphocytes hyperactive to T-helper cell lymphokines.[4]

Hyporeactivity of the immune system has been implicated in a number of investigations centering on loss of T-suppressor cell function or decreased percentage of T-suppressor cells. At specific times during the course of autoimmune disease, the number of circulating T-suppressor cells is diminished, but this does not seem to be consistent throughout the course of the disease. A relationship between the $CD4^+$ (T-helper) to $CD8^+$ (T-suppressor) cell ratio and these diseases has been suggested, as have differences in disease occurrence between male and female; however, these relationships have not yet been confirmed. T-suppressor cells can be depressed and can influence disease severity, but in themselves are not the etiologic factor for autosensitization.[4]

Another aspect of immune regulation that has been widely investigated in autoimmune disease is the role of idiotypic–anti-idiotypic antibodies in the remission–relapse cycles of certain disorders. Idiotypic–anti-idiotypic networks can be both suppressive and stimulatory to the immune system. Recent investigations suggest that there are cross-reactive monoclonal idiotypes found in lymphoproliferative disorders that are specific for DNA antibodies found in SLE. The implication is that the cells that produce the autoantibody are more subject to neoplastic transformation. This was found in a study of "naturally-occurring" autoantibodies that were monoclonal proteins.[4]

Another view of autoidiotypes suggests that the ability to produce certain autoantibodies is endogenous, although this in itself does not constitute the immunopathology. The shift from nonpathologic to pathologic autoantibody production occurs when a "minor" idiotypic antibody (Abl) expands into a major antianti-idiotypic antibody as a result of genetic alteration. The alteration occurs because the antianti-idiotypic antibody (Ab3) does not really "see" the originating antigen (immunogen), but instead responds to conformational idiotypes that are self antigens. Because of sharing in the idiotype of the originating antibody, the Ab1 and Ab3 become part of a regulatory idiotype. This suggests that autoimmune disease may be a multistep, multigene process in which there are specific etiologic factors or specific genetic factors that trigger autosensitization by a "minor" idiotypic response. The minor idiotype then shifts from a minor regulatory antianti-idiotype to a major idiotypic response that manifests or participates in immunopathologic tissue destruction. An example would be a bacterial antigen that stimulates production of an antibody sharing a common idiotype with a DNA antibody. The original Ab1 binds only the bacterial antigen, not DNA. However, the resultant antianti-idiotypic antibody (Ab3) binds DNA but not the original bacterial antigen because an idiotype is shared by the bacteria and the DNA. The anti-DNA is not necessarily immunopathologic unless there is a shift in production from a minor subpopulation of antibody-producing cells to a major population of antibody-producing cells.[4]

Another concept being explored is genetic modification of the variable regions of $CD3^+$ antigen receptors, which might enhance autoimmunization or at least modulate the response. The autoepitopes (autoantigens) seen by the immune response mechanism are unique substances. Their structure has to be easily accessible to the immune response, whether the antigen is a virus, a chemical modification, or a shared idiotype.[1, 3]

The autoepitopes found in the SLE/SLE-related groups are of interest. Suggested autoepitopes include the spectrum of histones—H1, H2A, H2B, H3, H4; histidyl-t-RNA synthetase (Jo-1); cyclin, snRNP, and the like. Some of these are autoepitopes of DNA bases, nucleic acid-binding proteins, or the Fc region of IgG. Because SLE is a multisystem disorder, multiple autoantibodies occur not just to nuclear-associated epitopes but to red blood cell antigens and to leukocyte antigens, either HLA- or granulocyte-specific.[4]

It has been suggested that autoantibodies are naturally-occurring mechanisms that function in the elimination of degraded antigens. The subsequent loss of immunoregulation could be from defective enzyme systems or defective immunoregulation, or any combination.[4]

Pathologic Effects

In autoimmune disease, the autoantibody itself may not be pathologic, but the resulting immune complexes may be, as in SLE, for example. In other instances, the autoantibody may be cytotoxic to cell-bound antigens that are then pathologic to the body. An example of this type is autoimmune hemolytic anemia or Goodpasture's syndrome. In other instances, the autoantibody can impair function of a cell, as in myasthenia gravis, in which the autoantibody inhibits the binding of the acetylcholine to its receptor in the neuronal synapse. Autoantibody can also be stimulatory, as happens with thyroid immunoglobulin (TIg). In this case, the autoantibody binds to the thyroid-stimulating hormone (TSH) receptor and functions as TSH to stimulate thyroxin (T4) production by the thyroid. Autoimmune diseases are not all autoantibody-mediated, but may be cell-mediated with destruction of target cells. Hashimoto's thyroiditis is an example of cellular proliferation and destruction of the target organ[1, 2, 3]

The common thread in autoimmune disease is the autoimmunization to self components with eventual immunologically-mediated injury. The mechanism of injury is as varied as are the target organs and tissues and symptoms. The immunopathologic injury may be antibody-mediated cytotoxic (Type II) reaction, immune complex deposition (Type III), or antibody-mediated enhancement or inhibitory reactions. The cell-mediated (lymphokine) disorders usually involve cellular cytotoxicity but occasionally may involve cellular proliferation.[1, 2, 3] The targets of autoimmune disease/disorders are widely varied and include cell receptors, specific cellular antigens and/or components, products of cells, catabolized fragments of cells, and organelles.

Autoimmune disorders can be categorized as nonorgan- (nontissue-) specific or organ- (tissue-) specific. Nonorgan-specific disease includes the systemic rheumatoid disorders: systemic lupus erythematosus, rheumatoid arthritis, ankylosing spondylitis, necrotizing angiitis (vasculitis), polymyositis, dermatomyositis, scleroderma, mixed connective tissue disease (MCTD), and Sjögren's syndrome.

Nonorgan/Nontissue-Specific Disease

SYSTEMIC LUPUS ERYTHEMATOSUS (SLE)

SLE is one of the most studied of the autoimmune systemic disorders. It affects females six to nine times more frequently than males, and is often a disease of young females, 20 to 30 years of age. Although the disease may have an insidious beginning, it can prove to be fatal at a very early age. The serious lesions of SLE are immune complex deposition involving the kidneys, blood vessels, and heart. Central nervous system (CNS) involvement occurs in about 50% of SLE patients. Fatalities are usually attributable to renal failure or cerebral hemorrhage.[1, 2, 3]

RHEUMATOID ARTHRITIS

Rheumatoid arthritis is frequently grouped with the SLE/SLE-like disorders because of the shared symptomatology of arthralgias. Unlike the other disorders in the group, rheumatoid arthritis usually results in bilateral joint involvement.

Organ-Specific Disease

The organ- or tissue-specific disorders frequently have a specific autoantibody, rather than the multiplicity of antibodies seen in the SLE/SLE-like group. In some of the endocrine disorders, however, multiple autoantibodies may be present. The antibody-mediated disorders involve cytotoxic injury with or without complement activation, and inhibitory or stimulatory responses of specific tissue. Cell-mediated (lymphokine) injury is also present.[4]

CYTOTOXIC REACTIONS

Cytotoxic reactions may be exhibited by some patients. Autoimmune hemolytic anemia with either warm or cold antibodies is an example of cytotoxic reactions with or without complement activation. If the autoantibody is non-complement-fixing and nonlytic, the destruction of red blood cells is due to splenic sequestration. The clinical results are anemia and spherocytosis.

Other examples with similar mechanisms occur with autoantibodies to platelets, granulocytes, lymphocytes, or other cellular components.

Other cytotoxic reactions may be directed at basement membrane to kidneys or lungs as in Goodpasture's syndrome, heart tissue as in the case of rheumatic fever, or desmosomes as in pemphigus vulgaris. The autoantibody involved is specifically targeted to the tissue. Cytotoxic reactions also occur in demyelinating disorders, with demonstrable autoantibodies to myelin; in thyroid disease, with autoantibodies to thyroglobulin and/or microsome; in gastric atrophy or pernicious anemia, with autoantibodies to intrinsic factor and/or parietal cells; in biliary cirrhosis, with microsomal autoantibodies and in other disorders.

Modifications of the cytotoxic type of immunologic injury are the enhancement autoantibody and the inhibitory autoantibody. Both are demonstrable in tissue-specific disorders. In myasthenia gravis, the autoantibody is to the acetylcholine receptor and inhibits the binding of acetylcholine to its natural receptor in the neuronal synapses. The acetylcholine is necessary for normal nerve impulse conduction. Occasional instances of myasthenia gravis have been shown to have an anti-idiotypic antibody that can mimic acetylcholine binding and facilitate continuation of low-level nerve impulses. As the disease progresses, the anti-idiotypic response is negated by increasing idiotypic antibody, and total impairment of nerve impulse occurs. Most of the idiotypic–anti-idiotypic antibodies described have been cross-reactive idiotypes, which suggests that they are not individual-specific but autoantibody-specific, *i.e.*, the anti-idiotypic antibody will inhibit the binding of idiotypic antibodies from several different individuals to the choline receptor in an *in vivo* test.[4]

ENHANCEMENT OR INHIBITORY REACTIONS

An enhancement reaction occurs when the autoantibody mimics the natural hormone, or peptide, by binding to a receptor and stimulating a specific response. Thyroid immunoglobulin (TIg), also known as LATS (long-acting thyroid stimulator), binds to the TSH receptor and mimics TSH stimulation of the thyroid. TIg as an autoantibody is present in a significant but small percentage of patients with hyperthyroidism. TIg is the specific autoantibody, but its mechanism is stimulatory to its receptor antigen rather than inhibitory or cytotoxic.[1, 3]

CELL-MEDIATED REACTIONS

One mechanism seen in organ-specific disorders is cell-mediated (lymphokine-mediated) rather than antibody-mediated. The proliferative and/or cytotoxic T lymphocytes with their lymphokine products are the causative factor in organ destruction. Hashimoto's thyroiditis is in part due to a mononuclear cell infiltrate that disrupts the organ structure and function. In Hashimoto's, the thyroid becomes enlarged, tender, and inflamed due to T-proliferative cells, their lymphokines, and the infiltrating macrophages. Allergic encephalomyelitis is similar, except that it is infiltration by T-proliferative cells into the central nervous system, specifically the meninges, with subsequent inflammation that causes the symptoms. The autoantigen in both of these disorders is a particulate cell-bound antigen that is more stimulatory to the cell-mediated system than to the antibody-mediated immune response. This does not mean, however, that there is not antibody-mediated response-associated injury just because the principal pathologic response is lymphokine-mediated.[1]

CLINICAL MANIFESTATIONS

Clinical symptoms of the nonorgan/non tissue-specific disorders are very similar. Common symptoms include joint pain, complaints associated with vasculitis and skin lesions. The organ- or tissue-specific disorders involve blood components, endocrine glands, kidney, gastrointestinal (GI) tract, central nervous system, skin, liver, lungs, muscle, and eye. The tissue-specific disorders are more easily defined because specific tissue or organ is the target. Examples are red blood cells in autoimmune hemolytic anemia, platelets in idiopathic thrombocytopenic purpura, and kidney and lung in Goodpasture's syndrome.[1, 2, 3]

Nonorgan-Specific Disease

The first symptoms of SLE may occur during puberty, with a common complaint of joint pain and/or sun sensitivity. A red rash across the upper cheeks and bridge of the nose that has a characteristic "butterfly" shape may be present. This rash is the origin of the name—lupus (wolf) and erythematosus (red).

Patients with rheumatoid arthritis or Sjögren's syndrome frequently present with arthralgias, and in Sjögren's with a possible sicca syndrome (dry eyes and/or mouth). Mixed connective tissue disease (MCTD) frequently exhibits arthralgias and esophageal dysphagia but no renal complications. Dermatomyositis has both skin and muscle complaints. Polymyositis has joint and muscle pain.[1, 2, 3, 4]

Organ-Specific Disease

In organ-specific disorders, whether cell-directed, membrane-directed, or receptor-directed, the clinical presentation is usually specific. For example, it may be muscle weakness as in myasthenia gravis or hyperthyroidism as in Graves's disease, or insulin-dependent diabetes as in the case of an islet cell antibody, and so forth.[1]

LABORATORY ANALYSES AND DIAGNOSIS

Most of the antibody-mediated autoimmune disorders will demonstrate a polyclonal gammopathy, usually of the IgG type; chronic inflammatory response; possible classic complement activation with circulating immune complexes; and altered function or numbers of autoantibody targets. Other components that may be affected include the immune regulatory system, such as decreased $CD8^+$ (T-suppressor) cells; the function of kidneys, lungs, blood flow, and the neuromuscular system; and multiple autoantibody activities.

SLE

Laboratory findings in SLE include a glomerular permeability type of proteinuria, polyclonal increase of IgG, complement activation via the classical pathway with decreased C3 and C4, a positive rheumatoid factor, possible positive cryoglobulins, circulating immune complexes, possible anemia and/or leukopenia, and a positive antinuclear antibody (ANA) test. The presence of ANA may be due to a number of autoantibody specificities to nuclear components, such as ds-DNA, DNP, SS-A, Sm, Ma, and others. The most definitive ANA specificity is ds-DNA and the Smith (Sm) autoantibody, which is a complement-fixing antibody and is particularly damaging. Sm antibody occurs in approximately 40% of all SLE patients. The ANA is not specific for SLE because approximately 3% to 7% of the normal population, 40% of the elderly population, and patients with other disorders such as rheumatoid arthritis can have positive reactions. High titers of ANA, especially those with solid and rim reaction patterns, however, are suggestive of SLE. The diagnosis can be established with more confidence if the ANA specificity can be attributed to ds-DNA and also to Sm (see Fig. 55-1).

Discoid lupus, a variant of SLE, may not exhibit proteinuria. Quite often patients are not ds-DNA-positive, although they frequently have SS-A antibodies. The finding of SS-A antibody in pregnant women has been associated with congenital heart disease of newborn and high-risk infants. The infant may or may not be positive for the SS-A antibody. In addition, spontaneous abortions have been related to antibodies of cardiolipin and to SS-A. SS-A antibodies usually result in a speckled ANA pattern when HEp-2 cells are used as the substrate.[5, 6]

ANA-negative SLE was originally reported to be associated with antibodies to ss-DNA. Many of the ANA-negative mouse kidney reactions may demonstrate weak-positive speckled ANA patterns on HEp-2 cells. Single-stranded DNA antibodies are frequently present in SLE, but usually in association with other nuclear-specific antibodies. The variation between substrates for ANA can often be correlated with differences in titer and to some extent with the pattern observed. For example, there are autoantibodies that are demonstrable on mouse kidney but not on HEp-2 cells, and vice versa. In addition, most autoantibodies that are disease-associated are usually IgG, but IgM and IgA classes of antibodies have been reported.[5, 6]

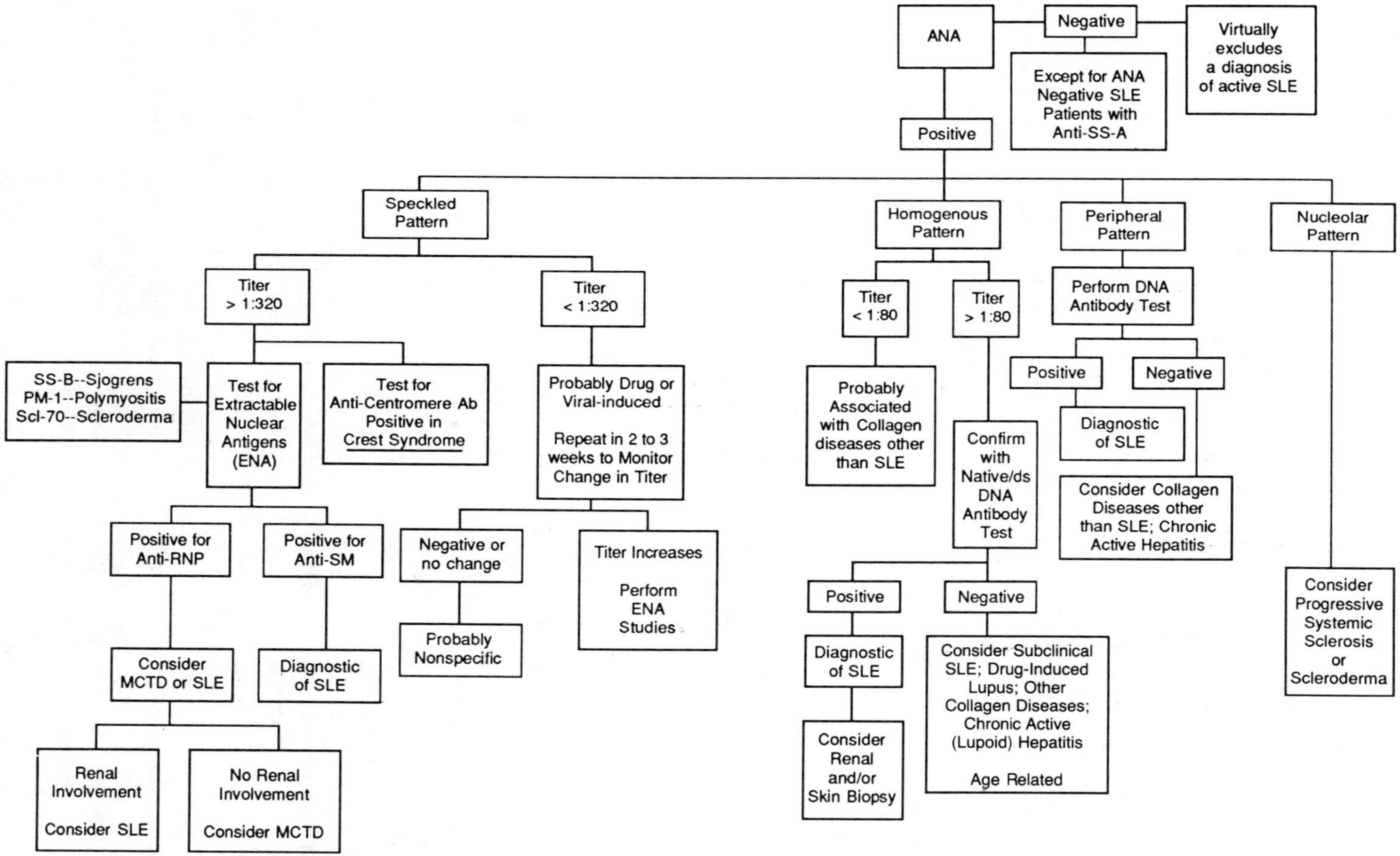

Figure 55-1 Algorithm for antinuclear antibodies (mouse or rat kidney substrate) as an aid in diagnosis.

SLE-Like Disorders

The SLE-like disorders have physical and clinical symptoms similar to those seen in SLE, but with specific physical–clinical variations and differences in autoantibody specificities. Another distinction is that complement activation is not as striking in the SLE-related disorders as it is in SLE. In mixed connective tissue disease (MCTD), the ANA is a high-titered speckled reaction with ribonucleoprotein (RNP) specificity.

The autoantibodies in Sjögren's syndrome are demonstrated as a speckled ANA of which the specificity is SS-B or SS-A and SS-B and an autoantibody to salivary duct.

In polymyositis the positive speckled ANA occurs in approximately 50% of the patients, with the specificity being PM-1 or Jo-1.

The ANA in dermatomyositis is frequently a nucleolar pattern with RNA specificity. Scleroderma also is characterized by an ANA nucleolar reaction, but may show a speckled or a centromere pattern. The CREST syndrome of scleroderma is characterized by a large speckled pattern that is actually the centromere antibody seen in dividing or mitotic cells. In addition, a spindle pattern has also been detected. One antibody specificity associated with scleroderma is the Scl-70.[5, 6]

The entire group of SLE-related diseases frequently exhibit speckled ANA patterns with specificities directed to what was originally called *extractable nuclear antigens (ENA)* because they were present in the saline wash of calf thymus extraction for DNA. Since their discovery, characterization of these substances has been continuing, with respect not only to their relationship to disease but also to their true specificity. RNP and Sm both appear to be endonucleases; PM-1 appears to be related to a polymerase; and Scl-70 is a 70 dalton ribosomal protein.[5] The type of autoantibody specificity and the manifestation of disease process are currently of great interest to researchers. Some have suggested that Z-DNA may be more "immunogenic" than normal B-DNA. There are also occasional reports of anti-idiotypic antibodies, both cross-reactive and individual, that have been demonstrated in SLE and SLE-like patients. This has led to speculation that these anti-idiotypes may be responsible for some of the cyclic patterns observed in patients in remission–relapse sequences.

Rheumatoid patients frequently have high titers of rheumatoid factor, a polyclonal gamma increase, and little or no complement consumption or circulating immune complexes. The serum protein pattern may reflect a chronic inflammatory response with increased alpha-1 and alpha-2 globulins. Rheumatoid patients do not all have classic rheumatoid factor (anti-IgM with IgG specificity), but may have an IgG or IgA class of rheumatoid factor (seronegative). Complement levels in the synovial fluid are reduced, compared to normal values of one-third of the serum value. The triggering event for rheumatoid arthritis may be Epstein-Barr virus (EBV). Whether it is EBV or some other event, the synovium becomes activated with mononuclear infiltrate, plasmacytosis, and antibody production. The antibody produced has been shown to have the capability of reacting as an EBV nuclear antigen, and reacts with an antigen called RANA (rheumatoid-associated nuclear antigen). RANA is demonstrable in a cell extract of Wil-2 cell line along with SS-A. RANA will demonstrate a speckled pattern when Wil-2 cells are used as the substrate for the ANA. Other laboratory findings are leukocytosis, decreased hyaluronidase, and increased protein in the synovial fluid.[4, 5]

Organ-Specific Disease

With patients exhibiting autoimmune hemolytic anemia, the antibody may be complement-fixing or hemolytic. In either case, the circulating red blood cells are lysed, resulting in intravascular hemolysis with decreased haptoglobin and hemopexin. The autoantibody may be detectable or nondetectable, depending on its specificity. Nonspecific autoantibodies can create significant clinical management problems in certain patients because compatible blood is not available. Specific autoantibodies such as those of the Ii system, however, can be defined, and compatible blood can be found.[1, 4]

In Goodpasture's syndrome, the autoantibody is usually of insufficient concentration or cross-reactivity to be detected in the patient's serum by the usual indirect fluorescent immunomicroscopy. A biopsy of the affected tissue for direct fluorescent immunomicroscopy or specific immunoassays using target tissue are the choice methods for demonstrating the presence of the autoantibodies (see Table 55-1). In analyzing these disorders via biopsy studies, usually the autoantibody is of the

Table 55-1 ***Autoantibody Detection***

Autoantibody	Substrate	Controls	Reaction Site	Disease Correlation
Nuclear (ANA)	Rat kidney	Negative ANA positive	Nucleus	Collagen vascular disease, age-related, drug-induced, malignancies
Mitochondrial (AMA)	Rat kidney	Negative AMA positive	Mitochondria	Primary biliary cirrhosis
Smooth muscle (ASMA)	Rat stomach	Negative ASMA positive	Actinomycin (smooth muscle)	Acute chronic or lupoid hepatitis (IgG), viral hepatitis, acute infectious mononucleosis (IgM)
Parietal cell (APCA)	Rat stomach	Negative APCA positive	Parietal cell microsomes	Pernicious anemia, atropic gastritis
Reticulin	Rat kidney	Negative	Reticulin	Malabsorption syndrome, sprue, celiac disease
Glomerular	Rat kidney	Negative	Basement membrane	Chronic active hepatitis, viral hepatitis
Bile duct	Rat liver	Negative	Epithelial cells of bile ducts	Primary biliary cirrhosis (70%–90%), alcoholic or post-necrotic cirrhosis (25%)
Adrenal	Human adrenal cortex (unfixed)	Negative	Adrenal cell cytoplasm	Primary adrenal atrophy (Addison's disease)
Striated muscle	Rat striated muscle	Negative	Myoid cell striations	Myasthenia gravis
Skin	Human skin	Negative	Epithelial basement membrane	Bullous, pemphigoid
Cardiac	Rat heart	Negative	Sarcolemma (GMP) Striations (AMP)	Postmyocardial infarction, SBE, pleural effusions

(*continued*)

Table 55-1 *Autoantibody Detection (continued)*

Autoantibody	Substrate	Controls	Reaction Site	Disease Correlation
Myelin	Rat sciatic nerve	Negative	Myelin sheath	Demyelinating disease
Colon	Human colon	Negative	Epithelial cells	Ulcerated colitis
Islet cell	Human pancreas blood group O	Negative	Islet cell cytoplasm	Diabetes
Salivary	Human salivary	Negative	Salivary duct cytoplasm	Sjögren's syndrome
Basement membrane	Monkey esophagus	Negative	Basement membrane between the dermis and the epidermis	Bullous, pemphigoid
Desmosomes (Intracellular)	Monkey esophagus	Negative	Intracellular epidermis	Pemphigus vulgaris
Ovarian	Human ovary	Negative	Ovary at follicular area	Sterility
dsDNA	Crithidea luciliae	Negative Antinative DNA Positive control	Kinetoplast	SLE
Histone	Acid-treated rat kidney	Negative Antinative DNA Positive control	Nucleus—no reaction indicates presence of histone antibody (if DNA and reconstituted histone are positive)	Drug-induced lupus

IgG class and there is no evidence of complement fixation.[1, 4]

Often there are several disorders that present with similar clinical—pathophysiologic pictures. The autoantibodies become useful, therefore, not only as a positive diagnostic indicator but as a tool to rule out disorders. In evaluating ANA reactions, it is well to remember that endocrine disorders may exhibit multiple antibodies, so that a positive parietal cell does not always mean gastric atrophy or pernicious anemia. Morever, certain autoantibodies require primate tissue for demonstration, *e.g.*, basement membrane in pemphigoid. If human tissue is used as the substrate, it is advisable to use tissue from O-negative individuals; otherwise reactions may be blood group-related rather than a "true autoantibody."[4, 5]

TREATMENT

Autoimmune disease/disorders are complex and sometimes frustrating. A variety of possibilities, many of which are still not understood, must be kept in mind. Most of the autoimmune disorders are currently treated with steroids to reduce antibody production, and possibly therapeutic plasmapheresis to remove immune complexes or autoantibody. If steroids do not prove useful, an immunosuppressive drug such as cytoxan may be used. In organ-specific disease, supportive therapy only may be used initially until cellular destruction or malfunction can be slowed down.[1, 4]

In drug-induced lupus, which mimics SLE in symptomatology, the patient is often being treated for cardiac arrhythmias with procainamide or phenylhydrazine. After removal of the drugs, the ANA titer will usually gradually disappear in relation to the half-life of IgG, and the symptoms will abate. A small number of these patients will not revert, however, and will exhibit symptoms and findings of SLE indefinitely.[4]

CASE STUDY

A 30-year-old woman saw her physician complaining of low-grade fever, anorexia, and joint pain. She reported a bout of severe flu a few weeks before. Otherwise her history and physical exam were not remarkable.

LABORATORY FINDINGS

Hemoglobin	12 g/dL (1.86 mmol/L)
WBC	$9 \times 10^3/mm^3$
Urinalysis	Normal
FANA	
1st week	Positive, 1:80, speckled pattern
4th week	Positive, 1:80, speckled pattern

Questions

1. What is the most likely condition the physician should expect?
2. Do laboratory findings support this diagnosis?

Discussion

1. In a woman in this age group with this symptomatology, SLE would be highly probable.
2. Laboratory data do not support that diagnosis. The most important findings are the FANA test results, in which the titer is lower than would be expected for SLE with a speckled reaction pattern. Moreover, on repeat testing the titer did not rise. With a normal urinalysis, WBC, and hemoglobin, this patient most likely does not have SLE. The ANA results indicate a nonspecific reaction, probably related to the flu episode reported by the patient.

REFERENCES

1. Stites D, Stobo J, Fudenberg H et al: Basic and Clinical Immunology, 5th ed. Los Altos, California, Lange Medical Publications, 1984
2. Bryant NJ: Laboratory Immunology and Serology, 2nd ed. Philadelphia, WB Saunders, 1986
3. Roitt I: Essential Immunology, 5th ed. Boston, Blackwell Scientific, 1984
4. Schwartz R, Rose N: Autoimmunity: Experimental and clinical aspects. Ann New York Acad Sci 475:1986
5. Nakamura R, Peebles C, Rubin R et al: Autoantibodies to Nuclear Antigens (ANA), 2nd ed. Chicago, American Society of Clinical Pathologists, 1985
6. Rose N, Friedman H, Fahey J: Manual of Clinical Laboratory Immunology, 3rd ed. Washington, D.C., American Society for Microbiology. 1986

BIBLIOGRAPHY

Stansfield W: Serology and Immunology. New York City, Macmillan, 1981

Part XII

INFECTIOUS DISEASES

Sharon L. Zablotney, Associate Editor

The infectious disease processes addressed by the chapters in this section are unique in a variety of ways. The more salient differences in these disorders include the fact that they generally are associated with no specific organ system or their etiology and/or pathogenesis are distinctive enough to warrant special attention and discussion apart from an organ system approach.

The infectious processes discussed here represent both common and uncommon prevalence and the gamut of morbidity and mortality. Nonetheless, as in any infectious disease process, the clinical laboratory plays an essential role in the accurate identification of the etiologic agent as well as the choice of effective treatment. The focus of these chapters is to enable the laboratory scientist to assist the clinician in achieving both accuracy and efficacy in the diagnosis and treatment of infectious disease and to do so within the context of cost-effective health care delivery.

Chapter 56

Sexually Transmitted Diseases

Madeline J. Ducate / Lauren A. Roberts

OVERVIEW

Sexually transmitted diseases (STDs) are considered as a group because of certain common clinical and epidemiologic features, but they encompass a much broader variety of specific illnesses caused by biologically dissimilar microbial agents. The term STD has come to replace the more classic "venereal disease" (VD) because the latter implied disease that spread only through sexual intercourse. The former term (STD) describes a diverse group of infections acquired by a broader range of heterosexual and homosexual behavior, including oral–genital, oral–anal, and genital–anal contact. Thus, during the past two decades physicians and health care practitioners have become concerned not only about the five "traditional" venereal diseases (gonorrhea, syphilis, chancroid, lymphogranuloma venereum, and granuloma inguinale) but also about approximately 20 additional disease entities. These include those caused by more recently identified and recognized organisms such as *Chlamydia trachomatis, Ureaplasma urealyticus,* herpes simplex virus, and human immunodeficiency virus (HIV). The major impact of these organisms has been on maternal and neonate morbidity, human reproduction and infertility, and irreversible, as yet, immunologic impairment.

Epidemiologic Considerations

Generally, most persons with active symptoms of STD will cease sexual activity and seek medical help; however, one of the major reasons for the current STD epidemic, and a critical issue in the management and control of these diseases, is a failure to ensure that the sexual partners of patients with STDs are examined and treated. Often these partners are asymptomatic or have only mild symptoms. The increase in incidence of STDs is compounded by the fact that many of the associated organisms are becoming more resistant to commonly used antimicrobial agents.

Anyone who is sexually active is at some risk of acquiring these infections. Frequent sexual contact with many different partners is a major risk factor for exposure to all types of STDs. For some organisms such as *Neisseria gonorrhoeae,* sexual transmission is the only important mode of transmission. Other diseases, such as hepatitis, giardiasis, shigellosis, and amebiasis, are perhaps acquired more frequently by nonsexual means, discussed elsewhere in this text. Homosexual and bisexual males are generally at higher risk for these enteric infections.

INCIDENCE/PREVALENCE

Although there are approximately 25 separate conditions identified as STDs, six major illnesses account for the vast majority of cases. They are gonorrhea, chlamydia, genital herpes, syphilis, viral hepatitis, and AIDS (see Table 56-1). Because of the serious problem of underreporting and the fact that some organisms such as non-lymphogranuloma venereum strains of chlamydia and genital herpes are not reportable diseases in most states, the true incidence of the STDs is not known.

MULTIPLE INFECTIONS

Specific pathogen identification is often complicated by the high frequency of multiple infections in the same patient. These multiple, sexually acquired infections probably reflect the multiplicity of sexual partners among patients seen in many of these studies and the frequency of the organisms in the general population. For example, concurrent *C. trachomatis* and *N. gonorrhoeae* infections have been reported in about 25% of men with gonorrhea and in as many as one-half of women with gonococcal cervicitis.[1, 2] In women with vaginitis, one study showed that 16% of cases were caused by mixed infection with various combinations of *Candida, Trichomonas,* and organisms associated with bacterial vaginosis.[3]

Table 56-1 ***Incidence of the Six Major STDs Seen in the United States, 1986***

Disease	Estimated Annual Incidence of Cases
Chlamydia	4,500,000
Gonorrhea	2,000,000
Genital herpes	500,000
Syphilis	90,000
Hepatitis B	30,000
AIDS	15,000

ETIOLOGY AND PATHOPHYSIOLOGY

Common Syndromes in Men

Urethritis is the most common clinical syndrome seen in males (see Table 56-2). It is generally classified as either gonococcal or nongonococcal (NGU), depending partly on the somewhat different clinical appearance of the two forms of the disease, but more often on the presence or absence of gonococci in the urethral discharge. About 40% of NGU is caused by *C. trachomatis,* with *U. urealyticus* implicated in about 50% of the *Chlamydia*-negative cases of NGU. It has been difficult to determine the significance of *Ureaplasma* infections in patients with urethritis because cultures for this organism are rarely performed. Moreover, it has been reported that up to 50% of asymptomatic sexually active persons are colonized with this organism.[4]

Postgonococcal urethritis is defined as the persistence or recurrence of urethritis after administration of penicillin alone in the treatment of gonococcal infections. Three of every four cases of postgonococcal urethritis are caused by *C. trachomatis.*[5]

Acute epididymitis is usually caused by *C. trachomatis* or *N. gonorrhoeae* in sexually active men under the age of 35. This condition must be differentiated from testicular torsion, tumor, and trauma and is usually, although not always, associated with overt or subclinical urethritis. Urinary pathogens such as *Escherichia coli* and *Pseudomonas aeruginosa* are the usual causes of acute epididymitis in older men.

Enteritis, proctitis, and proctocolitis are frequently encountered problems seen primarily in homosexual and bisexual men. The most important causes of these infections are *N. gonorrhoeae,* herpes simplex virus, *C. trachomatis, Treponema pallidum,* and *Campylobacter.* Proctitis can occur in men who practice passive rectal intercourse with a partner who has a urethral infection with one of these organisms. Proctocolitis, presumably acquired by oral–anal contact, is most often caused by *Entamoeba histolytica, Campylobacter* species, and *Shigella* species, whereas enteritis limited to the small intestine is generally due to *Giardia lamblia.* The microbiology of these infections is often complicated not only by the normal bacterial flora of the intestinal tract but also by the fact that asymptomatic carriage of enteric pathogens is not uncommon in this population. Up to 40% of homosexual men with gastrointestinal symptoms have more than one infection simultaneously.[5]

Table 56-2 ***Common STD Syndromes in Men***

Syndrome	Causative Agents
Urethritis	*Neisseria gonorrhoeae* *Chlamydia trachomatis* *Ureaplasma urealyticus*
Epididymitis	*C. trachomatis* *N. gonorrhoeae*
Hepatitis	Hepatitis A and B
Intestinal	
Proctitis	*N. gonorrhoeae* *C. trachomatis* Herpes simplex virus *Treponema pallidum* *Campylobacter* species
Proctocolitis	*Entamoeba histolytica* *Campylobacter* species *Shigella* species
Enteritis	*Giardia lamblia* *Entamoeba histolytica* *Shigella* species *Campylobacter* species

Common Syndromes in Women

As with men, *C. trachomatis* and *N. gonorrhoeae* are the leading causes of urethritis in women. Concomitant cervicitis may also be present (see Table 56-3).

Table 56-3 *Common STD Syndromes in Women*

Syndrome	Causative Agents
Urethral syndrome	*Chlamydia trachomatis* *Neisseria gonorrhoeae*
Vaginitis	*Gardnerella vaginalis*/anaerobes *Candida albicans* *Trichomonas vaginalis*
Cervicitis	*N. gonorrhoeae* *C. trachomatis* Herpes simplex virus
Endometritis	*C. trachomatis* *N. gonorrhoeae*
Salpingitis*	*N. gonorrhoeae* *C. trachomatis*

* Also referred to as pelvic inflammatory disease (PID)

Vaginitis, an inflammation of the vaginal mucous membrane, accounts for more than 7% of patient visits to gynecologists annually.[6] These infections are caused by a wide variety of microorganisms, including bacteria, fungi, viruses, and parasites. Some syndromes are caused by exogenous organisms, while others are caused by organisms of the patient's own normal vaginal flora. The type of infection and the causative agent are influenced by a number of factors, including sexual activity, contraceptive use, genital tract instrumentation, childbirth, and prior infection.[7] Most cases of infectious vaginitis can be placed into three categories: bacterial vaginosis (BV), formerly called nonspecific vaginitis or NSV, which causes 40% to 50% of cases; candidiasis, which accounts for 20% to 30% of cases; and trichomoniasis, which causes 20% to 30% of cases.[6, 8] *N. gonorrhoeae* is a less frequent cause of vaginal discharge, and is mainly associated with cervicitis.

Mucopurulent cervicitis is the most common major STD syndrome in women, and asymptomatic cases occur more frequently than symptomatic ones.[9] Cervicitis may accompany vaginitis due to *Candida albicans* or *T. vaginalis;* however, cervicitis without vaginitis is generally caused by *N. gonorrhoeae, C. trachomatis,* or both, or by herpes simplex virus. True cervicitis must be distinguished from cervical ectopy that presents with a red-appearing cervix and an increase in a mucoid vaginal discharge. A common sign of mucopurulent cervicitis (MPC) due to *C. trachomatis* is an edematous and friable cervix. Herpetic cervicitis, which often occurs in primary infections with this organism, appears as cervical vesicles and ulcers rather than being mucopurulent.

Chlamydial infections often ascend from the cervix into the endometrium, producing endometritis, which can then ascend into the fallopian tubes and produce salpingitis (inflammation of the fallopian tubes), parametritis, and/or peritonitis. Pelvic inflammatory disease (PID) is a less precise term used to describe this clinical syndrome. Many cases of PID are caused by more than one organism. The agents most often implicated in acute PID include *C. trachomatis* and *N. gonorrhoeae,* the primary causes of cervicitis. Also implicated are those organisms that can be regarded as abnormal components of the vaginal flora, namely, anaerobic bacteria including *Bacteroides* and gram-positive cocci, facultative organisms such as *E. coli, Actinomyces israelii,* and *Mycoplasma hominis.* These agents often cannot be detected in individual patients. Salpingitis is the most serious complication of female genital tract infections and is the major cause of ectopic pregnancies and infertility. Ectopic pregnancies, which cause 10% of all maternal deaths, are 8 to 10 times more likely to occur in women who have had salpingitis.[10, 11] Infertility occurs in as many as 20% of women who have had salpingitis.[12]

Genital Skin Lesions

Genital skin lesions can be classified as ulcerative or nonulcerative (see Table 56-4). The nonulcerative sexually transmitted infections include genital warts (condylomata acuminata), *Candida* balanitis or vulvitis, genital molluscum contagiosum, and infestation with scabies (*Sarcoptes scabiei*) or crab lice (*Phthirus pubis*). These nonulcerative infec-

Table 56-4 ***Genital Lesions: Ulcerative vs Nonulcerative***

Lesions	Causative Agents
Ulcerative	
Genital herpes	Herpes simplex virus
Syphilis	*Treponema pallidum*
Chancroid	*Hemophilus ducreyi*
Lymphogranuloma venereum	*Chlamydia trachomatis* serotypes L1, L2, and L3
Granuloma inguinale	*Calymmatobacterium granulomatis*
Trauma	
Nonulcerative	
Condylomata acuminata	Genital wart virus (human papillomaviruses)
Candida balanitis	*Candida albicans*
Molluscum contagiosum	Molluscum contagiosum virus
Scabies	*Sarcoptes scabiei*
Pubic (or crab) lice	*Phthirus pubis*

tions are frequently referred to as minor STDs because they often present as primary complaints or as findings incidental to other problems. They are readily amenable to therapeutic intervention.

The most common cause of ulcerative genital lesions in patients in the United States is herpes simplex virus (HSV). Other causes of genital ulcers include syphilis, chancroid, lymphogranuloma venereum (LGV), granuloma inguinale (GI), and trauma. LVG, GI, and chancroids are relatively uncommon in western nations.[13] Trauma resulting from sexual activity may produce abrasions and ulcer lesions that are occasionally infected with staphylococci or streptococci.

Systemic/Disseminated STDs

Untreated primary infection with some of the organisms that cause STDs can result in a variety of systemic and/or disseminated diseases.

N. gonorrhoeae usually invades the transitional and columnar epithelial surfaces of the genitourinary tract and its appendages; however, infection can be acquired through other mucosal sites such as the conjunctiva, pharynx, and anal canal. In addition, hematogenous dissemination can occur. Disseminated gonococcal disease, also called arthritis–dermatitis syndrome, is more common in women, and the risk is greatest during menstruation and in the second and third trimesters of pregnancy. Currently it is the most common cause of infectious arthritis in young adults. Differential diagnosis is extensive in all sexually active persons who have acute arthritis or polyarthralgias and skin rash. This is because the symptoms mimic other diseases such as serum sickness, acute hepatitis B, erythema multiforme, sarcoidosis with erythema nodosum, cutaneous vasculitis, and septicemia due to various organisms such as *Staphylococcus aureus*. Meningitis and endocarditis are also complications that can occur with untreated or inadequately treated gonococcal infections; however, they develop infrequently as a consequence of gonococcemia.

Syphilis is a subacute to chronic STD caused by the spirochete *T. pallidum,* and it is the second leading cause of genital ulcers in American men.[11] Primary chancres usually occur at or near the point of entry for the spirochetes into the body, including genital organs, rectum, and mouth. Because primary lesions of syphilis are self-limiting and generally painless, patients may not seek medical care until secondary symptoms of the disease appear. Untreated primary chancres are usually associated with regional lymphadenopathy. Secondary stages of this disease usually become manifest in about 4 to 8 weeks after the primary lesion. Although secondary syphilis may involve many organs of the body, it usually manifests on the skin and mucous membranes. These lesions are highly infectious and there are symptoms of systemic disease.

A latent stage, *i.e.,* a time during which no clinical signs of syphilis appear and the cerebrospinal fluid is normal, can occur sometime between the secondary and late stages. During the first 4 years of latency, the disease is again considered infectious. After this time, the disease is considered noninfectious except in the case of pregnancy, when the disease can be transmitted to the fetus. Late syphilis or tertiary syphilis is the most destructive and crippling phase of the disease, and includes late benign syphilis, cardiovascular syphilis, and neurosyphilis. Neurosyphilis occurs in about 8% of cases of untreated syphilis, and cardiovascular syphilis, primarily manifested as aortic insufficiency and aortic aneurysm, occurs in about 10% of cases. Gumma (histologically a granuloma) is the characteristic lesion of late benign syphilis.

Untreated lymphogranuloma venereum, caused by extremely virulent and invasive serotypes of *C. trachomatis,* progresses through three increasingly severe stages.

Perihepatitis manifests almost exclusively in women as upper abdominal pain with fever, tenderness, and spasms of the abdominal wall. Both *C. trachomatis* and *N. gonorrhoeae* can cause perihepatitis. This condition is spread to the surface of the liver from inflamed, infective fallopian tubes.[10]

Just as PID can result from an infection ascending into the upper genital tract of women, STDs usually associated with urethritis in young men, as well as the non-sexually transmitted form caused by Enterobacteriaceae or *Pseudomonas,* can ascend the genital tract and cause acute epididymo-orchitis in men.

HIV, the suspected causative agent of acquired immunodeficiency syndrome (AIDS), is the most devastating and fatal of all STDs to date. Although proportionately this disease is not as widespread as chlamydia or gonorrhea, the latter two conditions are treatable and do not take the same extensive toll on the human body. Because HIV causes severe immunosuppression, patients acquiring this disease are extremely susceptible to numerous opportunistic infections such as *Pneumocystis carinii* and disseminated fungal, mycobacterial, and viral infections. This blood-borne viral infection can be transmitted by nonsexual as well as sexual means (see Chap. 53).

Maternal/Neonate Transmission

Women who have or acquire an STD during pregnancy are likely to transmit the infection to the fetus. Table 56-5 lists the various STDs that can be transmitted from a mother to her newborn. Most of these diseases are transmitted at delivery when the infant passes through the birth canal. If the physician is aware of an active lesion or disease at the time of delivery, the infant is generally deliv-

Table 56-5 ***Maternal/Neonate Transmission of STD Organisms***

Disease in the Neonate	Causative Agents
Conjunctivitis	*Neisseria gonorrhoeae* *Chlamydia trachomatis*
Pneumonia	*C. trachomatis*
Otitis media	*C. trachomatis*
Sepsis, meningitis	*Streptococcus agalactiae* (group B)
TORCH syndrome*	Cytomegalovirus Herpes simplex virus *Treponema pallidum*

* TORCH (or STORCH) syndrome consists of various combinations of encephalitis with cognitive impairment and/or deafness, hepatitis, dermatitis, and disseminated intravascular coagulation. It is an acronym for syphilis, toxoplasmosis, rubella, cytomegalovirus, and herpes simplex virus.

ered by cesarean section. Pregnant women who receive adequate prenatal care should be examined and screened for STDs in their first and third trimesters.

CLINICAL MANIFESTATIONS AND LABORATORY EVALUATIONS

The clinical manifestations of STD typically include genital discharge, lesions, and/or pain. Appropriate collection and handling of the specimens for identification of the etiologic agent(s) are essential to obtain reliable results.

Gonococcal Disease

The presence of an inflammatory urethral exudate is required for the diagnosis of urethritis in either sex.

Infections of the lower genitourinary tract in women often present with overlapping symptoms but can be distinguished by relatively simple clinical observations and laboratory testing, and a precise microbial etiology can be established. Determination of the primary anatomic site of infection, *i.e.*, endocervix or vagina, urethra or bladder, is done by history and physical examination.

Because both urethral syndrome (urethritis in women) and bacterial cystitis present with dysuria, urinary frequency, and pyuria, they can usually be distinguished by performing a quantitative urine culture. If the colony count is at least 10^5 bacteria per mL of urine, the patient probably has cystitis with or without pyelonephritis, whereas a count of less than 10^4 bacteria per millimeter indicates probable urethritis.

In males (see Table 56-6), a discharge may not always be evident, and may require milking of the urethra or insertion of a small urogenital swab 1 to 2 cm into the urethra. A direct Gram-stained smear of the urethral exudate that reveals five or more polymorphonuclear cells (PMNs) per high-power field suggests urethritis. Demonstration of typical gram-negative diplococci that are inside the PMNs provides a tentative diagnosis of gonococcal urethritis. In smears of urethral exudates from men, the sensitivity and specificity of the Gram stain is greater than 90%.[14]

The diagnosis of mucopurulent cervicitis (MPC) is made by demonstrating purulent discharge from the cervical os or by demonstrating an increased number of neutrophils on Gram stain of endocervical discharge in women without visible mucous. Cervical smears from females may also be examined for *N. gonorrhoeae,* but the sensitivity is only 65%; thus, cultures should be performed to confirm the diagnosis.[7]

Specimens collected for the isolation of *N. gonorrhoeae* may be transported to the laboratory in a protective medium or, preferably, plated directly onto selective enriched media and incubated appropriately as soon as possible.

Table 56-6 ***Differentiation of Gonococcal vs Nongonococcal Urethritis in Men***

	Gonococcal	Nongonococcal
Incubation Period	2–7 days	~12 days
Discharge	Purulent, spontaneous	Less purulent, less spontaneous
Dysuria	Prominent	Prominent (may be the only sign)
Gram-Stained Smear	Numerous PMNs with gram-negative intracellular diplococci	Few to moderate PMNs with no gram-negative diplococci

Because the incidence of penicillin-resistant *N. gonorrhoeae* (the so-called PPNG—penicillinase-producing *N. gonorrhoeae*—and CMRNG—chromosomally-mediated resistant *N. gonorrhoeae*) has increased in recent years, all isolates should be tested for the enzyme β-lactamase and, when necessary, penicillin and ampicillin susceptibility.

The diagnosis of gonorrhea can also be made utilizing the enzyme-linked immunosorbent assay (ELISA) technique. The sensitivity and specificity of this method are comparable to that of the Gram stain in the male and more sensitive but less specific than the Gram stain for females.[15] This test can provide a more rapid result than culture and is useful for screening large populations. An additional advantage is that this method can detect nonviable organisms or those damaged by partial or inadequate treatment. Given the fragility of the organism in transport to a laboratory, additional cases of this disease can be confirmed by this method.

Nongonococcal Disease

Nongonococcal urethritis (NGU) and nongonococcal cervicitis are more common than gonococcal infections of the urethra and endocervix. The diagnosis of NGU has been based on the absence of *N. gonorrhoeae* and the presence of an inflammatory urethral discharge. Recently developed diagnostic tests are expected to improve the detection of this syndrome and the most likely cause, *C. trachomatis*. Suitable specimens for the detection of chlamydiae include epithelial cells from male or female urethral discharge and scrapings from conjunctiva or tissue biopsies. The quality of the specimen is critical to the detection of these organisms, and the material collected must contain epithelial cells because these organisms reside in the columnar epithelial cells. Special transport media are available that can help retain the viability of the organism while in transit. If chlamydiae are present, the epithelial cells will contain characteristic inclusion bodies. To improve the sensitivity of culturing for chlamydiae, sampling of multiple body sites such as urethra and endocervix, and/or multiple samples are recommended as well as serial passage in tissue culture.[16]

Fluorescein-conjugated monoclonal antibody test systems are now available for the direct detection of chlamydia antigen. The elementary bodies of *C. trachomatis* appear as apple-green fluorescing structures. This method requires 30 minutes to perform and is comparable to culture results in high-prevalence groups when the specimen is of good quality and is evaluated by a skilled laboratory scientist. False negatives occur when the infectivity in an individual is low.

Another alternative to culture is a recently introduced ELISA method that enables detection of viable and nonviable organisms within a few hours. It does not require expertise in fluorescent microscopy and is useful for screening large numbers of specimens.

Culture methods for *U. urealyticum* and *Mycoplasma hominis* are available but are not performed routinely in most laboratories. Specimens suggested for collection include urine, semen, prostatic secretions, urethral, vaginal, or cervical swabs, tissue, and blood. Wooden applicators should not be used as they contain substances toxic to ureaplasmas. Swabs may consist of calcium alginate, cotton, or rayon on plastic or aluminum shafts.[17] Specimens must be transported in special transport media designed to maintain viability of these organisms, and then inoculated to selective, enriched agar plates. After incubation, the agar surface is examined microscopically. An experienced microscopist can identify typical colonies after 24 hours of incubation.

Vaginitis

The causative agent of vaginitis can usually be determined by a microscopic examination of the vaginal discharge (see Table 56-7). A wet mount should be prepared and examined promptly for the presence of *T. vaginalis*. *T. vaginalis* may also be discovered during a routine urinalysis or in a Papanicolaou smear. Candidiasis can be diagnosed by

Table 56-7 ***Differential Diagnosis of the Major Causes of Vaginitis***

Vaginal Discharge	BV*	*Candida*	*Trichomonas*
*p*H	>5.0	<4.5	>5.0
Fishy (amine) odor**	Yes	No	No
Appearance	Homogeneous	Flocculent	Homogeneous
Consistency	Milklike to flour paste	Highly viscous	Watery
Color	White to gray	White	White to green
Wet prep	Clue cells	Yeast	Motile trichomonads

* Bacterial vaginosis (formerly nonspecific vaginitis—NSV)
** Odor enhanced by the addition of 10% KOH

the addition of 10% potassium hydroxide (KOH) to the wet mount, which will dissolve host cell protein and enhance the visibility of fungal elements. The presence of "clue cells" is indicative of bacterial vaginosis. A clue cell is an epithelial cell that is so heavily covered with coccobacillary organisms that the border of the cell is obscured. A Gram stain of vaginal secretions from a patient with BV would reveal epithelial cells loaded with gram-negative organisms producing a granular appearance, along with few to no PMNs and few to no lactobacilli (see Fig. 56-1). The use of culture for the diagnosis of BV is not recommended because either *Gardnerella vaginalis* or anaerobic bacteria can be isolated from 40% of asymptomatic women without evidence of vaginal infection.[18]

The *p*H of vaginal secretions is also helpful in determining the causative agent. In candidal vaginitis the *p*H is less than 4.5, while in bacterial vaginosis (BV) and trichomoniasis the *p*H is greater than 4.5. The addition of 10% KOH to vaginal secretions may elaborate a fishy aminelike odor in BV as well as in some cases of trichomoniasis. The diagnosis of BV is made when three out of four parameters are met: (1) a homogenous gray discharge, (2) the presence of clue cells, (3) a *p*H greater than 4.5, and (4) liberation of an amine odor after mixing vaginal secretions with 10% KOH.[19]

Genital Lesions

The most common causes of acute genital lesions in the United States are listed in Table 56-8.

When the exact etiology cannot be ascertained, the physician must rely on clinical presentation to differentiate the various conditions, based on epidemiologic knowledge and/or clinical experience.

HSV generally appears as painful, superficial, grouped vesicles that are quite diagnostic. Primary syphilis, on the other hand, presents as a single clean-based, nonpainful ulcer (chancre) with indurated margins. Pain is an important criterion in differentiating primary syphilis from HSV or chancroids.

GENITAL HERPES

The most sensitive and specific laboratory tool available to aid in the diagnosis of genital herpes is viral culture. Material from the base of ulcers or vesicles should be collected and placed into viral transport media for submission to the laboratory. Herpes cultures are usually positive within 2 to 3 days, and are approximately 95% accurate for di-

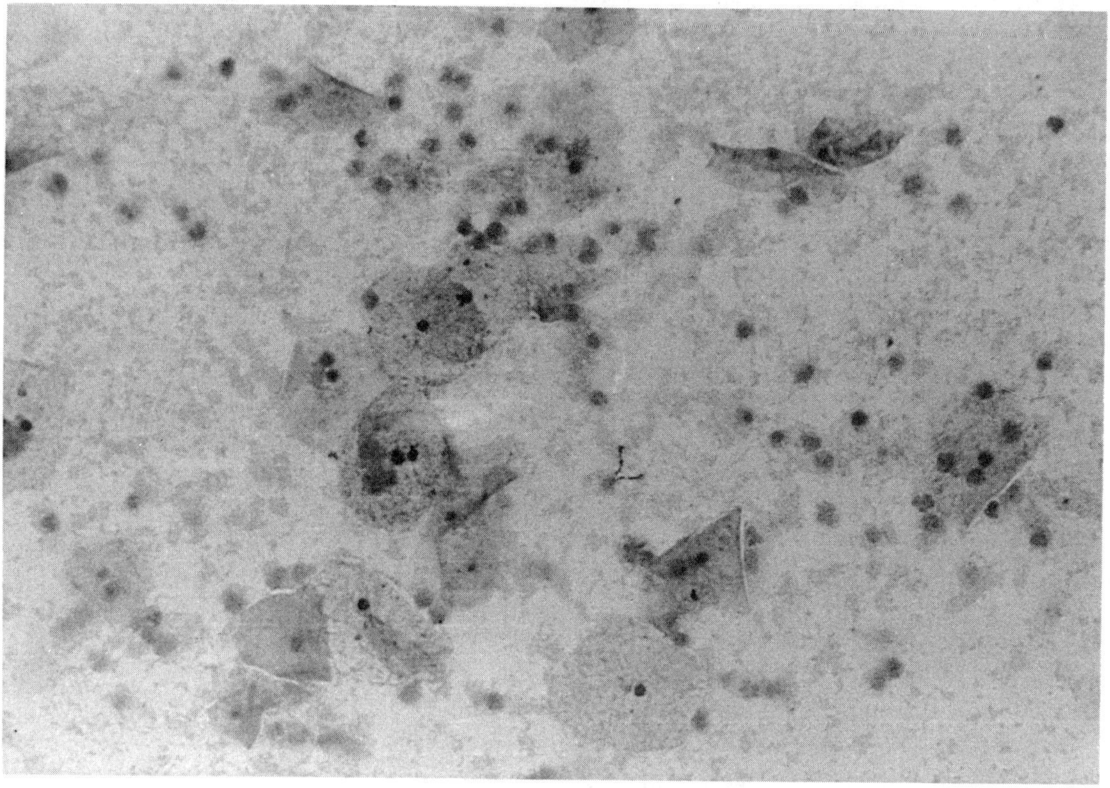

Figure 56-1 Gram stain of "clue cells" as seen in bacterial vaginosis.

Table 56-8 ***Clinical Presentations in the Differential Diagnosis of Acute Genital Ulcer***[13]

Presentation	Diagnosis
* Grouped vesicles	Genital herpes
* Onset during sexual activity	Traumatic ulcer
* Recurrences associated with same systemic medication	Fixed drug reaction
Deep ulcer with undermined border	Chancroid
Firm, rolled, elevated ulcer border	Granuloma inguinale
Painless, firm, indurated ulcer	Syphilis
Infiltrated papule or small erosion/discrete tender movable nodes	Lymphogranuloma venereum

* Pathognomonic

Data from reference number[13]

agnosis of the infection. If cultures are not available, the specimen can be spread on a slide for cytologic examination or immunofluorescent antibody-staining. The sensitivity of the cytologic examination is approximately 50% to 80%, and the findings are not entirely specific for the herpes virus. Herpes viral infections generally produce characteristic intranuclear inclusions and multinucleated giant cells. Immunofluorescent antibody stains and immunoenzymatic techniques (ELISA or immunoperoxidase assays) detect viral antigens and are useful in an emergency situation; however, the sensitivity and specificity of HSV detection varies according to the clinical stage of the lesion, and may range from 38% to 77%.[20] A latex agglutination test for the direct detection of HSV antigens is also available; however, clinical lesions must be "wet." For patients in very high-risk groups, the sensitivity and specificity have been shown to be 92% and 98% respectively when compared to cell culture.[21]

SYPHILIS

Genital ulcers that are suggestive of syphilis should be examined by dark field microscopy to detect the presence of the spirochetes. Treponemas are extremely sensitive to temperature and ambient air and are easily absorbed into porous materials such as swabs; thus, extreme care and close cooperation between the physician and the laboratory scientist are of utmost importance for successful identification of this organism. The diagnosis of syphilis cannot be excluded from a single negative examination; examinations should be repeated on several successive days before being considered conclusively negative. Dark field microscopy should not be performed on lesions from the oral cavity because of the presence of other treponemes. A simple fluorescent antibody test has been used for the identification of *T. pallidum* directly from clinical specimens.[22]

A serologic test for syphilis should be performed on all patients with genital ulcers. Nontreponemal tests such as the rapid plasma reagin (RPR) and the Venereal Disease Research Laboratory (VDRL) are rapid and inexpensive tests for screening large populations; however, they are nonspecific because the antibody measure is directed against diphosphatidyl glycerol (cardiolipin), which is a normal component of many tissues. False-positive tests can result from the serum of patients with atypical pneumonia, malaria, and other bacterial or viral infections, as well as after smallpox or other vaccinations. False positives are relatively common in autoimmune disorders such as systemic lupus erythematosus, in leprosy, in narcotic addicts, and in aged persons. A positive nontreponemal test result must be confirmed using a specific treponemal test such as the fluorescent treponemal antibody absorption (FTA-ABS) test or the microhemagglutination assay (MHA-TP) test. During the primary phase of this disease, nontreponemal tests are approximately 70% to 75% reactive when drawn 1 to 3 weeks after the chancre has disappeared, whereas the FTA is approximately 85% to 90% reactive. Secondary syphilis produces virtually 100% high titer-reactive nontreponemal and FTA testing, and symptoms such as malaise, fever, headache, and sore throat are often present. Again, these symptoms disappear spontaneously after several weeks to a year.

During the latent period of the disease, when there are no symptoms, the FTA has been found to be 97% reactive while the nontreponemal tests are approximately 72% reactive. During this time, cerebrospinal fluid (CSF) serology is generally negative. Late or tertiary syphilis, as demonstrated by a reactive CSF serology, is 77% reactive using the nontreponemal tests and 95% reactive using FTA.[23]

CHANCROIDS

The diagnosis of chancroid requires demonstration of the causative agent, *Hemophilus ducreyi.* A Gram stain of material from the base or edges of the lesion or bubo will reveal many small gram-negative coccobacillary organisms arranged in chains or groups. This organism can be isolated on an enriched chocolate agar containing vancomycin, and, if culture methods are available a more definitive identification is possible.

OTHER ULCERATIVE LESIONS

The diagnosis of LGV is usually made serologically, but can also be made by direct demonstration of the organisms in lesion material.

The primary lesion, which can appear as a painless papule, erosion, or ulcer, appears 3 to 30 days after sexual contact and disappears in days. The second stage is marked by regional lymphadenopathy, during which buboes appear that may suppurate and develop into draining fistulas. Rectal strictures and lymphatic obstructions occur in the last stage.

Complement fixation is the most common test performed. A titer of 1:16 is considered significant after 2 to 4 weeks. Material for direct immunofluorescent testing or for culture is obtained by inserting a needle into the affected lymph node and aspirating the viscous pus that will be present. The Frei test, a skin test using 0.1 mL of heat-killed organisms intradermally, is considered positive when an inflammatory nodule appears at the site of the injection and peaks at about 4 days.

Granuloma inguinale, caused by the gram-negative bacillus *Calymmatobacterium granulomatis,* is diagnosed by demonstrating Donovan bodies (dark-staining rod-shaped inclusions in macrophages) in a Wright or Giemsa-stained preparation of tissue from an infected lesion. Neither culturing nor serologic testing is practical or available at this time.

NONULCERATIVE GENITAL LESIONS

Condylomata acuminata (genital warts) result from infection with certain subtypes of the human papillomaviruses (HPV). They are usually diagnosed by their appearance as hyperplastic, verrucous lesions located in moist, mucocutaneous areas. The lesions begin as pinpoint papules and steadily enlarge, reaching diameters from a few millimeters to a centimeter or more in size. The warts are usually multiple, and in men are most commonly found on the prepuce, frenulum, and glans of the penis and, in homosexual males, around the anus. In the female, the warts may appear on the vagina, cervix, or anus. Confirmation of the diagnosis may be made by biopsy or typical findings on Papanicolaou smear.

Molluscum contagiosum is a self-limiting sexually acquired condition, resulting from infection with a pox virus that infects only keratinizing epithelial cells. These lesions, numbering anywhere from 1 to 20, are typically distributed over the lower abdomen, genitalia, and inner thighs. Caseous material may be expressed from these lesions with direct pressure. Although the diagnosis of molluscum contagiosum is usually based on clinical appearance, microscopic confirmation is demonstrated by characteristic cells containing large intracytoplasmic inclusions (Lipschütz cells).

Infestation with *P. pubis,* the pubic louse, is acquired through close contact usually coincident with sexual activity. This obligate human parasite adheres to the base of hair shafts and cannot survive for more than 24 hours without human contact. Most patients complain of itching; however, asymptomatic cases do occur. Diagnosis is made by the recognition and identification of the infecting lice.

Scabies, like infestation with lice, is spread through close contact of any sort. *Sarcoptes scabiei* is a burrowing mite that also cannot survive for long periods away from the host. Following primary infection, there is a delay of 4 to 8 weeks before the onset of clinical signs. Clinical disease develops after the patient becomes sensitized to the antigenic material produced by the mite. Individuals present with a variety of cutaneous lesions, resulting from both the presence of the organism and the intense scratching of pruritic lesions often secondarily infected with bacteria. Diagnosis is made by recognition of the primary sites of involvement and the secondary rash pattern. Areas on the margins of the inflamed sites are best searched or scraped for mites.

TREATMENT

Therapy is available for most sexually transmitted diseases, yet the incidence of these infections is rising.[24] Control of STDs is difficult for several reasons. Many patients are asymptomatic and do not seek medical attention. In some cases, inappropriate treatment may be administered based on clinical findings rather than on a specific etiologic diagnosis. Treatment of STDs should be administered after a thorough evaluation, including approriate laboratory tests, to establish the etiologic agent or agents, as multiple infection is not uncommon. Specimens should always be obtained before antimicrobial agents are administered.

A critical problem in controlling these diseases is proper treatment of the infected partner(s). Simultaneous treatment of infected partners will prevent reinfection or further transmission. A comprehensive guide to the treatment of STDs is published periodically by the Centers for Disease Control (MMWR, STD Treatment Guidelines). Table 56-9 summarizes the guidelines published in 1985.[24]

CASE STUDY

A 20-year-old male college student was seen in the campus clinic with complaints of dysuria and a mildly purulent discharge from his penis. A Gram stain revealed many intracellular gram-negative diplococci. He was treated with aqueous procaine penicillin G, and asked to identify sexual partners. Several weeks later the student returned, complaining of persistent urethritis. The discharge then appeared more watery and mucoid, and the Gram stain revealed many polymorphonuclear cells but no gram-negative intracelluar diplococci.

Questions

1. On what diagnosis was the treatment with penicillin G based?
2. What is the diagnosis several weeks post-treatment, and what organism is the most probable cause?
3. What are the next steps in eradicating the infection?

Discussion

1. Gonococcal urethritis was the diagnosis.
2. Postgonococcal urethritis is often the result of dual infection in a person who is treated only for gonorrhea. *N. gonorrhoeae* was eradicated, but the other pathogen persisted. Three out of four cases of postgonococcal urethritis are caused by *C. trachomatis*. Concurrent *C. trachomatis* and *N. gonorrhoeae* infections have been reported in 15% to 30% of men with gonorrhea. These patients represent a large group of chlamydial carriers, and virtually all men with

Table 56-9 ***STD Treatment Guidelines***

Disease/ Etiologic Agent	Recommended Treatment	Follow-up/Comments
Chlamydial infections and NGU caused by ureaplasmas	Tetracycline HCl or doxycycline	Test-of-cure may be omitted since treatment is highly effective. Test-of-cure may not become positive until 3–6 weeks after treatment.
Gonococcal infections	Amoxicillin, ampicillin, aqueous procaine penicillin G, or ceftriaxone plus tetracycline, doxycycline, or erythromycin	Follow-up cultures should be obtained from infected site(s) 3–7 days after completion of treatment. Rectal cultures should be collected from all women treated, regardless of whether rectal gonorrhea documented.

(continued)

Table 56-9 ***STD Treatment Guidelines (continued)***

Disease/ Etiologic Agent	Recommended Treatment	Follow-up/Comments
Penicillin-resistant *Neisseria gonorrhoeae*	Spectinomycin or ceftriaxone plus tetracycline, doxycycline, or erythromycin	Note: for proven cases of PPNG or CMRNG only
Genital herpes	Acyclovir	To reduce signs and symptoms only
Syphilis	Benzathine penicillin G or tetracycline HCl	Serologic followup
Trichomoniasis	Metronidazole	Resistance is rare
Bacterial vaginosis	Metronidazole	Treatment of asymptomatic carriers of *Gardnerella vaginalis* is not recommended.
Vulvovaginal candidiasis	Miconazole, clotrimazole, or nystatin	
Chancroid (*Hemophilus ducreyi*)	Erythromycin or ceftriaxone. Incision/drainage or excision of nodes is contraindicated.	Ulcers clinically improved after 7 days. Clinical resolution of lymph nodes is slower.
Lymphogranuloma venereum	Tetracycline. Fluctuant lymph nodes should be aspirated as needed. Incision and drainage of nodes are contraindicated.	Late sequelae such as strictures and/or fistulae may require surgical intervention.
Genital warts		
External	Cryotherapy or podophyllin	Since genital/anal warts are linked to squamous cell genital cancers, persistent warts should be biopsied.
Internal (cervical/vaginal)	Cryotherapy or 5-fluorouracil	
Pediculosis pubis (*Phthirus pubis*)	Lindane (1%) or pyrethrins and piperonyl butoxide (nonprescription)	Retreatment may be indicated after 7 days. Clothing and bed linen should be washed and dried by machine (hot cycle in each) or dry cleaned.
Scabies	Lindane (1%)	Pruritis may persist for several weeks after treatment. Additional weekly treatments may be warranted. Wash and dry clothing and bed linens as described above.

Data from reference number[24]

concomitant infections will develop postgonococcal urethritis if treated with penicillin alone.

3. This patient and his sexual partners should be examined and treated for *C. trachomatis*. Additionally, the specimen should be cultured again for *N. gonorrhoeae* to rule out reinfection or subclinical infection with penicillinase-producing *N. gonorrhoeae* (PPNG).

REFERENCES

1. Weisner PJ: Developing a national strategy for the control of chlamydial infections—U.S.A. In Mardh P-A et al (eds): Chlamydial infections. Proc Fifth International Symposium on Human Chlamydial Infections, Lund, Sweden, June 15–19, 1982, p 437. New York City, Elsevier Biomedical Press, 1982
2. McCormack WM, Mardh P-A: Fifth international symposium on human chlamydial infections. The American Venereal Disease Association 9:216, 1982
3. Josey WE, McKenzie WJ, Lambe DW Jr: *Corynebacterium vaginalis* (*Haemophilus vaginalis*) in women with leukorrhea. Am J Obstet Gynecol 126:574, 1976
4. Bowie WR, Wang S-P, Alexander ER et al: Etiology of nongonococcal urethritis: Evidence for *Chlamydia trachomatis* and *Ureaplasma urealyticus*. J Clin Invest 59:735, 1977
5. Oriel D: Infections of the male genital tract. In Mardh P-A et al (eds): Chlamydial infections. Proc Fifth International Symposium on Human Chlamydial Infections, Lund, Sweden, June 15–19, 1982, p 93. New York City, Elsevier Biomedical Press, 1982
6. Eschenbach DA: Vaginal infections. Clin Obstet Gynecol 26:186, 1983
7. Eschenbach D, Pollock HM, Schachter J: Laboratory diagnosis of female genital tract infections. In Cumitech 17, p 1. Washington, D.C., American Society for Microbiology, 1983
8. Fleury FJ: Adult vaginitis. Clin Obstet Gynecol 24:407, 1981
9. Westrom L, Mardh P-A: Genital chlamydial infections in female. In Mardh P et al (eds): Chlamydial infections. Proc Fifth International Symposium on Human Chlamydial Infections. Lund, Sweden, June 15-19, 1982, p 121. New York City, Elsevier Biomedical Press, 1982
10. Clair J, Kurtz JB: *Chlamydia trachomatis* and upper abdominal pain. Lancet 1: 1044, 1983
11. U.S. Department of Health, Education, and Welfare: Sexually transmitted disease: Summary and recommendations. 1980 Status Report, NIAID Study Group, USPHS, NIH Publication No. 81-2213
12. Taylor E, Barlow D, Blackwell AL et al: *Gardnerella vaginalis*, anaerobes, and vaginal discharge. Lancet 2:1376, 1982
13. Washington AE: Preventing complications of sexually transmitted disease: New treatment guidelines for an expanded spectrum of problems. Drugs 28:355, 1984
14. Jacobs NF, Kraus SF: Gonococcal and nongonococcal urethritis in men: Clinical and laboratory differentiation. Ann Intern Med 82:7, 1975
15. Manis RD, Harris B, Geiseler PJ: Evaluation of gonozyme, an enzyme immunoassay for the rapid diagnosis of gonorrhea. J Clin Microbiol 20:742, 1984
16. Jones RB, Katz BP, Van der Pol B et al: Effect of blind passage and multiple sampling on recovery of *Chlamydia trachomatis* from urogenital specimens. J Clin Microbiol 24:1029, 1986
17. Poulin SA, Kundsin RB, Horne HW Jr: Survival of *Ureaplasma urealyticum* on different kinds of swabs. J Clin Microbiol 10:601, 1979
18. Eschenbach DA: Diagnosis of bacterial vaginosis (nonspecific vaginitis): Role of the laboratory. Clin Microbiol Newsletter 6:134, 1984
19. Amsel R, Totten PA, Spiegel CA et al: Nonspecific vaginitis. Am J Med 74:14, 1983
20. Warford AL, Levy RA, Rekrut KA: Rapid laboratory diagnosis of herpes simplex virus. J Med Technol 2:496, 1985
21. Rawls WE: Herpes simplex virus types 1 and 2 and herpesvirus simiae. In Lennette EH, Schmidt NJ (eds): Diagnostic Procedures for Viral, Rickettsial, and Chlamydial Infections, 5th ed, p 309. Washington, D.C., American Public Health Association, 1979
22. Friedly G: Importance of bacterial stains in the diagnosis of infectious disease. J Med Technol 1:823, 1984
23. Berner JJ: Infectious diseases. In Effects of Diseases on Laboratory Tests, p 333. Philadelphia, JB Lippincott, 1983
24. Centers for Disease Control: 1985 STD Treatment Guidelines. MMWR 34(Suppl):4S–108S, 1985

BIBLIOGRAPHY

Centers for Disease Control: *Chlamydia trachomatis* infections: Policy guidelines for prevention and control, 1985. MMWR 34(Suppl): 3S–74S, 1985

Gibbs RS: Sexually transmitted diseases of the female. In Symposium on Infections in Office Practice. Med Clin North Am 67:221, 1983

Holmes KK, Handsfield HH: Sexually Transmitted Diseases. In Isselbacher KJ et al (eds): Harrison's Principles of Internal Medicine, p 889. New York City, McGraw-Hill, 1985

Hook EW, Stamm WE: Sexually transmitted diseases in men. In Symposium on Infections in Office Practice. Med Clin North Am 67:235, 1983

Lukehart SA: Syphilis diagnosis: What's on the horizon? Clin Microbiol Newsletter 8:151, 1986

Theis JH: Scabies. Clin Microbiol Newsletter 6:93, 1984

Thomason JL, Wilcoski LM, Lee GM et al: Pelvic inflammatory disease. Clin Microbiol Newsletter 8:181, 1986

Thomason JL, Wilcoski LM, McLaughlin CA: Trichomoniasis. Clin Microbiol Newsletter 8:9, 1986

Chapter 57

Skin and Soft Tissue Infection

Julia R. Crowley

Intact skin and its normal flora are effective barriers to infection, and very few organisms can cause infection unless there is some prior injury. Figure 57-1 illustrates the structure of normal skin. The dermis has a dense network of capillaries and lymphatic vessels that make immunoglobulins and other humoral defense factors available. Langerhans cells of the epidermis have the ability to process and present antigens to lymphocytes.[1] The lipids, acidity, and moisture content of the skin limit the survival of transient bacteria, while turnover of epithelial cells (desquamation) continually eliminates bacteria from skin surfaces. Normal flora of the skin can also be antagonistic to potential microbial colonizers. Such flora on the dry skin of adults consist primarily of *Staphylococcus epidermidis, Corynebacterium* species, *Micrococcus* species, and *Propionibacterium acnes.*[2] Gram-negative bacilli and yeast are rare on dry skin, but can appear on moist skin areas. Yeast are common normal flora of the scalp. Transient or colonizing flora reside for a limited time on the skin but then disappear. They may be harmless, or may cause disease under appropriate conditions. The overall health and immunologic competence of the host, as well as conditions in the immediate area of infection, are important factors in the development of both skin and soft tissue infections.

ETIOLOGY AND PATHOPHYSIOLOGY

Infections of the skin can be primary, in which there is no obvious underlying skin disease, or secondary to a previous skin disorder, trauma, or systemic infection. Primary infections are caused by a limited number of microorganisms, usually

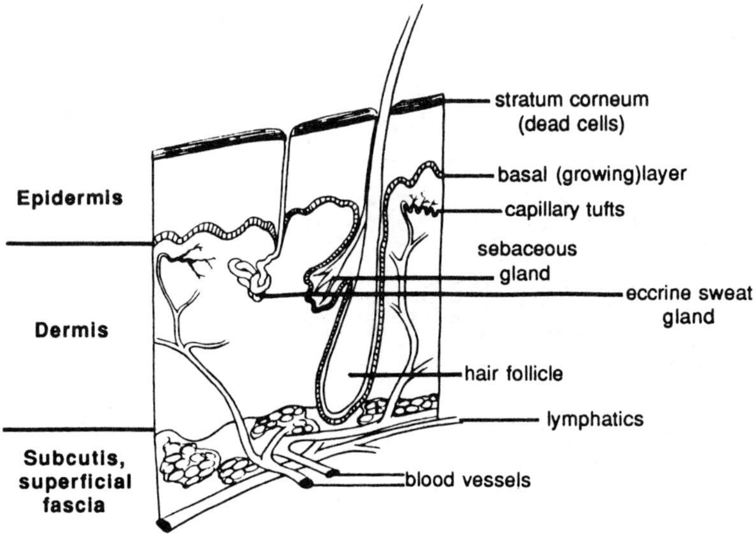

Figure 57-1 **Structure of the skin.**

Staphylococcus aureus, Streptococcus pyogenes (group A strep), and dermatophyte fungi.[2, 3] Secondary infections can be caused by a wide variety of bacteria, such as *S. aureus*, group A strep, *Proteus, Pseudomonas,* and *Escherichia coli,* as well as fungi and viruses.[4] It is not unusual to have several different kinds of bacteria present at the same time in wounds, burns, or skin damaged by previous disease. Some may be involved in the infectious process and some may be only colonizers.

Microorganisms or their products elicit an inflammatory response in the skin. Staphylococci, streptococci, enteric gram-negative bacilli, and pseudomonads frequently cause an acute inflammatory reaction, with polymorphonuclear leucocytes (PMNs) as the predominant cell. In some infections, such as those caused by mycobacteria, actinomycetes, and fungi, a chronic inflammatory response follows the acute phase due to the persistence of antigen in the area. Monocytes, macrophages,and lymphocytes replace PMNs as the predominant cell, and a granuloma is formed.[5] The ready presence of immunoglobulins and lymphocytes also makes the skin a prime location for manifestations of immediate and delayed hypersensitivity. The common skin lesions resulting from infection are described in Table 57-1.

S. aureus can colonize the anterior nares, and from that site or from the environment can colonize and infect the skin. Its potential virulence factors include hemolysins, leukocidin, epidermolytic toxins, coagulase, fibrinolysin, nuclease, lipases, hyaluronidase, and protein A, a cell-wall component that binds to the Fc portion of IgG. Primary infection usually begins with folliculitis, a pustular lesion that results when hair follicles are invaded. Furuncles, or boils, may occur if the organism spreads through the follicle walls into the dermis or if it is introduced following trauma. Large amounts of pus are formed, and pressure from the abscess and lytic enzymes can cause lateral spread through fibrous tissues. Deep suppurative lesions, cellulitis, lymphadenopathy, fever, and septicemia may result. Bullous impetigo, common in children, and staphylococcal scalded skin syndrome (toxic epidermal necrolysis), a serious disease of neonates, are caused by strains that produce exfoliatin, a toxin that splits layers of epidermis. *S. aureus* also colonizes streptococcal impetigo, but the staph is probably not an important contributor to the pathology of these lesions. Nasal carriage

Table 57-1 ***Types of Skin Lesions***

Term	Description	Example
Macule	Flat discoloration, usually smaller than 1 cm	Rash of measles
Papule	Solid, small, raised lesion	Nonpustular acne
Nodule	Solid, small, hard, raised lesion usually smaller than 2 cm, with depth into the tissue. Cellular proliferation	Enlarged lymph node
Tumor	Same as a nodule, but larger than 2 cm	Gumma of tertiary syphilis
Granuloma	A tumor characterized by a mass of tissue containing multinucleated giant cells, central necrosis resulting from hypersensitivity, and a peripheral zone of lymphocytes surrounded by fibrous tissue	Mycetoma
Vesicle	Small, blisterlike lesion of the epidermis filled with clear fluid, usually smaller than 1 cm	Chicken pox
Bulla	Same as a vesicle, but larger than 1 cm	Bullous impetigo
Pustule	A small elevation filled with thick, yellowish fluid	Pustules of folliculitis
Abscess	A localized collection of pus, fluid, and necrotic tissue	Traumatic abscess following injury
Ulcer	A necrotic, scooped-out lesion that can extend into the subcutaneous tissues	Sporotrichotic lesion

and skin colonization are common in patients with repeated staph infections, and are also associated with frequent use of needles, an important consideration in treatment failures.[2, 6]

Group A strep can be a transient skin colonizer that infects following some local trauma. These organisms can be further typed on the basis of their cell-surface M proteins, and types that cause skin infections are distinct from those that cause throat infections.[7] Some of these M types can be nephritogenic, causing a poststreptococcal glomerulonephritis. M proteins and lipotechoic acids of the cell surface are implicated in attachment of the bacteria to the skin surface,[8, 9] Other important antigens of group A strep that elicit antibody response in skin infections include deoxyribonuclease (DNAse) and hyaluronidase. Streptolysin O, on the other hand, elicits antibody response in throat infections but often not in skin infections. Streptococcal pyoderma, including impetigo, is associated with insect bites and other skin irritations. Dermatophyte fungi that cause breaks in the stratum corneum are common precursors to streptococcal cellulitis, a diffuse inflammation of the subcutaneous connective tissue. Erysipelas, a severe facial cellulitis with systemic toxicity, is less prevalent.

Dermatophytes of the genera *Microsporum, Epidermophyton,* and *Tricophyton* cause infection in the stratum corneum that is commonly referred to as *ringworm,* or *tinea.* These fungi often grow outward in a ring as they deplete the nutrients, especially iron, in the epidermal layers; therefore, viable organisms are more likely to be in the periphery of the lesion.[3] Anthropophilic species are least likely to cause severe reactions in humans, and may persist in the stratum corneum for years. *Candida albicans* and other normal flora yeast can cause cutaneous infections in moist or lacerated skin, especially in the compromised host, or can colonize preexisting skin conditions.

Infection of soft tissue, which is normally sterile, can result when organisms are introduced following external trauma or internal damage such as that caused by atherosclerosis or allergic vasculitis. Healthy living tissue has a high concentration of oxygen and a positive oxidation-reduction potential (Eh). Injuries that interfere with local blood flow lead to decreased oxygen, decreased Eh, tissue necrosis, and decreased activity of leukocytes. The environment becomes favorable for the growth of anaerobic and facultatively anaerobic organisms that produce gas and enzymes, leading to further necrosis and spread of infection. Necrotizing infections are of particular concern in surgical wounds. Skin and tissues can also become infected by extension from other foci or as a result of generalized systemic infection. Tissue infections that result from penetrating injury or burns are often polymicrobic. They may be inoculated with organisms from the environment, such as *Pseudomonas aeruginosa* in burn wounds, or may reflect the aerobic and anaerobic flora present on the surrounding skin and mucous membranes of the host.

Cellulitis, fasciitis, myonecrosis, and tissue necrotizing infections are types of soft tissue infection.[10] Some of the microorganisms that are isolated from wound and tissue infections are the anaerobes *Bacteroides fragilis, Clostridium perfringens* and other *Clostridium* species, and *Peptostreptococcus;* facultative anaerobes include *S. aureus, S. pyogenes,* and the enteric gram-negative bacilli. Facial cellulitis in children is most often caused by *Hemophilus influenzae,* type b. *P. aeruginosa,* various species of phycomycetes, and *Aspergillus* species can all cause gangrenous cellulitis in the compromised host. Sporotrichosis, chromomycosis, and mycetomas are subcutaneous tissue infections that follow abrasions or penetrating injury. *Sporothrix schenckii* infection progresses along the lymphatics. Chromomycosis, caused primarily by dematiaceous soil saprophytes, induces a host granulomatous response with a high degree of hyperplasia that can mimic carcinoma. Mycetomas, deep lesions that can progress to the bone, are caused by a wide variety of organisms. Actinomycetes and *Pseudallescheria boydii* are common isolates.

Skin and tissue infections can also be caused by a wide variety of other organisms. Although the more common are usually diagnosed by their clinical manifestations, laboratory tests are often needed to establish the etiology of infections that may be caused by viruses, rickettsia, mycobacteria, and systemic fungi and bacteria.

CLINICAL MANIFESTATIONS

Infections that trigger acute inflammatory reactions cause the tissues to become swollen, red, warm, and painful, and PMNs accumulate in the area. Different types of acute inflammation follow infection, depending upon whether exudates, cell proliferation, tissue necrosis, or a combination of these factors is present. For example, *S. aureus* strains can produce either acute pustular or bullous lesions, depending upon the virulence factors that they possess. Pus-filled boils characterize more invasive strains, while bullous impetigo lesions appear as fluid-filled vesicles that subsequently form varnishlike crusts. Reddening of the skin and large blistered areas that pull off easily are the responses to epidermolytic toxin in staphylococcal scalded skin syndrome. Large bullous gangrenous lesions can be caused by *Pseudomonas, Clostridium,* and gram-negative bacilli. Streptococcal impetigo lesions begin as pustular vesicles that develop into superficial or deep ulcers with a honey-colored crust. Cellulitis appears as tender, red, edematous areas, and invasion of bacteria, especially group A strep, into the lymphatics causes red streaking as the infection progresses.

The host response to soluble fungal antigens that diffuse into the epidermis and dermis varies from no reaction, to diffuse scaly patches, to defined rings of inflammation, to inflammatory exudative lesions. *C. albicans* lesions, usually found in skin folds, appear as red, weeping areas with scalloped edges, surrounded by satellite eruptions. The yeast can also cause a pustular folliculitis. Sporotrichosis is characterized by nodular ulcerations that progress along the lymphatics, chromomycosis by localized warty, cauliflowerlike lesions, and mycetomas by a swollen, deformed area of abscesses, draining sinuses, and granules containing the etiologic agent. Mycetomas are usually found on the hands or feet.

Indicators of tissue infection, especially anaerobic infection, are gas in the tissues, foul smell, black discoloration, and/or exudates with granules. The classic signs of inflammation may be absent.[4] In the case of any bacterial skin infection, fever may indicate septicemia and systemic spread of the organism.

Systemic viral and rickettsial diseases can produce rashes, vesicles, or other types of lesions. Herpes simplex virus causes a primary vesicular or bullous lesion; the virus is then established in ganglia and becomes latent, reactivating after various types of stress to the host. Mycobacterial skin infections usually present as granulomatous ulcers. Table 57-2 describes some of the typical lesions of skin infections.

LABORATORY ANALYSES AND DIAGNOSIS

Although diagnosis of common skin infections is usually based on the clinical appearance of the lesions, culture and sensitivity tests may be needed to confirm the diagnosis and guide therapy. Skin scrapings or other material from lesions should be collected after the lesion and surrounding area are carefully disinfected to eliminate irrelevant organisms. Any crusts and surface debris should also be removed. Specimens from the draining sinus tracts of mycetomas should be examined for granules that will contain the organisms. Because swabs contain trapped oxygen and cotton is toxic to some anaerobes, special anaerobic swabs and transport tubes should be used if anaerobic culture is needed. In most cases, material from the center of the lesion should be obtained, although material from the periphery of the lesions is necessary for isolation of dermatophytes. When fungi are suspected, a sterile scalpel can be used carefully to obtain skin scrapings. Swabs should not be used because fibers may be misleading when direct preparations are examined. Pus or fluid from closed lesions should be obtained with a needle and syringe, with all gas expelled from the syringe. Material collected in the syringe is suitable for aerobic and anaerobic culture and for viral culture. Specimens for viral culture or analysis should be collected and transported in special viral transport media and stored at $-70°$ C if processing cannot occur within 24 hours.

Culture of cellulitis is rarely useful,[11] but identification and sensitivity testing of organisms in other soft tissue infections can be important. Chronic localized infections, burns, necrotizing infections, and wounds may require biopsy. Histologic evaluation of granulomatous lesions helps to differentiate infection from neoplasm. For example, observation of brown sclerotic bodies in tissue is diagnostic of fungal chromomycosis rather than carcinoma. Quantitative culture of biopsy material may be requested, because knowledge of the number and type of organisms present helps the surgeon to determine the best time for wound closure or for skin grafts on burns. Culture may also help to establish the etiology of invasive infections by establishing the identity of the predominant organism.[11] Culture of abscesses should include methods to recover the variety of bacteria and fungi described above.

Several rapid direct methods can aid in the diagnosis of skin infection. Semiquantitative direct Gram stains can lead to presumptive identification, can help to guide test selection and culture methods, and can confirm final culture results. Acid-fast stains should be added for any granules or granulomatous specimens that may contain actinomycetes or mycobacteria. KOH preparations are necessary when fungi are suspected. Calcifluor white, a fluorescent compound, can be mixed with KOH to give good fungal contrast, but a fluorescence microscope is needed. A direct fluorescent antibody test is available for the identification of *B. fragilis* in clinical material. There are many direct test kits available for the detection of group A strep antigen in clinical specimens. Such

Table 57-2 ***Clinical Manifestations of Skin Infections***

Etiologic Agent/Disease	Lesion
Staphylococcus aureus	
Folliculitis	Pustules
Boils or furuncles	Circumscribed abscesses that become filled with pus
Carbuncles	Aggregates of boils
Impetigo	Bullous lesions with subsequent varnishlike crusts
Scalded skin syndrome	Large, flaccid bullae, epidermis separating into sheets with red, moist surface beneath
***Streptococcus pyogenes* (group A strep)**	
Impetigo	Pustular vesicles developing into ulcers with honey-colored crusts
Erysipelas	Red thickening of the skin
Cellulitis	Flat, reddened areas of the skin
Lymphangitis	Red streaks following the lymphatic channels
Pseudomonas aeruginosa	
Burn infection	Greenish discoloration
Ecthyma gangrenosum	Brown or black, spreading, bullous lesions
Folliculitis	Pustules
Anaerobic or mixed bacterial tissue infections	
Anaerobic cellulitis	Spreading necrosis of tissue, usually with gas formation (crepitation)
Gas gangrene	Severe form of spreading anaerobic cellulitis with dusky discoloration, surface bullae formation
Dermatophyte fungi	
Ringworm (tinea)	Scaly patches; ring of inflammation with healing center; persistent papules, pustules, abscesses
Candida albicans	
Intertriginous infection	Reddened areas with scalloped edges and pustules
Folliculitis and diaper rash	Pustules
Sporothrix schenckii	
Sporotrichosis	Ulcerating nodules progressing along lymphatic channels
Saprobic fungi	
Chromomycosis	Raised, warty lesions resembling cauliflower heads
Saprobic fungi, actinomycetes, bacteria	
Mycetoma	Massive swollen area with draining sinus tracts that discharge granules
Herpes simplex virus	Vesicles on a reddened base filled with clear fluid
***Mycobacterium* species**	Granulomatous ulcers, nodules

tests were developed to detect group A strep throat infection, but probably work as well with skin exudates.[12] Their specificity is high, around 95%, but sensitivity is much lower; therefore, negative direct strep test results should be confirmed by culture. Because glomerulonephritis may be among the sequelae of group A strep infection, the laboratory may perform serological tests to detect past infection. Skin lipids inhibit streptolysin O, and antibody response to this antigen, as measured by the ASO titer, occurs in less than half of patients with streptococcal skin infections. Anti-DNAse B or anti-hyaluronidase titers are more reliable than is ASO titer to indicate past infection with skin strains of group A strep.[9, 13] Sensitivity testing is generally not performed because most group A strep are susceptible to penicillin G, the drug of choice.

S. aureus is commonly identified from culture by conventional coagulase tests; however, latex agglutination tests are available that rapidly detect both staphylococcal-bound coagulase and protein A. Rapid enzymatic and biochemical methods are available for same-day identification of the more common Enterobacteriaceae, anaerobes, streptococci, and staphylococci from culture.[14] *S. aureus* should be tested for resistance to penicillin G, because this is the antibiotic of choice for treatment. Enterics and pseudomonads have unpredictable sensitivities and should be tested for antibiotic resistance.

Because viruses and rickettsia reproduce only

Table 57-3 ***Treatment for Skin and Tissue Infection***

Organism	Therapy
Staphylococcus aureus	Penicillin G, if *S. aureus* is susceptible Penicillin with clavulanic acid* or ceftriaxone alone if *S. aureus* is a β-lactamase producer Clindamycin or erythromycin for penicillin-allergic patients Vancomycin for severe hospital infection Rifampin or topical neomycin for nasal carriers
Group A strep	Penicillin G Clindamycin or erythromycin for penicillin-allergic patients
Anaerobes, mixed infection	Penicillin with clavulanic acid Metronidazole with gentamicin
Dermatophytes	Topical miconazole alone or with anti-inflammatory agent Topical triclosan Griseofulvin for severe infection
Candida	Topical miconazole Ketoconazole
Sporothrix	Topical and oral potassium iodide
Agents of chromomycosis	5-flucytosine Thiabendazole
Pseudallescheria boydii	Miconazole
Nocardia, Actinomyces	Sulfamethoxazole-trimethoprim with streptomycin
Herpes simplex	Acyclovir for primary lesions only

* Clavulanic acid is a β-lactamase inhibitor.

within living cells, they often produce inclusions or cause distinctive cytopathic effects (CPE). For example, cells obtained from vesicles of herpes and chickenpox may be large and multinucleated. These inclusions can sometimes be seen in Tzanck preparations, a type of Giemsa stain. Infected cells will contain viral or rickettsial antigen that may react in various direct immunodiagnostic tests, or elicit detectable humoral antibody response.

TREATMENT

Treatment of skin infections can include draining pus-filled abscesses, débridement of necrotic tissue, topical agents, and systemic antibiotics. Table 57-3 (page 737) indicates recommended treatment for various agents causing infection.[14–21]

Staphylococcal abscesses may heal following drainage or, in severe infections, require systemic antibiotics. Penicillin and methicillin resistance can be a problem. Penicillin G is the antibiotic of choice for susceptible organisms because it is 10 to 100 times more active than the beta-lactamase (penicillinase)-resistant penicillins. Topical therapy supresses but does not cure the carrier state, and must be continued for prolonged periods to be effective.[15] Followup blood cultures may be necessary if the patient develops symptoms of bacteremia. Nasal cultures may also be ordered to determine whether or not the carrier state has been eliminated.

In soft tissue infections, abscesses should be drained and foreign material and necrotic tissue removed. Because many of the bacteria present in mixed infections have different antibiotic sensitivities and some, especially the *B. fragilis* group, can produce β-lactamase, these infections have been successfully treated with combinations of antibiotics. Burn wounds are never sterile, and their bacterial population should be monitored by culture throughout healing because septicemia is a serious consequence of uncontrolled bacterial populations in burns.

Antibacterial antibiotics are not effective against fungi, and specific antifungal drugs are necessary. In fungal infections, topical treatments of antibiotics combined with antiinflammatory agents are often used, but systemic antibiotics may be needed for severe infections. For effective therapy for mycetoma, the etiologic agent must be determined. Mycotic mycetomas are very difficult to treat because drugs do not penetrate into the extensive cystic and fibrotic areas of the lesions. Actinomycotic mycetomas may respond better to treatment with antibacterial antibiotics. In herpes simplex infections, initial lesions respond to acyclovir, but there is no effective treatment for recurrent herpes.[16]

CASE STUDY #1

A four-year-old child was brought to the emergency room with swollen eyes, lethargy, and back pain. His mother reported crusted lesions on his legs for the past week. Urinalysis revealed moderate red blood cell casts and moderate leukocytes and red blood cells. Other laboratory findings included increased serum BUN and creatinine, and increased sedimentation rate and α-2-globulin level. Whole serum complement and C3 were decreased, throat culture was negative, but group A strep was cultured from one active lesion. ASO titers were normal but anti-DNAse B was elevated. The child was treated with penicillin, and followup cultures 10 days later were negative. Urinalysis revealed a few red and white blood cell casts, and the urinalysis results did not become normal for 2 months.

Questions

1. What is the most likely diagnosis in this case?
2. What laboratory findings support this conclusion?
3. Of what use was treatment with penicillin G?

Discussion

1. The diagnosis was probably streptococcal glomerulonephritis that developed while the child had active skin lesions.
2. A diagnosis of glomerulonephritis is supported

by the urinalysis findings and increased serum BUN and creatinine. A positive skin lesion culture for group A strep and an increased level of anti-DNAse B confirm streptococcal origin. A normal ASO titer is consistent with streptococcal skin lesions. Other laboratory findings suggest the presence of an acute inflammation and an active immunologic process.

3. Treatment of the skin lesions in this disease does not usually alter the course of nephritis, but helps to prevent chronic disease.

CASE STUDY #2

A 45-year-old diabetic man was seen by his family physician because of multiple boils and abscesses on his thighs. He also reported flulike symptoms and inability to eat for the past 12 hours. Except for a temperature of 101° F, the physical examination was normal. A glucose test done immediately in the office showed that the patient's glucose was 185 mg/dL. The patient controlled his diabetes with insulin injections in his thighs, and the abscesses appeared to be located at the injection sites. The abscesses were drained and a pus specimen was sent to the local hospital laboratory for culture and sensitivity, along with a nasal swab to be cultured for *Staphylococcus aureus*. A course of oral dicloxacillin was given during the next 24 hours. The next day the patient's temperature was normal and fasting glucose was 130 mg/dL. Antibiotic therapy was changed to penicillin G when the laboratory reported that S. *aureus* had been isolated and was sensitive to that antibiotic. The nasal culture was positive for S. *aureus* also, and the physician added rifampin to the penicillin therapy. One month following treatment the patient's nasal culture was negative, his fasting blood sugar was 120 mg/dL, and the abscesses had healed.

Questions

1. What is the likely explanation for the development of S. *aureus* skin lesions in this patient?
2. What further complication might be suspected from the physical findings?
3. Why was rifampin added to the therapeutic regimen?

Discussion

1. Diabetics whose treatment needs adjustment often develop boils of the sort described in this case. Moreover, persons who use needles regularly, such as diabetics receiving insulin injections, have an increased nasal carrier rate of S. *aureus*. The organisms are thus readily available for invasion of the injection sites.
2. A temperature of 101° F and the symptoms reported by the patient suggested bacteremia. The course of dicloxacillin resulted in a normal temperature within 24 hours.
3. Rifampin is effective in eliminating the nasal carrier state, which otherwise could be a source of recurrent episodes of staph infection for this patient.

REFERENCES

1. Roitt I, Brostoff J, Male D: Immunology, p 114. St Louis, CV Mosby, 1985
2. Leyden JJ: Pathophysiology of Certain Bacterial Diseases. In Soter NA, Baden HP (eds): Pathophysiology of Dermatologic Diseases, pp 347–359. New York City, McGraw-Hill, 1984
3. Gonzalez: Pathophysiology of Certain Fungal Diseases. In Soter NA, Baden HP (eds): Pathophysiology of Dermatologic Diseases, pp 376–385. New York City, McGraw-Hill, 1984
4. Aly R: Microbiology of Skin and Nails. In Baron S (ed): Medical Microbiology, 2nd ed, pp 1185–1195. Menlo Park, California, Addison-Wesley, 1986
5. Marchesi VT: Inflammation and Healing. In Kissane JM (ed): Anderson's Pathology, 8th ed, vol 1, pp 22–59. St Louis, CV Mosby, 1985
6. Sheagren JN: *Staphylococcus aureus:* The persistent pathogen. Medical Progress. N Engl J Med 310(21): 1368–1373, 1984
7. Anthony BF, Kaplan EL, Wannamaker LW et al: The diagnosis of streptococcal infections in a defined population of children: Serotypes associated with skin and respiratory infections. Am J Epidemiol 104:652–666, 1976
8. Ellen RP, Gibbons RJ: M protein-associated adherence of S. pyogenes to epithelial cells: Prerequisite

for virulence. Infection and Immunity 5:826–830, 1972

9. Slade HD: Group A Streptococci. In Youmans GP, Paterson PY, Sommers HM (eds): The Biologic and Clinical Basis of Infectious Disease, pp 165–172. Philadelphia, WB Saunders, 1985
10. Mader JT: Bone and Necrotizing Soft Tissue Infections. In Baron S (ed): Medical Microbiology, 2nd ed, pp 1207–1216. Menlo Park, California, Addison-Wesley, 1986
11. Isenberg HD, Washington JA II, Balows A et al: Collection, Handling and Processing of Specimens. In Lennette EH, Balows A, Housler WJ Jr et al (eds): Manual of Clinical Microbiology, 4th ed, pp 73–98. Washington, D.C., American Society for Microbiology, 1985
12. Facklam RR, Carey RB: Streptococci and Aerococci. In Lennette EH, Balows A, Housler WJ Jr et al (eds): Manual of Clinical Microbiology, 4th ed, pp 154–175. Washington, D.C., American Society for Microbiology, 1985
13. Berner JJ: Effects of Diseases on Laboratory Tests, p 124. Philadelphia, JB Lippincott, 1984
14. D'Amato RF, McLaughlin JC, Ferraro MJ: Rapid and Mechanized/Automated Systems in Microbiology. In Lennette EH, Balows A, Housler WJ Jr et al (eds): Manual of Clinical Microbiology, 4th ed, pp 52–65. Washington, D.C., American Society for Microbiology, 1985
15. Leyden JJ, Kligman AM: Topical Antibiotic in the Prophylaxis of Experimental *S. Aureus* and *S. Pyogenes* Infections in Humans. In Maibach H, Aly R (eds): Skin Microbiology: Relevance to Clinical Infection, pp 269–274. New York City, Springer-Verlag, 1981
16. Finegold DS, Taplin D: Infections and infestations of the skin. J Am Acad Dermatol 11(5, part 2): 971–974, 1984
17. Blumer JL, O'Brien CA, Lemon E et al: Skin and soft tissue infections: Pharmacologic approaches. Pediatr Infect Dis 4(3):336–341, 1985
18. Davis JM, Dineen P: Antibacterial Drugs. In Modell W (ed): Drugs of Choice 1984/1985, pp 150–169. St Louis, CV Mosby, 1984
19. Rosenblatt JE: Antimicrobial Susceptibility Testing of Anaerobes. In Lorian V (ed): Antibiotics in Laboratory Medicine, 2nd ed, pp 159–180. Baltimore, Williams & Wilkins, 1986
20. Graybill JR, Drutz DJ: Ketoconazole for Management of Mucocutaneous Candidiasis Syndrome. In Maibach H, Aly R (eds): Skin Microbiology: Relevance to Clinical Infection, pp 333–341. New York City, Springer-Verlag, 1981
21. Rippon JW: Medical Mycology: The Pathogenic Fungi and Pathogenic Actinomycetes, 2nd ed, pp 85, 86, 185, 259, 287. Philadelphia, WB Saunders, 1982

Chapter 58

Parasitic Infections

JoLynne Campbell

For many years the study of parasites was considered the domain of public health practitioners. Parasites were believed by many to be found only in tropical areas where sanitation was inadequate and the people were poor. Often parasitology was brought to public awareness only in times of war.

Today, the study of parasitic infections is well established within the area of infectious diseases. With increased travel to and immigration of populations from countries all over the world, the physician can see a variety of parasitic diseases. Parasites can and do invade all the body systems; therefore, the physician should include them in the differential diagnosis, especially if the patient has a history of travel, is a foreign student studying in the United States, or is a recent immigrant.

It should be noted that, in the laboratory diagnosis of any infectious disease involving serological tests, cross-reactions sometimes occur, test results can be affected by interfering substances such as abnormal protein levels, and immunosuppressive therapy can lower titers. Serological titers, in addition, will gradually decrease over time.

In many infectious processes, the liver function tests are abnormal. After treatment, however, the results should return to normal.

ETIOLOGY AND PATHOPHYSIOLOGY

Gastrointestinal Disorders

Diarrheal diseases are one of the leading causes of morbidity and mortality worldwide. In the U.S. they are the third most common complaint seen by general practitioners.[1] Although the majority of such disorders in the U.S. are caused by bacteria and viruses, parasites should not be overlooked. There are a variety of helminths and protozoa that can cause acute to chronic illness, manifesting symptoms from mild to severe. (See also Chap. 24.)

The pathophysiology seen in gastrointestinal parasitic disorders is as varied as are the etiologic agents. The intestinal protozoa, for example, have diverse habitats and means of pathogenesis.

Giardia lamblia, a flagellate, resides in the small intestine. The attachment sucker can cause mechanical irritation to the local mucosa, and the organism may penetrate the mucosal surface and invade the secretory tubules. Hypogammaglobulinemia, achlorhydria, reduced levels of IgA, and other immunosuppressive conditions can predispose individuals to infection.

Entamoeba histolytica, an ameba, infects the large intestine. Ulceration of the intestinal wall occurs, caused by proteolytic enzymes and cytotoxins produced by the organism. Extraintestinal infections can occur in untreated cases.

Cryptosporidia, a sporozoan, has recently been found in severe diarrheal diseases of immunosuppressed persons, but it has also been implicated as a cause of self-limited "traveler's" diarrhea in the immunocompetent individual.

Of the intestinal helminths, *Ascaris lumbricoides,* a nematode, causes anatomical rather than physiological damage to the host's intestinal tract. Due to their large size, the adult worms are able to maintain their position within the lumen and do not attach to the intestinal wall. However, in heavy infections the worms often coil together, causing intestinal obstruction. They may also undergo "abnormal migrations," perforating the intestinal wall and/or migrating up the alimentary canal. (See Table 58-1.)

Hepatobiliary Disorders

Many parasites cause disorders of the hepatobiliary system. Both the helminths and the protozoa are represented as agents of hepatobiliary disease, as indicated in Table 58-2.

The ameba *E. histolytica,* is the protozoan representative. Because the organism is endemic in about 5% of the U.S. population, complications from asymptomatic intestinal infections are not uncommon. If left untreated, amebae infecting the intestinal tract can penetrate the submucosa, enter the circulation, and be filtered out in the liver, where most, but not all, of the ameba will be destroyed. Those surviving undergo multiplication leading to abscess formation, usually in the right lobe. Some liver abscesses erode through the diaphragm, infecting the lung tissue (see p. 745).

The helminths that produce hepatobiliary disease most frequently are the nematode of dogs and cats, *Toxocara canis* or *cati;* the trematodes, *Schistosoma mansoni, Clonorchis sinensis,* and *Fasciola hepatica;* and the cestode *Echinococcus granulosus.*

Toxocara causes visceral larva migrans in humans, a condition that occurs because humans are not the parasite's preferred host, and the life cycle is incomplete. When the nematode larvae become trapped within the liver tissue, the organism's metabolites produce a tissue reaction, resulting in local hemorrhages, necrosis, and infiltration of the lymphatic ducts. Over time, granulomas are formed around the trapped larvae.

Table 58-1 ***Gastrointestinal Disorders***

Clinical Manifestations	Etiologic Agents	Diagnostic Tests	Treatment	Comments
Diarrhea with or without blood and/or mucus Abdominal pain with or without cramping Flatulence Anorexia Fatigue (chronic) Steatorrhea Malabsorption syndrome Intestinal obstruction Worm migration	*Entamoeba hystolytica* *Cryptosporidia* *Giardia lamblia* *Ascaris lumbricoides*	*Microbiological* O and P (all) (modified acid-fast for *Cryptosporidia*) Duodenal aspirate or Entero-Test (*Giardia*) *Other Tests* Sigmoidoscopic biopsy (amebiasis) Intestinal mucosal biopsy (*Cryptosporidia*) Radiographic studies (*Ascaris, Giardia,* and *E. histolytica*)	*Amebiasis* Iodoquinol Metronidazole Dehydroemetine *Giardiasis* Quinacrine HCl or Metronidazole *Cryptosporidia* Spiramycin *Ascariasis* Mebendazole or Pyrantel pamoate	*Amebiasis* Extraintestinal infections can occur in untreated cases. *Giardiasis* Hypogammaglobulinemia, achlorhydria, reduced levels of IgA, and other immunosuppressive conditions can predispose a person to infection. *Cryptosporidiosis* Can cause severe diarrhea in immunocompromised host *Ascariasis* Abnormal migrations of adult worms can occur (during fever, chemotherapy, or anesthesia).

S. mansoni is second only to malaria as the leading cause of morbidity and mortality throughout the world. The organism is endemic in Africa, Asia, South America, and portions of the West Indies. Although the life cycle is not completed in the United States, the blood fluke is seen in the Puerto Rican population.

Although they live in the inferior mesenteric vein of the lower colon of humans, the adult worms have little to do with the pathological process. The eggs that are swept by the venous portal system to the liver are the primary cause of disease; eggs trapped within the liver tissue trigger granuloma formation. In heavy infections, periportal fibrosis occurs, producing characteristic "clay-pipestem" fibrosis. Salmonellosis often accompanies *Schistosoma* infections.

Clonorchis sinensis is a trematode commonly known as the "Chinese liver fluke." Humans become infected by eating raw or poorly cooked fish. The adult worms establish themselves in the biliary tree and cause thickening and dilation of the bile ducts. Only in heavy infections do they spill over into liver tissue. Hyperplasia of the bile duct mucosa is common. Adenocarcinomas have been associated with *Clonorchis* infections.[2]

Fasciola hepatica, known as the "sheep liver fluke," occurs when humans ingest the encysted larvae located either on aquatic vegetation or in water. Once ingested, the larvae migrate through the liver to the bile ducts. As the infection moves from the acute to the chronic phase, there is often an absence of symptoms. However, obstruction of the bile ducts can occur.

Table 58-2 ***Hepatobiliary System Disorders***

Clinical Manifestations	Etiologic Agents	Diagnostic Tests	Treatment	Comments
Hepatitis, with or without jaundice (often with fever and diarrhea) Hepatomegaly, with or without tenderness Referred pain, often to right scapula Abscesses with elevation and fixation of right diaphragm Cirrhosis with accompanying ascites, splenomegaly, and portal hypertension Space-occupying lesions of liver Biliary obstruction with cholecystitis Hypereosinophilia (20%–70%)	*Entamoeba histolytica* *Clonorchis sinensis* *Schistosoma mansoni* *Toxocara canis* or *cati* *Echinococcus granulosus* *Leishmania donovani* *Fasciola hepatica*	*Microbiological* O and P Giemsa-stained smears *Serological* IFA or ELISA for *Toxocara* and leishmaniasis IFA, IHA, gel diffusion precipitation test for extraintestinal amebiasis CF, IHA, IIF, and ELISA for schistosomiasis IHA, LA, IE for hydatid disease *Other Tests* Gallium scan, ultrasonography, laparoscopy, and liver biopsy CBC Intradermal test Rectal biopsy Casoni skin test Hatching tests *Liver Function Tests* (Urine urobilinogen and bilirubin are excellent screening tests.)	*Extraintestinal Amebiasis* Metronidazole *plus* Iodoquinal *Clonorchis, Fasciola,* and *Schistosoma* Praziquantel *Visceral Larva Migrans* Diethylcarbamazine* or Thiabendazole* *Hydatid Disease* Surgery Mebendazole* *Kala-azar* Stibogluconate sodium	*Amebiasis* Extraintestinal infections are often the result of untreated infections. *Hydatid disease* Rupture of cysts may cause anaphylaxis. Spilled cyst material is also highly infective and can cause secondary cyst formation. *Toxocara* Retinitis, chorioretinitis, epilepsy, and myocarditis can be complications of infection. Malaria can also cause hepatosplenomegaly. *Fasciola* Spurious infections often occur from ingesting infected (egg-containing) livers.

* Experimental

Echinococcus granulosus is a cestode common in sheep-raising areas where humans can act as intermediate hosts in the parasite's life cycle. The larval stage of the organism penetrates the intestinal wall, enters the circulation, and ends up in the liver. Within the liver tissue a hydatid cyst is formed. The infection is asymptomatic until the cyst becomes large. At that time, the cyst is like a space-occupying tumor, producing pressure necrosis of surrounding tissue. If leaks occur, a pronounced eosinophilia is produced. With rupture, anaphylaxis can occur.

Leishmania donovani complex is the agent of visceral leishmaniasis or kala-azar. The organism is endemic in many areas of Africa, India, Asia, Southern Europe, and South and Latin America, where it is transmitted to humans by the bite of the sandfly (*Phlebotomus*). The organism infects cells of the reticuloendothelial system, especially the liver and spleen, and often the bone marrow.

Respiratory Tract Disorders

The parasite that primarily infects the lungs of humans is the trematode *Paragonimus westermani.* Other parasites may appear in the lungs as a part of their life cycle, or may infect the lungs by accident (see Table 58-3).

Paragonimus westermani matures in the lungs. Humans become infected by ingesting metacercaria from the fluids of freshwater crabs, or crayfish in the U.S. The adult worms live near a bronchus in a cystlike structure, releasing their eggs into bronchi or bronchioles. The metabolites produced by the worms cause hemorrhages and leukocyte infiltration into the tissue surrounding the "cystic" structure. With time, tissue fibrosis occurs.

E. histolytica can infect the lungs if a liver abscess is adjacent to the diaphragm. The organisms can erode the diaphragm, and then invade the lung tissue by the mechanisms described above.

Strongyloides stercoralis is a nematode that resides in the gastrointestinal tract. Like other nematodes such as *Ascaris* and hookworm, it undergoes a lung migration in its larval stage. The larvae usually remain in the lungs, feeding and growing, for about 2 weeks. The metabolites produced by the larvae, especially in cases of reinfection, cause an allergic response in the host, and pneumonitis

Table 58-3 ***Respiratory Tract Disorders***

Clinical Manifestations	Etiologic Agents	Diagnostic Tests	Treatment	Comments
Inflammatory reaction in lung Cough, with or without blood-flecked sputum Shortness of breath Chronic bronchitis Pleurisy, with or without pleural effusion Pneumonia, right lower lobe	*Paragonimus* *Strongyloides* *Entamoeba histolytica*	*Microbiological* O and P (all) Duodenal aspirate Sputum examination *Serological* CF for *Paragonimus* or IIF and ID IHA, IIF, and ELISA for amebiasis IHA, IFF (an experimental test) for *Strongyloides*	*Paragonimus* Praziquantel or Bithional *Strongyloides* Thiabendazole *Amebiasis* Mexonidazole followed by iodoquinol (plus chloroquine if the source is a liver abscess)	*Strongyloides* Hyperinfection may cause serious tissue infection in immunocompromised hosts due to autoinfection. *E. histolytica* Extraintestinal infections often result in untreated intestinal infections. *Pneumocystis carinii* The parasite causes interstitial plasma cell pneumonia in immunocompromised children and adults. It is a common cause of infection in AIDS patients. (See Chaps. 10, 53, 61.)

may result. In an immunosuppressed patient, the larvae of *Strongyloides* often "flood" the alveolar spaces.

Nervous System Disorders

The most common parasite, endemic in the United States, causing nervous system disorders is *Toxoplasma.* The organism is ubiquitous in nature, and human immunity to this organism increases with age. There is only one species, *T. gondii,* and all strains appear to be antigenically similar. The forms of the parasite include tachyzoites, tissue cysts, and oocysts. The oocyst is produced only in the intestines of members of the cat family, and is the form that maintains the life cycle of *T. gondii.* Humans are exposed by contact with infected meat, soil, or litter boxes. Once within the host, the organism can infect any tissue of the body and can remain asymptomatic within the tissue for years. The latent nature of the infection can have serious consequences in persons who become immunosuppressed. If pregnant women without antibodies are exposed to Toxoplasma, the organisms can result in congenital infection of the fetus. Within the tissue, the organism causes focal areas of necrosis and cellular infiltrates, with calcification of the cysts in the retina and brain.

Naegleria, and more rarely *Acanthamoeba,* are free-living protozoa that can cause primary amebic meningoencephalitis. The onset of symptoms is short, and the course of infection is fulminant. A history of swimming and diving in warm, aerated water is consistent with the infection. Edema and hemorrhage are usual and extend into the gray matter. Death occurs within 2 to 5 days.

Cysticercosis is an infection caused by the larval stage of *Taenia solium.* The infection is rare in the United States but common in Latin America. When the egg hatches in the intestine the larval stage enters the circulation and has a predilection for human brain tissue. Within the tissue, the larvae form a fluid-filled bladder that acts upon tissue like a space-occupying lesion. These structures may be found in the ventricles, subarachnoid spaces, and parenchyma of the brain.

Strongyloides larvae may invade the central nervous tissue of immunosuppressed persons. Usually the invasion is a consequence of an undiagnosed intestinal infection.

Trypanosoma brucei (gambiense and *rhodesiense)* are hemoflagellates that are transmitted to humans by the bite of the tsetse fly (*Glossina*). The organisms are agents of a form of African sleeping sickness. The trypomastigote, the flagellated form of the organism, is found in the circulating blood, lymphatics, and lymph nodes, and within the spinal fluid. As the organisms multiply, hyperplasia of lymphoid tissue occurs. As the organisms invade the central nervous system, the antigen–antibody complexes cause a variety of physiological reactions, including kinin release and destruction of fibroblasts.

Trypanosoma cruzi, the South American hemoflagellate, can cause nervous system disorders in children.

(See Table 58-4.)

Heart Disorders

In the western hemisphere, a major cause of parasitic heart disorders is the hemoflagellate *T. cruzi.* The African trypanosomes can also cause some cardiac dysfunctions; however, the mechanism of pathogenesis is not known. Chagas's disease should be considered if the patient has a history of living or visiting in Central or South America, and has had contact with the reduviid (or "kissing") bug.

The reduviid bug usually bites humans at night, feeding at the corners of the mouth and eyes. An acute inflammatory reaction often occurs at the site of the bite, which can develop into the characteristic chagoma. The trypomastigote stage of the organism is found in the blood and lymphatics, where the flagellated form is carried throughout

Table 58-4 *Nervous System Disorders*

Clinical Manifestations	Etiologic Agents	Diagnostic Tests	Treatment	Comments
Headache and fever Drowsiness Meningoencephalitis Retinochoroiditis Hydrocephalus Seizures Disorientation and/or dementia Winterbottom's sign	*Naegleria fowleri* *Toxoplasma gondii* *Taenia solium (Cysticercus cellulosae)* *Trypanosoma brucei (gambiense)* *T. brucei (rhodesiense)* *T. Cruzi* *Strongyloides stercoralis*	*Microbiological* O and P (*Strongyloides* and *T. solium*) Duodenal aspirate (*Strongyloides*) Spinal fluid (*Strongyloides* and *Naegleria*) *Serological* IHA, IgG and IgM, IIF, ELISA, and FIAX (titer of ≥1:256 significant with IIF and ELISA) (*Toxoplasma*) IIF, IHA, and ELISA (trypanosomiasis) IHA and ELISA with limited success for cysticercosis *Other Tests* Radiography CT scans CSF analysis Serum protein increased (over 50 mg/dL) WBC increased (mainly neutrophils) IgM increased	*Naegleria* Amphotericin B *Toxoplasmosis* Pyrimethamine *plus* Trisulfapyrimidine *Cysticercosis* Praziquantel *Trypanosomiasis* Early stage: suramin CNS involvement: melarsoprol	*Naegleria* Infections have a sudden onset and run a fulminant course. *Toxoplasma* Can cause serious congenital infections leading to mental and motor retardation Cerebral disorders also may be caused by *Plasmodium falciparum* and *Schistosoma japonicum*

the body. The amastigote stage is the intracellular form that can multiply in any cell of the body. The organism, however, prefers cells of the reticuloendothelial system, striated muscle, and neuroglia cells. The organism produces pseudocysts in the heart. In the chronic stages of the disease, inflammation and fibrosis of the myocardium occur, with a marked cellular infiltrate. Heart-muscle loss occurs due to hypertrophy of the muscle layers. (See Table 58-5.)

Table 58-5 *Heart Disorders*

Clinical Manifestations	Etiologic Agents	Diagnostic Tests	Treatment	Comments
Myocarditis Tachycardia Fever Romaña's sign Abnormal EKG Megaesophagus and/or megacolon	*Trypanosoma cruzi* (South American trypanosomiasis, Chagas's disease)	*Microbiological* Giemsa-stained blood smears *Serological* CF (significant titer ≥1:8) RIA, IHA, and direct agglutination *Other Tests* EKG Biopsy of lymph nodes (touch prep procedure)	Nifurtimox	*T. cruzi* Can cause acute CNS infection in children

Vascular System Disorders

The primary parasitic infection implicated in disorders of the vascular system is malaria, which is considered by the World Health Organization to be the number one worldwide health problem.

Other parasitic infections that can cause vascular system disorders are filariasis, *Babesia, Diphyllobothrium,* and trypanosomiasis.

There are four malarial parasites that cause disease in humans: *Plasmodium vivax, P. malariae, P. falciparum,* and *P. ovale.* Each parasite begins its infectious stage in humans in the liver parenchymal cells, where the exoerythrocytic cycle may be short-lived or prolonged, depending on the species. If the organism maintains a resting stage within the liver, then relapses of the infection may occur.

Whatever the species, the basic pathophysiology is the same in the erythrocytic stage. During the erythrocytic cycle, the erythrocytes and/or the visceral capillaries become infected. As the organisms are released from the cells, both infected and noninfected erythrocytes are lysed. Plugging of the capillaries can cause ischemia in affected tissue.

Babesiosis is an infection transmitted to humans by ticks. The organism within the erythrocyte has a ringlike stage that resembles malaria. As in malaria, the rupturing of erythrocytes occurs. The infection in the U.S. occurs primarily in southern New England.

Filariasis is no longer endemic in the U.S. The infection has a wide distribution, however, in many tropical areas. *Wuchereria bancrofti, Brugia malayi,* and *Brugia timori* are the filariae most often implicated in vascular system disorders.[3] The adult worms live within the lymph nodes, releasing microfilariae into the circulation. The worms cause inflammatory reactions and fibrosis of the lymph node tissue; with time, disruption of the lymph flow can occur.

Diphyllobothrium latum is the fish tapeworm that can infect humans. It has been a problem in cool lake areas of the U.S.; however, with the control of raw sewage, the incidence of the infections has decreased around the Great Lakes area. The infection is asymptomatic in most people, although, in some, a deficiency of B_{12} occurs that resembles pernicious anemia.

Trypanosomiasis has been discussed above.

Table 58-6 ***Vascular System Disorders***

Clinical Manifestations	Etiologic Agents	Diagnostic Tests	Treatment	Comments
Paroxysm, with or without periodicity Hepatosplenomegaly Anemia Lymphadenitis and/or lymphangitis Hematuria B_{12} deficiency Disseminated intravascular coagulation (DIC)	*Plasmodium* *vivax* *ovale* *malariae* *falciparum* *Wuchereria bancrofti* *Brugia* *malayi* *timori* *Babesia microfti* *Trypanosoma*	*Microbiological* O and P (D. latum) Blood smears (malaria, filariae, *Babesia*, trypanosomiasis) *Serological* IHA, ELISA, IIF (titer of 1:64 is significant) (malaria) IIF, IHA, and ELISA (trypanosomiasis) IIF (*Babesia*) *Other Tests* Serum albumin transaminase (*Babesia*) Radiography (filariae) CBC Sedimentation rate	*Malaria* *Uncomplicated* Chloroquine phosphate *Uncomplicated, with resistant strain* Quinine sulfate *plus* Pyrimethamine *plus* Sulfadiazine *Severe illness* Quinine dihydrochloride *Relapses* Primaquine phosphate *Filariae* Diethylcarbamazine *Diphyllobothrium* Niclosamide *Trypanosoma* Suramin	*P. falciparum* Considered a medical emergency since it can cause cerebral disease and death Acute hemolysis often causes "Blackwater fever."

The organisms can and do cause changes in lymphoid tissue and in the reticuloendothelial tissue. (See Table 58-6.)

Skin and Mucous Membrane Disorders

Skin and mucous membrane disorders are seen more commonly in tropical climates than in temperate ones. Therefore, the parasites implicated in these types of disorders are, in general, not endemic in the United States. The exception is the agent of cutaneous larva migrans. (See Table 58-7.)

Leishmania tropica, a complex of organisms, is transmitted to humans via the bite of the sandfly (*Phlebotomus*). The infective stage is the promastigote, which becomes an amastigote upon entering humans. The amastigote infects the macrophages and endothelium of the vessels. As granulomas are formed around the infected foci, nodules are produced.

Leishmania braziliensis produces ulcers of the oral or nasal mucosa. Cutaneous tracts are also produced, which are larger than those of *L. tropica.* Often the lesions become secondarily infected with bacteria.

The filaria *Onchocerca volvulus* is transmitted to humans through the bite of the blackfly (*Simulium*). The adult worms, often in groups, become encapsulated in the subcutaneous tissues. Nod-

Table 58-7 ***Skin and Mucous Membrane Disorders***

Clinical Manifestations	Etiologic Agents	Diagnostic Tests	Treatment	Comments
Lesions, either dry or wet, on face or limbs Nodules on limbs, trunk, or head Serpiginous tunnels Lymphadenitis or "hanging groin"	*Leishmania tropica braziliensis mexicana* *Onchocerca volvulus* *Ancylostoma braziliense*	*Microbiological* Urine (*Onchocerca*) Touch preps (*Leishmania*) *Serological* DAgg (significant titer of 1:64) (*Leishmania*) IFA and ELISA (*Onchocerca*) *Other Tests* Biopsy (*Leishmania, Onchocerca*) Skin snip (*Onchocerca*) Urine examination for microfilariae	*Leishmaniasis* Stibogluconate sodium *Onchocerciasis* Diethylcarbamazaine *Cutaneous Larva Migrans* Thiabendazole	*Leishmania* Many of the lesions can leave disfiguring scars when infected with bacteria.

ules are formed due to the fibrous tissue produced by the allergic response of the host.

Ancylostoma braziliense, the agent of cutaneous larva migrans or "creeping eruption," is the hookworm of dogs. When humans become exposed to larvae from dog feces in soil, they can become infected. Because humans are not the normal host, the larvae become trapped in the subcutaneous tissue. As the larvae begin to migrate through the tissue, a severe reaction occurs to the worms and their metabolites. Often the tracts become secondarily infected with bacteria.

Urinary Tract Disorders

Infectious urinary tract disorders are caused most commonly by bacterial infections. There is only one parasite, *Schistosoma haematobium,* that has the urinary tract as an intrinsic part of its life cycle. (See Table 58-8.)

The adult worms of *S. haematobium* reside in the vesical plexus. As the eggs work their way into the urinary bladder from the bladder wall, they often cause an acute inflammatory reaction and hematuria. With time, granulomas may form around trapped eggs. Hyperplasia, fibrosis, and ulcerations of the tissue occur. Often carcinoma of the bladder is a result of chronic infection.[4] Obstruction of ureters occurs in some cases, causing damage to the upper urinary tract similar to that seen in other types of obstructive disease (see Chap. 16).

P. falciparum, as described above, causes an intravascular hemolysis that results in a hematuria known as "Blackwater fever."

Genital Tract Disorders

With the one exception of *Trichomonas,* parasites are not normal inhabitants of the genital tract. *Trichomonas* infections should be considered with any case of acute vaginitis. (See Table 58-9.)

Table 58-8 ***Urinary Tract Disorders***

Clinical Manifestations	Etiologic Agents	Diagnostic Tests	Treatment	Comments
Hematuria Proteinuria Nephrotic syndrome Renal failure	*Schistosoma haematobium* *Plasmodium falciparum*	*Microbiological* Urine centrifugation–sedimentation (*Schistosoma*) Stained blood smears (malaria) *Serological* IHA, ELISA, and IIF (malaria and schistosomiasis) *Other Tests* Hatching test Urine microscopic examination for eggs Biopsy of bladder wall	*S. haematobium* Praziquantel *P. falciparum* Chloroquine phosphate or Quinine sulfate *plus* Sulfadiazine *plus* Pyrimethamine or Quinine dihydrochloride	*S. haematobium* Often accompanied by carcinoma of bladder wall

Trichomonas vaginalis is a flagellate that inhabits the genital tract of some men and women. The infection in men is usually asymptomatic. The organism is transmitted mainly by sexual intercourse. When infected, the vaginal mucosa becomes highly irritated due to the metabolites of the organism, the tissue becomes hyperemic, and often lesions are produced. (See also Chap. 56.)

Enterobius vermicularis has been reported as a rare cause of vaginitis and salpingitis in young girls. The infections are the result of the female worms going astray during their migration phase.

Table 58-9 ***Genital Tract Disorders***

Clinical Manifestations	Etiologic Agents	Diagnostic Tests	Treatment	Comments
Vaginitis, with or without discharge Dysuria Salpingitis	*Trichomonas vaginalis* *Enterobius vermicularis* *Wuchereria bancrofti*	*Microbiological* Direct smear (*Trichomonas*) Scotch tape (*Enterobius*) Blood smear (*Filariae*)	*Trichomoniasis* Metronidazole *Enterobiasis* Pyrantel pamoate *Wuchereria* Diethylcarbamazine	*Trichomonas* The most common parasitic cause of genital tract disorders *Enterobius* and *Wuchereria* The rarest causes of genital infections

Wuchereria bancrofti in endemic areas is a cause of elephantiasis of the scrotum. The consequences of lymphadenitis and fibrosis of the lymphatics occurs in only a small portion of the endemic population.

CLINICAL MANIFESTATIONS

Patients with parasitic infections of the gastrointestinal tract may present with one or more of the following symptoms: diarrhea, with or without blood or mucus; abdominal pain and cramping; flatulence; anorexia; chronic fatigue; steatorrhea; malabsorption syndrome; intestinal obstruction; and passage of worm in stool, or occasionally from the nose or mouth.

Within the hepatobiliary system, clinical manifestations of parasitic infection include hepatitis, with or without jaundice, often with fever and diarrhea; hepatomegaly, with or without tenderness; referred pain, often to right scapula; abscesses with elevation and fixation of right diaphragm; cirrhosis with accompanying ascites, splenomegaly, and portal hypertension; space-occupying lesions of the liver; biliary obstruction with cholecystitis; and hepatosplenomegaly.

Clinical manifestations of parasitic infection of the respiratory tract include inflammatory reaction in the lung; cough, with or without blood-flecked sputum; shortness of breath; chronic bronchitis; pleurisy, with or without pleural effusion; and right lower lobe pneumonia.

Patients with parasitic infections affecting the nervous system present with one or more of the following: headache and fever; drowsiness; meningoencephalitis; retinochoroiditis; hydrocephalus; seizures; disorientation and/or dementia; and in Gambian sleeping sickness, Winterbottom's sign (swelling of posterior cervical lymph nodes).

Manifestations of parasitic heart disorders include myocarditis; tachycardia; fever; unilateral edema of the eyelid (Romaña's sign); abnormal EKG; and megaesophagus and/or megacolon.

The effects of parasitic infection of the vascular system include paroxysm (sudden onset of shaking chills followed by a period of fever and sweating), with or without periodicity; hepatosplenomegaly; anemia; disseminated intravascular coagulation; lymphadenitis and/or lymphangitis; and B_{12} deficiency.

Clinical manifestations of parasitic skin disorders include lesions, either dry or wet, on the face or limbs and nodules on the trunk, limbs, or head. Serpiginous tunnels formed by creeping tracks made by larvae are a feature of "creeping eruption." All of these lesions often become secondarily infected by bacteria. "Hanging groin" due to lymphadenitis may also occur.

With *S. haematobium* infection of the urinary tract, hematuria and proteinuria are prominent findings. An associated nephrotic syndrome sometimes occurs and, with progressive obstruction, renal failure ensues.

Trichomonas infections are characterized by vaginitis, with or without discharge. Dysuria may occur. Vaginitis and salpingitis are associated with *E. vermicularis* when it rarely invades the genital tract.

LABORATORY ANALYSES AND DIAGNOSIS

An examination of stool for ova and protozoa (O and P) should be performed when parasitic infection of the gastrointestinal tract is suspected. A concentration procedure and permanent-stained smear on three stool specimens collected 2 to 3 days apart are the minimum procedures recommended for meaningful results. If the stool results remain negative while the index of suspicion of infection is high, a purged specimen should be collected.[5] Oil or magnesium laxatives and barium enema interfere with the examination of stool for parasites. Because it takes ten days to 2 weeks for barium to clear from the intestinal tract, it is important that stool samples for laboratory evaluation be collected before such substances are administered to the patient. Collection should also be delayed if the patient has received antibiotics, antimalarial drugs, or antidiarrheal medications.[6]

Due to the nature of *Giardia* infections, the

organisms often appear in the stool in "showers," and therefore can be missed with stool examinations alone. Examination of wet preparation or permanent-stained smears of duodenal material is often helpful.

Serological tests are helpful only in the case of extraintestinal infections of *E. histolytica.* Other tests such as radiographic studies may be useful in cases of amebiasis and ascariasis. Sigmoidoscopic biopsy may prove useful with intestinal and extraintestinal amebiasis, while intestinal mucosal biopsy with routine histological studies may be helpful with *Giardia* and *Cryptosporidium* infections.

When the hepatobiliary system is affected, examinations of stool for O and P should be ordered as described above. If trematodes are suspected, the zinc flotation procedure should be avoided because the ova of *Schistosoma, Clonorchis,* and *Fasciola* do not float well in the preparation.

When leishmaniasis is suspected, blood, bone marrow, liver, and spleen biopsy material can be stained and examined for presence of the intracellular organism. If the preparations are negative, the material can be cultured on a diphasic blood medium that will enhance the development of flagellar stages.

Because many of the parasites causing hepatobiliary disease actually invade tissue, they are able to produce serological responses in humans (see Table 58-2). *Toxocara* infection is a clinical diagnosis; however, the primary means of confirming the diagnosis is through serological methods because the life cycle is not completed in humans and no adult worms appear in the intestinal tract. The indirect immunofluorescence (IFA) or enzyme-linked immunosorbent assay (ELISA) tests for both IgG and IgM antibodies are the methods of choice. An ELISA diagnostic titer is considered to be ≥1:32.

Extraintestinal amebiasis is detected fairly well using serology. Some procedures used are the gel diffusion precipitation test (GDP), the indirect fluorescent antibody test (IFA), and the indirect hemagglutination test (IHA).[7] The IHA method is the most sensitive, with 90% to 100% of the positive cases giving a titer ≥1:128.[8] A significant IHA titer is considered to be ≥1:256.

Several serological methods are available for the diagnosis of trematode infections. The complement fixation (CF) test, indirect hemagglutination (IHA), indirect immunofluorescence (IIF), and ELISA procedures can be used for schistosomiasis. Both the CF and IHA tests are useful in the diagnosis of fascioliasis and clonorchiasis.

Hydatid disease can be diagnosed quite readily using serology. The tests of choice are IHA, latex agglutination (LA), and immunoelectrophoresis. With the IHA method, a titer ≥1:256 is diagnostically significant.

Visceral leishmaniasis can be diagnosed using the FA and ELISA procedures. The IHA is not species-specific, however.

The patient with a hepatobiliary disorder usually has an enlarged and tender liver, an elevated temperature, and leukocytosis. Leukocytosis with an increased eosinophilia is highly suggestive of a parasitic infection. For example, eosinophils are the predominant cell type seen in *Toxocara* infections. If the WBC is less than $4.0 \times 10^3/mm^3$ with a predominance of monocytes, leishmaniasis should be suspected. There is usually an elevation in total serum protein of 10 g/dL (100 g/L). Urine urobilinogen and bilirubin are excellent screening tests for hepatobiliary disorders because any increase over normal values is significant.

Other tests that may be helpful in establishing a diagnosis are listed in Table 58-2. Gallium scan and ultrasonography may be useful in the detection of extraintestinal amebiasis. Examination of biopsy material may help in the diagnosis of visceral larva migrans (liver nodules) and schistosomiasis (rectal biopsy).[9]

Hatching tests for *S. mansoni* are helpful in detecting mild or light infections, and in determining the viability of eggs recovered in the stool specimen. Intradermal tests may be useful in screening for schistosomiasis and *E. granulosus* (Casoni skin test).

Laboratory analyses most useful in parasitic infections of the respiratory tract include an O and

P examination of feces for *Strongyloides* larvae, *E. histolytica* trophozoites and/or cysts, and for *Paragonimus* ova. Duodenal aspirates, in addition, could be helpful in the case of *S. stercoralis* infection. Examination of sputum may be useful in detecting *Strongyloides* in immunosuppressed patients, and in cases of *Paragonimus.* If a lung abscess due to *E. histolytica* is suspected, aspirate material may be cultured.

The complement fixation test is at present the serological method of choice for *Paragonimus* infections. A titer of ≥1:8 is considered diagnostic. The indirect immunofluorescent (IIF) and immunodiffusion (ID) tests are experimental tests, and therefore are not commercially available.

If helminths are suspected in a nervous system disorder, a stool specimen for O and P examination should be ordered (see Table 58-4). Giemsa-stained smears of blood, lymph node aspirate material, and spinal fluid should be examined if trypanosomiasis is suspected.

Spinal fluid examination is also recommended for disseminated *Strongyloides* infection. In cases of primary amebic meningitis (PAM), spinal fluid is often purulent, with more than 20×10^3 white cells per cubic mm. Neutrophils are the predominant cell type, and the protein may be slightly elevated.

Serology is the method of choice for the diagnosis of toxoplasmosis. Several methods are available, such as IHA, IIF, ELISA, and the fluoroimmunoassay (FIAX). A titer of 1:256 is significant with both the IIF and the FIAX tests.

Serological tests are often negative in central nervous system (CNS) infections, although the IHA and ELISA methods are available for the diagnosis of cysticercosis.

African trypanosomiasis can be diagnosed using IIF, IHA, and ELISA tests, while radiography and CT scans are helpful in the differential diagnosis of CNS infections.

The laboratory detection of *T. cruzi* is often by means of Giemsa-stained blood smears. They should be examined for the presence of the trypomastigote. Serology is helpful in the diagnosis of the disease—mainly the complement fixation test (CF) (see Table 58-5). A significant CF titer is 1 : 8. A specialized CF test available for *T. cruzi* infection, the Machado test, is used mainly in endemic areas.[10] RIA, IHA, and direct agglutination tests are other sensitive methods used in the diagnosis of Chagas's disease. Electrocardiogram and biopsy of lymph nodes can also be useful tests in the differential diagnosis of the disease.

Thick and thin blood smears stained with Giemsa or Wright's stain should be examined for malaria, *Babesia, Trypanosoma,* and filariae infections. If the blood smears are negative, new smears should be made every 6 to 12 hours for a period of 2 to 3 days. Negative smears may be due to suppressive therapy.

Serology is not useful in the diagnosis of acute malaria, but the IIF test can be used in the case of a longstanding infection. A titer of 1:64 is diagnostic (see Table 58-6). The IHA and ELISA procedures are also used. An IIF test is available for *Babesia.* Serology results for trypanosomiasis vary. The IIF and ELISA procedures may be of help in the diagnosis; however, false-negative results do occur. In evaluating the patient with vascular system disorders, WBC, RBC, platelet counts, and sedimentation rate are useful. In malaria, the patient has a normocytic anemia, increased sedimentation rate, and decreased platelet count. The serum albumin and transaminases in *Babesia* are increased. Lymphangiography can be helpful in filariasis.

In the diagnosis of skin disorders due to parasites, stained touch preparations of biopsy material from the edge of lesions should be examined for the presence of the amastigote of *L. tropica* (see Table 58-7). If the smears remain negative, culturing the buffy coat from the patient's blood specimen is often helpful.

Examination of urine for the presence of the microfilariae of *O. volvulus* may be useful, especially after the patient has received an oral dose of diethylcarbamazine.

Serology may be helpful in the diagnosis of leishmaniasis. A direct agglutination titer of ≥1 : 64 is considered significant. *Onchocerca* infections can be diagnosed using IFA and ELISA methods. The examination of skin-snip material for microfilariae is the definitive method of diagnosis.

The examination of urine sediment for the eggs of *S. haematobium* is the definitive method for its diagnosis (see Table 58-8). Giemsa-stained blood smears should be examined as described above if *P. falciparum* is suspected.

Serological tests as described above are available for the diagnosis of malaria and schistosomiasis. In the case of *S. haematobium,* other useful tests include urinalysis for the presence of blood and protein in urine, examination of biopsy material from the bladder wall, and a hatching test to detect the presence of eggs in the urine.

A wet preparation of vaginal material should be examined for the presence of *Trichomonas* (see also Chap. 56). If a pinworm infection is suspected, a Scotch tape preparation or a swube (a sticky paddle in a tube) should be examined. The specimen should be collected in the morning before the patient has gone to the bathroom, bathed, or dressed.

The serological tests of choice for *Trichomonas* infections are IHA and gel diffusion.[10]

TREATMENT

Treatment for parasitic infections of the GI tract is quite varied, as is shown in Table 58-3. *E. histolytica* infections are treated according to the clinical picture. In the case of asymptomatic disease, the drug of choice is iodoquinol, with metronidazole (Flagyl) the alternative choice. Because Flagyl has a prophylactic effect against the spread to extraintestinal sites, it is preferred by some physicians. In mild to moderate and severe intestinal disease, the treatment of choice is Flagyl *plus* iodoquinol. To guard against the development of resistant strains, some authorities have suggested the addition of chloroquine to the treatment regimen. When amebiasis is suspected by the physician, corticosteroids and immunosuppressive drugs should be avoided because they can lead to severe invasive infections.

For infections with *G. lamblia,* the drug of choice is quinacrine hydrochloride; Flagyl is the alternative choice, especially for children, because it is less toxic.

Cryptosporidiosis is a self-limited infection in the immunocompetent host. If treatment should be deemed necessary, however, Spiramycin has been found effective.

Infections with *Ascaris lumbricoides* are treated with mebendazole (Vermox). Alternative choices are pyrantel pamoate (Antiminth) or piperazine citrate. If *Ascaris* is present in a mixed infection, it is important that the *Ascaris* should be treated first. Otherwise, some drugs may disturb the adult worms and bring about abnormal migrations.

Followup stool examinations 2 to 4 weeks post-treatment are important to the successful management of gastrointestinal disorders due to infections with intestinal parasites.

Treatment for infections of the hepatobiliary system and respiratory tract is outlined in Tables 58-2 and 58-3.

Treatment for nervous system disorders is varied. For example, for *Naegleria* infections, which have been almost uniformly fatal, only amphotericin B has shown any success. The recommended treatment for toxoplasmosis is pyrimethamine plus a trisulfapyrimidine. For cysticercosis, treatment is praziquantel and/or surgery. In the early stages of African trypanosomiasis when the organism is in the blood and lymphatic tracts, the drug of choice is suramin; with CNS involvement it is melarsoprol (Arsobae).

The treatment of choice for South American trypanosomiasis is Nifurtimox (Lampit), which is available through the Centers for Disease Control.

The treatment for malaria is based on the severity of the illness and whether resistant strains are the causative agent. For treating liver stages of *P. vivax* and *P. ovale,* the drug of choice is primaquine phosphate. For filariae, the drug of choice is diethylcarbamazine; for *Babesia,* the drug of choice is niclosamide; and for trypanosomiasis, the drug of choice for the blood and lymph stages is suramin.

The drug of choice for leishmaniasis is stibogluconate sodium. Onchocerciasis is treated with diethylcarbamazine. Cutaneous larva migrans is treated with thiabendazole.

Treatment for skin and mucous membrane and urinary tract infections is outlined in Tables 58-7 and 58-8.

CASE STUDY #1

A 35-year-old white man visited the dermatology clinic for evaluation of a lesion on his left cheek. He was an agricultural missionary in Colombia, South America, home on leave. The facial lesion has been enlarging in size progressively over a 3-month period. The examination showed a 3-cm ulcerated lesion with a scaly base. Small lesions were also present in a linear arrangement on his left arm. The lymph nodes in the left axilla were enlarged.

The laboratory workup showed a leukopenia ($3.0 \times 10^3/mm^3$) with lymphocytes and monocytes as the predominant cell types. Other test results included a total serum protein of 11.5 g/dL (115 g/L) with an increase in IgG levels; an alanine aminotransferase of 120 U/L; a total bilirubin of 5.0 mg/dL (85.8 μmol/L), and an alkaline phosphatase of 198 U/L. Examination of peripheral blood smears and bone marrow aspirates showed 10% to 15% eosinophilia.

Questions

1. What is/are the possible diagnoses, given this patient's history and laboratory findings?
2. What additional tests would you recommend?
3. What tests are the most nearly diagnostic, and why?

Discussion

1. The possible differential diagnoses could be leishmaniasis first, sporotrichosis, mycetoma, and cutaneous manifestations of a number of bacterial infections.
2. A serology workup should be performed, plus histological examination of biopsy material.
3. The most nearly diagnostic test for leishmaniasis would be the biopsy because the definitive method is finding the amastigotes within the macrophages. The direct agglutination test is very sensitive; however, cross-reactions do occur.

Laboratory and Therapeutic Followup

The serological workup gave a direct agglutination titer of 1 : 2048 to *Leishmania donovani* antigen and 1 : 512 to *L. tropica.* No agglutination occurred with *L. braziliensis* antigen. A biopsy specimen from the edge of the lesion contained organisms consistent with *Leishmania* species. The specimen also showed evidence of an inflammatory infiltrate, with many of the macrophages containing amastigotes of *Leishmania.* The patient was treated with stibogluconate sodium over a seven-week period. His response to therapy was dramatic. By the tenth day of treatment, the facial lesion had healed and the arm lesions were nonpalpable.

CASE STUDY #2

A 22-year-old woman was seen in the emergency room with shaking chills, nausea, vomiting, and diarrhea. While being treated, her chills subsided and she began to have a fever, which quickly reached 104°F (40°C). Laboratory analyses showed a leukocytosis, a decreased platelet count, an increased sedimentation rate, an alanine aminotransferase of 65 U/L, an aspartate aminotransferase of 42 U/L, and a lactate dehydrogenase of 340 U/L. The young woman had recently spent her vacation touring Southeast Asia.

After admission to the hospital, the patient experienced a profuse sweating episode, after which she slept normally. Blood was drawn when she awakened, and the findings included a slight leukopenia, an increased sedimentation rate, and decreased liver function test results.

Questions

1. What is/are the possible diagnoses?
2. What additional tests would you recommend?

3. What tests are the most nearly diagnostic, and why?

Discussion

1. The possible differential diagnoses could be malaria, kala-azar, typhoid, and hepatitis. Nausea, vomiting, diarrhea, chills, and fever are symptomatic of these diseases.

2. Additional tests that should be ordered include thick and thin blood smears, stool culture, and a serological test.

3. The most nearly diagnostic test, given the patient's symptoms, would be examination of Giemsa- (or Wright's)-stained blood smears. Because the patient had experienced a paroxysm with subsequent return to normal of her liver function test, malaria should be suspected.

Laboratory and Therapeutic Followup

The hematology lab reported many red cells of normal size infected with the trophozoites of *Plasmodium.* Due to the cell morphology, number of cells infected, and presence of "ring" stages only, the diagnosis of *P. falciparum* was made. Because such infections can produce severe intravascular hemolysis and disseminated intravascular coagulation (DIC), treatment was begun immediately. The patient was treated with oral quinine sulfate, and responded favorably.

REFERENCES

1. Guerrant RL: Gastrointestinal infections and food poisoning: Principles and definition of syndromes. In Mandell GL, Douglas RG, Bennett JE (eds): Principles and Practice of Infectious Diseases, 2nd ed, p 636. New York City, John Wiley & Sons, 1985
2. Flavell DJ: Liver-fluke infection as an aetiological factor in bile duct carcinoma of man. Trans R Soc Trop Med Hyg 75:814–824, 1981
3. Mahmoud AAF: Trematodes (Schistosomiasis, other flukes). In Mandell GL, Douglas RG, Bennett JE (eds): Principles and Practice of Infectious Diseases, 2nd ed, p 1575. New York City, John Wiley & Sons, 1985
4. Mathews HM, Healy GR: Evaluation of two serological tests for *Trichomonas vaginalis* infection. J Clin Microbiol 17:840–843, 1983
5. Reisberg B: Amebiasis and Giardiasis. In Youmans GP, Paterson PY, Sommers HH (eds): The Biologic and Clinical Basis of Infectious Diseases, p 532. Philadelphia, WB Saunders, 1985
6. Goldsmith RS: Infectious diseases. In Krupp MA, Chatton MJ, Tierney LM Jr (eds): Current Medical Diagnosis and Treatment 1986, p 905. Los Altos, California, Lange Medical Publications, 1986
7. Patterson M et al: Serologic testing for amoebiasis. Gastroenterology 78:136–141, 1980
8. Rusberg B: Amebiasis and giardiasis. In Youmans GP, Paterson PY, Sommers HM (eds): The Biologic and Clinical Basis of Infectious Diseases, p 532. Philadelphia, WB Saunders, 1985
9. Marsden PD: Other nematodes. Clin Gastroenterol 7:219–229, 1978
10. Markell EK, Voge M, John DT: Intradermal tests and serologic methods. In Markell EK, Voge M, John DM: Medical Parasitology, 6th ed, p 361. Philadelphia, WB Saunders, 1986

Chapter 59

Septic Shock

Patricia Collins

Septic shock may be defined as a state of impaired cellular function and altered hemodynamics that develops secondary to sepsis. It is a very serious clinical entity in which the mortality rate is substantial, although it can be reduced by early diagnosis. The progression from one stage to another is influenced not only by early recognition but also by appropriate antibiotic therapy, careful monitoring, prompt removal of any septic foci, and supportive treatments. Septic shock has a mortality rate of approximately 40%, which has not decreased significantly over the years.[1, 2] The number of deaths attributed to septic shock is reported to be more than 100,000 annually.[3]

Although the appearance of septic shock is a medical emergency, patients are rarely admitted to the hospital with this diagnosis but rather develop the condition during a hospital stay. Treatment of sepsis may not be satisfactory if the origin of infection is not identified and cultured.

ETIOLOGY AND PATHOPHYSIOLOGY

The number of etiologic agents responsible for septic shock is diverse. Gram-positive bacteria such as *Staphylococcus aureus* and *Streptococcus pyogenes* are capable of producing shock, but the majority of cases of bacteremic shock are due to gram-negative bacilli. Organisms implicated include members of the Enterobacteriaceae such as *Escherichia coli, Enterobacter aerogenes,* and *Serratia marcescens. Enterobacter sakazakii*[4] and other more recently identified microorganisms have been implicated, as well as *Pseudomonas aeruginosa.* Viruses, fungi, and rickettsiae may also be involved in a small number of cases.

Historically it was thought that there was little similarity in the clinical pictures of gram-positive and gram-negative septic shock.[5] Research, however, has revealed that the response of the host to sepsis is independent of the type of invading microorganism, but rather depends on several host-related factors.[6] One important factor is how the individual acquires septicemia. Epidemiologically, the bacteria may invade the blood stream by endogenous means, for example, through a urinary tract infection or by trauma involving the biliary, gastrointestinal, or genital tract. It has been reported that 58% of all cases of septic shock originate in the urinary tract, followed by biliary tract at 17% and the gastrointestinal tract at 12%.[7] Catheterization, bronchoscopy, inhalation equipment, intravenous equipment, and surgical intervention are some examples of exogenous sources of the invading bacteria. A breakdown of skin integrity seen with burns, ulcers, fistulas, or abscesses may also be a source of infection. Another contributing factor to host response is the presence of immunosuppressive therapy, with subsequent decreased antibody formation and impaired granulocytic and lymphocytic activity. A number of underlying diseases that may also affect the host's ability to respond to bacterial invasion are listed at the top of the right hand column. Another host-related factor that may play a part in the picture of septic shock is the age of the patient. Infants younger than a year old and adults older than 65 years are at the greatest risk due to immature or impaired cellular and humoral immunity.

The stimulus that triggers the chain of events leading to septic shock is the subject of much controversy. Most patients who develop shock secondary to sepsis have underlying conditions with their own hemodynamic effects. These may profoundly affect cardiovascular and other responses to sepsis.

Nevertheless, host responses are initiated immediately following the invasion of the organism and are affected by the condition of the host as described above. The onset of sepsis apparently initiates defects in normal metabolism. One of the earliest metabolic defects seen is abnormal glucose metabolism. Glucose intolerance with hyperglycemia stimulated by the release of catecholamines has been noted in approximately 40% of patients with sepsis. Fat metabolism is also altered with the release of free fatty acids and a decreased ability of the body to use long-chain free fatty acids as an energy source. As the septic process progresses, protein becomes unavailable as an energy source.

Underlying Disease States

Chronic renal disease
Cirrhosis or liver disease
Coronary disease
Diabetes mellitus
Leukemia
Malnutrition
Metastatic carcinoma

Other changes occur related to the entrance of the bacterium into the blood stream. The complement system is activated by the alternate pathway, either by the lipopolysaccharide portion of the bacterium, by immune complexes, or by the surfaces of the invading organism itself. Attention has focused on the role of the lipid A core of the lipopolysaccharide (LPS), a major component of the outer membrane of gram-negative bacteria, as a trigger mechanism. Although complement activation is vital to the normal host defense mechanism, the release of C3a and C5a in the process has some adverse effects. C3a provokes release of vasodilators, which enhance contraction of smooth muscle and increase capillary permeability. These vasodilators are histamine, prostaglandins, bradykinin, and serotonin from mast cells and basophils. While C5a mobilizes and directs the migration of leukocytes, it also stimulates neutrophil aggregation, which in turn leads to tissue ischemia through the formation of microemboli. C5a is also active in endothelial cell destruction, which leads to peripheral vascular injury.

The initial directed migration of polymorphonuclear leukocytes (PMNs) to an inflammatory site requires adherence to the endothelium and diapedesis through the cell wall. The enhanced adherence observed in septic shock and subsequent degranulation of phagocytes may contribute to the toxic shock syndrome by promoting the release of enzymes into the vascular space, producing endothelial damage.[1, 8]

Traditionally, the progression of hemodynamic changes has been linked to high and low cardiac output phases. In early sepsis, a high cardiac output or hyperdynamic state is seen. It is characterized by an increased heart rate and increases in cardiac index, myocardial contractility, and oxygen consumption. The release of histamine by the mast cells contributes to vasodilation, affecting both the arterial and the venous circulation. Vasodilation in turn contributes to the reduction of systemic vascular resistance and subsequent lowering of the blood pressure. Hypotension activates compensatory mechanisms to increase cardiac output in an attempt to maintain the blood pressure. Also associated with the decrease in systemic vascular resistance in experimental animal models is the release of prostaglandins.[3] Whether there is a similar effect in humans has yet to be determined. If so, treatment in this early stage with aspirin and indomethacin may improve survival, as it has done in the animal model. Some persons have postulated that the release of leukocyte endogenous mediator (LEM), endogenous pyrogen (EP), or lymphocyte-activating factor (LAF) contributes to endorphin release, which may play a part in myocardial depression and hypotension.[9]

With the heart and lungs working hard to keep up with the increased need for oxygen, stimulated by the invading organism, there is arteriovenous shunting, with a narrowing of the difference between arterial and venous oxygen content. This lowers the PaO_2 and the amount of oxygen in circulation. Anoxia occurs in selective capillary beds with capillary leakage of fluid into interstitial spaces, and less venous return is seen. Hypovolemia results in metabolic acidosis, disseminated intravascular coagulation (DIC), and respiratory acidosis. Profound hypotension occurs, despite a normal or increased cardiac output. Vasoconstriction in the pulmonary and renal areas causes hyperventilation and decreased urine output.

The late hypodynamic stage of septic shock includes low cardiac output, high systemic vascular resistance, and reduced oxygen consumption. Patients with preexisting cardiac disease progress rapidly to this stage. Increased anaerobic metabolism increases metabolic acidosis and hypovolemia. Acute respiratory distress syndrome (ARDS) leads to respiratory failure, and vasoconstriction gives way to vasodilation followed by circulatory collapse.

Some authorities suggest that following the course of cardiac output by measuring the cardiac index may not accurately determine the patient's status.[3] New technology that enables measurement of the left ventricular ejection fraction (EF) and wall motion abnormalities using radionuclide imaging is a much more accurate predictor of the patient's progress. These studies should be performed in conjunction with right-sided heart catheterization and thermodilution cardiac outputs. Cardiac index, left cardiac work index, oxygen delivery, and oxygen consumption have been measured to define physiological patterns associated with outcome in septic shock patients. The results suggest that patterns of survival may be determined in critically ill septic patients before the hypotensive phase of shock.[10]

CLINICAL MANIFESTATIONS

The development of septic shock occurs in an orderly progression, and early recognition enhances chances for survival. Initially there is a hyperdynamic stage or warm, pink shock, followed by the normodynamic stage or cool shock. The third and last stage is the hypodynamic stage or cold shock.

The first clinical sign is usually mental confusion, haziness, or inappropriate behavior and delayed response stimuli. This may not be noticeable in some elderly patients who may be suffering from loss of memory, confusion, or an underlying condition that evokes these symptoms. Fever is usually present as the body temperature rises to 101° F or above in response to the invading microorganism. Shaking chills and sweating may occur. Because of the requirements for increased oxygen, tachycardia and hyperventilation, with respirations greater than 20, are seen. At this point cardiac output is adequate, so the skin is warm and dry and may be flushed due to peripheral vasodilatation. Blood pressure and urine output are normal.

As shock progresses, respiratory acidosis becomes evident with a decrease in blood *p*H. Respiration becomes shallow. In response to bacterial endotoxins or LPS, the fluid going to capillary beds is trapped, resulting in decreased return flow of blood through the veins. Hypotension results as the systolic blood pressure begins to fall below 90 mm Hg. As the capillary fluid leaks into the interstitial spaces, urine volume begins to decrease. The patient may become disoriented and combative, and may exhibit thirst. Tachycardia continues, with a heart rate of 100–150.

As classical signs of shock begin to appear, cardiac output is decreased and arterial blood pressure is reduced to below 80 mm Hg. As the latter decreases, an imbalance between the oxygen delivered by the heart and the oxygen required by the heart is created, resulting in further impairment of cardiac output. The continuing decrease in blood pressure enhances the activities of the sympathetic nervous system, with the subsequent release of catecholamines. Catecholamines attempt to raise the blood pressure through vasoconstriction of the peripheral, renal, and gastrointestinal circulations. This results in the cold, clammy skin phenomenon seen with an advanced shock state. Bacterial endotoxins and cellular enzymes increase anaerobic metabolism and increase metabolic acidoses, with the final result being circulatory collapse. The pulse becomes rapid, weak, and thready. Unexplained petechiae and jaundice are features that may be present in this stage. Small emboli released from leaking capillaries may result from disseminated intravascular coagulation (DIC). Pulmonary congestion is manifested by shortness of breath, rales, and wheezes. The level of consciousness continues to deteriorate and, unless responsive to treatment, the patient expires.

LABORATORY ANALYSES AND DIAGNOSIS

The importance of laboratory support in the diagnosis and monitoring of septic shock cannot be overemphasized. Once the cascade of septic shock has begun, it will continue unless treatment and supportive measures are instituted. Often clinical signs are not recognized until the patient enters the hypodynamic or cold stage of shock, when chances of recovery are greatly diminished. Laboratory data can alert the clinician to earlier stages of the syndrome.

Patients who are at risk should be monitored for possible complications during their hospital stay, because timely detection of bacteria or fungi in the blood stream remains vital in preventing septic shock. The rapid fulminant nature of septicemia makes initiation of antibiotic treatment essential for survival. Although not all patients who have bacteremia or septicemia go into septic shock, septic patients whose resistance is lowered by underlying disease, immunosuppressive agents, or age require prompt, specific antibiotic therapy in order to reduce the probability of complications and enhance chances for a more favorable outcome. Blood cultures should be performed routinely on patients who are at high risk, as well as on those individuals who have an altered level of consciousness and/or fever. Although fever is a classical response to the entrance of microorganisms into the blood, occasionally a subnormal temperature may occur instead.[9]

The clinical pattern of bacteremia can be transient, intermittent, or continuous. Transient bacteremia is usually associated with manipulation of infected tissues, instrumentation involving microbial colonized tissues (*e.g.*, dental procedures), or surgery (*e.g.*, transurethral resection of the prostate). Intermittent bacteremia is associated with undrained abscesses, and continuous bacteremia is a feature of acute and subacute endocarditis or is a complication of the use of intravenous catheters.[11] For these reasons, the number and timing of blood cultures as well as the interpretation of a positive culture should be considered in light of clinical findings. For adults, the collection of two to three separate blood culture samples, approximately 60 minutes apart, with a minimum of ten mL of blood or a 1:10 blood/ broth ratio is recommended (see Chap. 61). Studies have shown, however, that collection of samples larger than ten mL will increase the number of bacteremias detected.[1, 12]

In many instances, it is impossible to obtain a culture prior to the initiation of antibiotics; however, technology developed in recent years enables the removal of most of the commonly used antibiotics, using resins or physical separation methods.[13]

Because of the time required for detection of growth in most blood culture systems and the fact that some microorganisms lack the ability to grow in the culture media commonly used, noncultural methods are being developed. Flow cytometry, limulus assay for endotoxin, DNA hybridization, radioimmune assay (RIA), enzyme-linked immune assay (ELISA), gas liquid chromatography, and antigen detection procedures are being investigated, refined, and developed for possible use in the clinical laboratory. The last two have limited use currently in some laboratories as an adjunct to cultural procedures.[1] Antimicrobial susceptibility testing of the isolates is important, and can be performed either by dilution methods or by agar diffusion tests (see Chap. 63).

During the early or warm phase of shock, it is necessary to monitor blood gases when cellular oxygen delivery and/or utilization decreases. Arterial blood gases begin to reflect respiratory and metabolic acidosis as well as hypoxemia. The $PaCO_2$ rises above 48 mm Hg in a male or 45 mm Hg in a female (sea level values). If there is normal lung function, the depth of respiration maintains a $PaCO_2$ level that serves to maintain the normal blood *p*H around 7.40. In early sepsis, the blood *p*H begins to fall below 7.35. A decrease in the $PaCO_2$ in the arterial blood results in an attempt to compensate by increasing both cardiac output and blood pressure. The latter subsequently falls, resulting in clinically noticeable hypotension. In later stages of shock, when metabolic acidosis increases, the *p*H continues to fall, $PaCO_2$ decreases, and PaO_2 becomes normal. Other conditions that may alter blood gas exchange include diabetes, pulmonary disorders, carcinoma, sarcoidosis, and congestive heart failure. The hypoxemia may become more severe in the latter stages of septic shock despite oxygen administration. If this occurs, the prognosis is poor.

Due to abnormalities in the microcirculation and increased platelet adhesiveness, disseminated intravascular coagulation (DIC) may occur. Normally this process is held in check by naturally-occurring inhibitors. However, vascular changes may override the ability of these inhibitors to control hemostasis. Early laboratory findings include (1) thrombocytopenia, (2) decreased fibrinogen, (3) decreased clotting factors, and (4) increased degradation products. These products are formed as a result of the fibrinolytic system being activated. In suspected DIC, Sirridge recommends the tests listed below.[14]

Thrombocytopenia is primarily associated with bleeding problems, but may also be caused by a lack of production in the bone marrow or destruction due to infectious agents and drugs. Direct

Initial Screening Tests for Disseminated Intravascular Coagulation

Activated partial thromboplastin time
Fibrin degradation product tests
Fibrinogen concentration
Paracoagulation tests
Platelet count
Prothrombin time
Thrombin time

counts of platelets rather than estimation of platelets are usually done. Laboratory values of coagulation tests vary, depending upon the condition of the patient and the stage of the disease. Results may change by the hour as the situation gets worse or improves. The activated partial thromboplastin time (APTT), prothrombin time (PT), and thrombin time (TT) are all ways to measure the speed by which clotting occurs. A shortened APTT, increased TT, and normal to slightly prolonged PT suggest DIC. All three tests are usually prolonged in severe disease. Decreases in other coagulation factors are often seen in late DIC. Thrombin time may be prolonged because of decreased fibrinogen or increased fibrin degradation products. Fibrinogen levels decrease as the severity of the disease increases.

Leukopenia is a characteristic seen in early stages of septic shock because of the margination of PMNs. White blood cell counts then rise to $15.0–20.0 \times 10^3/mm^3$ or greater. Continued leukopenia is associated with poor prognosis.

Increases in the excretion of catecholamines due to the stress associated with shock occur. There is a migration of lipids, but the triglycerides are not affected. Plasma glucose levels go up, however, in response to the lactic acid (anaerobic) metabolism. As the patient approaches the hypodynamic state, poor renal perfusion causes changes in kidney function tests. Decreased urine volume is accompanied by low specific gravity and proteinuria.[15] The blood urea nitrogen (BUN) begins to rise above the high normal of 20 mg/dL (7.1 mmol/L), and the creatinine remains at the normal level of around 1.2 mg/dL (106 μmol/L), an indication of prerenal azotemia. Mild dehydration, a high-protein diet, increased protein catabolism, and massive blood loss are other conditions that may also account for these results.[16] Hepatic enzymes also increase as tissue ischemia increases. Alanine aminotransferase (ALT), aspartate aminotransferase (AST), and lactate dehydrogenase (LD) levels increase to more than 1½ times the upper limit of the reference range, more than 2 times the upper limit of the reference range, and more than 2 to 2½ times the upper limit of the reference range respectively. In an attempt to show relationships between hepatic dysfunction, the duration of shock, and the clinical course of septic shock, one study found that there was no statistical difference between survivors and nonsurvivors with respect to the AST, ALT, alkaline phosphatase, total protein (TP), and serum bilirubin levels. It was found that clinical jaundice was evident in 63% of the patient population studied, and that jaundice was seen twice as often in nonsurvivors as in survivors.[17] Because of increasing oliguria and abnormal exchange of fluids, electrolytes should be monitored to ensure normal balance.

Pancreatic changes also occur, due to ischemia. Elevations in amylase may be seen with aortic aneurysm or biliary or pancreatic dysfunction, or after surgery. The lipase activity may also be elevated and, in contrast to amylase, which is present in both the pancreas and the parotid glands, lipase is present only in the pancreas. Thus, elevations in this enzyme are more specific for pancreatic involvement.

TREATMENT

Although it has been reported that no beneficial effect from administration of an appropriate antibiotic could be demonstrated in patients with rapidly fatal underlying diseases, immediate therapy for septic shock is directed toward eradication of the cause of sepsis, along with correction of abnormal hemodynamic parameters, acidosis, and electrolyte imbalance.[18] Surgical drainage of the focus of the infection may be required if it can be located.

Due to the emergency nature of septic shock, it is inadvisable to wait for microbiological culture results prior to the administration of antibiotic therapy. Standard antibiotic therapy prior to the identification of the agent has traditionally included the administration of an aminoglycoside such as gentamicin or amikacin sulfate, along with a β-lactam antibiotic. Combination therapy kills microorganisms at a more rapid rate than does either agent alone. This combination also works better when there is either multiorgan involvement or mixed infection, because of the varying peak level of activity and modes of action. For the patient in septic shock, the first dose of antibiotic is likely to be crucial, particularly if the patient is in the late hypodynamic phase. The maximum amount that the patient can tolerate should be administered intravenously. This is another reason for the use of combined therapy, as the range between efficacy and toxicity is narrow for aminoglycosides.

Once the cause of sepsis has been identified by the laboratory, specific therapy can be instituted. Most studies indicate that gram-positive bacteria respond effectively to a combination of nafcillin and ampicillin or to vancomycin alone. Most gram-negative bacteria respond well to an aminoglycoside in combination with a third-generation cephalosporin. Caution must be used, however, if renal function is impaired. Careful monitoring of the serum creatinine is suggested in order to monitor dosage.[19] Even this procedure is not without problem, as the BUN or creatinine may not always reflect the renal status of the elderly.[2] Specific antibiotic therapy will eradicate the microorganism from the blood, but repeated blood cultures may not become negative until the crisis of septic shock has passed.

Supportive measures include the administration of fluids. Initially fluids can be given by mouth but, if the signs of shock continue, intravenous administration of lactated Ringer's solution, fresh-frozen plasma, or other colloids or crystalloids is begun. The administration of fluids is used to restore fluid balance and to ensure that the electrolytes are within normal limits. Hemodynamic changes can be monitored by measurements in arterial pressure, wedge pressure, blood pressure, heart and respiratory rates, and urine output. In the hyperdynamic stage of shock, ventilatory support may be necessary. Arterial blood gases are useful to monitor the maintenance of PaO_2 at above 70 mm Hg with normal pressure in order to avoid adult respiratory distress syndrome.[9] Patients with septic shock appear to have a more rapid course of events with respect to this syndrome than those who develop shock as a result of trauma.[20]

Urine output should be monitored carefully to prevent fluid overload. It may be necessary to use a mild diuretic. Concomitant with recovery is a return to normal urine specific gravity and a decrease in proteinuria.

To counteract the peripheral vasodilatation and subsequent hypotension, an inotropic agent or vasoactive drug such as dopamine is recommended. This drug causes an increase in heart rate and cardiac output. Effectiveness is dose-dependent, so careful evaluation of dosage is necessary. Excess dosage may also dispose the patient to cardiac arrhythmias.

Heparin, platelets, or specific clotting factors are administered if there is laboratory evidence of DIC. Other therapy, such as corticosteroid or naloxone administration, is sometimes initiated; however, there continues to be debate concerning the efficacy of these agents.[21] Return to normal values of the PT, TT, and APTT is indicative that the therapy used to counteract DIC has been successful.

The therapeutic measures described above continue in the hypodynamic or late phase of shock. The patient may respond to treatment and recover, or the patient's condition may deteriorate despite therapy. Clinical jaundice may be evident, and the BUN and creatinine may continue to rise. Metabolic acidosis with a continuing *p*H drop, decrease in blood pressure, and oliguria are likely to result in death.

CASE STUDY #1

A 56-year-old woman was admitted to the hospital complaining of shortness of breath. Physical examination revealed a woman in acute respiratory distress with warm, dry skin, slight tachycardia, temperature 38° C, respirations 22, and blood pressure 100/70. She had been admitted to the hospital 3 years previously with carcinoma of the colon and had been placed on a course of chemotherapy.

Radiographic examination of the chest revealed an opacity in the right lung, along with pulmonary edema. All laboratory tests were normal except for a slight leukopenia, 4+ proteinuria, and slightly increased blood urea nitrogen (BUN) and serum creatinine. Blood gas results showed a decrease in both PaO_2 and oxygen saturation.

Four days later the patient was placed in the intensive care unit because of hyperventilation, continued fever, and hypoxia. Multiple blood cultures taken at admission were negative at this time. Sputum culture showed normal respiratory flora. Both hematocrit and platelets were low, while both BUN and creatinine continued to increase. Although she continued to spill large amounts of protein in the urine, her urine output diminished. Antimicrobic therapy of clindamycin and tobramycin had been initiated because of suspected sepsis. However, despite vigorous oxygen administration her PaO_2 remained under 30 mm Hg, and 6 days after admission she expired. On that same day *Cryptococcus neoformans* was isolated from her blood culture.

Questions

1. What were the first clinical signs of septic shock?
2. Which laboratory data supported the diagnosis?
3. Why did it take so long to isolate the causative organism?
4. Why did the patient fail to respond to treatment?

Discussion

1. Clinical signs of the hyperdynamic stage of septic shock were present. Fever, warm, dry skin, hyperventilation, and tachycardia are all early warning signs. In addition, the blood pressure was slightly low for a 56-year-old female.
2. Leukopenia is a common symptom in early shock, although this usually changes as the condition progresses to reflect the body's response to the invading microorganism. The presence of immunosuppressive agents may be responsible for the failure of a patient to develop subsequent leukocytosis. The fall in hematocrit and platelets suggests the beginning of disseminated intravascular coagulation (DIC). Proteinuria, along with rising kidney function test results, reveals the extent of urinary tract involvement.
3. This study illustrates that, while most cases of septic shock are bacterial in origin, the possibility of other types of microorganisms should not be overlooked. This is particularly true with someone who has been on immunosuppressive drugs. It is probable that the source of the microorganism causing the sepsis is in the right lung, and that the *C. neoformans* was overgrown by the faster-growing bacteria in the sputum culture. Apparently there was no request for a fungal culture on the sputum. While most yeasts are detected in the blood culture during the first 4 days of incubation, this strain did not appear until later. The presence of chemotherapeutic agents probably affected the growth rate of the organism. Frequently these cultures appear negative upon gross examination, and growth is retarded if the bottle is not properly vented.
4. Death was due to circulatory collapse brought about by inadequate antimicrobic therapy. Had antifungal therapy such as amphotericin B been administered early in the course of sepsis, the outcome might have been different. This case illustrates the rapid and fulminant nature of the disease and the importance of early microbial detection.

CASE STUDY #2

A 75-year-old man was admitted to the hospital for a transurethral resection (TUR) of the prostate. Two days postoperatively he complained of shaking chills. Temperature was 39.9° C, respirations were 20, and blood pressure was 120/84. Blood cultures were drawn, and a combined antibiotic therapy of cefoxitin and gentamicin was begun. The following day the patient became disoriented and flushed. Tachycardia was noted. The blood pressure fell to 90/60. Results of the laboratory tests taken at this time are seen in the following table.

LABORATORY FINDINGS (3 DAYS POSTOPERATIVELY)

	Reference Values	**Patient Values**
Blood		
Platelet count	150–400 × 10^3/mm^3	112 × 10^3/mm^3
White blood cell count	5–10 × 10^3/mm^3	18 × 10^3/mm^3
Hematocrit	40%–54%	38%
Serum		
Urea nitrogen	10–20 mg/dL (3.6–7.1 mmol/L)	22 mg/dL (7.9 mmol/L)
Creatinine	0–1.0 mg/dL (88.4 μmol/L)	1.2 mg/dL (106 μmol/L)
Alanine amino-transferase	6–24 U/L	38 U/L
Aspartate amino-transferase	10–25 U/L	42 U/L
Lactate dehy-drogenase	45–100 U/L	260 U/L
Amylase	12–125 U/L	110 U/L
Lipase	10–180 U/L	18 U/L

Urine output decreased slightly, but urinalysis was normal. *Escherichia coli* and *Pseudomonas aeruginosa* were isolated from the blood. The patient was given intravenous fluid therapy, oxygen, and methylprednisolone. The antibiotic therapy continued, and the patient became afebrile within 48 hours. Monitoring of the patient continued until all laboratory values returned to within normal limits.

Questions

1. What factors accounted for the recovery of this patient?
2. How did the laboratory aid in the treatment of this patient?

Discussion

1. Early recognition of possible septic shock is important in recovery. Although this patient had a normal blood pressure and his respirations were just within normal limits, the elevated temperature indicated a probable septic process. Prompt administration of combined antibiotic therapy after drawing blood for culture was appropriate. Septic shock must be considered in a patient who demonstrates probable sepsis, disorientation, and tachycardia. This was confirmed by a lowering of blood pressure and the subsequent laboratory data.
2. Polymicrobic involvement occurs in about 6% of cases of septic shock. In this case, the selection of antibiotics was appropriate because the *E. coli* was susceptible to the cephalosporin, while the *P. aeruginosa* was susceptible to the aminoglycoside. Given the blood culture results, the physician could have chosen to use a single antibiotic such as ticarcillin but, because of the patient's thrombocytopenia and elevated ALT/AST values, chose to remain with the initial drug therapy.

   BUN and creatinine values and decreased urine output indicated that there was kidney involvement, even though the urinalysis was normal. Normal amylase and lipase indicated that there was no pancreatic involvement.

   The patient feels better when the temperature returns to normal. However therapy, both antibiotic and supportive, should be continued until all laboratory results return to within normal limits.

REFERENCES

1. Root RK, Sande ML: Septic Shock. New York City, Churchill Livingstone, 1985
2. Holloway WA, Rheinhardt J: Septic shock in the elderly. Geriatrics 39:48–54, 1984
3. Parker MM, Parrillo JE: Septic shock: Hemodynamics and pathogenesis. JAMA 250:3324–3327, 1983
4. Jimenez EB, Gimenez CR: Septic shock due to Enterobacter sakazakii. Clin Microbiol Newsletter 4:26, 1982
5. Barber HR, Gaber EA: Septic Shock on OB and GYN. Springfield, Illinois, Charles C Thomas, 1971

6. Mizock B: Septic shock: A metabolic perspective. Arch Intern Med 144:579–585, 1984
7. Lamb LS: Think you know septic shock? Nursing 12:34–43, 1982
8. Venezio FR, Westenfelden GO, Phaio JP: The adherence of polymorphonuclear leukocytes in patients with sepsis. J Infect Dis 145:351, 1982
9. Rice V: The clinical continuum of septic shock. Crit Care Nurse 4:86–109, 1984
10. Abraham E, Baird RD, Cobo JC et al: Sequential cardiorespiratory patterns associated with outcome in septic shock. Chest 85:75–80, 1984
11. Reller LB: Blood cultures. In Washington JA II (ed): Cumitech 1A. Washington, D.C., American Society for Microbiology, 1982
12. Ilsrup DM, Washington JA II: The importance of volume of blood cultured in the detection of bacteremia and fungemia. Diagn Microbiol Infect Dis 1:107, 1983
13. Wallis C, Melnik JL, Wende RD et al: Rapid isolation of bacteria from septicemic patents receiving antibiotics with the antimicrobial removal device. J Clin Microbiol 11:462, 1980
14. Sirridge MS, Reaner S: Laboratory Evaluation of Hemostasis and Thrombosis. Philadelphia, Lea & Febiger, 1983
15. Berner JJ: Effects of Diseases on Laboratory Tests. Philadelphia, JB Lippincott, 1983
16. Teitz NW: Textbook of Clinical Chemistry. Philadelphia, WB Saunders, 1986
17. Banks JG, Foulis AK, Lendingham IMA et al: Liver function in septic shock. J Clin Pathol 35:1249–1252, 1982
18. Bryant RE, Hood AF, Hood CE et al: Factors affecting mortality of gram-negative bacteremia. Arch Intern Med 127:I120, 1971
19. Cavanaugh D, Knoppel RA, Shepherd JH et al: Septic shock and the obstetrician/gynecologist. South Med J 75 (7):809–813, 1982
20. Modig J, Borg T, Wegenius G et al: The value of variables of disseminated intravascular coagulation in the diagnosis of adult respiratory distress syndrome. Acta Anesthesiol Scand 27:369–375, 1983
21. Sprung CL, Caralis PV, Marcail EH et al: The effects of high-dose corticosteroids in patients with septic shock: A prospective controlled study. N Engl J Med 311:1137–1143, 1984

Chapter 60

Nosocomial Infections

Mary J. R. Gilchrist / Linda H. Brooks

Nosocomial (noso = disease, and *komeo* = hospital) refers to an infection that results from an exposure during hospitalization, even though the infection may not clinically appear until after discharge. Patients already incubating an infection may be admitted to a hospital, yet not show any clinical manifestations of the infection until a day or more after admission. This is not a nosocomial infection but a *community-acquired infection,* and care must be taken not to confuse the two. Figure 60-1 illustrates the relationship of incubation period, date of admission, and date of onset with respect to community- and hospital-acquired infections. In this decade, changes in reimbursement patterns for medical care have encouraged home and outpatient care rather than inpatient care. *Iatrogenic* (*iatros* = physician, *genic* = producing) infections are those that are a result of any clinical intervention, whether it occurs in the hospital or in another clinical setting. As the number of clinical pro-

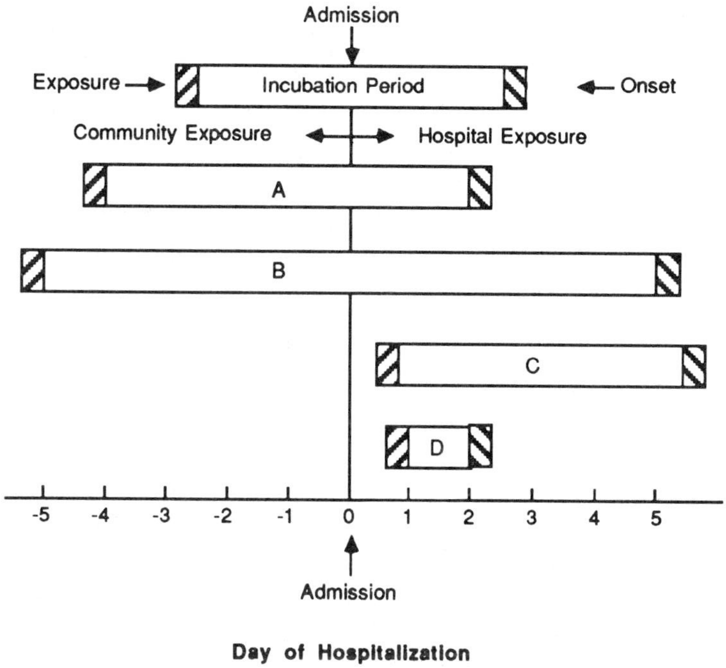

Figure 60-1 Hospital-acquired versus community-acquired infection. Patients A and D had disease onset on Day 2 of hospitalization. As they had different diseases, the incubation periods were 6 and 1 day(s) respectively. Patients B and C had disease onset on Day 5 of hospitalization, with incubation periods of 10 and 4 days respectively. Only C and D had hospital-acquired (nosocomial) infections as their exposures occurred after hospitalization.

cedures performed on an outpatient basis increases, iatrogenic infections will present greater challenges.

ETIOLOGY AND PATHOPHYSIOLOGY

In order for an infection to occur, three requirements must be met satisfactorily: susceptibility of the host; pathogenicity of the etiologic agent; and transmission of agent to host. With regard to hospital-acquired infections, there are unique circumstances related to each of these requirements.

Susceptibility of the Host

In the normal host, resistance to infection occurs by means of physical barriers, mechanical removal, chemical or immunologic interference, or microbial competition. Although intact skin and mucous membranes present physical barriers to infection by microorganisms, breaching these barriers is a common circumstance among hospitalized patients. The loss of integrity of the skin due to surgical wounds or to burns often leads to subsequent infection. Patients who are hospitalized are often fitted with devices that produce long-term breaks in the integrity of the skin. For example, intravascular cannulae (catheters) are placed to administer treatment and monitor patient status. The cannula bridges the skin barrier and enters the sterile intravascular space. Microorganisms on the surface of the skin may thus gain access to the intravascular space, as shown schematically in Figure 60-2. Physical devices that are implanted wholly within sterile spaces are also potential sources of nosocomial infections. Prosthetic heart valves and prosthetic joints may become contaminated during surgery or may be seeded long after surgery by organisms involved in transient bacteremia. Materials that cannot be subjected to autoclaving for sterilization, such as heart valves of animal origin and some synthetic substances, have been the sources of nosocomial infection by organisms not removed by disinfection of these devices.

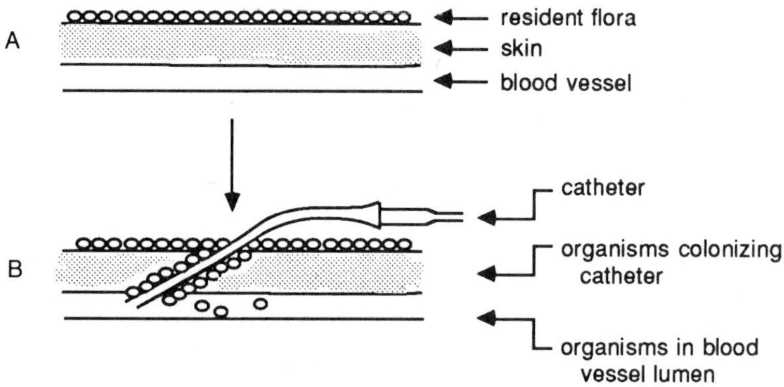

Figure 60-2 Breach of skin barrier by catheter potentiates infection. (*A*) Organisms residing on the skin surface have relatively little tendency to cross this barrier. (*B*) When an indwelling line is in place, organisms from the skin surface colonize the interface and have ready access to the vessels into which the catheter extends.

In either case, the presence of the foreign body often reduces the host's ability to combat colonization and subsequent infection. In many cases, cure can be effected by removal of the foreign body, but cannot be accomplished by application of aggressive antimicrobial chemotherapy alone unless the foreign body is removed.

Mechanical removal of organisms at the surface of mucous membranes is an effective way to reduce the entry of these organisms into susceptible sites. For example, tears, cilia and mucus, and urine flow all play a role in flushing organisms from internal sites. Devices that compromise mechanical removal of organisms may potentiate nosocomial infections. An indwelling urinary catheter reduces the efficiency of flushing of the urethra. This, among other mechanisms, may help potentiate the acquisition of nosocomial urinary tract infections among patients at risk.

The normal host is protected by chemical and immunologic barriers to infection. For instance, the low *p*H of the gastric contents drastically reduces the number and variety of microorganisms that gain access to the intestine via the oral route. Patients with reduced gastric acidity may be at increased risk for acquisition of such infections. Chemical imbalances in hospitalized patients, such as elevated blood and body fluid glucose in diabetics, may lead to nosocomial infections. Overwhelming fungal infections are not uncommon in patients with uncontrolled glucose levels. The cellular and humoral immune mechanisms of the host are critical to infection resistance. Immunologic predisposition to infection may be innate, either congenital or acquired, or may be iatrogenic, due to the administration of immunosuppressive agents such as steroids or chemotherapeutic agents. An immature immunologic system in neonates and a senescent one in the aged are responsible for age-related immunocompromise. In developed countries, the population most at risk for nosocomial infection is the immunocompromised patient. Infections of immunocompromised patients, usually nosocomial, are discussed in Chapter 61.

Many body sites are colonized with normal flora that effectively compete for residence at the site and thus minimize the number of pathogens that may colonize the site. The mechanisms of this "colonization resistance" are not entirely understood, but probably include the production of metabolites (*e.g.*, fatty acids) that inhibit the growth of or kill other competitors. A variety of other mechanisms, such as competition for binding sites or for metabolic substrates, may also play a role. Administration of antibiotic therapy may remove some flora and abolish colonization resistance, allowing other organisms to find a niche and produce a deleterious effect. Pseudomembranous colitis is thought to involve such a mechanism. When certain antibiotics are administered, the composition of the intestinal flora is altered both quantitatively and qualitatively. Subsequent proliferation of the bacterium *Clostridium difficile* and production of toxins result in the patient symptomatology characteristic of pseudomembranous colitis.

Pathogenicity of the Etiologic Agent

Pathogenicity of the etiologic agent is the second requirement for an infection to occur. The microorganism must be able to survive in the environment, colonize the host, invade across physical barriers, and evade host immune mechanisms. Common pathogenic bacteria possess enzymes and toxins that allow them to cross physical barriers and inflict physiological damage to tissues. Furthermore, many of these microorganisms produce capsules that render them resistant to opsonization and phagocytosis in the absence of specific antibody. These common pathogenic microorganisms are often involved in nosocomial infections.

In developed countries, however, another subset of microorganisms plays a far more prevalent role in nosocomial infections. The "normal flora" of the skin and mucous membranes are a group of bacteria that are distinguished by their relative lack of invasive and toxic properties. In the normal host they rarely cause infections, although they maintain constant contact. In the hospitalized patient whose skin and/or mucous membranes are compromised by indwelling lines or hardware, these agents can gain access to sterile spaces and can colonize these spaces in the presence of foreign bodies. Recent research suggests that some agents possess superior characteristics in this regard. For example, certain strains of *Staphylococcus epidermidis* are slime producers[1] and may have a survival advantage in the ecologic niche at the surface of catheters in intravascular spaces. Further research will elucidate the mechanisms of pathogenesis of these opportunistic agents; however, their marginal pathogenic potential is perhaps best illustrated by the fact that they cannot easily persist if the foreign body that facilitated their colonization is removed.

Transmission of Agent to Host

A mechanism of transmission is the third requirement for establishment of an infection. The transmission of agents to hosts is shown schematically in Figure 60-3. In hospitals in developed countries, the most common transmission mechanism is the hand. Primarily involved are health care providers who fail to wash their hands when passing from patient to patient. Some agents are transmitted from patient to patient by the hands or by fomites contaminated with the infectious agent. Patients may be placed in isolation to control such transmission. Isolation of patients is often most efficiently accomplished using categories to define the type of precautions necessary.[2] A summary of the most recent isolation precaution category recommendations is shown in Table 60-1.

Drainage-secretion precautions, which call for handwashing by personnel and for appropriate discard of contaminated dressings and fomites, are most often instituted for most agents that infect wounds.

If the nature of the etiologic agent is serious and thus the outcome of widespread dissemination is potentially more serious—for example, the methicillin-resistant *Staphylococcus aureus* (MRSA)—*contact precautions* may be considered necessary to contain the agent.

Strict precautions include coverage for agents that are spread both by air and by contact. For example, varicella, the agent of chicken pox, can cause devastating disease in immunocompromised hosts and is contained in a hospital setting by strict isolation.

Agents of diarrhea (*e.g., Salmonella, Shigella,* rotavirus) are transmitted by the fecal/oral route, and *enteric precautions* will minimize their transmission. Fecal/oral transmission is not limited to agents of diarrhea. For example, the picornaviruses that cause polio, aseptic meningitis, and hepatitis are also transmitted by this route. Therefore, appropriate isolation conditions for such diseases include enteric precautions.

Many agents are transmitted by the respiratory

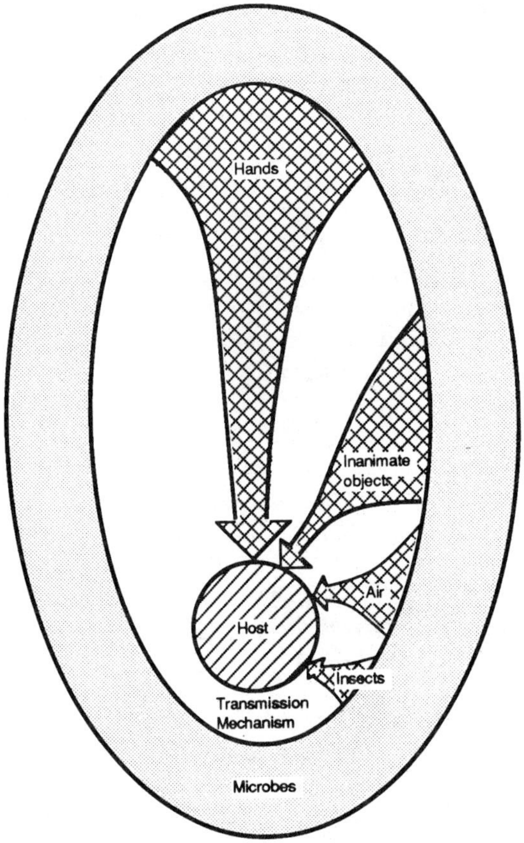

Figure 60-3 Mechanisms of transmission of nosocomial infections in developed countries. The relative contribution of transmission mechanisms is depicted schematically. In developed countries, where hospitals have filtered air systems and many objects are sterilized before use, hands play a major role in transmission of organisms. Handwashing is generally the most effective means of further reducing the rates of nosocomial infection. In developing countries, where hospitals exert less control over the environment, insect vectors, air, and inanimate objects likely play a relatively larger role in infection.

route. *Bordetella pertussis,* the agent responsible for whooping cough, is commonly transmitted by introduction of respiratory secretions into a susceptible host. The respiratory secretions do not always need to be introduced into the respiratory tract. With respiratory syncytial virus (RSV), for example, it is known that the respiratory secretions are effective in transmitting infection if introduced into the mucous membranes of the eye.[3] Control of transmission of these agents in hospitals is effected when *respiratory isolation* is implemented. Hand washing, masks (and goggles for RSV), and containment of respiratory secretions minimize transmission to hospital personnel and patients.

Some agents survive very poorly in the environment and/or are noninvasive. These are agents that normally require the introduction of the body fluids of the affected patient into the candidate host; alternatively, these body fluids may transmit the agent if they gain intimate contact with mucous membranes of the candidate host. In developed countries, where it is not routine practice to reuse devices without intervening sterilization, nosocomial infections with such agents are less common. However, some practices in developed countries, such as hemodialysis, reuse of probes for neurological exams, acupuncture, and allergy testing, have led to acquisition of nosocomial infections such as hepatitis B. *Blood and body fluid precautions* are employed to control such infections. These are particularly important for health care givers, who often expose themselves accidentally via puncture with contaminated needles. Furthermore, intentional introduction of body fluids via such mechanisms as blood transfusion or organ transplants is a commonly known potential source of nosocomial infections. Agents transmitted include hepatitis B, hepatitis nonA-nonB, cytomegalovirus (CMV), and the agent of acquired immunodeficiency syndrome (AIDS). Judicious practices minimize these problems. For example, detection of these agents or antibodies to these agents in the donor may disqualify that donor.

Blood and body fluid precautions can only be successful in containing transmission if they are applied to all patients capable of transmitting the disease. Because not all carriers can be identified, the Centers for Disease Control have recently

Table 60-1 ***Summary of Category-Specific Isolation Precautions***

Category	Mode of Dissemination	Precautions Specified					
		ROOM	*GLOVES*	*GOWNS*	*MASKS*	*HANDS*	*DISPOSE*
Strict	Air and contact	PC	R	R	R	R	R
Contact	Contact	PC	a	b	c	R	R
Respiratory	Air	PC			c	R	R
AFB	Air (adult pulmonary and laryngeal)	PC		b	d	R	R
Enteric	Fecal/oral	PIC	a	b		R	R
Drainage/secretion	Contact		a	b		R	R
Blood and body fluid	Parenteral/mucous	PIC	a	b		R	R

P = private; **C** = cohort with patients with same infection; **I** = private if patient hygiene is poor; **a** = indicated if contact with infected material; **b** = indicated if clothing may become soiled; **c** = indicated if close to patient; **d** = indicated if patient is coughing and does not cover mouth; R = required.

In all cases, hand washing and proper disposal of contaminated materials are required. With blood and body fluid precautions, take special care to avoid needle-stick injuries; clean up all body fluid spills with a 1:10 dilution of 5.25% sodium hypochlorite.

Another category of isolation, *Protective,* serves to minimize introduction of infectious agents *to* a compromised host rather than dissemination *from* an infected host.

advocated the institution of universal body fluid precautions. These involve the routine protection of health workers from skin and mucous membrane exposure whenever exposure to body fluids of *any* patient is anticipated. In implementing universal body fluid precautions many hospitals will substitute them for most other categories of precautions except respiratory where both will be observed when necessary.[3a]

There exists a large group of agents, in particular many parasites, for which there is no known transmission mechanism in the hospital setting. For example, if the intermediate host is a snail or a mosquito, then, in the controlled environment of a hospital in a developed country, the agent cannot be transmitted because it cannot complete its life cycle in the absence of the intermediate host. Thus there are no isolation conditions for many parasitic agents, although it is conceivable that isolation conditions would be necessary in a hospital lacking vector control.

Where nosocomial infections are concerned, transmission does not always play a role. For example, immunocompromised patients become infected with their own flora. Moreover, resident flora of hospitalized patients are often quite antibiotic-resistant; therefore, exchange of these microorganisms from patient to patient must be minimized. Occasionally it is necessary to place such patients in *protective isolation,* a set of practices that protects the individual in isolation rather than the other patients and staff.

CLINICAL MANIFESTATIONS

The clinical manifestations of nosocomial infections are commonly typical of the disease in question, with the exception that patients who are immunocompromised may not always demonstrate all the characteristic symptoms. If neutropenic, the immunocompromised patient may not produce pus at a wound site or have the leukocytosis characteristic of a bacterial infection. In addition, for such patients there are often ongoing symptoms that mask the symptoms of a nosocomial infection. For example, fever without infection is a common complication in patients suffering from cancer or undergoing anti-cancer chemotherapy. Thus, it is often difficult to determine whether fever is a harbinger of infection, a symptom of underlying disease, or an outcome of treatment.

In many special cases, nosocomial infections can be detected early by careful monitoring. For example, when indwelling lines are in place, routine care should include daily examination of the site for evidence of infection.[4] Similar precautions apply to patients with surgical wounds.[5] With indwelling urinary catheters, special precautions are known to minimize the risk of nosocomial infection. These include hygienic care of the perineum, maintenance of a closed system to minimize introduction of organisms, and reduction in length of time in place. To monitor for infection, urine is sampled and cultured quantitatively. Similar precautions apply to patients undergoing chronic ambulatory peritoneal dialysis (CAPD).

In certain settings, special tests may be applied for the detection of nosocomial infections. Patients undergoing hemodialysis are at special risk for the acquisition of hepatitis B, and thus may best be monitored routinely for serologic evidence of the infection. In the immunocompromised, in whom purulent discharge, blood counts, and fever may not be reliable indices of infection, it may be useful to institute a routine of surveillance cultures.[6] For example, blood cultures for bacteria, viruses, and fungi may be the only reliable indicators of the need for specific therapeutic intervention.

LABORATORY ANALYSES AND DIAGNOSIS

In most hosts there are certain chemical or physiological signs of infection. Fever, leukocytosis, elevated erythrocyte sedimentation rate, and altered liver function test results are nonspecific signals of the onset of a condition that may include infection. In many cases it is possible to establish a differential diagnosis that may include as few as a half dozen microorganisms and a short list of noninfectious causes. Thus, empiric therapy with antimicrobial agents directed at the most likely agents is often instituted at onset of symptoms. In order to institute specific antimicrobial therapy directed at the actual agent, however, it is necessary to isolate and identify the agent.

Specialized tests may be necessary for nosocomial infections. Infection of intravenous catheter sites can be documented by culturing both the blood and the catheter itself. Special procedures may be required to quantitate the microorganisms because it is not uncommon for a few skin flora to contaminate the catheter at or near the site of insertion through the skin.[7] For patients undergoing peritoneal dialysis, it may be necessary to culture the spent dialysis fluid. In such cases, the concentration of organisms in the fluid may be below the limits of detection of the test unless the organisms are concentrated by filtration or centrifugation or unless a large volume is cultured.[8, 9]

Clinical laboratory scientists are often asked to perform specialized tests to detect organisms in the environment as potential sources of nosocomial infections. Several decades ago it was popular to perform routine environmental surveillance cultures in hospitals; that practice is now discouraged.[10] There is no demonstrable relationship between the infection rate and the level of organisms in the environment[11] because animate rather than inanimate sources of infection are the usual case. Some hospitals are reverting to the outdated philosophy of environmental sampling by culturing cooling towers and potable water in a search for *Legionella*. Unless there is a demonstrated problem, this practice should be actively discouraged as wasteful and nonproductive. As with other environmental culturing, it is only useful if performed as part of a rationally formulated epidemiological investigation of an outbreak of nosocomial disease. Careful surveillance of patients and the risk factors that they share can minimize the work of culturing and enhance the potential for success. If all affected patients had blood drawn into a certain type of tube, for example, it may be useful to culture other samples of that lot of tubes for contamination by a common agent. If they were all receiving routine urine specific gravity tests, it may be useful to culture the device that was used in common. These examples are detailed in the case studies at the end of the chapter. In each case the laboratory scientist can contribute perspective and expertise. For example, many organisms have a predilection for water environments (*e.g.,* the Pseudomonadaceae) and are not likely to be found in air or on dry surfaces. On the other hand, an outbreak of aspergillosis in immunocompromised patients is likely to be precipitated by introduction of air currents contaminated by organisms during renovation or construction. In the first case, moist surfaces and water would be the best culture sources. In the second case, all air sample cultures would tend to yield *Aspergillus.* Thus, if an investigation is undertaken it is necessary to quantitate levels of organisms per volume of air, using an air sampling device, a procedure normally reserved for those engaged in research.

Specialized Laboratory Procedures to Identify Outbreaks

In many cases the laboratory may be asked to assist in the determination of whether two organisms infecting two different patients have been acquired from a common source. It is very important that the laboratory and the infection control officer work closely together. In such cases all laboratories have at hand certain limited resources to aid in this determination. For example, it is useful to completely speciate the organisms. If both are of the same species, then it may be useful to evaluate the biotypes of the two organisms. Most laboratory identification schemes provide a profile number with the species name. This number indicates the reactions of the various *bio*chemicals, and is thus termed a *bio*type. Organisms of the same species with very similar biotypes are more likely to be from a common source than those with very dissimilar biotypes.

In addition to speciation and biotyping, it may be useful to examine the antibiograms of the two organisms. The minimal inhibitory concentration (MIC) of a single organism for a given drug may vary by plus or minus one two fold dilution. Thus, two organisms can be judged dissimilar only if very substantial differences in MICs are detected. Moreover, if these differences are not limited to antibiotics for which, for example, levels of induction of the enzyme β-lactamase might render highly variant MICs, then the organisms can be judged to be different.

Serotyping is available on a limited basis in most laboratories, depending upon their size and particular emphasis. Most laboratories are prepared to distinguish among the major serogroups of *Salmonella.* If isolates of *Salmonella* from two different patients on the same nursing unit were found to be of different serogroups, group B and group D, one could surmise they were not from a common source. If the two isolates were both from group B, however, a public health reference laboratory could further serotype to document the similarity or dissimilarity of members of the serogroup.

Other specialized tests are usually limited to public health or other specialized research or reference laboratories. For example, the spectrum of susceptibility to a variety of bacteriophage strains (phage typing) can be useful to document subtypes of *S. aureus,* and the spectrum of susceptibility to a variety of bacteriocins can be useful to document subtypes of *Pseudomonas aeruginosa.* Plasmid and membrane protein analyses may be selectively applied to the evaluation of organism similarities (see Fig. 60-4).

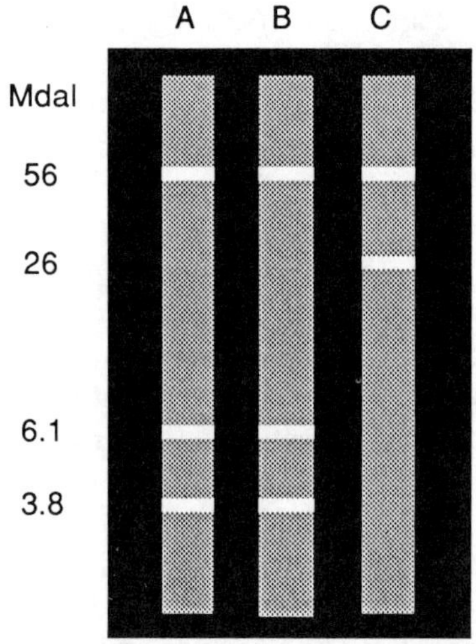

Figure 60-4 Plasmid analysis. Schematic depiction of the separation of plasmid DNA on the basis of size. In each of lanes A, B and C, DNA extracted from three different strains of bacteria is subjected to electrophoresis. The location of the bands in the lane is determined by the mobility of the DNA in the electrical field, primarily a function of the molecular weight (size) of the plasmids. Thus, the plasmid profile (the total content of plasmids and the size of those plasmids) of a microorganism may be determined. Such plasmid profiles may be useful to distinguish strains from one another. Even though two bacterial isolates are of the same species and serotype, they may not necessarily have a common source in the environment. In the example depicted, A and B both show plasmids of 56, 6.1 and 3.8 Mdal, while C has plasmids of 56 and 26 Mdal. Very different plasmid profiles would usually suggest that the bacterial isolates were not from a common source. However, similar plasmid profiles do not confirm a common source, since certain plasmid compositions may be widespread and stably distributed within a species. With the application of appropriate limitations in interpretation, plasmid analysis may be useful in the investigation of outbreaks.

During the next decade, it is expected that nucleic acid probes for the identification and detection of microorganisms will be utilized on a more routine basis. Understanding the limits and applications of these agents will be important if their potential is to be utilized most accurately to distinguish among similarities and differences in microorganisms.

PREVENTION OF NOSOCOMIAL INFECTIONS

Evolution of Infection Control Programs

Nosocomial infections have plagued hospitals since their inception. For most of that time, hospital-acquired infections were assumed to be an inevitable outcome for most hospital patients. With the practices introduced by Semmelweiss and Lister and refined by Florence Nightingale and many others, nosocomial infections were no longer an inevitable result of hospitalization.[12] During part of this century, patients suffering from infectious diseases were segregated into hospitals designed solely for "Communicable Diseases." As understanding of microbiology increased, so did a complacency toward nosocomial infections. The widespread application of vaccines to prevent the most dramatic infectious diseases contributed to the reduced interest in infection control. This complacency peaked with the development of antibiotics and the feeling that it was just a matter of time before all infections were eradicated.

Complacency was shattered in the late 1950s when there was an alarming increase in nosocomial infections caused by a highly resistant strain of *S. aureus.* The Communicable Disease Center (now Centers for Disease Control [CDC]) and the American Hospital Association (AHA) jointly developed strategies for hospitals to improve their control over these infections. Over time there evolved a specialized function of infection control practitioner, and a committee of the medical staff to monitor the infections in the hospital and develop strategies to control them. In the mid1970s, the

Joint Commission for Accreditation of Hospitals (now the Joint Commission for Acceditation of Health Care Organizations [JCAHCO]) published standards for the infection control function in a hospital, thus firmly establishing the practice of infection control in American hospitals.

Current measures for the prevention and control of nosocomial infection minimize emphasis on the physical environment and rely on studying the pattern of emerging infections, using epidemiological methods. Institutional policies for infection control mandated by the JCAHCO embody several important functions. Surveillance and monitoring involve the collection of data. Initially, surveillance is performed to establish the baseline endemic nosocomial infection rate. Once this is accomplished, epidemics are readily detected through monitoring of rates. Control strategies vary with the type of infection, but in all cases include intensive staff education on hand washing and asepsis. Isolation of the patient is often used to prevent the spread of a particular infection. The absolute value of isolation is not always documentable, but posting of precautions does serve as an important reminder of appropriate techniques.

Extent and Impact of Nosocomial Infections

The extent of nosocomial infections is difficult to determine absolutely because there is no reporting system for this information, and it is not a topic hospitals are eager to discuss.[13] According to data from the Study on the Efficacy of Nosocomial Infection Control (SENIC) and reports from a small group of hospitals enrolled in the National Nosocomial Infections Survey (NNIS), approximately 5% of all hospital patients develop nosocomial infections. As a basis of comparing hospitals, however, this figure is of very little use in assessing the relative value of an institution's infection control program. More valuable for this purpose is a set of observations that has been developed from a variety of studies: large hospitals tend to have higher infection rates than small hospitals; hospitals with heavier surgical schedules and more complex surgical procedures have higher rates than those which do less surgery; teaching hospitals tend to have higher rates than nonteaching hospitals; and hospitals in the Northeast and West have higher rates than do those in the rest of the country. The linkage among these hospitals with the higher rates is the relative risk of their patient populations and the intensity of the services offered. Large hospitals and teaching hospitals are usually referral centers for patients too ill to be treated at small community hospitals. Such hospitals also tend to perform more high-risk, invasive diagnostic and treatment procedures, which offer more opportunity for infection. Seriously ill patients are more likely to require prolonged treatment with drugs that alter immune response, which can increase risk of hospital-acquired infection. Antineoplastic drugs and steroids are two classes of drugs that compromise immune function. Any surgical procedure carries risk of infection; the longer and more complex the procedure, the higher the risk. The type of surgery also influences risk. A "clean" procedure, *e.g.*, joint surgery, is less at risk for infection than a "dirty" one, *e.g.*, abdominal gunshot wound repair.

Nosocomial infections have an impact on both the patient and the institution. Typically, there is an increase in the length of stay. The most common type of nosocomial infection is a urinary tract infection,[13] which averages 1 extra hospital day per infection. The next most common infection is a surgical wound infection, averaging 7 extra days of hospitalization per infection. For the patient, this increase in morbidity means greater discomfort, increased time away from family, and increased loss of work. Serious surgical wound infections may also result in disfiguring scars. For the institution, the financial implications are enormous. The average 250-bed hospital has approximately 2000 extra patient days each year that are attributable to nosocomial infection, resulting in an annual cost of $1 million. Under current strategies for reimbursement to a hospital, much of these costs are not recoverable by the institution. The impact of nosocomial infections on patient mortality is also great. The CDC has shown that 10% of patients with nosocomial infections die while in the hospital. Of these deaths, one out of ten is a direct result of the infection, and in three of the ten deaths the infection is a significant factor. In the other six deaths, the presence of the infection is not significant. This results in approximately 20,000 deaths per year directly attributable to nosocomial infection, and another 60,000 in which the infection is a significant factor.[13]

Efficacy of Infection Control Programs

Recent studies have indicated that infection control programs that are the most sophisticated, are optimally staffed, and have the full cooperation of all staff are able to prevent 32%[14] of nosocomial infections. This reduction in infection rate would bring about a significant reduction in patient morbidity and mortality, and have a favorable financial impact on hospitals. Nevertheless, some nosocomial infections are an inevitable outcome of certain hospitalizations.

CASE STUDY #1

One ward of a hospital was found to have experienced a number of infections due to *Serratia marcescens* during a brief time period. Among these were infections of the urinary tract and bacteremias. Upon investigation by the epidemiologist and clinical laboratory scientist, orders were noted that all patients were to be monitored for urine specific gravity. Patients were told to save their urine and that the nurse would remove it for testing on the instrument in the utility room.

Questions

1. What is the most likely source of the outbreak?
2. What steps should be taken to minimize the chances of recurrence?
3. What is the role of the laboratory in controlling such nosocomial outbreaks?

Discussion

1. The most likely source of the outbreak is the urine collection containers and the specific gravity devices. (Cultures from both yielded *S. marcescens.*)
2. The epidemiologist and the microbiologist should conduct a nursing in-service program to explain how the organism may be transmitted from patient to patient on hands and how standing reservoirs of urine can increase the quantities of the organism. Nurses should be instructed not to reuse the urine collection devices, to clean the specific gravity devices after each use, and to wash their hands after handling each patient sample. To illustrate the points, nurses should be shown samples of cultures of *S. marcescens* with colony counts so they can understand the magnitude of bacterial contamination. The nurse epidemiologist should continue to monitor for reappearance of the organism and for recurrence of previous nursing practices. If it is discovered that some staff have reverted to previous practices, additional in-service programs should be conducted.
3. The role of the laboratory includes reporting all isolates to the epidemiologist, devising optimized culture techniques to detect the agent in question, providing guidance to the epidemiologist on the selection of sites to be cultured, assisting in the teaching about the organism and its transmission, and continued monitoring for the agent in the future.

CASE STUDY #2

A series of isolations of *Staphylococcus aureus* from cerebrospinal fluid (CSF) occurred on a nursing unit housing patients with no known underlying disease. The nurse epidemiologist evaluated the situation and could find no evidence that a single physician performed the lumbar puncture in all cases or that a single assistant was present in all cases. Two different kinds of lumbar puncture trays were utilized. There was a common bottle of antiseptic solution for skin preparation. Bottles with the same lot number were removed and examined.

Although no etiologic agents were cultured from the skin preparation agent, removal of the lot was temporally associated with subsidence of isolation of the microbial agent in CSF cultures.

Questions

1. What appears to be the source of this outbreak?
2. What steps should the laboratory take to increase the possibility of isolating an organism from this source?
3. What explanations might account for the failure to isolate organisms from the solution?
4. How typical are the results of this investigation?

Discussion

1. The common bottle of antiseptic solution used for skin preparation is the most likely source.
2. The skin preparation should be filtered to concentrate the organisms and its antibacterial activity neutralized prior to culture.
3. Microbial agents are sometimes present in a "damaged" form, *i.e.,* their cell walls or other mechanisms for growth *in vitro* are not capable of functioning unless they are cultured under appropriate conditions. Alternatively, the organism was not in the skin preparation container, but rather another practice was in place that was discontinued by an individual who learned from the questions asked during the investigation.
4. This story illustrates a common pattern in the investigation of outbreaks. Sound epidemiologic principles were applied, a minimum of culturing endeavor was undertaken, no organism was isolated, the outbreak subsided, and further investigation was not possible.

REFERENCES

1. Davenport DS, Massanari RM, Pfaller MA et al: Usefulness of a test for slime production as a marker for clinically significant infections with coagulase-negative staphylococci. J Infect Dis 153:332, 1986
2. Garner JS, Simmons BP: CDC Guideline for Isolation Precautions in Hospitals. Infect Control 4:249, 1983
3. Hall CB, Douglas RG Jr, Steinhoff MC: Infectivity of respiratory syncytial virus (RSV) by various routes of inoculation. Pediatr Res 13:461, 1979

3a. MMWR 36:25, August 21, 1987

4. Simmons BP: CDC guidelines for prevention and control of nosocomial infections: Guidelines for prevention of intravascular infections. Am J Infect Control 11:183, 1983
5. Garner JS: CDC Guidelines for the prevention and control of nosocomial infections: guidelines for prevention of surgical wound infections. Am J Infect Control 14:71, 1986
6. Schimpff SC: Surveillance cultures. J Infect Dis 144:81, 1981
7. Maki DG, Weiss CE, Sarafin HW: A semiquantitative method for identifying intravenous catheter-related infection. N Engl J Med 296:1305, 1977
8. Vas SI, Law L: Microbiological diagnosis of peritonitis in patients on chronic ambulatory peritoneal dialysis. J Clin Microbiol 21:522, 1985
9. Dawson MS, Harford AM, Garner BK et al: Total volume culture technique for the isolation of microorganisms from chronic ambulatory peritoneal dialysis patients with peritonitis. J Clin Microbiol 22:391, 1985
10. Committee on Infections Within Hospitals, American Hospital Association: Statement on microbiologic sampling in the hospital. Hospitals 48:125, 1974
11. Maki DG, Alvarado CJ, Hassemer CA et al: Relation of the inanimate hospital environment to endemic nosocomial infections. N Engl J Med 307:125, 1982
12. Semmelweis IP: Childbed fever. In Classics in infectious diseases. Rev Infect Dis 3:808, 1981
13. Haley RW, Schaberg DR, Crossly KB et al: Extra days and prolongation of stay attributable to nosocomial infections: A prospective interhospital comparison. Am J Med 70:51, 1981
14. Haley RW, Culver DH, White JW et al: The efficacy of infection surveillance and control programs in preventing nosocomial infections in U.S. hospitals. Am J Epidemiol 121:182, 1985

BIBLIOGRAPHY

Hughes JM: Nosocomial infection prevention and control. In Lennette EH et al (eds): Manual of Clinical

Microbiology, 4th ed. Washington, D.C., American Society for Microbiology, 1985

Isenberg HD, Smith JK: The epidemiology and control of nosocomial and opportunistic infections. In Balows A, Hausler WJ Jr (eds): Diagnostic Procedures for Bacterial, Mycotic, and Parasitic Infections, 6th ed. Washington, D.C., American Public Health Association, 1981

McGowan JE Jr: The role of the laboratory in control of nosocomial infection. In Stratton CW (ed): Topics in clinical microbiology. Infect Control 5:144, 1984

Soule BM (ed): APIC Curriculum for Infection Control Practice. Association for Practitioners of Infection Control. Dubuque, Iowa, Kendall-Hunt, 1983

Chapter 61

Infections in the Immunocompromised Host

Holly Alexander

The human immune system is an extremely complex system composed of a carefully balanced interaction of nonspecific and specific factors that have evolved to distinguish "self" from "nonself." They protect the body during its constant exposure to microorganisms, both those that colonize the body and those in the environment.

Although it is common to refer primarily to patients with neoplastic disease, especially those receiving cytotoxic or immunosuppressive therapy, as "immunocompromised," a patient may be considered to be immunocompromised when any component of the immune system is depressed due to any one of a number of underlying problems. When any part of the immune system does not function properly, the host may become more susceptible to infection. The types of infections seen in such patients are usually related to the type of underlying immune defect (see Table 61-1). (See also Chap. 53.)

HOST DEFENSE MECHANISMS

The first line of defense against microbial infections involves a large number of nonspecific host factors. These include anatomic barriers, microbial antagonism, metabolic factors, and the phagocytic cells of the immune system. Specific host defenses such as antibody responses and cell-mediated immunity

Table 61-1 ***Immune Defects and Infecting Organisms in Patients with Neoplastic Diseases***

Neutropenia	Immunoglobulin Defects	Impaired Cell-Mediated Immunity
Bacteria		
Enterobacteriaceae	*Streptococcus pneumoniae*	*Listeria monocytogenes*
Pseudomonas aeruginosa	Enterobacteriaceae	*Salmonella* species
Staphylococcus aureus	*Pseudomonas aeruginosa*	*Nocardia asteroides*
	Streptococcus pyogenes	*Mycobacterium* species
	Hemophilus influenzae	
Fungi		
Aspergillus species		*Cryptococcus neoformans*
Mucor/Absidia/Rhizopus		*Candida* species
Candida species		*Histoplasma capsulatum*
		Coccidioides immitis
Parasites		
	Pneumocystis carinii	*P. carinii*
		Toxoplasma gondii
		Strongyloides stercoralis
Viruses		
	Vaccinia virus	Herpesviruses
		Cytomegalovirus
		Herpes simplex
		Varicella-zoster
		Vaccinia virus

Adapted from reference number[4]

must be acquired, and therefore take longer to develop.

Anatomic barriers are the first line of host defense against the constant exposure to microorganisms. Intact skin and mucous membranes, although colonized by large numbers of microorganisms, are rarely invaded. Bacteria found on the skin and along mucous membranes produce metabolic end-products and secrete factors that often make it difficult for other more pathogenic microorganisms to become established.

Cellular immunity, consisting primarily of the white blood cells, is highly complex and also contains both nonspecific and specific factors. Nonspecific factors are the polymorphonuclear leukocytes (PMNs or neutrophils) and the monocytes. The specific component of cellular immunity is the T lymphocytes. Cytotoxic T cells destroy cells that are covered with the target antigen. Helper T cells promote maturation of antigen-stimulated cells, especially the lymphocytes. Suppressor T cells regulate the immune response by blocking the activity of helper T cells. The functions of these and other subsets of cells are highly interrelated and regulate the immune response through a variety of positive and negative feedback mechanisms. The term *cell-mediated immunity* (CMI) refers to this specific response, which is important in controlling infections due to intracellular bacteria, fungi, parasites, and viruses.

The third component of host defense is humoral immunity, which consists of soluble immune factors that play an important role in controlling extracellular organisms. Some of these, such as the components of the complement system and chemotactic factors, are nonspecific defense mechanisms, but the most important is the production of specific antibodies by B lymphocytes. Antibodies promote phagocytosis by neutrophils of organisms, especially encapsulated bacteria, such as *Streptococcus pneumoniae, Hemophilus influenzae,* and *Neisseria meningitidis*. Lymphokines, a soluble product produced by lymphocytes, activate macrophages to enhance their ability to kill intracellular organisms.[1, 2] (See also Chap. 53.)

Endogenous Microorganisms

There is a life-long commensal and sometimes symbiotic relationship between humans and microorganisms. Infants are colonized with maternal and environmental organisms immediately after birth.

Microorganisms have evolved to fill specialized ecological niches on the skin and along all mucous membranes. Coagulase-negative staphylococci, *Corynebacterium,* and *Propionibacterium* are the most common organisms found on the skin of a normal host. Coagulase-negative staphylococci and *Corynebacterium* may also be isolated in small numbers from the conjunctiva. The mouth and upper respiratory tract are colonized by viridans-group streptococci, coagulase-negative staphylococci, *Neisseria* species (other than *N. gonorrhoeae* and *N. meningitidis*), *Corynebacterium,* yeast, nonpathogenic mycoplasmas and spirochetes, and anaerobes such as the *Bacteroides melaninogenicus* group and *Fusobacterium* species. There may also be small numbers of bacteria that may be considered pathogenic under other circumstances, including *Staphylococcus aureus, H. influenzae, S. pneumoniae,* Enterobacteriaceae, and *Streptococcus pyogenes* (Group A). The intestinal tract contains predominantly anaerobes including *Bacteroides* species, *Fusobacterium* species, *Clostridium* species, *Eubacterium* species, *Veillonella* species, *Peptostreptococcus,* and *Peptococcus*. Some of the Enterobacteriaceae are present in large numbers, and many other types of bacteria and fungi are present as well. Both the male and female genital tracts are colonized with microorganisms; however, the female genital tract contains much larger numbers. Lactobacilli predominate in the healthy vagina, but coagulase-negative staphylococci, viridans-group streptococci, and small numbers of Enterobacteriaceae, yeast, and anaerobes may also be present. Some microorganisms, once acquired, are not eliminated but remain dormant, often in host macrophages. Examples of such organisms are mycobacteria, *Cryptococcus neoformans, Pneumocystis carinii,* and viruses of the herpes groups: herpes simplex, herpes zoster, and cytomegalovirus, and Epstein-Barr virus. They rarely cause severe disease during the initial infection. Most of these organisms are controlled by CMI and remain latent in normal hosts. They may reactivate in immunocompromised patients with defective CMI, and cause serious infections.[1, 3]

Microorganisms that make up the normal flora are a dynamic population that respond rapidly to environmental changes. Patients who are admitted to the hospital become colonized with organisms prevalent in the hospital environment. These include *Pseudomonas* species and *Acinetobacter* species as well as antibiotic-resistant strains of Enterobacteriaceae and staphylococci. Seriously-ill hospitalized patients have less than optimal host defenses, and are therefore susceptible to hospital-acquired infections caused by these organisms. Use of antibiotics, whether prophylactic or therapeutic, disrupts the normal flora and may allow the overgrowth of resistant organisms.[3]

Although the immunocompromised host is as susceptible as the normal population to microorganisms with primary virulence, these patients are more likely to develop infections with endogenous or environmental microorganisms. These organisms, which rarely cause infections in healthy persons with intact immunity, are therefore called "opportunistic" pathogens. (See also Chaps. 53 and 60.)

TYPES OF IMMUNOCOMPROMISED PATIENTS

The immune system may be depressed due to any one of a number of underlying conditions. Patients may have a decrease in the absolute number of leukocytes, or the number of leukocytes may be normal but one or more types of leukocytes may be functionally defective. Although normal neutrophil counts range from 1.5 to 7.0×10^3 cells/mm^3, the danger of infection is not usually severe until the absolute number of neutrophils decreases to less than 500 cells/mm^3. In rare cases, there may be a deficiency in antibody production or in components of the complement system due to congenital defects.

Use of cytotoxic drugs, corticosteroids, and radiation therapy exacerbates the immunocompromised condition in patients with malignancies and in organ transplant patients. Cytotoxic drugs such as methotrexate, cytosine arabinoside, and cyclophosphamide destroy replicating cells and lead to granulocytopenia. Corticosteroids have numerous effects on the immune system, including suppression of the inflammatory responses and delayed type hypersensitivity. Radiation leads to granulocytopenia and damages anatomic barriers as well.

Neoplastic Conditions

Patients with neoplastic disease are the most common group considered to be immunocompromised. Immunosuppression may be due to the type of cancer, the type of treatment, or both. Advances in treatment and supportive care have extended the life expectancy for patients with many types of cancer, but infection continues to be a major cause of morbidity and mortality.[1, 2, 3]

HEMATOLOGIC MALIGNANCIES

Patients with leukemia are treated aggressively with cytotoxic drugs to induce remission. During this induction period, the number of granulocytes in the peripheral blood falls below 1.0×10^3/mm^3. These patients are highly susceptible to infection, usually with gram-negative bacilli such as the Enterobacteriaceae and *Pseudomonas aeruginosa;* however, staphylococci, *Candida,* and *Aspergillus* are also common. Bacteremia, often associated with a perirectal lesion, and pneumonia are the most common infections seen at this stage of the disease. After remission occurs and patients are placed on maintenance chemotherapy, the danger of infection remains, but the type of organism changes due to a defect in the cellular immune system. Infections in this instance are most often caused by viruses of the herpes family, especially herpes zoster, parasites such as *Pneumocystis carinii,* bacteria such as *Legionella* species and *Listeria monocytogenes,* and fungi such as *Cryp-*

tococcus neoformans and *Nocardia* species (see Table 61-2). Patients who receive multiple blood transfusions are at risk for nonA-nonB hepatitis.

Patients with Hodgkin's disease are not granulocytopenic; however they have a defect in cell-mediated immunity. The most common infections in these patients are due to organisms such as *C. neoformans, L. monocytogenes,* and mycobacteria. Although many Hodgkin's patients undergo splenectomy, they usually have only a slightly increased risk of infection with encapsulated organisms such as *S. pneumoniae.*

Patients with other types of lymphoma have infections similar to those in patients with Hodgkin's, which are most commonly due to aerobic bacteria. However, these patients have a higher incidence of infection, especially bacteremia, pneumonia, and urinary tract infection, because they are treated aggressively with cytotoxic drugs and radiation.

Table 61-2 *Organisms Most Commonly Associated with Hematologic Malignancies*

	Leukemia					
	*ANLL**	*ALL*[†]	*CLL*[‡]	**Lymphoma**	**Hodgkin's**	**Myeloma**
Bacteria	Enterobacteriaceae *Pseudomonas aeruginosa* *Staphylococcus aureus* *Staphylococcus epidermidis* *Corynebacterium* group JK	Enterobacteriaceae *P. aeruginosa* *S. aureus*	Enterobacteriaceae *P. aeruginosa* *S. aureus* *Streptococcus pneumoniae* *Hemophilus influenzae* *Legionella*	Enterobacteriaceae *P. aeruginosa* *S. aureus* *S. pneumoniae*	*Listeria monocytogenes* Mycobacteria *S. pneumoniae*	Enterobacteriaceae *P. aeruginosa* *S. pneumoniae* *H. influenzae* *Neisseria meningitidis*
Fungi	*Candida* species *Aspergillus* species *Mucor/Rhizopus*		*Cryptococcus neoformans* *Nocardia* species *Histoplasma capsulatum*		*C. neoformans* *H. capsulatum* *Coccidioides immitis*	*Candida* species *Aspergillus*
Parasites		*Pneumocystis carinii*			*P. carinii* *Toxoplasma gondii*	
Viruses		Herpes zoster Herpes simplex Cytomegalovirus	Herpes zoster	Herpes zoster	Herpes zoster Cytomegalovirus	

* Acute nonlymphocytic leukemia

[†] Acute lymphocytic leukemia, predominantly in children

[‡] Chronic lymphocytic leukemia

SOLID TUMORS

Solid tumors *per se* do not lead to an increase in infections. However, these patients are usually treated with cytotoxic drugs, corticosteroids, radiation, or combination therapy. While one type of treatment alone will somewhat increase host susceptibility to infection, patients treated with both drugs and radiation are at major risk for developing opportunistic infections. They have damaged immune systems with decreased leukocytes as well as damaged skin and mucous membranes. The infections most commonly acquired are due to both aerobic and anaerobic gram-negative bacilli, and to staphylococci and streptococci. *Candida* and *Aspergillus* are found much less often in patients with solid tumor, compared to incidence in patients with hematologic malignancies.[4]

Other Leukopenic Conditions

Patients may be leukopenic for reasons other than malignancies and related treatment. Congenital deficiencies in one or more of the leukocyte subpopulations may lead to an increased incidence of infection.[1, 5]

Acquired immunodeficiency syndrome (AIDS) is caused by infection with the human immunodeficiency retrovirus (HIV), which specifically decreases the population of helper T cells and leads to a severe suppression of cell-mediated immunity. Infections in these patients resemble those seen in other patients with diminished CMI. Infections due to fungi, *P. carinii, Cryptosporidium,* mycobacteria (especially *Mycobacterium avium-intracellulare*) and the herpes family of viruses cause severe problems in these patients.[6]

Nonleukopenic Conditions

Patients who are not leukopenic may nonetheless be immunocompromised due to a functional defect in one or more components of the immune system. Patients with disruption of anatomic barriers, metabolic abnormalities, or autoimmune disease, neonates, and the elderly may all be considered to be immunocompromised (see list opposite).

Nonleukopenic Immunocompromised Patients

Disrupted anatomic barriers
- Burns
- Trauma
- Indwelling catheters
  - Urinary
  - Central venous access (Hickman and Broviac)

Metabolic abnormalities
- Malnutrition
- Diabetes mellitus
- Alcoholism
- Drug abuse
- Pregnancy

Autoimmune disease
- Rheumatoid arthritis
- Systemic lupus erythematosus

Organ dysfunction
- Hepatic insufficiency
- Functional or anatomic asplenia
- Uremia/hemodialysis

Organ transplant
- Renal
- Cardiac
- Liver

Organ Transplant

Another important category of immunocompromised patients is those with organ transplants. Virtually all of these patients develop infections because they are treated aggressively with corticosteroids and other drugs that depress CMI.

Renal transplantation is now a relatively common procedure because of medical advances such as improved use of immunosuppressive drugs. Bone marrow, cardiac, and liver transplantation are becoming more common. Patients with cardiac and liver transplants have infections similar to patients with renal transplants. Patients with bone marrow transplants are at risk for all types of infections because they are given drugs to destroy all leukocytes, both those circulating and those in the bone marrow.

Patients with renal transplants acquire infections due to a wide variety of microorganisms. There is a definite relationship between the organism(s) causing infection and the length of time after transplantation that the infection occurs (see Fig. 61-1). Cytomegalovirus is a particular problem in these patients, and may not only cause disease but lead to allograft dysfunction.[7] (See also Chap. 15.)

CLINICAL MANIFESTATIONS

The presentation of infectious diseases may be modified in the immunocompromised patient, who may be unable to respond normally to the infection because of the underlying disease. In the neutropenic patient, there may be no increase in the peripheral white blood cell count. In pulmonary infections, there may be little infiltrate to arouse the suspicion of the clinician. In some cases, fever may be the most visible symptom that an infectious process is developing.

Fever/Bacteremia

Fever in the immunocompromised patient may be a manifestation of underlying malignancy or a sign of infection. Febrile patients in whom infection is suspected must be treated aggressively, especially if they are neutropenic, because delays may be fatal. The abrupt appearance of fever or the detection of bacteremia should trigger a search for an underlying source of microorganisms. Perirectal lesions, the lung, and the urinary tract are common sources. It is thought that the gastrointestinal tract may be the source of organisms in a large number of cases in which no other source is identi-

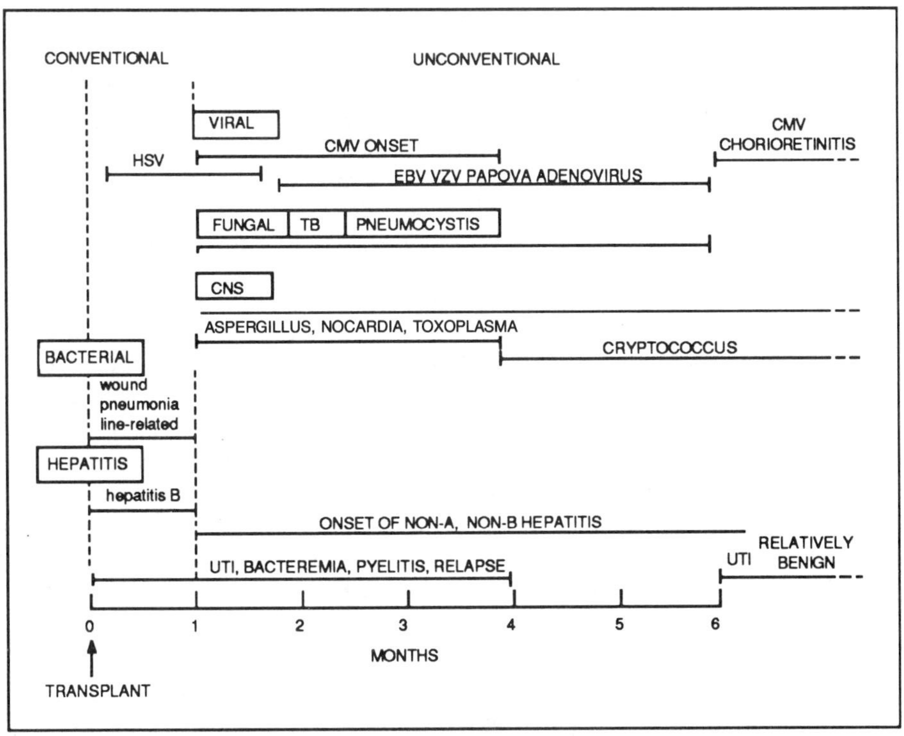

Figure 61-1 Timetable for the occurrence of infection in the renal transplant patient.

fied. Infections with Enterobacteriaceae, staphylococci, *Pseudomonas, Candida,* and *Bacteroides* may be associated with shock and lead to increased mortality. No organism may be isolated in as many as 50% of patients who appear septic. However, many of these patients respond to a course of antibiotic therapy.

Pneumonia

Pneumonia is a major cause of mortality in immunocompromised patients. Symptoms may be minimal and may not reflect the severity of disease. Fever and cough are almost always present, but sputum production may be minimal if the patient is neutropenic. The pattern of infiltrate on x-ray may not be particularly useful in determining the type of pathogen present. In general, however, bronchopneumonia with consolidation and occasional cavitation is associated with bacterial pneumonia. Interstitial pneumonia due to *Pneumocystis* or cytomegalovirus is often found. A nodular infiltrate may be associated with fungal disease. The wide variety of microorganisms that may cause disease in these patients are listed in the left hand column.

In immunocompromised patients, it is important to remember that not all radiologic evidence of pneumonia has an infectious etiology. Pneumonitis may also be present due to tumor, radiation or drug-induced injury, pulmonary hemorrhage, or edema.[2]

Organisms Causing Pneumonia in Immunocompromised Patients

Bacteria
Enterobacteriaceae
Pseudomonas aeruginosa
Staphylococcus aureus
Legionella species
Mycobacterium species

Fungi
Nocardia species
Aspergillus species
Mucor/Rhizopus
Cryptococcus neoformans

Parasites
Pneumocystis carinii
Strongyloides stercoralis (rare)

Viruses
Cytomegalovirus

Central Nervous System (CNS)

Meningitis, meningoencephalitis, and brain abscess are manifestations of CNS disease seen in immunocompromised patients. Symptoms may be minimal, such as fever and lethargy, or may be typical and include headache, stiff neck, and focal neurologic signs.

These patients, especially those who are hypogammaglobulinemic, are susceptible to meningitis caused by the same organisms that infect the normal population: *S. pneumoniae, H. influenzae,* and *N. meningitidis.* Aerobic gram-negative bacilli are a cause of meningitis in neutropenic patients, and can usually be found concurrently in the blood stream. Coagulase-negative staphylococci are the most common cause of meningitis in patients with implanted foreign bodies, such as ventriculoatrial or ventriculoperitoneal shunts or Ommaya reservoirs. Other skin flora, such as *Corynebacterium* species or viridans-group streptococci, are found less often (see list at the top of the opposite page).

In patients with defective CMI, meningitis is commonly caused by *L. monocytogenes* and *C. neoformans. Cryptococcus* infection probably occurs initially through the respiratory tract and spreads through the blood stream to the CNS. *Toxoplasma gondii* and herpes zoster may reactivate and cause meningoencephalitis in these patients. *T. gondii* and HIV are common causes of CNS disease in AIDS patients.

Fungi, such as *Aspergillus* species and *Mucor/Rhizopus* may cause both meningitis and brain abscess in immunocompromised patients. These di-

Organisms Causing CNS Disease in Immunocompromised Patients

Bacteria
Enterobacteriaceae
Pseudomonas aeruginosa
Listeria monocytogenes
Coagulase-negative *Staphylococcus* species (patients with VA or VP shunts)

Fungi
Cryptococcus neoformans
Aspergillus species
Mucor/Rhizopus

Parasites
Toxoplasma gondii
Strongyloides stercoralis (rare)

Viruses
Herpes zoster
HIV (AIDS patients)

agnoses are more often made at postmortem examinations.

Urinary Tract

Immunocompromised patients who have an indwelling urinary catheter have increased risk of developing urinary tract infection. However, this risk is due to the presence of the catheter rather than to the underlying disease, and is no different from that of other catheterized patients.

Aerobic gram-negative bacilli are isolated most commonly from urine culture. The source of the organism is usually the gastrointestinal tract. Therefore, if the patient is colonized with hospital microflora, the bacteria may be resistant to some antibiotics. It is often difficult to determine the significance of *Candida* species isolated from urine, because patients may be colonized, rather than infected with yeast, and are often asymptomatic. On the other hand, presence of *Candida* in the urine may be a manifestation of disseminated candidiasis, and these patients must be treated aggressively if they are to survive.

Other Infections

Skin infections are not an uncommon problem in immunocompromised patients. Children with leukemia are at risk for severe disseminated varicella infection. Adults with defects in CMI who have previously had chickenpox often develop zoster (shingles), a reactivation of the latent herpes zoster virus. Other types of skin lesions may be a manifestation of disseminated disease, such as the appearance of discrete maculopapular lesions in patients with disseminated candidiasis.

Gastroenteritis may be the result of therapy the patient is receiving as well as of an infectious cause. Cytotoxic drugs as well as antibiotics may cause a disturbance in bowel flora and allow overgrowth of *Clostridium difficile.* This organism produces toxin-causing diarrhea that may progress to pseudomembranous colitis. *Cryptosporidium* is a coccidian parasite that causes diarrhea and is a particular problem in AIDS patients.

LABORATORY ANALYSES AND DIAGNOSIS

When infection is suspected in the immunocompromised patient, specimens should be collected without delay because in most cases the physician must start the patient on empiric therapy as soon as possible. Direct smears should be prepared from appropriate specimens. Special histologic stains may be necessary to reveal parasites. Immunofluorescent (or immunoperoxidase) reagents are useful for detecting *Legionella* species and some viruses, especially herpes simplex and herpes zoster. Depending on the site of infection, material should be cultured for bacteria, fungi, mycobacteria, and viruses. Antimicrobial susceptibility tests should be performed on bacteria that are isolated, but it may be necessary to confer with the physician to determine which organisms are significant. Organisms that may be considered normal flora in other patients may be significant pathogens in the immunocompromised host.

Serologic studies are rarely useful in immunocompromised patients, with the exception of tests for antibodies to *Legionella pneumophila, Coccidioides immitis, Histoplasma capsulatum,* and specific serology for Epstein-Barr virus. Testing for antibodies to organisms that remain latent after initial infection is rarely useful except to establish that the patient has been exposed to the organism. Determination of IgG antibodies to herpes simplex and cytomegalovirus is not useful unless the patient is initially seronegative and becomes seropositive during an illness. It is not clear at the present time if testing for IgM antibodies will be more useful.

Fever/Bacteremia

Multiple bacterial and fungal blood cultures should be obtained on all patients with suspected bacteremia (see Chap. 59). Cultures may be collected at different times or from two different sites at the same time if there is urgency. To assess the possibility of a contaminated central venous catheter, one culture may be drawn through the catheter and another drawn through a peripheral vein. It may be difficult to assess the significance of cultures that yield organisms commonly considered contaminants, such as *Corynebacterium* species or coagulase-negative staphylococci. If these organisms are isolated from multiple cultures, they should be speciated if possible to provide additional information to aid the clinician in determining their significance. Viral blood cultures should be collected from patients at risk for CMV. Isolation of this virus from the buffy coat correlates better with presence of disease than does detection of virus shedding in urine or saliva.

Pneumonia

Sputum is the most common specimen submitted for detection of pulmonary pathogens. If the patient is neutropenic, these specimens should be evaluated microscopically by criteria that do not require the presence of neutrophils, because these may be absent due to the underlying disease. Specimens should be rejected for culture only if they contain 25 squamous epithelial cells per low-power field.

It is often difficult to assess the significance of the organisms isolated because the culture may also contain significant numbers of organisms with which the patient is colonized. More invasive procedures are often necessary to obtain diagnostic specimens. Fiberoptic bronchoscopy has all but replaced transtracheal aspiration as a method of obtaining specimens for culture and cytology. Unfortunately, bronchial wash specimens are also contaminated with oral pharyngeal flora. Specimens obtained with a catheter-protected brush theoretically may be more valuable, but in practice are also often contaminated. Transbronchial biopsies are usually more useful, especially in obtaining material for stained smears. Needle aspirates have also been used, but they may not provide adequate specimens, especially in fungal disease. Open-lung biopsy may be performed in patients when other methods of obtaining specimens do not yield a diagnosis. This provides an optimal specimen that is not contaminated by oropharyngeal flora, but the procedure is not undertaken lightly because these patients are seriously ill and may be at risk for hemorrhage.

Blood cultures should be collected when bacterial pneumonia is suspected. Pleural fluid, if present, should also be cultured.

Central Nervous System

Bacteria causing meningitis are usually isolated from cultures of cerebrospinal fluid (CSF) or ventricular fluid without difficulty unless the patient has received prior antibiotic therapy. Bacteria are often seen in the direct gram-stained smear prepared in a cytocentrifuge or from the pellet of a centrifuged specimen. Blood cultures should be collected, because these patients may be bacteremic. It is more difficult to identify the etiologic agent of meningoencephalitis or brain abscess.

Radiolabeled scans and computerized tomography may aid in discriminating between tumors and infectious processes. The etiologic agent is rarely detected in CSF, and more invasive procedures such as brain biopsy are usually required. Tissue should be obtained both for culture and for histologic examination.

In case of gastroenteritis, stool specimens should be submitted for bacterial culture because these patients may be infected with the usual stool pathogens. *Salmonella* can be a particular problem in patients with a defect in CMI, and may also be found in the blood. A test for *C. difficile* toxin should be performed if the patient has received antibiotics or chemotherapy. Stool from AIDS patients with diarrhea should be examined for *Cryptosporidium.*

Urinary Tract

Clean-catch urine specimens should be collected from uncatheterized patients. In catheterized patients, urine must be collected from the catheter, not from the bag. Specimens should be transported to the laboratory rapidly and cultured quantitatively, as with urine specimens from any patient.

Other Infections

Specimens for direct smear and culture should be collected from the affected site. Herpes zoster skin lesions are usually diagnosed clinically, but in atypical presentations fluid for virus culture should be collected from the vesicles. Material for smears may be obtained by scraping cells from the base of the lesion. It may be necessary to obtain punch biopsies from other types of skin lesions for culture and histology.

Other Laboratory Testing

It is important to monitor the hematologic status of immunocompromised patients. They will frequently be anemic and/or thrombocytopenic. Hemorrhage is a serious complication in patients with hematologic malignancies. Other laboratory analysis may be useful, depending on the organ system involved in the infection.[5]

TREATMENT

After a patient has been placed on appropriate antibiotic therapy, response to therapy should be monitored with additional cultures. If the pathogen continues to be present, antimicrobial susceptibility tests should be repeated to ensure that the organism has not acquired resistance to the antibiotic during therapy. If the organism persists during appropriate therapy, the physician should search for an underlying source of infection such as an abscess or infected catheter.

Antibiotic levels should be monitored in patients who receive the aminoglycosides gentamicin, tobramycin, and amikacin. These antibiotics have a narrow therapeutic ratio, *i.e.,* a narrow concentration range that is high enough to be inhibitory to bacteria without being so high as to cause toxicity. Although this is rarely a problem with other antibiotics, the physician may wish to monitor therapy to ensure that adequate antibiotic levels have been achieved.

In serious infections, it may be useful to monitor the level of bacteriostatic or bactericidal activity present in a patient's serum. This measures the sum of specific and nonspecific factors present, including antibiotics, in the serum. However, there are no well-defined guidelines as to necessary levels, especially in immunocompromised patients. (See also Chap. 63.)

CASE STUDY

A 61-year-old man had been diagnosed as having a mesothelioma six months prior to his present hospital admission. At that time a central venous catheter had been inserted for intravenous access. Ten days ago he had received a course of chemotherapy and had been hospitalized since then. He developed a fever of 102° F, chills, and sweats. He had no other symptoms except a mild cough. There was no dysuria, hematuria, or flank pain.

The total white blood cell count was 1.0×10^3 cells/mm^3 with three segs and the remainder lymphocytes and monocytes. The urinalysis was unremarkable. Blood cultures were drawn, one from the access line and two from peripheral veins. The patient was started on vancomycin and ceftazidime pending results of the culture.

Coagulase-negative staphylococci were isolated from all three cultures. The organisms were later identified as *Staphylococcus warnerii.* Susceptibility tests showed the organism to be resistant to penicillin, oxacillin, and erythromycin, and sensitive to vancomycin.

Ceftazidime was discontinued, and the patient was treated with vancomycin for 10 days. Two days later, the patient again developed a fever of 102° F and chills. Blood cultures again yielded coagulase-negative staphylococci identified as *S. warnerii.*

Questions

1. What is the most likely source of the infection, and what laboratory results confirm this conclusion?
2. Explain the white blood cell findings.
3. After finding the organism persisting after antibiotic therapy, what steps should be taken?

Discussion

1. The central venous catheter is a likely source of infection with skin flora such as coagulase-negative staphylococci. The isolation of the same species from the catheter site as well as from peripheral veins confirms this conclusion.
2. Immunosuppression due to chemotherapy is often characterized by granulocytopenia. In this event white cell counts are not high, even when infection exists.
3. The patient should be treated again with vancomycin, and the central venous catheter should be replaced. Blood cultures obtained after treatment should remain negative.

REFERENCES

1. Grieco MH (ed): Infections in the Abnormal Host. New York City, Yorke Medical Books, 1980
2. Rubin RH, Young LS (eds): Clinical Approach to Infections in the Immunocompromised Patient. New York City, Plenum, 1981
3. Young LS: Nosocomial infections in the immunocompromised adult. Am J Med 70:398–404, 1981
4. Singer C, Kaplan NH, Armstrong D: Bacteremia and fungemia complicating neoplastic disease. Am J Med 62:731–742, 1977
5. Sculier JP, Klastersky J: Significance of serum bactericidal activity in gram-negative bacillary bacteremia in patients with and without granulocytopenia. Am J Med 76:429–435, 1984
6. Gottlieb MS, Groopman JE: Acquired Immune Deficiency Syndrome. New York City, Alan R. Liss, 1984
7. Rubin RH, Wolfson JS, Cosimi AB et al: Infection in the renal transplant recipient. Am J Med 70:405–411, 1981

Chapter 62

Osteomyelitis

Louis B. Caruana

Although *osteomyelitis* refers to an inflammation of the bone and bone marrow, the term is also popularly used to refer to infection of the bone marrow cavity and the bone itself. The infection is usually caused by gram-positive cocci such as *Staphylococcus aureus,* but a variety of gram-negative bacteria, fungi, rickettsiae, and viruses may be implicated as the etiologic agent. The number of unusual organisms that have been found to cause osteomyelitis is expanding. *Staphylococcus* is the most commonly isolated infectious agent in pyogenic osteomyelitis, however. Pyogenic osteomyelitis was a major orthopedic problem before the introduction of chemotherapeutic and antimicrobial agents in the 1940s.

ETIOLOGY AND PATHOPHYSIOLOGY

Osteomyelitis may affect any age group or either sex, but the disease is usually found in children and adolescents in whom bone is still growing. Pyogenic vertebral osteomyelitis is uncommon in children under the age of 10 years. From ages 10 to 19 there is increased frequency in this form of the disease, but the majority of cases occur in males after the age of 50. Diabetics, as well as other compromised hosts such as heroin addicts, appear to have a predilection for vertebral osteomyelitis. Infections of the bones are usually the result of blood-borne (hematogenous) spread to the infected site, but may also result from trauma with secondary infection. Osteomyelitis may also arise by spread of infection from a contiguous abscess; however, involvement of the bone in addition to subcutaneous or surrounding tissues must be confirmed.[1] Increasingly common forms of this disease are vertebral osteomyelitis, seen in immunocompromised adults,[2, 3, 4] and clavicular osteomyelitis, a complication of subclavian catheter usage.[5] Osteomyelitis of the pubis has been reported after surgical procedures such as prostatectomy, bladder resection, and urethral suspension.[6] Osteomyelitis of the skull bones has been reported, but is a relatively rare disease.[7] Today acute osteomyelitis occurs less frequently because of effective antimicrobial treatment. However, if treatment is not adequate in amount or duration, chronic osteomyelitis will result.[8]

The onset of acute osteomyelitis is usually abrupt but can be insidious. If the infected bone or bones are left untreated or inadequately treated, chronic osteomyelitis results in avascular necrosis of the affected site. No specific criteria separate acute from chronic osteomyelitis. Clinically, newly diagnosed bone infection is considered acute, whereas recurrent infection, characterized by the presence of a large area of dead bone (sequestrum), is considered the chronic stage of the disease. The high frequency of infection of the metaphyses of the bone suggests that this site is susceptible to bacterial infection. It is possible that the decreased blood flow with subsequent decreased numbers of phagocytes favors the growth of organisms at this site, and consequently their spread to the entire bone. Because children with rich red-marrowed bones are affected more commonly than adults, it has been suggested that bones rich in red marrow favor bacterial colonization.

Etiologic agents responsible for osteomyelitis reach the bones through one of three routes: (1) by hematogenous spread, (2) by extension from a contiguous site of infection, and (3) by direct penetration through the overlaying skin as a result of trauma or surgery.

Hematogenous Causes

S. aureus causes 60% to 90% of acute hematogenous bone infections in children under the age of 12, although adults can be affected as well.[9, 10, 11] Acute hematogenous osteomyelitis in children frequently localizes in the diaphyseal end of the long bones, especially the femur and tibia. The infection originates in the metaphyseal sinusoidal veins, where blood flow is diminished and the lack of phagocytic leukocytes favors the growth of infectious organisms. *Streptococcus pyogenes* and *Staphylococcus* species other than *aureus,* as well as gram-negative bacilli, may be implicated. The number of unusual organisms found to cause osteomyelitis is expanding, possibly due to better isolation and identification methods. Gram-negative bacilli are responsible for vertebral infections in adults, while Group B streptococci are emerging as an agent frequently found in neonatal osteomyelitis.[8] Osteomyelitis is a well-recognized complication of sickle cell disease; although its etiologic agent is usually *Salmonella,* it may be caused by other gram-negative organisms such as *Escherichia coli* or *Hemophilis influenzae*[12, 13] and anaerobes such as *Bacteroides* species or *Actinomyces* species.[14]

A single microbic organism is usually responsible for the infection in hematogenous osteomyelitis. Polymicrobic hematogenous osteomyelitis is rare.

Contiguous Focus

Bone infections from a contiguous abscess can have a wide range of etiologic agents and, according to some reports, may even be polymicrobic. *S. aureus* is the organism isolated most commonly in these cases, but a variety of gram-negative organisms may be implicated, especially in the immunocompromised patient.[15] Novel routes of bone infection should not be overlooked. For example, sneakers were found to be the source of *Pseudomonas aeruginosa* in children with osteomyelitis of the foot following puncture wounds.[16, 17] Human bites, if deep enough, may result in osteomyelitis due to indigenous anaerobic mouth flora. The pathogen most frequently isolated from wounds inflicted by domestic animal bites is *Pasteurella multocida,* but other species such as *P. pneumotropica, P. ureae, P. haemolytica,* and *Eikenella corrodens* may be isolated in cases of contiguous focus etiology.[18, 19] Because the infection develops as a direct extention of the local infection, multiple aerobic and anaerobic bacteria may be isolated from the infected bone.

Direct Penetration via Trauma or Surgery

Penetrating trauma or surgery, in which local infection gains access to traumatized bone, offers another focus route of infection. Insertion of prostheses in or adjacent to the bone and other surgical procedures for nontraumatic bone or joint disorders offer additional routes of infection. The likely organism implicated is *S. aureus,* but aerobic gram-negative bacilli may be the causative agent as well.[20]

CLINICAL MANIFESTATIONS

Acute Osteomyelitis

Acute osteomyelitis should be suspected in febrile patients with localized bone pain. Generally it is characterized by local pain, fever, and tenderness to palpitation over the affected site. Infections usually occur in the hip, vertebrae, sacroiliac joints, or other deep-seated bones.[21, 22] The clinician should suspect osteomyelitis in cases of rheumatic fever, rheumatoid arthritis, septic arthritis, cellulitis, and tumor. Hematogenous infection of a long bone in children or a vertebra in adults may be more easily overlooked than an infected peripheral joint.

The abrupt onset of pain of increasing severity and fever are the cardinal signs of osteomyelitis. Irritability, lethargy, and often dehydration are present as well. The symptoms are both local and general, depending upon the bones affected. The local symptoms are pain and tenderness at the end of a long bone, with acute inflammation. Back pain may be a diagnostic clue to vertebral osteomyelitis if other causes of the pain are ruled out.[4]

Back and neck pain, with or without rigidity, is a common complaint, and is seen in at least 90% of cases. Atypical symptoms include occipital, arm, chest, abdominal, or leg pains.

Pubic bone pain or tenderness should alert the clinician to possible osteomyelitis of the pubis. This is a rare but serious infection resulting from bacteremia following pelvic surgery or trauma.[6]

Chronic Osteomyelitis

Chronic osteomyelitis is usually seen in adults and is associated with underlying predisposing factors such as vascular disease, history of postoperative infection, heroin addiction, hemodialysis, or hemoglobinopathy. Some patients tolerate chronic osteomyelitis well, with symptoms that are nonspecific but may include local swelling and pain in the affected bone. Sequestrum formation is frequent, and sinuses may develop that drain the bone abscess to the surface.

LABORATORY ANALYSES AND DIAGNOSIS

Although radiographic or radionuclide studies may be helpful, definitive diagnosis of osteomyelitis rests on the isolation and identification of the etiologic agent from blood cultures or from a biopsy of the bone lesion itself. *S. aureus* is the leading pathogen, but other microbes may be identified as well. *Mycobacterium tuberculosis,* for example, can produce a chronic vertebral osteomyelitis. Blood cultures should include both aerobic and anaerobic phases, and should include methods to isolate unusual etiologic organisms such as *Aspergillus, Candida,* and *Rhizopus.* Multiple blood cultures may be necessary to isolate and identify the etiologic agent; however, if they are negative, bone biopsy material should be cultured to establish the diagnosis.[21, 23] Culture of sinus tract drainage is not reliable and should not be recommended.[20]

Bone scanning often shows positive results before roentgenographic findings appear; however, bone scans may give false-negative results, especially in neonates. Bone biopsy remains the procedure of choice for establishing a definitive diagnosis in patients suspected clinically of having osteomyelitis who have negative roentgenographic or bone scans.[22, 24]

Often the erythrocyte sedimentation rate (ESR) is elevated in pyogenic vertebral osteomyelitis, and this may be of value in both diagnosis and followup studies.[25] The ESR may or may not be elevated in other sites of infection and, therefore, has limited diagnostic value there. Acute phase reactants, *e.g.*, C-reactive protein, may also be elevated.[17] Routine blood counts are frequently of no value, but leukocytosis is often present in children with acute osteomyelitis. Serologic tests, *e.g.*, teichoic acid antibody, have recently been evaluated for *S. aureus* osteomyelitis and have been found to be a useful diagnostic tool.[26]

TREATMENT

Antimicrobial susceptibility studies should be performed on all organisms isolated from specimens appropriately collected from legitimate sites of the bone or from blood cultures. Precise bacteriologic identification is essential for appropriate antimicrobial therapy.[27] Acute hematogenous osteomyelitis is often a life-threatening disease in children, and thus early treatment with antibiotics is essential to obviate the need for surgery.[9] Surgical débridement is necessary if radiologic evidence of bone destruction is present or if there is soft tissue fluctuance, indicating abscess formation.

Treatment may be difficult because the identity of the etiologic organism may be unresolved. If the causative agent cannot be determined in a patient with clinical symptoms, empiric antimicrobial therapy should be instituted. Its spectrum should include *S. aureus* as well as gram-negative bacilli and anaerobes. Clindamycin, oxacillin, or penicillin G, depending on β-lactamase results, and tobramycin may be an effective battery; however, susceptibility studies should be considered first.[6, 8, 28] Under current federal regulations there are incentives to reduce the length of hospital stays; thus outpatient treatment for some cases of osteomyelitis may be indicated.[29]

Prophylactic use of antimicrobial agents might be useful in cases of contiguous infection. Osteomyelitis associated with a prosthesis generally requires the removal of the appliance and the initiation of appropriate antimicrobial therapy.

CASE STUDY #1

A 67-year-old white man was admitted to the hospital for coronary bypass surgery. On the third postoperative day he developed fever (39° C) and complained of dysuria and persistent back pain. Conservative treatment with gentamycin was instituted. After a few days, the patient improved and was discharged. Five days later he was readmitted with low back pain and chills. Urinalysis was within normal limits, the WBC count was $11.0 \times 10^3/mm^3$, and the ESR was 136 mm/hr (Westergren). Open vertebral biopsy was performed, and culture of disc material revealed *Pseudomonas aeruginosa.* Treatment with tobramycin was begun, and the patient subsequently improved.

Questions

1. What is the most likely source of this organism, and how was it disseminated?
2. What is the relationship between vertebral osteomyelitis and this source of the infection?

Discussion

1. Clinical findings suggest a urinary tract infection from which the organism spread by hematogenous means.
2. Review of the literature reveals that 28.5% of genitourinary tract infections result in vertebral

osteomyelitis. The onset of spinal or vertebral osteomyelitis is usually insidious, with symptoms of back pain and muscle rigidity. Delayed diagnosis is believed to be the most important reason for 7% incidence of neurologic complications secondary to vertebral osteomyelitis.[4] Further review of the literature documents two cases of adult vertebral osteomyelitis secondary to *Hemophilus influenzae,* serotypes b and c respectively. Symptomatology for both cases was similar to that in the above case; however, no source of or predisposing factor for the infection could be identified. Both patients recovered following specific antimicrobial treatment.[3]

CASE STUDY #2

A two-week-old neonate was referred to the hospital by a health visitor because the baby disliked passive movement of the left arm. The mother reported that the patient had been feverish and was not feeding well. Radiographic films of the left shoulder excluded a fracture, and a consultant pediatrician diagnosed Erb's palsy. One week later the physical therapist, at an outpatient session, noticed that the girl cried when the left arm was moved. Repeat x-ray films revealed an osteolytic lesion of the humerus with a periosteal reaction. A bone scan was normal, however.

Questions

1. What organism is a likely cause of osteomyelitis in this age group?
2. What steps should be taken, and how often will this condition be encountered?

Discussion

1. *Streptococcus agalactiae,* grown in pus from the shoulder joint, is a likely cause of the osteomyelitis.
2. The patient should be placed on specific antimicrobial treatment until symptoms clear.

Neonatal osteomyelitis is rare. Early diagnosis is essential for effective treatment. Neonatal osteomyelitis should be considered in the differential diagnosis of neonates presenting postnatally with limb palsy. Group B streptococcus and *S. aureus* are two of the microbes commonly isolated in these cases.[30]

REFERENCES

1. Schmid FR: Infections: Arthritis and osteomyelitis. Prim Care 2(2):295, 1984
2. Modic MT et al: Vertebral osteomyelitis: Assessment using MR. Radiology 157 (1):157, 1985
3. Holzgang J et al: Adult vertebral osteomyelitis caused by *Haemophilus influenzae.* Clin Microbiol 3 (3):261, 1984
4. William MR, Berry PH: *Pseudomonas* vertebral osteomyelitis following open heart surgery: Case report. Texas Med 80:47, 1984
5. Joklik WK, Willett HP, Amons DB (eds): Zinsser Microbiology, 18th ed, p 456. Norwalk, Connecticut, Appleton-Century-Crofts, 1984
6. Hoyme UB et al: Osteomyelitis pubis after radial gynecologic operations. Obstet Gynecol 63(3 suppl):475, 1984
7. Balm AJM et al: Osteomyelitis in the head and neck. J Laryngol Otol 99 (10):1059, 1985
8. Waldvogel FA, Vasey H: Osteomyelitis: The past decade. N Engl J Med 303:360, 1980
9. Morrey BF, Peterson HA: Hematogenous pyogenic osteomyelitis in children. Orthoped Clin North Am 6:935, 1975
10. Mollan RAB, Piggot J: Acute osteomyelitis in children. J Bone Joint Surg [Br] 59:2, 1977
11. Turck M, Counts GW: Staphylococcal infections. In Isselbacher KJ et al (eds): Harrison's Principles of Internal Medicine, 10th ed, p 925. New York City, McGraw-Hill, 1983
12. Barter SJ, Hennessy O: Actinomycetes as the causative organism of osteomyelitis in sickle cell disease. Skeletal Radiol 111:271, 1984
13. Mallouh A, Talab Y: Bone and joint infection in patients with sickle cell disease. J Pediatr Orthoped 5:158, 1985
14. Vichinsky EP, Lubin BH: Sickle cell anemia and related hemoglobinopathies. Pediatr Clin North Am 27:429, 1980
15. Fierer J et al: The fetid foot: Lower extremity infections in patients with diabetes mellitus. Rev Infect Dis 1:210, 1979

16. Fisher MC et al: Sneakers as a source of *Pseudomonas aeruginosa* in children with osteomyelitis following puncture wounds. J Pediatr 106(4):607, 1985
17. Crosby LA, Powell DA: The potential value of the sedimentation rate in monitoring treatment outcome in puncture-wound-related *Pseudomonas* osteomyelitis. Clin Orthop 188:168, 1984
18. Gadberry JL et al: *Pasteurella pneumotropica* isolated from bone and joint infections. J Clin Microbiol 19(6):926, 1984
19. Shimizu K et al: *Eikenella corrodens* tenosynovitis and osteomyelitis of the hand: A case report. Arch Jpn Chir 53(6):800, 1984
20. Andreoli TE, Carpenter CCJ, Plum F et al (eds): Osteomyelitis, p 596. Philadelphia, WB Saunders, 1986
21. Norden CW: Osteomyelitis. In Stein JH (ed): Internal Medicine, p 1226. Boston, Little, Brown & Co, 1983
22. Wheat J: Diagnostic strategies in osteomyelitis. Am J Med 78(6B):218, 1985
23. Dich VQ et al: Osteomyelitis in infants and children: A review of 163 cases. Am J Dis Child 129:1273, 1975
24. Fletcher BD et al: Osteomyelitis in children: Detection by magnetic resonance. Pediatr Radiol 150:57, 1984
25. Kern RZ, Houpt JB: Pyogenic vertebral osteomyelitis: Diagnosis and management. Can Med Assoc J 130:1025, 1984
26. Wheat LJ et al: Serological diagnosis of *Staphylococcus aureus* osteomyelitis. J Clin Microbiol 21:764, 1985
27. Ray CG: Bone and joint infections. In Sherris JC (ed): Medical Microbiology: An Introduction to Infectious Diseases, p 562. New York City, Elsevier, 1984
28. Hirschmann JV: Osteomyelitis. In Isselbacher KJ et al (eds): Harrison's Principles of Internal Medicine, 10th ed, p 1972. New York City, McGraw-Hill, 1983
29. Tomczak RL: Outpatient treatment of osteomyelitis. J Am Podiatr Med Assoc 75(5):261, 1985
30. Isaacs D, Bower DB, Moxon ER: Neonatal osteomyelitis presenting as nerve palsy. Br Med J 292:1071, 1986

BIBLIOGRAPHY

Bannatyne RM, Saunders EF: Anaerobic osteomyelitis in sickle cell disease: Associated pathophysiology. Am J Pediatr Hematol Oncol 7:301, 1985

Barnwell PA et al: *Aspergillus* osteomyelitis: Report of a case and review of the literature. Diagn Microbiol Infect Dis 3:515, 1985

Bar-Ziv J et al: Rib osteomyelitis in children: Early radiologic and ultrasonic findings. Pediatr Radiol 15:315, 1985

Bracikowski JP et al: *Campylobacter* osteomyelitis. South Med J 77:1611, 1984

Burns JR, Gregory JG: Osteomyelitis of the pubic symphysis after urologic surgery. J Urol 118:803, 1977

Cole WG, Dalyiel RE, Leitl S: Treatment of acute osteomyelitis in childhood. J Bone Joint Surg 64B:218, 1982

del Busto R, Quinn EL, Fisher EJ: Osteomyelitis of the pubis. JAMA 248:1498, 1982

Duszynski DO et al: Early radionuclide diagnosis of acute osteomyelitis. Radiology 117:337, 1975

Emslie KR, Fenner LM, Nade ML: Acute haematogenous osteomyelitis: II. The effect of a metaphyseal abscess on the surrounding blood supply. J Pathol 142:129, 1984

Fitzgerald RH, Kelly PJ: Recurrent sepsis, malignant change, and sarcoidosis following posttraumatic osteomyelitis. In Hierholzer G, Lob G (eds): Posttraumatic Osteomyelitis. New York City, Springer-Verlag, 1980

Gillespie KM, Mayo KM: The management of acute haematogenous osteomyelitis in infants and children. Am J Dis Child 129:1273, 1975

Goldenberg OL, Reed JI: Bacterial arthritis. N Engl J Med 312:764, 1985

Hall BB, Rosenblatt JE, Fitzgerald RH: Anaerobic septic arthritis and osteomyelitis. Orthop Clin North Am 15(3):505, 1984

Javaloyas M et al: Bilateral and symmetrical osteomyelitis due to gram-negative bacilli: A report on two cases. Scand J Rheumatol 14:289, 1985

Keeley K, Buchanon GR: Acute infarction of long bones in children with sickle cell anemia. J Pediatr 101:170, 1982

Koch SE, Wintroub BU: Pott's puffy tumor: A clinical marker for osteomyelitis of the skull. Arch Dermatol 121:548, 1985

Lang AG, Peterson HA: Osteomyelitis following puncture wounds of the foot in children. J Trauma 16:993, 1976

Levine AM, Meier P, Dorfman HA: Case report 329 (osteomyelitis of humerus bone). Skeletal Radiol 14:152, 1985

Lewis RP, Sutter VL, Finegold SM: Bone infections involving anaerobic bacteria. Medicine (Baltimore) 57:279, 1978

Lindenbaum S, Alexander H: Infections simulating bone tumors: A review of subacute osteomyelitis. Clin Orthop 184:193, 1984

Musher DM et al: Vertebral osteomyelitis: Still a diagnostic pitfall. Arch Intern Med 136:105, 1976

Nathan C: Cryptococcal osteomyelitis treated with 5-fluorocytosine. Am Rev Respir Dis 110:78, 1974

Osborn R et al: Osteomyelitis of the mandible in a patient with malignant osteopetrosis. J Oral Med 40(2):76, 1985

Schmid FR: Principles of diagnosis and treatment of bone and joint infections. In McCarty DJ (ed): Arthritis and Allied Conditions, 10th ed. Philadelphia, Lea & Febiger, 1984

Siebert WT, Dewan S, Williams TW: *Pseudomonas* puncture wound osteomyelitis in adults. Am J Med Sci 283:83, 1982

Skevis XA: Primary subacute osteomyelitis of the talus. J Bone Joint Surg (Br) 66B:101, 1984

Slagel SA, Skiendzielewski JJ, McMurry FG: Osteomyelitis of the cervical spine: Reversible quadriplegia resulting from Philadelphia collar placement. Am Emerg Med 14(9):912, 1985

Varros PN et al: Chronic plasma cell osteomyelitis. J Am Pediatr Med Assoc 75:258, 1985

Worsaae N, Reibel J, Rechnitzer C: Tuberculous osteomyelitis of the mandible. Br J Oral Maxillofac Surg 22:93, 1984

Chapter 63

Antimicrobials

Janice M. Klaassen

One of the primary functions of the microbiology laboratory is to guide the physician in the choice of the appropriate antimicrobial therapy, when and if such therapy is indicated. To perform this service, the laboratory must have sufficient information about the patient's history and condition, the infecting organisms, possible antimicrobial agents for treatment, and relative cost of treatment.

In order to make the most efficient choice of antimicrobial drugs for testing, a clear understanding of the pharmacology and pharmacokinetics of the agents is necessary. Many antimicrobial agents are effective only in certain areas of the body, against a narrow group of organisms, or under very specific conditions of *p*H and temperature. Because of these circumstances, there is no reason to test the agent when the situation precludes its use. Reporting results when this occurs may in fact give misleading information to the physician, inappropriately indicating the possibility of the agent's effectiveness or sanctioning its use. Just as most laboratories calculate a "normal range" in chemistry and hematology for their patient populations, each laboratory should select the most appropriate antimicrobial agents for susceptibility testing in its own special setting. This will enable the laboratory to report the most useful information for the type of infection, site of infection, and patient conditions, including age or underlying disease states.

CLASSES OF ANTIMICROBIALS AND MODES OF ACTION

Penicillins

The antimicrobial agent penicillin was discovered by Fleming in 1929, but was not widely used until World War II. Its mechanism of action is to inhibit the cell wall synthesis of bacteria. There are many steps in this synthesizing process, and the penicillins may act on more than one.[1] Because mammalian cells lack cell walls, penicillins are among the least toxic antimicrobial agents. They are the drug of choice whenever the infecting organism is susceptible and the patient has no history of adverse reactions.[2]

The basic structure of the penicillins contains two rings (thiazolidine and β-lactam) and a variable side chain. Each change in the structure of the side chain forms a new penicillin and accounts for the different characteristics of the individual penicillins. The β-lactam ring provides penicillin with its bactericidal activity, and is also the target of the majority of resistance mechanisms.

The primary means of resistance to the penicillins is a plasmid-induced production of β-lactamase, an enzyme that splits the β-lactam ring, rendering the penicillin molecule inactive. This enzyme can be an exogenous product of the organism conveying "resistance" to the surroundings (*e.g., Staphylococcus aureus*) or incorporated into its cell wall (some gram-negative bacilli). Other gram-negative organisms may be resistant due to the inability of the penicillin molecule to break through the protein outer coat to reach the cell wall.[3]

The penicillins can be divided into three major categories: natural, penicillinase-resistant, and increased-spectrum penicillins (see list below). The natural penicillins, including penicillin G and V, are useful for treatment of most infections caused by gram-positive organisms and gram-negative cocci.[4] The penicillinase-resistant penicillins, *e.g.,* methicillin, are active against β-lactamase-produc-

Classifications of Penicillins

Natural Penicillins
Penicillin G
Penicillin V
Phenbenicillin
Phenethicillin
Propicillin

Penicillinase-Resistant Penicillins
Cloxacillin
Dicloxacillin
Methicillin
Nafcillin
Oxacillin

Increased-Spectrum Penicillins
Amoxicillin
Ampicillin
Azlocillin
Carbenicillin
Hetacillin
Mezlocillin
Piperacillin
Ticarcillin

ing *S. aureus* in addition to the organisms mentioned. The increased-spectrum penicillins are active against gram-negative bacilli because of the ability to cross the protein barrier outside their cell wall. Some of these agents (*e.g.*, carbenicillin) are also active against *Pseudomonas aeruginosa,* but most are sensitive to β-lactamase.[5]

Cephalosporins

The cephalosporins have many characteristics in common with the penicillins: they were originally derived from molds; they contain a β-lactam ring, providing the same general mechanism of antimicrobial activity; they are bactericidal; and the side chain confers the functional differences. Instead of a thiazolidine ring, however, the cephalosporins contain a dihydrothiazine ring, which may account for some increased activity against gram-negative organisms.

The cephalosporins are grouped on the basis of their general activity (see list opposite). The spectrum of the "first-generation" cephalosporins is very similar to that of the penicillinase-resistant penicillin group, which has activity against most gram-positive organisms and only minimal activity against gram-negatives.[6] The "second-generation" cephalosporins have an increased spectrum of activity against gram-negatives, with similar activity against gram-positives.[6] The "third-generation" cephalosporins have an even larger spectrum of activity against gram-negative organisms, but have decreased activity against the gram-positives. Some of the third-generation cephalosporins are even active against *P. aeruginosa.*[7] Even with their high margin of therapeutic safety, third-generation cephalosporins are most often reserved for severe and/or life-threatening infections or when the alternative is multiple antibiotic therapy, due to their relatively high cost compared to that of other agents with similar spectrums of activity.[8, 9]

Resistance mechanisms to the cephalosporins are similar to those found with the penicillin group. Like the penicillins, the cephalosporins have a very high therapeutic index for safety and are the drug of choice when the organisms are susceptible. The cephalosporins are excreted by the kidney, achieving very high urinary tract levels, but patients with renal disease may need a modified course of treatment.[7] First- and second-generation cephalosporins do not cross into the cerebrospinal fluid (CSF) even in the presence of inflammation. Third-generation cephalosporins are well absorbed into the CSF; this, coupled with their activity against gram-negative organisms, makes third-generation

Classifications of Cephalosporins

First-Generation Cephalosporins

Cefadroxil
Cefazolin
Cephalexin
Cephalothin
Cephapirin
Cephaloridine
Cephradine

Second-Generation Cephalosporins

Cefaclor
Cefamandole
Cefmetazole
Cefonicid
Ceforanide
Cefotiam
Cefoxitin
Cefuroxime

Third-Generation Cephalosporins

Moxalactam
Cefbuperazone
Cefmenoxime
Cefoperazone
Cefotaxime
Cefotetan
Cefpiramide
Cefsulodin
Ceftazidime
Ceftizoxime
Ceftriaxone

cephalosporins the treatment of choice for most cases of gram-negative meningitis.[7]

Aminoglycosides/Aminocyclitols

The aminoglycoside/aminocyclitol group of antimicrobial agents has been among the antimicrobials most commonly used since the first was discovered in 1943. They are active against a wide variety of gram-negative and gram-positive organisms, both aerobic and facultative. The transport mechanism required to enter the bacterial cell relies on oxidative phosphorylation; therefore, anaerobes and other strictly fermentative bacteria are generally resistant. The mechanism of action is inhibition of protein synthesis by attacking one or more of the binding sites on the bacterial ribosomes.[10] Aminoglycosides are selective for bacterial cells because they are not actively transported into eukaryotic cells, nor do they act on eukaryotic ribosomes. Bacterial resistance to the aminoglycosides can involve the inability of the drug to gain access into the cell, *e.g.*, anaerobes, or can be due to plasmid-mediated enzymes produced by the bacterium that modify an essential portion of the molecule, rendering it inactive, *e.g.*, enzymes that acetylate.[11, 12]

The aminoglycosides (see list below) differ by the number and type of the amino-sugars that are attached to an aminocyclitol ring core. These sugars are bound by a glycosidic bond—hence the name aminoglycoside. Streptomycin, isolated from *Streptomyces griseus*, is of historical interest and was originally used for the treatment of tuberculosis. Gentamicin, derived from *Micromonospora* species, is the aminoglycoside most commonly used for infections due to gram-negative bacilli, including *Pseudomonas* species. It is relatively inexpensive compared to other aminoglycosides and "third-generation" cephalosporins. Tobramycin, derived from *Streptomyces* species, is similar to gentamicin in spectrum of activity and has slightly more resistance to inactivating enzymes. For this reason, tobramycin should not be used unless the organism is resistant to gentamicin. Amikacin is a semisynthetic aminoglycoside with less activity against *Pseudomonas* species but also less susceptibility to the inactivating enzymes than other aminoglycosides. Like tobramycin, it should be reserved for situations where it is absolutely needed. Spectinomycin is not a true aminoglycoside but an aminocyclitol ring compound. It has an inhibitory mechanism of action similar to that of the aminoglycosides, but has a different pattern of toxicity. Spectinomycin is primarily used for the treatment of *Neisseria gonorrhoeae*.[13]

Aminoglycosides and Aminocyclitols

Amikacin
Gentamicin
Kanamycin
Neomycin
Netilmicin
Spectinomycin
Streptomycin
Tobramycin

Aminoglycosides, given parenterally, are well distributed throughout the body, but only by intrathecal administration can therapeutic levels be attained in CSF.[14, 15] Aminoglycosides are not metabolized but are eliminated unchanged, primarily by the kidney. For this reason, patients with diminished renal function must have modified treatment schedules. Toxic side-effects of the aminoglycosides are usually dose-related.[16]

Damage to the eighth cranial nerve, either the auditory or the vestibular portion, and the kidney can be seen with any of these agents.[17] Lower levels of an aminoglycoside can often be used when coupled with a β-lactam antimicrobial agent, which facilitates the transport of the aminoglycoside into the bacterium by causing cell wall defects. The combination of β-lactam and aminoglycoside agents is also used for the initial treatment of life-threatening infections before susceptibility testing can be performed. In general, the use of aminoglycosides should be limited to situations in which infections are life-threatening, when susceptibility testing indicates the organism is resistant to other less toxic agents, or when these resistant organisms are expected.

Tetracyclines

Tetracyclines, like the aminoglycosides, are inhibitors of protein synthesis by ribosome interference, but are transported into the cells by a different mechanism.[18] They are effective against a very broad spectrum of organisms, but are bacteristatic. Tetracyclines can be divided into two (or three) groups, based on rate of clearance from the serum (see list below). Distribution in the tissues and serum varies with the individual tetracycline, as does the method of inactivation and excretion.[19] Most tetracyclines are excreted by the kidney in the active form, although some are inactivated by the liver or other nonrenal mechanisms. Patients with poor renal function may require modification of dosage or another antimicrobial agent.[20]

The primary means of resistance against the tetracyclines is an inhibition of transport into the bacterial cell, and heavy use of these compounds has made resistant strains common.[21] Toxic side-effects of the tetracyclines are usually related to gastrointestinal upset. All tetracyclines are chelated by divalent cations: Ca^{2+} or Mg^{2+}. For this reason, tetracyclines are not absorbed well when taken with a meal containing milk or other dairy products, or with antacids.[22] Tetracyclines are easily bound to calcium and actively deposited in new bone and teeth, causing a yellowish discoloration. They should not be given to children developing adult teeth or to women during the last 25 weeks of pregnancy.[23, 24, 25]

Classification of Tetracyclines

Short-Acting Tetracyclines
Oxytetracycline
Tetracycline

Intermediate-Acting Tetracyclines
Methacycline
Demeclocycline

Long-Acting Tetracyclines
Doxycycline
Minocycline

Chloramphenicol

Chloramphenicol's mechanism of action is inhibition of protein synthesis by reversibly binding to ribosomes, preventing attachment of the next amino acid. Because this binding is reversible, its action is bacteristatic.[26] Chloramphenicol is available for parenteral or oral use and is well distributed throughout the body, including the CSF. It is active against a broad spectrum of both gram-positive and gram-negative organisms, *Chlamydia, Rickettsia,* and *Mycoplasma* species. Given all of these factors, it is unfortunate that the fact that this agent may have very negative side-effects has limited its use.

The major side-effects of chloramphenicol are usually divided into two categories.[27, 28, 29] The first is a dosage-dependent, reversible bone marrow depression that can be seen in long-term or high-dosage protocols. Once treatment has been stopped, the bone marrow recovers and the peripheral blood picture returns to normal. For this reason, patients on chloramphenicol should have their peripheral white blood cell count monitored periodically. The other type is not dosage-dependent, but has shown some genetic predisposition. In these patients a severe aplastic anemia develops, weeks or even months after therapy has been stopped. This side-effect is associated with a high mortality rate, and as yet there is no way to predict which patients will be affected.

Resistance to chloramphenicol can be caused by the inability of the agent to permeate the bacterial cell wall or by bacterial enzymes that convert the agent to an inactive form.[30, 31]

Chloramphenicol is metabolized by the liver to an inactive form, and then excreted by the kidney. Patients with renal disease, therefore, do not usually require any modification of dosage. Patients with poor liver function may need changes based on the degree of liver impairment. Chloramphenicol can also greatly prolong the half-life of many common therapeutic agents, causing toxic buildup.

Because of its extreme effects on bone marrow metabolism, the use of chloramphenicol is limited to severe or life-threatening infections caused by susceptible organisms or initial therapy for encephalitis or meningitis.

Sulfonamides and Trimethoprim

The sulfonamides inhibit a number of bacterial cell processes. They act as a chemical analog competing with *p*-aminobenzoic acid (PABA), which is used in the bacterial cell production of folic acid. Folic acid is essential in several stages of the synthesis of nucleic acids and proteins. The competition with PABA is reversible, causing a bacteristatic effect.[32]

Sulfonamides, like the tetracyclines, are separated into three groups, based on their serum half-life (see list opposite). They are active against a broad range of both gram-positive and gram-negative organisms. Primarily available for oral dosage, they are all well distributed throughout the body and into the CSF in the presence of inflammation.[33] A small percentage of the drug is metabolized by the liver, but the majority is excreted intact by the kidney, resulting in very high urine levels.[34] The long-acting sulfonamides were responsible for side-effects such as kidney damage due to sulfa crystal precipitation; however, they are no longer routinely used. The reactions seen with treatment include fever, rash, and perhaps minor bone marrow depression. Because of the high percentage of resistance among common infectious organisms, most sulfa drugs are presently used only for urinary tract infections.[35]

Trimethoprim is a synthetic analog of a portion of the folic acid molecule. Like the sulfa drugs, it causes a competitive inhibition of protein and nucleic acid synthesis, but its action involves a different step in the process.[36] Trimethoprim can be used alone as an antimicrobic, but when used in conjunction with a sulfonamide (*e.g.*, sulfamethoxazole) it has an excellent synergistic effect.[37]

Classification of Sulfonamides

Short-Acting Sulfonamides
Sulfisoxizole
Sulfadiazine
Sulfamerazine
Sulfamethazine
Sulfamethizole

Intermediate-Acting Sulfonamides
Sulfamethoxazole

Long-Acting Sulfonamides
Sulfamethoxydiazine

Erythromycin

Erythromycin is an excellent alternative antimicrobial agent for patients who are allergic to penicillin. Erythromycin, derived from *Streptomyces* species, belongs to a group of antibiotics called *macrolides,* which are high-molecular-weight compounds composed of large lactone rings attached to sugars. Erythromycin acts against a wide spectrum of both gram-positive and gram-negative organisms, *Chlamydia, Rickettsia,* mycoplasmas, and treponemes, and is relatively nontoxic. Erythromycin, like chloramphenicol, inhibits protein synthesis by binding to ribosomes, blocking transpeptidation.[38] It is bacteristatic in normal doses, but can be bactericidal in high concentrations.[39] It is metabolized by the liver and is not active in urine.

Clindamycin and Lincomycin

Clindamycin and lincomycin, although not chemically related to the macrolides or chloramphenicol, have very similar mechanisms of action inhibiting the same ribosomal units.[38] Clindamycin tends to be more bactericidal than erythromycin, and also has increased activity against anaerobic organisms, especially *Bacteroides* species.[40] As with erythromycin, the majority of the adverse reactions are mild. Clindamycin, however, has been associated with pseudomembranous colitis and the large intestine overgrowth of *Clostridium difficile.*[41] Clindamycin and lincomycin are also metabolized by the liver, and are inactive in the urine.[42]

Polypeptides

The polymyxins A, B, C, D, and E are polypeptide compounds derived from a species of *Bacillus.* Polymyxin B and polymyxin E are the only ones used for systemic therapy because of the extreme neuro- and nephrotoxicity of this group.[43] Polymyxin B is used primarily to treat severe infections caused by strains of *P. aeruginosa* that are resistant to other less toxic agents. Polymyxin E, also known as colistin, is primarily used for highly resistant organisms infecting the urinary tract. The polymyxins modify the permeability of the bacterial cell membrane, causing a loss of cellular contents and eventual cell death.[44, 45]

Vancomycin is a glycopeptide that inhibits cell wall and membrane synthesis and is therefore bactericidal for gram-positive organisms.[46] It is well distributed throughout the body, but reaches marginally therapeutic values in CSF only with inflammation. Vancomycin is excreted by the kidney, the majority of the agent still active.[47] It is only available for IV therapy, and is primarily used for treatment of methicillin-resistant *S. aureus* infections, severe enterococcal infections, and patients who are allergic to penicillin.

Like the polymyxins, bacitracin was derived from a species of *Bacillus.*[44] It contains a thiazolidine ring, like the penicillins, but not a β-lactam ring. Its activity and mechanism are similar to those of vancomycin. Bacitracin's use is limited to topical application because of its nephrotoxicity.

Other Clinically Important Antibacterials

Nitrofurantoin, methenamine, and the organic acids, *e.g.*, nalidixic acid, are antimicrobial agents used solely for treatment of urinary tract infections. They are quickly excreted by the kidney, and therefore do not actually reach "therapeutic" levels in serum. For this reason they are often called "urine antiseptics." Nitrofurantoin is useful against a wide spectrum of gram-positive and gram-negative organisms.[48] Nalidixic acid is active against enteric gram-negative bacilli. Its mechanism is thought to be an ability to inhibit bacterial DNA synthesis without affecting the host cells.[49] Compounds related to nalidixic acid, fluorinated quinolones, *e.g.*, norfloxacin, have increased gastrointestinal absorption. This results in higher serum and tissue levels, which may allow their use for infections outside the urinary tract.[50] Methenamine itself is not active against microorganisms, but is converted to formaldehyde in the presence of the acid *p*H of the urine. It is therefore active against most organisms infecting the urinary tract.[51] It is not helpful against organisms that tend to alkalize urine, *e.g.*, *Proteus* species, which split urea to ammonia. Because it takes approximately 1 hour for conversion of methenamine to formaldehyde in the bladder, it cannot be used for patients with indwelling catheters.

Metronidazole interferes with anaerobic metabolism and is therefore not active against aerobic or facultative organisms.[52] It is active against a number of anaerobic bacteria, especially *Bacteroides fragilis,* as well as several parasites: *Entamoeba histolytica, Giardia lamblia,* and *Trichomonas species.*[53] Metronidazole is metabolized by the liver, and caution should be used when treating patients with impaired liver function.

Carbapenems (imipenem) and monobactams (aztreonam) are relatively new β-lactam antimicrobial agents. Imipenem is active against a wide variety of aerobic gram-positive and gram-negative organisms as well as anaerobic organisms, including *B. fragilis.*[54] It is well distributed throughout the body with the exception of the meninges in the absence of inflammation, and the urine. Aztreonam, a monocyclic β-lactam agent, has excellent activity against the Enterobacteriaceae and other gram-negative organisms including *Pseudomonas,* but little or no activity against gram-positive or anaerobic organisms.[55] Clavulanic acid, derived from a *Streptomyces* species, is a β-lactamase inhibitor. Synergistic activity is seen when clavulanic acid is combined with many drugs from the penicillins and cephalosporins.[56] Amoxicillin combined with clavulanic acid is released under the name "Augmentin."

Antimycobacterial Agents

Therapeutic agents for the treatment of mycobacterial infections are classified on the basis of their use—for *Mycobacterium tuberculosis,* "atypical" mycobacterial infection, or leprosy—and of their efficacy and toxicity at therapeutic levels. Agents with good bactericidal effects and relatively low toxicity are labelled "first-line drugs." Agents with lower levels of effectiveness and/or higher toxicity are labelled "second-line drugs" (see the list in the opposite column).

Most of the first-line drugs for *M. tuberculosis* infections are bactericidal, but they vary in their activity based on the location of the infection and the rate of multiplication of organisms at that site.[57]

Second-line drugs for treatment of *M. tuberculosis* infections are usually reserved for situations in which resistance is found and/or when a second regime of therapy is required. A number of other agents have been used alone or in combination with varying degrees of success.

"Atypical mycobacterial" infections present a special problem to the clinician and to the laboratory. The levels and types of resistance are not predictable, even with first-line drugs. In the case of pulmonary infection caused by an atypical *Mycobacterium* species, susceptibility testing is essential. Treatment has been effective with isoniazid, rifampin, and the aminogylosides, individually or in combination.[58]

Leprosy (*Mycobacterium leprae*) has been effectively treated with a sulfonamide compound, Avlosulfone (Dapsone).

Antimycobacterial Agents

First-Line Drugs
Ethambutol
Isoniazid
Rifampin
Streptomycin

Second-Line Drugs
Cycloserine
Ethionamide
Para-aminosalicylic acid

Atypical Mycobacterial Agents
Aminoglycosides
Augmentin
Capreomycin
Erythromycin
Isoniazid
Rifampin
Tetracycline
Viomycin
or combinations of the above

Anti-Leprosy Agents
Acedapsone
Avlosulfone
Clofazimime
Rifampin

Antifungal Agents

The individual antifungal agents currently in use in the United States can be divided by the chemical groups from which they are derived and by their use as therapy for either superficial or systemic mycoses (see the list on p. 808).

The antifungal agents from the polyene macrolide group, Amphotericin B and Nystatin, derived from *Streptomyces* species, attach to the ergosterol portion of the fungus cell membrane, causing increased permeability of the cell membrane.[59] This results in a loss of cellular contents and eventual cell death. During systemic treatment, however, there is a tendency for these agents to attach also to cholesterol in kidney cells. Nystatin is used only as a topical agent for superficial yeast infections because of its extreme renal toxicity when given

Antifungal Agents

Polyene Macrolides
Amphotericin B
Nystatin

Imidazoles
Miconazole
Ketoconazole
Clotrimazole

Other Agents
Griseofulvin
5-fluorocytosine

systemically. Amphotericin B, despite its nephrotoxic side-effects, is the treatment of choice for most systemic mycoses because of its excellent fungicidal abilities.

The imidazoles—miconazole, ketoconazole, and clotrimazole—when given systemically are generally less toxic than the antifungal agents of the polyene group. Their mechanism of action, which is fungistatic, seems to be an inhibition of ergosterol synthesis in the fungal cell membrane.[60] Miconazole and clotrimazole are usually limited to use as topical agents for superficial fungal infections caused by yeast or dermatophytes. Ketoconazole has shown considerable promise for use against systemic mycoses. Recently there have been reports of serious liver toxicity with its use, although ketoconazole is still considered less toxic than amphotericin B.[61] Benefits have been seen in the use of amphotericin B and ketoconazole in combination, decreasing the toxic side-effects of each.

Griseofulvin is an antifungal agent derived from *Penicillium* species that acts by inhibiting cell wall synthesis of fungi. It is used primarily for dermatophyte infections, and can be given either topically, systemically, or in combination. Long-term therapy is required for this agent. With treatment it is incorporated into the new, healthy keratin layers which come in contact with the fungus as these layers grow to the surface.

5-Fluorocytosine, an analogue for cytosine, was originally developed for use as an anti-cancer agent with mixed success. It was later found to show activity against *Candida* species by inhibiting the yeast's DNA synthesis. Disadvantages are its toxic effects on developing blood cells in the bone marrow and its unpredictable pattern of resistance, even in primary therapy.

Antiviral Agents

As with other infectious diseases, there are three basic approaches to treatment of viral infections: physical elimination or neutralization, increasing the patient's immune response, and interference with the growth of the infectious agent.

Antiviral therapies that inactivate the virus directly are usually limited to discrete or mucocutaneous viral infections. These include treatment by cryotherapy, cautery, UV light, or topical treatment with detergents or chemical solvents such as chloroform and ether. Other antiviral treatments may attempt to stimulate the host's immune response (interferon treatment). The most promise is seen in the development of antiviral chemotherapeutic agents that interfere with various stages in viral replication.

There has been considerable difficulty in developing agents that inhibit the virus without harming the host cells, because the replication process and metabolism of viruses is so closely linked to host cell function. Because testing in the clinical laboratory for susceptibility to these agents is not yet practical, this discussion will be limited to a listing and brief outline of their actions.

The majority of these agents have been developed for the larger, complex DNA viruses (see list on p. 809). Acyclovir inhibits the DNA polymerase of herpesviruses.[62] Idoxuridine and trifluorothymidine (thymidine analogues) inactivate viral DNA in pox- and herpesviruses.[63] Vidarabine, an adenine deoxyriboside analogue, is active against herpes simplex virus (HSV)1 and 2, Epstein-Barr virus, varicella, variola, some rhabdoviruses, and RNA tumor viruses.[64, 65] It has also shown activity to viral strains of HSV that are resistant to

Antiviral Agents

Acyclovir
Amantidine
Idoxuridine
Methisazone
Ribavirin
Rimantadine
Trifluorothymidine
Vidarabine

acyclovir. Amantadine and rimantadine are synthetic amines active against influenza A virus, but not influenza B.[66] Both agents inhibit the uncoating of the virus, and have been used as preventives in immunocompromised or debilitated hosts, such as the aged. Methisazone, used in the treatment of poxviruses, acts by inhibiting viral protein synthesis, causing assembly of incomplete viruses.[67] Ribavirin is a synthetic nucleoside that inhibits viral nucleic acid synthesis, showing activity against a wide variety of RNA and DNA viruses, including herpesviruses, poxviruses, adenoviruses, and arenaviruses.[68]

As with other infectious agents, viruses are beginning to show natural, and sometimes induced, resistance to these new chemotherapeutic agents.[69]

LABORATORY ASSISTANCE IN THE SELECTION AND MONITORING OF ANTIMICROBIAL AGENTS

Susceptibility Testing

Many factors affect the need for susceptibility testing and the choice of antimicrobial chemotherapy. If the disease process requires antimicrobial treatment, the first consideration is whether the causative organism has a highly predictable pattern of susceptibility. Many organisms do not require routine testing because of their predictable susceptibility patterns, such as *Streptococcus pyogenes.* However, even this organism may require testing when the patient's history precludes use of the agent of choice, as in allergy to penicillin, or when previous therapy has failed. The identity of the organism, or suspected organism, can give clues to appropriate treatment. If the organism is not yet confirmed, certain clinical situations may indicate the most likely organisms and/or treatment of choice. Additional information, such as a Gram stain, used with the clinical history, can help predict the most useful antimicrobial agent. Otitis media in preschool children is often caused by *Streptococcus pneumoniae* or *Hemophilus influenzae.* If, in addition to this statistical information, a Gram stain of the fluid from the infected ear reveals gram-positive cocci, an excellent choice in antimicrobial therapy can be made before or without susceptibility testing. Other rapid methods that aid in the determination of the optimal agent include direct fluorescent antibody testing, ELISAs, or other immunoassays such as latex agglutination or counter-immunoelectrophoresis. Each of these rapid methods, in combination with the clinical history, may provide enough information for choosing appropriate therapy until susceptibility test results are available.

Second, the conditions and history of the patient affecting the choice of antimicrobial agent must be considered. That is, does the patient have an underlying disease or condition that makes the use of certain agents contraindicated? Relative cost for the "entire" treatment process must also be considered, not just the cost of one dose of an antimicrobial agent. The cost of administration and the length of treatment must also enter into the analysis of cost. Finally, agents that are only available for IM or IV administration may not be appropriate for outpatient treatment regimes.

Most initial isolates of *M. tuberculosis* do not require susceptibility testing since they are usually sensitive to the first-line agents. However, if the patient has a history of previous treatment or if the isolate is an atypical *Mycobacterium* species testing should be performed because the susceptibility pattern is not predictable. Diffusion tests used for other bacteria are not suitable for Mycobacteria because of the slow growth rate. Several procedures are available, including quadrant plates/paper disk and radiometric assays. Studies comparing the radiometric method and conventional testing have shown good correlation with much faster results by the radiometric assay.[70] The disadvantages to the radiometric method are cost of equipment, volume of samples needed for cost effectiveness, and expertise required for optimal performance.

Many laboratories that routinely perform testing for Mycobacteria are now re-evaluating their requirements. Decreased numbers of new cases of mycobacterial infection have made the expense of performing cultures and susceptibility tests prohibitive for the majority of laboratories. It may also be more efficient to send testing to a reference laboratory that maintains the level of expertise necessary for optimum test reliability. Even with testing sent to reference laboratories, the clinical laboratory scientist has an obligation to aid the physician in the choice of appropriate testing and their interpretations.

The majority of laboratories may not be performing susceptibility testing for antifungal agents. However, each laboratory should be able to aid the physician in interpreting the report from the reference lab. Susceptibility testing for antifungal agents can be accomplished by broth or agar dilution methods or disk diffusion. The broth dilution method is used primarily for yeasts and can provide a minimal inhibitory or cidal level. The agar dilution method can also be adapted for fungi, but variable results may be seen unless the inoculum size is well controlled.[71] Disk diffusion testing for antifungal agents is still experimental and is limited by the lack of stability of polyene compounds and the diffusion characteristics of the imidazoles.[72] The primary consideration, regardless of the method of testing, is the site of infection, as some agents are only licensed for topical use. As with other agents with low safety margins, the patient's kidney and liver function should be tested at the beginning of treatment and carefully monitored during the course of therapy. If 5-fluorocytosine is used, the patient should have a WBC and platelet count done periodically to monitor bone marrow function.

Even with appropriate testing, not all infections should be treated with systemic antimicrobial agents. It is essential that the benefits of treatment be considered in the context of possible side-effects. On the other hand, the patient with a depressed immune system may require treatment for infections caused by organisms usually considered normal flora. In addition to the effects of the agent on the infectious organisms, these agents affect the patient's entire balance of normal microflora and may cause an emergence of resistant strains. Careful consideration must be given to the relative risk to the patient from both the infecting organisms and the chosen antimicrobial agent.

Third, when treatment is necessary, the possibility of attaining the level of antimicrobial agent needed to inhibit the organism at the site of infection must be considered, and the appropriate routes of administration. The assignment by the laboratory of "sensitive," "intermediate," or "resistant" labels to the susceptibility pattern is based on the levels necessary to inhibit the organism versus attainable levels in the serum of the patient, following recommended doses and under normal conditions. If the inhibition level is within the range of what is considered a safe serum level, the result is labelled "sensitive." If the inhibition level is in the toxic range of serum levels, the result is "resistant." These attainable serum levels may be quite different when an alternate route of administration is used, or if the patient has liver or kidney dysfunction. In addition, even when the required *serum* levels are reached, it may not be possible to attain the necessary levels of antimicrobic at the site of infection, because each area of the body has different perfusion rates for each antimicrobial agent (see Table 63-1).[73] As indicated in this table, the same 2-gram IV dose of ceftazidime yields vastly different levels in the bile, pleural fluid, and skeletal muscle. For this reason, each susceptibility test report must be analyzed for treatment feasibility based on the site of infection, regardless of the assignment of a "sensitive"

Table 63-1 ***Typical Peak Concentration of Ceftazidime in Tissue Fluids After Administration of 2 g Intravenously***

Tissue or Tissue Fluid	Peak Concentration (mg/L or mg/kg)
Bile	36.4
Organic bone	31.1
Pleural fluid	28.0
Lymph	24.0*
Uterine muscle	18.9
Heart muscle	12.7
Skeletal muscle	9.4
Aqueous humor	11.0
Breast milk	5.2
Sputum	3.5†

* l-g dose
† Intramuscular dose

or "resistant" label to a result. Testing the "minimal inhibitory concentration" (MIC) or the "minimal bactericidal concentration" (MBC) of the antimicrobial agent for the organism in question may provide more quantitative information with which to assess the possibility of successful treatment. A report of "sensitive" usually correlates with an attainable site level of three to five times the MIC by normal dosages,[74] but this will not always assure successful treatment. It is often necessary, therefore, to discuss susceptibility test results with respect to these factors and their influence on the choice of appropriate therapy with the attending physician.

In the discussion on the pharmacology of the antimicrobial agents, considerable overlap can be seen in their range of activity, indicating little reason to test routinely more than one agent in each category; moreover, certain antimicrobial agents are of little use except for urinary tract infections. With this in mind, the National Committee for Clinical Laboratory Standards (NCCLS) has made recommendations for appropriate antimicrobial agents to test and report for various groups of pathogenic organisms (see Table 63-2).[75] These agents have been selected on the basis of proven activity against the organisms listed. Many laboratories may not perform sufficient numbers of susceptibility tests to keep a battery on hand for each group of organisms. An alternative is to maintain a panel of antimicrobials for gram-positive organisms, one for gram-negative organisms, and one for urinary tract infections of either Gram reaction (see Table 63-3). With this method, the reporting of these agents that are not applicable for a particular isolate can be restricted. This will prevent the assumption that an antimicrobial agent is "useful" against the organisms in question when, in fact, it is not. Such a report could be very misleading, implying sanction of the agent's use and resulting in incorrect therapy and possible loss of life. Reporting should also be restricted for those antimicrobial agents that are considered secondary or backup, unless resistance is seen in the primary agent. This will help prevent overuse or inappropriate use of newer drugs, which could lead to resistant strains of bacteria.

The laboratory can be most helpful by maintaining a spectrum of antibiotics, in addition to the routine selection, that can be used in a variety of clinical situations. To gain the most information from each susceptibility report, the antimicrobials must be chosen carefully. One method of selecting the panels involves the laboratory, the physicians who use the laboratory results, physicians from the infectious disease department in the hospital, and the pharmacy that provides these medications. A survey of the physicians and pharmacists in the hospital or laboratory service area to determine which antimicrobials are most commonly used can be very helpful. From this information and the NCCLS charts, a list of the antimicrobial agents that should be used in the laboratory to provide the most meaningful information can be compiled. Physicians in the area can then be informed about which antimicrobial agents will be tested on a routine basis and those the laboratory has available for special request. This information will also help the hospital pharmacists by providing them with guidelines for inventory stock.

Table 63-2 ***Suggested Groupings of Antimicrobials That Should Be Considered for Routine Testing and Reporting by Clinical Microbiology Laboratories***

Enterobacteriaceae	*Pseudomonas*	*Staphylococcus*	Enterococci
Amikacin	Amikacin	Amikacin or	Penicillin or
Ampicillin	Azlocillin or	Gentamicin or	Ampicillin
Augmentin	Piperacillin	Kanamycin or	Erythromycin
Aztreonam or	Aztreonam	Netilmicin or	Nitrofurantoin
Cefotaxime or	Carbenicillin or	Tobramycin	Norfloxacin
Ceftazidime or	Mezlocillin or	Augmentin	Tetracycline
Ceftizoxime or	Ticarcillin	Cephalothin	Vancomycin
Ceftriaxone or	Cefoperazone	Chloramphenicol	
Moxalactam	Ceftazidime	Clindamycin	**Other Streptococci**
Carbenicillin or	Cefotaxime or	Erythromycin	
Ticarcillin	Ceftriaxone or	Imipenem	Cephalothin
Cefamandole or	Moxalactam	Methicillin or	Chloramphenicol
Cefonicid or	Chloramphenicol	Nafcillin or	Clindamycin
Cefuroxime	Gentamicin	Oxacillin	Erythromycin
Cefazolin	Imipenem	Penicillin G	Penicillin
Cefoperazone	Netilmicin	Tetracycline	Tetracycline
Cefoxitin	Tobramycin	Trimethoprim/	Vancomycin
Cephalothin	Trimethoprim/	Sulfameth	Nitrofurantoin
Chloramphenicol	Sulfameth	Vancomycin	Norfloxacin
Gentamicin	Ceftizoxime	Nitrofurantoin	
Imipenem	Norfloxacin	Norfloxacin	
Kanamycin	Sulfisoxazole	Sulfisoxazole	
Mezlocillin or	Tetracycline	Trimethoprim	
Piperacillin			
Netilmicin			
Tetracycline			
Tobramycin			
Trimethoprim/			
sulfamethoxazole			
Cinoxacin or			
Nalidixic Acid			
Nitrofurantoin			
Norfloxacin			
Sulfisoxazole			
Trimethoprim			

Data from reference number[75]

It may also be helpful to maintain a chart or listing of the antimicrobial agent disks tested in the laboratory. This chart should include the generic and trade names of the antimicrobial agents that these disks represent. If possible, it should also include the same information for other disks that are commercially available but not tested on site. This will enable the laboratory staff to become better informed and to provide improved consultation to other members of the health care team.

Table 63-3 ***Suggested Alternate Groupings of Antimicrobials for Routine Testing***

Gram-Positive Organisms	Gram-Negative Organisms	Urinary Tract Isolates (G+ or G−)
Amikacin or	Amikacin	Ampicillin
Gentamicin or	Ampicillin	Ceftizoxime
Kanamycin or	Carbenicillin or	Erythromycin
Netilmicin or	Piperacillin or	Nalidixic acid or
Tobramycin	Azlocillin or	Cinoxacin
Ampicillin	Mezlocillin or	Nitrofurantoin
Augmentin	Ticarcillin	Norfloxacin
Cephalothin	Augmentin	Sulfisoxazole
Clindamycin	Aztreonam or	Tetracycline
Chloramphenicol	Cefotaxime or	Trimethoprim
Erythromycin	Ceftazidime or	Trimethoprim/
Methicillin or	Ceftizoxime or	Sulfamethoxazole
Nafcillin or	Ceftriaxone or	
Oxacillin	Moxalactam	
Penicillin	Cefamandole or	
Tetracycline	Cefonicid or	
Trimethoprim/	Cefuroxime	
Sulfamethoxazole	Cefoperazone or	
Vancomycin	Ceftazidime	
	Cefazolin	
	Cefoxitin	
	Cephalothin	
	Chloramphenicol	
	Gentamicin	
	Imipenem	
	Tetracycline	
	Tobramycin or	
	Netilmicin	
	Trimethoprim/	
	Sulfamethoxazole	

Therapeutic Drug Monitoring

Once appropriate antimicrobial therapy has been chosen, according to the susceptibility test results, it is often necessary to monitor closely the actual levels of antimicrobial agent achieved. These measurements allow modification or maintenance of dosage to achieve more appropriate therapy levels. For some antimicrobial agents, such as aminoglycosides, therapeutic and toxic levels are close, and individual patient metabolism may cause significant differences in actual levels with the same dose (see list on p. 814). In patients with liver or renal impairment, normal doses may cause higher than expected serum levels because of decreased excretion or metabolism of the drug.

The concentration of antimicrobial agents can be determined by a variety of methods. Most often these levels are performed on serum, but urine and CSF may also be assayed. The bioassay involves testing the patient's serum, against known levels of the antimicrobial agent, for its ability to inhibit a

Antimicrobial Agents for Therapeutic Drug Monitoring

Aminoglycosides
- Amikacin
- Gentamicin
- Kanamycin
- Netilmicin
- Tobramycin

Chloramphenicol
Vancomycin
Trimethoprim

control test organism with a known MIC. High pressure liquid chromatography (HPLC), a chemical assay, involves extraction and separation of the antimicrobial agent from other compounds in the patient's serum, for determination of the concentration by comparison to controls. This method is accurate but is usually too complicated and lengthy for the average laboratory.

The immunoassays are the method most commonly used today. Radioimmunoassay (RIA), enzyme immunoassay (EIA), enzyme multiplied immunoassay technique (EMIT), and fluorescence polarization immunoassay (FPIA) involve competitive assays of serum antimicrobial concentrations with control levels for test antibody.[76] These methods are relatively accurate, are simple, and provide rapid results for monitoring patient therapy.

Occasionally the antimicrobial activity of serum, also known as the Schlicter or serum killing-power test, is used to guide antimicrobial therapy for patients with bacterial endocarditis.[77] This test measures the ability of serial dilutions of serum to inhibit or kill standard concentrations of the infecting agent. Assessing the overall antimicrobial activity of serum has advantages over measuring the levels of individual antibiotics. With this assay a number of additional factors can be taken into account, including the innate antibacterial properties of serum and the combined or synergistic effects of multiple antibiotics (*e.g.*, aminoglycosides and β-lactam agents together). However, this test is not always a good predictor of therapeutic success or failure unless the method is well-standardized.[78]

Regardless of the method chosen, the laboratory has an obligation to provide explicit directions for patient sample collection. For these assays, accurately timed and properly collected specimens are absolutely essential for meaningful results.

REFERENCES

1. Yocum RR, Waxman DW, Strominger JL: The mechanism of action of penicillin. J Biol Chem 255:3977, 1980
2. Saxon A: Immediate hypersensitivity reactions to β-lactam antibiotics. Rev Infect Dis 5(suppl 2):368, 1983
3. Sukes RB, Matthew M: The β-lactamases of gram-negative bacteria and their role in resistance to β-lactam antibiotics. J Antimicrob Agents Chemother 2:115, 1976
4. Neu HC: Structure-activity relations of new β-lactam compounds and *in vitro* activity against common bacteria. Rev Infect Dis 5(suppl):319, 1983
5. Verbist L: Comparison of the activities of the new ureido-penicillins—piperacillin, mezlocillin, azlocillin, and Bay K4999—against gram-negative organisms. Antimicrob Agents Chemother 16:115, 1979
6. Lentnek AL, Sohn CA, Wikler MA et al: A national comparative study of antimicrobial susceptibility of common gram-negative and gram-positive isolates: I. Comparison of the first-generation cephalosporins cefazolin, cephalothin, and cephapirin; II. Comparison of the first-generation cephalosporin cefazolin with the second-generation agents cefamandole and cefoxitin. Adv Therapy 1:299, 307, 1984
7. Thornsberry C: Review of *in vitro* activity of third-generation cephalosporins and other new β-lactam antibiotics against clinically important bacteria. Am J Med 79(suppl 2A):14, 1985
8. Moellering RC: Can the third-generation cephalosporins eliminate the need for antimicrobial combinations? Am J Med 79(suppl 2A):104, 1985
9. Britton HL, Schwinghammer TL, Romano MJ: Cost containment through restriction of cephalosporins. Am J Hosp Pharm 38:1897, 1981

10. Hancock REW: Aminoglycoside uptake and mode of action, with special reference to streptomycin and gentamicin. II. Effects of aminoglycosides on cells. J Antimicrob Chemother 8:429, 1981
11. Davies JE: Resistance to aminoglycosides: Mechanism and frequency. Rev Infect Dis 5(suppl):3261, 1983
12. Benveniste R, Davies J: Enzymatic acetylation of aminoglycoside antibiotics by *E. coli* carrying an "R" factor. Biochemistry 10:1787, 1971
13. Ward ME: The bactericidal action of spectinomycin on *Neisseria gonorrhoeae.* J Antimicrob Chemother 3:323, 1977
14. Kaiser AB, McGee GA: Aminoglycoside therapy of gram-negative bacillary meningitis. N Engl J Med 293:1215, 1975
15. Gyselynck A-M, Forrey A, Cutler R: Pharmacokinetics of gentamicin: Distribution and plasma and renal clearance. J Infect Dis 124(suppl):570, 1970
16. Silverblatt F: Pathogenesis of nephrotoxicity of cephalosporins and aminoglycosides: A review of current concepts. Rev Infect Dis 4(suppl):S360, 1982
17. Bodey GP, Feld R, Burgess MA: β-Lactam antibiotics alone or in combination with gentamicin for therapy of gram-negative bacillary infection in neutropenic patients. Am J Med Sci 271:179, 1976
18. Craven GR, Gavin R, Fanning T: The transfer RNA binding site of the 30s ribosome and the site of tetracycline inhibition. Symposium Quant Biol 34:129, 1969
19. Fabre J, Milek E, Kalfopoulos P et al: The Kinetics of Tetracyclines in Man: Digestive Absorption and Serum Concentrations. In Doxycycline (Vibramycin), A Compendium of Clinical Evaluation. New York City, Pfizer Laboratories, 1973
20. Whelton A: Tetracyclines in renal insufficiency: Resolution of a therapeutic dilemma. Bull NY Acad Med 54:223, 1978
21. Sompolinsky D, Zemira S: Plasmid-determined resistance to tetracycline. Microbios 30:109, 1981
22. Bar WH, Adir J, Garrettson L: Decrease of tetracycline in man by sodium bicarbonate. Clin Pharmacol Ther 12:779, 1971
23. Witkop CJ, Wolf RO: Hypoplasia and intrinsic staining of enamel following tetracycline therapy. JAMA 185:1008, 1963
24. Grossman ER, Walcheck A, Freedman H: Tetracycline and permanent teeth: The relationship between doses and tooth color. Pediatrics 47:567, 1971
25. Whalley PJ, Adams RH, Combes B: Tetracycline toxicity in pregnancy: Liver and pancreatic dysfunction. JAMA 189:357, 1964
26. Rahal JJ, Simberkoff MS: Bactericidal and bacteristatic action of chloramphenicol against meningeal pathogens. Antimicrob Agents Chemother 20:281, 1979
27. Yunis AA: Chloramphenicol-induced bone marrow suppression. Sem Hematol 10:225, 1973
28. Scott JL, Finegold SM, Belkin GA et al: A controlled double-blind studyof the hematologic toxicity of chloramphenicol. N Engl J Med 272:1137, 1965
29. Daum RS, Cohen DL, Smith AL: Fatal aplastic anemia following apparent "dose-related" chloramphenicol toxicity. J Pediatr 94:403, 1979
30. Okamato S, Suzuki Y: Chloramphenicol-, dihydrostreptomycin-, and kanamycin-inactivating enzymes from multiple drug-resistant *Escherichia coli* carrying episome "R." Nature 208:1301, 1965
31. Butler T, Linh NN, Arnold K et al: Chloramphenicol-resistant typhoid fever in Vietnam associated with R-factor. Lancet 2:983, 1973
32. Woods DD: Relation of *p*-aminobenzoic acid to mechanism of action of sulfanilamide. Br J Exp Pathol 21:74, 1940
33. Anand N: Sulfonamides and Sulfones. In Corcoran JW, Hahn FE (eds): Antibiotics III: Mechanism of Action of Antimicrobial and Antitumor Agents, pp 667–669. Berlin, Springer-Verlag, 1975
34. Craig WA, Kunin CM: Trimethoprim/sulfamethoxazole: Pharmacodynamic effect of urinary *p*H and impaired renal function. Ann Intern Med 78:491, 1973
35. Then RL: Mechanisms of resistance to trimethoprim, the sulfonamides, and trimethoprim/sulfamethoxazole. Rev Infect Dis 4:261, 1982
36. Bushby SRM, Hitchings GH: Trimethoprim, a sulfonamide potentiator. Br J Pharmaco Chemother 33:72, 1968
37. Bushby SRM: Sensitivity Patterns and Use of Combined Disc of Trimethoprim/sulfamethoxazole. In Bernstein LS, Salter AJ (eds): Trimethoprim/Sulfamethoxazole in Bacterial Infections, pp 29, 30. Edinburgh, Churchill Livingstone, 1973
38. Oleinick NL: The Erythromycins. In Corcoran JW, Hahn FE (eds): Mechanism of Action of Anti-

microbial and Antitumor Agents, p 396. New York City, Springer-Verlag, 1975
39. Haight TH, Finland M: Observations on mode of action of erythromycin. Proc Soc Exp Biol Med 81:188, 1952
40. Sutter VL: *In vitro* susceptibility of anaerobes: Comparison of clindamycin and other antimicrobial agents. J Infect Dis 135 (suppl):S7, 1977
41. Tedesco FJ: Clindamycin and colitis: A review. J Infect Dis 135 (suppl):S95, 1979
42. Panzer JD, Brown DC, Epstein WL et al: Clindamycin levels in various body tissues and fluids. J Clin Pharmacol 12:259, 1972
43. Jawetz E: Polymyxin, colistin, and bacitracin. Pediatr Clin North Am 8:1057, 1961
44. Goodwin NJ: Colistin and sodium colistimethate. Med Clin North Am 54:1267, 1970
45. Hoeprich PD: The polymyxins. Med Clin North Am 54:1257, 1970
46. Wantanakunakorn C: The antibacterial action of vancomycin. Rev Infect Dis 3(suppl):S210, 1981
47. Moellering RC, Krogstad DJ, Greenblatt DJ: Pharmacokinetics of vancomycin on normal subjects and in patients with reduced renal function. Rev Infect Dis 3(suppl):S230, 1981
48. Kucers A, Bennett NM: Nitrofurans. In Kucers A, Bennett NM (eds): The Use of Antibiotics, pp 748–780. Philadelphia, JB Lippincott, 1979
49. Goss WA, Deitz WH, Cook TM: Mechanism of action of nalidixic acid on *Escherichia coli.* II. Inhibition of deoxyribonucleic acid synthesis. J Bacteriol 89:1068, 1965
50. Barry AL, Jones RN, Thornsberry C et al: Antibacterial activity of ciprofloxacin, norfloxacin, oxolinic acid, cinoxacin, and nalidixic acid. Antimicrob Agents Chemother 25:633, 1984
51. Scudi JV, Reinhard JF: Absorption, distribution, and renal excretion of Mandelamine (methenamine mandelate). J Lab Clin Med 33:1304, 1948
52. Lindmark DG, Muller M: Antitrichomonad action, mutagenicity, and reduction of metronidazole and other nitroimidazoles. Antimicrob Agents Chemother 10:476, 1976
53. Wolfe MS: Giardiasis. JAMA 233:1362, 1975
54. Neu HC: Clinical perspectives on imipenem. J Antimicrob Chemother 12(suppl D):149, 1981
55. Neu HC, Labthavikul P: Antibacterial activity of a monocyclic β-lactam SQ 26, 776. J Antimicrob Chemother 8(suppl E):111, 1981
56. Reading C, Cole M: Clavulanic acid: A β-lactamase-inhibiting β-lactam from *Streptomyces clavuligerus.* Antimicrob Agents Chemother 11:852, 1977
57. Stead WW, Dutt AK: Chemotherapy for tuberculosis today. Am Rev Respir Dis 125(3)(suppl):94, 1982
58. Zimmer BL, DeYoung DR, Roberts GD: *In vitro* synergistic activity of ethambutol, isoniazid, kanamycin, rifampin, and streptomycin against *Mycobacterium Avium-Intracellulare* complex. Antimicrob Agents Chemother 22:148, 1982
59. Hamilton-Miller JMT: Chemistry and biology of the polyene macrolide antibiotics. Bacteriol Rev 37:166, 1973
60. Borgers M, Bossche HV, Brabender MD: The mechanism of action of the new antimycotic ketoconazole. Am J Med 74:2, 1983
61. Dismukes WE, Stamm AM, Graybill PC et al. The treatment of systemic mycoses with ketoconazole: Emphasis on toxicity and clinical response in 52 patients. Ann Intern Med 98:13, 1983
62. Biron KK, Elton GB: *In vitro* susceptibility of varicellazoster virus to acyclovir. Antimicrob Agents Chemother 18:443, 1980
63. Spector SA, Tyndall M, Kelly E: Inhibition of human cytomegalovirus by trifluorothymidine. Antimicrob Agents Chemother 23:113, 1983
64. Bryson YJ, Connor JD: *In vitro* susceptibility of varicella zoster virus to adenine arabinoside and hypoxanthine arabinoside. Antimicrob Agents Chemother 9:540, 1976
65. Coker-Vann M, Dolin R: Effect of adenine arabinoside on Epstein-Barr virus *in vitro.* J Infect Dis 135:447, 1977
66. Browne MJ, Moss MY, Boyd MR: Comparative activity of amantadine and ribavirin against influenza virus *in vitro:* Possible clinical relevance. Antimicrob Agents Chemother 23:503, 1983
67. Kucers A, Bennett NM: Methisazone. In Kucers A, Bennett NM (eds): The Use of Antibiotics, p 965. Philadelphia, JB Lippincott, 1979
68. Hall CB: Ribavirin: Beginning the blitz on respiratory viruses? Pediatr Infect Dis 6:668, 1985
69. Crumpacker CS, Schnipper LE, Marlow SI et al: Resistance to antiviral drug of herpes simplex virus isolated from patients treated with acyclovir. N Engl J Med 306:343, 1982
70. Middlebrook G, Reggiardo Z, Tigert GP: Automatable radiometric detection of growth of *Mycobac-*

terium tuberculosis in selective media. Am Rev Respir Dis 115:1066, 1977

71. Brass C, Shainhouse JZ, Stevens DA: Variability of agar dilution-replicator method of yeast susceptibility testing. Antimicrob Agents Chemother 15:763–768, 1979
72. Grendahl JG, Sung JP: Quantitation of imidazoles by agar-disk diffusion. Antimicrob Agents Chemother 14:509, 1978
73. Harding SM: Pharmacokinetics of the third-generation cephalosporins. Am J Med 79 (suppl 2A):21, 1985
74. Hewitt WL, McHenry MC: Blood level determinations of antimicrobial drugs: Some clinical considerations. Med Clin North Am 62:1119, 1978
75. National Committee for Clinical Laboratory Standards: Performance Standards for Antimicrobial Disk Susceptibility Tests, 3rd ed. Approved Standard. NCCLS Publication M2-A3. Villanova, Pennsylvania, National Committee for Clinical Laboratory Standards, 1984
76. Buchanan AG, Witwicki E, Albritton WL: Serum aminoglycoside monitoring by enzyme immunoassay, biological, and fluorescence immunoassay procedures. Am J Med Technol 49:437, 1983
77. Schlicter JG, MacLean H: A method of determining the effective therapeutic level in the treatment of subacute bacterial endocarditis with penicillin. Am Heart J 34:209, 1947
78. Weinstein MP, Stratton CW, Ackley A et al: Multicenter collaboration evaluation of a standardized serum bactericidal test as a prognostic indicator in infective endocarditis. Am J Med 78:262, 1985

Part XIII

NUTRITIONAL AND METABOLIC DISORDERS

Glenda D. Price, Associate Editor

Included in this section are a number of disorders that are linked by virtue of their etiology, deriving from genetic defects or nutritional deficits. There is no common pathway or physiological process or body system associated with all of the disorders; however, their consistent pattern of defective or missing enzymes, dietary intolerance, or dietary requirements is sufficient to group them in this section.

It is recognized that several metabolic disorders are found in other sections of this text. When appropriate to a specific system or other common process, the disorder has been discussed in that section. It is believed that the reader will benefit most from this approach.

With the exception of malnutrition and starvation, the role of the laboratory in these disorders is to assist in the identification of the defect that is the cause of the patient's symptoms. By such identification, unnecessary therapeutic and diagnostic activities are minimized and dietary management can be instituted. Until such time as a mechanism exists to incorporate a missing gene or correct a defective one, there is no other contribution that the laboratory can make to assist the clinician.

Chapter 64

Osteoporosis

Robert M. Shoemaker

Osteoporosis is a generic term referring to a state of diminished mass per unit volume of normally mineralized bone. It is the most common skeletal disorder, second only to arthritis as a leading cause of skeleto-muscular morbidity in the geriatric population. There is frequently a prodromal period before clinical symptoms or complications are manifested. Initial symptoms occur when bone mass is so depleted that the skeletal frame can no longer withstand the physical stresses of daily life. Compression fractures of the vertebrae and fractures of the proximal femur, humerus, distal radius, and ribs commonly occur with minimal trauma.

Presently a cure is not available; however, early detection and treatment can be of great value in halting the progression of the disease. Prevention of fractures in susceptible individuals is the principal goal of intervention. Strategies include adequate dietary supplementation, weight-bearing exercise, and estrogen replacement in postmenopausal women. There are no laboratory tests for identifying patients at risk or those with mild osteoporosis.

CLASSIFICATION OF OSTEOPOROSIS

Postmenopausal and age-related bone loss are the most common conditions contributing to osteoporosis. Sedentary, postmenopausal caucasian women with life-long dietary calcium deficiency are among those most likely affected with osteoporosis. The average American woman lives for about 25 years beyond menopause. Among those over 50 years of age, more than half are likely to have radiographically detectable evidence of osteopenia in the spine, and more than one-third develop major orthopedic problems related to osteoporosis. Furthermore, the majority of approximately 200,000 hip fractures and 80% of the one million fractures sustained by women over age 50 are secondary to osteoporosis.[1]

A large-scale epidemiologic study disputes the theory that menopause is the singular event in the pathogenesis of osteoporosis that results in an increased incidence of hip fractures among white females. The data show a sharp increase in the rate of hip fractures for caucasian women between the ages of 40 and 44, approximately 15 to 20 years earlier than generally believed. Moreover, the data reveal a gradual increase in fractures, with no apparent inflection indicative of accelerated risk around the time of menopause or thereafter.[2, 3]

Age-related ("senile") osteoporosis occurs in both men and women, and is caused by bone loss that normally accompanies aging. Endocrine-mediated osteoporosis can occur in conjunction with postmenopausal or age-related factors.

Heritable Osteoporosis

Heritable osteoporosis is a group of diseases that are often congenital and are referred to collectively as *osteogenesis imperfecta,* with either autosomal dominant or recessive inheritance. All of these disorders seem to be associated with defective bone matrix formation, with specific disorders in collagen metabolism having been identified in some cases.

Osteoporosis associated with homocystinuria due to cystathionine-β-synthase deficiency is a very rare condition, with an autosomal recessive inheritance. The cause of osteoporosis in homocystinuria remains unclear, but the anomaly is thought to be associated with normal collagen metabolism.

Endocrine-Mediated Osteoporosis

Numerous hormones affect skeletal development and skeletal mass. Any young or middle-aged individual with osteoporosis should be evaluated for possible endocrine-mediated osteoporosis.

Primary or secondary hyperthyroidism accelerates bone turnover and remodeling, and bone resorption surpasses bone formation, resulting in a net decrease in bone mass. Signs and symptoms of hyperthyroidism, including determination of the T_3 uptake (T_3U) and thyroxine (T_4) levels, should be assessed in osteopenic patients, especially among those on long-term thyroid hormone replacement therapy.

Primary and secondary hyperparathyroidism also increase bone turnover, resulting in increased bone resorption. Increased parathyroid hormone secretion induces a hypercalcemia.

Endogenous and iatrogenic hyperadrenalism result in a refractory state of diminished bone mass. Chronic glucocorticoid excess reduces bone mineral and connective tissue metabolism. Because of their atrophic effect on the jejunum, excess glucocorticoids decrease intestinal absorption of calcium. The resultant stimulation of the PTH–vitamin D axis increases the serum ionized calcium level, resulting in increased bone resorption. Consequently, the effects of glucocorticoids decrease the bone mass, resulting in symptomatic osteoporosis. Symptoms are commonly more severe in the axial rather than the appendicular skeleton.

Diet-Related Bone Loss

Chronic dietary deficiencies of calcium, vitamin C, and protein can lead to decreased bone loss. Chronic alcoholism is the most common cause of bone loss in young men, and is related to the typically poor nutritional status of chronic alcoholics. Furthermore, ethanol has been implicated as a cause of decreased intestinal calcium absorption.

Drug-Induced Bone Loss

Long-term anticoagulation with heparin leads to osteopenia. Although the cause remains unclear, it may be related to mucopolysaccharide metabolism. Methotrexate has likewise been reported as inducing osteopenia.

Disuse Osteoporosis

Both focal and generalized immobilization result in rapid and profound decrease in bone density, with a proportionate loss of bone matrix and mineral content. Spinal cord injury resulting in paraplegia and quadriplegia is characterized by marked osteopenia.

Symptoms of disuse bone loss are common in degenerative lower motor neuron diseases. Although ambulation alone does not protect against osteoporosis, use of antigravity muscle and weight-bearing activity are essential to skeletal health.

Idiopathic Osteoporosis

Both juvenile and adult forms of idiopathic osteoporosis are rare. The juvenile form presents in late childhood or early adolescence with an onset of symptomatic osteopenia and skeletal fragility. The disease may be severe, and may result in vertebral compression fractures, kyphosis, and loss of height. Although remission occurs spontaneously, residual disability remains, and peak adult bone mass is seldom achieved. Idiopathic adult osteoporosis occurs in middle-aged males in whom symptomatic axial osteopenia is evident.

Disease-Related Bone Loss

Regardless of etiology, chronic illness commonly leads to osteopenia, with malnutrition and disuse the major contributors. Frequently, glucocorticoid treatment required for management of many chronic illnesses increases bone loss, as described above.

Osteopenia is a common complication of most bone marrow tumors. Multiple myeloma may be associated with marked generalized axial and appendicular osteopenia. Myeloma cells produce an osteoclast-activating substance that is a potent stimulator of bone resorption. Myeloma should be suspected in an adult over age 50 who has symptomatic osteopenia.

Approximately 1% of myelomas are nonsecretory, and a definitive diagnosis in all patients is made by bone marrow biopsy. Furthermore, leukemia, lymphoma, and the rare mast cell tumor may be associated with osteoporosis.

PREDISPOSING FACTORS

Race and Heredity

In the caucasian population, the incidence of symptomatic osteoporosis is lower in persons from Southern Europe and the Mediterranean area than in those of Northern European descent. Although black persons have a greater bone mass at all ages, they generally have a lower incidence of symptomatic disease.

Osseous cells are endowed with genetic information that determines their ability to form, resorb, or maintain bone. While genetic information may be crucial to the understanding of osteoporosis, the relationship between genetic factors and other determinants of bone physiology requires further research.

Age and Sex

In the mature skeleton, bone mass remains fairly constant until the fifth decade, when it begins to decline. Bone loss is approximately 0.5%/year after age 40, and follows a more rapid course in women than in men. This age-related phenomenon occurs in both sexes and in all societies. At any given age, bone mass in men is greater than that in women. After age 40, men lose about 0.5% to 0.75% yearly, whereas women lose bone at twice that annual rate. Among postmenopausal women, some may temporarily lose 3% annually.

Nutrition

Adequate calcium intake is essential to the attainment and maintenance of maximal bone mass. Moreover, the body's need for calcium increases with age. The recommended daily allowance for a young adult approved by the National Research Council of the National Academy of Sciences is 800 mg. Dietary surveys of women with osteoporosis indicate a daily calcium consumption of less than 500 mg. The resultant calcium deficiency causes an increased mobilization of calcium from the skeletal reserve by increasing the secretion of parathyroid hormone and 1,25 - Dihydroxycholecalciferol (calcitriol) in order to restore calcium homeostasis.

The efficiency of calcium absorption from the upper gastrointestinal tract declines with age; thus, older persons need more dietary calcium to maintain a positive balance. Healthy premenopausal women over age 30 need about 1000 mg of calcium daily. In pregnant women and those over age 50, approximately 1500 mg of calcium/day is recommended. 2000 Mg of calcium are required for lactating women to prevent premature catabolism of bone.

Protein consumption is directly related to renal excretion of calcium. The high-protein diet typical of many affluent Western countries may be a major contributor to accelerated osteopenia among these populations.

1,25-Dihydroxycholecalciferol (an active vitamin D metabolite) helps to regulate normal blood calcium and phosphate levels by increasing both their absorption from the gastrointestinal tract and their resorption from bone.

Both dietary sources and sunlight provide the required amount of vitamin D. The elderly, however, are commonly deficient in vitamin D because of decreased consumption of vitamin D-fortified milk (and other dairy products). Infrequent exposure to sunlight coupled with decreased intestinal absorption of vitamin D also contributes to a deficiency.

Exercise and Weight-Bearing Stress

Daily weight-bearing exercise (*e.g.*, brisk walking) is crucial to skeletal maintenance. Mechanical weight-bearing stress is probably the most significant exogenous factor influencing bone development and remodeling. A sedentary individual is more likely to develop osteoporosis than is an active person who engages daily in some form of physical exercise. Common causes of osteoporosis resulting from decreasing the muscular forces acting on bone include immobilization of a limb, degeneration of a peripheral nerve of the spinal cord, and prolonged bed rest.

CLINICAL MANIFESTATIONS

Clinical manifestations of osteoporosis in the axial skeleton include vertebral compression fractures, causing continuous or intermittent back pain from the midthoracic to the midlumbar (occasionally to the lower lumbar) regions. Furthermore, progressive spinal deformity associated with compression fractures of the thoracic vertebrae leads to loss of height and progressive thoracic kyphosis ("dowager's hump"). Lower ribs eventually rest on the iliac crests, with the resultant downward pressure on the viscera causing abdominal protrusion. In the appendicular skeleton, fractures caused by minimal trauma are commonly associated with the intertrochanteric and intracapsular areas of the proximal femur, proximal humerus, and distal radius.[1, 4]

The manifestation of acute pain in the mid- to lower thorax or high lumbar areas of the spine while at rest or during routine daily activity is probably the earliest symptom of osteoporosis. The onset of pain is sudden. Most patients can recall the exact moment of occurrence, and can usually identify the exact locus from which the pain originates.

Spinal movement is drastically restricted. Pain intensifies with sitting or standing, with relief experienced with bed rest in a fully recumbent position.

Coughing, sneezing, and straining to move the bowels can cause excruciating pain. Anorexia, abdominal distention, and ileus associated with retroperitoneal bleeding may accompany lower thoracic and upper lumbar compression fractures. Persons with vertebral compression fractures in the midthoracic spine are relatively asymptomatic except for mild kyphosis, minor height loss, and discomfort along the rib cage. Clinically, the most common symptom is back pain associated with vertebral compression fractures or fractures of the proximal femur or distal radius sustained after little or no trauma.

Osteoporosis due to hyperparathyroidism is characterized by a variety of signs and symptoms, including bone pain, pseudogout, peptic ulcer, nephrolithiasis, fatigue, thirst, constipation, pancreatitis, and central nervous system disturbances. Whenever several of these conditions are manifested in an osteopenic patient with hypercalcemia and hypophosphatemia, further investigation of hyperparathyroidism is warranted.

LABORATORY ANALYSES AND DIAGNOSIS

Although postmenopausal osteoporosis is the most common form of bone loss, other causes must be systematically excluded. The history may suggest bone loss secondary to hyperparathyroidism, excess cortisol secretion, myeloma, or osteomalacia. A thorough history is necessary, therefore, in making a differential diagnosis, and should include history of acute illness, review of related symptoms, medical history, family history, and physical examination.

Laboratory Analyses

An extensive history facilitates the judicious selection of appropriate baseline laboratory tests. The most useful laboratory analyses include a complete blood count, an erythrocyte sedimentation rate, and measurement of serum calcium, phosphate, urea nitrogen, and creatinine levels and alkaline phosphatase activity. Measurement of urinary calcium, phosphorus, and creatinine excretion/24 hours may be informative. In uncomplicated postmenopausal disease, laboratory test results are usually within normal reference ranges and do not measure the extent or rate of progressive bone loss. Commonly, serum calcium, inorganic phosphate, and alkaline phosphatase levels are normal even in severe postmenopausal disease, although an elevated alkaline phosphatase may occur after a fracture. Thus, laboratory results generally do not contribute to assessment of the prognosis in uncomplicated postmenopausal osteoporosis.

In order to evaluate osteopenia secondary to conditions other than age-related and postmenopausal osteoporosis, other laboratory analyses are necessary. For those with suspected hyperthyroidism, measurement of the T_3 uptake, T_4, and free thyroxine index (FT_4I) is indicated. Serum protein electrophoresis or urine immunoelectrophoresis is performed when multiple myeloma is suspected. In patients with hypercalcemia, C-terminal immunoreactive parathyroid hormone is recommended.

Osteomalacia must be considered in the differential diagnosis of osteopenia. Osteomalacia is a qualitative rather than a quantitative disorder of bone characterized by an increased, decreased, or normal mass of insufficiently mineralized bone matrix. Abnormalities in vitamin D absorption and metabolism contribute to the pathogenesis of the disease. The diagnosis is corroborated by fluorescent microscopic examination of undecalcified trabecular bone tissue obtained by transiliac bone biopsy after time-separated double tetracycline labeling. Measurement of active vitamin D metabolites (*i.e.*, serum calcidiol and calcitriol) is useful in the evaluation of osteomalacia.

Radiographic Findings

Presently, radiologic procedures are the methods of choice for the diagnosis and evaluation of osteoporosis. Standing anteroposterior and lateral radiographs of the thoracic and lumbar spine should be obtained for any individual suspected of having a compression fracture. X-rays of the thoracic and lumbar spine affected by postmenopausal osteoporosis show evidence of decreased bone density, giving the vertebral column a "washed-out" appearance. Generally, as much as 30% to 50% of bone mass must be lost before radiographically-detectable findings occur. The two most useful techniques for assessing the bone mineral content in the axial skeleton are dual-photon absorptiometry and dual-energy quantitative computed tomography (CT).

Transiliac Bone Biopsy

Bone biopsy involves three steps: dynamic labeling, biopsy technique, and histomorphologic examination. Dynamic labeling uses orally-administered tetracycline as a time-delayed fluorescent marker to facilitate measurement of appositional bone formation. Tetracycline is absorbed by bone and deposited in areas of active mineralization. A bone sample is obtained by closed transiliac bone biopsy, using strict asepsis. Histomorphologic analysis of undecalcified sections of bone permits examination of the relationship between fully mineralized, hypomineralized, and nonmineralized portions of bone.[5, 6]

Histologic examination of corticocancellous bones from transiliac biopsies indicates that postmenopausal osteoporosis is a heterogeneous disorder with wide-ranging skeletal kinetics and bone remodeling activity. This finding is not surprising, because net loss of bone mass occurs in a number of ways when formation and resorption are not balanced. Clinical and biochemical findings, however, fail to predict histologic changes. Some physicians consider bone biopsy to be an essential part of a diagnostic workup in order to tailor therapy to the fundamental pathophysiologic processes. Others resort to transiliac biopsy reservedly. Because of regional sampling error, bone biopsy should be used to exclude a diagnosis of osteomalacia or osteitis fibrosa, and not to establish a diagnosis of osteoporosis.

TREATMENT AND PREVENTION

Management of osteoporosis has two facets: treatment of acute symptomatic disease and its complications, and maintenance of skeletal mass and integrity.

Treatment of Acute Symptoms

The goals of therapy are to relieve pain, provide comfortable mechanical support for the spine, provide assistance in daily activities, coordinate a physical rehabilitation program, and provide encouragement and support to both patient and family. Treatment of complications of spinal osteoporosis involves a regimen consisting of bed rest, administration of analgesics and muscle relaxants, and application of hot compresses. A second phase consists of gradual mobilization over two to five weeks, with assisted ambulation and the use of thoracic hyperextension orthosis as tolerated. As soon as acute pain has subsided, a daily program of active spinal extension exercises is prescribed.[7]

Maintenance of Skeletal Integrity

The incidence of hip fractures is lower in women with adequate calcium intake than in those with deficient consumption. Inasmuch as many elderly women are on low-sodium diets that are concurrently low in calcium, adequate supplementation is indicated. All patients receiving dietary calcium supplementation should be encouraged to maintain a high urine volume. Although hypercalcemia, hypercalciuria, nephrolithiasis, and urolithiasis are not common in uncomplicated postmenopausal osteoporosis, a 24-hour urine collection to measure calcium, phosphate, and creatinine excretion should be performed prior to the initiation of supplementation. Prolonged bed rest or immobilization, sarcoidosis, metastasis, multiple myeloma, primary hyperparathyroidism, hypercalciuria, and hypervitaminosis D can account for either transient or sustained hypercalcemia. Once these conditions are excluded, dietary calcium supplementation can be administered. Nonprescription oral calcium supplements include calcium carbonate, phosphate, lactate, and gluconate. Natural food sources with a high calcium content include dairy products, green leafy vegetables, and sardines. An 8 oz glass of whole milk supplies about 250 mg of calcium.

Those patients deficient in vitamin D may be prescribed supplementation within recommended guidelines. Treatment of postmenopausal osteoporosis with massive quantities of vitamin D can lead to dangerous hypercalcemia. If vitamin D supplementation is prescribed, regular measurement of the serum calcium level is recommended.

Estrogens are increasingly regarded as effective for preventing or arresting the progression of osteoporosis. Estrogen therapy following menopause inhibits bone resorption and helps maintain axial and appendicular bone integrity. Estrogen therapy is most effective in the perimenopausal period before bone loss becomes severe, and may be indicated to prevent untimely bone loss in women in whom menopause has been surgically induced. The increased risk of endometrial cancer associated with estrogen therapy must be assessed with each patient. Those taking estrogens must have frequent gynecologic examinations.[8, 9]

Regular weight-bearing activity is necessary for maintenance of bone mass. The amount of weight bearing necessary to maintain skeletal mass throughout adult life is not known; however, a daily program of spinal extension exercise (*e.g.*, a 30-minute walk) is advocated.

Fluorides may be beneficial in the treatment of osteoporosis. There is evidence of a decreased incidence in vertebral body compression fractures in patients taking fluoride as compared with untreated controls. Calcium treatment must be adequate during fluoride therapy to prevent an osteomalacialike condition with brittle bones. The efficacy and safety of fluoride usage are presently being assessed in extensive longitudinal studies, and it currently remains experimental. Likewise, the peptide hormone calcitonin and the anabolic steroid stanozolol are being investigated to ascertain their effectiveness in inhibiting bone resorption.[1]

CASE STUDY

A 66-year-old Caucasian woman was admitted to the hospital after sustaining a fall at home. Initial assessment disclosed facial lacerations and multiple contusions on the arms, legs, thighs, hips, and upper chest. Vital signs showed a temperature of 98.5° F, pulse 65, respirations 15, and blood pressure 115/78. X-rays obtained on admission revealed a simple fracture of the intertrochanteric area of the right proximal femur, and a lateral radiograph of the thoracic and lumbar spine showed visible loss of bone density. Personal and medical history indicated that the patient is a widow with two children and four grandchildren. She resides alone and has had relatively good health, with no history of chronic illness. The patient reported a simple fracture of the left distal radius 5 years prior to this admission.

LABORATORY FINDINGS

	Admission	*Postoperative*
WBC	N	N
RBC	sl ↓	sl ↓
Hgb	sl ↓	sl ↓
Hct	sl ↓	sl ↓
Differential	N	
Platelets	N	
PT	N	
APTT	N	
ESR	N	
Glucose	N	sl ↑
BUN	N	N
Creatinine	N	N
Na	N	N
K	N	N
Cl	N	N
CO_2	N	N
Ca	N	N
PO_4	N	N
Mg	N	N
Alk Phos		↑

Questions

1. What is the most likely diagnosis? Why?
2. What tests would confirm the diagnosis?
3. Do the laboratory findings support this diagnosis?
4. What treatment is likely?

Discussion

1. Uncomplicated postmenopausal osteoporosis is the most likely diagnosis because it is most commonly found in white women of this age group. The type of fracture sustained by this patient and her history support this diagnosis.
2. Radiologic procedures such as dual photon absorptiometry or dual energy quantitative CT should confirm the diagnosis.
3. The laboratory findings support the diagnosis. Except for alkaline phosphatase, which is expected to be elevated after a fracture, laboratory findings in uncomplicated postmenopausal osteoporosis are usually normal, even when bone loss has been extensive. Slightly elevated glucose is associated with postoperative IV infusion of 5% dextrose in water (D5W).
4. A treatment regimen consisting of a 7 to 10 day period of bed rest, and gradual mobilization over 3 to 5 weeks with assisted ambulation, followed by a daily program of active spinal extension exercise, would be prescribed. Oral calcium would also be recommended as a daily supplement.

REFERENCES

1. Kaplan FS: Osteoporosis. Clin Symp 35(5):1983
2. Brody JA, Farmer ME, White LR: Absence of menopausal effect on hip fracture occurrence in white females. Am J Pub Health 74:1397–1398, 1984
3. National Institutes of Health: Looking at menopause's role in osteoporosis. JAMA 254:2379–2380, 1985
4. Consensus Conference: Osteoporosis. JAMA 252:799–802, 1984
5. Fallon MD, Teitelbaum SL: The interpretation of flourescent tetracycline markers in the diagnosis of metabolic bone diseases. Human Pathol 13:416–417, 1982
6. Frost HM: Tetracycline-based histological analysis of bone remodeling. Calcif Tissue Res 3:211–217, 1969
7. Sinaki M: Postmenopausal spinal osteoporosis: Physical therapy and rehabilitation principles. Mayo Clin Proc 57:699–703, 1982
8. Carr BR, McDonald PC: Estrogen treatment of postmenopausal women. Adv Int Med 28:491–508, 1983
9. Whedon GD: Osteoporosis. N Engl J Med 305:397–399, 1981

Chapter 65

Cystinuria / Homocystinuria

Benjamin J. Andrusaitis

CYSTINURIA

Etiology and Pathophysiology

Amino acids in the plasma are completely filtered through the glomerulus. Subsequently, they are reabsorbed in the renal tubules by several transport mechanisms. A genetic defect in one such transport mechanism in the proximal convoluted tubules results in large increases in the urinary excretion of the dibasic amino acids lysine, arginine, ornithine, and cystine. Due to the solubility characteristics of cystine, overexcretion tends to result in precipitation and renal calculi formation. The renal calculi are responsible for the clinical manifestations, and thus the disease is called *cystinuria.* Cystinuria is inherited as an autosomal recessive trait, with a prevalence in the United States of approximately 1 in 15,000.[1]

Clinical Manifestations

Cystinuria affects both sexes, with males having more severe clinical symptoms. The peak age of onset is in the second and third decade. Onset can occur, however, from early childhood through old age.[2]

Pain from the passage of renal calculi through the ureter (renal colic) is the most common initial symptom. Growth retardation due to renal insufficiency, recurrent infections, and high blood pressure are typical clinical findings. Untreated cystinuria can result in renal failure.[3]

Laboratory Assessment

The diagnosis of cystinuria is a possibility in any patient with urinary calculi. One of the simplest diagnostic tools in assessing cystinuria is microscopic examination of the urine sediment for cystine crystals. For cystine crystals to become apparent, however, cystine concentration must exceed the level that will produce the clinical manifestations of cystinuria. Approximately one-half of cystinuric patients have stones of mixed composition, and 10% have stones composed of substances other than cystine.[3]

Any patient with urolithiasis should have a urinary cyanide-nitroprusside test performed to rule out cystinuria.[4] This test is a sensitive indicator of cystine concentrations that will produce stone formation; a negative result excludes the diagnosis of cystinuria. The test is not, however, specific for homozygous stone formers. Some heterozygotes, which do not require treatment, will test positive. Homocystine and acetone will also produce false-positive results.

In patients with a positive nitroprusside test, the diagnosis of cystinuria can be established by identifying the specific amino acids present in excess in the urine with thin-layer chromatography or high-voltage electrophoresis. Quantitation of amino acids can be performed by ion-exchange chromatography or by colorimetric assay. Quantitation is used to differentiate homozygotes from heterozygotes and in monitoring therapy designed to lower urine cystine concentration. Cystine excretion is also seen in Wilson's disease, Fanconi's syndrome, and cystinosis as part of general aminoacidurias.[5]

HOMOCYSTINURIA

Etiology and Pathophysiology

Homocysteine is an intermediate in the metabolism of methionine to cystine. The main intermediate in this pathway is cystathionine, formed from homocysteine and serine and catalyzed by cystathionine-β-synthase. Homocysteine may also be reconverted to methionine by the action of N^5-methyltetrahydrofolate reductase. Normally, there is very little accumulation of homocysteine in the plasma or urine. Homocysteine is unstable in aqueous solutions and is converted to homocystine when present.[6]

The most common cause of homocystinuria is cystathionine-β-synthase deficiency. The enzyme deficiency may be partial or complete. Decreased levels of this enzyme result in increased levels of methionine, homocystine, and other sulfur-containing amino acids in body fluids. The accumulation of homocystine results in abnormalities in the vascular endothelium and in thrombus formation. Decreased cystine production affects collagen synthesis and results in skeletal and ocular changes.[7]

A much rarer cause of homocystinuria is N^5-methyltetrahydrofolate reductase deficiency due to defects in folate metabolism or to a genetic defect in enzyme synthesis. The clinical symptoms of these conditions are generally milder and easier to manage.

Clinical Manifestations

Homocystinuria produced by cystathionine-β-synthase deficiency typically appears by age five. Nearly all patients present with impaired vision from dislocated optic lenses, which can result in glaucoma. Osteoporosis may be present, but rarely is clinically significant. Vascular complications are the most serious clinical manifestation, caused by damaged vascular endothelium. Arterial occlusion can be lethal before age 10. Mental retardation is present in a minority of cases.[3] The presence of connective tissue abnormalities and dislocated lenses are causes for suspecting cystathionine-β-synthase deficiency.

Laboratory Assessment

The biochemical findings in cystathionine-β-synthase deficiency include homocystinuria, marked elevation in plasma methionine and homocystine concentrations, and reduced or absent plasma cystine levels.

Neonatal screening can be performed with the Guthrie bacterial inhibition assay. Bacterial growth, which requires large amounts of methionine in the presence of patient blood, is a semiquantitative indicator of methionine concentration.[8] Liver disease, tyrosinosis, and hepatic S-adenosyl methionine synthetase deficiency can also produce positive results.[6] A positive Guthrie assay and homocystinuria are indicative of cystathionine-β-synthase deficiency. The Guthrie assay is a relatively nonsensitive test, and thus a negative result does not rule out the enzyme deficiency.

Homocystinuria can be assessed with the cyanide-nitroprusside test, as described above. Although a negative result can rule out homocystinuria, a positive result must be verified to rule out the presence of other disulfides.

Verification of homocystinuria can be performed by thin-layer chromatography or high-voltage electrophoresis. Quantitation of homocystine, to verify the diagnosis and to follow the effect of treatment, can be performed with column chromatography.[2]

Confirmation of cystathionine-β-synthase deficiency as the underlying cause of homocystinuria can be accomplished by measuring plasma amino acid levels. Increased plasma methionine levels and homocystine and reduced levels of cystine indicate cystathionine-β-synthase deficiency. Normal or low levels of methionine with homocystinuria are indicative of N^5-methyltetrahydrofolate reductase deficiency.

TREATMENT

Treatment for these disorders is discussed in Chapter 30.

CASE STUDY #1

A thirty-five-year-old white man complained of intense pain on urination, recurrent lower back pain, and fever. The patient's body temperature was 38.3° C (101° F). Routine blood tests indicated a slight leukocytosis, but no other abnormalities. A urinalysis showed a cloudy specimen with cystine crystals, 3+ bacteria, and 3+ white blood cells, 2+ hematuria, 3+ proteinuria, and 3+ nitrite. A urine culture indicated a colony count greater than 100,000/mL, with an identification of *Escherichia coli.* As a followup, a cyanide-nitroprusside test was positive.

Questions

1. Based on the urinalysis findings, what condition appears to exist in this patient?
2. How would cystinuria be confirmed?
3. How would zygosity be determined?

Discussion

1. Recurrent pain, a positive urine culture, and other abnormal urinalysis findings indicate a urinary tract infection. This is often the initial presenting symptom of cystinuria. The presence of cystine crystals in the urine and a positive cynaide-nitroprusside test are indicative of the disease.
2. To confirm cystinuria, a urine amino acid analysis should be performed by thin-layer chromatography; excretion of cystine, lysine, arginine, and ornithine should be demonstrated.
3. Amino acid quantitation by column chromatography should indicate that the patient is homozygous for cystinuria.

CASE STUDY #2

The parents of a 14-month-old white male reported their child's vision problems and failure to develop physically at a normal rate. Examination indicated slowed physical and mental development, bilateral dislocated lenses, and fine, sparse hair. Laboratory tests indicated a positive cyanide-nitroprusside test.

Routine blood chemistries, urinalysis, and CBC were normal.

Questions

1. What disorder do the clinical findings suggest?
2. What laboratory findings would you expect?
3. What is the significance of finding elevated levels of methionine?

Discussion

1. The clinical findings suggest homocystinuria.
2. Followup studies by thin-layer chromatography should indicate homocystinuria. Plasma amino acid analysis should indicate the presence of homocystine and elevated levels of methionine.
3. A diagnosis of cystathionine-β-synthase deficiency leading to homocystinuria should be made, based on the elevated levels of methionine.

REFERENCES

1. Thier SO: Cystinuria. In Wyngaarden JB, Smith LH (eds): Cecil Textbook of Medicine. Philadelphia, WB Saunders, 1985
2. Thier SO, Segal S: Cystinuria. In Stanbury JB, Wyngaarden JB, Fredrickson DS (eds): The Metabolic Basis of Inherited Disease. New York City, McGraw-Hill, 1978
3. Rosenberg LE, Short EM: Inherited defects of membrane transport. In Petersdorf RG, Adams RD et al (eds): Harrison's Principles of Internal Medicine. New York City, McGraw-Hill, 1983
4. Bradley M, Schuman GB: Examination of the urine. In Henry JB (ed): Clinical Diagnosis and Management by Laboratory Methods. Philadelphia, WB Saunders, 1984
5. Eberlein WR: Aminoaciduria in childhood: Cystinuria and cystinosis. Am J Med Sci 225:677, 1953
6. Silverman LM, Christenson RH, Grant GH: Amino acids and proteins. In Tietz NW (ed): Textbook of Clinical Chemistry. Philadelphia, WB Saunders, 1986
7. Kelly TE: Diseases of genetic origin. In Kaplan LA, Pesce AJ (eds): Clinical Chemistry: Theory, Analysis, and Correlation. St Louis, CV Mosby, 1984
8. Guthrie R: Screening for "inborn errors of metabolism" in the newborn infant—a multiple test program. Birth Defects 4:92, 1968

Chapter 66

Malnutrition and Starvation

Deborah T. Firestone / Craig A. Lehmann

Public interest in nutrition has been increasing over the years, as people have become better informed about the short- and long-term effects of the food that they eat. This increased attention has led a number of investigators to study the nutritional status of various populations, and to identify those that are malnourished. Such studies have drawn attention to the prevalence of malnourished patients in hospitals and nursing homes.[1, 2]

Malnutrition describes a condition of poor nourishment. Prolonged intake of a diet that is nutritionally deficient or the abrupt or gradual withdrawal of food can lead to starvation. The identification of patients who are malnourished or those at risk of becoming malnourished is important, because studies have shown that these patients have an increased rate of morbidity and mortality.[3, 4] The nutritional assessment of a patient is the first step in identifying malnutrition and starvation, and the clinical laboratory plays a central role in this evaluative process.

PATHOPHYSIOLOGY OF NUTRITIONAL DEFICIENCIES

Nutritional deficiencies can develop over a short or a long period of time, and may involve one or, more commonly, many nutrients. The way in which the body adapts to these changes depends on (1) whether there are reserves of the nutrient, (2) the difference between the amount of intake of the nutrient and the amount needed by the body, and (3) the amount of time over which the reduced intake of the nutrient continues.

The physiological response of the body to a nutritional deficiency occurs in three stages. In stage one, the body responds to the insufficient intake of nutrients by utilizing reserves of the nutrient, if any. Stage two results if the deficient intake of the nutrient continues. It is characterized by altered serum and/or urine concentrations of the nutrient or its metabolites. In this stage, although the patient may be asymptomatic, the nutritional deficiency may be detected using appropriate laboratory tests. The final physiological response of the body, the development of stage three, is determined by the available stores of fat in the body. When the available stores of lipid are depleted, protein in the body is used as a last source of energy, which leads to the ultimate demise of the patient. In stage three, the patient is symptomatic and the nutritional deficiency can be detected using a number of laboratory tests.

Vitamin deficiencies can be either primary, due to inadequate intake, or secondary as the result of various disease processes. Vitamins can be divided into two groups, fat-soluble (A, D, E, and K) and water-soluble (C and B-complex). They perform a variety of physiological functions, for example, as cofactors in numerous enzymatic reactions. The body's adaptation to vitamin deficiency is diverse, and depends on the particular function that is being compromised.

Minerals are necessary for many normal functions within the body, *e.g.*, cellular and humoral immunity. Although the body is able to compensate over a period of time for deficiencies in the mineral content of the diet, if the deficiency continues for a prolonged period, compensatory mechanisms are no longer adequate, and serious diseases such as iron-deficiency anemia or osteomalacia can result.

Studies of hospitalized patients in the United States have shown that nutritional deficiency is associated with compromised immunity and may be a significant contributor to severe infections.[4, 5] In undernourished children and adults, lymphoid tissues, such as the tonsils, spleen, and thymus, atrophy in response to nutritional deprivation. There is a decrease in the number of T lymphocytes, impairment in delayed hypersensitivity skin reactions to various antigens, and a decrease in the serum concentration of many complement components. The primary antibody response to most antigens is depressed, although the secondary antibody response is usually unaffected. The bactericidal activity of polymorphonuclear leukocytes (PMNs) is reduced, and breaks in the integrity of the mucocutaneous junction may be caused by deficiencies in specific vitamins and minerals, thus making the patient more susceptible to infections.

CLINICAL SYNDROMES

Acute malnutrition, due to any one of many clinical syndromes, may lead to a state of starvation in the patient. Patients with *anorexia nervosa,* an eating disorder most often seen in teenage girls, suffer from a distorted body image that makes them preoccupied with losing weight and being thin. Weight loss is accomplished by either fasting or eating small amounts of food, and may be accompanied by self-induced vomiting. Anorexia nervosa may be life-threatening because of the medical complications of starvation. Patients with *bulimia* show poor control over their intake of food. These patients indulge in binge eating, or the ingestion of large quantities of food, followed by induced vomiting in order to avoid a gain in weight. The compulsive overeating that occurs in bulimia may also occur to varying degrees in other clinical conditions. Patients may also be classified as bulimic anorexics, persons who normally fast or ingest small quantities of food, but periodically gorge themselves, and then vomit to maintain their low weight.

Cancer patients often experience a condition of acute malnutrition, as a result of the disease process itself or as a result of treatment modalities such as chemotherapy and radiation. In fact, one of the first symptoms of cancer in a patient may be an unexplained weight loss.

Conditions of protein-calorie malnutrition (PCM) can also lead to a state of starvation. PCM in children is most prevalent in areas of the world that are undeveloped. The two most common classifications of PCM are kwashiorkor and marasmus. *Marasmus,* generally being more severe in nature, is characterized by a diet that is deficient in protein and calories. This results in a depletion of the adipose tissue and skeletal muscle (somatic) protein, leading to a general wasting of the patient. *Kwashiorkor,* on the other hand, can vary from a mild to a severe syndrome, and is characterized by a diet that is low in protein with carbohydrates being the major source of calories. In kwashiorkor, the somatic protein stores are generally maintained, while the visceral protein stores are depleted. Patients with marasmic kwashiorkor exhibit symptoms of both.

There are syndromes in which chronic malnutrition, over a period of time, may lead to starvation. This may occur in drug addicts and alcoholics due to prolonged ingestion of diets rich in "empty calories," such as ethanol. These individuals may have an unbalanced diet to begin with, and the presence of drugs and/or alcohol can compound the problem by interfering with the normal absorption and utilization of ingested nutrients. Chronic malnutrition with eventual starvation may also be present in cancer patients, as well as in patients who fail to eat well-balanced meals because of inadequate or inferior nutrients supplied from the environment, or because of a diet regime.

There are patient populations that may be suffering from acute or chronic malnutrition that does not progress to conditions of starvation. This population includes the increasing number of elderly patients, who for financial, emotional, or physical reasons do not consume foods that supply the proper nutritional requirements. Patients with malabsorption syndromes or diets deficient in a specific nutrient or metabolite may exhibit clinical signs and symptoms indicative of acute or chronic malnutrition. These patients, although they are malnourished, do not have deficiencies in their diets that are severe enough to lead to starvation.

CLINICAL MANIFESTATIONS

While the syndromes of malnutrition and starvation are complex in their etiology, so too are the clinical signs and symptoms of the disorders. The clinical picture of patients with any one of these disorders is variable and will depend on the degree, type, and duration of the eating disorder. A patient may present with symptoms that are specific enough to suggest a possible deficiency in a class of nutrients, such as bleeding tendencies (vitamin K deficiency) or hypochromic anemia (iron deficiency). On the other hand, symptoms that may reflect a combination of nutritional deficiencies include bradycardia, hypotension, hypothermia, dry skin, amenorrhea, hyperactivity, abdominal pain, lethargy, weight loss, wasting, muscle weakness, anorexia, growth retardation, desquamation and pigmentation of the skin, diarrhea, and hepatomegaly.

Clinical assessment of patients with nutritional disorders can be made using a combination of history-taking, evaluation of signs and symptoms, and anthropometric measurements (measurements of the size, weight, and proportions of the human body). A nutritional history should include questions that establish whether there have been any recent weight losses or gains, illnesses, changes in dietary habits, and medications taken. An assessment of food intake, which can be obtained through either the patient's recall of food eaten or a diary of food intake over a period of time, can at best provide only an estimate of the nutritional status of the patient, due to the variability in methodologies.

Anthropometric measurements, if interpreted correctly, can be used to monitor the nutritional status of a patient. Changes in body weight, as well as rapidity of weight loss, can be an accurate indicator of a change in the nutritional status of nonedematous patients. Measurements of height can be a more sensitive indicator of malnutrition in children than in adults, because children frequently exhibit a retardation in growth in response to malnutrition. Triceps skinfold measurements (SF) are frequently used to estimate body fat. In cases of severe malnutrition, subcutaneous body fat disappears. Mid-upper-arm circumference measurements (MAC) of the nondominant arm have been used to evaluate changes in skeletal muscle mass. SF and MAC measurements are useful tools in the identification of severe malnutrition, but values must be interpreted carefully when distinguishing mild to moderately malnourished patients from lean, healthy individuals.

LABORATORY ANALYSES AND DIAGNOSIS

Routine Laboratory Tests for Assessing Nutritional Status

Laboratory tests used as part of the initial nutritional evaluation of a patient will vary, depending on the patient population under study.

The anemia, leukopenia, and decreased hemoglobin and hematocrit associated with malnutrition can be detected by a complete blood count. Because the immune defenses of undernourished children and adults are impaired, total lymphocyte counts are decreased and cell-mediated immunity, as determined by delayed hypersensitivity responses, is frequently abnormal in these patients. Studies have shown a correlation between the degree of anergy and the severity of the nutritional deficiency in a patient. The degree of anergy has also been used as an indicator of prognosis, sepsis, and mortality.[2, 3, 4]

Triglyceride and cholesterol determinations can be used to determine whether the fat content of the diet is appropriate and whether fat is being absorbed properly.

Albumin is one of the biochemical markers most frequently used in assessing the protein status of an individual. However, the long half-life of albumin (18 days) and the equilibration of extravascular albumin with the intravascular stores[6] limit its usefulness as a marker of recent protein changes in the diet.[7] Albumin has been identified as a predictor of patients who will develop postoperative complications.[3]

While there is little value in measuring the individual levels of minerals, unless a patient history dictates otherwise, decreases in sodium, potassium, chloride, bicarbonate, calcium, phosphate, and magnesium could corroborate a diagnosis of malnutrition in the absence of other disease.

Blood urea nitrogen (BUN) determinations are increased, reflecting the breakdown of protein in the body. Twenty-four-hour urinary creatinine can be used to measure the somatic protein status (muscle mass) of a patient. Creatinine, a breakdown product of skeletal muscle, is excreted into the urine in decreasing amounts as the degree of malnutrition becomes more severe.[7] An accurate determination of urinary creatinine is dependent on proper sample collection. The creatinine height index (CHI) is obtained by dividing the 24-hour creatinine excretion of a patient by the 24-hour creatinine excretion of a control matched by height and weight.[8] The CHI is affected by changes in creatinine excretion due to age and by variability in the standards, and therefore must be interpreted carefully in evaluating cases of PCM.

The total iron-binding capacity (TIBC), an indirect measurement of transferrin, can serve as an overall indicator of protein nutrition. Interpretation of TIBC values, however, must take into consideration limiting factors, such as iron stores of the patient.

Nonroutine Tests for Assessing Nutritional Status

The determination of rapid turnover visceral proteins, such as thyroxine-binding prealbumin (2-day half-life) and retinol-binding protein (10-hour half-life), has proved to be particularly useful in evaluating the short-term effects of nutritional therapy with respect to protein. In addition, these proteins are the first of the visceral proteins to respond to total parenteral nutrition. The plasma levels of these proteins are low during periods of protein depletion, and increase rapidly when the nutritional deficiency is corrected.[9] Inflammatory conditions can also have a direct effect on levels of thyroxine-binding prealbumin and retinol-binding protein.[10]

Transferrin determinations can also be used as an indicator of visceral protein depletion. Transferrin has a half-life of approximately eight days, and the levels of this protein correlate with short-term changes in protein deficiency. Transferrin levels have been shown to predict accurately which patients will develop post-operative complications.[3]

The serum concentration of many of the complement components is decreased in conditions of protein-calorie malnutrition. The decrease may be due to a reduced rate of synthesis and to an increased rate of consumption in antigen–antibody reactions (*e.g.*, infections). The extent to which C3 levels are reduced correlates with morbidity.[5]

Leukocyte terminal deoxynucleotidyl transferase (TdT) is present in large amounts in immature thymocytes, and levels of the enzyme decrease as T cells mature. In PCM, there is a decreased activity of thymic hormone, which results in defects in the normal maturational sequence of T lymphocytes.[11] This results in an increase in "null" cells, which may be immature T cells.[12] Determination of TdT can, therefore, be used as an indirect measurement of nutritional deficiency and of defects in the maturational sequence of T lymphocytes.

Deficiencies in the essential fatty acids (EFA) are most often a result of the side-effects of treatment modalities, such as fat-free parenteral feeding, or of certain disease processes, such as fat malabsorption in Crohn's disease. Total lipid analysis can be performed to assess the EFA status of a patient. This test, however, does not separate the classes of lipids, and the performance of more sophisticated procedures, such as 5, 8, 11-eicosatrienoic levels and the eicosatrienoic acid/arachidonic acid ratio (the triene/tetrane ratio), can be used to accomplish such a classification.[13]

The reasons for nutritional deficiencies in vitamins and trace elements are varied. They include inadequate dietary intake, and impaired absorption, metabolism, or excretion due to disease, medical treatments, or increased nutritional demands, *e.g.*, pregnancy, surgery. Indications for the measurement of a specific vitamin or trace element most commonly are based on information obtained from a patient's dietary history or clinical symptoms that the patient presents, for example, xerophthalmia due to vitamin A deficiency.

Factors Influencing Laboratory Analyses

The laboratory tests used as part of a nutrition profile can be affected by a patient's diet and intake of drugs. It is, therefore, imperative that laboratory scientists become familiar with the various factors that can influence the interpretation of a particular laboratory analysis. Drugs can reduce food intake and digestibility, impair absorption, increase excretion, inhibit synthesis, and interfere with the utilization of nutrients. These interactions can result in mineral and electrolyte imbalances and affect the levels of vitamins in laboratory assays. Clinical laboratory scientists must evaluate test results in the light of these interfering factors, in order to avoid the reporting of erroneous or misleading results.

TREATMENT

Treatment of patients with nutritional deficiencies can be accomplished by a change in diet, oral supplementation, enteral feeding, or parenteral feeding. The laboratory plays a critical role in the monitoring of patients on enteral and parenteral feedings, and the laboratory scientist should be aware of the complications that may develop. These include fluid and electrolyte imbalance, acid–base imbalance, glycosuria, hyperglycemia, and hepatic and hematologic abnormalities. Prolonged use of total parenteral nutrition may result in vitamin (folic acid, vitamin A, vitamin E, biotin) and mineral (zinc) deficiencies.[14]

CASE STUDY

A 17-year-old female was seen by her physician at her mother's request. The mother reported that the girl was chronically tired and had trouble concentrating in school; she had previously been on a diet and had lost 30 pounds, but appeared to be eating well now.

A physical examination was performed and a detailed medical history was taken. Both proved to be unremarkable.

After an overnight fast, blood was drawn for a routine 20 chemistry profile and a complete blood count.

The complete blood count was within normal limits, and the only abnormalities on the 20 chemistry profile were an elevated bicarbonate level and a decreased plasma potassium and chloride concentration. Based on these results, the patient appeared to be in metabolic alkalosis, and was both hypokalemic and hypochloremic. Because no finding pointed to a diagnosis, the patient was seen on a followup visit.

On further investigation, the patient revealed that she felt tremendous social pressures from her peers at school. All of her friends were very fashion-conscious, with great emphasis on being thin. She felt particular pressure because of a previous weight problem, and she was afraid of gaining back the weight she had lost.

When questioned about how she was keeping her weight off, the patient reluctantly revealed that, although she enjoyed eating and therefore ate whatever she liked, she was vomiting and taking laxatives at least once a day in order to avoid a gain in weight.

Questions

1. Given this patient's history, what disorder is probable?
2. Are the reported laboratory findings consistent with this diagnosis?
3. What next step is warranted in the treatment of this patient?

Discussion

1. Bulimia is the probable disorder in this case.
2. There are many disorders that can cause hypochloremia (*e.g.*, renal disorders, prolonged vomiting), hypokalemia (*e.g.*, chronic starvation, gastrointestinal loss), and metabolic alkalosis (*e.g.*, prolonged diuretic use, loss of HCl from the stomach). Using a combination of the patient's medical history, physical examination, and laboratory results, it is possible to rule out some of the causes, thereby limiting the number of possibilities.

The most common laboratory findings in bulimia are metabolic alkalosis, hypokalemia, and hypochloremia. In cases involving dehydration, BUN may be elevated, and serum amylase may be elevated when gastric dilatation is present.

3. At this point, the patient should be referred to an eating disorders center.

REFERENCES

1. Bistrian BR, Blackburn GL, Vitale J et al: Prevalence of malnutrition in general medical patients. JAMA 15:1567–1570, 1976
2. Shaver HJ, Loper JA, Lutes RA: Nutritional status of nursing home patients. J Parenter Enteral Nutr 4:367–370, 1980
3. Mullen JL, Gertner MH, Buzby GP et al: Implications of malnutrition in the surgical patient. Arch Surg 114:121–125, 1979
4. Harvey KB, Ruggiero JA, Regan CS et al: Hospital morbidity and mortality risk factors using nutritional assessment. Clin Res 26:581A, 1978
5. Chandra RK: Serum complement and immunoconglutinin in malnutrition. Arch Dis Child 50:225–229, 1975
6. Hoffenberg R, Black E, Brock JF: Albumin and γ-globulin tracer studies in protein depletion states. J Clin Invest 45:143–151, 1966
7. Forbes GB, Bruining GJ: Urinary creatinine excretion and lean body mass. Am J Clin Nutr 29:1359–1366, 1976

8. Viteri FE, Alvarado J: The creatinine height index: Its use in the estimation of the degree of protein depletion and repletion in protein-calorie-malnourished children. Pediatrics 46:696–706, 1970
9. Shetty PS, Watrasiewicz KE, Jung RT et al: "Rapid-turnover transport proteins: An index of subclinical protein-energy malnutrition." Lancet 2:230–232, 1979
10. Ramsden DB, Prince HP, Burr WA et al: The inter-relationship of thyroid hormones, vitamin A, and their binding proteins following acute stress. Clin Endocrinol 8:109–122, 1978
11. Chandra RK: Serum thymic hormone activity in protein-energy malnutrition. Clin Exp Immunol 38:228–230, 1979
12. Chandra RK: T- and B-lymphocyte subpopulations and leukocyte terminal deoxynucleotidyl-transferase in energy-protein undermalnutrition. Acta Paediatr Scand 68:841–845, 1979
13. Holman RT: The ratio of trienoic: tetranoic acids in tissue lipids as a measure of essential fatty acid requirement. J Nutr 70:405, 1960
14. Howard L, Bigaonette J, Chu R et al: Water-soluble vitamin requirements in home parenteral nutrition patients. Am J Clin Nutr 37:421–428, 1983

BIBLIOGRAPHY

Burritt MF, Anderson CF: Laboratory assessment of nutritional status. Hum Pathol 15:130–133, 1984

Carpentier YA, Barthel J, Bruyns J: Plasma protein concentration in nutritional assessment. Proc Nutr Soc 41:405–417, 1982

Durnin JVGA, Fidanza F: Evaluation of nutritional status. In Somogyi JC, Wenger R (eds): Principal aspects of clinical nutrition. Bibl Nutr Dieta 35:20–30, 1985

Groer ME, Shekleton ME: Basic Pathophysiology—A Conceptual Approach, pp 309–343. St Louis, CV Mosby, 1979

Labbe RF (ed): Symposium on laboratory assessment of nutritional status. Clin Lab Med 1(4):605–796, 1981

Mitchell JE: Medical complications of anorexia nervosa and bulimia. In Anorexia Nervosa and Bulimia: Diagnosis and Treatment, pp 48–77. Minneapolis, University of Minnesota Press, 1985

Tomaiolo PP: Malnutrition in the elderly: Its recognition and treatment. Compr Ther 11:54–58, 1985

Truswell AS: Malnutrition in the third world—I. Br Med J 291:525–528, 1985

Woods HF: Biochemical methods in nutritional assessment. Proc Nutr Soc 41:419–424, 1982

Chapter 67

Disorders of Carbohydrate Metabolism

H. Elise Galloway

SIMPLE SUGARS

The sugars of interest in the simple sugar category are lactose, galactose, fructose, and pentose. Although there are others that may present problems, their incidence is quite low, and they will not be considered here. See Chapter 38 for discussion of impaired glucose metabolism.

The inability of the body to use monosaccharides and disaccharides can be attributed directly to lack of the specific enzyme for a particular sugar. This lack is manifested in one of two ways: it results either in a malabsorption problem or in a metabolic pathway defect that causes an increased amount of pathway precursors. Malabsorption is addressed elsewhere (see Chap. 21) and will be discussed only briefly here.

Etiology and Pathophysiology

Lactose or milk sugar is a disaccharide composed of galactose and glucose. *Lactase,* an enzyme produced in the brush borders of the intestinal mucosal cells, splits lactose into its two monosaccharides. As mammals mature, the ingestion of lactose normally decreases, which parallels a decrease in the production of lactase. Adults normally have a low level or absence of lactase[1] and, in some, this may result in an acquired lactose intolerance.

The more serious dysfunctions of sugar metabolism are due to the lack of specific enzymes involved in metabolic pathways. These disorders involve the metabolism of fructose, galactose, and the pentose sugar, xylulose. Occasionally infants are not able to manufacture lactase, which results in congenital lactose intolerance. All of these disorders are autosomal recessive defects, and the incidence of occurrence is low (see Table 67-1).

Fructose intolerance can result if any one of three enzymes is missing: fructokinase, fructose-1-phosphate aldolase B, and fructose-1,6-diphosphatase.[2] Galactosemia is most often seen due to the lack of galactose-1-phosphate uridyltransferase. This deficiency results in the accumulation of galactose-1-phosphate and galactitol, the metabolite implicated in the development of cataracts. Two other enzymes involved in galactose metabolism have been associated with intolerance. They are galactokinase and, very rarely, uridine diphosphate galactose-4-epimerase.[3] Pentosuria is a relatively benign autosomal recessive defect of the glucuronic acid oxidation pathway resulting from a decrease in the activity of L-xylulose reductase.[4] It is found primarily in persons of Jewish extraction. Congenital lactose intolerance, first described in 1959 by Hoezal,[5] results from the absence of lactase in infants. It is a rare condition that can prove fatal if not diagnosed and treated.

Clinical Manifestations

Sugar intolerances present with similar clinical symptoms. Diarrhea or loose stools after eating, abdominal pain, cramps and/or distention, and failure to thrive are all relatively nonspecific signals either of malabsorption or of enzyme deficiencies. However, it is possible for there to be no clinical signs initially.

Children who present with cataracts should be considered for galactose intolerance because galactokinase patients have no aversion to milk and are asymptomatic except for the development of cataracts. Uridyltransferase-deficient patients, on the other hand, present with vomiting, hepatomegaly, diarrhea, edema, and lethargy—symptoms that frequently do not appear until several days after milk feeding begins. Cataracts may also be observed within a few days of milk ingestion.[3] Fructokinase deficiencies are relatively benign and may be undetected. Hereditary fructose intolerance (HFI or aldolase B deficiency) is manifested when sucrose or fructose, in fruits for instance, become part of the diet. It can present as a severe, acute reaction with vomiting, convulsions, and coma, or in a milder, chronic form with failure to thrive, vomiting, hepatomegaly, and jaundice.[2] Fructose-1,6-diphosphatase deficiency can be life-threatening, and should be suspected in full-term newborns of normal weight who begin to hyperventilate and go into convulsions and/or coma after eating a fortified diet.

Laboratory Analyses and Diagnosis

There are several simple screening tests that yield presumptive evidence of these defects. Because glucose is the primary circulating carbohydrate, it is the one generally seen in the urine when the renal threshold is exceeded. The presence of a reducing substance that is not glucose provides preliminary evidence of other sugar defects. Galactose, fructose, xylulose, and lactose are all reducing substances that will give a positive result with a test for reducing substances such as Benedict's and a negative test with a specific glucose method such as glucose oxidase (dipstick method). All newborns should be checked by this procedure and should be followed for several days, as the sugar may not be present at all times. Any child with clinical symptoms, especially jaundice, should be checked for reducing sugars. In infants, the

Table 67-1 ***Summary of Simple Sugars***

Disorder	Substrate	Incidence	Screening Tests	Presumptive Diagnosis	Definitive Diagnosis
Lactose Intolerance					
Acquired: no lactase	Lactose → galactose and glucose	Low in Caucasians High in Blacks and Orientals	Reducing substances in urine (for all of the intolerances)	Lactose tolerance test or Hydrogen breath test	Biopsy of mucosal cells of intestine
Congenital: no lactase		Low		Thin-layer chromatography (TLC)	
Fructose Intolerance					
Fructokinase	Fructose → fructose-1-phosphate	One in 130,000		Fructose tolerance test	Demonstration of block or decrease in activity of affected cells (liver, intestine)
Fructose-1-phosphate aldolase B	Fructose-1-phosphate → glyceraldehyde and dihydroxyacetone phosphate	One in 20,000 (Switzerland)		TLC	
Fructose-1, 6-diphosphatase	Key enzyme in gluconeogenesis	Less than 50 cases reported			
Galactose Intolerance					
Galactose-1-phosphate uridyltransferase	Galactose-1-phosphate → UDP galactose	One in 62,000		Inhibition test or	Demonstration of decrease in enzyme activity in red cells or amniotic fluid cells
Galactokinase	Galactose → galactose-1-phosphate	Less than one in 100,000		Enzyme activity by fluorescent technique	
Uridine diphosphate galactose-4-epimerase		Unknown		TLC	
Pentosuria					
L-xylulose reductase		One in 50,000		TLC	

presence of reducing substances in feces and an acid *p*H of the stool suggests a congenital lactose deficiency.[6] This is not the case in adults, however, so this is not a useful screening procedure for acquired lactose intolerance.

Acquired lactose intolerance may be more common than had been previously suspected. Medical record reviews and interviews with elderly people have revealed that many people put themselves on self-limiting diets by removing lactose products or using lactase pills to relieve diarrhea and abdominal discomfort. When they do this, symptoms disappear.

Changes in blood analytes can also be helpful in diagnosis. In HFI there may be a pronounced hypoglycemia and decrease in phosphate levels due to the accumulation of fructose-1-phosphate in the liver.[2] Levels of methionine and tyrosine may be increased in the blood. Fructose-1,6-diphosphatase deficiency may present with hypoglycemia and ketoacidosis. Increased levels of lactate, ketones, alanine, and uric acid are seen in the blood and appear in the urine. Galactosemia due to the transferase defect frequently presents with a decrease in blood glucose. In many states, infant screening procedures for galactosemia are now mandatory.[7, 8] These are usually performed by a direct flourescent measurement of galactose-1-phosphate uridyltransferase activity or by an inhibition test.

Presumptive tests include chromatography, which can be used to identify the specific sugar present in the urine or blood.[9] Tolerance tests for fructose and lactose are also used to assess the patient's ability to metabolize these substances. According to some authorities, the hydrogen breath test for lactose intolerance has, to date, not proved to be of any greater value than the tolerance test.[1, 10]

Definitive tests are necessary to obtain a confirmed diagnosis of lactose and fructose intolerance. Intestinal mucosal biopsy is necessary to determine the exact defect in enzyme activity. However, galactose enzyme defects are present in the red blood cell and can be determined from enzyme activity of red cell hemolysates. They can also be detected in cultured cells of amniotic fluid. A gas–liquid chromatographic method for the detection of galactitol in amniotic fluid has been reported,[11] which correlates well with cell culture results. This provides a more rapid method for prenatal diagnosis because it eliminates the time needed for cell culture growth.

Treatment

In all of these defects, diet provides the best therapy. Absence of the sugar from the diet results in complete recovery in most instances. This is accomplished in HFI by removal of all food containing sucrose and fructose. It is sometimes necessary to provide supportive measures such as infusion of fresh plasma or exchange transfusions. The prognosis is good if the sugar is removed, and these patients generally put themselves on self-imposed diets that avoid foods containing sucrose and fructose.

With fructose-1,6-diphosphatase deficiency, removal of the two sugars fructose and sucrose proves effective. Correction of the hypoglycemia and acidosis by intravenous measures is sometimes necessary.

In galactokinase deficiency, removal of galactose from the diet generally results in complete recovery, and the cataracts will regress.

With galactose-1-phosphate uridyltransferase deficiency, it is necessary to eliminate galactose from the diet. Failure to do so will result in liver damage and eventually death. Both mental retardation and cataracts are consequences of this disease. A galactose-free diet results in regression of symptoms if it is begun in time. This disorder, although not as severe as phenylketonuria (PKU), is important to diagnose early to avoid mental retardation.

Lactose intolerance can be managed by removal of lactose from the diet. Lactase is available in pills and liquid and can be taken with meals to help to alleviate symptoms that result from ingestion of milk products.

Genetics

Genetic counseling and prenatal diagnosis are important in galactosemia. This is the only one of these disorders that can be assessed prior to birth.[8] Mothers who have fetuses with the defect should avoid lactose in their diets. Prior knowledge of the condition provides information needed to properly manage the neonate.

GLYCOGEN STORAGE DISEASES

Glycogen storage diseases are disorders resulting from an enzyme deficiency. In most cases the clinical laboratory plays a relatively minor role. All are autosomal recessive defects except for Type VIII, which is probably sex-linked.[12] The eight types and their associated enzyme defects and incidence are given in Table 67-2.[13]

Clinical Manifestations

Type I presents with hepatomegaly, xanthomas, and renal enlargement. There may be bleeding due to impaired platelet function, and diarrhea may be present. Type II is seen in three forms.[14] The classic case is seen in infants who present with hypotonia, muscle weakness, and congestive heart failure. The symptoms appear within six months after birth, and average life expectancy is one year. The disease may not be manifested until childhood, when symptoms of muscle weakness and hypotonia appear. Death is frequently due to pneumonia and respiratory failure. In adults the primary symptom is muscle weakness. Hypoglycemia, increased lipid levels, and mild cirrhosis are frequently present. Type IV should be suspected in infants who fail to thrive and have little weight gain. There is an increase in the size of the liver and spleen, and cirrhosis with early death is not uncommon. People with Type V frequently are normal, well-developed individuals who have no problem at rest but have a limited ability to perform strenuous exercise. This defect usually manifests later in life, typically between 20 and 40 years of age. Type VI is difficult to diagnose clinically, as there may be few symptoms. It is a milder form of Type I. Type VII presents like McArdles's (Type V). Type VIII patients may have a mild hepatomegaly due to increased liver glycogen.

Laboratory Analyses and Diagnosis

Type I is diagnosed by liver biopsy. Patients have hypoglycemia after a 2-hour fast, and sometimes hyperlipidemia, increased uric acid, and increased lactic acid are found. An oral glucose tolerance test will demonstrate a diabetic-type response. In Type II a muscle biopsy will show an increase in the concentration of glycogen and a decrease in enzyme activity. Activity may be assayed in leukocytes, and fibroblast culture allows for prenatal diagnosis.[15] There is no therapy. Type III shows an increase in lipid levels and hypoglycemia. The clini-

Table 67-2 ***Types of Glycogen Storage Disease***

Type	Name	Enzyme Deficiency	Incidence[12]
I	Von Gierke's	Glucose-6-phosphatase, Type 1a[13]	1/100,000
II	Pompe's	Lysosomal α1,4-glucosidase (acid maltase)	1/100,000
III	Cori's	Amylo-1,6-glucosidase	1/100,000
IV	Andersen's	α1,4-glucan : α1,4-glucan 6-glucosyl transferase	1/500,000
V	McArdle's	Muscle phosphorylase	1/500,000
VI	Hers's	Liver phosphorylase	1/200,000
VII	Tauri's	Muscle phosphofructokinase	1/500,000
VIII		Phosphorylase-b-kinase	1/100,000

cal course is similar to that in Type I, but milder. Type IV presents with a normal glucose tolerance test and increased serum transaminase levels. The treatment is for liver failure and ascites. Fibroblasts can be cultured for prenatal diagnosis, but prognosis is poor. Type V occasionally results in myoglobin in the urine. Lactic acid levels are not elevated after exercise. Diagnosis can be made by measuring lactic acid levels both before ischemic exercise and afterwards, when there is a two- to three-fold increase over basal levels. In McArdle's defect this increase does not occur. Type VI is difficult to diagnose. Assays do not distinguish phosphorylase from phorylase-b-kinase. Type VII may also present with myoglobin in the urine. In Type VIII, liver test results associated with hepatomegaly are found, and fibroblasts can be cultured.

Treatment

In those types of glycogen storage disease that can be treated, diet has proved effective in some instances. In Types I and III, frequent feeding with continuous nasogastric feeding at night has been successful. Type I responds to high-carbohydrate ingestion, while Types III and V[16] have been more successfully managed with a high-protein intake. All of these defects are best managed through medical treatment of symptoms and diet, with monitoring of therapy by the laboratory as appropriate.

Genetics

Genetic counseling can be very helpful with the glycogen storage disorders. Heterozygous screening is available for Types II, III, IV, VI and VII. Prenatal diagnosis is possible with Type II, IV, and VIII.[8]

Case Study

A 65-year-old white woman was admitted with a tentative diagnosis of irritable bowel syndrome manifested by episodic diarrhea and chronic left upper quadrant abdominal pain. She had a long history of abdominal complaints, having had watery bowel movements at various times since age 18. Approximately 2 years prior to admission she had had recurrent diarrhea and abdominal pain with weight loss. She was seen by a gastroenterologist, who found no organic etiology for either symptom. Diarrhea is currently controlled with Metamucil, paregoric, and other similar agents.

Routine laboratory findings were normal except for an elevated bicarbonate level (32 mEq/L[32 mmol/L]). A lactose tolerance test was performed, using 50 grams of lactose given orally. This resulted in five to six loose, watery bowel movements within 2 hours of ingestion. Glucose levels remained close to the fasting result of 69 mg/dL (3.82 mmol/L). With a 100-gram fat, high-residue diet her weight stabilized, and stool studies were normal.

Questions

1. For what two conditions was this patient evaluated?
2. What condition is suggested by the laboratory findings?
3. What treatment is likely to be effective?

Discussion

1. The patient was evaluated for malabsorption and lactose intolerance.
2. The laboratory findings suggest lactose intolerance, because ability to metabolize lactose is apparently absent.
3. Diet modification to eliminate lactose should be effective treatment. The patient should be instructed regarding a lactose-free diet and told to try a high-carbohydrate, high-residue, lactose-free diet with several small feedings per day.

REFERENCES

1. Taylor RH: Clinical tests for hypolactasia, lactose malabsorption, and lactose tolerance. Lancet 2: 766, 1982
2. Gitzelmann R, Steinmann B, von den Bughe G: Essential Fructosuria, Hereditary fructose intol-

erance, and fructose 1,6 diphosphatase deficiency. In Stanbury et al: The Metabolic Basis of Inherited Disease, 5th ed, p 118. New York City, McGraw-Hill, 1983

3. Segal S: Disorders of galactose metabolism. In Stanbury et al: The Metabolic Basis of Inherited Disease, 5th ed, p 167. New York City, McGraw-Hill, 1983
4. Hiott H: Pentosuria. In Stanbury et al: The Metabolic Basis of Inherited Disease, 5th ed, p 192. New York City, McGraw-Hill, 1983
5. Editorial: When does lactose malabsorption matter in adults? Br Med J 2:351, 1975
6. Savilaliti E, Lauviola K, Kiutunen P: Congenital lactose deficiency: A clinical study on sixteen patients. Arch Dis Child 58:246–252, 1983
7. Lyson M, Russo PJ: Normal initial blood galactose levels in a newborn with galactosemia. Am J Dis Child 136:747–748, 1982
8. McCormack MK: Screening for genetic traits and diseases. Am Fam Physician 24 (4): 153–166, 1981
9. Bhatti T, Clamp J: Identification and estimation of monosaccharides and disaccharides in urine by GLC. Clin Chem Acta 22:563–567, 1968
10. Berg A Erikson M, Barany F et al: Hydrogen concentration in expired air analyzed with a new hydrogen sensor. Scand J Gastroenterol 20:815–823, 1985
11. Allen J, Holton J, Gillets M: Gas–liquid chromatographic determination of galactitol in amniotic fluid for possible use in prenatal diagnosis of galactosemia. Clin Chem Acta 110:59–63, 1981
12. Howell RR, Williams JC: Glycogen storage diseases. In Stanbury et al: The Metabolic Basis of Inherited Disease, 5th ed, p 141. New York City, McGraw-Hill, 1983
13. Otomo YI, Narisaiwa K, Torda K: A new variant of glycogen storage disease Type 1a. J Inherited Metab Dis 2:45–49, 1979
14. Matsuiski T, Yoshino M, Terasawa K et al: Childhood acid maltase deficiency. Arch Neurol 41:47–52, 1984
15. Midorihawa, Okada, Kato et al: Diagnosis of Pompe's disease using pyridylamino-maltosligosaccharides as substrates of 1,4 glucosidase. Clin Chem Acta 147:97–102, 1985
16. Slovim AE, Goan PJ: Myopathy in McArdle's syndrome: Improvement with a high protein diet. N Engl J Med 312:355–359, 1985

Chapter 68

Gout

Benjamin J. Andrusaitis

ETIOLOGY AND PATHOPHYSIOLOGY

Gout is a disease produced either by an increased rate of purine catabolism or by a decreased renal excretion of uric acid. The resultant hyperuricemia can lead to precipitation of monosodium urate. Precipitation is most common in the joints of the lower extremities and the kidneys. The crystals in the joints are phagocytized by leukocytes, resulting in the release of lysosomal enzymes that can damage the surrounding tissue and produce a recurrent, acute arthritis, the clinical hallmark of gout. Kidney deposition of crystals can result in nephropathy, acute intratubular uric acid deposition, and nephrolithiasis.[1]

Biochemistry

In the first step of purine synthesis, the enzyme phosphoribosylpyrophosphate synthetase catalyzes the production of phosphoribosylpyrophosphate (PRPP) from ribose-5-phosphate. In the second, rate-limiting step, phosphoribosylamine is produced from PRPP and glutamine. The reaction is catalyzed by PRPP-aminotransferase. The enzyme is regulated by feedback inhibition by the end-products of the pathway, the nucleotides adenosine monophosphate (AMP) and guanosine monophosphate (GMP), which are subsequently incorporated into nucleic acids.[2]

Nucleic acids are catabolized to the nucleotides AMP, GMP, and inosine monophosphate (IMP), and subsequently to nucleosides. The nucleosides, inosine and guanosine, are converted to the free bases hypoxanthine and guanine, which are converted to xanthine. Uric acid is produced from xanthine through the action of xanthine oxidase.

The free bases are reutilized by the action of salvage pathways. Hypoxanthine and guanine undergo phosphoribosylation, which is catalyzed by hypoxanthine-guanine phosphoribosyl transferase (HPRT) to reform the nucleotides IMP and GMP respectively. Adenine is reconverted to AMP by the action of adenine phosphoribosyl transferase.[3] Thus, purines are conserved by a less energetically demanding process than *de novo* synthesis. Dietary nucleic acids are converted directly to uric acid; however, the major source of uric acid is the catabolism of endogenous purines.

Hyperuricemia

Uric acid is a weak acid with a *p*Ka of 5.75. In plasma with a *p*H of 7.4, uric acid exists almost entirely in the form of urate, which has a solubility limit of 7.0 mg/dL (0.42 mmol/L).[4] While values above this are used as a general indicator of hyperuricemia, caution must be used in assessing suspected cases of gout on the basis of serum uric acid levels. The relationship of hyperuricemia to the development of clinical symptoms is complex. While hyperuricemia correlates with the risk of developing gout, it is not a definitive diagnostic indicator.[4]

CLASSIFICATION OF GOUT

Primary and Secondary

In establishing a prognosis and determining treatment, it is useful to distinguish the etiology of gout as primary or secondary in nature. In primary gout, the hyperuricemia is of unknown origin or directly related to purine metabolism or uric acid excretion. Secondary gout is a consequence of any number of conditions that affect uric acid production or excretion.

Production and Excretion

Also helpful in the diagnostic evaluation is the determination of the underlying biochemical mechanism responsible for the hyperuricemia. Gout may result from an overproduction of uric acid, an underexcretion of uric acid, or a combination of the two defects.[5]

OVERPRODUCERS

Two-thirds of patients with primary gout show some degree of overproduction.[4] Approximately 10% of cases of primary gout involve idiopathic overproduction.[6]

A rare form of primary gout is an X-linked genetic deficiency in or absence of the enzyme HPRT. Decreased levels of this enzyme result in decreased activity of the free base salvage pathway and an increased rate of uric acid production. Complete absence of HPRT results in the Lesch-Nyhan syndrome. Clinically, this syndrome is characterized by nephropathy, nephrolithiasis, growth and mental retardation, and lack of muscle control.[7] Death from renal failure usually occurs before the teenage years without therapy.[4]

Patients with a partial deficiency in HPRT show milder neurologic dysfunction and typical gout-associated physical findings early in adulthood. Serum and urine uric acid values are greatly elevated.

Primary overproduction of uric acid may also result from rare X-linked mutations in the enzyme PRPP-synthetase. This genetic variant produces increased enzyme activity, resulting in increased intracellular levels of PRPP and excessive uric acid production. Clinically, these patients resemble those with partial HPRT deficiency, but do not show neurologic symptoms.[4] Conditions that increase cellular turnover will accelerate purine metabolism. The result is a secondary increase in uric acid production, and the possible development of gout. These conditions include lymphoproliferative and myeloproliferative diseases, tumors, red cell disorders, multiple myeloma, psoriasis, and administration of cytotoxic drugs.

Uric acid-induced acute renal failure is a common complication of lympho/myeloproliferative disorders, the risk of which increases with chemotherapy.[1]

UNDEREXCRETORS

Underexcretion of uric acid is the result of abnormal renal handling of uric acid, resulting in hyperuricemia. Nearly all plasma uric acid is filtered by the glomerulus. The filtered uric acid is reabsorbed in the proximal convoluted tubules and secreted back into the lumen in the distal portion of the proximal tubule. There is some reabsorption of uric acid in the distal tubule.[8] Alterations in any of these mechanisms can produce underexcretion of uric acid and result in hyperuricemia. Underexcretors are characterized by hyperuricemia and normal or decreased values for 24-hour uric acid excretion.[1, 6]

Approximately 90% of cases of primary gout involve idiopathic underexcretion of uric acid, with or without overproduction.[6] In cases in which overproduction is present, a larger portion of uric acid is excreted via the gastrointestinal tract. This can lead to an underestimation of uric acid production based on the 24-hour uric acid excretion value. In this situation, any increase in the uric acid excretion value indicates overproduction.[6]

Secondary underexcretion of uric acid can result from chronic renal insufficiency, chronic alcohol ingestion, chronic diuretic use, lead-induced renal disease, organic aciduria, and endocrinopathies.[8]

UROLITHIASIS

Renal calculi formation is a complication in a small minority of the cases of primary or secondary gout.[9] Urine becomes saturated with uric acid at a *p*H below 5.5. Thus, an acidic *p*H and the degree of hyperuricemia are major factors in stone formation. Adjusting the *p*H to above 6.0 and maintaining a high urine output prevents stone formation.

HYPOURICEMIA

Hypouricemia is rare. The most common cause is uricosuric drug treatment. Hypouricemia may also be seen in genetic defects of purine metabolism, such as xanthine oxidase deficiency and liver disease.[8] Hypouricemia is also seen in renal reabsorption defects, such as Fanconi's syndrome and Wilson's disease.[10]

CLINICAL MANIFESTATIONS

Ninety percent of the cases of gout affect men, with the incidence among women after menopause approaching that of men. In men, the peak age of onset is 45 years.[4] Gout is a possible diagnosis if the patient presents with recurrent attacks of acute arthritis, most commonly in the lower extremities. The first metatarsal-phalangeal joint is typically the first and most common site of clinical symptoms. The joint is swollen, inflamed, and very tender. The etiology of onset of acute attacks is unknown; they may occur with normal serum uric acid values.

Recurrent attacks of acute gout are indicative of chronic gout. Such patients tend to show visible deposits of urate crystals (tophi), renal abnormalities, and urolithiasis, and tend to be resistant to therapy.[4]

Patient history plays an important role in the diagnosis of gout. A careful history will usually rule out other causes of joint inflammation, such as trauma or infection. Gout is commonly associated with obesity, chronic alcohol intake, a high-protein diet, and chronic thiazide diuretic use. A family history of gout indicates a genetic component to the disease and suggests a diagnosis of primary gout. If the initial clinical picture does not rule out gout, a more thorough diagnostic assessment is indicated.

LABORATORY ANALYSES AND DIAGNOSIS

The serum uric acid value may be used only as a general guide in the diagnosis of gout. High serum uric acid levels tend to confirm a diagnosis of gout, while consistently low uric acid values tend to exclude it.[10] Serum glucose, creatinine, urea nitrogen, and 24-hour urine uric acid and creatinine values will help in differentiating the underlying biochemical mechanism as either overproduction or underexcretion of uric acid. The usual indicators of tissue inflammation (leukocytosis, elevated erythrocyte sedimentation rate) will be apparent.

A definitive diagnosis of gout is established by examination of the synovial fluid from the affected joint. The presence of intracellular, negatively birefringent sodium urate crystals is diagnostic for gout. The synovial fluid examination will rule out pseudogout, a crystal-induced arthritis produced by calcium pyrophosphate dihydrate. The synovial fluid white blood cell count will be elevated. A Gram stain and a culture should be done to rule out infection.

Overproduction of uric acid is characterized by marked hyperuricemia and 24-hour uric acid excretion values greater than 600 mg in patients on low purine diets with normal creatinine clearance values.[1, 6]

The differential diagnosis of uric acid-induced acute renal failure can be made if the ratio of the concentration of uric acid to creatinine in urine is greater than 1.0.[11] In children, this ratio is normally greater than 1.0.[1] In general, 24-hour uric acid excretion values greater than 800 mg are associated either with a primary overproduction due to an enzymatic defect or with a secondary overproduction.[4]

Table 68-1 ***Reference Ranges***[12]

	Phosphotungstic Acid Methods	Uricase Methods
Women	3.0–6.5 mg/dL (0.18–0.38 mmol/L)	2.6–6.0 mg/dL (0.15–0.35 mmol/L)
Men	4.5–8.2 mg/dL (0.27–0.48 mmol/L)	3.5–7.2 mg/dL (0.21–0.42 mmol/L)

TREATMENT

The goal of treatment for attacks of acute gout is to alleviate the symptoms of the attacks as quickly as possible. Generally, treatment is assessed by the response to therapy.

In chronic gout, the goal of treatment is to decrease the body's uric acid load and prevent subsequent complications. The type of therapy employed is dependent upon the underlying mechanism of hyperuricemia, as assessed by the 24-hour uric acid excretion value. Overproducers are treated with drugs that decrease uric acid synthesis (such as xanthine oxidase inhibitors). Underexcretors are treated with uroscopic drugs. In both cases, the goal is to attain a serum uric acid level within the normal range (see Table 68-1).

CASE STUDY

A 55-year-old white man sought medical attention complaining of an extremely sore right large toe. The patient's history indicated chronic alcohol use. Upon examination, the affected toe was swollen, red, warm, and extremely tender. The pain was recurrent and had become progressively worse. The patient complained that he was "twisting" his ankles frequently. There was no history of other joint or bone problems. Body temperature was slightly elevated. There were no other unusual physical findings.

Routine blood chemistries were normal except for the following:

LABORATORY FINDINGS

	Patient Value	Normal Value
Serum uric acid	10.5 mg/dL (0.62 mmol/L)	3.5–7.2 mg/dL (0.21–0.42 mmol/L)
White blood cell count	$21 \times 10^3/mm^3$	$4.5–11.0 \times 10^3/mm^3$
Erythrocyte sedimentation rate	50 mm/hr	0–15 mm/hr

As a followup, a creatinine clearance assay and a 24-hour urine uric acid were ordered, with the following results:

	Patient Value	Normal Value
Creatinine clearance	95 mL/min	90–130 mL/min
24-hour urine uric acid	300 mg/dL (17.7 mmol/L)	Less than 500 mg/dL (29.5 mmol/L)

At this point, a synovial fluid analysis was performed. The sample was cloudy and viscous, with a volume of 5.0 mL. The white blood cell count was 620 cells/mm^3 (normal = less than 200 cells/mm^3). A Gram stain and a culture were negative. Intracellular, negatively birefringent sodium urate crystals were reported.

Questions

1. What is this patient's diagnosis, and what laboratory finding is definitive?
2. What etiology do the laboratory findings suggest?
3. Explain the other laboratory findings.

Discussion

1. Due to the presence of sodium urate crystals in the synovial fluid, this patient should be diagnosed as having gout.
2. From the hyperuricemia and urine chemistries, the etiology is assessed as idiopathic underexcretion. This is aggravated by chronic alcohol ingestion, resulting in an acidosis that interferes with renal excretion.
3. The leukocytosis and elevated erythrocyte sedimentation rate are nonspecific responses to inflammation.

REFERENCES

1. Boss GR, Seegmiller JE: Hyperuricemia and gout classification, complications, and management. N Engl J Med 300:1459, 1979
2. Wood AW, Wyngaarden JE: Properties of 5-phosphoribosyl-1-pyrophosphate glutamine aminotransferase from human lymphoblasts. J Biol Chem 248:138, 1973
3. Watts RWE: Purines and nucleotides. In Brown SS, Mitchell FL, Young DS (eds): Chemical Diagnosis of Disease. Amsterdam, Elsevier, 1979
4. Wyngaarden JB: Gout. In Wyngaarden JB, Smith LH (eds): Cecil Textbook of Medicine. Philadelphia, WB Saunders, 1985
5. Klinenberg JR: Hyperuricemia and gout. Med Clin North Am 61:299, 1977
6. Palella TD, Kelley WN: An approach to hyperuricemia and gout. Geriatrics 39(11):89, 1984
7. Nyhan WL: The Lesch-Nyhan syndrome. Adv Nephrol 3:59, 1974
8. Rock RC, Walker WG, Jennings CD: Nitrogen metabolites and renal function. In Tietz NW (ed): Textbook of Clinical Chemistry. Philadelphia, WB Saunders, 1986
9. Woo J, Cannon DC: Metabolic intermediates and inorganic ions. In Henry JB (ed): Clinical Diagnosis and Management by Laboratory Methods. Philadelphia, WB Saunders, 1984
10. Whitby LG, Percy-Robb IW, Smith AF: Lecture Notes on Clinical Chemistry. Oxford, Blackwell Scientific Publications, 1984
11. Kelton J, Kelley WN, Holmes EW: A rapid method for the diagnosis of acute uric acid nephropathy. Arch Intern Med 138:612, 1978
12. Tietz NW (ed): Clinical Guide to Laboratory Tests. Philadelphia, WB Saunders, 1983

Chapter 69

Total Parenteral Nutrition

Maria Luisa J. Morsi

Health practitioners appreciate the fact that good nutrition plays a major role in health maintenance, wound healing, and heightened resistance to infection. Clinical experience has demonstrated the value of optimal nutritional states in resisting the effects of trauma and disease as well as in improving response to medical and surgical therapy. Trauma, injury, or extensive debilitating disease creates malnutrition, present or potential, and hypermetabolic nutritional demands. If the patient's condition is further complicated by the inability to eat or take enteral feedings, nutritional status can be improved and maintained over extended periods solely through nutritional support. The most sophisticated and dramatic method of nutritional support is total parenteral nutrition. It is the complete sustaining of increased nutritional requirements through intravenous feedings. New techniques and products have been developed that greatly enhance the ability to provide this nutritional support to the patient.

CHARACTERISTICS OF TOTAL PARENTERAL NUTRITION (TPN) AND INTRAVENOUS HYPERALIMENTATION

Total parenteral nutrition is the administration, usually through a central venous catheter, of protein hydrolysates or amino acids plus glucose and other essential nutrients, in amounts sufficient to meet normal calorie and nitrogen needs.[1]

Intravenous hyperalimentation is the administration through a central venous catheter of simple essential nutrients such as protein hydrolysates or amino acids plus glucose, vitamins, and minerals, in a calorie concentration in excess of normal requirements.[1, 2]

PURPOSE OF TPN AND INDICATIONS FOR USE

The primary nutritional goals of TPN are to conserve lean body mass and to maintain nutritional equilibrium. Reversal of growth arrest in children is possible if intake is sufficient to establish a substantial positive kilocalorie and nitrogen balance.

Situations in which TPN should be strongly considered include the following:

1. Unavailability of the gastrointestinal tract
2. Anticipation of unavailability of the normal gastrointestinal tract due to need to maintain patient in anabolic state
3. Need to minimize intestinal activity during periods of limited function
4. Critical situations, as an alternative to enteral feeding in order to avoid uncertainties of nutrient uptake or utilization

COMPOSITION OF TPN SOLUTIONS

Solutions utilized in total parenteral nutrition should be formulated to meet the nutritional needs of the individual. In general, 30 kcal/kg of body weight/day are necessary to maintain the ideal weight of the adult with restricted activity. Infants require 100 to 130 kcal/kg of body weight/day.[1, 2] Kilocalories should be increased appropriately to permit weight gain in individuals who are significantly underweight or to meet other needs. Providing 2500 to 3000 kcal/day supplied by three liters of 25% dextrose in water will satisfy maintenance needs for many stable hospitalized adults. While in the catabolic stress of severe trauma, the need may well rise to 5000 to 7000 kcal/day, which is approximately 50 to 60 kcal/kg.[3] Frequent determination of body weight and other anthropometric parameters are important guides.

Glucose is the most effective and most frequently used carbohydrate source in TPN solutions, while a synthetic crystalline L-amino acid solution is the usual nitrogen source. Recommended dietary allowances (RDAs) are approximately 0.8 g protein/kg of body weight for healthy adults, but in practice TPN should provide 1 to 1.5 g/kg/day of protein to most adults to assure that positive N balance will be achieved.[1] Adequate calorie intake is also necessary to achieve positive nitrogen balance and anabolism. Fat is a highly desirable energy source because it has a high caloric density and provides essential fatty acids. Recently, a 10% soybean oil emulsion stabilized with egg yolk phospholipid has been proven to be safe and effective.[4] These substances, normally used as a supplement to the main TPN solution, are provided separately according to need—usually one to two 500-mL bottles a week for adults.

Precise knowledge of principles of correct vitamin, mineral, and trace element supplementation for patients on TPN is meager.[5] Commercial multivitamin preparations are available for use in TPN solutions, as are individual vitamins for formulating the solution according to patient's needs. No specific recommendations can be made for electrolyte prescription. It is usually based on the requirement for normal electrolyte balance, with adjustments according to individual patient monitoring. Solutions containing trace elements are also now commercially available.

COMPLICATIONS: PREVENTION, MANAGEMENT, AND LABORATORY MONITORING

A knowledge of potential complications associated with the administration of TPN can reduce their frequency. The development of multidisciplinary nutritional support teams—qualified individuals who follow established techniques, remain alert to potential complications, and intervene quickly to minimize the morbidity associated with complications—has made TPN a safe and effective adjunct in clinical management.[6, 7] Potential complications are largely avoided by adhering to basic metabolic principles of nutrient administration and anatomic requirements of catheter insertion as well as through precise monitoring of a patient's response to TPN infusion.[8]

Technical Complications

Studies of insertion of subclavian catheters have indicated complication rates of between 3% and 6%. The types of complications related to catheter insertion are pneumothorax, hydrothorax, arterial injury, hematomas, thoracic duct laceration, air embolism, embolization of severed catheter tips, cardiac arrhythmias, cardiac perforations, and pericardial tamponade, which is a compression resulting from the accumulation of excess fluid in the pericardium.[9]

Septic Complications

In TPN, the entire nutritional system is vulnerable, and any break in its integrity and sterility may permit the direct access of pathogenic microorganisms to the patient's circulation. This danger is compounded by the high nutritional properties of the infused fluids, and by the debility and anergy of a large proportion of these patients. In recent years, TPN has been administered with very low rates of infection. This improving trend is evidently due to increasing experience with this relatively recent modality of treatment, adherence to rigid protocols of practice, and the development of a multidisciplinary team approach to TPN.

Gram-positive cocci and fungi are the predominant organisms causing TPN-related sepsis. *Staphylococcus epidermidis, Staphylococcus aureus,* and *Candida albicans* are the organisms most commonly isolated. Gram-negative bacteria are isolated relatively infrequently, especially in comparison to the frequency with which they cause septicemia due to primary infection at a site other than the TPN catheter.[10]

Fever is the hallmark of TPN-related sepsis. Chills and tachycardia may also be prominent features. Increased glucose intolerance with hyperglycemia and glycosuria, a manifestation of sepsis-induced insulin resistance, may be the earliest clue to impending sepsis.[11]

The TPN system becomes suspect immediately when fever develops that is not clearly attributable to the patient's underlying disease. The sequence of decisions in the management of TPN patients developing sepsis is detailed in Figure 69-1.[12]

Metabolic Complications

Increased knowledge of the metabolism of substrates, electrolytes, vitamins, and trace minerals has defined requirements for patients with various disease states, and improved patient monitoring has reduced the occurrence of metabolic complications. Close biochemical and clinical monitoring, as seen in Tables 69-1 and 69-2, can prevent serious complications. Early detection of abnormalities allows for correction by minor adjustments in nutrient solutions without the need to resort to radical measures.

GLUCOSE METABOLISM

Blood glucose concentrations depend on glucose supply, utilization, and excretion. Utilization of glucose is maximal in infants and decreases with advancing age. Disease states could decrease glucose utilization. A normal adult can tolerate infusions of up to 400 to 500 grams of glucose over 24 hours with little difficulty. By gradually increasing glucose infusion over several days, up to 1500 grams a day can be mobilized.

Blood glucose concentrations during TPN will normally be less than 130 or 140 mg/dL (7.2 or 7.8 mmol/L), with no more than 2^+ glycosuria. Any episode of hyperglycemia with concentrations greater than 200 mg/dL (11.1 mmol/L) or 4^+ gly-

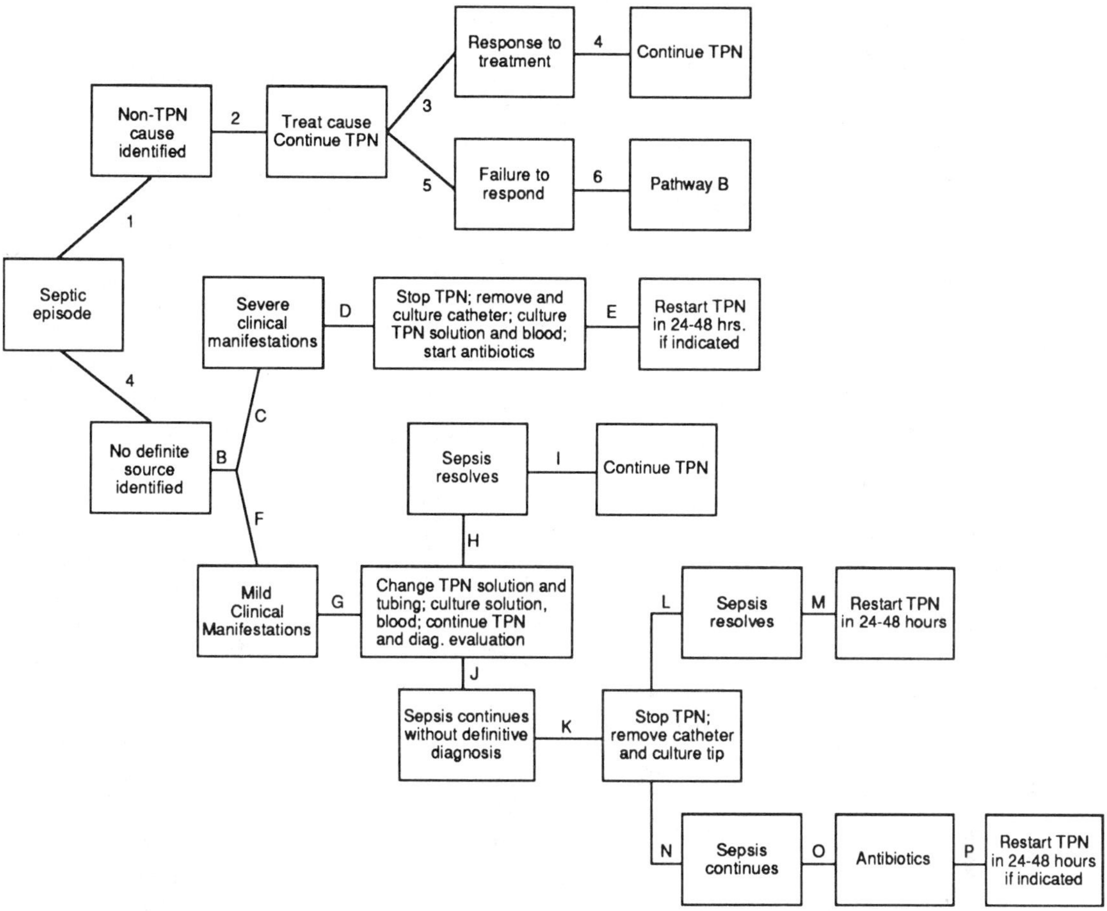

Figure 69-1 **Sequence of decisions in the evaluation and management of sepsis occurring in patients receiving TPN. (From Silverman H, Eisenberg D: Parenteral and Enteral Nutrition for the Hospitalized Patient. East Norwalk, Appleton-Century-Crofts, 1982)**

cosuria must be evaluated immediately and treated appropriately.

A complication commonly reported during the development of TPN support was the syndrome of hyperglycemic, hyperosmolar, nonketotic coma. This problem has become less common with improved understanding and close monitoring of glucose metabolism in patients receiving TPN.

A rise in serum insulin occurs rapidly with carbohydrate infusion, reaching a steady state of four to six times basal secretion within 6 hours. Initial insulin secretion is proportional to infused glucose load. With time, both blood sugar and serum insulin concentration decline. Hypoglycemia may occur when the infusion is interrupted for as little as 15 to 30 minutes. In the interest of safety, even though experimental data show a rapid decrease in serum insulin, it is advised that patients receiving more than 2000 mL/day of TPN be tapered to 2000 mL daily, in decrements of 1000 mL, and then given 5% dextrose at 100 to 125 mL/hour for 12 to 24 hours before the subclavian catheter is removed.[13]

Table 69-1 *Suggested Monitoring Schedule of Pediatric Patients on TPN*

Variable Monitored	Suggested Frequency	
	*Initial Period**	*Later Period†*
Serum electrolytes	3–4 times/wk	2–3 times/wk
Serum urea nitrogen	3 times/wk	2 times/wk
Serum calcium, magnesium, phosphorus	3 times/wk	2 times/wk
Serum glucose	‡	‡
Serum acid-base status	3–4 times/wk	2–3 times/wk
Serum ammonia	2 times/wk	Weekly
Serum protein (electrophoresis or albumin/globulin)	Weekly	Weekly
Liver function studies	Weekly	Weekly
Hemoglobin	2 times/wk	2 times/wk
Urine glucose	Daily	Daily
Clinical observations (*e.g.*, activity, temperature)	Daily	Daily
WBC count and differential count	As indicated	As indicated
Cultures	As indicated	As indicated
Serum triglyceride	As indicated	As indicated

* Initial period is period before full glucose intake is achieved, or any period of metabolic instability.

† Later period is period during which patient is in a metabolic steady state.

‡ Blood glucose should be monitored closely during period of glucosuria (to determine degree of hyperglycemia) and for two to three days after cessation of parenteral nutrition (to detect hypoglycemia). In latter instance, frequent Dextrostix determination constitutes adequate screening.

(From Academy of Pediatrics Committee on Nutrition: Commentary on parenteral nutrition. Pediatrics 70:4, 1983)

AMINO ACID METABOLISM

Prerenal azotemia results when excessive amounts of protein hydrolysate or amino acid are infused, and is aggravated by underlying dehydration. Patients usually present with signs of dehydration and an elevation of serum blood urea nitrogen (BUN). Close monitoring of body weight, fluid balance, and serum BUN prevents this complication.[14]

Hyperammonemia is a problem that occurs when casein or fibrin hydrolysates are infused, because these solutions contain up to 40,000 ug of free ammonia/dL. With the advent of crystalline amino acid solutions, in which free ammonia is absent, this problem has become much less prevalent, except in pediatric patients. This complication is probably related to a deficiency of arginine, an important substrate in the Krebs-Henseleit cycle. In infants receiving TPN, serum ammonia levels should be closely monitored. Treatment is again preventive, with daily administration of arginine.[15]

FATTY ACID METABOLISM

Long-term TPN with fat-free hypertonic dextrose–amino acid solutions might be expected to lower serum cholesterol and elevate triglyceride concentrations. In several studies, however, no change in triglyceride concentration was seen during TPN, but there were marked decreases in serum cholesterol, sometimes to less than half the original concentration. The lowest concentration occurs during the second to fourth week. Occasionally, a gradual recovery of cholesterol was seen in spite of continued fat restriction.[16, 17] No harmful metabolic effects of cholesterol depression are known. Perhaps a beneficial effect might be anticipated in patients with severe familial hypercholesterolemia.[18]

Patients maintained on preparations of glucose and amino acids without supplemental fat for 3 to 6 weeks will eventually develop essential fatty acid deficiency.[19, 20] This is diagnosed by characteristic serum biochemical changes, including low serum levels of linoleic and arachidonic acids, and an in-

Table 69-2 ***Suggested Monitoring Protocol for Adults on TPN***

Baseline Tests

CBC:	Hbg	Nitrogen balance	AST
	Hct	Fe and TIBC	Alkaline phosphatase
	RBC indexes	FBS	Serum osmolality
	WBC differential count	BUN	Cholesterol
	Platelets	Creatinine	Triglycerides
Na^{2+}	Ca^{2+}	Uric acid	Urinalysis
K^+	PO_4	PT	Chest x-ray
Cl^-	Mg^{2+}	PTT	ECG
CO_2		Albumin	Body weight (kg)
Skin tests (PPD, mumps, cocci)		Total protein	Height (cm)
		Bilirubin	

Stabilization Tests (daily first 5–7 days)

Fractional urines (sugar and acetone) every 6 hours; simultaneous blood sugars first and second days
Body weight
Intake and output record
Nitrogen balance
Serum electrolytes
Blood glucose

Followup Routine

Daily	Fractional urines (sugar and acetone)		
	Body weight		
	Intake and output		
Three times a week	Electrolytes (Na^+, K^+, Cl^-, CO_2)		
Once a week	CBC: platelets	PT	Mg^{2+}
	RBC indexes	Ca^{2+}	
	Creatinine	PO_4	
	BUN		
Once a month	Repeat baseline tests		
	Add serum vitamin B_{12}, folate, Zn^{2+}		

Data from reference number[3]

crease in serum triene/tetraene ratio (eicosatrienoic acid/arachidonic acid ratio), which is normally 0.4.[21] Other abnormal laboratory findings include elevated serum liver function tests, increased red blood cell fragility, anemia, thrombocytopenia, and decreased levels of serum prostaglandin. Deficiency is prevented by administering fat emulsions (500 mL of a 10% solution) to patients on TPN at least twice weekly.[22]

VITAMIN METABOLISM

Currently, most available multivitamin formulas do not include Vitamin K, which therefore must be added to the TPN solution in order to prevent prothrombin deficiency and potential bleeding. Biotin is another vitamin that is included only in certain preparations. Its deficiency symptoms are thinning of the hair and dermatitis, which may be apparent in cases of long-term TPN.

MINERAL METABOLISM

The early hypophosphatemia seen with parenteral nutrition was due to a rapid influx of phosphorus into the body muscle mass at the initiation of anabolism after a period of catabolism. Clinical signs and symptoms of hypophosphatemia usually appear when serum inorganic phosphate concentrations fall below 1 mg/dL (0.323 mmol/L).[23] Hypophosphatemia is generally an iatrogenic condition. Phosphate requirements are dictated by the degree of malnutrition before TPN is initiated, the presence of predisposing medical conditions, and the amount of glucose calories in the solution being administered. Treatment of hypophosphatemia should primarily be preventive. Maintenance phosphate may be administered in routine TPN solutions. To avoid a precipitous fall in serum calcium and possible tetany, additions of phosphate should be accompanied by calcium supplementation as calcium gluconate.

In patients receiving TPN, the requirements for magnesium are increased because of new tissue synthesis. Clinical symptoms due to hypomagnesemia develop when the serum concentration falls below 1 mEq/L (0.5 mmol/L).[24] In addition to producing neuromuscular symptoms, magnesium deficiency has a significant effect on potassium, calcium, and phosphorus metabolism. Urinary potassium losses can increase markedly, resulting in significant and progressive hypokalemia. All clinical symptoms are reversible with magnesium replacement, and can be avoided by maintenance administration.

In the patient with impaired renal function, as suggested by a creatinine clearance of less than 30 mL/minute, hypermagnesemia should be avoided.[25] In TPN patients generally, weekly monitoring of serum magnesium levels should enable prevention of this condition, but levels should be monitored at least twice weekly in patients with impaired renal function. There are two possible causes of hypermagnesemia, which alone or in combination can contribute to impaired trace mineral nutriture during TPN: preexisting, underlying disorders may predispose to depletion of one or more trace minerals, and some factor(s) intrinsic to the TPN regimen itself may impair trace mineral nutriture. Experience has shown, however, that a reduction in intake of minerals due to a lack of sufficient delivery from the intravenous alimentation solutions is by far the leading cause of trace mineral deficiency during TPN. A conscious prospective program of clinical and laboratory assessment, including serial evaluation of the signs, symptoms, biochemical parameters, and functional tests for iron, zinc, copper, selenium, chromium, and molybdenum, should be instituted in each individual undergoing TPN.[26]

LIVER FUNCTION

Patients who are maintained on TPN for one to three weeks often develop abnormalities in serum liver function tests.[27, 28] The etiology of the elevation of serum liver enzymes and bilirubin levels remains obscure. Caution is necessary because of the possibility of inducing further hepatic damage and perhaps liver failure. Patients with suspected hepatic disease should undergo liver function tests prior to infusion of TPN. Premature and newborn infants may be especially susceptible to hepatic toxicity, and should be observed carefully during TPN.[12]

Almost all components of the nutrient solutions have been implicated in liver dysfunction in patients receiving TPN. Patients should be given balanced TPN solutions according to their caloric requirements. Serum liver enzymes levels should be monitored at least once a week during TPN administration.[8]

CASE STUDY

A 29-year-old woman was thrown from a car as it went off the road. She sustained head injury, blunt chest trauma with rib fractures and severe pulmonary contusions, and multiple pelvic and vertebral fractures. Because ileus will most likely occur due to her injuries and reoccur when she undergoes instrumentation of her spine, total parenteral nutrition was initiated. The total calories provided were approximately 2600 kcal.

Questions

1. What tests would indicate that the patient is not able to tolerate the high glucose load of the TPN?
2. Which parameters could be used to assess the adequacy of nutritional support with regard to protein and vitamins?
3. Immobilization would result in losses of which specific nutrients? What would be indications of these losses?
4. Antimicrobial drugs such as amphotericin or carbenicillin accentuate magnesium loss from the body. How could this be measured?

Discussion

1. The two test results that would indicate that the patient is not tolerating the high glucose load are the elevation of blood glucose levels and the presence of glucose in the urine. Any episode of hyperglycemia with concentrations greater than 200 mg/dL (11.1 mmol/L) or 4^+ glycosuria must be evaluated immediately and treated appropriately.
2. The use of changes in body weight, serum albumin, and anthropometric parameters to assess the adequacy of protein content of the nutritional support could be complicated by changes in the fluid compartment of the body. Nitrogen balance studies should also be done, with a 24-hour urinary urea nitrogen determination. A positive nitrogen balance would indicate that the patient is anabolizing more than she is catabolizing.

   For evaluation of vitamin nutriture, clinical laboratory assessments of the different vitamins would indicate either vitamin deficiency or overdose.
3. Nitrogen, calcium, and sulfur are usually excreted in large amounts during prolonged immobilization. Increased urinary excretion of nitrogen, calcium, and cystine would be indicative of negative balance for these three nutrients.
4. Urinary balance studies of magnesium would be used to measure the magnesium loss from the body.

REFERENCES

1. Shils ME: Total parenteral nutrition. In Goodhart RS, Shils ME (eds): Modern Nutrition in Health and Disease. Philadelphia, Lea & Febiger, 1973
2. Shils ME: Guidelines for total parenteral nutrition. JAMA 220:1721, 1972
3. Williams SR: Nutrition and Diet Therapy. St Louis, Times Mirror/Mosby College Publishing, 1985
4. Wilmore DW, Moylan JA, Helmkamp GM et al: Clinical evaluation of a 10% intravenous fat emulsion for parenteral nutrition in thermally injured patients. Ann Surg 178:503, 1973
5. Meng HC: Parenteral nutrition: Principles, nutrient requirements, and techniques. Geriatrics 30:97, 1975
6. Layden T, Rosenberg J, Nemchausky B et al: Reversal of growth arrest in adolescents with Crohn's disease after parenteral alimentation. Gastroenterology 70:1017, 1976
7. Weinster RL, Butterworth CE: Handbook of Clinical Nutrition. St Louis, CV Mosby, 1981
8. Rombeau JL, Caldwell MD: Parenteral Nutrition. Philadelphia, WB Saunders, 1986
9. Ryan JA, Abel RM, Abbott WM et al: Catheter complications in total parenteral nutrition. N Engl J Med 290:757, 1974
10. Allen JR: The incidence of nosocomial infection in patients receiving total parenteral nutrition. In Johnson IDA (ed): Advances in Parenteral Nutrition, p 339. Baltimore, University Park Press, 1978
11. Sanders RA, Sheldon GF: Septic complications of total parenteral nutrition: A five-year experience. Am J Surg 132:214, 1976
12. Silberman H, Eisenberg D: Parenteral and Enteral Nutrition for the Hospitalized Patient. Norwalk, Connecticut, Appleton-Century-Crofts, 1982
13. Grant JP: Handbook of Total Parenteral Nutrition. Philadelphia, WB Saunders, 1980
14. Dudrick SJ, MacFadden BV, Van Buren CT et al: Parenteral hyperalimentation: Metabolic problems and solutions. Ann Surg 176:259, 1972
15. Heird WC, Nicholson JR, Driscoll JR Jr et al: Hyperammonia resulting from intravenous alimentation using a mixture of synthetic L-amino acids: A preliminary report. J Pediatr 81:162, 1972

16. Abbott WM, Abel RM, Fischer JE: The effects of total parenteral nutrition upon serum lipid levels. Surg Gynecol Obstet 142:565, 1976
17. DeBesten L, Reyna RH, Conor WE et al: The different effects on the serum lipids and fecal steroids of high-carbohydrate diets given orally or intravenously. J Clin Invest 52:1384, 1973
18. Torsvik H, Fischer JE, Feldman HA et al: Effects of intravenous hyperalimentation on plasma-lipoproteins in severe familial hypercholesterolemia. Lancet 1:601, 1975
19. Fleming CR, Smith LM, Hodges RE: Essential fatty acid deficiency in adults receiving total parenteral nutrition. Am J Clin Nutr 29:976, 1976
20. Paulsrud JR, Pensler L, Whitten CF et al: Essential fatty acid deficiency in infants induced by fat-free intravenous feeding. Am J Clin Nutr 25:896, 1972
21. Richardson TJ, Sgoutas O: Essential fatty acid deficiency in four adult patients during total parenteral nutrition. Am J Clin Nutr 28:258, 1975
22. Goodgame JT, Lowry ST, Brennan MF: Essential fatty acid deficiency in total parenteral nutrition: Time course of development and suggestions for therapy. Surgery 84(2):271, 1978
23. Hill GL, Guinn EJ, Dudrick SJ: Phosphorus distribution in hyperalimentation-induced hypophosphatemia. J Surg Res 20:527, 1976
24. Shils ME: Experimental human magnesium depletion. Medicine 48:61, 1969
25. Randall RE Jr, Cohen MD, Spray CC Jr et al: Hypermagnesium in renal failure: Etiology and toxic manifestations. Ann Intern Med 61:73, 1964
26. Solomons NW: On the assessment of trace mineral nutriture in patients on total parenteral nutrition. Nutr Support Serv 1:3, 1981
27. Grant JP, Cox LE, Kleinman LM et al: Serum hepatic enzyme and bilirubin elevations during parenteral nutrition. Surg Gynecol Obstet 145:573, 1977
28. Sheldon GF, Peterson SR, Sanders R: Hepatic dysfunction during hyperalimentation. Arch Surg 113:504, 1978

Chapter 70

Hyperlipoproteinemias

Craig Lehmann/Deborah T. Firestone

Hyperlipoproteinemias were first classified in 1965 by Fredrickson, who placed them into five major categories.[1] Since then, laboratory methodologies and research have provided a better understanding of these disorders, and have shown that the term hyperlipoproteinemia is not fully representative. The term *dyslipoproteinemia* better describes these abnormalities, because it accounts for decreases in some lipoproteins that occur, and for physiological variations in the phenotype.

Fredrickson's classification accounts for all variations of hyperlipoproteinemias except for the newly discovered hyperalphalipoproteinemia.[2, 3] Hyperalphalipoproteinemia is usually primary (familial), and involves autosomal dominant inheritance. Patients with it present increased concentrations of plasma high-density lipoproteins (HDLs). Because increased HDLs have not been shown to have harmful effects on health, no further discussion of them will be presented here, except to say that research has shown that increased HDLs appear to be related to decreased risk of coronary artery disease.

The primary clinical interest in hyperlipoproteinemias centers on their association with increased risk of coronary artery disease and pancreatitis. This association requires that an accurate distinction be made between primary disorders, which are familial, and secondary disorders, which are associated with other disease processes, so that the proper treatment may be administered. This distinction can only be made through careful evaluation of patient and family history and of clinical signs and symptoms, use of appropriate sampling methods, and proper utilization, interpretation, and correlation of laboratory tests.

ETIOLOGY AND PATHOPHYSIOLOGY

Type I

Type I hyperlipoproteinemia is very rare, almost exclusively primary, and acquired by autosomal recessive inheritance. The abnormality is manifested by an inability to clear chylomicrons. This is due to a decreased activity of lipoprotein lipase (LPL) or a deficiency in apolipoprotein C-II.[4, 5] The presence of plasma chylomicrons results in increases in triglyceride levels that are among the highest within the hyperlipoproteinemias. These high concentrations inflame the pancreas and result in recurring episodes of pancreatitis. For these reasons, a diagnosis is generally made early in life.

Although most primary disorders are diagnosed early in life, secondary conditions must be ruled out, especially in the adult. Secondary conditions that can present lipid abnormalities resembling type I are lupus erythematosus, pancreatitis, dysglobulinemia, oral contraceptive therapy, hypothyroidism, and uncontrolled diabetes mellitus.

Type II

Fredrickson's type II, a common hyperlipoproteinemia, has been divided into two subclasses, IIa and IIb. Type IIa is primary heterozygous, and acquired by autosomal dominant inheritance. It leads to hypercholesterolemia and increased low-density lipoproteins (LDLs). Type IIb is almost always primary, with a possibility of being either autosomal dominant or derived from a combination of genetic causes that leads to a combined hyperlipoproteinemia of very low-density lipoproteins (VLDLs) and low-density lipoproteins (LDLs). Type IIb is almost exclusively heterozygous and rarely appears in the homozygous state. Patients with type IIa either lack sufficient LDL receptors or have a defect in the receptors or a defect in LDL metabolism within the cell.[6] Homozygous patients demonstrate much higher levels of LDL cholesterol than do heterozygous patients. Patients with type IIb familial combined hyperlipoproteinemia present increased plasma LDLs and VLDLs. The exact defect has not yet been resolved. The increase in VLDLs may be polygenic and/or involve a variety of secondary conditions. Family studies usually reveal other family members with types IIa or IV.

Patients with lipid elevations that resemble primary type II patterns are those who have diabetes mellitus, myxedema, hypothyroidism, nephritic syndrome, hepatic disease, anorexia nervosa, treatment for another disease with numerous drugs, stress, or high-cholesterol/fat diets.

Type III

Hyperlipoproteinemia type III is very rare, almost exclusively primary, and acquired by autosomal recessive inheritance. The primary condition is due to dys-β-lipoproteinemia, resulting in plasma increases of VLDLs that are high in cholesterol. Type III hyperlipoproteinemias are apolipoprotein E^2 homozygotes. Normal individuals possess the apolipoprotein in the E^3 genotype form. Other variations have been reported that involve apolipoprotein E.[7, 8, 9] A primary role of apolipoprotein E is to clear chylomicron remnants and intermediate-density lipoproteins (IDLs). The site of its involvement is the liver receptors, where chylomicron remnants and IDLs are taken up. It appears that the apolipoprotein E^2 homozygote lacks the ability to bind the remnants to the receptors.

Although most dys-β-lipoproteinemias are primary, there are secondary disorders that can present lipid abnormalities resembling Type III. These include hypothyroidism, diabetes mellitus, myxedema, biliary cirrhosis, systemic lupus erythematosus, and gout.

Type IV

Type IV is a very common hyperlipoproteinemia, sometimes referred to as endogenously-induced hyperlipoproteinemia, that may be primary by autosomal dominant inheritance. The precise biochemical defect involved in Type IV is not known. It appears that the lipid increase is caused by a decrease in VLDL catabolism and/or an increase in the synthesis of VLDLs. Patients can present either a familial hypertriglyceridemia or a familial combined hyperlipoproteinemia. Research has demonstrated an association between apolipoprotein A-I and C-III genes for hypertriglyceridemia.[10]

Often, moderate alcohol ingestion may cause a lipoprotein pattern consistent with type IV lipoproteinemia. Other secondary conditions that may present lipid abnormalities resembling those of type IV are stress, estrogens, oral contraceptives, diet, thiazides, beta blockers, diabetes mellitus, and lipid storage diseases (*e.g.*, Gaucher's, Niemann-Pick).

Type V

Type V is a rare form of mixed familial hypertriglyceridemia that appears to be heterozygous or homozygous for an uncommon apolipoprotein $E^{4, 11}$ and/or may have elevations in sialylated apolipoprotein C-III 2.[11, 12] These defects produce elevated VLDLs and chylomicrons. The lipoprotein elevations cause inflammation of the pancreas.

As with type IV, secondary forms are numerous and common, and thus a careful effort must be made to distinguish them from the primary form. Common secondary disorders are alcoholism, myeloma, pancreatitis, diabetes mellitus, obesity, exogenous estrogens, and hyperuricemia.

CLINICAL MANIFESTATIONS

Early and frequent occurrence of abdominal pain and pancreatitis are key factors in making a diagnosis of a type I condition. Patients who consistently present triglyceride levels greater than 1500 mg/dL (17 mmol/L) may also exhibit eruptive xanthomas, lipemia retinalis, splenomegaly, and hepatomegaly. Patients generally complain of abdominal pain after the intake of a fatty meal. This is due to the increased chylomicrons and their effect on the pancreas. The episodes of pancreatitis are the most serious complications of type I for the patient, as there is no increased risk of coronary artery disease.

Type II hyperlipoproteinemias are associated with a high incidence of coronary artery disease. Heterozygotes tend to develop coronary artery disease as early as the third decade of life. Type IIa generally results in higher cholesterol levels than does the familial combined type IIb. Homozygotes tend to have very high plasma cholesterol levels and to develop coronary artery disease before the second decade of life. Planar and tuberous xanthomas are usually present on the patient's elbows, knees, and hands. Type IIb patients tend to be overweight and have elevated plasma VLDLs in addition to their LDLs. It is very rare that type IIb patients present xanthomas.

Patients with dys-β-lipoproteinemia (type III) present unique tubero-eruptive and palmar xanthomas *(xanthoma striatum palmare)*. These xanthomas appear in various hues of yellow and orange. Many patients have glucose intolerance and are obese. Coronary artery disease, ischemic vascular disease, and peripheral vascular diseases are prevalent. Clinical signs and symptoms vary with age, sex, and related secondary forms.

Most patients with type IV hyperlipoproteinemia are obese and present no xanthomas. They are generally adults, and may have an additional secondary disorder such as hypertension, diabetes mellitus, or hyperuricemia. Familial hypertriglyceridemia seems to have little correlation to coronary artery disease, which is not the case for the combined hyperlipoproteinemia.[13]

Patients with type V disease are generally obese and describe dryness of eyes and mouth, along with numbness of distal extremities. Patients usually present with pancreatitis and eruptive xanthomas, but not as early in life as in type I because type V usually occurs in adults.

LABORATORY ANALYSES AND DIAGNOSIS

Patient history is very important in order to interpret laboratory results properly. Patients should be questioned for a family history of hyperlipoproteinemia and/or coronary heart disease. They should also be questioned about alcohol consumption, because of its association with hypertriglyceridemia. Other circumstances may affect the results of laboratory tests used to assist in the diagnosis of hyperlipoproteinemia. There should not have been a recent record of surgery or of myocardial infarction within the previous month. Recent illness, present drug therapy, such as contraceptives, or dietary habits altered within the previous 2 weeks may also interfere with the interpretation of test results.

Blood samples for analysis must be collected from fasting patients, and analysis should not be delayed. For very short delays (2–4 hours), samples should be stored at 4° C. For electrophoresis, samples can be stored at 4° C with EDTA up to 5 days.[14]

Although cholesterol and triglyceride analyses still remain the primary tests for screening hyperlipoproteinemias, a recently described method involving precipitation of VLDL and LDL may prove to be helpful, especially in the screening of large populations.[15, 16]

Once cholesterol and triglycerides have been estimated and one or both are demonstrated to be elevated in at least two samples on different occasions, preliminary phenotype classification should be established by the 18-hour 4° C plasma observation test, as shown in Figure 70-1. After preliminary classification has been made and secondary factors have been ruled out, additional information for phenotyping and coronary artery disease risk can be obtained by the series of tests shown in Figure 70-1.

Although there is debate about the relevance of lipoprotein electrophoresis as a routine clinical tool, it is useful in detecting the presence of chylomicrons in types I and V, and of a lipoprotein X band, a marker of obstructive jaundice. Electrophoresis also helps to distinguish between types III and IV by revealing the presence of a broad beta band, present in type III. Therefore, electrophoresis for selected samples is still appropriate. On a routine basis, many laboratories include HDL, LDL, and VLDL cholesterol tests as a lipid profile. The LDL and VLDL cholesterol levels are generally calculated from relationships among total cholesterol, triglycerides, and HDL cholesterol values. Although there have been suggestions to measure apolipoproteins, such as apolipoprotein B (the primary protein in LDL) and apolipoprotein A1 (the primary protein in HDL), their clinical importance has not been fully demonstrated. In addition, most clinical laboratories are unprepared for these analyses at this time. Their potential role as diagnostic tests and predictors of coronary artery risk remains to be seen.

Most hyperlipoproteinemias can be classified by the tests previously described. However, other measurements and measurement ratios have been helpful in their classification and/or in the prediction of coronary artery disease risk. The ratios most widely used for this purpose are cholesterol/triglycerides, LDL cholesterol/HDL cholesterol, and VLDL cholesterol/triglycerides. For example,

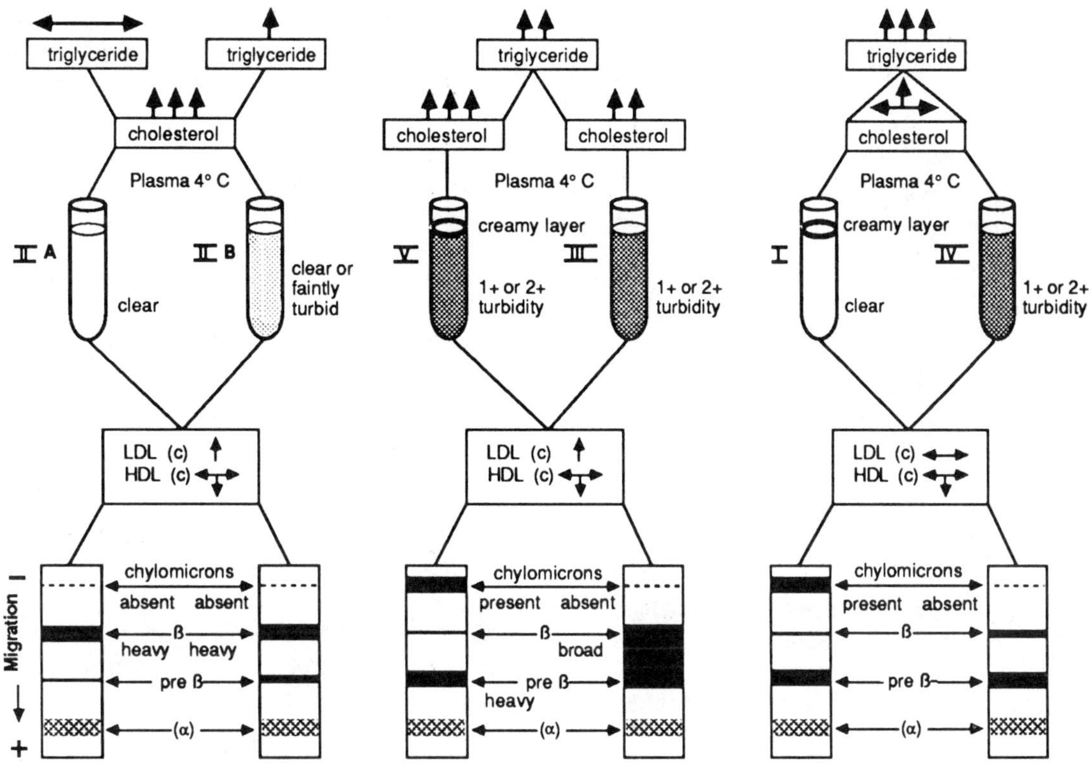

Figure 70-1 Plasma observation test.

type III demonstrates a ratio of VLDL cholesterol/triglycerides greater than 0.30. A more involved procedure, useful in separating phenotype I from type V, is postheparin lipase activity (PHLA). Lipoprotein lipase levels in type I do not rise following the infusion of heparin.

Laboratory analyses that are helpful in assessing secondary conditions include those for glucose intolerance and hepatic, renal, and/or endocrine function.

TREATMENT

Type I

Presently, there is no effective drug for type I patients; however, diet works well in controlling the condition and in preventing the occurrence of pancreatitis, a major objective of the therapy. Such diets consist of less than 20 grams of fat per day. In addition to diet changes, patients are counseled to restrict alcohol and to supplement their diet with fat-soluble vitamins.

Types IIa and IIb

Both subclasses of type II respond well to diet alterations. The diet should include low-fat and low-cholesterol intake. Type IIb responds well to niacin and gemfibrozil, while IIa responds best to colestipol and niacin. It should be noted that homozygous familial hypercholesterolemia is far more difficult to treat, as patients respond poorly to diet and drugs. When patients cannot tolerate standard drugs, probucol is an effective alternative.

Type III

Patients with type III respond well to cholesterol and caloric restrictions. Generally, to normalize lipid levels, drug intervention is also required. The drug most widely prescribed is niacin but, for patients who cannot tolerate this drug, gemfibrozil and clofibrate are excellent alternatives.

Type IV

Most patients with type IV respond well to diets that restrict fats, cholesterol, and calories. The avoidance of certain drugs as well as alcohol is imperative. If drugs become necessary, niacin, gemfibrozil, and clofibrate are recommended.

Type V

Patients with type V respond to diets that include low-fat and low-cholesterol intake. Restriction of alcohol and exogenous estrogens is imperative. For patients who do not respond well to dietary changes, the drug gemfibrozil is effective. (See Table 70-1.)

CASE STUDY

A routine physical examination of a 45-year-old male accountant revealed that the patient was overweight for his height and frame size. In addition, the patient's blood pressure was elevated (165/90). Fasting blood samples were drawn for a 20 chemistry profile, complete blood count, and urine analysis. The laboratory tests were all normal except for a moderate elevation in cholesterol and a major elevation in triglycerides.

During a followup visit to his physician, the patient was questioned for a family history of hyperlipoproteinemia and/or coronary heart disease. To rule out secondary complications, the patient was also questioned about dietary habits, drug therapy, recent illness, and alcohol consumption. All responses were negative and these factors were considered noncontributory to the lipid elevations.

Laboratory tests performed at this time were cholesterol, triglycerides, high-density lipoprotein cholesterol (HDLc), low-density lipoprotein cholesterol (LDLc), and 18-hour 4° C refrigeration observation. The laboratory was also directed to hold an additional sample for possible lipoprotein electrophoresis.

The cholesterol and triglyceride analyses were consistent with the previous data, moderately elevated cholesterol and extremely elevated triglycerides. The HDLc and LDLc were normal. The 18-hour, 4° C refrigeration observation showed a 2^+ turbidity. There was no creamy layer at the surface.

Questions

1. What hyperlipoproteinemia types can be eliminated in light of the initial laboratory test results?
2. Considering the additional laboratory findings, what hyperlipoproteinemia type is most likely?
3. What treatment is most effective for this type?

Discussion

1. Hyperlipoproteinemia types IIa and IIb can be ruled out immediately because they involve extremely elevated cholesterol levels and normal to slightly elevated triglycerides, as demonstrated in Figure 70-1.
2. The absence of a creamy layer at the surface after refrigeration rules out phenotypes I and V, as indicated in Figure 70-1. This leaves two possibilities, phenotypes III and IV. Of these two, the laboratory data present more supportive evidence for phenotype IV, because the LDLc is normal. This is not the case with phenotype III (see Fig. 70-1). The slight elevation in cholesterol with phenotype IV is due to the increased cholesterol found in the increased VLDL fraction and not in the LDL fraction. This can be confirmed by electrophoresis. The electrophoretic pattern should reveal no broad beta band, as seen in phenotype III, but a heavy prebeta band that is consistent with phenotype IV.

Table 70-1 ***Drug Therapy for Hyperlipoproteinemias***[17]

Drug	Phenotype	Effect	Adverse Effect	Laboratory Monitoring
Nicotinic Acid (Niacin)				
(Mechanism for lipid reduction unknown)	II, III, IV, V	↓ Triglyceride ↓ VLDL cholesterol ↓ LDL cholesterol ↑ HDL cholesterol	Hepatic Peptic ulcers	HDL cholesterol Liver function tests Glucose Cholesterol Triglyceride LDL cholesterol Uric acid
Cholestyramine and Colestipol				
(Anion-exchange resin that binds intestinal bile acids)	IIa	↓ LDL cholesterol	Constipation Nausea Hypoprothrombinemia (<Vitamin K)	Cholesterol Triglyceride Prothrombin time LDL cholesterol HDL cholesterol
Clofibrate				
(Mechanism not yet clear)	III, IV	↓ Triglyceride ↓ VLDL cholesterol ↓ LDL cholesterol ↑ HDL cholesterol	Myositis Hepatic Gastrointestinal Many additional effects	HDL cholesterol Cholesterol Triglyceride Liver function tests Complete blood count Protein Creatine kinase
Gemfibrozil				
(Mechanism not yet clear; research has demonstrated that the drug inhibits peripheral lipolysis and decreases hepatic extraction of free fatty acids)	IIa, IIb, III IV, V	↓ VLDL ↓ LDL ↑ HDL	Myositis Hepatic Many additional effects	Cholesterol Triglyceride K Levels Complete blood count HDL cholesterol LDL cholesterol Liver function tests
Probucol				
(Increased rate of fractional catabolism of LDL also inhibits cholesterol synthesis)	II	↓ LDL ↓ HDL	Hepatic Diarrhea Nausea	Cholesterol Triglyceride HDL cholesterol Liver function tests Glucose Urea nitrogen Uric acid LDL cholesterol

3. The patient should be placed on dietary restrictions of fats, cholesterol, and calories, because most patients with phenotype IV respond well to this regimen. However, if drug therapy becomes necessary, tests other than cholesterol and triglycerides should be included as part of the monitoring process. Drug therapy can cause such adverse side-effects as hepatic and gastrointestinal problems and peptic ulcers, as seen in Table 70-1.

REFERENCES

1. Fredrickson DS, Lees RS: Editorial: A System for phenotyping hyperlipoproteinemia. Circulation 31:321–327, 1965
2. Glueck CJ, Fallat RW, Millet F et al: Familial hyperalphalipoproteinemia. Metabolism 24:1243, 1975
3. Fredrickson DS, Levy RI: Familial hyperlipoproteinemias. In Wyngaarden JB, Fredrickson DS (eds): The Metabolic Basis of Inherited Disease, 3rd ed, pp 545–614. New York City, McGraw-Hill, 1972
4. Fredrickson DS, Levy RI, Lees RS: Fat transport in lipoproteins—An integrated approach to mechanisms and disorders. N Engl J Med 276:1967
5. Breckenridge WC, Little JA, Steiner G et al: Hypertriglyceridemia associated with a deficiency of apolipoprotein C-11. N Engl J Med 298:1265–1273, 1978
6. Tolleshaug H, Hobgood KK, Brown MS et al: The LDL receptor focus in familial hypercholesterolemia: Multiple mutations disrupt transport and processing of a membrane receptor. Cell 32:941–951, 1983
7. Rall SC Jr, Weisgraber KH, Innerarity TL: Identification of a new structural variant of human apolipoprotein E, E2 (Lys 146 Gln) in a type III hyperlipoproteinemic subject with E3/2 phenotype. J Clin Invest 72:1288–1297, 1983
8. Gregg RE, Ghiselli G, Brewer HB Jr: Apolipoprotein E bethesda: A new variant of apolipoprotein E associated with type III hyperlipoproteinemia. J Clin Endocrinol Metab 57:969–974, 1983
9. Havel RJ, Kotite L, Kane JP et al: Atypical familial dys-β-lipoproteinemia associated with apolipoprotein phenotype E3/3. J Clin Invest 72:379–387, 1983
10. Karathansis SK, McPherson J, Zannis VI et al: Linkage of human apolipoproteins A1 and C-111 Genes. Nature 304:371–373, 1983
11. Ghiselli G, Schaffer EJ, Zech LA et al: Increased prevalence of apolipoprotein E4 in type V hyperlipoproteinemia. J Clin Invest 70:474–477, 1982
12. Holdsworth G, Stocks J, Dodson P et al: An abnormal triglyceride-rich lipoprotein containing excess sialylated apolipoprotein C-111. J Clin Invest 69:932–939, 1982
13. Sniderman AD, Wolfson C, Teng B et al: Association of hyperapobetalipoproteinemia with endogenous hypertriglyceridemia and atherosclerosis. Ann Intern Med 97:833–839, 1982
14. Ballantyne CF: Role of the clinical biochemistry laboratory in the assessment of dyslipoproteinemias. Ann Clin Biochem 21:166–175, 1984
15. Lehmann CA, Rosenfeld MH, Danielson LA: A rapid, reliable screening method for hyperlipidemia. Lab Med 14:782–784, 1983
16. Lehmann CA, Treanor WJ, Malchiodi L: Efficacy of a simplified screening procedure for hyperlipoproteinemias. J Med Technol 2:174–176, 1985
17. Barnhart ER: Physicians' Desk Reference, 40th ed. Oradell, New Jersey, Medical Economics Books, 1986

BIBLIOGRAPHY

Brensike JF, Levy RI, Kelsey SF et al: Effects of therapy with cholestyramine on progression of coronary arteriosclerosis: Results of the NHLBI Type II Coronary Intervention Study. Circulation 69:313–324, 1984

Coronary drug project research group: Clofibrate and niacin in coronary heart disease. JAMA 231:360–381, 1975

Ghiselli G, Schaefer EJ, Gascon P et al: Type III hyperlipoproteinemia associated with apolipoprotein E deficiency. Science 214:1239–1241, 1981

Glueck CJ, Levy RI, Glueck HI et al: Acquired type I hyperlipoproteinemia with systemic lupus erythematosus, dysglobulinemia, and heparin resistance. Am J Med 47:318–325, 1969

Goldstein JL, Schrott HG, Hazzard WR et al: Hyperlipidemia in coronary heart disease. II. Genetic analysis of lipid levels in 176 families and delineation of a new inherited disorder, combined hyperlipidemia. J Clin Invest 52:1544–1568, 1973

Grundy SM: AHA special report: Recommendations for the treatment of hyperlipidemia in adults—a joint statement of the Nutrition Committee and the Council on Arteriosclerosis of the American Heart Association, Arteriosclerosis 4:445A–468A, 1984

Holdsworth G, Stocks J, Dodson P et al: An abnormal triglyceride-rich lipoprotein containing excess sialylated apolipoprotein CIII. J Clin Invest 69:932–939, 1982

Kashyap ML, Hynd BA, Robinson K et al: Abnormal preponderance of sialylated apolipoprotein CIII in triglyceride-rich lipoproteins in type V hyperlipoproteinemia. Metabolism 30:111–118, 1981

Levy RI: Drugs used in the treatment of hyperlipoproteinemia. In Goodman AS, Goodman LS, Gilman A (eds): The Pharmacological Basis of Therapeutics, pp 834–847. New York City, Macmillan, 1980

Levy RI, Fredrickson DS, Shulman R et al: Dietary and drug treatment of primary hyperlipoproteinemia. Ann Intern Med 77:267–294, 1972

Mellies MJ, Gartside PS, Glotfelter L et al: Effects of probucol on plasma cholesterol, high- and low-density lipoprotein cholesterol, and apolipoproteins A1 and A2 in adults with primary familial hypercholesterolemia. Metabolism 29:956–964, 1980

Norum RA, Lakier JB, Goldstein S et al: Familial deficiency of apolipoproteins A1 and C-III and precocious coronary artery disease. N Engl J Med 306:1513–1519, 1982

Schaefer EJ: Dietary and drug treatment. In Brewer HB Jr (moderator): Type III hyperlipoproteinemia: Diagnosis, molecular defects, pathology, and treatment. Ann Intern Med 98:623–640, 1983

Specher DS, Schaefer EJ, Kent KM et al: Cardiovascular features of homozygous familial hypercholesterolemia: Analysis of 16 patients. Am J Cardiol 54:20–30, 1984

W.H.O. cooperative trial on primary prevention of ischaemic heart disease using clofibrate to lower serum cholesterol: Mortality followup. Report of the Committee of Principal Investigators. Lancet 2:379–385, 1980

Zannis VI, Breslow JL: Characterization of a unique human apolipoprotein E variant associated with type III hyperlipoproteinemia. J Biol Chem: 1759–1762, 1980

Part XIV

TOXICOLOGY AND DRUG MONITORING

Janet Duben-Von Laufen
Associate Editor

Chapter 71

Toxicology and Drug Monitoring

Thomas Spillman

EMERGENCY TOXICOLOGY AND DRUG MONITORING

Drug analysis provides the physician with valuable insight in planning emergency treatment for the toxic patient. Treatment of the unconscious or obtunded (dull or confused) patient with unknown, inaccurate, or incomplete history requires differentiation among almost unlimited possibilities of toxicity and disease. Even when history or symptoms indicate the presence of a particular drug, detection of other unsuspected substances may require special measures or alter management of the patient.

The Comatose or Convulsing Patient

Guidelines have been established for immediate treatment of the comatose or convulsing patient, addressing a critical condition if it exists but introducing minimal risk if it does not.[1] Specifically, glucose (for hypoglycemic coma), thymine (for alcoholic or dietary chronic deficiency crisis), and naloxone (for opiate toxicity) are administered routinely. Also provided are respiratory support including intubation, maintenance of blood pressure with pressor drugs, seizure control with anticonvulsants, and correction of acidosis by alkalinization with intravenous bicarbonate.

Minimizing Absorption of the Toxic Oral Drug Dose

Following initial stabilization of the patient, oral ingestion of a toxic drug may warrant emesis (induction of vomiting) if the patient is awake. This is accomplished by the administration of syrup of ipecac, the extract of the root of a South American plant. Alternatively, gastric lavage may be used when the patient is comatose or seizing and at risk for choking on the gastric contents after emesis. Activated charcoal is often given orally after emesis to adsorb the remaining traces of the drug. Charcoal adsorption is effective for most drugs, both acidic and basic, but not for organic liquids such as alcohols. Once the lavage is completed, absorption of drug remaining in the intestinal tract is sometimes further decreased by administration of cathartics such as sodium sulfate.

Identification of the Toxic Drug(s)

Identification of the toxin is required for selection of an antidote or a method to enhance its removal from the body. A broad, all-purpose drug screen, if immediately available, will require several hours to provide this identification. History, clinical symptoms, and routine laboratory tests may narrow the possibilities in the meantime. Opiates, barbiturates, alcohol, methaqualone, and benzodiazepines, for example, tend to produce slowed respiration, hypotension, drowsiness, or coma. Stimulants such as amphetamines, theophylline, and cocaine produce agitation, convulsions, hypertension, and rapid respiration. Additional specific clinical characteristics may provide more specific information, for example, the pinpoint pupils often seen with opiate use.[2]

Once the toxin is identified, blood levels may be useful in determining the need for special clinical measures. Nomograms have been developed to predict risk of delayed toxicity from specific blood levels of aspirin and acetaminophen at known periods of time after ingestion. The relationship of circulating levels to the known risk of immediate reaction is available in reference sources for other drugs with pronounced toxicities. Although urine is the specimen of choice for detecting accumulated drugs and metabolites, drug quantitation is meaningful only when performed on blood. For drugs of habitual use, interpretation even of blood levels to account for behavior is sometimes complicated by individual tolerance. Behavioral tolerance to barbiturates, opiates, and alcohol is well known, although lethal thresholds do not increase appreciably in parallel with behavioral response. It should be noted that interpretation of blood levels requires knowledge of the state of absorption and distribution of the drug at the time of sampling.

Other Laboratory Analyses

Important laboratory tests involved in a rapid assessment of the patient include electrolytes and blood gases, which will reveal an anion-gap metabolic acidosis in the presence of several toxins including ethanol, methanol, ethylene glycol, and salicylates. For alcohols, an osmolal gap will also be expected (see p. 884 below).

Treatment to Reduce Drug Levels

The net result of the processes of absorption, distribution, and clearance of a drug is an increase and subsequent decline in circulating drug levels in a complex but reasonably predictable pattern. Levels first rise during absorption of the drug from the site of administration and its distribution into the circulation. Following this rise, blood levels decline as the drug begins to be partitioned into any tissue spaces in addition to the blood and cleared from the blood by metabolism and/or excretion. During a simple excretion phase of decline, the circulating level decreases by half of the existing level during each fixed period of time, called the *circulating half-life.*

A steady-state level is established by giving a second dose of the drug before the first dose is completely eliminated from the body. The result is a new level higher than that seen after the initial dose, because the new dose is superimposed on the old one. When the total level is higher, the absolute amount cleared during the same time period is also greater. This sequence of increasing peak followed by increasing rate of elimination continues until the two effects offset one another (after 5–6 cycles) and a steady state is reached in which peak and trough levels, respectively, are the same after each dose. Whenever this process achieves steady-state levels too slowly for the clinical need, a loading dose may be given intravenously, followed by smaller regular maintenance doses. The time required for a toxic drug level to subside to safety may be calculated from the known half-life, although the patient's hepatic and renal integrity, use of other drugs, and possible saturation of the normal pathways of drug clearance must be considered.

If life-threatening levels of toxic drugs are not cleared quickly enough for the clinical need by physiological means, invasive measures may be useful. All such measures require that the toxin exist largely in the blood rather than in other tissue compartments.

The simplest invasive procedure is *peritoneal dialysis,* in which cycles of dialysis fluid are introduced through an incision into the peritoneal cavity and left for 1 to 2 hours before draining. *Hemodialysis* is a higher-risk procedure involving continuous-flow removal of blood from the body, incubation of the blood with dialysis fluid across a semipermeable membrane, and return of the blood to the body. The procedure introduces a volume of fluid equal to the volume of the dialysis apparatus, which must be filled initially with fluid to prevent decrease of blood volume on initiation of treatment. Hemodialysis and also *hemoperfusion,* in which the blood flows through a column filled with charcoal or ion-exchange resin, require the patient to be treated with heparin to prevent coagulation of the blood in the apparatus, and both reduce platelet counts.[3] *Plasmapheresis* is a similar process that separates the blood cells from the plasma and returns them to the body suspended in a buffered electrolyte solution.[4] Drug located in the blood but bound to protein is not removed by dialysis, but may be removed by hemoperfusion due to competition for binding by the charcoal or resin, and will be removed efficiently by plasmapheresis or the more radical measure of exchange transfusion.

Examples of drugs for which overdose may justify invasive removal include digoxin, with cardiotoxic action and a long circulating half-life, and phenytoin, which can induce lethal seizures, particularly when its clearance by the liver has been oversaturated. Invasive measures may also be used for phenobarbital, salicylates, and theophylline. Even if removed from the circulation by invasive measures, most drugs will rebound as the portion compartmentalized in the extracellular fluid, tissues, or membranes reequilibrates with the blood. Repeated cycles of treatment may be necessary.

Few specific antidotes are available for treatment of toxic patients. A specific antagonist (blocker), naloxone, is available for opiates; N-acetylcysteine can be given to reduce toxicity of acetaminophen overdose; deferoxamine chelates and promotes renal excretion of toxic levels of iron; and controlled ethanol administration competitively reduces the metabolism and subsequent toxicity of methanol and ethylene glycol.[5]

GENERAL PATHOPHYSIOLOGY OF DRUG ABSORPTION, DISTRIBUTION, AND CLEARANCE

Absorption

The absorption of a drug and its distribution through the tissues and fluids of the body are highly dependent on its solubility in the body fluids and its diffusion through biological membranes under prevailing local conditions. These properties are influenced by the *p*H-dependent state of ionization, and they determine which route of administration, oral or parenteral, is the more effective with respect to drug absorption.

The *p*K of a drug indicates the relationship for that drug between *p*H and ionization; it is the *p*H at which half of a population of drug molecules is ionized. At one *p*H unit from the *p*K, the distribution of the ionized form is 1 : 9 or 9 : 1, and at two *p*H units from the *p*K, the ratio is 1 : 99 or 99 : 1. A basic drug with a *p*K of 4.3 would be more than 99% ionized in the stomach at *p*H 1.0, but would be only 10% ionized in the duodenum at *p*H 5.3, and thus be more rapidly absorbed as it moved out of the stomach. Morphine, for example, exhibits a basic ionization with a *p*K (*p*Kb) of 6.1, so that in the stomach it would be more than 99% ionized, and in the duodenum somewhat less than 90% ionized. The consequently inadequate gastrointestinal absorption is generally overcome by parenteral administration: intramuscular or intravenous routes.

Rapid hepatic metabolism of a drug is another process limiting the potency of orally-administered drugs. Because the blood flow from the intestinal tract passes through the liver before reaching the central venous system, drugs that that organ metabolizes efficiently reach the peripheral circulation in reduced concentrations. An example is cocaine, which is extremely ineffective if taken by mouth due to rapid first-pass liver metabolism as well as extensive hydrolysis in the blood before reaching the brain.

Distribution

Gastrointestinal absorption or direct introduction of a drug into the circulation is followed by distribution of the substance throughout the body. The pattern of distribution of a drug is determined by its chemical properties, and information is available regarding these patterns for each drug. Whereas some substances are highly water-soluble and are distributed through the vascular and extracellular spaces, others tend to accumulate in body lipids or bind to circulating protein, especially albumin. The protein-bound portion of a drug is a temporarily inactive reservoir, with only the unbound or free portion exerting biological activity. For especially toxic drugs such as phenytoin, which may be more than 90% protein-bound, fluctuations in drug binding by protein as seen in uremia may profoundly alter the biologically active levels without changing total blood levels, so that determination of the amount of *free* or *unbound* drug in the blood is of use.

The *volume of distribution* is the apparent volume into which a drug is distributed, based on calculation from blood levels. If the drug is accumulated in tissues outside the blood, the appearance will be that of distribution into a large volume, sometimes larger than the entire body volume. When drugs undergo such distribution into theoretical compartments in the body other than the blood, clearance from the body will be slow.

Clearance

Clearance of drugs from the circulation usually occurs by metabolism in the liver followed by excretion of the metabolites in the urine, although some drugs are primarily excreted without metabolism. Many chemical modifications occur in the hepatic microsomal system, including oxidation, hydroxylation, deamination, methylation, acetylation, and conjugation with glycine, sulfate, and glucuronic acid.[6] These reactions most often reduce the biological activity and increase the solubility of the parent drug, although a few metabolites are known to be active or toxic.

The capacity of these metabolic pathways is stimulated or induced by the presence of many substances on which they act, and is usually adequate to process circulating levels of drugs at a constant percentage of the total each hour (first-order kinetics). Aspirin, theophylline, and phenytoin, however, are three important exceptions for which hepatic metabolic pathways become saturated at high concentration, resulting in a leveling-off of metabolism at a maximal rate despite increasing blood levels.

In cases in which excretion of the parent drug in the urine is a significant pathway for elimination, enhancement of that process will improve the rate of patient recovery. Tubular resorption of a drug involves passage across biological membranes, and is blocked by ionization of the drug. For acidic drugs with *p*Ks between 3.0 and 7.5, or for basic drugs with *p*Ks between 7.5 and 10.5, appropriate adjustment of urine *p*H favors the ionization and excretion of the drug in the urine. Within these ranges, the *p*K is close enough to the typical urine *p*H that the drug is not already fully ionized, but still within the range in which attainable changes of urine *p*H will increase the degree of ionization.[7] Commonly encountered drugs for which ion-trapping with sodium bicarbonate or ammonium chloride effectively enhances elimination are amphetamines, imipramine, phencyclidine, and quinidine in acidic urine, and barbiturates and salicylates in alkaline urine.

MAJOR CLASSES OF SPECIFIC PHARMACOLOGICALLY ACTIVE AGENTS ASSAYED IN THE LABORATORY

Nonnarcotic Analgesics

Aspirin is the acetate ester of salicylic acid, the parent compound of the salicylates, a family of analgesic (pain-relieving), antiinflammatory, and antipyretic (fever-reducing) compounds (see Fig. 71-1). Therapeutic levels of these drugs act primarily by inhibiting prostaglandin synthesis, which is directly involved in generation of inflammation, fever, and pain. Aspirin is the least toxic and most commonly used of the salicylates. After oral ingestion, aspirin is absorbed from the stomach and small intestine, and levels peak in the blood in 2 hours. Metabolism occurs mainly in the liver, with excretion of the metabolites and a small amount of the unmetabolized drug in the urine.

The circulating half-life of aspirin is only 15 minutes, but two important mechanisms may prolong the action of the drug. First, salicylic acid, a major metabolite of aspirin, is also biologically active and has a longer circulating half-life (2–3 hours). Second, the enzyme pathways for liver metabolism of aspirin are easily saturable, and with increasing doses the circulating lifetime of aspirin itself becomes much greater. Chronic aspirin use may lead to serious salicylate poisoning, particularly in children, by gradually overburdening the metabolic capacity of the liver. Symptoms of aspirin toxicity include nausea, vomiting, tinnitus (ringing in the ears), hyperpnea (exaggerated respiration), coma, and convulsions. Direct stimulation of the central nervous system (CNS) causes

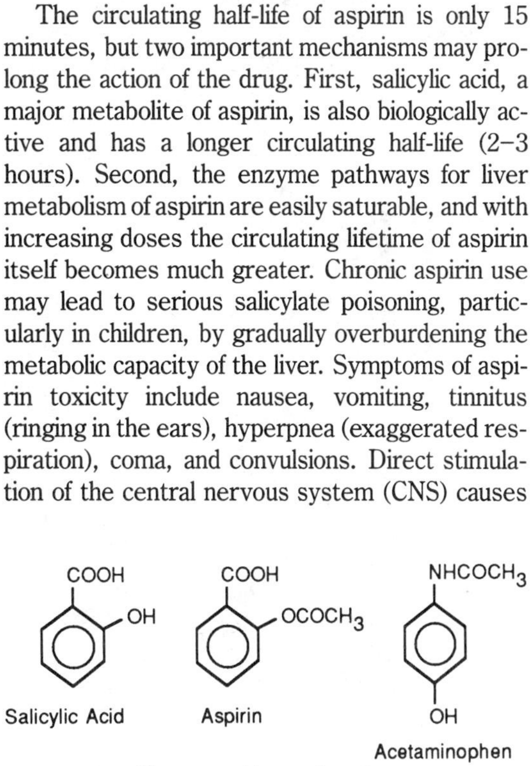

Figure 71-1 **Nonnarcotic analgesics.**

hyperventilation and respiratory alkalosis. Uncoupling of oxidative phosphorylation causes a compensatory increase in glycolysis, which may cause hypoglycemia and increased production of lactic and pyruvic acids. Direct inhibition of Krebs cycle enzymes by salicylate prevents normal metabolism of these acids and can lead to severe metabolic acidosis, requiring clinical intervention.[8]

When acute aspirin poisoning is suspected, a rapid semiquantitative test for aspirin may be performed in the laboratory. If aspirin toxicity is confirmed, standard measures to minimize uptake of the drug remaining in the gastrointestinal tract are taken, followed by a period of 6 hours of observation and medical support. Quantitative salicylate levels can then be obtained for prediction of the ultimate severity of the poisoning. The nomogram constructed by Done (see Fig. 71-2) predicts the ultimate toxicity based on the circulating levels at a specific time after ingestion.[9]

Acetaminophen (Tylenol) is an aminophenol compound with analgesic and antipyretic action similar to that of the salicylates, although its anti-inflammatory activity is minor (see Figure 71-1). The drug is absorbed from the gastrointestinal tract more rapidly than aspirin, and peak blood levels occur within 1 hour. Elimination occurs by hepatic metabolism to a number of conjugates and hydroxylated forms, and the serum half-life is 1 to 4 hours.

As with aspirin, laboratory analysis is primarily performed only for suspected acute toxic overdose. The initial symptoms of acetaminophen toxicity are nonspecific and include nausea, vomiting, and sweating. Following this initial toxic phase, the symptoms resolve. However, potentially fatal liver injury may have already occurred. The hepatotoxicity results from accumulation of a highly toxic metabolite of acetaminophen normally inactivated by liver stores of glutathione. In overdose, the metabolite may deplete glutathione reserves and injure the liver. As with testing for aspirin, a rapid spot test may be performed to confirm the presence of acetaminophen. Chemical reducing poten-

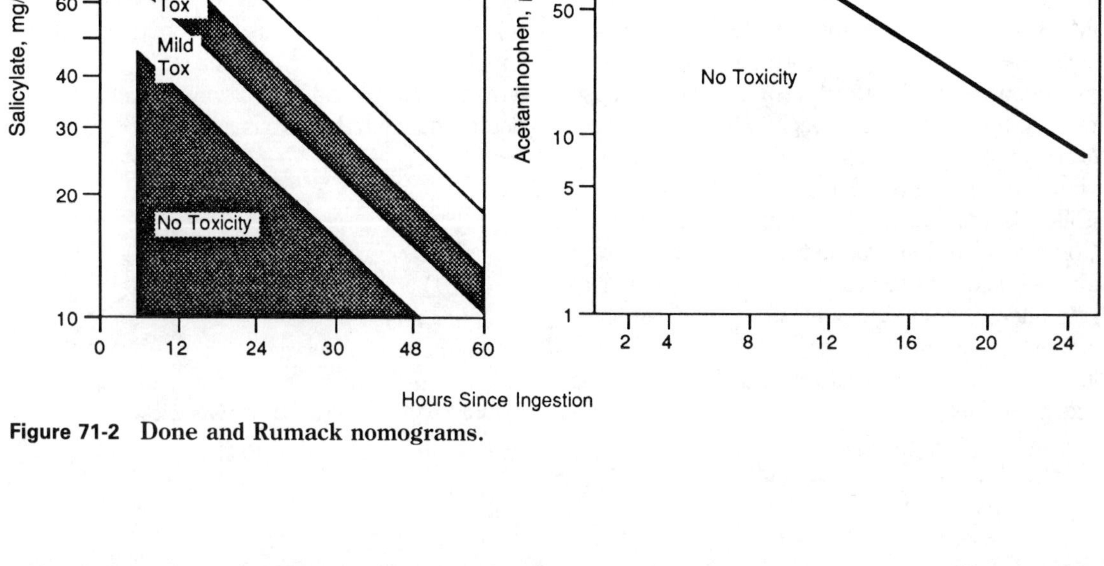

Figure 71-2 Done and Rumack nomograms.

tial in the body may be reestablished by administration of N-acetylcysteine, within the first 16 hours after ingestion of a toxic overdose and at 4-hour intervals for 3 days. As with the Done nomogram for salicylates, the Rumack nomogram for acetaminophen toxicity (see Fig. 71-2) predicts hepatotoxicity and indicates the need for N-acetylcysteine therapy and hospitalization based on serum levels determined 4 hours or more after ingestion.[10] Serum bilirubin and enzymes will reflect hepatotoxicity, with aspartate aminotransferase (AST) levels peaking 72 hours postingestion.[11]

Opiates (Narcotics)

Opiates are drugs and analogs of drugs obtained from the opium poppy. The major natural opiates are morphine and codeine. Heroin is a synthetic derivative of morphine that is about three times more potent due to increased lipid solubility and ease of passage into the CNS. Other important synthetic opiatelike drugs include meperidine (Demerol), methadone, and the opiate blocker naloxone (Narcan) (see Fig. 71-3). The major clinical uses of the opiates are in relief of pain, coughing, and diarrhea.[12] They act on the CNS to suppress pain impulses and the cough stimulatory mechanism, and to induce hypertonic contraction of the intestinal walls and reduce peristalsis. With the exception of methadone, the uptake of opiates in the gastrointestinal tract is slow, incomplete, and variable, so that for analgesia or recreational use they are commonly administered by injection. Opiates are vaporized by heat, so smoking is another efficient route of administration that rapidly produces high circulating levels of the drugs.

The opiates are cleared mainly by hepatic me-

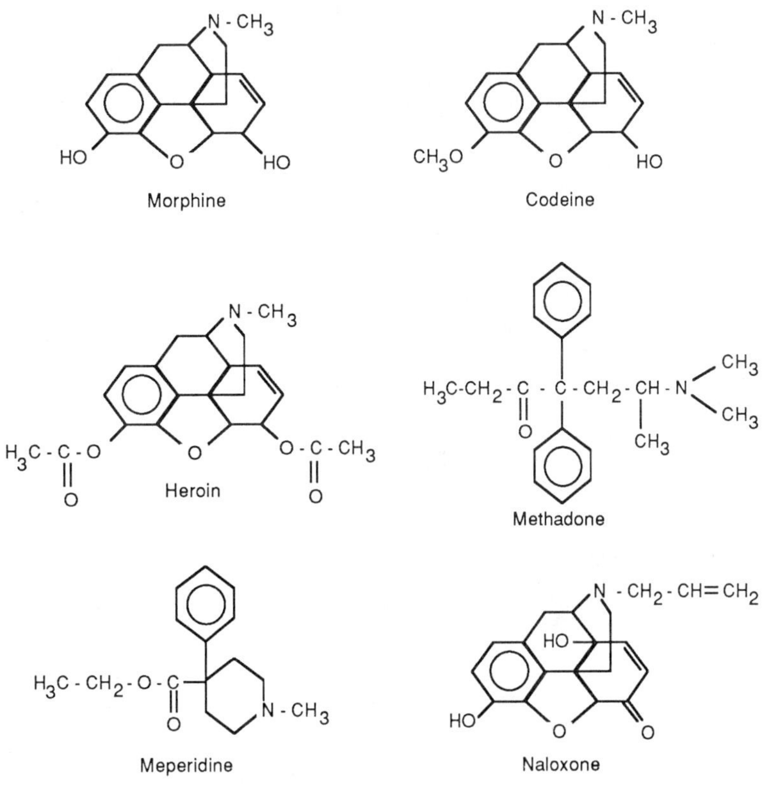

Figure 71-3 Natural and synthetic opiates.

tabolism and renal excretion of the metabolites, largely as the glucuronides, with a duration of action of 4 to 5 hours. Opiate overdose leads to potentially lethal respiratory depression. Miosis (contraction of the pupils) is usually noted after opiate use, a reaction sometimes useful in recognizing opiate intoxication although respiratory depression itself may cause dilation of the pupils.[13] Regular use of opiates leads to tolerance, due both to induction of liver microsomal enzyme levels and to decreased response of the CNS to the drug.

The withdrawal syndrome following opiate addiction is a clinically important state in itself. Symptoms include elevation of heart rate and blood pressure, sweating, severe aching, diarrhea, anxiety, respiratory stimulation, vomiting, fever, and chills. This state develops within 8 to 12 hours after morphine withdrawal and requires several days for resolution.

Opiates are often detected with a urine screen to identify the source of a toxic overdose. In acute toxicity with respiratory depression, the inactive synthetic analogue of the opiates, naloxone (Narcan), may be administered to block the opiate receptor. Naloxone is capable of inducing rapid and severe opiate withdrawal symptoms in the addict, however, so that the use of a second opiate, methadone, may be required. Methadone itself is capable of producing physical addiction, respiratory depression at toxic doses, and withdrawal symptoms when discontinued, although these effects are milder than those for morphine.[14] In long-term drug rehabilitation programs, methadone is substituted for other recreational opiates to provide a transitional substance from which later withdrawal will be more easily accomplished. In these programs, the laboratory may be used to verify the presence of urinary methadone and its major metabolite to ensure compliance. The latter will not be present if the methadone tablet was dissolved directly in the urine specimen.

Behavioral Depressants

The sedative-hypnotics, most notably the barbiturates, alcohol, methaqualone, glutethimide, and methyprylon, depress the CNS, an effect that differs depending on the dosage. At low doses, these agents depress anxiety and inhibition and generate a euphoria, giving the impression of CNS stimulation. As the dosage is increased, however, they progressively produce sedation, hypnosis (sleep), general anesthesia, coma, and death from respiratory depression.[15]

Barbiturates are the derivatives of barbituric acid (see Fig. 71-4). They are used mainly as sedatives or hypnotics, although the sleep they produce is an abnormal state in which rapid-eye-movement (REM) sleep is reduced. In contrast to the opiates, the barbiturates produce sedation without relief of pain. Certain rapidly cleared barbiturate derivatives are also used as anesthetics, and phenobarbital is used as an anticonvulsant at subsedative concentrations. Recreational use of the barbiturates is mainly directed at the low-dose euphoria.[16]

Barbiturates are highly lipophilic and easily absorbed from the gastrointestinal tract, so that, unlike for the opiates, oral administration is effective and common. The barbiturates are rapidly distributed to the brain and cross the blood–brain barrier easily. As the drug equilibrates with more remote body lipids, however, it is shifted rapidly out of the brain. The degree of side-chain hydrophobicity determines the distribution and action of the barbiturates, which are classified as ultrashort-acting (thiopental), short-acting (secobarbital, pentobarbital), intermediate-acting (amobarbital), or long-acting (phenobarbital). Clearance of barbiturates from the blood occurs through metabolism by microsomal liver enzymes, production of which is increased by barbiturate exposure.

Barbiturate toxicity includes loss of judgment and motor coordination, followed by respiratory failure at high doses. The depressant effects of alcohol are additive to the barbiturates, and toxicity may occur with amounts of the two combined that would not be toxic for either if taken alone. As with opiate tolerance, barbiturate tolerance develops with consistent use and increasing dosages are required to attain constant effects.

Serious physical dependence, characteristic of

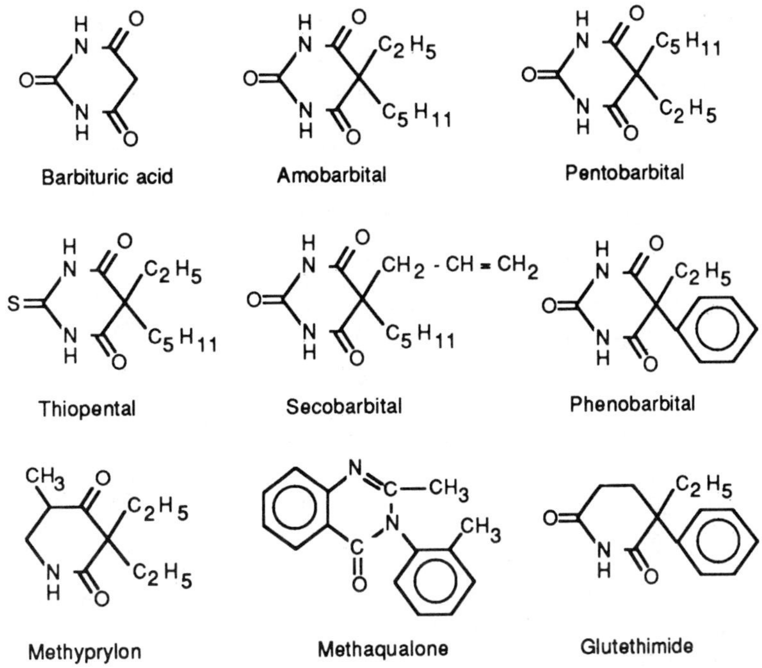

Figure 71-4 Barbiturates and related central nervous system (CNS) depressants.

chronic depressant abuse, also develops. Withdrawal symptoms develop over about a day and, like those for the opiates, run their course in several days to a week. Barbiturate withdrawal produces hypotension, weakness, tremors, and, in extreme cases, convulsions. A state of delirium may develop, leading to exhaustion, cardiovascular collapse, and death.[14] This state and the similar state seen with alcohol withdrawal are often treated with the benzodiazepines chlordiazepoxide (Librium) or diazepam (Valium).

Laboratory analysis of the barbiturates is generally for detection of barbiturates in suspected abuse or addiction or in quantitation of levels of phenobarbital when it is used as an anticonvulsant. Currently, no specific antidote or blocker analogous to naloxone for the opiates is available for the barbiturates.

Alcohol. The mechanism of action of ethanol on the CNS is not known, although nonphysiologic concentrations have been shown to inhibit ion pumps responsible for electrical nerve impulse generation. Ethanol, as well as methanol and ethylene glycol, the other alcohols that are often ingested, is readily absorbed from the stomach and the small intestine due to its small molecular dimensions and lipid solubility. While alcohols other than ethanol possibly have direct CNS effects, their toxicities are predominantly due to their metabolic products.[17]

Withdrawal from ethanol addiction is a potentially fatal state similar to that of barbiturate withdrawal, although seizures are somewhat less common. The patient experiences agitation, increasing for 1 to 2 days to a state known as delirium tremens (DTs). The agitation may be counteracted by phenothiazines, particularly chlorpromazine (Thorazine), but reversal of the syndrome is better accomplished with benzodiazepines, especially chlordiazepoxide (Librium).[14]

Metabolism of ethanol is mostly by oxidation in the liver to acetyl CoA, which is normally oxidized to carbon dioxide and water. The first two metabolic reactions for ethanol, however, consume the enzyme cofactor nicotinamide adenine dinucleotide (NAD). The eventual shortage of NAD blocks aerobic metabolism and limits the progression of metabolism of carbohydrates and amino acids to the final product of glycolysis, lactic acid. Lactic acid accumulates in the blood, creating metabolic acidosis. Methanol and ethylene glycol both share the metabolic pathway of ethanol and also induce anion-gap metabolic acidosis, although the actual metabolic products of these alcohols are different.[18] These metabolites are considerably more toxic than the alcohols themselves. For this reason, ethanol may be given therapeutically to compete for the metabolic processes of the liver and allow the usually minor pathways of renal or respiratory clearance to remove these alcohols instead.

Whereas metabolic acidosis has many nontoxicologic causes, the existence of an osmolal gap specifically indicates large amounts of nonionized substances such as alcohol in the blood. The *osmolal gap* is the difference in the measured and calculated serum osmolalities. Serum osmolality is measured by determination of its freezing point. Normally, the osmolality value obtained by this process corresponds to that calculated from the serum sodium, glucose, and urea (BUN) concentrations (the major contributors to the ionic content or osmolality of the serum) by the following formula:

$$\text{Osmolality} = 2 \times \text{Na} + \frac{\text{Glucose}}{18} + \frac{\text{BUN}}{2.8}$$

When any of the alcohols is present in intoxicating concentrations, this calculated result will be different from the measured value. For example, for each 10 mg/dL (2.17 mmol/L) of ethanol, the osmolal gap increases by 2.2 mOsm/kg.[19] Where direct assays of alcohols are not available, this approximation is useful, although it does not identify the nonionized substance specifically.

Methaqualone (Quaalude) is a nonbarbiturate sedative-hypnotic (see Fig. 71-4), and is popularly abused for a barbituratelike euphoria with less drowsiness. Administered orally, the drug is completely absorbed in 2 hours. Clearance is by hepatic metabolism, with excretion of most metabolites in the urine and a minor portion in the bile. Toxic effects include delirium, convulsions, and coma, with cardiovascular and respiratory depression only slightly less severe than those caused by the barbiturates.[20] The effects are additive with the barbiturates and alcohol. Methaqualone detection in screening is used to confirm the source of toxicity.

Psychedelic Anesthetics/Sedatives

Phencyclidine (PCP) was developed as an anesthetic, but its clinical use was discontinued as a result of its hallucinogenic properties (see Fig. 71-5). These properties and its low cost have in turn popularized its illicit use. PCP creates an unresponsive state characterized by a blank stare, in which the subject can communicate and appears to be awake but is detached and unresponsive to pain. PCP may be injected, smoked, inhaled, or ingested, and is often taken inadvertently with other drugs that have been diluted with inactive fillers, to which it has been added to create the impression of potency. PCP is hydroxylated in the liver before excretion of the metabolites in the urine. Toxic reaction consists mainly of several hours of aberrant behavior in which the most common cause of death is violent or delusional acts.[21] PCP is detected in the urine for identification of the cause of drug-induced delirium. Myoglobinuria may also be pronounced due to intense muscle contractions, even in the absence of seizures. This is important because acidification of the urine is often used to enhance PCP excretion by ion-trapping, and may cause serious renal damage by precipitating the myoglobin.[22] Diazepam (Valium) and chlorpromazine (Thorazine) are often used to treat the state of agitation.

Cannabinoids (marijuana). Δ-9-tetrahydrocannabinol (see Fig. 71-5) is the psychoactive agent in the marijuana plant, which may be smoked or ingested directly or used as a concentrated extract called *hashish.* This primarily recreational drug is a mild sedative-hypnotic at low levels, at which anxiety and inhibitions are relieved. Higher

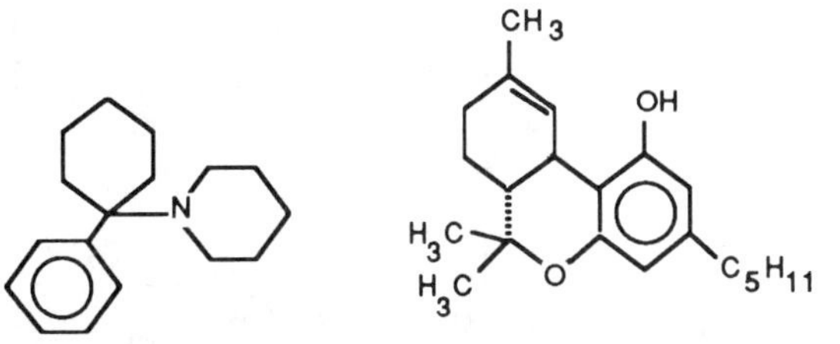

Phencyclidine Tetrahydrocannabinol

Figure 71-5 Psychedelic anesthetic/sedatives.

doses, however, result not in coma or death but rather in hallucinogenic effects.[23] The role of the laboratory in its detection is generally for evaluation of behavioral influences. Metabolism occurs primarily in the liver, after which the poorly defined metabolites are excreted half in the urine and half in the feces, mostly over a period of a few days. Due to apparent distribution of small amounts of the drug or lipophilic metabolites into body tissues, low levels of the urinary metabolites have been reported for weeks after cessation of use by chronic users.[24]

Antianxiety Drugs (Minor Tranquilizers)

Benzodiazepines constitute a family of commonly used sedatives with effects similar to those of the barbiturates and alcohol (see Fig. 71-6). Three of the most common are chlordiazepoxide (Librium), diazepam (Valium), and oxazepam (Serax). The ability of the benzodiazepines to suppress anxiety is much stronger than their induction of sleep, and they depress respiration much less than do the barbiturates.[25] Although they are commonly used in suicide attempts, overdose with benzodiazepines alone is rarely fatal. The effects are additive with alcohol and barbiturates, and such combinations in overdose may be lethal.

Absorption of benzodiazepines is slow at the acid *p*H of the stomach and occurs mainly in the small intestine, with maximum blood levels occurring 8 to 24 hours after ingestion. This slow absorption may cause quantitation to lead to underestimation of the actual dose if obtained too soon after a toxic ingestion. In addition to contributing to benzodiazepine-induced CNS depression, ethanol also increases the rate of benzodiazepine absorption. Clearance of the benzodiazepines from the blood takes place by oxidation and conjugation in the liver, followed by renal excretion. This metabolism occurs in a nonsaturable mode so that, unlike with aspirin or phenytoin, even massive overdoses of benzodiazepines are cleared rapidly by natural processes.

Toxicity may manifest as minor respiratory depression, hypotension, and coma. Hemoperfusion will rarely be useful in the comatose patient, unless with suspicion of concomitant barbiturate ingestion. No antidote for the benzodiazepines is currently available.

Anticonvulsant/Antiepileptic Drugs

Anticonvulsant/antiepileptic drugs reduce seizure activity in a wide range of epileptic disorders, although each is most effective with a certain type of seizure. (See Chap. 48.) The major drugs for treatment of seizure disorders share some limited structural similarity (see Fig. 71-7). Phenytoin

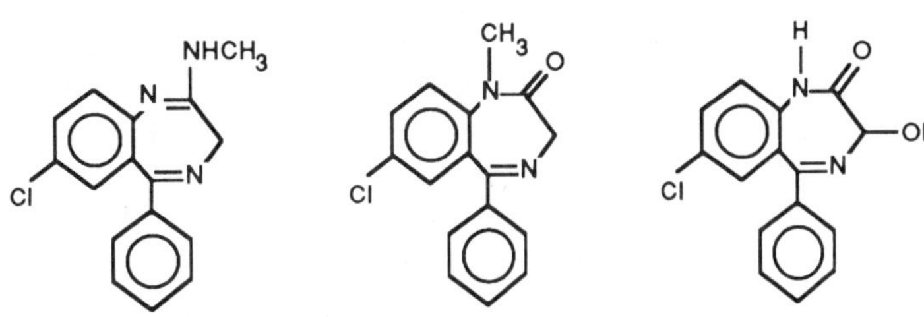

Chlordiazepoxide Diazepam Oxazepam

Figure 71-6 Benzodiazepines.

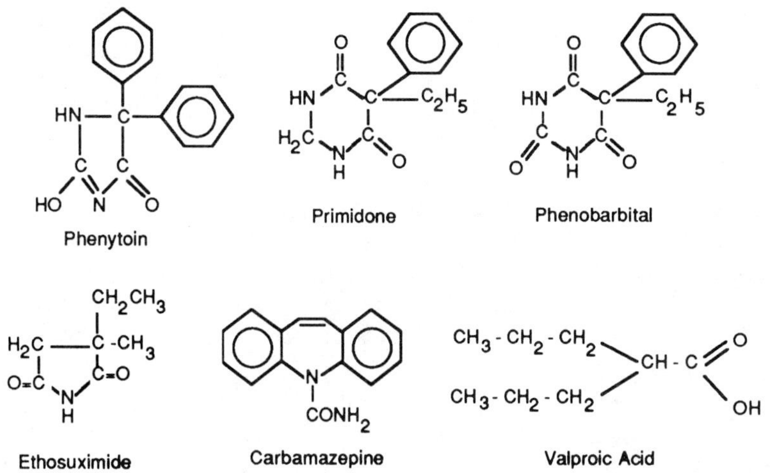

Figure 71-7 Anticonvulsant/antiepileptic drugs.

(Dilantin), primidone (Mysoline), phenobarbital, ethosuximide (Zarontin), and carbamazepine (Tegretol) share amounts of structure around the ring nitrogen, while valproic acid (Depakene) has no apparent structural similarity.

Phenytoin, primidone, phenobarbital, and carbamazepine are all effective to variable degrees in both simple and complex partial as well as general tonic–clonic seizures, and are used individually or in combination.[26] (These drugs are much less effective in the absence of myoclonic types of general seizures, for which ethosuximide and valproic acid are selectively effective and most often used.)

With the exception of acute seizure emergency (status epilepticus) and neonatal seizure control, the antiepileptics are generally administered as oral preparations. Peaks of circulating drug typically occur 1 to 8 hours after oral administration, with phenobarbital and phenytoin being absorbed more slowly and peaking as late as 18 to 24 hours after ingestion. Dosage intervals are typically 8 hours for drugs in this group, circulating half-lives of which range around 20 to 40 hours. Exceptions are phenobarbital, with a longer half-life of 4 days, and valproic acid, with a shorter half-life of 8 to 15 hours that requires slightly more frequent dosing intervals.

Clearance of these drugs is mainly by hepatic metabolism. The metabolic pathway for phenytoin is particularly sensitive to saturation at high levels, and intestinal reabsorption (enterohepatic recirculation) of the biliary excretion products slows its excretion. A third of carbamazepine excretion takes place directly into the stool without hepatic metabolism, and half of phenobarbital and a third of ethosuximide are excreted in the urine without metabolism. Otherwise, clearance of hepatic metabolites in the urine is the final mechanism of disposition.

Antipsychotic/Neuroleptic Drugs (Major Tranquilizers)

Psychosis refers to a mental state of dissociation from reality and lack of the ability to communicate with one's surroundings, as contrasted to simple feelings of anxiety, tenseness, depression, or frustration. The sedatives or minor tranquilizers (above) are used to treat these latter conditions, whereas the antipsychotics or neuroleptics are used to manage psychotic behavior.

Phenothiazines are the largest group of antipsychotic drugs, including chlorpromazine (Thorazine), fluphenazine (Prolixin), and promethazine (Phenergan) (see Fig. 71-8). The mechanism of action of this group is thought to be blockage of

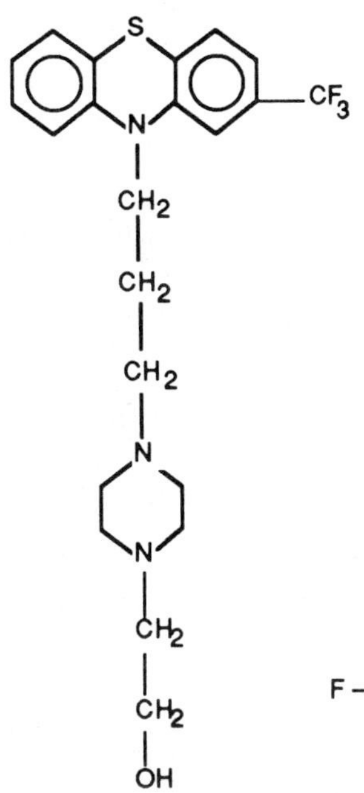

Fluphenazine

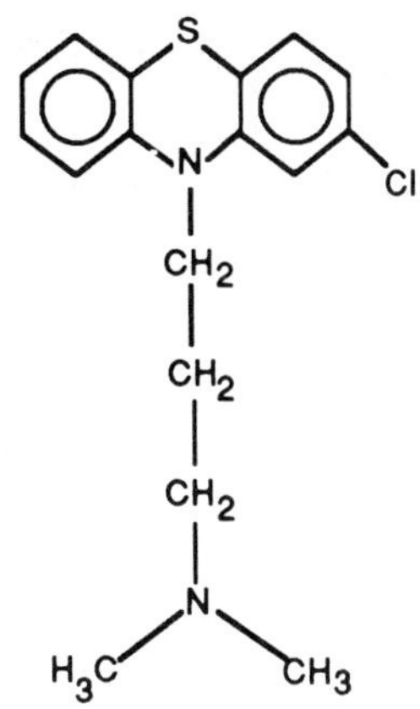

Chlorpromazine

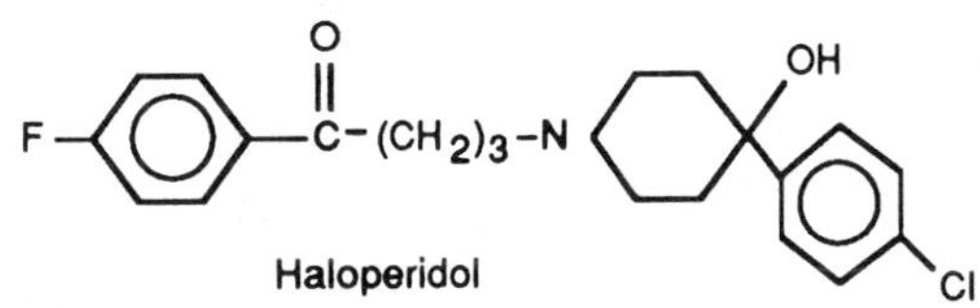

Haloperidol

Figure 71-8 Antipsychotic/neuroleptic drugs.

dopamine receptors in the brain.[27] The phenothiazines are usually administered orally and absorbed slowly. The drugs are metabolized by the liver, and the metabolites excreted in the urine. Clearance of these drugs is among the slowest of any group, with metabolites reported in the urine a year after discontinuation of the drug. Side-effects, in addition to sexual dysfunction, include muscular tremor and twitching, increased heart rate, dry mouth, blurred vision, constipation, and hepatotoxicity.

These side-effects may discourage compliance, so that monitoring of serum drug levels serves both to adjust the dose and to verify compliance. Overdose of phenothiazines is also common, due to their use in a patient population with a high tendency for suicide attempts. Urine screening for metabolites may be useful in identification in toxic overdose. The usual expression of phenothiazine overdose is a state of lethargy or sedation compounded by episodes of restlessness, tremors, or spasms. Coma is encountered mostly in accidental overdose in children.

Haloperidol (Haldol) is a butyrophenone (see Fig. 71-8), structurally different from the phenothiazines but pharmacologically similar.[27] Haloperidol differs in being less hepatotoxic but more apt to cause involuntary muscle tremors. It is metabolized more rapidly than are the phenothiazines. Determination of serum levels of the drug serves the same purpose as for the phenothiazines.

Clinical Antidepressants

The major *tricyclic antidepressants* (see Fig. 71-9) include amitriptyline (Elavil), nortriptyline (Pamelor), imipramine (Tofranil), desipramine (Norpramin), doxepin (Sinequan), and protriptyline (Vivactyl). These drugs are used in the control of depression, both for autonomous forms in which no specific external events trigger the state, and also

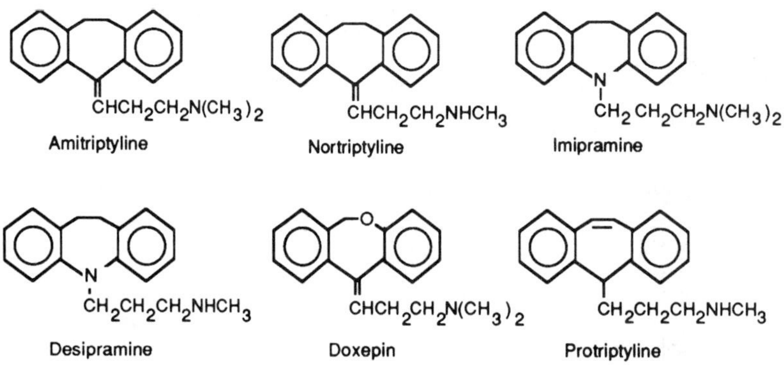

Figure 71-9 Tricyclic antidepressants.

in conditions such as terminal illness.[28] Standard oral doses are increased in slow stepwise fashion, guided by blood levels and observed clinical response, which is maximal after a delay of 2 to 3 weeks. Oral administration is used for convenience, although extensive first-pass clearance by the liver impairs absorption from the intestine into the peripheral circulation. Peak levels are obtained in 4 to 8 hours. Side-effects include dry mouth, urinary retention, blurred vision, hypotension, and constipation (anticholinergic action). At toxic levels, confusion, agitation, irritability, difficulty in speaking, respiratory depression, coma, convulsions, and cardiac arrhythmias can occur. Physostigmine is used for reversal of the anticholinergic effects.

The mechanism of action of *lithium* salts in stabilizing mood is unknown. There is no known role of lithium in normal physiology, and therapeutic levels of the substance do not alter the mood of the normal individual.[29] Its close chemical relationship to potassium and sodium ions has led to experimentation, suggesting a possible influence on membrane polarization in neurologic transmission. Lithium carbonate is administered orally in treatment of mood disorders, particularly manic–depressive states. The salt is readily absorbed from the gastrointestinal tract, with peak blood levels occurring in 2 to 4 hours. One- to two-thirds of the dose is excreted in the urine in the first 6 to 12 hours, after which excretion continues slowly for 10 to 14 days. Toxicity in overdose consists of nausea and vomiting, ataxia, seizures, coma, and cardiac arrhythmias. Renal clearance of lithium is reduced by sodium depletion and, with the typically rapid rate of clearance of lithium, a change in lithium clearance may quickly create toxic levels. Regular monitoring of therapeutic blood levels is important in maintaining the drug in the therapeutic range.

Behavioral Stimulants

Behavioral stimulants act on the nervous system to alter chemical transmission of nerve impulses in complex and only partially understood ways. For some drugs, such as cocaine, the best understood influences are secondary to the main purpose of the drug. The distinction among the types of chemical nerve transmitters involved is important to understanding what is known regarding the actions of these drugs.

Transmission of nerve impulses at adrenergic synapses between nerve cells is generally accomplished by release of either catecholamines (epinephrine, norepinephrine) or acetylcholine.[30] After release, catecholamines are reabsorbed by the transmitting nerve cell, to return the synapse to the resting state. Because large amounts of catecholamines are produced by the adrenals, epinephrine is also known as adrenaline and these catecholamine-reactive nerve endings are known as *adrenergic synapses*. The skeletal muscle (somatic) system and part of the visceral (autonomic) nervous system are equipped with nerves using acetylcholine rather than norepinephrine (NE) as neurotransmitters. That portion of the autonomic nervous system using only acetylcholine is known as the *parasympathetic* system, while the other portion, using catecholamine transmission, is the *sympathetic* nervous system. Drugs stimulating catecholamine synapses or mimicking the action of norepinephrine are thus known as *sympathomimetic amines.* The effects of stimulation of NE synapses include general vasoconstriction, increased heart rate, sweating, increased body temperature, increased mental activity, dilation of the pupils, and decreased intestinal peristalsis.

Amphetamines/sympathomimetic amines constitute a family of analogues to NE, of which the prototype drug of abuse is amphetamine (see Fig. 71-10). Amphetamine is thought to both stimulate the release of NE into the adrenergic synapse and have a direct effect on the postsynaptic receptor. The effect of amphetamine is to stimulate a physiological response like that to NE, and it has found clinical applications in the treatment of absence seizures and hyperactivity in children. An amphetamine analogue, methylphenidate (Ritalin), (see Fig. 71-10) has also been used in hyperactivity, although the mode of action is not understood. The widest uses of sympathomimetic amines are as weight control drugs, decongestants (due to vasoconstrictive properties), inducers of wakefulness and alertness, and euphoriants.[31]

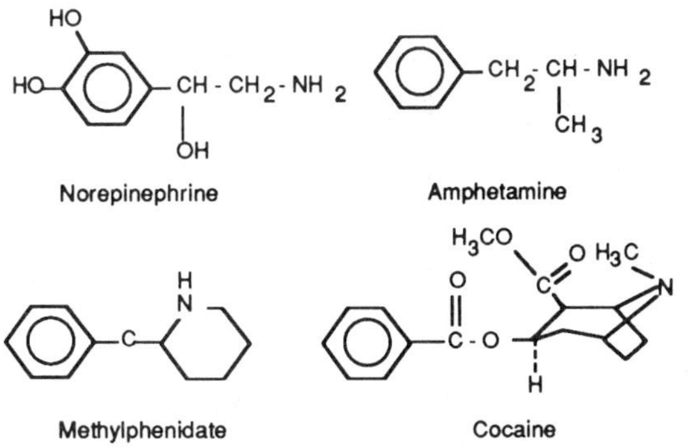

Figure 71-10 **Norepinephrine and behavioral stimulants.**

Sympathomimetic amines are taken orally to obtain the moderate-dose stimulatory effects, which, in addition to increased alertness, energy, and sense of wellbeing, include the undesired side-effects of sweating, dry mouth, increased blood pressure, and increased respiration. Intravenous use induces an intensely pleasurable sensation or "rush" that is associated with a manic paranoia. The high lipid solubility of the sympathomimetic amines promotes their ready absorption across nasal, lung, and gastrointestinal membranes. Blood levels peak within 3 hours of oral ingestion, and the half-life in the blood is 7 to 34 hours. Hepatic metabolism includes hydroxylation, dealkylation, deamination, and oxidation, before excretion of these metabolites into the urine.

Acute toxicity is associated with nausea, vomiting, headache, palpitations, confusion, dizziness, and even seizures and coma. Pupils are dilated but reactive. Hypertension and ventricular tachyarrhythmias are of particular concern, as cerebral vascular and cardiac events are often responsible for death in amphetamine toxicity.

Cocaine is a naturally-occurring alkaloid from the South American plant *Erythroxylon coca* that has limited medical but widespread social usage.[32] (See Fig. 71-10.) Cocaine exerts many of the same effects as sympathomimetic amines, not by acting directly on the NE receptor, but by inhibiting the uptake of norepinephrine from the synapse once it is secreted. The accumulation of NE leads to sympathetic stimulation. This effect is responsible for the increased heart rate and blood pressure experienced with cocaine use.

The euphoria created by cocaine, however, is a result not primarily of the sympathetic stimulation but rather of the interaction with dopamine receptors in the brain. Additionally, cocaine acts as a local anesthetic at the area of membrane absorption, leading to its medical application as a local anesthetic for ophthalmologic procedures. Rapid hydrolysis in the blood and liver minimizes the effect of orally-administered cocaine. The highly hydrophobic nature of the drug promotes its passage across membranes in the oral, nasal, and bronchial passages, thus gaining access to a shorter circulatory pathway to the brain. The hydrochloride salt is often snorted, and the nonionized or free-base form, also known as "crack," is vaporized by smoking and absorbed directly through the lungs. While the vasoconstrictive activity of cocaine progressively reduces absorption through the nasal passages, sympathetic stimulation actually opens bronchial passages for better absorption and passage to the brain.

Cocaine toxicity proceeds through a biphasic process of increasing CNS stimulation followed by CNS depression. Symptoms similar to those of amphetamine toxicity, including nausea, vomiting, and seizures with increased blood pressure and respiration rate later give way to paralysis, respiratory failure, circulatory failure, and loss of vital functions. Cocaine is eliminated with a short half-life of 75 minutes, with the pleasurable effects lasting for a shorter period. Cocaine is metabolized rapidly in the blood by pseudocholinesterase and liver enzymes before excretion in the urine. The parent drug is excreted only when high levels are present. Laboratory testing consists of detection of the cocaine or metabolites, particularly benzoylecgonine, in the urine in monitoring cocaine use or in confirming the etiology of a toxic crisis.

Cardiac Drugs

Neurologic stimulation of the heartbeat occurs by means of nerve impulses, the timing of which is normally controlled by the design and arrangement of the conduction pathways.[33] The sino–atrial (S–A) node at the junction of the venous sinus and the atrium transmits a natural rhythmic pulse throughout the atrial walls. A second nerve bundle at the junction of the atria and ventricles, the A–V node, passes the impulse to the ventricles. At the A–V node, the impulse is delayed to allow the ventricles to fill before the impulse is finally transmitted rapidly throughout the ventricles, leading to an abrupt contraction and ejection of the blood out of the heart.

Much of the heart is subject to self-excitation and is capable of initiating uncoordinated heartbeats. The S–A node normally controls the heartbeat because it discharges more frequently than the rest of the pathway, and each impulse from the S–A node depolarizes the nerves, overriding their tendencies to self-excitation. An abnormal site of impulse initiation may develop due to increased excitability of the heart, which can result from local lack of blood flow (ischemia), lack of sleep, anxiety, or overuse of stimulants such as caffeine.

Quenching of the excitation of each heartbeat once it has been completed is accomplished by the existence of a refractory period, in which the nerves cannot be stimulated. All nerves are stimulated during the contraction and then enter the refractory period at once, so that the nerve impulse dies. If the refractory period is shortened, as in response to an increase of epinephrine, some pathways may recover their excitability before the previous impulse has been terminated, and a continuous cycle of contraction may begin to move around the heart (circus movements), resulting in flutter or fibrillation in which the heart does not function as a pump.

Flutter or fibrillation in the atria is much less serious than that in the ventricles because the movement of the blood is primarily driven by the ventricular beats. Despite atrial fibrillation, transmission of impulses from the atria to the ventricles is still controlled by the A–V node, which causes stimulation to pass to the ventricles only periodically and along the proper pathways. Ventricular fibrillation, in contrast, causes immediate cessation of blood flow throughout the body. Once initiated, flutter or fibrillation may be terminated by application of an intense electric current through the heart to cause all the nerves to become refractory at once. Otherwise, within 60 to 90 seconds the heart muscle itself is so weak from lack of perfusion that correction of the nerve impulse pattern alone can no longer reinitiate the heartbeat. Cardiac massage in conjunction with recoordination of nerve impulses is required for resuscitation.

Quinidine, procainamide/N-acetyl procainamide, and disopyramide (see Fig. 71-11) act to slow

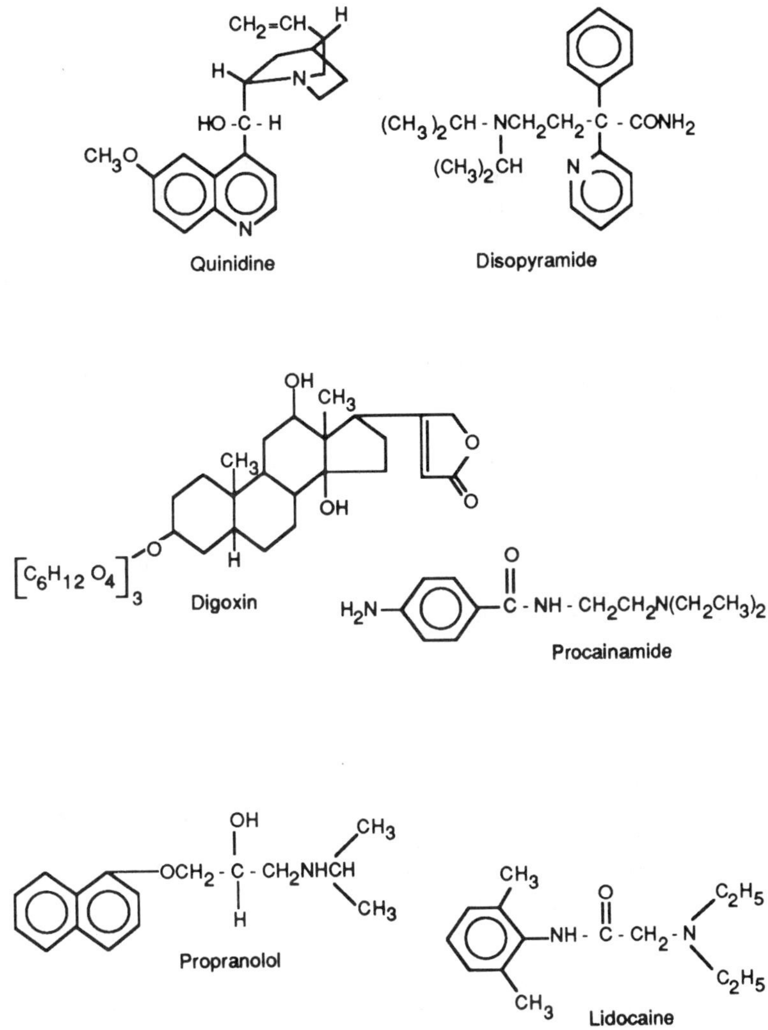

Figure 71-11 Cardiac drugs.

the high-velocity conduction rates and prolong the refractory period of the high-velocity pathways throughout the heart, ensuring the complete termination of each impulse.[34] They are favored for use in atrial flutter, fibrillation, and tachycardia. The drugs are cardiotoxic in overdose, resulting in depression of nodular conduction. They are absorbed rapidly from the gastrointestinal tract, with peak blood levels occurring at 1 to 2 hours after administration. Clearance is by hepatic metabolism and renal clearance, with half-lives of 3 to 6 hours. Laboratory monitoring is used to adjust the dosage to maintain therapeutic levels. One major metabolite of procainamide, N-acetyl procainamide, is biologically active, and requires quantitation in procainamide therapy.

Lidocaine (see Fig. 71-11) and *phenytoin (Dilantin)* (see Fig. 71-7) both reduce abnormal initiation of nerve impulses, particularly in the ventricles, and depress high-velocity conduction, altering the kinetics of nerve fiber voltage development.[34] First-pass inactivation by the liver renders oral administration of lidocaine ineffective. When administered intravenously, it is cleared by the liver with a half-life of 1 to 2 hours. Lidocaine overdose results in convulsions, coma, and respiratory arrest. Phenytoin, an established anticonvulsant, has similar electrophysiological actions and is particularly useful in counteracting digoxin toxicity.

Propranolol and other beta-adrenergic blockers specifically counteract the increased excitability and spontaneous discharges promoted by epinephrine (adrenaline), and act to slow conduction and prolong the refractory period at the A–V node[34] (see Fig. 71-11). Clearance is hepatic, with a circulating half-life of 3 to 6 hours. Toxicity may include A–V node block and circulatory collapse.

The *digitalis* family of drugs—digoxin (see Fig. 71-11), digitoxin, and ouabain—slows the heart rate by influencing vagal nerve activity, slowing conduction and prolonging the refractory period of the A–V node.[34] These drugs are particularly useful for ventricular control in atrial tachyarrhythmias. Whereas the majority of digoxin and ouabain is excreted by the kidneys, digitoxin is eliminated nearly entirely by hepatic metabolism. The circulating half-lives of these drugs are long: 2 to 5 days. A narrow therapeutic index requires periodic monitoring of blood levels. Toxicity includes premature ventricular beats, ventricular tachycardia, and even ventricular fibrillation, which may be counteracted by lidocaine and phenytoin. Accidental overdose occurs most often with children, and the long half-life of the drug indicates intervention. Digoxin-specific Fab antibody fragments are available on a limited basis to bind and inactivate the circulating drug, and charcoal hemoperfusion is also effective.

Antibiotics (See also Chap. 63.)

The *aminoglycoside* antibiotics—gentamicin, tobramycin, amikacin, kanamycin, streptomycin, and neomycin (see Fig. 71-12)—exert their biological activity by binding directly to the ribosomes of gram-negative bacteria and inhibiting protein synthesis.[35] Their highly polar nature limits passage across biological membranes, and absorption from the gastrointestinal tract is minimal. Administration is parenteral, either intramuscular or intravenous, with peak blood levels occurring in 30 to 90 minutes. Clearance is almost totally renal, with a half-life of 2 to 3 hours, and 50% to 60% of the dose is excreted in 24 hours. Toxicity consists of permanent ototoxicity (loss of hearing) and reversible nephrotoxicity, primarily acute tubular necrosis, due to high concentrations of the drug in the urine. Clearance of the drugs varies ten-fold with renal status, so that regular monitoring of drug levels is important in limiting the incidence and severity of renal damage.

Vancomycin is a complex glycopeptide not structurally related to the aminoglycosides but similar in many respects. The drug is active mainly against gram-positive bacteria, and acts by inhibiting cell wall synthesis.[36] Like the aminoglycosides, vancomycin is poorly absorbed from the gastrointestinal tract and is therefore administered intravenously. Excretion is mainly renal, with ototoxicity and nephrotoxicity similar to and additive to that of the aminoglycosides. Monitoring serves to minimize renal damage.

Chloramphenicol is a bacteriostatic agent that inhibits growth of a fairly broad spectrum of organisms, including many strains of gram-negative bacteria and all anaerobic species[37] (see Fig. 71-12). The drug is lipophilic and readily crosses biological membranes including the blood–brain barrier, but is only slightly soluble in water. Oral absorption is consequently rapid, with peak concentrations 1 to 2 hours after dosing. The limited solubility of chloramphenicol causes it to be 50% bound to blood proteins. Intravenous administration is in the form of an inactive but highly water-soluble succinate ester, which is hydrolyzed to the active drug. Metabolism occurs mainly by glucuronidation in the liver followed by renal excretion of the glucuronide, with a half-life in the normal adult of 1.5 to 3.5 hours.

Chloramphenicol has induced aplastic anemia in rare cases of chronic use, although this phenome-

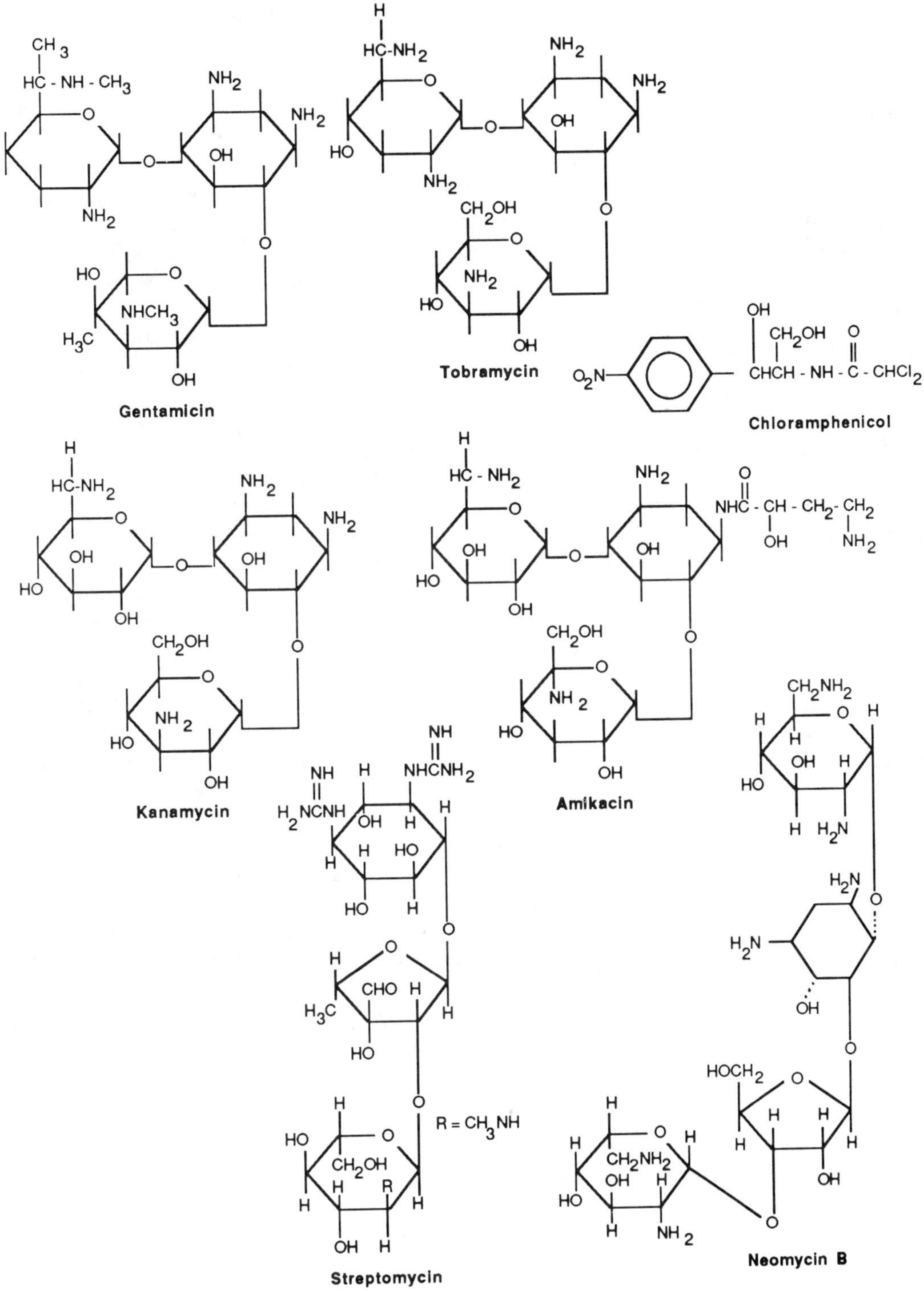

Figure 71-12 Antibiotics

non is not related to dose. More importantly, potentially fatal acute toxicity can develop in overdose or accumulation due to inadequate hepatic metabolism, a particular risk with neonates.[38] The drug inactivates the bacterialike mitochondrial ribosomes and causes circulatory collapse (gray baby syndrome). Circulating levels require frequent monitoring to avoid accumulation.

Other Drugs and Toxins

Theophylline is a xanthine (see Fig. 71-13), chemically related to caffeine and theobromine, consumed in large amounts in coffee, tea, and chocolate. The xanthines stimulate respiration, heart rate, and to some extent mental alertness, while relaxing certain smooth muscle and systemic blood vessels. Theophylline has found clinical application in stimulating respiration in apnea of the newborn and relaxation of the bronchi in chronic asthma.[39] Absorption after oral dosage is rapid, with maximal blood levels attained within 2 hours. Elimination is primarily by hepatic metabolism, followed by urinary excretion of the metabolites. The circulating half-life in children is 3.5 hours, and in adults 8 to 9 hours. Toxic reaction includes headache, palpitation, dizziness, nausea, hypotension, tachycardia, and seizures. Clearance of theophylline, like that of salicylates and phenytoin, is saturable at high circulating levels, and due to its toxicity may require hemoperfusion while seizure control is exerted with diazepam. Quantitation of blood levels in the laboratory is useful in adjusting dosage and evaluating suspected or documented toxicity.

Organophosphorus compounds are used widely as insecticides, including in home aerosol products. Their mechanism of both insect and human toxicity is tight binding to and inhibition of cholinesterase, the enzyme-destroying acetylcholine in the synapse after each discharge of a cholinergic neuron. The consequence of this inhibition is interruption of the conduction of normal nerve impulses.[40] The organophosphorus compounds may be inadvertently inhaled, ingested, or absorbed through the skin, especially by children. The onset of the symptoms, known as a cholinergic crisis, is rapid, and includes a syndrome with the acronym of SLUDGE: salivation, lacrimation (watering of the eyes), urination, defecation, gastrointestinal cramping, and emesis (vomiting). Respiratory or cardiac arrest may be induced.

Organophosphorus toxicity may be inferred from a low serum pseudocholinesterase level. Inhibition of this circulating enzyme to half or less of the normal range indicates serious inhibition of synaptic cholinesterase as well. Organophosphorus poisoning is treated by respiratory support and the administration of the acetylcholine receptor blocker atropine at 10- to 30-minute intervals for 24 to 48 hours. Atropine binds to the muscarinic class of acetylcholine receptors, counteracting the high acetylcholine concentration and reversing the cardiac and bronchoconstricting effects of the drug. Atropine does not bind to the nicotinic class of acetylcholine receptor to relieve the respiratory depression. A second antidotal substance, pralidoxime, displaces the organophosphorus compound from the cholinesterase and will gradually

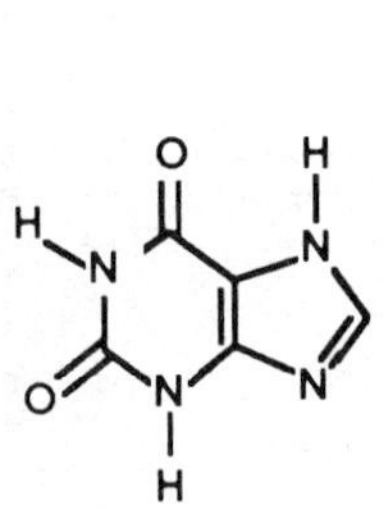

Xanthine

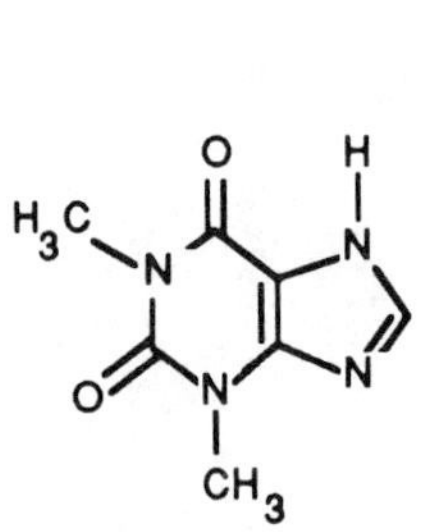

Theophylline

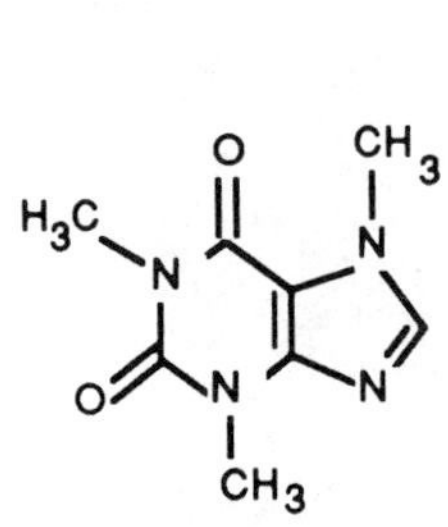

Caffeine

Figure 71-13 Xanthines.

reverse the poisoning. Plasma pseudocholinesterase levels may not return to normal for 1 to 4 weeks after recovery.

Iron is commonly encountered in accidental overdose by children.[41] Although the regulation of uptake of iron in the intestine normally prevents dietary iron overload, in extreme overdose the iron induces hemorrhagic gastroenteritis, and damage to the gastric mucosa is so severe that absorption can no longer be controlled. In turn, the iron-binding capacity of the blood is overloaded, and toxic circulating levels of free iron develop. Intestinal damage occurs within 2 hours, but other symptoms do not appear for several more hours. After that period, hypotension, metabolic acidosis, pulmonary edema, and liver and kidney failure develop, with a high incidence of death in the absence of treatment. Laboratory evaluation of the serum iron and total iron-binding capacity (TIBC) are important in determining the severity of the excess of free iron. An iron chelator, deferoxamine, is given to complex the iron and allow it to be excreted into the urine, where it creates a pink color that is useful in monitoring the course of therapy.

CASE STUDY #1

A 30-year-old white woman was found by her husband, obtunded, at 9 pm. A nearby bottle that had contained 40 to 50 100-mg tablets of phenobarbital was empty. She was taken to a local community hospital, where gastric lavage was performed and pill fragments were recovered. Lavage was followed by instillation of activated charcoal, but the patient's condition continued to deteriorate and she was nearly comatose. Following a failed endotracheal intubation for respiratory support, she was transported by helicopter to a tertiary care trauma center where she arrived at midnight, comatose, and was successfully intubated. Gastric lavage was repeated. Tachycardia was noted (110–115) in compensatory reaction to falling blood pressure, which was maintained at 130/80 mm Hg. Pupils were sluggishly reactive, indicating the absence of midbrain injury. A STAT urine drug screen was performed, which revealed only phenobarbital. At 2:30 AM, the serum phenobarbital was 106 ug/mL (457 μmol/L) (Toxic: >30 ug/mL [129 μmol/L]). Blood ethanol was 225 mg/dL (48.8 mmol/L) (Toxic: >100 mg/dL [21.7 mmol/L]). The patient was heparinized and charcoal hemoperfusion was initiated at 3:30 am. Within 30 minutes, the patient was noted to be more alert. Perfusion was continued for a total of 2 hours. Seventy-five minutes after the completion of the treatment, the phenobarbital level was 51 ug/mL (220 μmol/L). The patient was observed for the next 24 hours, and psychiatric consultation was requested.

Questions

1. The first serum level of phenobarbital was obtained more than 2 hours after the patient's arrival at the trauma center. Should it have been obtained sooner?
2. If the urine drug screen had shown the presence of barbiturates as a class and the identification of phenobarbital had not been known from the history, would differentiation among the barbiturates by the laboratory have been important in determining treatment?
3. What alternative methods of increasing the elimination rate for phenobarbital exist, and why would they be better or worse than the method used?

Discussion

1. There was no need to obtain the serum phenobarbital level sooner. Gastric lavage was performed again upon arrival, and continued absorption of the drug seemed probable. Peak blood levels of phenobarbital normally occur 6 to 18 hours after ingestion, so that deferring the blood testing until the moment of decision for hemoperfusion gave a higher level and better indication of the degree of toxicity to be expected. The maximum blood levels expected from the information available were calculated

as 5 g phenobarbital distributed in 0.9 L/kg body weight (standard volume of distribution for phenobarbital) in a 50-kg individual: 111 ug/mL (478 μmol/L). This toxic level, confirmed by the blood testing, in conjunction with the additive effects of ethanol was considered to justify the hemoperfusion.

2. Barbiturate differentiation would have been important. Properties of barbiturates vary enormously. The normal serum half-life for phenobarbital is about 3 days and may be increased by the induced hypotension, which impairs kidney function. By contrast, the next most slowly cleared, pentobarbital, has a serum half-life of about 30 hours, and the other barbiturates, 12 to 24 hours. Further, short- and ultrashort-acting barbiturates (pentobarbital, secobarbital, and thiopental) are rapidly sequestered in adipose tissue and, while not eliminated from the body, are largely partitioned out of the CNS, where they are no longer dangerous. Thus, phenobarbital overdose requires more aggressive intervention than does overdose of the other barbiturates.
3. Renal clearance of phenobarbital accounts for a significant portion (25%) of the total clearance. Phenobarbital is an acidic drug with a *p*Ka of 7.24, within the range in which alkalinization of the urine enhances excretion. Ion-trapping is effective for phenobarbital, although less so than is hemoperfusion. Like hemoperfusion, ion-trapping would not enhance ethanol removal. Hemodialysis would be better for the removal of alcohol, but is of limited use with drugs as highly protein-bound as phenobarbital, which is 50% associated with protein. Plasmapheresis or exchange transfusion would be ideal for removal of both the protein-bound drug and the alcohol, although hemoperfusion is simpler and was effective in this case.

CASE STUDY #2

An 1100-g premature female infant whose delivery was associated with foul-smelling amniotic fluid developed a fever of 102° F with a white cell count on day of life (DOL) 5 of $6.7 \times 10^3/mm^3$ (Reference Range: $10–30 \times 10^3/mm^3$ at birth). A lumbar puncture (LP) was performed; the cerebrospinal fluid (CSF) protein was determined to be 324 mg/dL (3240 mg/L) (RR: up to 150 mg/dL [1500 mg/L] during the first month of life), and CSF glucose 34 mg/dL (1.89 mmol/L) (RR: 45–70 mg/dL [2.50 to 3.89 mmol/L]). CSF cultures were initiated, and ampicillin and gentamicin were administered empirically.

On DOL 7, the white cell count was $58 \times 10^3/mm^3$ and the infant developed seizure activity, which was controlled with phenobarbital. LP was performed again: CSF protein was 452 mg/dL (4520 mg/L); CSF glucose was 5 mg/dL (0.28 mmol/L); CSF cell count was 903 /mm^3, indicating persistent bacterial infection. *Gardnerella vaginalis* was isolated from the earlier CSF specimen, and chloramphenicol (CM) therapy was initiated on DOL 9. Daily blood levels of CM were 23, 32, and 16 ug/mL (71, 99, and 49 μmol/L) on the next three days, respectively (RR: Therapeutic 10–20 ug/mL [31–62 μmol/L]). Total bilirubin had peaked on DOL 4 at 7.2 mg/dL (123 μmol/L) (RR: Less than 1.0 mg/dL [17 μmol/L]), and even after discontinuing phototherapy was only 2.3 ug/mL (39 μmol/L) on the day before CM was initiated.

On the 4th day of CM therapy (DOL 13), the infant developed a pallor described as dusky or cyanotic, and blood pressure began to decline. Metabolic acidosis developed, with a CO_2 level of 12 mEq/L (12 mmol/L) (RR: 24–32 mEq/L). A CM level, drawn at 7:25 AM, was 120 ug/mL (371 μmol/L). STAT analysis of a second specimen drawn at 10:30 AM was 223 ug/mL (689 μmol/L).

The apparently misformulated IV solution was stopped immediately, and dopamine was administered to improve tissue perfusion. One hour after a complete exchange transfusion, the CM level was 149 ug/mL (460 μmol/L). Seven hours later, a second transfusion was performed. Two hours after that transfusion, the CM level was 114 ug/mL (352 μmol/L). Two hours after a third complete exchange transfusion, the blood level was 83 ug/mL (256 μmol/L). On the 2 subsequent days, CM levels were 33 and 14 ug/mL (102 and 43 μmol/L).

Further CSF cultures were negative, and the infant recovered without apparent secondary effects.

Questions

1. Why did a complete exchange transfusion not remove the CM altogether?
2. Should CM levels be performed more than once a day?

Discussion

1. This case illustrates the "rebound" phenomenon seen with lipid-soluble drugs, which are distributed extensively into the tissues of the body and diffuse back into the blood over a period of time. Although chloramphenicol is administered as a highly water-soluble ester, it is hydrolyzed rapidly in the blood to the poorly soluble active form. This water-insolubility reflects a lipophilic nature that allows free passage across the blood–brain barrier, promoting effectiveness in the CSF but also causing a pronounced rebound effect. The determination of blood levels of the drug was delayed for 1 to 2 hours after each transfusion to allow some degree of reequilibration and to avoid overestimation of the benefit of the transfusion.
2. CM levels should not usually be performed more than once a day. The particular need for CM monitoring in neonates is due to the importance of the late-developing hepatic enzyme, which allows elimination of the drug through the kidneys by converting it into the water-soluble glucuronide. This enzyme also conjugates bilirubin, so that neonatal jaundice parallels and reflects the limitation of the liver's capacity to eliminate the drug. The usual reason for CM toxicity in the neonate, which typically develops on the fourth day of treatment, is gradual accumulation of unmetabolized drug, so that daily monitoring is usually adequate. In this case, bilirubin metabolism had already developed and CM metabolism was probably not a critical factor. Misformulation is a rare, unforeseeable event that first became evident in the characteristic gray pallor (gray baby syndrome) that was recognized by the alert medical staff. CM levels served to confirm the situation and monitor therapy.

REFERENCES

1. Hanenson IB: General principles in the management of acute poisoning. In Hanenson IB (ed): Quick Reference to Clinical Toxicology, p 1. Philadelphia, JB Lippincott, 1980
2. McCarron MM: The use of toxicology tests in emergency room diagnosis. J Anal Toxicol 7:131, 1983
3. Rosenbaum JL, Kramer MS, Raja RM et al: Current status of hemoperfusion in toxicology. Clin Toxicol 17:493, 1980
4. Jones JS, Dougherty J: Current status of plasmapheresis in toxicology. Ann Emerg Med 15:474, 1986
5. Gelman CJR, Conner CS: Rational use of antidotes in toxicology. In Bayer MJ, Rumack BH, Wanke LA (eds): Toxicologic Emergencies, p 69. Bowie, Maryland, RJ Brady, 1984
6. Gram TE: Metabolism of drugs. In Craig CR, Stitzel RE (eds): Modern Pharmacology, p 37. Boston, Little, Brown & Co, 1982
7. Wanke LA, Bennett WM: Enhancement of elimination: Diuresis, peritoneal dialysis, hemodialysis, and hemoperfusion. In Bayer MJ, Rumack BH, Wanke LA (eds): Toxicologic Emergencies, p 53. Bowie, Maryland, RJ Brady, 1984
8. Gossel TA, Bricker JD: Nonnarcotic analgesics. In Principles of Clinical Toxicology, p 227. New York City, Raven Press, 1984
9. Done AK: Salicylate intoxication: Significance of measurements of salicylate in blood in cases of acute ingestion. Pediatrics 26:800, 1960
10. Rumack BH, Matthew H: Acetaminophen poisoning and toxicity. Pediatrics 55:871, 1975
11. Rumack BH, Kulig K: Acetaminophen overdose. In Bayer MJ, Rumack BH, Wanke LA (eds): Toxicologic Emergencies, p 99. Bowie, Maryland, RJ Brady, 1984
12. Wald PH, Weisman RS, Goldfrank L: Opioids. Top Emerg Med 7:9, 1985
13. Jaffe JH, Martin WR: Opioid analgesics and antagonists. In Gilman AG, Goodman LS, Gilman A (eds): The Pharmacological Basis of Therapeutics, p 494. New York City, Macmillan, 1980
14. Jaffe JH: Drug addiction and drug abuse. In Gilman

AG, Goodman LS, Gilman A (eds): The Pharmacological Basis of Therapeutics, p 535. New York City, Macmillan, 1980
15. Julien RM: Sedative-hypnotic compounds. In A Primer of Drug Action, p 38. New York City, WH Freeman, 1985
16. Baltarowich LL: Barbiturates. Top Emerg Med 7:46, 1985
17. Kulig K, Duffy JP, Linden CH et al: Toxic effects of methanol, ethylene glycol, and isopropyl alcohol. Top Emerg Med 7:14, 1985
18. Wanke LA: Methanol and ethylene glycol poisoning. In Bayer MJ, Rumack BH, Wanke LA (eds): Toxicologic Emergencies, p 207. Bowie, Maryland, RJ Brady, 1984
19. Glasser L, Sternglanz PD, Combie J et al: Serum osmolality and its applicability to drug overdose. Am J Clin Pathol 60:695, 1973
20. Harvey SC: Hypnotics and sedatives. In Gilman AF, Goodman LS, Gilman A (eds): The Pharmacological Basis of Therapeutics, p 339. New York City, Macmillan, 1980
21. Hartness CC, Buchan JE, Bayer MJ: Phencyclidine. Top Emerg Med 7:33, 1985
22. Rowland LP, Penn AS: Myoglobinuria. Med Clin North Am 56:1233, 1972
23. Julien RM: Marijuana: The ancient drug of cannabis. In A Primer of Drug Action, p 170. New York City, WH Freeman, 1985
24. Dackis CA, Pottash ALC, Annitto W et al: Persistence of urinary marijuana levels after supervised abstinence. Am J Psychiatry 139:9, 1982
25. Schauben JL: Benzodiazepines. Top Emerg Med 7:39, 1985
26. Gerson B: Antiepileptic agents. In Gerson B (ed): Essentials of Therapeutic Drug Monitoring, p 175. New York City, Igaku-Shoin, 1983
27. Gossel TA, Bricker JD: Antipsychotic agents. In Principles of Clinical Toxicology, p 274. New York City, Raven Press, 1984
28. Gerson B: Tricyclic and tetracyclic antidepressants. In Gerson B (ed): Essentials of Therapeutic Drug Monitoring, p 149. New York City, Igaku-Shoin, 1983
29. Baldessarini RJ: Drugs and the treatment of psychiatric disorders. In Gilman AG, Goodman LS, Gilman A (eds): The Pharmacological Basis of Therapeutics, p 391. New York City, Macmillan, 1980
30. Julien RM: Synaptic transmission and transmitters. In A Primer of Drug Action, p 231. New York City, WH Freeman, 1985
31. Linden CH, Kulig KW, Rumack BH: Amphetamines. Top Emerg Med 7:18, 1985
32. Grinspoon L, Bakalar JB: Cocaine: A Drug and Its Social Evolution. New York City, Basic Books, 1976
33. Guyton AC: Rhythmic excitation of the heart. In Textbook of Medical Physiology, p 165. Philadelphia, WB Saunders, 1981
24. Bump TE: Clinical pharmacology of conventional and newer antiarrhythmic drugs. In Das Gupta DS (ed): Principles and Practice of Acute Cardiac Care, p 348. Chicago, Year Book Medical Pub, 1984
35. Frame P: Antibiotics. In Hanenson IB (ed): Quick Reference to Clinical Toxicology, p 111. Philadelphia, JB Lippincott, 1980
36. Sande MA, Mandell GL: Antimicrobial agents: Miscellaneous antibacterial agents; antifungal and antiviral agents. In Gilman AG, Goodman LS, Gilman A (eds): The Pharmacological Basis of Therapeutics, p 1222. New York City, Macmillan, 1980
37. Sande MA, Mandell GL: Antimicrobial agents: Tetracyclines and chloramphenicol. In Gilman AG, Goodman LS, Gilman A (eds): The Pharmacological Basis of Therapeutics, p 1181. New York City, Macmillan, 1980
38. Burns LE, Hodgman JE, Cass AB: Fatal circulatory collapse in premature infants receiving chloramphenicol. N Engl J Med 261:1318, 1959
39. Rall TW: Central nervous system stimulants: The xanthines. In Gilman AG, Goodman LS, Gilman A (eds): The Pharmacological Basis of Therapeutics, p 592. New York City, Macmillan, 1980
40. Gossel TA, Bricker JD: Pesticides. In Principles of Clinical Toxicology, p 128. New York City, Raven Press, 1984
41. Banner W, Tong TG: Iron poisoning. Pediatr Clin North Am 33:393, 1986

Part XV

GERIATRICS

Glenda D. Price, Associate Editor

Chapter 72

Geriatric Changes in Laboratory Results

Joan E. Aldrich

The prolongation of life expectancy during the twentieth century has been a testimony to the advances made in medicine and biology. The average age of the population of the United States has been increasing steadily, and the major cause of the increased average has been a decrease in morbidity and mortality during the first six decades of life.[1] Once a person has reached age 60, remaining life expectancy is not remarkably different from what it was at the turn of the century.[2] Indeed, it has been postulated that there is a maximum number of years beyond which "normal humans" cannot expect to survive; this limit is estimated to be about 110 to 120 years.[3] Major emphasis in basic and clinical medicine is now being directed toward defining the physiological and pathological effects of aging, toward prevention and treatment of those effects, and toward improving the quality of extended life.

The phenomenon of aging is a continuum beginning at birth. Many age groupings have been defined, usually based on some external parameters. For example, differing diseases or differing nutritional needs can be used to classify pre-adults into perinatal, infant, child, pre-adolescent, and adolescent age groups. However, no such fundamental, widely accepted criteria are obvious for grouping adults in their later years. In fact, the traditional concept of an "old person" as frail or unhealthy more accurately describes the average person who is over 75 rather than one who is younger than 75.[2] There are stereotypes for a 50-year-old, a 70-year-old, and a 90-year-old, but how does one person change while aging from one group to the next? What makes one person who is 70 years old resemble another who is 90 years old? Are there objective criteria for classifying the elderly that are more closely related to physiology than is chronological age? So far these questions have not been answered. Most of the changes in laboratory results that reflect the physiological aging process are also a continuum.

Because of the constraints of our retirement and insurance systems, age 65 is the minimum age upon which most of the demographic data concerning the aged is based. Although these data are reflected in this chapter, for those aspects that deal with physiology and pathology, the span 50 to 60 years of age will be treated as the end of the adult period and the beginning of old age. This definition will incorporate at least a few years of lead time in considerations of the disorders that become threatening to the health of those who are at or beyond the average life expectancy.

The percentage of the U.S. population that is at least 65 years old has increased steadily during the twentieth century and is now estimated at over 11%[4] (see Fig. 72-1). This percentage will increase at a more rapid rate in the early part of the next century as members of the 1947 to 1957 baby boom reach age 65 and beyond. Approximately one in six U.S. citizens may be over 65 years old by the year 2030.[3] Moreover, an increasing number of the aged are living a longer life.[1] Men who are now 65 years old can expect (on average) to live 13 more years, and women an additional 18 years. Men who are now 75 years old can expect (on average) to live 9 more years, and women an additional 12 years.[3] The group showing the largest percentage increase in survival is 85 years old and older (see Table 72-1).

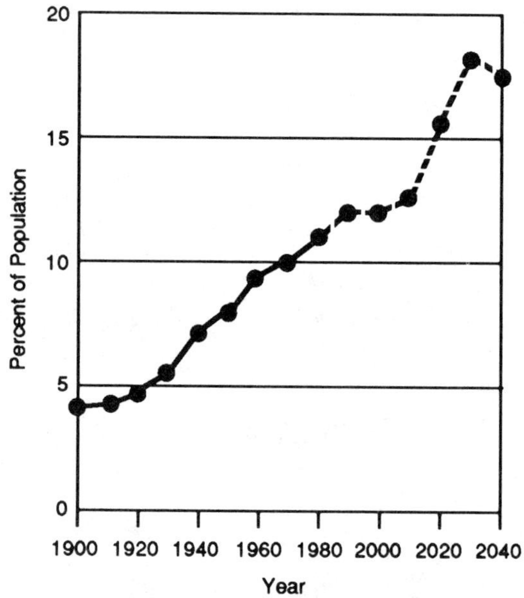

Figure 72-1 **Percent of US population that is age 65 and over. Data beyond 1980 are estimates. (Adapted from Applewhite SR: Disadvantaged elderly. In Ernst NS, Glazer-Waldman HR [eds]: The Aged Patient, p 65. Chicago, Year Book Medical Pub, 1983)**

These figures are based on previous census data and projected birth rates. A breakthrough in the treatment of heart disease, cancer, or stroke—the leading causes of death in all adult age groups—would have a profound effect on the distribution of age groups and on the health care system in the United States.

It is well known that the health care needs of the elderly are great in proportion to their percentage of the population.[5] Representative figures for 1982 (see Table 72-2) show that 27.7% of hospital admissions were accounted for by the 11.5% of the population over 65 years old.[6] This is a reflection not only of the increase in incidence of illness that occurs with increased age, but also of the increase in incidence of concurrent, multiple illnesses[1] that complicate both the progress and treatment of disease. Thus, the frequency of hospitalization and the average length of stay (11 hospital days per

Table 72-1 ***Estimated US Population (in Thousands) of the Aged and Decennial Increases 1900–1980***

	65 Years & Over		75 Years & Over		85 Years & Over	
Year	*Number*	*% Increase*	*Number*	*% Increase*	*Number*	*% Increase*
1900	3,099	–	899	–	122	–
1910	3,986	28.6	1,170	30.1	167	36.9
1920	4,929	23.7	1,449	23.8	210	25.7
1930	6,705	36.0	1,945	34.2	272	29.5
1940	9,031	34.7	2,664	37.0	370	36.0
1950	12,397	37.3	3,904	46.5	590	59.5
1960	16,675	34.5	5,621	44.0	940	59.3
1970	20,085	20.4	7,598	35.2	1,432	52.3
1980	25,544	27.2	9,967	31.2	2,240	56.4

(Data from reference number[1])

year vs 5.8 for all younger people) are increased in the elderly.[1] Even those who maintain independent (nonnursing-home) living status require more physician visits (6.3 per year) than do younger people (4.6 visits per year)[1] and use three times as many prescriptions.[3]

Both the frequency of hospitalization and the severity of illness in the elderly lead to utilization of laboratory tests. The changes in the test results that are associated with aging *per se,* and not with illness in addition to aging, are the subject of this chapter.

PHYSIOLOGICAL AGING

Old age is associated with the development of limitations in many body parameters, among them decreased renal blood flow, cardiac output, lean body mass, vital capacity, glucose tolerance, and cellular immunity.[3] The aging of specific body systems of an individual is greatly influenced by the interaction of inheritance with hormonal and immunologic regulation and environmental stresses. Thus King *et al*[7] distinguish between "diseases of aging, diseases commonly associated with aging, and lesions often seen in the elderly" that correlate with the three major influences, inheritance, regulation, and stress. This is a useful classification because it enables understanding of the sequence of events for an individual, *i.e.,* a person's genetic inheritance defines functional and regulatory capacity at any age, which in turn determines the amount of reserve available for response to external stress at that age.

Many organs decrease in size with increasing age, most notably the thymus, spleen, kidney, liver, and brain.[7] Because this change in organ size is universal, it is probably determined by species inheritance and is only fine-tuned by the genes of a specific individual. The varying degree of limitation in the reserve capacity in each organ of the individ-

Table 72-2 ***Hospital Admissions in the U.S. in 1982***

Age Group (years)	Number of Admissions
<15	3,654,000
45–64	8,688,000
>65	10,697,000

(Data from reference number[6])

ual then predisposes to the effect of that decreased organ size. For example, the liver is well known for its ability to increase its function many-fold, and thus is unlikely to become a limiting factor due to loss of size alone. This view is supported by the fact that drug regimens for elderly patients differ from those for young patients mostly on the basis of altered absorption, distribution, and excretion, and not because of failure (limitation) of the hepatic detoxification systems related to the smaller size of the liver. In contrast, the major loss of thymus gland tissue with age overcomes any reserve capacity that it has, and thus immune functions become limiting in old age both in the absence of external factors (*e.g.*, autoimmune disease, some diabetes mellitus) and in their presence (*e.g.*, infections, some malignancies).

The etiology of some other age-related phenomena apparently relates to regulatory changes without a concurrent change in organ size. Examples include osteoporosis and atherosclerosis.[7] Although the specific deficiency in these disorders is not known, their gradual and irrevocable onset appears to be a failure to resist or recover from the effects of stresses that have existed throughout life, *e.g.*, upright posture and dietary lipid in these examples. Lesions of specific cell types may also depend on the regulation of mitotic capacity. Organs rich in cells with active or potential mitosis are associated with hyperplastic, metaplastic, and neoplastic changes in the elderly.[7] These organs include the skin, bone marrow, endocrine gland, and liver, and the respiratory, gastrointestinal, and genitourinary tracts.

The environmental stresses that each individual withstands during an average life span are extremely variable. Furthermore, the specific diseases or disorders that occurred much earlier in one lifetime may contribute to compromised regulatory capacity during old age. This variability in personal history also provides an explanation for the wider variation in most laboratory results that is found in healthy older people, compared to that in younger adults.

The combined influences of these factors (inheritance, regulation, and exogenous stress) on cause of death is reflected in Table 72-3. The major contribution of cardiovascular and renal diseases to shortened life span is most likely due to the limited reserve of functional capacity in these organ systems, while malignancies, the class that makes the next greatest contribution, may depend more on altered regulation or exogenous stress.

Table 72-3 ***Gain in U.S. Life Expectancy if Selected Causes of Death Were Eliminated***

Cause of Death	Years Gained *At Birth*	Years Gained *At Age 65*
Major cardiovascular–renal diseases	10.9	10.0
Heart diseases	5.9	4.9
Vascular diseases affecting the central nervous system	1.3	1.2
Malignant neoplasms	2.3	1.2
Accidents (excluding vehicular)	0.6	0.1
Motor vehicle accidents	0.6	0.1
Influenza and pneumonia	0.5	0.2
Other infectious diseases	0.3	0.1
Diabetes mellitus	0.2	0.2

(Data from reference number[7])

Whichever etiologies cause the complex of changes referred to as "aging," measurable changes in several laboratory test results occur in elderly people, and many of the changes relate to the functional or regulatory changes mentioned above.

CHANGES IN FUNCTION AND REGULATION

Kidney and Urinary Tract

It is well documented that glomerular filtration rate decreases with increasing age. A study of 548 healthy males, aged 30 to 80 years, demonstrated that *creatinine clearance* is stable in adults until age 34, then decreases steadily until age 65, and then decreases markedly after age 65.[8] These data were confirmed with inulin clearance studies that demonstrated that the alteration was due to change in glomerular filtration and not in tubular secretion or reabsorption. Across the age group studied, average creatinine clearance decreased from 140 mL/min/1.73 m^2 (1.34 mL/sec/m^2) at 30 years of age to 97 mL/min/1.73 m^2 (0.93 mL/sec/m^2) at 80 years of age. In the same study, the average *serum creatinine* values did not change significantly, but values for intermediate age groups were not reported. Because muscle creatine is the endogenous source of creatinine, this constant serum creatinine concentration may be explained by a decrease in muscle mass with increased age, which lessens the load of creatinine to be cleared by the kidneys.

Blood urea nitrogen (BUN) is reported to increase with age. Data obtained on 4800 adults attending a well population screening center[9] showed that the greatest difference in BUN exists between persons in their forties (mean 14.4 mg/dL [5.14 mmol/L]) and those in their sixties (mean 16.4 mg/dL [5.85 mmol/L]). At even greater ages the BUN decreases slightly, which may be explained by decreased protein intake by the elderly. It is notable that other serum constituents known to depend on renal excretion, such as *uric acid* and *inorganic phosphate,* show patterns similar to that of BUN (see Table 72-4).

Uric acid and inorganic phosphate are known to be reabsorbed by the renal tubules to a significant extent, and yet their changes with age parallel the change in creatinine at levels at which tubular reabsorption and secretion of creatinine are insignificant. This indicates that glomerular filtration rate, and not renal tubular function, is gradually approaching the limit of compromise over this age span. The decrease in mean serum value of uric

Table 72-4 ***Serum Constituents that Reflect Glomerular Filtration Rate***

Age Group (years)	Sex	Serum Value*†			
		Creatinine	*Urea-Nitrogen*	*Uric Acid*	*Inorganic Phosphate*
20–29	M	1.01 (0.16)	15.18 (2.83)	6.29 (1.13)	3.51 (0.61)
	F	0.79 (0.17)	13.96 (3.18)	4.89 (1.00)	3.65 (0.54)
30–39	M	1.02 (0.17)	15.54 (2.74)	6.54 (1.17)	3.56 (0.62)
	F	0.83 (0.14)	13.90 (2.42)	4.63 (1.05)	3.62 (0.51)
40–49	M	1.04 (0.17)	15.52 (2.60)	6.52 (1.20)	3.50 (0.60)
	F	0.83 (0.16)	14.42 (2.79)	4.66 (1.02)	3.60 (0.61)
50–59	M	1.04 (0.19)	15.95 (2.83)	6.53 (1.20)	3.51 (0.60)
	F	0.84 (0.15)	15.47 (2.96)	5.11 (1.13)	3.82 (0.55)
60–69	M	1.05 (0.18)	16.80 (3.08)	6.45 (1.21)	3.56 (0.57)
	F	0.89 (0.17)	16.39 (3.01)	5.58 (1.15)	3.85 (0.55)
70–79	M	1.10 (0.22)	16.87 (3.51)	6.41 (1.67)	3.62 (0.69)
	F	0.84 (0.16)	15.33 (2.64)	5.22 (1.26)	3.91 (0.61)

*Mean (standard deviation); mg/dL

†Conversion to SI units may be made as follows:

Creatinine: mg/dL × 88.4 = µmol/L

Urea nitrogen: mg/dL × 0.357 = mmol/L

Uric acid: mg/dL × 0.059 = mmol/L

Inorganic phosphate: mg/dL × 0.323 = mmol/L

(Adapted from reference number[9])

acid (especially in women) during the eighth decade remains unexplained. It may reflect a larger proportion of reabsorption due to relatively sluggish flow of renal filtrate, or a separate, specific change in uric acid metabolism.

Painful, frequent, or incomplete urination is a problem for many of the elderly. It may be caused by a general loss of muscle tone in the bladder or urethra or, in men, by prostatitis or prostatic hypertrophy. Partial obstruction of the urethra is found in 20% to 30% of men over 65 and in 11% to 14% of incontinent women.[10] The consequent stagnation of urine in the bladder predisposes these individuals to an abrupt increase in urinary tract infections after ages 65 to 70.[7] This is not only a source of discomfort but, combined with the decline in immune function that occurs with aging, poses the threat of infection ascending to the kidney.[10] The presence of more than five *leukocytes* per high-power field in the sediment of a *routine urinalysis* correlates with significant bacteriuria.[10] The small increases in the amount of *albumin* or *glucose* in the urine, which are frequently seen in the urine of the elderly, remain unexplained. This may reflect an unspecified renal tubular reabsorption deficit, or may be the result of the increased frequencies of subclinical renal disease and of glucose intolerance seen in the elderly.

Glucose Intolerance

Elderly subjects tend to have a slightly higher fasting level of serum glucose (FBS) than do younger adults. They also have altered insulin response to a glucose load, which results in diagnostically significant changes in postabsorptive glucose level.[11] The magnitude of the change depends on the challenge; fasting blood glucose increases 2 mg/dL (0.11 mmol/L) per decade throughout adult life, while blood glucose level after a meal increases 4 mg/dL (0.22 mmol/L) per decade.[12] As little as a 50-gram oral dose of glucose leads to significant changes in the pattern of the glucose tolerance test[13] (see Fig. 72-2). This relative intolerance for glucose is a consistent finding even in healthy old people. In addition, the incidence of type II (maturity onset) diabetes mellitus is increased in the elderly.[14] Coupled with the apparent decline in the renal threshold for glucose, diabetes mellitus is more difficult to diagnose in the elderly, and its treatment is more difficult to monitor.

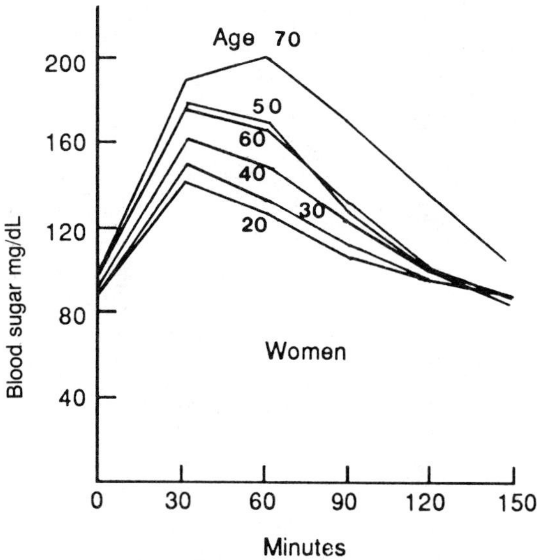

Figure 72-2 Responses of women to a 50-gram oral glucose load. (From Jackson RA: Blood sugar and diabetes. In Hodkinson M [ed]: Biochemistry of the Elderly, p 209. New York, Churchill Livingstone, 1984).

An alternative for monitoring blood glucose control is measurement of *glycosylated hemoglobin* (HbA_{1C}). However, glycosylated hemoglobin increases from about 7% in healthy 25-year-olds to over 9% in healthy people above age 70. This increase appears to verify that a continual glucose intolerance develops with age,[15] and decreases the sensitivity of using the HbA_{1C} level to monitor the success of treating type II diabetes mellitus in the elderly.

The relatively large changes in glucose level that follow oral intake, compared to the clinically insignificant changes in FBS, would seem to point toward insulin response as the causative factor. However, no changes between the young and the elderly have been found in the results of fasting insulin, C-peptide, ratio of insulin to proinsulin, insulin half-life, or insulin–glucagon relationships.[13] The post-absorptive increase in glucose is properly accompanied by an increase in *insulin* level. Evidence for the mechanism of the limitation supports the hypothesis that peripheral tissues or their receptors become less sensitive to the effect of insulin. Thus a higher insulin level, which results from a higher glucose level, is required for adequate stimulation of peripheral glucose uptake.[13] The postulated change in peripheral receptors for insulin is further supported by data showing that suppression of *free fatty acids* and stimulation of *human growth hormone* parallel the changes expected from the alteration in glucose tolerance.[11] (See also Chap. 38.)

Anemia

The frequency with which the whole blood hemoglobin level is used as a screening test for anemia has prompted many studies investigating this criterion for detecting anemia in the elderly. These have involved mainly the study of factors related to synthesis of hemoglobin and erythrocytes, because there is no evidence for altered erythrocyte destruction in the healthy aged population.[16] There is a slight increase (approximately 4.5 mOsm/kg of water) required for 50% hemolysis in an *osmotic fragility* test,[17] indicating the presence of spherocytes in the blood of elderly people. On the other hand, there is a gradual tendency toward a slightly increased average cell size as measured by the *mean cell volume* (MCV). These findings are not mutually exclusive. They may indicate increased variability in the size of circulating erythrocytes.

Intestinal absorption of iron from the gut is not impaired with age,[16] although it can be compromised by the commonly found decrease in gastric hydrochloric acid.[8, 18] Nevertheless, serum *iron* level decreases with age,[19] and serum *ferritin*[20] as well as *bone marrow iron* stores[8] increases, which indicate impaired uptake of iron by erythrocyte precursors. In patients with iron deficiency anemia, decreased serum iron usually stimulates an increased serum transferrin level, but *transferrin* is decreased in the elderly in spite of their low iron level. This may be due to limited hepatic synthesis of transferrin or to development of a new set-point for regulation that perhaps is mediated by altered membrane receptors.

The mean level of *vitamin* B_{12} in serum is distinctly lower in aged adults than in younger adults, as shown by Hayes *et al*[21] in their study of 213 healthy volunteers between the ages of 60 and 86 years. Remarkably, the B_{12} level was stable during that age span, indicating that the change from the level in younger donors occurs prior to age 60. In the same study, *folate* in serum and erythrocytes showed no change between values in young and old adults.

Bone marrow cellularity decreases 50% during the first 30 years of life, then stabilizes until age 70, and subsequently decreases an additional 40% during the following decade.[16] This is thought to reflect an increase in bone marrow fat rather than an absolute decrease in hematopoietic cells, and thus probably does not reflect any true decrease in potential erythrocyte production rate. Nevertheless, *hemoglobin* level and *erythrocyte count* (RBC), which are both constant in adult males until age 40, gradually decrease until age 70, when a marked decrease[22] parallels the change in bone marrow cellularity. After a rise in values following menopause, females follow the same pattern of change as do men. The significance of these changes is obscured by the fact that there are also increases in the variances of hemoglobin and RBC in older age groups, which result in no change in the average values (per red blood cell) of *MCH* and *MCHC*.[19] Thus Htoo *et al*[23] have rejected the necessity for age-adjusted reference values for erythrocyte parameters in the elderly, based on the results of their study of 292 subjects between the ages of 65 and 100 years, in which exclusion of only 17 donors from the data pool resulted in identical ranges for RBC, hemoglobin, hematocrit, and red cell indices in the elderly and in younger adults.

Dybkaer *et al*,[19] in an attempt to reconcile these

findings, reviewed 90 publications and derived relative median values of erythrocyte parameters using 30-year-old males as the basis for comparison. This is a useful method for comparison because it removes the effects of altitude on the subjects and minimizes the effects of analytical variations on the laboratory results. Dybkaer confirmed the tendency for age-related decreases in RBC, hemoglobin, hematocrit, iron, and transferrin for males, and for females after menopause.

Cardiovascular and Respiratory Systems

There are few tests available in the routine clinical laboratory that specifically measure pulmonary function. However, blood gas results accurately reflect the decrease in vital capacity that is found in the elderly. Thus *arterial* pO_2 decreases approximately 5% every 15 years starting in the thirties, and pCO_2 increases approximately 2% per decade after age 50.[19] There is also a corresponding, compensating slight increase in bicarbonate with age,[24] such that arterial *p*H does not change.

Cardiovascular diseases and their sequelae are the largest single cause of death in the United States. Coronary atherosclerosis, with or without symptoms, occurs in a major proportion of the elderly. Age-related organ changes affecting the cardiovascular system are mostly anatomical and include fibrosis, calcification, and the deposition of lipofuscin, amyloid, and cholesterol in arteries and arterioles and in the heart muscle, its lining and covering, and valves.[7]

Some laboratory tests are used almost exclusively for monitoring the pathological consequences of atherosclerosis, *e.g.*, enzyme tests for the diagnosis and prognosis of myocardial and cerebral infarctions. The sequence and predictive value of elevated serum levels of *creatine kinase* (CK), *aspartate aminotransferase* (AST), and *lactate dehydrogenase* (LD) following myocardial infarction are well known. While fewer than 25% of patients with cerebral infarction show elevation of these serum enzymes, levels of CK, AST, and hydroxybutyrate dehydrogenase (a measure of LD isoenzyme 1) correlate inversely with survival time.[25] Remarkably, there is a weakly positive correlation between the levels of these serum enzymes and the time-to-discharge for survivors of cerebral infarctions. Because of these findings, it is important to note that serum creatine kinase (CK) in women decreases from teen-age years until menopause, followed by a small but distinct postmenopausal rise.[26] These results were found while searching for a marker for carriers of X-linked muscular dystrophy; the magnitude of the postmenopausal rise was sufficient to confound the desired interpretation in the study. In men CK has a linear, although clinically insignificant, increase with age.[24] There is a small but steady increase with age in AST and in LD.[19] None of these changes in enzyme levels is sufficient to interfere with their interpretation following either cardiac or cerebral infarction.

Serum lipid measurements reflect the propensity for development of atherosclerosis, although they are not direct measurements of the magnitude of arterial plaque formation. The proposal for age-adjusted reference ranges for serum *cholesterol* has been made for many years,[27] and the magnitude of the average increase with age is significant (see Fig. 72-3). A representative study[24] of cholesterol levels in fasting healthy adults between ages 25 and 79 showed an increase of approximately 40 mg/dL in median serum cholesterol level between ages 60 and 79. A similar increase was observed in a large study of healthy men and women, in the same age range, in which there was no standardization of fasting by the subjects.[9] This study also confirmed the decrease in average cholesterol of people in their seventies that is shown in Figure 72-3.

Interestingly, median *high-density lipoprotein (HDL) cholesterol* level increases significantly for men aged 60 to 79 years, compared to the levels in men 25 to 44 years and 45 to 59 years, but the value for women is essentially constant in all three age groups[28] (see Table 72-5). These data suggest that losing the "protective effect" of the childbearing years in women negates the "protective

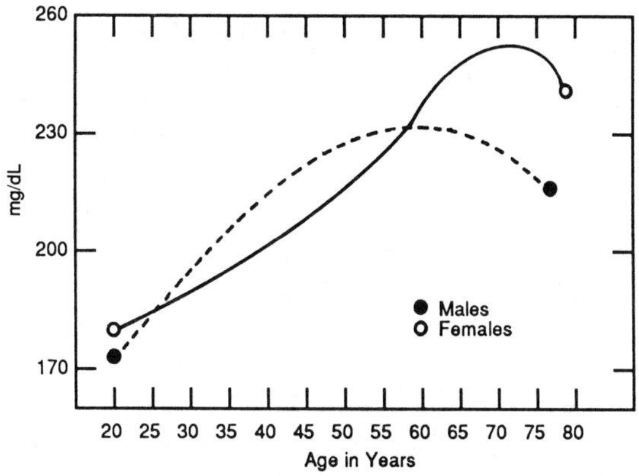

Figure 72-3 Change in cholesterol level with age. (From Winsten S: The ecology of normal values in clinical chemistry. CRC Crit Rev Clin Lab Sci 7:319, 1976)

effect" of rising HDL cholesterol in old age, an hypothesis that is consistent with the increased morbidity and mortality from cardiovascular disease seen in postmenopausal women.

The median *triglyceride* level also shows a tendency to increase with age, although to a lesser extent than the cholesterol level. The study of West and Ash[28] was performed on fasting home-living (presumably healthy) donors selected by age and sex to represent their elderly patient population. Although the number of subjects in each age group was relatively small, the study showed a shift to increased median triglyceride values as well as an increased range of values (see Table 72-5).

The development of methods for fractionating different *lipoproteins* and for measuring their *apolipoproteins* has improved the specificity of age-related changes in serum lipid levels. Another study of healthy, fasting men between ages 20 and 76 years, by Alaupovic *et al,*[29] confirmed the peak in cholesterol and triglyceride values during the 40- to 60-year-old age span, and the gradual rise with age in HDL cholesterol values. Furthermore, by measuring the apolipoprotein markers of lipoproteins, this study explained that the inverse relationship between *very-low-density lipoprotein* (VLDL) and *high-density lipoprotein* (HDL) is an indicator of successful conversion of VLDL into HDL, and thus successful metabolism of VLDL triglyceride and VLDL cholesterol. VLDL and HDL, which both contain apolipoproteins C and E, were measured in heparin-Mn^{+2}-precipitated serum. The amount of cholesterol contained in the

Table 72-5 ***Median and Range of Serum Lipids***

Age Group (years)	Sex	Serum Values*†		
		Total Cholesterol	*HDL Cholesterol*	*Triglycerides*
25–44	M	188 (130–277)	44 (15–70)	114 (46–296)
	F	186 (125–224)	60 (18–98)	82 (40–256)
45–59	M	181 (87–272)	47 (13–89)	114 (60–422)
	F	188 (108–337)	62 (28–95)	110 (44–350)
60–79	M	228 (146–303)	59 (32–80)	150 (62–338)
	F	223 (164–306)	59 (15–94)	137 (56–572)

*Median (range); mg/dL
†Conversion to SI units may be made as follows:
Total cholesterol: mg/dL × 0.0259 = mmol/L
HDL cholesterol: mg/dL × 0.0259 = mmol/L
Triglycerides: mg/dL × 0.0113 = mmol/L

(Adapted from reference number[28])

precipitated VLDL particles was sharply higher in age-matched patients with angiographically demonstrated cardiovascular disease than in normal donors. The concentrations of *apolipoproteins B, C-III,* and *E* followed the same pattern as VLDL cholesterol. These findings may result in a laboratory test in which abnormality predates the occurrence of symptoms of atherosclerotic disease or predicts the presence of arterial plaques or the severity of vascular occlusion.

Leukocytes, Immunity, and Infection

The number of *total leukocytes* and the proportions of *monocytes* and *eosinophils* are virtually constant from ages 30 to 80.[19] *Neutrophils* increase slightly in men and decrease slightly in women during the same age interval, and it is not yet certain whether their function changes with age. The relative constancy of total *lymphocyte count* with aging is not indicative of the significant changes in lymphocyte subsets that occur.

The involution of the thymus during early adulthood and the corresponding decreases in its hormones are well documented. Thymopoietin begins to decline at age 30 and reaches undetectable levels after age 60.[30] Using recently developed monoclonal antibodies to the T3 lymphocyte antigen, there are conflicting reports of whether *total T lymphocytes* ($OKT3^+$) decrease with age.[31, 32] However, there is evidence for decreased T-cell differentiation into *helper-* ($OKT4^+$) and *suppressor-* ($OKT8^+$) cell types, which may account for the observed decrease in number and mitogenic responsiveness of T cells.[33] The magnitude of this phenomenon, which begins at about age 40, results in only half as much response to mitogens added to T-cell cultures in the 80- and 90-year age groups as is found in cells from young adult donors. This lack of differentiation into helper and suppressor T cells also accounts for the decrease seen in *sheep red blood cell rosette* formation, because this test is a measure of mature T cells.[30]

Circulating levels of *natural antibodies, e.g.,* blood group antibodies, begin to decline in young adulthood and reach 50% levels or less at age 80.[33] Formation of *antibodies to new antigens, e.g.,* pneumococcal polysaccharide, parainfluenza virus, and tetanus toxoid, is also impaired in the elderly (see Fig. 72-4), which contributes to their increased susceptibility to infection.[30] Fortunately, proper booster sequence and strain-matching do result in protective active immunization for the elderly in epidemics.

On the other hand, the incidence of *autoantibodies, e.g,* rheumatoid factor, antinuclear protein, and antithyroglobulin, increases markedly with age.[30] Both the lack of appropriate (natural and acquired) antibodies and the presence of inappropriate (autoimmune) antibodies are thought to reflect lack of T-cell helper and suppressor influences on B cells, rather than an intrinsic age-related change in B cells. Nevertheless, serum

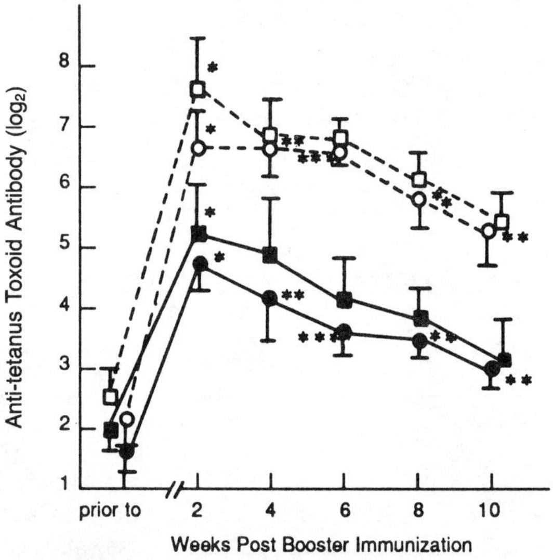

Figure 72-4 Serum anti-tetanus toxoid antibody responses boosted 6 weeks after primary immunization. Symbols represent titer ± 1 se of total (filled squares) and IgG antibodies (filled circles) in aged subjects, and total (open squares) and IgG antibodies (open circles) in younger adults. (From Bentley DW: Immunisation. In Fox RA [ed]: Immunology and Infection in the Elderly, p 333. New York, Churchill Livingstone, 1984)

IgG and *IgA* levels increase with age, and *IgM* levels decrease.[34] The IgM decrease corresponds to the decrease in blood group antibodies and the relative lack of an initial response to immunogens, while the IgG increase may reflect the ability to maintain responsiveness to antigens previously encountered. Total serum *globulins* in men tend to be very slightly higher after age 55, while values for women tend to increase until menopause and then level off.[35]

Infections are less likely to produce fever in the aged.[36] This may be a failure in the leukocyte protection system that prohibits release of pyrogens from invading organisms. This is consistent with depressed *neutrophil* function, which is implied by their decreased chemiluminescence.[37] However, results of other tests of neutrophil function that measure chemotaxis and phagocytosis, and of the nitroblue-tetrazolium test, have not conclusively shown depression of the inflammatory response in the elderly.[37, 38]

An alternative explanation for lack of fever is depression of the specific hypothalamic response to endogenous pyrogen (interleukin I),[36] or a generalized suppression of the hypothalamus or the autonomic system.[36, 39] In any case, this suppression is consistent with the inverse relationship between body temperature and infectious morbidity, and also contributes to the well-known increase in sensitivity and vulnerability to cold seen in the elderly.

Hepatic Function

The liver performs two basic types of functions: synthesis and deactivation/excretion. The synthetic function is reflected in the concentration of plasma proteins. A gross indicator of plasma protein concentration is the *erythrocyte sedimentation rate* (ESR), which increases in adults at a rate of 0.22 mm/hr per year due to the corresponding small increases in globulins and *fibrinogen*.[8] The change in ESR is not related to mortality,[8] and has little clinical value due to large inter-person variation.[40]

Total serum protein concentration is virtually constant after age 55[35] because the increase in globulins is offset by a decrease in *albumin* of approximately 1 g/dL (10 g/L) compared to that in younger adults.[19] While this decrease is insufficient to be symptomatic, it may reflect decreasing reserve capacity of the liver and may relate to altered carrier capacity of albumin, *e.g.*, protein-bound drugs or calcium. Decreased concentrations of other carrier proteins are also seen with aging, *e.g.*, transferrin and apolipoproteins. Decreased albumin level is also a frequent, nonspecific finding in many illnesses, and the elderly when ill show a decrease to lower levels than younger adults,[41] which may be significant for adjustment of dosages of therapeutic drugs used to treat the illness. Decreased albumin causes an increase in the degree of competition among different drugs for the remaining protein-binding sites, and tends to increase the active (non-protein-bound) fraction of a drug. Because this is coupled with a decrease in hepatic blood flow, which reduces the rate of inactivation of a drug, decreased renal filtration, and significantly decreased volume of distribution,[42] *therapeutic drug monitoring* is especially important in the elderly.[43]

The deactivation/excretion function of the liver can be monitored by the hepatobiliary enzyme *alkaline phosphatase* (ALP). The serum levels of hepatic parenchymal enzymes do not change significantly with age,[8] although AST and LD increase slightly in older women.[9, 19] ALP in older women, but not in men, shows a significant increase during the years spanning the menopause,[9] attaining values $1\frac{1}{2}$ times the upper limit of the younger reference range.[44] The *liver isoenzyme* of ALP increases sufficiently to account for this change (see Fig. 72-5), but it is not accompanied by a change in *gamma-glutamyl transpeptidase* (GGT), which is a more sensitive indicator of hepatobiliary dysfunction. This dichotomy remains unexplained, although it may be related to uncertainty in the algorithms used to compute the proportion of each isoenzyme of ALP from the results of multiple chemical inhibition assays. ALP in men, but not in

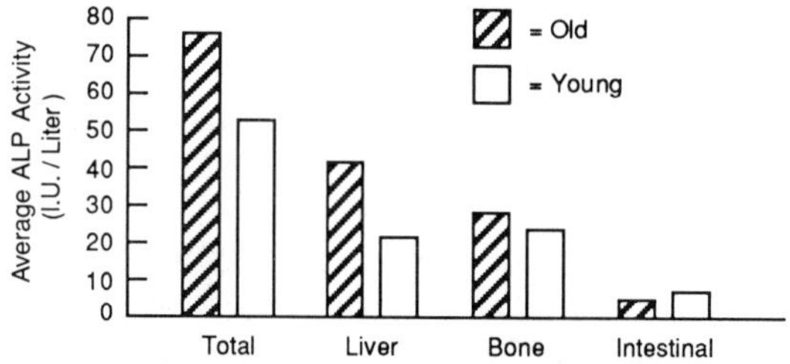

Figure 72-5 Calculated ALP isoenzyme fractions in two age groups of healthy individuals. (From O'Carroll D, Statland BE, Steele BW, Burke MD: Clinical inhibition method for alkaline phosphatase isoenzymes in human serum. Am J Clin Pathol 63:564, 1975)

women, shows a small but distinct drop after age 70 (see Table 72-6). *Bilirubin* levels, which also reflect the excretory function of the liver and hepatobiliary integrity, do not change with age.[19]

Musculoskeletal System

The volume of muscle is decreased in the elderly, but the loss is apparently so gradual that the serum levels of the muscle enzymes *creatine kinase* (CK), AST, and LD do not change remarkably with age. The change in serum *creatinine* is minimal (see Table 72-4), and there is no overt muscle pathology. In contrast, the loss of bone mass with age, which eventually results in osteoporosis, constitutes an important threat to health and independence, especially of elderly women. Although not a direct cause of significant mortality,[45] chronic bone and joint diseases, and trauma, including fractures, are significant contributors to hospitalization of the elderly.[46]

The laboratory indicators of bone disease most commonly used are *calcium, inorganic phosphate,* and *alkaline phosphatase.* However, the dependence of these analytes on other body systems presents a confusing picture. As noted above, the rise in ALP in aged women corresponds to the increase in liver isoenzyme, although there is also a slight increase in the *bone isoenzyme* (see Fig. 72-4). The rise in inorganic phosphate that is seen in elderly women is thought to reflect altered renal function (see Table 72-4). Furthermore, the level of total calcium depends not only on bone metabolism but also on the decrease in its protein-bound fraction that is secondary to decreased albumin. Nonetheless, after reaching a peak level in the 60s, total calcium drops to premenopausal levels in older women[9] (see Table 72-6). In contrast, men have only a very slightly decreasing level during their entire adult life.

Because both men and women are presumably undergoing the same gradual, age-related changes in hepatobiliary and renal function, which are reflected in ALP, albumin, and inorganic phosphorus, and because the incidence of osteoporosis increases most markedly in women following menopause, there must be an underlying change in bone homeostasis in elderly women. The paradox of high incidence of osteoporosis in the presence of calcium levels that are found in normal women in their 30s and 40s remains a source of frustration because of the inability to detect or monitor the disease by laboratory screening tests.

Thyroid Function

The incidence of both hypo- and hyperthyroidism increases in the elderly; they present a difficult diagnostic problem[25] because of more subtle clinical presentation, *e.g.*, mental clarity, heat and cold intolerance, and neuromuscular irritability are commonly altered in these individuals.

Thyroxine (T_4) levels are virtually constant across the age span 30 to 80 years, but *triiodothyronine* (T_3) shows a significant decrease between ages 50 and 65 that accelerates in the following 15 years and amounts to a total drop of 20%.[19] A major portion of T_3 normally arises from peripheral deiodination of T_4; thus the lower T_3 level may be secondary to peripheral body changes and may not indicate a change in the thyroid gland itself. The amounts of *thyroid-binding globulin* (TBG), *free T_4,* and *reverse T_3* do not change with age, but *thyroid-stimulating hormone* (TSH) increases slightly.[47] This change in TSH may be simply a normal response to the depressed T_3 level

Table 72-6 ***Serum Constituents Related to Bone Metabolism***

Age Group (years)	Sex	Serum Values*†		
		Calcium (mg/dL)	*Phosphate (mg/dL)*	*Alkaline Phosphatase (KA units‡)*
20–29	M	10.03 (0.38)	3.51 (0.61)	9.41 (2.34)
	F	9.97 (0.42)	3.65 (0.54)	7.28 (1.82)
30–39	M	9.98 (0.42)	3.56 (0.62)	9.50 (2.65)
	F	9.85 (0.37)	3.62 (0.51)	7.11 (2.22)
40–49	M	9.94 (0.41)	3.50 (0.60)	9.79 (2.69)
	F	9.85 (0.43)	3.60 (0.61)	7.75 (2.57)
50–59	M	9.91 (0.39)	3.51 (0.60)	9.98 (2.92)
	F	9.98 (0.40)	3.82 (0.55)	9.87 (3.13)
60–69	M	9.89 (0.41)	3.56 (0.57)	10.21 (3.25)
	F	10.05 (0.42)	3.85 (0.55)	10.66 (3.47)
70–79	M	9.90 (0.49)	3.62 (0.69)	8.64 (3.31)
	F	9.88 (0.40)	3.91 (0.61)	10.51 (3.42)

*Mean ± (standard deviation)

†Conversion to SI units may be made as follows:
Calcium: mg/dL × 0.25 = mmol/L
Phosphate: mg/dL × 0.323 = mmol/L
Alkaline phosphatase: KA units × 7.1 = U/L

‡King Armstrong units
(Adapted from reference number[9])

mediated through negative feedback between the thyroid and the pituitary and hypothalamus. If this is the case, the physiological integrity of the thyroid–pituitary axis is maintained in the elderly. Interestingly, the response to a *thyrotropin-releasing hormone stimulation* test is suppressed in older men, although it is not in older women,[19] possibly reflecting a sexual difference in set-point because women have a T_4 level about 10% higher than that in men throughout life.

PROBLEMS IN DEFINING REFERENCE RANGES FOR THE ELDERLY

Major problems exist in defining reference ranges for the elderly. On the one hand, most studies are cross-sectional rather than longitudinal, and thus only survivors are available to be studied at advanced age. This may skew the data toward apparent better health. On the other hand, the occurrence of multiple disorders, many of which have atypical presentation or are clinically silent in the elderly, may contaminate a data collection and skew it toward apparently poorer health. The combination of these two opposing possibilities probably contributes to the wider range of values for results that are seen for many laboratory tests performed on the elderly. An additional point of contention is whether it is appropriate to apply reference ranges determined on healthy, ambulatory people to the interpretation of results from sick, hospitalized patients irrespective of their ages. Moreover, despite their increasing proportion in the population, it is difficult to recruit elderly people for reference studies. Large longitudinal population studies are underway in a few sites,[40, 46, 48] but they are logistically difficult.

In addition, it is very difficult to define reference sets of donors so that changes in laboratory values that are due to aging can be separated from the changing incidence of a disease that occurs with aging. One approach is to compare the data between groups of people who are known to have different incidences of the relevant disease in the population. Using this approach, Larson and Wilson[14] compared the incidence of glucose intolerance in Australians (in whom it is fairly common in the general population) to its incidence in Eskimos (in whom it is much less common in the general population). Because elderly groups from both populations showed decreased tolerance to glucose, the study concluded that this change is due to age. Obviously it is not possible to do such comparison studies for all laboratory tests.

Another approach is to use regression analysis to measure the change in analyte level with age. Ash *et al*[24] collected data on 60 laboratory tests from fasting men whose ages spanned 62 years. The results of each test were regressed on age, and the magnitude of the change was compared to the standard error as a measure of the significance of the change. Only 15 routine chemistry and hematology tests were found to change significantly with age. Only four tests changed enough to affect their clinical relevance (serum albumin, cholesterol, inorganic phosphate, and ESR). While this is an interesting and significant approach to defining reference values in the context of diagnosis, it is unfortunate that their study included only men and had relatively few subjects in the elderly age groups. This approach also tends to conceal some sudden changes that occur over brief age spans (*e.g.*, the changes in glucose tolerance, urea, and ALP between ages 60 and 70), which decreases its usefulness for following the changes occurring in one individual.

Other investigators have examined the shape of the distribution of values for an analyte and compared Gaussian statistics, with and without transformation, to percentiles.[9, 24] Their final choice of recommended reference ranges included consideration of the clinical utility of the test, which confirms that neither of these statistical techniques used alone successfully meets the application needs.

All of the arguments about reference ranges apply to the elderly as well as they do to the young. The discussion here of trends and changes has attempted to point out age-related alterations in laboratory test results that appear to be independent of specific diseases. Combined with the diagnostic criteria cited in other chapters of this book, these data may improve the understanding of laboratory results obtained from elderly patients.

REFERENCES

1. Fairchild TJ, Burton BS: Aging in the year 2000. In Ernst NS, Glazer-Waldman HR (eds): The Aged Patient, p 84. Chicago, Year Book Medical Pub, 1983
2. Eisenberg S: Medical health problems and health care issues. In Ernst NS, Glazer-Waldman HR (eds): The Aged Patient, p 101. Chicago, Year Book Medical Pub, 1983
3. Besdine RW: Geriatric medicine. In Heckler RM (ed): The Merck Manual, p 2224. Rahway, New Jersey, Merck Sharp and Dohme Research Laboratory, 1982
4. Applewhite SR: Disadvantaged elderly. In Ernst NS, Glazer-Waldman HR (eds): The Aged Patient, p 65. Chicago, Year Book Medical Pub, 1983
5. Libow LS: Genral concepts of geriatric medicine. In Libow LS, Sherman FT (eds): The Core of Geriatric Medicine, p 1. St Louis, CV Mosby, 1981
6. Boeckx RL: Pediatric Clinical Chemistry: ASCP Teleconference. Chicago, American Society of Clinical Pathology, 1986
7. King DW, Pushparaj N, O'Toole K: Morbidity and mortality in the aged. Hosp Pract 17:97, 1982
8. Gambert SR, Csaka ME, Duthie EH Jr et al: Interpretation of laboratory results in the elderly. Postgrad Med 72:147, 1982
9. Wilding P, Rollason JG, Robinson D: Patterns of change for venous biochemical constituents detected in well population screening. Clin Chim Acta 41:375, 1972
10. Fox RA, Horan MA: Genitourinary infection. In Fox RA (ed): Immunology and Infection in the Elderly, p 109. New York City, Churchill Livingstone, 1984
11. Sandberg H, Yoshine R, Maede S et al: Effects of oral glucose levels on serum immunoreactive insu-

lin, free fatty acid, growth hormone, blood sugar levels in young and adult subjects. J Am Geriatr Soc 121:433, 1973
12. O'Sullivan JB: Age gradient in blood glucose levels. Diabetes 23:713, 1974
13. Jackson RS: Blood sugar and diabetes. In Hodkinson M (ed): Biochemistry of the Elderly, p 209. New York City, Churchill Livingstone, 1984
14. Larsen LH, Wilson M: Age- and sex-specific reference limits for carbohydrate tolerance. Med J Aust 2:672, 1979
15. Graf RJ, Halter JB, Porte D: Glycosylated hemoglobins in normal subjects and subjects with maturity onset diabetes: Evidence for a saturable system in men. Diabetes 27:834, 1978
16. Freedman ML: Anemia in the elderly: Physiologic or pathologic? Hosp Pract 17:121, 1982
17. Bowdler AJ, Dougherty RM, Bowdler NC: Age as a factor affecting erythrocyte osmotic fragility in males. Gerontology 27:224, 1981
18. Fox RA: Diarrhoea. In Fox RA (ed): Immunology and Infection in the Elderly, p 157. New York City, Churchill Livingstone, 1984
19. Dybkaer R, Lauritzen M, Krakauer R: Relative reference values for clinical chemical and haematological quantities in "healthy" elderly people. Acta Med Scand 209:1, 1981
20. Qvist I, Norden A, Olofsson T: Serum ferritin in the elderly. Scand J Clin Lab Invest 40:609, 1980
21. Hayes AN, Williams DJ, Skelton D: Vitamin B_{12} (cobalamin) and folate blood levels in geriatric reference group as measured by two kits. Clin Biochem 18:56, 1985
22. Kelly A, Munan L: Haematologic profile of natural populations: Red cell parameters. Br J Haematol 35:153, 1977
23. Htoo MSH, Kofkoff RL, Freedman ML: Erythrocyte parameters in the elderly: An argument against new geriatric normal values. J Am Geriatr Soc 27:547,1979
24. Ash KO, Clark SJ, Sandberg LB et al: The influences of sample distribution and age on reference intervals for adult males. Am J Clin Pathol 79:574, 1983
25. Denham MJ, Hodkinson HM: Serum enzymes and prognosis in cerebral infarction. Age Ageing 2:86, 1973
26. Bundey S, Crawley JM, Edwards JH et al: Serum creatine kinase levels in pubertal, mature, pregnant, and postmenopausal women. J Med Genet 16:117, 1979
27. Keys A: Serum cholesterol and the question of "normals." In Benson ES, Strandjord PE (eds): Multiple Laboratory Screening, p 169. New York City, Academic Press, 1969
28. West DW, Ash O: Adult reference intervals for 12 chemistry analytes: Influences of age and sex. Am J Clin Pathol 81:71, 1984
29. Alaupovic P, Knight C, Downs D: Age-related changes in the plasma apolipoproteins of normolipidemic men and male patients with angiographically documented coronary artery disease. In Schneider J, Kaffarnik H (eds): Lipoproteins and Age: International Symposium in Marburg, 1980, p 20. New York City, Thieme-Stratton, 1982
30. Weksler ME: The senescence of the immune system. Hosp Pract 16:53, 1981
31. Nagel JE, Chrest FJ, Adler WH: Evaluation of T-lymphocyte subsets by monoclonal antibodies in young and aged humans. J Immunol 127:2086, 1981
32. Hallgren HM, Jackola DR, O'Leary JJ: Unusual pattern of surface marker expression on peripheral lymphocytes from aged humans suggestive of a population of less differentiated cells. J Immunol 131:191, 1983
33. Hallgren HM: Immune response alterations during human aging. J Med Technol 2:685, 1985
34. Bentley DW: Immunisation. In Fox RA (ed): Immunology and Infection in the Elderly, p 333. New York City, Churchill Livingstone, 1984
35. McPherson K, Healy JJR, Flynn FV et al: The effect of age, sex, and other factors on blood chemistry in health. Clin Chim Acta 84:373, 1978
36. Fox RA: The clinical response to infection. In Fox RA (ed): Immunology and Infection in the Elderly, p 3. New York City, Churchill Livingstone, 1984
37. Puxty JAH, Fox RA: The phagocytic system. In Fox RA: Immunology and Infection in the Elderly, p 310. New York City, Churchill Livingstone, 1984
38. Phair JP, Reisberg BE: Nosocomial infections. In Fox RA (ed): Immunology and Infection in the Elderly, p 70. New York City, Churchill Livingstone, 1984
39. Dihman VM: Age-associated elevation of hypothalamic threshold to feedback control and its role in development, ageing, and disease. Lancet 1:1211, 1971
40. Landahl S, Jagenburg R, Svanborg A: Blood compo-

nents in a 70-year-old population. Clin Chim Acta 112:301, 1981
41. Hodkinson M: Test disturbances due to illness or medication. In Hodkinson M (ed): Clinical Biochemistry of the Elderly, p 24. New York City, Churchill Livingstone, 1984
42. Gray J: Clinical pharmacology of antimicrobial agents in the elderly patient. In Fox RA (ed): Immunology and Infection in the Elderly, p 204. New York City, Churchill Livingstone, 1984
43. Sherman FT, Libow LS: Pharmacology and medication. In Libow LS, Sherman FT (eds): The Core of Geriatric Medicine, p 92. New York City, Churchill Livingstone, 1984
44. O'Carroll D, Statland BE, Steele BW et al: Chemical inhibition method for alkaline phosphatase isoenzymes in human serum. Am J Clin Pathol 63:564, 1975
45. Agner E, Damm P, Hanse PF et al: Causes of hospitalization in different age intervals. Dan Med Bull 29:140, 1982
46. Agner E, Agner T, Damm P et al: Hospitalization and medical diagnoses in an aged population. Dan Med Bull 29:145, 1982
47. Ray RA, Howenitz P: RIA in thyroid function testing. Diagn Med 7:55, 1984
48. Shock N: Normal Human Aging: The Baltimore Longitudinal Study of Aging. Washington, D.C., U.S. Department of Health and Human Services, 1984

Part XVI

THE NEONATE

Virginia Sullivan Randolph
Associate Editor

Pediatric patients are a group of varied, changing individuals who are linked together in medicine but who are as different from each other as they often are from adults or geriatric patients. Pediatric patients can be divided into several subgroups based on the physiological changes occurring. The neonate is one subgroup. In fact, this group is a collection of patients who are quite varied: the newborn of 0 to 6 hours will differ physiologically from the newborn of 36 hours. This group, however, has some unique problems that are the major focus of this section. Some common problems, such as infectious diseases, endocrinopathies, and anemias, are covered in other sections of this text, and the reader is encouraged to refer also to those sections.

When evaluating the pediatric patient it is important to remember that the individual is in a dynamic growth process. Because each child may develop at a rate different from others, general concepts concerning development are important. The newborn will have very different laboratory results from those of a 1-year-old child, and results for both will differ from those of a 14-year-old; however, to expect two 13-year-olds to have reached the same developmental level can lead to false interpretation of results.

The process of birth alters analytes and fluid volume in the circulatory system and the concentration of cells, and therefore the newborn will have values for chemistry and hematology test results that will change each hour after birth for the first few days. Because of the common occurrence of a less than completely developed liver at birth, the results of liver function, enzyme, and protein tests will reflect this phenomenon. In general, enzymes and proteins will be found in lower concentrations in the neonate than in the older patient. The neonate has a fairly rapid metabolic rate, and changes occur quickly with these patients, making interpretation of laboratory results and the identification of significant changes a difficult task at times. The laboratory scientist must always be prepared to differentiate among error, normal variation, and significant change with any group of patients; however, because of the dynamic neonatal period these decisions become especially important in newborns.

Once the child has stabilized after birth, there is a gradual change in cellular and chemical composition of the venous blood specimen. The neonate will also have a developing immune system, with development stages reflected in laboratory tests. From the age of 2 years to puberty, the laboratory results for a number of chemistry analytes are a direct reflection of the growth spurts that occur. Prior to puberty, the endocrine changes will result in changes in chemistry values for proteins, lipids, and analytes transported by proteins.

In addition to some of the conditions not covered in other areas of the text, this section provides information concerning the congenital or hereditary conditions most relevant for clinical laboratory evaluation. For these conditions, it is important to recognize that seemingly incompatible laboratory results at various times may only represent different stages of the condition.

Chapter 73

Screening for Congenital Disorders

Lucy J. Randles

The detection of certain disease processes early in infancy is critical to the treatment, normal growth, and successful maturation of the infant. The purposes of diagnostic screening procedures are to detect disease in its preclinical state, *i.e.*, the point at which symptoms are not evident or recognizable, and to restrain progression of the disease to an advanced stage that may result in irreversible and/or untreatable manifestations.

In order for screening tests to accomplish these purposes in a cost-effective manner, certain criteria regarding the test procedure and the disease to be identified must be met:

1. The disease must be life-threatening or likely to affect very seriously the future of the patient.
2. Treatment must be available.

3. There must be a high incidence of the disease in its preclinical state.
4. The test should be highly sensitive and reveal all individuals who have the disease, thereby minimizing the number of results that might be considered falsely negative due to interfering substances or low concentrations of analyte.
5. The test should be specific enough to result in relatively few false-positive results to minimize the number of persons apparently detected as having the disease in whom the disease is not present.
6. The test should be inexpensive and convenient to run.
7. The test should not cause discomfort or harmful side-effects to the patient.

Several of the congenital disorders discussed below lend themselves to effective diagnostic screening. Some, although test procedures are currently available to detect them do not warrant broadscale screening for reasons that are discussed.

CONGENITAL HYPOTHYROIDISM

Hypothyroidism is defined as a syndrome characterized by a deficiency in thyroid hormones. Classic symptoms in adults result from slowed metabolic processes that are regulated by thyroid hormones. In the neonate, hypothyroidism presents with characteristics similar to those associated with cretinism. Cretins typically demonstrate sparse hair, narrow forehead, puffy eyes, depressed nasal bridge, puffy cheeks, protruding tongue, thick neck, distended abdomen, umbilical hernia, and short legs.[1] In addition, brain development is slowed, leading to mental retardation, and overall growth is slowed, leading to dwarfism.

At birth, the clinical signs and symptoms may not be present or may be difficult to observe. However, the most common symptoms include prolonged jaundice, edema, gestation beyond 42 weeks, abdominal distention, and poor feeding.[2]

By the first 10 to 12 weeks of gestation, the fetal thyroid gland is capable of synthesizing thyroid hormones.[3] The biosynthesis of thyroid hormones occurs in several steps, which have been described in Chapter 35. Hypothyroidism in the newborn can occur as a result of a problem involving any of these steps, and hypothyroidism can occur in a transient or permanent form.

Permanent

Permanent hypothyroidism is most frequently caused by thyroid dysgenesis, in which thyroid glands are hypoplastic, absent, or ectopic. In many of these neonates, some thyroid tissue is present, with the degree of hormone deficiency varying.

The second most frequent cause of congenital hypothyroidism is a hereditary defect in thyroid hormone synthesis. These cases may include defects in thyroid stimulating hormone (TSH) responsiveness, in which patients have a small gland and low radioiodine uptake and lack response to exogenous TSH. A defect in iodide transport results in patients having a low radioiodine uptake and a low thyroid iodine. In organification defects, the patient has rapid and high uptake of radioiodine, but the radioiodine is not oxidized nor organically bound because of a deficiency in the peroxidase enzyme system. Patients with a mild form of this defect experience nerve deafness. The combination of nerve deafness and goiter is called *Pendred's syndrome.* In defects involving iodotyrosine coupling, patients cannot form iodothyronines, and iodine exists in forms other than as triiodothyronine (T_3) and thyroxine (T_4). Problems with iodoprotein secretion result in patients' exhibiting an iodinated albumin in their blood. Thyroglobulin synthesis defects result in goiter, high radioiodine uptake, and absent or greatly diminished thyroglobulin.[1] Patients with inborn defects usually exhibit a goiter and may be cretinous, hypothyroid, or euthyroid depending on the severity of the defect.

Other causes of permanent hypothyroidism in the newborn include TSH deficiency, which may be associated with a variety of syndromes including familial hypopituitarism, hypothalamic hypothyroidism, and congenital absence of the pituitary, and thyroxine-binding globulin (TBG) deficiency, in which patients are euthyroid with normal free T_4 and TSH, high T_3, and low T_4.[4]

Transient

Transient neonatal hypothyroidism can occur as a congenital goiter produced by maternal excessive iodine intake,[5] abnormalities related to amniofetography,[6] or maternal thyroid-stimulating-hormone-binding inhibitor immunoglobulins.[7] The transient nature of these disorders is evidenced by the low T_4 and high TSH levels at birth, which return to normal and stay normal for approximately three years after withdrawal of therapy.[8]

Transient hypothyroidism has also been found in infants after exposure to antithyroid compounds via the placenta and in infants exposed to iodine containing contrast agents during fetal life or to iodine containing antiseptic agents in postnatal life.[5, 9] Neonatal Graves's disease has been found in infants delivered from mothers with active or recently active Graves's disease, possibly from the placental transfer of thyroid-stimulating immunoglobulins.[4]

Laboratory Screening

Because of the brain's normally rapid growth in the first 6 months of life, infants not treated for hypothyroidism in the first 3 months of life may incur severe retardation. If diagnosis and treatment occur before 3 months of age, 75% of children achieve an IQ above 90. If diagnosis and treatment occur at 3 to 6 months of age, only 50% of children achieve this level.[10] Neonatal hypothyroidism is one of the most common endocrine metabolic causes of mental retardation, with an incidence of 1:3000–1:5000 live births. Consequently, many states have adopted laws that mandate screening of newborns for hypothyroidism.

Screening protocol may involve one or more of the following test combinations:

Primary T_4 and TSH
Primary T_4 and supplemental TSH
Primary T_4 and supplemental TSH and TBG
Primary TSH alone
Primary TSH and supplemental T_4

Results expected in the various disorders can be seen in Table 73-1.

Neonatal hypothyroidism resulting from thyroid dysgenesis may demonstrate normal T_4 levels and normal or slightly elevated TSH levels because of the residual tissue that is present. Such hypothyroidism might be compensated for initially. Low T_4 levels will also be seen in premature infants as well as in those with a congenital deficiency in TBG, and thus use of the T_4 test alone may cause a number of false positives. Hypothyroidism due to pituitary or hypothalamic disease will result in a normal TSH. It should also be noted that newborns typically exhibit a TSH surge within 24 hours of birth, so that an elevated TSH is not necessarily diagnostic of congenital hypothyroidism.[11] For these reasons, neither T_4 nor TSH testing alone provides a satisfactory screening protocol.

One recommended protocol tests all newborns for T_4 and performs TSH tests on all newborns with T_4 values of <6.5 μg/dL (83.9 nmol/L). A second specimen is obtained 4 to 6 weeks later, and both T_4 and TSH tests are performed. Testing a second specimen will reveal compensated hypothyroidism and late onset of TSH increases.[12]

Specimens for hypothyroidism screening may

Table 73-1 ***Laboratory Findings in Hypothyroid Disorders***

	T_3	T_4	Free T_4	TSH
Thyroid dysgenesis	N	N or ↓	–	↑
Defective thyroid hormone synthesis	N	N or ↓	–	↑
TSH deficiency	↓	↓	↓	Sl ↑
Thyroid hormone unresponsiveness	↑	↑	↑	↑
TBG deficiency	↑	↓	N	N

be obtained from cord blood or capillary heel punctures. Dried capillary blood from a heelstick has been the most common source of specimen, largely because it is routinely used for the screening of other neonatal metabolic disorders. If capillary blood is used, the specimen should not be drawn until the infant is at least three days old to avoid the effects of the normal surge of TSH. It is also important that the circles on the filter paper be completely filled and fully saturated so that the blood samples flow through to the back side of the filter paper, thus ensuring that a sufficient specimen volume has been obtained.

Although samples of cord blood have not been used routinely in testing, there are advantages to doing so. The TSH surge can be prevented by clamping the umbilical cord immediately after delivery, the analysis can be performed immediately rather than after waiting three days, a liberal volume of blood is available, and there is no potential risk of injury to the infant's heel.[13]

T_4 and TSH testing routinely uses radioimmunoassay (RIA) methodologies, although earlier methods did not demonstrate adequate sensitivity and specificity limits; T_4 testing methods have become relatively simple, convenient, and cost-effective to perform. The same cannot be said for TSH measurement, as lack of needed test sensitivity in the low range of values continues to be a problem, unless "ultrasensitive" TSH procedures are used (see also Chap. 35).

Confirmatory Testing

Newborns with abnormalities revealed by initial screening require followup clinical and laboratory evaluation. This should include venous serum T_4, T_3 uptake, and TSH testing. T_4 and T_3 uptake values must be assessed relative to the normally high values seen in the first few months of life (see Table 73-2). Serum TSH values >10 μU/mL (10 mIU/L) in infants older than 10 days are abnormal, and compatible with either transient or permanent hypothyroidism.[13]

Thyroid scans, serum thyroglobulin assays, and bone-age studies are helpful in classifying the type

Table 73-2 ***Reference Ranges for Thyroid Function Tests Based on Age***

Age	T_4 (μg/dL)	T_3 (ng/dL)	TSH (μU/mL)
At birth (cord)	10.8 (6.6–7.5)	50 (14–86)	9.0 (2–40)
2 to 5 days	*15.1 (8.5–22)	*180 (115–235)	*<20
3 to 12 months	*11.2 (7.2–15.6)	*175 (105–245)	*<10
1 to 5 years	*10.5 (7.3–15)	*168 (105–269)	*<10
11 to 15 years	*8.1 (5.6–11.7)	*133 (83–213)	*<10

Conversion to SI units is as follows:
T_4 μg/dL × 12.9 = nmol/L
T_3 ng/dL × 0.0154 = nmol/L
TSH μU/mL × 1 = mIU/L

Mean values are preceded by *. Reference ranges appear in parentheses.

and severity of the disease. Followup testing at 1- or 2-month intervals is recommended to evaluate the adequacy of replacement therapy with thyroxine, using immediate full-maintenance doses and later adjusting the dosage.[14]

Because of the nature of the procedures and the equipment that is needed to perform thyroid function tests adequately, screening should be conducted only in regional centers. Although screening tests may be available for use in physicians' offices or small laboratories, their accuracy and precision must be continually monitored with sensitive quality control systems and sophisticated equipment. Consequently, the only way in which thyroid testing can remain cost-effective is for a test site to maintain an adequate volume of tests to offset equipment, reagent, and quality control costs.

CYSTIC FIBROSIS

Cystic fibrosis, although not strictly a disease of neonates, often manifests itself at birth or within the first month of life. It has been described as the most common hereditary lethal disease within the U.S. Caucasian population, but is seen rarely in people of Mongolian descent or in North African Negroes. The gene for cystic fibrosis is located on the long arm of chromosome 7, and transmission occurs as an autosomal recessive trait. Occurrence of the disease is approximately 1 in 2500 births.

The disease is also referred to as *fibrocystic disease of the pancreas* and as *mucoviscidosis*. Clincally, it can be very difficult to identify, particularly in early life, because its effects vary in severity and impact on a number of body systems. A biochemical defect results in fibrosis or fatty replacement of the exocrine parenchyma of the pancreas, and ultimate obstruction of the ducts. The islets of Langerhans are not usually affected. Although the exocrine cells of the pancreas are affected, it is important to note that 10% of diagnosed cystic fibrosis patients exhibit normal overall pancreatic function.

The disease generally affects any mucus-producing organs, glands, and tissues. The physiochemical abnormality and excessive volume of the mucous secretions result in obstruction of organ passages, and ultimately are responsible for the manifestations associated with the disease. As the disease progresses, bronchial obstruction occurs and patients develop chronic pulmonary disease with repeated infections.

Two clinical expressions of the disease have been described: one that involves the GI system only, and one that involves both the respiratory system and the GI system.[15] The child who presents with GI disease can usually be diagnosed more readily. GI manifestations include intestinal obstruction at birth that results from an abnormal accumulation of meconium (meconium ileus). Although meconium ileus is always associated with cystic fibrosis, as many as 25% of patients with this complication may not have pancreatic involvement, which suggests that the meconium ileus results from the abnormal physiological nature of intestinal secretions.[16]

Other manifestations of the GI form include atresia of the small intestine and pancreatic achylia (inability of the pancreas to digest fats), which results in steatorrhea accompanied by malnutrition because of the loss of liposoluble vitamins, protein, and nutrients through the stools. Malnutrition has been demonstrated in children less than 2 months of age.[16, 17] Iron-deficiency anemia has been indicated with a decreased hemoglobin, decreased serum ferritin, decreased vitamin E, and increased carboxyhemoglobin.[18]

Within only a few days after birth, the child who presents with the respiratory form of the disease will exhibit persistent coughing, generalized bronchial obstruction, and eventually obstructive emphysema. Repeated generalized bronchial infections follow. The most common organism isolated prior to antibiotic therapy has been *Staphylococcus aureus*. After repeated antibiotic treatment, the organism most commonly isolated is the mucoid form of *Pseudomonas aeruginosa*. Cystic fibrosis patients are generally immunocompetent when tested, although they exhibit an obvious susceptibility to pulmonary infections.

Other complications that appear later in life include nasal polyps, glucose intolerance, cirrhosis, pancreatitis and pancreatic lithiasis, and infertility due to azoospermia.

Laboratory Screening

There has been and continues to be considerable debate as to the value of diagnostic screening for cystic fibrosis. Several tests have been proposed, but none provides the degree of diagnostic sensitivity and specificity that is required to instill confidence in those interpreting the tests.

The screening test most frequently suggested is the meconium albumin test. Although the test is easy to perform, its results are questionable. It is based on the presence of albumin, which is presumed to be present because of the absence of pancreatic secretions that normally contain a proteolytic enzyme. However, albumin often is present from the swallowing of amniotic fluid and/or from a blood-contaminated stool specimen. In addition, pancreatic function is not always affected in cystic fibrosis patients.

The dried immunoreactive trypsin test (IRT) has undergone widespread consideration as a screening test. The specimen is easy to obtain by saturating marked circles on filter paper with capillary blood and allowing it to dry. The circles are then cut out, and trypsin is measured by RIA. The units of measurement are designated "Arbitrary Units" (AU), in which 1 AU represents the immunoreactivity of 1 μg of purified trypsin extract. A value of >220AU/L suggests further confirmatory testing for cystic fibrosis.[19, 20, 21] Because the IRT measures only a manifestation of the disease, rather than its gene product, it should be remembered that the pathophysiology of other diseases might result in an elevated trypsin. Also, if the pancreatic function is normal, the trypsin level will not be elevated.

The remaining screening tests are based on a unique phenomenon that is characteristic of cystic fibrosis patients and serves as one of the three major criteria for diagnosis. Sweat glands, being a type of exocrine gland, secrete a "presweat" upon stimulation. The presweat normally undergoes a resorption process whereby electrolytes are resorbed. Patients with cystic fibrosis do not resorb the electrolytes, which appear elevated in sweat specimens.[22]

Either sodium (Na) or chloride (Cl) can be measured in sweat specimens. Although Cl has been utilized most, the Cystic Fibrosis Foundation recommends that both Na and Cl be measured to check the quality of the specimen. It is important that a sufficient volume (at least 60 mg) of specimen be obtained for accurate interpretation of the results. A commercial semiquantitative test is available that is both highly specific and highly sensitive. It is based on a silver-phosphate-impregnated patch that is used to absorb sweat following pilocarpine iontophoresis. Silver ions react with chloride ions to form a white AgCl precipitate, which appears in a ring form on the patch. The interpretation of the test is based on the "degree of break" around the perimeter of the indicating region. No break is normal and represents a chloride of <40 mEq/L (<40 mmol/L), a partial break indicates possible CF and represents a chloride level of between 40 and 60 mEq/L (40–60 mmol/L), and a complete break indicates classic CF and represents a chloride level of >60 mEq/L (>60 mmol/L).[23, 24] Patients demonstrating borderline or questionable results should undergo repeated testing. This test is relatively new and it has not undergone correlation studies against the reference method for confirmatory diagnosis. Until that time, its value to and acceptance by the communities of interest are questionable. It does offer, however, a major advantage over other sweat testing procedures in that it requires a smaller volume of specimen.

Osmolality measurement of sweat has been considered both a screening and a confirmatory test for cystic fibrosis. The test is based on the premise that elevated sweat osmolality, measured by vapor pressure osmometry, will be the result of

Table 73-3 ***Reference Ranges for Sweat Osmolality***

Age	Range
4–9 days	121 ± 23 mmol/Kg
10 days–2 months	109 ± 13 mmol/Kg
2 months–12 months	86 ± 13 mmol/Kg
12 months–23 years	105 ± 14 mmol/Kg

high concentrations of electrolytes. Reference ranges based on age appear in Table 73-3. Cystic fibrosis patients will have a value of >210 mmol/Kg.[25, 26, 27]

A major advantage of vapor pressure osmometry is that it allows sweat testing to be done on infants who are 8 days old. All other sweat testing procedures require the infant to be 6 to 8 weeks old. Diagnosis, therefore, can be made far earlier. The test should not be run on infants less than eight days old, as the values will be too high. The infant cannot be underweight or dehydrated, as the values will be falsely elevated.

Carrier Status/Prenatal Tests

Carriers of cystic fibrosis, who number approximately one in 20 Caucasians and who are unaffected by the disease, are detectable utilizing the principles of DNA linkage analysis. The technology involves analyzing blood samples from several family members for the presence of specific DNA markers that are sufficiently close to the CF gene to permit tracking of the gene in families.[28] At least one family member must be an individual who has been previously diagnosed as having cystic fibrosis. Without the prior history of cystic fibrosis in the family, the carrier status for the CF gene cannot be detected. The number of carriers in the U.S., who have no clinically recognizable symptoms, has been projected to be 5% of the entire population.

DNA linkage analysis can be used to detect cystic fibrosis prenatally for couples who have had a CF child, by testing fetal DNA from amniotic cells or chorionic villi along with blood samples from the mother, father, and previously affected child. The accuracy of the information gained from testing and the resulting prenatal prediction is related to the distance between the marker loci and the CF gene.[28]

Confirmatory Tests

The only confirmatory test for cystic fibrosis is sweat Na or Cl using Gibson and Cooke's quantitative pilocarpine iontophoresis. It is the only method recommended by the Cystic Fibrosis Foundation, and all CF centers are required to use it to meet the Foundation's accreditation requirements. Because there are so many sources of error if proper technique is not used, it is important that only experienced and knowledgeable persons perform the test.[24]

Diagnostic screening for cystic fibrosis will not likely become a reality because available tests do not possess the needed levels of sensitivity and specificity; they are inconvenient, not easily performed, and costly; and their value in prolonging the life of the child is questionable. There are conflicting opinions as to whether or not early treatment of the disease is helpful in prognosis, because complications are not always predictable and are treated as they occur. The majority of patients are diagnosed within the first year of life, while others may not be diagnosed until the teen years or even adulthood.

The Cystic Fibrosis Foundation has discouraged screening because of the effects that an erroneous diagnosis can have on the parent–child–family relationship. If a definitive diagnosis cannot be made promptly after a presumptive diagnosis because the classic manifestations of the disease do not appear, the negative effects of anticipatory grief may be experienced.[29, 30]

The primary benefits of screening for cystic fibrosis are to provide an opportunity for reproductive counseling and to provide data for research. The majority of concerned individuals have said that money should not be spent on screening tests, which are invalid and not meaningful. Instead, they advise that the dollars should be spent on research to identify the underlying etiology. When that is found, a cure will be forthcoming.

PHENYLKETONURIA (See also Chap. 30.)

Phenylketonuria (PKU) is an inherited metabolic disorder resulting from an inability to convert phenylalanine to tyrosine. The hydroxylation of phenylalanine, by action of the enzyme phenylalanine hydroxylase, is demonstrable only in the liver, with no measurable activity in the brain, lung, kidney, or muscle. The system is complex and requires a cofactor, tetrahydrobiopterin, and another enzyme, dihydropteridine reductase, which maintains the cofactor in its active form. Defects may occur in any part of the system, but the most common error occurs as a result of a deficiency in phenylalanine hydroxylase.

Phenylketonuria is an autosomal recessive trait in which the heterozygote parents exhibit no clinical manifestations. Approximately 1 in 60 persons is a heterozygous carrier of the PKU gene. Carriers are identified by the small differences in the rate of increase of phenylalanine levels after meals and in the production of tyrosine. The ratio of phenylalanine to tyrosine in blood is greater in PKU-gene carriers than in normal people. The PKU locus has been identified on the 12th chromosome.[31, 32]

In classic PKU, phenylalanine accumulates in blood urine, and cerebrospinal fluid. Blood levels of 20 mg/dL (1210 μmol/L) or greater are associated with classic PKU.[33] Phenylpyruvic acid, a phenylalanine metabolite, and o-hydroxyphenylacetic acid, a phenylpyruvic acid metabolite, are both normally undetectable, but are demonstrable in urine with classic PKU. Their presence is indicated by a characteristic musty or "mousy" odor of the urine.

Untreated classic PKU causes severe mental retardation, but the mechanism by which phenylalanine and its metabolites cause brain damage is unknown. Treatment consists of restricting the dietary intake of phenylalanine. This is effective because phenylalanine is an essential amino acid and cannot be synthesized by the human body. The controlled diet also provides extra tyrosine to substitute for the tyrosine that cannot be made by the child with PKU.

The diet includes both a special formula and low-protein foods. The inclusion of the special formula is critical, and provides the PKU patient with additional amino acids that are needed to prevent the depletion of protein that would occur if low-protein foods are given alone. Blood phenylalanine levels should be kept at between 2 and 10 mg/dL (121–605.0 μmol/L) to allow normal brain development.[33] However, values outside this range can occur in certain situations. Acute febrile illnesses can result in phenylalanine levels greater than 20 mg/dL (1210 μmol/L). Blood phenylalanine levels should be obtained weekly in infants to allow for the earliest possible detection of PKU.

Variant forms of PKU and related defects in phenylalanine metabolism have been identified and are distinguishable from classic PKU by the blood phenylalanine levels and the presence or absence of phenylalanine metabolites in the urine. It is critical that the infant be on a normal diet to determine which defect is present and whether treatment is indicated. Infants with atypical PKU have blood phenylalanine levels between 12 mg/dL and 20 mg/dL (726–1210 μmol/L), demonstrate phenylalanine metabolites in the urine, and require diet therapy. A level between 2 mg/dL and 12 mg/dL (121–726 μmol/L) is usually a nonPKU hyperphenylalaninemia. These infants do not have detectable metabolites in their urine and do not require therapy, as it appears that brain damage does not occur unless the blood phenylalanine level is persistently greater than 12 mg/dL (726 μmol/L).[33]

Hyperphenylalaninemia can also occur occasionally in infants who have a deficiency in phenylalanine hydroxylase cofactor, tetrahydrobiopterin (BH_4). BH_4 deficiency occurs as a result of one of several disorders in a group known as *pterin defects*. Blood phenylalanine levels will not be useful in distinguishing the pterin defects from classic PKU because they both result in high blood phenylalanine levels.

Pterin defects must be diagnosed correctly because, if they are misdiagnosed and treated as PKU, children with pterin defects will sustain severe neurologic damage. The damaging factor in pterin defects appears to be a marked deficiency in monoamine neurotransmitters in the brain, which affect phenylalanine metabolism and the formation of tyrosine. Therefore, appropriate therapy includes replacement of these neurotransmitters.[33]

The fetal effects of maternal PKU are quite extensive. Infants delivered from mothers with hyperphenylalaninemia have demonstrated increased frequencies of mental retardation, microcephaly, congenital heart disease, and low birthweight.[34, 35] However, it has also been determined that a high maternal blood phenylalanine level does not necessarily mean that the baby has PKU.[36]

Laboratory Screening

Diagnostic screening for PKU has been performed for 20 years, and is routinely conducted in all states and in many other areas of the world.

More than 90% of infants with PKU are identified by newborn screening. Some are missed, however, because of failure to obtain a specimen, failure to obtain an adequate amount of specimen, loss of specimen, laboratory error when testing is done on a limited basis without appropriate quality control procedures, and failure to follow up on original reports of positive or questionable results.

Blood specimens are collected on filter paper 24–48 hours after birth and sent to PKU test centers, frequently state Departments of Health. The American Association of Pediatrics Committee on Genetics has stated that cord blood specimens cannot be utilized for screening, and that infants initially screened before 24 hours of age should be rescreened before the third week of life. Premature babies and infants receiving parenteral feeding or being treated for illness should be screened at or near the seventh day of life.[36] Blood screening tests are based on the growth inhibition of *Bacillus subtilis* by β-2-thienylalanine and phenylalanine's ability to overcome the inhibition. Dipstick testing for urinary phenylpyruvic acid is available but not recommended, as plasma phenylalanine levels must exceed 15 mg/dL (907.5 μmol/L) before detectable amounts of phenylpyruvic acid will appear in the urine, resulting in a delayed diagnosis. The screening tests will identify all persons with hyperphenylalaninemia, including those with transient and persistent forms.

Patients with hyperphenylalaninemia detected by screening should have a repeat screening or a quantitative amino acid analysis using a venous blood specimen. A phenylalanine level of <2 mg/dL (<121 μmol/L) indicates transient hyperphenylalaninemia. If the infant appears well, no further testing is necessary. However, the infant's mother should be tested for maternal PKU, as the transient elevation of phenylalanine in the baby could have come from the mother. If the second test is positive, the patient should be referred to a pediatric metabolic center. A list of these centers is available from the National Center for Education in Maternal and Child Health, 3520 Prospect Street, NW, Washington, D.C. 20057, telephone (202) 625-8400.

GALACTOSEMIA

Galactosemia is also inherited as an autosomal recessive disease. Clinical manifestations occur as a result of the body's inability to convert galactose to glucose because of a missing or deficient enzyme or enzymes. The normal metabolic pathway of galactose in humans is illustrated in Figure 73-1. (See also Chap. 67.)

The most common deficiency is that of galactose-1-phosphate uridyltransferase, and infants with this deficiency are said to have classic galactosemia. The disease has severe consequences for affected infants who are on milk diets. The infant may appear normal at birth, but within a few days may develop jaundice and hepatomegaly, which eventually lead to cirrhosis, cataracts, and mental

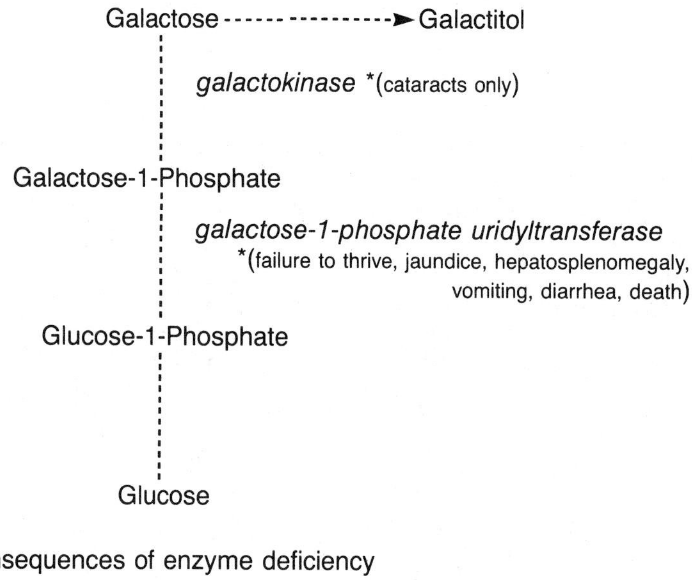

Figure 73-1 Normal metabolic pathway of galactose in humans.

retardation in untreated infants. Variants of classic galactosemia, which demonstrate only a partial deficiency in transferase, have been reported without any clinical findings. Black persons classically demonstrate milder forms of the disease.[37]

Galactokinase deficiency results in the early formation of cataracts. The increased levels of galactose in the blood result in an accumulation of galactose in the lens. The reduction of galactose to galactitol by aldolase reductase results in damage to the lens.

Laboratory Screening

Diagnostic screening for galactosemia can be accomplished by measuring the accumulated metabolites of galactose or by measuring the enzyme directly. The Paigen galactose assay uses disks of dried filter paper blood specimens that are surrounded by a bacterial growth of epimerase-deficient *Escherichia coli.* Galactose-1-phosphate can be measured by adding alkaline phosphatase to the medium. Cord blood can be used for assay by this method.[38]

In the Beutler enzyme assay, transferase activity is detected by the fluorescence of NADPH, after a 3-hour period in which the dried blood disk is incubated with galactose-1-phosphate and NADP. The test is considered negative for galactosemia if fluorescence occurs. False positives can occur after exposure of the specimen to heat and humidity.[38] The variant states, which are not clinically significant, are also detected using this procedure.

The normal blood galactose level is less than 5 mg/dL (0.28 mmol/L). Galactosemic infants who drink milk may have levels of 200–300 mg/dL (11.1–16.7 mmol/L). Normal urinary galactose is less than 50 mg/dL (2.8 mmol/L). Galactosemic infants may have urinary levels of from 500–2,000 mg/dL (27.8–111.0 mmol/L).[39]

Galactose in the urine can be measured by the galactose dipstick method and/or the Clinitest for reducing substances. Glucose-specific dipsticks will be negative, and the Clinitest will be positive.

CASE STUDY

A fair-complected, blond, blue-eyed child 1 year of age was brought to a hospital emergency room by his mother because the child had fallen from a sofa. The mother described the child as "always difficult, irritable, and never able to sit still for a minute." She expressed concern that the child had been "slow to learn the things that a 1-year-old child should be able to do." She complained that the child's diapers smelled "musty" all of the time.

Further questioning of the mother revealed that the child had been born at home and that no postnatal urine or blood testing had been performed, although state law required blood and urine screening for neonatal disorders.

Physical examination of the child revealed minor bruises to the trunk of the body resulting from the fall. Further neurologic evaluation indicated that the child was mentally retarded for his chronological age.

Questions

1. Given the history and physical findings, what is the most likely diagnosis?
2. What laboratory analyses should be performed and what results would be expected for this diagnosis?
3. What treatment and followup are appropriate?

Discussion

1. Phenylketonuria is the likely diagnosis.
2. A blood sample should be drawn and a urine specimen collected—both for amino acid analysis. Serum phenylalanine level would be >20 mg/dL (1210 μmol/L) and the serum tyrosine level would be decreased. High levels of phenylalanine and phenylpyruvic acid would be detected in the urine.
3. A special diet low in phenylalanine should be prescribed. Periodic serum phenylalanine levels should be ordered to monitor the child's progress. The family should be referred to a pediatric metabolic center for counseling and followup care.

REFERENCES

1. Hershman JM et al: Thyroid disease. In Endocrine Pathophysiology, 2nd ed, p 45. Philadelphia, Lea & Febiger, 1982
2. LaFranchi S: Newborn screening for congenital hypothyroidism. Pediatr Ann 9:390, 1980
3. Fisher DA, Keim AH: Thyroid development and disorders of thyroid development in the newborn. N Engl J Med 304:702, 1981
4. Howanitz JH, Howanitz PJ: Disorders of the endocrine system. In symposium on perinatal diagnosis. Clin Lab Med 1(2):399, 1981
5. Casswell F, Kerr MM: Congenital goiter and hypothyroidism produced by internal ingestion of iodides. Lancet 1:1241–1243, 1970
6. Stubble P, Heidemann P et al: Transient congenital hypothyroidism after amniofetography. Eur J Pediatr 135:97–99, 1980
7. Takasu N, Mori T et al: Transient neonatal hypothyroidism due to maternal immunoglobulins that inhibit thyrotropin-binding and post-receptor processes. J Clin Endocrinol Metab 59(1):142–146, 1984
8. Nose O, Harada T et al: Transient neonatal hypothyroidism probably related to immaturity of thyroidal iodine organification. J Pediatr Apr: 573–576, 1986
9. Fisher DA, Klein AH: Thyroid development and disorders of thyroid function in the newborn. N Engl J Med 304(12):702–712, 1981
10. Committee of Genetics: Screening for congenital metabolic disorders in the newborn infant: Congenital deficiency of thyroid hormone and hyperphenylalaninemia. Pediatrics 60:389, 1977
11. Wilson DP, Coldwell JG: Newborn hypothyroid screening: The private sector. Am J Dis Child 139(7):662, 1985
12. LaFranchi SH, Hanna CE et al: Northwest regional screening program. Pediatrics 76(11):734, 1985
13. Walfish PG: The best way to screen for neonatal hypothyroidism. Diagn Med 7(2):67–75, 1984
14. Guyda HJ: Therapy of congenital hypothyroidism: Evolution of biochemical parameters. In Burrow

GN, Dussault (eds): Neonatal Thyroid Screening, p. 247. New York City, Raven Press, 1980

15. Barbero GJ: Editor's column: Commentary: The clinical forms of cystic fibrosis. J Pediatr 100(6):914, 1982
16. Di Sant'agnese PA, Farrell PM: Neonatal and general aspects of cystic fibrosis. In Young DS, Hicks JM (eds): The Neonate, pp 204–213. New York City, John Wiley & Sons, 1976
17. Reardon MC, Hammond KB et al: Nutritional deficits exist before 2 months of age in some infants with CF identified by screening tests. J Pediatr 105:271, 1984
18. Ater JL, Herbst JJ et al: Relative anemia and iron deficiency in cystic fibrosis. Pediatrics 71(5):810, 1983
19. Wilcken B, Brown AR et al: Cystic fibrosis screening by dried blood spot trypsin assay: Results in 75,000 newborn infants. J Pediatr 102:383, 1983
20. Crossley JR, Elliott RB et al: Dried bloodspot screening for cystic fibrosis in the newborn. Lancet 1:472, 1979
21. Crossley JR, Smith PA et al: Neonatal screening for cystic fibrosis using immunoreactive trypsin assay on dried blood spot. Clin Chim Acta 113:111, 1981
22. Sedor FA: Body fluid analysis. In Bishop ML, Duben-Von Laufen J et al (eds): Clinical Chemistry: Principles, Procedures, Correlations, p 490. Philadelphia, JB Lippincott, 1985
23. Cystic Fibrosis Foundation: Editorial; correspondence: Screening for cystic fibrosis. J Pediatr 106(3):527, 1985
24. Hammond K: Problems in diagnosing cystic fibrosis: Will new tests help? Diagn Med 8:35–41, 1985
25. Schoni MH, Kraemer R et al: Early diagnosis of cystic fibrosis by means of sweat microosmometry. J Pediatr 104(5):691, 1984
26. Webster HL, Barlow WK: New approach to cystic fibrosis diagnosis by use of an improved sweat inducer/collection system and osmometry. Clin Chem 27:385–387, 1981
27. Gibson LE, Cooke RE et al: A test for concentration of electrolytes in sweat in cystic fibrosis of the pancreas utilizing pilocarpine by iontophoresis. Pediatrics 523:545–549, 1959
28. Technical Bulletin: Cystic Fibrosis. Integrated Genetics Reference Laboratory, 31 New York Avenue, Framingham, Massachusetts 01701, February, 1986
29. Cystic Fibrosis Foundation Committee Report: Position paper: Neonatal screening for cystic fibrosis. Pediatrics 72(11):741, 1983
30. Holtzman NA: Commentary: Routine screening of newborns for cystic fibrosis: Not yet. Pediatrics 73(1):98, 1984
31. Berry HK: Screening newborns for genetic disease: The PKU model. Diagn Med 7(1):50–54, 56, 58, 1984
32. McKusick VA: The human gene map. Clin Gen 10:25–89, 1984
33. Levy HL: Phenylketonuria—1986. Ped in Rev 7(9):269–274, 1986
34. Levy HL et al: Maternal phenylketonuria. DHHS Publication (HSA) p 5299, 1981
35. Lenke RR et al: Maternal phenylketonuria and hyperphenylalaninemia: An international survey of the outcome of untreated and treated pregnancies. N Engl J Med 303:1202, 1980
36. Committee on Genetics, American Academy of Pediatrics: Maternal phenylketonuria. Pediatrics 76(8):313, 1985
37. Levy HL et al: Newborn screening for galactosemia and galactose-related defects. J Pediatr 92:871, 1978
38. Mamunes P: Newborn screening for metabolic disorders. Clin Perinatol 3(1):238–240, 1976
39. Berry HK: The spectrum of metabolic disorders. Diagn Med 7(3):39–55, 1984

Chapter 74

Congenital Heart Disease

Michael W. Sullivan

Congenital heart disease (CHD) affects approximately 8–9 infants/1000 live births. Over half of patients with CHD will die before the age of 1 year if they are not accurately diagnosed and treated. After careful evaluation of a symptomatic child's history, physical examination, x-ray, and electrocardiogram, the primary care physician must determine not only if the child has a heart disorder but also if the heart disorder requires immediate specialized cardiac care. Many congenital heart defects do not cause problems to the patient until early childhood or adolescence. Infants with multiple cardiac defects that present with severe cardiac symptomatology (*e.g.*, congestive heart failure) at birth should receive specialized and aggressive treatment.

ETIOLOGY AND PATHOPHYSIOLOGY

In most cases of CHD, isolated causes cannot be found, and they may be genetic or environmental. A single gene mutation can account for about 3% of cases, as in Ullrich-Noonan syndrome. About 5% of cases are associated with chromosomal aberrations. For example, about one-third of patients with Down's syndrome also have a ventricular septal defect, endocardial cushion defect, or others. Ventricular septal defect is also seen in cases of trisomy 18 and trisomy 13. Turner's syndrome is associated with coarctation of the aorta.[1–8] It has also been found that families that have had children with CHD have a much higher incidence of having more children with heart disease.[9] Although environmental factors such as rubella, maternal diabetes, and maternal drug abuse account for some CHD cases, it appears that most cases are a result of a genetic–environmental interaction.[10, 11, 12]

Congenital heart diseases are classified as cyanotic or acyanotic. *Cyanosis* is defined as having 4–5 g/dL (0.62–0.78 mmol/L) of reduced hemoglobin in the systemic circulation. A patient classified with cyanotic CHD has a right-to-left cardiac shunt, although some patients may not actually appear cyanotic. With a right-to-left cardiac shunt, unoxygenated blood flows from the right side to the left side of the heart without being circulated through the pulmonary vasculature for oxygenation. Patients without a right-to-left cardiac shunt, even if they are cyanotic for some other reason (*e.g.*, low cardiac output), are classified as acyanotic.[13] (See Table 74-1.)

Cyanosis develops due to decreased peripheral circulation. Decreased peripheral capillary blood flow causes a higher percentage of oxygen to be released from the red cells to the tissues, resulting in a higher percentage of deoxygenated hemoglobin.[14] The degree of cyanosis is dependent not only on the severity of the congenital heart defect but also on the amount of hemoglobin present. If the degree of anemia is severe and the infant is hypoxic, cyanosis may not be seen. If it does appear, the mere presence of cyanosis does not necessarily indicate CHD. The underlying cause of cyanosis could be central nervous system disorders or pulmonary disorders rather than CHD.

In cases of cyanotic CHD, unoxygenated blood bypasses the lungs and is sent back to the systemic circulation. In this event, not only will the extremities appear cyanotic, but the trunk and mucous membranes will also be involved. The presence of central cyanosis is consistent with CHD and pulmonary diseases in which inadequate oxygen exchange in the lungs occurs. An "oxygen challenge test" is used to differentiate cardiac from pulmonary etiologies; administration of pure oxygen does not cause a change in the cyanosis if it is cardiac in origin.

Table 74-1 ***Common Cyanotic and Acyanotic Congenital Heart Defects***

Cyanotic CHD	Tetralogy of Fallot
	Transposition of the great arteries
	Hypoplastic left heart
Acyanotic CHD	Ventricular septal defect
	Patent ductus arteriosus
	Atrial septal defect
	Pulmonary stenosis
	Aortic stenosis
	Coarctation of the aorta

CLINICAL MANIFESTATIONS

Patients with CHD may exhibit certain symptoms, listed in Table 74-2.[15, 16] The symptoms by themselves may not be diagnostic of a particular congenital heart defect, but should alert the physician to include CHD as a possible diagnosis. Many patients with CHD are asymptomatic unless the defect is severe. In severe cases of CHD, symptoms occur at a very early age. Symptoms that are indicative of CHD are easy fatigability, (*e.g.*, the infant falls asleep before feeding is complete), dyspnea on exertion, tachypnea, slow growth, and cyanosis. Central cyanosis is best evaluated by examining the mucous membranes around the mouth and lips. If central cyanosis is present, they will appear blue (perioral cyanosis). In cases of prolonged cyanosis, the nailbeds will also appear cyanotic and clubbing of the nailbeds will occur. Clubbing usually does not occur before the age of 1 year.[17, 18]

Table 74-2 *General Signs and Symptoms Associated With CHD*

Infants	Children
Dyspnea	Dyspnea
Difficult feeding	Poor physical development
Tachypnea	Decrease in exercise tolerance
Recurrent respiratory infections	Recurrent respiratory infections
Heart murmur	Heart murmur and thrill
Cyanosis	Cyanosis
Hypoxemic spells	Clubbing of fingers and toes
Failure to gain weight	Squatting

Congestive heart failure (CHF) is defined as the failure of the heart to maintain adequate blood circulation. The presentation of CHF will depend on the severity of the cardiac defect. Three cardinal signs of CHF are cardiomegaly, tachypnea, and hepatomegaly. *Cardiomegaly* is a result of the heart's attempt to maintain adequate cardiac output. Prior to the development of cardiomegaly, tachycardia will be evident. The cardiac rate is increased to compensate for the decreased stroke volume brought about by the cardiac defect.[19] *Tachypnea* is the result of congestion in the lungs in which the body compensates by hyperventilation, and is a cardinal sign of left-sided cardiac failure. *Hepatomegaly* occurs secondarily to systemic venous congestion.[20] The liver traps edematous fluid, which causes it to enlarge. This is a hallmark of right-sided cardiac failure, especially in infants. In older children, classic signs of cardiac failure, such as the distended neck vein and peripheral edema, are evident. Peripheral edema is seen in infants only in severe cases of CHF.[21]

LABORATORY ANALYSES AND DIAGNOSIS

Prompt and accurate diagnosis of symptomatic patients is dependent on information the physician obtains from an accurate history, performance of a physical examination, and accurate interpretation of electrocardiograms, arterial blood gas analyses, echocardiogram, and cardiac catheterization.

Specimens for Blood Gas Analysis

Blood for arterial blood gas (ABG) analysis for the pediatric patient can be obtained from the radial or brachial arteries. Finger punctures are not recommended for PaO_2 determinations.[22] In some cases, it may be adequate to obtain arterialized capillary blood from an earlobe puncture.[23] However, in cases of severely decreased cardiac output, vasoconstriction, or systolic pressure of less than 95, the results from capillary blood from an earlobe puncture will be unreliable.[24, 25, 26, 27]

In neonates and infants, a heel stick may be performed. This type of specimen will be adequate for measurements of pH but not of PaO_2. By far the best method for collection of an arterial specimen is via an indwelling umbilical artery catheter. Meticulous records must be kept on the amount of blood that is removed for laboratory testing in order to prevent the child from becoming hypovolemic. Radial and temporal arteries may also be used for arterial blood gas analysis.[28]

The consistent laboratory finding in the neonate, with respect to conditions characterized by right-to-left shunt, is a PaO_2 value of < 50 mm Hg, indicating severe hypoxemia. Hypercapnia ($PaCO_2 > 45$ mm Hg) is usually also present, with a resulting acidemia ($pH < 7.25$). Respiratory acidosis often occurs after about one month of age.

Specimens for Other Laboratory Determinations

Blood for electrolytes, calcium, blood urea nitrogen, creatinine, and glucose can be obtained by venipuncture, capillary puncture, or arterial puncture. It should be kept in mind that some analytes vary in concentration between venous and arterial specimens and between serum and plasma.[29, 30, 31]

If necessary, the monitoring of glucose can be accomplished by the nursing staff through the use of test strips that measure glucose in a drop of whole blood. Because reliability of these methods varies greatly, the laboratory *must* have a major role in selecting test methodologies, in training the nursing staff in the proper use of the chosen method, and in conducting the quality assurance activities necessary for the proper interpretation of these methods. (See also Chap. 38.)

In the older pediatric patient, a urine specimen can be obtained using the clean-catch method if the patient can move about. If not, an indwelling catheter can be inserted and specimens obtained from it can be used for analysis. In the neonate and infant, it may be necessary to place a plastic bag around the genitalia for collection.

Congestive Heart Failure

If severe cyanotic CHD with congestive heart failure is present, adequate oxygenation of the tissues is of the utmost importance, and administration of oxygen will be necessary. Because isolated arterial blood gas measurements only reflect the oxygenation status of the patient at the moment of the drawing of the specimen, and because the PaO_2 can be altered rapidly due to stress to the patient, it is ideal to monitor the PaO_2 continuously. This can be accomplished through the use of a transcutaneous PaO_2 ($tcPaO_2$) monitor. The principle of operation of the monitor is based on the fact that oxygen diffuses through the skin. The monitor consists of a small heating device and an oxygen electrode. The heating element causes vasodilation, and thus there is increased local capillary blood flow. Oxygen from the capillaries diffuses through the skin and into the sensor, where it is electrochemically reduced with a modified Clark electrode. When maximum capillary blood flow is achieved, the $tcPaO_2$ values will closely reflect the arterial PaO_2.[32] The advantage of this method over drawing blood for analysis is that it does not deplete the blood volume, there is no chance of accidental introduction of heparin or air bubbles into the circulation, and there is no waiting for results.[33]

Transcutaneous PaO_2 sensors are not meant to replace arterial blood gas sampling, but are to be used in conjunction with them. Arterial blood gases should be drawn occasionally in order to ensure the accuracy of the $tcPaO_2$ monitor. Correlation of $tcPaO_2$ and ABG PaO_2 levels is good except in cases of hypothermia, hypovolemia, hypoxemia, septicemia, low birth weight, and acidemia.[34]

Transcutaneous CO_2 ($tcPaCO_2$) monitors have also been developed. Transcutaneous CO_2 measurements do not always correspond well with arterial $PaCO_2$ values. Some studies have shown that the $tcPaCO_2$ values are considerably higher than arterial $PaCO_2$ values.[35, 36] Presently, $tcPaCO_2$ monitors are good for estimating arterial $PaCO_2$ levels, but should not be used as a replacement for them.

TREATMENT

Medications

Although congenital heart defects cannot be corrected through the use of medications, support and improvement of cardiac and pulmonary function can be achieved. A major diagnostic feature of CHD is congestive heart failure. Treatment of the patient in CHF centers on improving cardiac function, eliminating edema, providing oxygen, and reducing the patient's energy requirements.[37]

The medication of choice for improving cardiac function is digoxin, which increases the force of the systolic contraction and thus increases cardiac output. If adequate cardiac compensation cannot be accomplished through the use of digoxin, diuretics should be added to the therapeutic regimen to decrease cardiac afterload by reducing accumulated fluids.[38] Depending on the severity of the CHF and pulmonary involvement, oxygen may be required to ensure adequate tissue oxygenation. The patient should be allowed to rest and in some cases be sedated, so that the energy needed for cardiac performance is conserved.

LABORATORY MONITORING OF MEDICATION

Toxicity levels vary somewhat in infants and adults, but generally, digoxin levels over 3.5 ng/

mL (4.5 nmol/L) in the pediatric patient should be considered toxic. Toxicity manifests itself by slowing of the heart rate and development of cardiac arrhythmia.

Specimens drawn for digoxin levels should be drawn 6 to 8 hours after the last oral dose. This time period allows for absorption of the drug and tissue equilibrium.[39] (See also Chap. 71.)

Because diuretics such as furosemide are given when digoxin treatment alone does not satisfactorily alleviate the symptoms of congestive heart failure, serum electrolytes should be monitored. The patient on diuretics may become hyponatremic or hypokalemic, or may develop hypochloremic alkalosis.[40] Arterial blood gas results should be analyzed to monitor the patient's acid-base balance.

Surgery

Depending on the severity of the heart lesion(s), surgery may be performed. There are two types of surgery, palliative and corrective. Palliative surgery involves reducing or increasing pulmonary blood flow, depending on how the pulmonary blood flow has been altered by the cardiac lesion. This type of surgery will not correct the cardiac lesion, but it will help to relieve congestive heart failure symptoms. Corrective surgery, as the name implies, will repair the actual cardiac defect. If possible, palliative surgery will be performed on the symptomatic infant and corrective surgery will be delayed until the child is older, when operative mortality is lower.[41, 42]

POSTOPERATIVE LABORATORY MONITORING

The patient's pulmonary function should be monitored with frequent arterial blood gas analyses and/or transcutaneous PaO_2 measurements. Electrolytes should be monitored in an effort to detect hyponatremia and hypokalemia, which may result in cardiac arrhythmias. Serum creatinine and blood urea nitrogen determinations should be performed to monitor renal function. Hematologic parameters and coagulation studies should be monitored closely, especially if there was significant blood loss during surgery or if postsurgical bleeding is noted. It may be necessary to transfuse some patients to correct the hematologic and coagulation abnormalities. Packed red cells should be infused if anemia has developed. The hematocrit should be kept above 35% in the acyanotic child, and above 45% in the cyanotic child who has undergone a palliative procedure.[43] When bleeding problems exist, fresh-frozen plasma, cryoprecipitate, and platelet transfusions may be needed.

CASE STUDY

A term infant was delivered vaginally with no complications and was taken to the newborn nursery. At about the 36th hour of life, during a bath, the infant began screaming and became cyanotic. Evaluation of the cyanosis revealed it to be peripheral and central. An audible murmur was also noted, and the infant was transferred to the neonatal intensive care unit for further evaluation.

Upon her arrival in the intensive care unit, blood was drawn for an arterial blood gas, hematocrit, and hemoglobin in order to evaluate the cyanosis further. The blood gas results were normal except for a PaO_2 of 30 mm Hg. The hematocrit was 52%, and the hemoglobin was 17 g/dL (2.6 mmol/L). Because of the cyanosis and decreased PaO_2, a cardiologist was consulted to determine the exact nature of the cardiac lesion.

Questions

1. How are the blood gas, hemoglobin, and hematocrit results helpful in evaluating the cyanosis in this patient?
2. How can the PaO_2 be used to differentiate between cardiac and pulmonary disorders as the cause of cyanosis?
3. What types of testing should be performed to diagnose congenital heart diseases accurately?

Discussion

1. In a normal infant, peripheral cyanosis of the hands and/or feet may appear after the infant is exposed to the cold or after crying. In this infant's case, central and peripheral cyanosis

was noted. Central cyanosis is caused by inadequate oxygen transport to the tissues due to abnormalities in the heart, lungs, or hemoglobin, (*e.g.*, congenital methemaglobinemia). The exact cause must be identified so that proper treatment can be initiated. Initially, a chest x-ray should be performed to determine if the cyanosis is due to disorders of the heart or lungs. Other more specific procedures such as an echocardiogram may be needed if the chest x-ray does not reveal anything conclusive. In this case, the decreased PaO_2 supported the observation of central cyanosis.

In cases of polycythemia (hyperviscosity syndrome), infants may appear cyanotic when they are really plethoric and ruddy. In polycythemia, the PaO_2 would be normal but the hematocrit would be greater than 65%. This is not the situation with this infant.

2. Although the response is not always predictable, the infant's response to the administration of 100% O_2 can sometimes help to differentiate between cardiac and pulmonary causes of cyanosis. If lung disease is present, the PaO_2 after administration will go up significantly and the infant will lose the cyanotic appearance. In cardiac disease, the PaO_2 will remain about the same and the cyanosis will persist.

3. Diagnosis is not made based on clinical laboratory testing, but based on results of the physical examination, chest x-ray, and ECG; the exact cardiac defect is determined by echocardiography and cardiac catheterization. Once the cardiac lesion is identified, the appropriate form of treatment will be established. Depending on the defect, surgery may be an alternative. The clinical laboratory's primary role in cases of congenital heart disease is to provide clinical information for monitoring the patient's condition to maintain homeostasis before and after the diagnosis is made.

REFERENCES

1. Wolfe RR: Cardiovascular diseases. In Kempe CH, Silver HK, O'Brien D (eds): Current Pediatric Diagnosis and Treatment, 6th ed, p 334. Los Altos, California, Lange Medical Publications, 1980
2. Levin AR: Heart diseases. In Wasserman E, Gromisch DS (eds): Survey of Clinical Pediatrics, p 250. New York City, McGraw-Hill, 1981
3. Cullum L, Liebman J: The association of congenital heart disease with Down's syndrome (mongolism). Am J Cardiol 24:354, 1969
4. Tandon R, Edwards JE: Cardiac malformations associated with Down's syndrome (clinicopathologic correlations). Circulation 47:1349, 1971
5. Laursen HB: Congenital heart disease in Down's syndrome. Br Heart J 38:32, 1976
6. Taylor AI: Autosomal trisomy syndrome: A detailed study of 27 cases of Edwards's syndrome and 27 cases of Patau's syndrome. J Med Genet 5:227, 1968
7. Smith DW: The No. 18 trisomy and D1 trisomy syndromes. Pediatr Clin North Am 10:389, 1963
8. Nora JJ, Tomes FG, Sinha AK et al: Characteristic cardiovascular anomalies of XO Turner syndrome XX and XY phenotype and XO/XX Turner mosaic. Am J Cardiol 25:639, 1970
9. Moller JH, Neal WA: Heart Diseases in Infancy, p 19. New York City, Appleton-Century-Crofts, 1981
10. Rowe RD: Letter to the Editor: Cardiovascular lesions in rubella. J Pediatr 68:147, 1966
11. Hastreiter AR, Joorbchi B, Pkujatti G et al: Cardiovascular lesions associated with congenital rubella. J Pedriatr 71:59, 1967
12 Levin AR: Heart Diseases. In Wasserman E, Gromisch DS (eds): Survey of Clinical Pediatrics, p 250. New York City, McGraw-Hill, 1981
13. Wolfe RR: Cardiovascular diseases. In Kempe CH, Silver HK, O'Brien D (eds): Current Pediatric Diagnosis and Treatment, 6th ed, p 334. Los Altos, California, Lange Medical Publications, 1980
14. Oehler JM: Family-Centered Neonatal Nursing Care, p 195, Philadelphia, JB Lippincott, 1981
15. Wolfe RR: Cardiovascular diseases. In Kempe CH, Silver HK, O'Brien D (eds): Current Pediatric Diagnosis and Treatment, 6th ed, p 318, Los Altos, California, Lange Medical Publications, 1980
16. Moller JH, Neal WA: Heart Diseases in Infancy, pp 15–18. New York City, Appleton-Century-Crofts, 1981
17. Moller JH, Neal WA: Heart Diseases in Infancy, pp 16, 23. New York City, Appleton-Century-Crofts, 1981

18. Goldman HI, Maralit A, Sun S et al: Neonatal cyanosis and arterial oxygen saturations. J Pediatr 82:319, 1973
19. Oehler JM: Family-Centered Neonatal Nursing Care, p 222. Philadelphia, JB Lippincott, 1981
20. Oehler JM: Family-Centered Neonatal Nursing Care, p 222. Philadelphia, JB Lippincott, 1981
21. Wolfe RR: Cardiovascular diseases. In Kempe CH, Silver HK, O'Brien D (eds): Current Pediatric Diagnosis and Treatment, 6th ed, p 330. Los Altos, California, Lange Medical Publications, 1980
22. Jung RC, Balchum OJ, Massey FJ: The accuracy of venous and capillary blood for the prediction of arterial *p*H, pCO_2, and pO_2 measurements. Am J Clin Pathol 45: 129, 1966
23. Langlands JHM, Wallace WFM: Small blood samples from earlobe puncture. Lancet 2:315, 1965
24. Laughlin DE, McDonald JS, Bedwell GN: A microtechnique for measurement of pO_2 in "arterialized" earlobe blood. J Lab Clin Med 64:330, 1964
25. Koch G: The validity of pO_2 measurements in capillary blood as a substitute for arterial blood. Scand J Clin Invest 21:10, 1968
26. Sadove MS, Thompson RD, Jobsen E: Capillary versus arterial blood gases. Anesth Analg 52:724, 1973
27. Lapinski MW: Collection, processing, and measurement of blood gases. In Henry JB (ed): Clinical Diagnosis and Management, 17th ed, pp 99–102. Philadelphia, WB Saunders, 1984
28. Oehler JM: Family-Centered Neonatal Nursing Care, p 162. Philadelphia, JB Lippincott, 1981
29. Young DS, Bermes EW: Specimen collection and processing; Sources of biological variation. In Tietz NW (ed): Textbook of Clinical Chemistry, p 487. Philadelphia, WB Saunders, 1986
30. Kupke IR, Kather B, Zeugner S: On the composition of capillary and venous blood serum. Clin Chem Acta 112: 177–185, 1981
31. Ladenson JR, Tsai L-MB, Michael JM et al: Serum versus heparinized plasma for 18 common chemistry tests. Am J Clin Pathol 62:545–552, 1974
32. Lubbers DW, Grossmann U: Gas exchange through the human epidermis as a basis of $tcpO_2$ and $tcpCO_2$ measurements. In Huch R, Huch A (eds): Continuous Transcutaneous Blood Gas Monitoring, p 30. New York City, Marcel Dekker, 1983
33. Kazmucha-Kinne S, Kisling JA: Continuous blood gas monitoring. In Schreiner RL, Kisling JA (eds): Practical Neonatal Respiratory Care, pp 279–286. New York City, Raven Press, 1982
34. Versmold HT, Linderkamp O, Holzmann M et al: Transcutaneous monitoring pO_2 in newborn infants: Where are the limits? Influence of blood pressure, blood volume, blood flow, viscosity, and acid–base state. Birth Defects 15:285, 1979
35. Hansen TN, Tooley WH: Skin surface CO_2 tension in sick infants. Pediatrics 64:942–945, 1979
36. Huch R, Fallenstein F, Seiler D et al: $tcpCO_2$—state of development. Birth Defects 15:413–419, 1979
37. Sackster S, Gildea JH, Dassy C: Common congenital cardiac defects. Am J Nurs 78:266, 1978
38. Caldwell RL: Congenital heart disease. In Schreiner RL, Kesling JA (eds): Practical Neonatal Respiratory Care, pp 178–180. New York City, Raven Press, 1982
39. Howanitz PJ, Howanitz JH: Therapeutic drug monitoring and toxicology. In Henry JB (ed): Clinical Diagnosis and Management, 17th ed, p 351. Philadelphia, WB Saunders, 1984
40. Caldwell RL: Congenital heart disease. In Schreiner RL, Kesling JA (eds): Practical Neonatal Respiratory Care, p 179. New York City, Raven Press, 1982
41. Oehler JM: Family-Centered Neonatal Nursing Care, pp 240–242. Philadelphia, JB Lippincott, 1981
42. Caldwell RL: Congenital heart disease. In Schreiner RL, Kesling JA (eds): Practical Neonatal Respiratory Care, p 180. New York City, Raven Press, 1982
43. Caldwell RL: Congenital heart disease. In Schreiner RL, Kesling JA (eds): Practical Neonatal Respiratory Care, p 180. New York City, Raven Press, 1982

Chapter 75

Hyaline Membrane Disease (Respiratory Distress Syndrome)

Michael W. Sullivan

Respiratory distress syndrome (RDS) due to deficient surfactant production (hyaline membrane disease—HMD) is the most common cause of respiratory distress in term and premature infants, and causes the highest rate of mortality and morbidity. Approximately 12,000 infants will die each year as a result of HMD.[1, 2] Severe and progressive pulmonary insufficiency and the highest mortality rate occur over the first 72 hours. If the infant survives, spontaneous recovery ensues. HMD is the direct result of inadequate surfactant (dipalmitoyl phosphotidylcholine) production by alveolar type II pneumocytes in the lung.[3] Surfactant is necessary for the maintenance of adequate surface tension in the alveoli to prevent alveolar collapse and to permit gas exchange throughout the respiratory cycle. Storage of the surfactant begins at 24 weeks of gestation, but delivery of the surfactant to the alveolar surface does not occur until about 30 weeks.[4] Fetal lung maturity is not reached until approximately 35 weeks of gestation. Mortality and morbidity due to RDS have decreased due to determination of fetal lung maturity via amniocentesis and determination of the lecithin–sphingomyelin (L–S) ratio (see Chap. 41), administration of glucocorticoid to the mother prior to delivery, and administration of natural and artificial surfactant to the infant after birth.[5]

ETIOLOGY AND PATHOPHYSIOLOGY

HMD is seen in approximately 10% of all preterm infants. As the gestational age increases, the risk of HMD decreases, and HMD is rare in full-term infants. Recently, a protein has been identified that interferes with surfactant production and function. The inhibitor appears in the alveoli due to an abnormal protein leak in the lungs of infants with RDS.[6] The frequency of HMD in the premature infant is increased in cases of maternal diabetes, maternal hypotension, acute fetal distress, sibling with HMD, being the second-born of twins, and emergency cesarean section.[1]

In the high-risk infant there is inadequate surfactant production. This leads to progressive alveolar collapse (atelectasis), which decreases lung compliance and increases the work of breathing. Atelectasis leads to hypoxemia and hypoventilation with hypercapnia. Hypoxemia is a potent vasoconstrictor and results in decreased pulmonary blood flow, causing a reversion to fetal circulation (a right-to-left shunt). Decreased pulmonary blood flow enhances hypoxemia, and the amount of lactic acid is increased due to anaerobic metabolism. The resulting acidosis inhibits enzymes necessary for production of surfactant, and the cycle continues. A simplified explanation of the pathogenesis of HMD is summarized in Figure 75-1.[4] Pulmonary hypoperfusion and hypoxemia lead to alveolar epithelial damage and increased capillary permeability, with plasma leakage into the alveolar spaces. In the alveoli, fibrinogen is converted to fibrin, resulting in what are described as hyaline membranes.[7] The effect of the membranes is that they further inhibit oxygen–carbon dioxide diffusion.

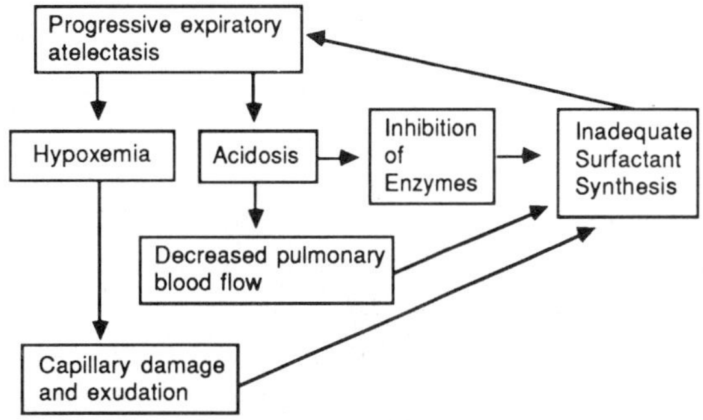

Figure 75-1 **Overview of pathogenesis of HMD. (From Phelan PD, Landau LI, Olinsky A: Respiratory Illness in Children, 2nd ed, p 12. Boston, Blackwell Scientific Publications, 1982)**

CLINICAL MANIFESTATIONS

Signs and symptoms of respiratory distress are evident within 2 hours after birth. The predominant symptoms are tachypnea (usually greater than 60 breaths/minute), expiratory grunting, prominent retractions of the sternum, and nasal flaring. As the disease progresses, central cyanosis on room air occurs. The infant becomes inactive and hypotonic.

LABORATORY ANALYSES AND DIAGNOSIS

Antepartum

Under certain circumstances it may be necessary for the physician to deliver an infant prematurely. Assessment of the pulmonary maturity of the fetus will aid the physician in that decision, because the more premature the infant, the more probable it is that HMD will develop. Evaluation of the amniotic fluid can be used to determine pulmonary maturity. There are a number of tests to evaluate fetal maturity, but the most accurate test is the determination of the lecithin–sphingomyelin ratio. As the fetal lung matures, the quantity of lecithin (phosphatidylcholine) relative to that of sphingomyelin increases.[8] An L–S ratio of greater than 2 indicates mature lungs, except in cases of maternal diabetes (IDM) and hemolytic disease of the newborn (HDN), and essentially eliminates the chances of HMD. In cases of infants of diabetic mothers, in whom HMD has been seen even with L–S ratios greater than 2.0, some researchers feel that to minimize the risk of HMD the gestational age should be at least 36 weeks and the L–S ratio at least 2.5.[9, 10] Some institutions use an L–S ratio of 3.5 to indicate lung maturity in IDM.[11] Delayed lung maturity is also seen in some cases of infants affected with HDN.[12, 13] (See Chap. 41.) Decreased indexes are associated with decreased pulmonary maturity, and thus with a greater risk that the infant will develop HMD.

Currently, the use of ultrasonography, a noninvasive technique, has been shown to have promise in estimating fetal pulmonary maturity.[14] Some studies have shown that evaluating placental morphology through the use of ultrasonography correlates well with the L–S ratio.[15]

Postpartum

Laboratory results do not play a primary role in the initial diagnosis of HMD; however, arterial blood gases and electrolytes indicate an initial respiratory acidosis followed by a metabolic acidosis. If not determined antepartum in amniotic fluid, an L–S ratio can also be determined using a gastric aspirate of the affected infant in the first 6 hours after birth. Hematocrit and glucose are also important.

The chest x-ray is usually diagnostic in severe cases of HMD. The classic appearance of the lungs is a diffuse, fine, reticulogranular pattern involving both lungs, with prominent air bronchograms extending beyond the heart border and into the periphery of the lungs to give a ground glass appearance.[1]

TREATMENT

Antepartum

Administration of glucocorticoids to the mother prior to delivery is often utilized. Glucocorticosteroids prevent HMD by accelerating pulmonary maturation of the fetus. Studies have shown that the incidence of respiratory distress is significantly decreased when the mother is treated with steroids prior to delivery.[1, 16–21]

Postpartum

Treatment after delivery is directed at the symptoms produced by the disease, although use of direct endotracheal administration of artificial and natural surfactant to treat the disorder is currently under evaluation.[16, 22, 23]

Laboratory results are very important in monitoring treatment, and the keystone treatment of the hypoxemia in HMD is oxygen. The extent of oxygenation will depend on the severity of the disease. The PaO_2 should be maintained at levels between 50 and 80 mm Hg. Frequent PaO_2 measurements should be made so that hyperoxygenation does not occur, as this may cause retrolental fibroplasia and blindness.[24] Frequent PaO_2 measurements can be made from arterial blood collected from indwelling umbilical artery catheters or through the use of transcutaneous PaO_2 monitors ($tcPaO_2$). The advantages of the $tcPaO_2$ monitor are described in Chapter 74. When blood for arterial blood gases is drawn, meticulous records of the amount and time of collection must be kept in order to determine the amount of blood that must be replaced via transfusion. The $tcPaO_2$ monitors are not meant to replace arterial blood gas analyses, but to be used in conjunction with them. When dealing with an infant with respiratory distress, it is essential to monitor blood gases for the presence and subsequent treatment of metabolic and/or respiratory acidosis.

The hematocrit should be monitored after withdrawal of blood for arterial blood gases, and its level should be maintained at between 45% and 55% with transfusion of packed red cells to ensure adequate hemoglobin for oxygenation of the tissues. If the infant has previously been ABO- and Rh-typed and has had a negative antibody screen, then group O, Rh(Du)-negative packed cells may be used for the duration of the infant's hospital stay without further ABO and Rh typing or crossmatching.[25] It may be necessary to infuse red cells or plasma to ensure a normal blood pressure and adequate tissue perfusion. Decreases in blood pressure with subsequent decreases in tissue perfusion could result in metabolic acidosis.[1]

Another complication is hypothermia, which causes increased oxygen consumption as the infant's body tries to maintain a normal temperature. The increased oxygen consumption may be enough to cause or contribute to hypoxia. Stress of any kind, *e.g.*, pain or physical manipulation, can cause increased energy consumption, preventing the infant from using available energy for pulmonary functions.

Because the infant in respiratory distress has high energy demands but only a small glycogen reserve, intravenous feeding of glucose is essential to keep the infant from becoming hypoglycemic. The glucose must be monitored frequently. A venous puncture, heel stick, or withdrawal of blood from an umbilical catheter can be performed to obtain a specimen for glucose determinations. Some intensive care units use "dip stick" glucose screening tests that require only a drop of whole blood. These methods can be very unreliable if not utilized properly, and the precautions discussed in Chapter 74 must be followed.

To monitor the infant's fluid and electrolyte balance adequately, both serum electrolytes and urine output with specific gravity determinations should be measured. The purpose of these determinations is to ascertain the infant's state of hydration and renal function.

CASE STUDY

An infant was delivered by emergency cesarean section at 26 weeks of gestation. A detailed maternal obstetric and medical history were not immediately available; however, it was known that the mother's previous pregnancy had terminated in a premature delivery. Within a few minutes after birth, the infant became tachypneic (respirations of 85/min) and began to exhibit sternal retractions, expiratory grunting, nasal flaring, and peripheral cyanosis. The infant was intubated and given oxygen, and taken to the neonatal intensive care unit. Arterial blood gas, hematocrit, and glucose tests and a chest x-ray were performed.

LABORATORY FINDINGS
(Reference Values, Neonates)

*p*H: 7.13 (7.32)
PaO_2: 35 mm Hg (59.5)
$PaCO_2$: 50 mm Hg (47.3)
Base excess: −14 (−3.7)
Glucose: 70 mg/dL
Hematocrit: 52%
Chest x-ray: Granular or ground glass appearance

Questions

1. What is the significance of the fact that a previous child had also been born prematurely?
2. Explain the significance of the laboratory data.

Discussion

1. The risk of delivering a premature infant is greater if there is a past history of delivering a premature infant. The incidence of hyaline membrane disorder (HMD) is increased in premature infants, primarily because of fetal lung immaturity, due to inadequate surfactant production.
2. The chest x-ray is one of the most helpful diagnostic tests in this case. It should be noted, however, that the ground glass appearance of the lung, while characteristic of HMD, is not seen in every case.

   The arterial blood gases in this case show evidence of respiratory acidosis. This is evidenced by the increased $PaCO_2$ and decreased *p*H. It will be important to monitor the $PaCO_2$. As the infant fatigues due to the amount of work that is expended to breathe, he will begin to hypoventilate, which will exaggerate the hypoxemia and hypercapnia. Ventilatory support will be needed as the $PaCO_2$ exceeds 60 mm Hg.

   The decreased PaO_2 may be explained in two ways. The first is reduction in the ventilation–perfusion ratios (a low V/Q, or alveolar underventilation). Because of inadequate surfactant production with subsequent alveolar collapse, adequate oxygen–carbon dioxide exchange does not occur. However, the main cause of the hypoxemia is right-to-left shunting, due to increased pulmonary vascular resistance at the ductus arteriosus and foramen ovale. Oxygen therapy aids in reducing the right-to-left shunting by improving pulmonary vascular resistance, because oxygen is a potent pulmonary vasodilator. If hypoxemia and hypoventilation persist, eventually a mixed respiratory–metabolic acidosis may occur. Acidosis contributes to increased pulmonary vascular resistance and reduces the amount of surfactant production. The obvious course for this patient is to maintain his PaO_2 level at between 60 and 80 through the administration of oxygen, and to monitor the PaO_2 with arterial or capillary blood gas analysis or a $tcPaO_2$ monitor. If the $PaCO_2$ continues to rise, ventilation support should be instituted.

To prevent hypovolemia, the hematocrit should be checked regularly throughout the infant's stay, especially if arterial blood gases and other laboratory tests are drawn frequently. To prevent dehydration and hypoglycemia due to insensible water loss and the infant's limited glycogen reserves and increased metabolic demands, glucose and fluids should be administered. Blood glucose and electrolytes should be monitored at least daily. Any abnormalities in these values should be reported to the intensive care unit immediately.

REFERENCES

1. Escobedo MB: Hyaline membrane disease. In Schreiner RL, Kisling JA (eds): Practical Neonatal Respiratory Care, pp 87–94. New York City, Raven Press, 1982
2. Farrell PM, Wood RE: Epidemiology of HMD in the U.S.: Analysis of national morbidity statistics. Pediatrics 58: 167–176, 1976
3. Brumley GW, Hodson WA, Avery ME: Lung phospholipids and surface tension correlations in infants with and without hyaline membrane disease and in adults. Pediatrics 40: 13, 1967
4. Phelan PD, Landau LI, Olinsky A: Respiratory Illness in Children, 3rd ed, pp 3–11. Boston, Blackwell Scientific Publication, 1982
5. Loper DL: Surfactant replacement therapy. J Neo Nat 4(5): 14, 1986
6. Ikegami M, Jobe A, Berry D: A protein that inhibits surfactant in respiratory distress syndrome. Biol Neonate 50: 121–129, 1986
7. Oehler JM: Family-Centered Neonatal Nursing Care, p 195. Philadelphia, JB Lippincott, 1981
8. Gluck L, Kulovich MV, Borer RC Jr et al: Diagnosis of the respiratory distress syndrome by amniocentesis. Am J Obstet Gynecol 109: 440, 1971
9. Mueller-Heubach E: Lecithin–sphingomyelin ratio in amniotic fluid and its value for the prediction of neonatal respiratory distress in pregnant diabetic women. Am J Obstet Gynecol 130: 28–43, 1978
10. Cruz A, Buhi W, Birk S et al: Respiratory distress syndrome with mature lecithin–sphingomyelin ratios: Diabetes mellitus and low Apgar scores. Am J Obstet Gynecol 126: 78–82, 1976
11. Greene MF, Montserrat deMF, Tulchinsky D: Biochemical Aspects of Pregnancy. In Tietz NW (ed): Textbook of Clinical Chemistry, p 1776. Philadelphia, WB Saunders, 1986
12. Morrison JC: The lecithin–sphingomyelin ratio in cases associated wtih fetomaternal disease. Am J Obstet Gynecol 127: 363–368, 1970
13. Harding P: Amniotic fluid phospholipids and fetal maturity. J Obstet Gynecol 115: 298–306, 1973
14. Golde SH, Platt LD: The use of ultrasound in the diagnosis of fetal lung maturity. Clin Obstet Gynecol 27(2): 391–401, 1984
15. Kazzi GM, Gross TL, Sokol RJ et al: Noninvasive prediction of hyaline membrane disease: An optimized classification of sonographic placental maturation. Am J Obstet Gynecol 67(5): 161–165, 1985
16. Relier JP, Eggermont E: Hyaline membrane disease—recent developments. Eur J Obstet Gynecol Reprod Biol 15: 409–424, 1983
17. Ballard RA, Ballard AL: Use of prenatal glucocorticoid therapy to prevent respiratory distress syndrome. Am J Dis Child 130: 982–987, 1976
18. Ballard P, Benson B, Brehier A: Glucocorticoid effects in fetal lung. Am Rev Respir Dis 115(Suppl): 29–36, 1977
19. Block MF, Kling OR, Crosby WM: Antenatal glu-

cocorticoid therapy for the prevention of respiratory distress syndrome in the premature infant. Obstet Gynecol 50: 186–190, 1977

20. Caspi E, Sehreyer P, Weinraub Z et al: Changes in amniotic fluid lecithin–sphingomyelin ratio following maternal dexamethasone administration. Am J Obstet Gynecol 122: 327–331, 1975
21. Dluholucky S, Babic J, Taufer I: Reduction of incidence and mortality of respiratory distress syndrome by administration of hydrocortisone to mothers. Arch Dis Child 51: 420–423, 1976
22. Gitlin JD, Parad R, Taeusch HW Jr: Exogenous surfactant therapy in hyaline membrane disease. Semin Perinatol 8(4): 272–282, 1984
23. Fujiwara T, Chida S et al: Artificial surfactant therapy in hyaline membrane disease. Lancet 1:55–59, 1980
24. Kempe CH, Silver HK, O'Brien D: Current Pediatric Diagnosis and Treatment, 6th ed, p 69. Los Altos, California, Lange Medical Publications, 1980
25. Schmidt PJ (ed): Standards for Blood Banks and Transfusion Services, 11th ed, p 27. Arlington, Virginia, American Association of Blood Banks, 1984

Chapter 76

Hemolytic Disease of the Newborn

Michael W. Sullivan

Hemolytic disease of the newborn (HDN) is the direct result of fetal red cell destruction by maternal IgG antibodies. The number of severe cases of Rh HDN has dramatically decreased with the advent of Rh immune globulin (RhIG), but cases of HDN due to other IgG red cell antibodies and mild cases of ABO HDN still do occur. Mortality and morbidity have decreased due to the refinement of treatment. Depending on the antibody associated with the hemolytic process, there is a marked degree of variability in the severity of the disease, ranging from intrauterine death to the absence of clinical symptoms.

ETIOLOGY AND PATHOPHYSIOLOGY

Origin of Maternal Antibodies

For HDN to occur, there must first be an antigen present on the fetal red cells that is not present on the maternal red cells. Second, the mother must be sensitized to produce an IgG antibody against that antigen. Third, the maternal antibody must be able to cross the placenta and bind to the fetal red cells. Finally, the red cells coated with antibody are destroyed by the reticuloendothelial cells of the fetus. (See Chap. 41.)

HDN may be classified by the maternal IgG antibody involved. The categories follow, in descending order of severity:

1. Rh hemolytic disease, due to anti-D alone or in combination with anti-C or anti-E
2. "Other" HDN, due to antibodies against other antigens in the Rh system, such as anti-C or anti-E, or to antibodies in other systems, such as anti-K, anti-Fy^a, and many others
3. ABO HDN, due usually to anti-A,B in group O women, but rarely to anti-A or anti-B[1]

HDN will not occur with the first pregnancy due to antibodies in the first two categories if the mother has not been sensitized to foreign red cell antigens via transfusion. The first pregnancy serves as the source of primary sensitization, and subsequent pregnancies provide the stimulus for the secondary immune response and the production of the IgG antibody. The probability of HDN occurring increases as the number of pregnancies increases. HDN due to ABO incompatibility may occur in the first pregnancy because the antibody is already present.

Effects of the Destruction of Fetal and Newborn Red Cells

When the fetal red cells are destroyed *in utero,* the hemoglobin that is released is converted to bilirubin, which crosses the placenta, enters the maternal circulation, and is conjugated in the liver and excreted. In severe cases of HDN, there is an increase in the demand for fetal red blood cells. Extramedullary hematopoiesis in the liver and spleen ensues, with a subsequent increase in nucleated red cells and hepatosplenomegaly. If there is extensive fetal red cell destruction, severe anemia will occur. Eventually, the severity of the anemia will result in increased cardiac output and generalized edema. Death may occur *in utero.*

If intrauterine death does not occur and the fetus is delivered, continued red blood cell destruction occurs, and the level of unconjugated bilirubin increases. This is due to the inability of the newborn liver to conjugate bilirubin so that it can be excreted. If the amount of unconjugated bilirubin increases to the level of 20 mg/dL (342 μmol/L), it will eventually cross the blood–brain barrier and cause brain damage (kernicterus). Prevention of kernicterus is the goal of treatment for HDN.

CLINICAL MANIFESTATIONS

The live-born infant suffering from classic HDN is pale and edematous with an enlarged liver and spleen and jaundice, as described above for the fetus.

LABORATORY ANALYSES AND DIAGNOSIS

Prenatal Testing

The goal of prenatal testing and history is to identify women who are at risk of having a child who could be affected with HDN and to follow the extent of fetal red cell destruction that may exist. (See Chap. 41.)

Postnatal Testing

IMMUNOHEMATOLOGY

In all cases in which there is suspicion that the infant may have been affected by a maternal IgG antibody, an ABO and Rh type should be performed on the cord blood. A direct antiglobulin test (DAT) should be performed on the cord blood if the mother is known to be immunized.[2] (See Table 76-1.) It is always beneficial to have a maternal specimen to test also, but if that is not possible an accurate medical history is essential. It is not advisable to perform a DAT on the cord blood from a

Table 76-1 ***Laboratory Studies Recommended for Maternal and Cord Bloods in Cases of Suspected HDN***

Maternal Blood	Cord Blood
ABO group	ABO group
Rh group	Rh group
D^u, if apparently Rh-negative	D^u, if apparently Rh-negative
Antibody screening test	Direct antiglobulin test
Identification of antibody, if present	Eluate from red cells, if direct antiglobulin test is positive and clinical circumstances warrant
	Identification of antibody in eluate

nonimmunized mother because such testing could result in a false positive in 5% of the cases. In this event, observation of the newborn for pathologic jaundice is a better way to identify ABO HDN than a DAT on a cord blood.[3, 4]

Special problems in typing cord cells arise, depending on the severity of the hemolytic process. If the DAT is strong, the cells may spontaneously agglutinate in the high-protein media used in testing. Also, it must be kept in mind that cells may be heavily coated with antibody, and false negatives may occur. Laboratories offering testing under these circumstances must be prepared to take appropriate steps to mitigate these technical problems. Otherwise, misleading results may be provided to clinicians. Figure 76-1 gives an example of how to proceed with cord blood testing.

The most important test in assessing the presence of Rh HDN is the DAT, although the strength of the DAT does not correlate perfectly with the severity of the disease. If the DAT is positive, an elution should be performed and the antibody identified. Not all the antibodies present in the mother's serum will necessarily be present on the newborn red cells. This should be kept in mind when determining which specimens to use for crossmatch if an exchange transfusion is necessary.

An antibody screen and panel should be performed on the cord serum in cases of HDN due to antibodies other than ABO. The antibodies present should be the ones identified in the mother's serum, unless all the antibody had been absorbed onto the cord cells.

HEMATOLOGY

Although hematologic review of cord blood is not alone diagnostic of HDN, the results are helpful in determining the severity of the disease. In cases of severe Rh HDN, numerous nucleated red blood cells (NRBC) will be seen in the infant's peripheral blood. There may also be a macrocytic anemia with reticulocytosis. The cord hemoglobin will yield direct information on the severity of the disease. Normal cord hemoglobin is between 14 and 20 g/dL (2.2–3.1 mmol/L), but in moderate to severe cases of HDN the cord hemoglobin may fall as low as 8 g/dL (1.2 mmol/L) or less. The medical staff may have established criteria regarding the levels of cord hemoglobin and bilirubin to assist in decisions concerning the need for immediate exchange transfusions. In ABO HDN, the cord hemoglobin is usually mildly decreased, and spherocytes may be seen on the peripheral blood smear.

CHEMISTRY

The unconjugated bilirubin concentration in the cord blood also serves as a useful guide in determining the severity of the disease, and thus the need to perform an exchange transfusion. It should be emphasized that cord blood should be delivered to the laboratory as soon as possible after collection if it is to be analyzed for bilirubin. If it cannot be delivered immediately, it must be stored away

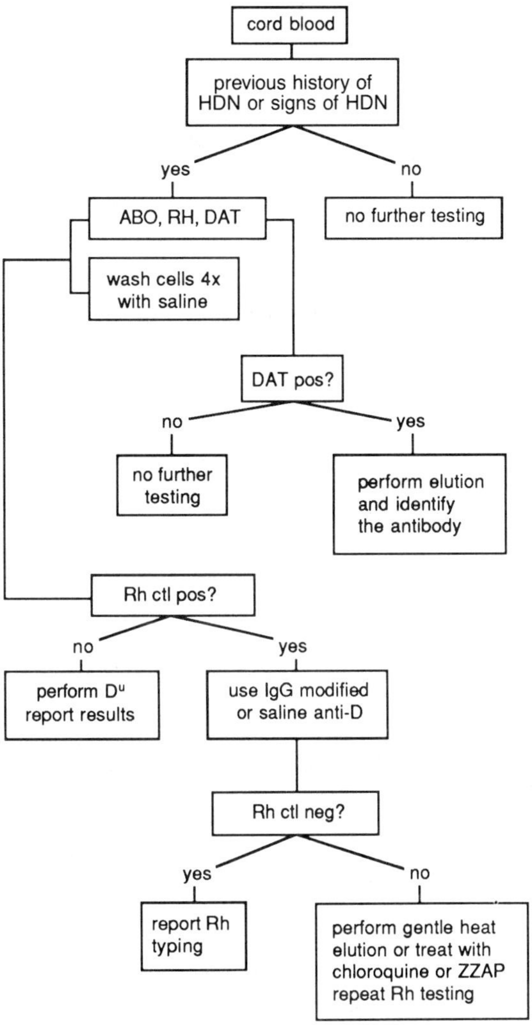

Figure 76-1 Testing of cord blood in suspected cases of HDN.

from light to prevent the deterioration of bilirubin. The significance of the unconjugated bilirubin level depends on the weight of the infant. Generally, an unconjugated cord bilirubin level of 6 mg/dL (102.6 μmol/L) or greater is an indication to perform an exchange transfusion.[5] However, it should be noted that various institutions set their own criteria with respect to bilirubin levels as an indicator for exchange transfusion. The occurrence of kernicterus depends on the level of unconjugated bilirubin, the degree of hypoalbuminemia, the gestational age, and the general condition of the infant. Table 76-2 shows a comparison of results found in normal infants with those in infants with ABO and Rh HDN.[6]

TREATMENT OF HDN

Antepartum

After an amniocentesis has determined that the fetus's life is endangered but the fetus is not mature enough to deliver, the decision to perform an intrauterine transfusion (IUT) may be made, as described in Chapter 41.

To crossmatch blood for an IUT, the mother's serum should be used and testing should include techniques that will detect clinically significant IgG antibodies. The blood must be negative for the antigens against which the mother has antibodies.

Blood to be used for IUT should be group O, D^u-negative, and less than five days old. Deglycerolized blood is the product of choice because it contains minimal amounts of plasma, platelets, anticoagulant, and leukocytes. Depending on the institution, blood sero-negative for cytomegalovirus (CMV) may be required. It may be necessary to adjust the hematocrit to 80% to prevent volume overload. It has been suggested that blood used for IUT be irradiated to reduce the possibility of graft-host disease. IUTs are performed at two-week intervals until conditions are suitable to induce labor.

There may be problems in ABO and Rh typing of cord cells from an infant who has had an IUT because of the presence of the transfused cells. In this event, an accurate ABO and Rh type may not be possible until the transfused cells are gone. The strength of the DAT may be very weak or negative depending on the number of IUTs. Therefore, the DAT will not be helpful in assessing the severity of the hemolytic disease process.

Table 76-2 *Comparison of ABO, RH, and "Other" Antibodies Associated with HDN*

Diseases Due to		
Anti-D	*"Other" (e.g., anti-c, E, Kell)*	*ABO Incompatibility*
Maternal Blood Type		
D negative	Negative for involved antigen	90% group O
Infant Blood Type		
D positive	Positive for involved antigen	90% A_1 or B
Maternal Antibody		
Anti-D	Anti-c, E, Kell, and others	Immune anti-A_1, anti-B, and/or anti-A,B
Onset of Bilirubinemia		
Variable, usually 24 hr	Same as for Rh disease	Avg. 24–36 hr
Anemia		
Variable, can be severe	Same as for Rh disease	Usually absent, occasionally mild to moderate
DAT		
Positive	Positive	Occasionally positive, usually negative
Cord Hemoglobin		
Mild: >13 g/dL Mod.: 8–13 g/dL Sev.: <8 g/dL	Same as for Rh disease	Mild: >13 g/dL Mod.: 8–13 g/dL
Blood Smear		
Macrocytosis and hypochromia; greatly increased NRBC	Same as for Rh disease	Occasionally microspherocytes, moderately increased NRBC

Conversion to SI units is as follows:
Hemoglobin g/dL × 0.155 = mmol/L

Postpartum

Depending on the severity of the hemolytic process, an exchange transfusion may be necessary. An exchange transfusion accomplishes several therapeutic objectives:

1. It removes excess bilirubin from the newborn circulation to prevent kernicterus.
2. It removes the antibody-coated red cells to prevent further hemolysis.
3. It reduces the amount of circulating maternal antibody.
4. It introduces antibody-free red cells that will have a longer life span and will contain HbA, which has a lower oxygen affinity than HbF.
5. It expands the pool of albumin that will be available to carry excess bilirubin.

Ideally, it is best to have a maternal blood specimen available for crossmatching because it has the highest concentration of antibody. When the maternal specimen is not available, the next choice for crossmatch would be to use the eluate from the cord cells or the cord serum. Because there may be maternal IgG antibodies present in the cord serum that do not have antigenic sites on the newborn red cells to react with, blood must be selected that is negative for those antigens. The eluate is preferred over the cord serum if time permits.

The selection of ABO-type blood will depend on

the ABO type of the infant and the mother. Blood selected for transfusion should be compatible with the mother's ABO type and lack any other antigens to which the mother has antibody(ies). If the mother and infant have different ABO types, group O blood should be used. It is not necessary to use Rh-negative blood if anti-D is not the cause of the hemolytic process. It is necessary that the blood lack the antigen to which the mother has an antibody. If group O blood is used and the infant is group A, B or AB, then the plasma must be removed and replaced with either group AB fresh-frozen plasma or plasma that is compatible with the infant. The donor blood must be less than 5 days old, and can be deglycerolized red cells or fresh red cells. Addition of fresh-frozen plasma or 5% albumin is needed to adjust the hematocrit of the unit to between 40% and 50%.

Depending on the size of the infant, enough blood is prepared to provide a 2-volume exchange, although all the bilirubin, antibody-coated cells, or maternal antibody present in the infant's circulation will not be removed. When bilirubin is removed from the infant's circulation, the bilirubin present in the tissues enters the circulation to reestablish equilibrium. Thus, after the exchange transfusion, the bilirubin in the plasma will increase due to this process and due to the continued destruction of newborn red cells that were not removed by the exchange. The bilirubin must be closely monitored, and if it continues to increase at greater than 0.5 mg/dL/hour (8.6 μmol/L/hour) or if the level approaches 20 mg/dL (342 μmol/L), repeat exchange transfusions will be necessary.[7]

Postexchange Laboratory Monitoring

Postexchange laboratory monitoring may include the following:

1. The infant's acid–base balance should be monitored frequently to include arterial blood gases and electrolytes. A transcutaneous PaO_2 monitor ($tcPaO_2$) is very helpful in the continuous monitoring of the infant's PaO_2.
2. Because there may be few platelets present in the units of blood used for exchange transfusion, the platelet count should be monitored; if a count of less than $25 \times 10^3/mm^3$ occurs, platelet transfusions may be necessary.
3. Hypoglycemia may develop, and thus, to prevent sequelae due to hypoglycemia, blood glucose should be monitored. This may be carried out effectively in the intensive care unit through the use of whole blood glucose reagent strips that utilize a reflectance photometer to determine the quantity of glucose present, provided that the precautions noted in Chapters 38 and 74 are followed.
4. The indirect bilirubin should be monitored closely postexchange to determine if subsequent exchanges may be needed.[8]

It should be noted that, in all cases involving premature and term infants in which multiple laboratory tests are required, the volume of the specimen must be kept to a minimum to prevent volume depletion and the subsequent need for replacement blood therapy. The total blood volume in infants (especially premature infants) is small, and removing even 3–5 mL of blood each time testing is needed will be harmful to the infant; therefore, instruments that utilize micro-sampling techniques are essential. The use of $tcPaO_2$ monitors and whole blood reagent strips for determining glucose levels has risen in popularity in response to the need to minimize the amount of iatrogenic blood loss.

Prevention of HDN Due to Anti-D

The number of cases of HDN due to anti-D has decreased dramatically since the development of Rh immune globulin (RhIG). The purpose of RhIG is to suppress the maternal immune system production of anti-D and thus prevent the possibility of HDN in future pregnancies, as is described in Chapter 41. An Rh (D^u)-negative mother who delivers an ABO-compatible Rh-positive infant and does not receive RhIG has about a 7% to 8% chance of developing anti-D. This figure drops to about 1% when the mother is administered a single dose of RhIG postpartum. If RhIG is given ante- and postnatally, the incidence decreases to about 0.1%.[9]

Because of the increased use of antepartum RhIG, the physician (or nurse) in charge of the patient during delivery must notify the blood bank that the mother received antepartum RhIG. Otherwise, the blood bank may detect anti-D in the mother's serum and therefore not recommend administration of postpartum RhIG. If there is a significant fetal–maternal bleed and postpartum RhIG is not given, Rh sensitization could occur. Additionally, when antenatal RhIG is administered, 1% to 2% of infants develop a positive DAT due to the RhIg (anti-D), and the maternal antibody screen may be negative. Thus, it is important that the blood bank know if the mother received antenatal RhIg.

TESTING OF THE MATERNAL SPECIMEN PRIOR TO ADMINISTRATION OF RhIG

Prior to administration of postpartum RhIG to a mother who has delivered an Rh-positive infant, the following tests may be performed on the postpartum maternal specimen. It should be noted that AABB Standards require that the maternal Rh status be determined during admission for delivery, abortion, or amniocentesis.[10]

1. ABO and Rh type including D^u.
2. Antibody screen and antibody identification panel if necessary
3. AABB Standards require that the specimen be tested to detect a fetal–maternal bleed, which would require more than one dose of RhIG for effective prophylaxis.[11]

METHODS OF DETECTING THE FETAL–MATERNAL HEMORRHAGE (FMH)

Some institutions use the microscopic D^u test as a screening test to determine the presence of a significant number of fetal cells in the maternal circulation. This method cannot be performed on patients with a positive DAT. This test is specific for Rh-positive cells, but is not very sensitive.[12] The occurrence of an FMH of greater than 30 mL is estimated at only 0.3% of all deliveries. However, failure to detect an FMH greater than 30 mL, due to the use of insensitive screening techniques such as the microscopic D^u procedure, is a contributing factor to the "failure rate of RhIG."[13] Subsequent to a positive microscopic D^u procedure, a quantitative test would need to be performed to determine the number of vials of RhIG to administer.

A screening test utilizing the erythrocyte rosetting test has been shown to be more sensitive than the microscopic D^u, and the results are more reproducible.[14, 15] This technique uses Rh-positive indicator cells that form easily detectable rosettes around fetal Rh-positive red cells. The procedure does not use the antiglobulin phase, so it can be performed on a patient with a positive DAT. It can detect FMHs as low as 5 mL. The entire procedure may take up to 45 minutes to perform. Because this is only a qualitative test, a quantitative Kleihauer-Betke test must be performed to determine the number of vials of RhIG to administer.

QUANTIFICATION OF FMH

The Kleihauer-Betke technique is considered the reference method in determining the amount of FMH and in calculating the dose of RhIG to administer. The test is based on the principle that fetal hemoglobin (HbF) is resistant to elution from the red cell at an acid *p*H, whereas adult hemoglobin (HbA) will be eluted. The percent of fetal cells counted is multiplied by 50 to determine in mL the volume of fetal cells in the maternal circulation. This value is divided by 30 (which is the amount of fetal cells that will be neutralized by one vial of RhIG), and the result is the number of vials of RhIG to administer. This procedure is difficult to standardize, and reproducibility is poor. Because of the imprecision, the actual volume of the FMH may vary from one-half to twice the value determined by the procedure. This must be taken into account when determining the number of vials of RhIG to administer. It is far better to overtreat than to undertreat, so it is recommended that more vials of RhIG be added to the calculated number of vials.[16]

ADMINISTRATION OF RhIG

RhIG is administered intramuscularly, usually in the buttocks, within 72 hours after delivery. RhIG is the only type of immune prophylaxis offered in order to prevent HDN. It must be kept in mind that HDN due to other IgG red cell antibodies can and does occur, but is not very common.

CASE STUDY

A woman who was 33 weeks pregnant had fallen down a flight of stairs and then gone into active labor. She was unconscious at the time of delivery, and delivered a girl who weighed 1600 g. A detailed history of the mother revealed that she had been transfused with five units of blood three years earlier, after an automobile accident. She had delivered her first child two years after the accident. Her prenatal history revealed that she had anti-K. The child had no complications. The Kell genotype of the father was Kk. During this pregnancy, the titer of the anti-K had risen from 1:8 to 1:64. An amniocentesis was performed at 28 and 29 weeks to determine the status of the fetus. The change in absorbance was not high enough to warrant any immediate action.

At birth, a cord blood specimen was taken from the baby girl and a venous specimen from the mother. Both specimens were sent to the blood bank for testing. The results of the initial workup for both patients are outlined below:

LABORATORY FINDINGS
(Baby girl—cord blood)

Cell typing (cells washed 4 times)

Anti-A	Anti-B	Anti-A,B	Rh control	Anti-D
0	0	0	4^+	3^+

Direct Antiglobulin Test
Polyspecific AHG 4^+

The mother typed O, D^u-negative. She had a positive antibody screen at 37°C (albumin) and AHG. Anti-Kell and anti-D were identified. The anti-D reacted 1^{+w} (weak) with R_1R_2 cells, and was not enhanced with enzyme-treated cells. The titer of the anti-D was 1:2. The mother's cells were Kell-negative.

Questions

1. How can the Rh typing be resolved for the baby?
2. What additional blood tests should be performed on the infant?
3. Explain why the mother's anti-D reacted so weakly.
4. Based on the above information, is the mother a candidate for Rh immune globulin?
5. If blood for an exchange transfusion is needed, what blood type should be selected?

Discussion

1. The original Rh typing had been performed with anti-D suspended in a high-protein solution along with the appropriate negative control. Cells that are heavily coated with antibody may spontaneously agglutinate in a high-protein medium. This was probably the case with this baby. In this case, the Rh typing should be repeated, using IgG-modified anti-D or saline reactive (IgM) anti-D. These antisera should be used because the antibody is not suspended in a high-protein media. The appropriate negative control should also be run. The D^u test should not be performed when using either of these two reagents because (1) the saline reactive anti-D is IgM, and cannot react with AHG, and (2) if the cells are already coated with IgG antibody, as in this case, a false positive will be seen with the D^u test. If, after testing with IgG-modified or saline-reactive anti-D, the Rh control is still positive, a gentle heat elution (45°C) or elution with chloroquine or ZZAP can be performed to remove the antibody. It should be noted that treatment of the cells with chloroquine may weaken the expression of the D anti-

gen. The Rh testing should then be repeated. In this case the baby was Rh(D)-positive.

2. It is important to identify the antibody that is causing the positive DAT. In this case, ABO antibodies can be eliminated as possibilities because the mother and infant have the same blood type. Although the identity of the mother's antibody is known, identification of the antibody coating the infant's cells is still necessary. An elution should be performed on the infant's cells and the eluate tested against selected panel cells to confirm that the antibody is anti-K. It is important to save a sample of the saline from the last wash of the cells to test parallel to the eluate. The last wash should not react with any of the cells. This negative reaction ensures that all unattached antibody had been washed free from the cells before the elution, and that the positive reaction with the eluate is actually the result of the antibody eluted from the cells. If the identity of the antibody had not been known, an entire antibody identification panel would need to be performed on the eluate. In this case, anti-K was the only antibody eluted from the infant's cells.

   If possible, Kell antigen typing should also be performed on the infant's cells. Because Kell typing requires an indirect antiglobulin technique, any antibody attached to the cells must be removed. ZZAP cannot be used for this purpose as it has been shown to denature the Kell blood group system antigens. Chloroquine may be used, but it may not render the cells antibody-free, especially if the DAT is strong (4^+). In this case, it seems academic that the infant's cells are Kell-positive because anti-K was eluted from them and anti-K was identified in the maternal serum. For the sake of completion, however, if Kell typing of the infant's cells is needed, one could wait until the antibody-coated cells were removed from the infant's circulation and then retype the antibody free cells.

   It would be helpful to have a hemoglobin and bilirubin performed on the cord blood also. In this case, the baby had a cord hemoglobin of 12 g/dL (1.9 mmol/L) and a total bilirubin of 4 mg/dL (68.4 μmol/L).

3. In cases like this, in which the reaction of the anti-D is so weak, one must be suspicious that the presence of the anti-D is due to antepartum, prophylactic administration of Rh immune globulin and is not the result of immunologic stimulation. It is important that the mother's history be explored to determine if she received antepartum Rh immune globulin. If she has not received it, the presence of the anti-D would suggest active immunization. In this case, her history revealed that she had received a dose of Rh immune globulin after each amniocentesis.

4. Because the mother meets the criteria for receiving Rh immune globulin (she is D^u-negative, she delivered an Rh(D)-positive baby, and she has no history of active immunization), she is a candidate to receive Rh immune globulin. Again, it was particularly important in this case to determine that she had received antepartum Rh immune globulin.

5. If blood is needed for an exchange transfusion, the maternal specimen should be used for the crossmatch. In this case, because the mother has anti-D, although it is due to Rh immune globulin, group O, Rh(D)-negative, Kell-negative blood must be selected for crossmatch if it is to be compatible with her serum.

REFERENCES

1. Widmann FK (ed): AABB Technical Manual, 9th ed, p 249. Washington, D.C., American Association of Blood Banks, 1985
2. Widmann FK (ed): AABB Technical Manual, 9th ed, p 305. Washington, D. C., American Association of Blood Banks, 1985
3. Vengelen-Tyler V: The serologic investigation of hemolytic disease of the newborn caused by antibodies other than anti-D. In Garraty G (ed): Hemolytic Disease of the Newborn, pp 145–172. Arlington, Virginia, American Association of Blood Banks, 1984
4. Walker RH: Relevancy in the selection of serologic

tests for the obstetric patient. In Garraty G (ed): Hemolytic Disease of the Newborn, pp 173–203. Arlington, Virginia, American Association of Blood Banks, 1984

5. Wennberg RP, Goetzman BW: Neonatal Intensive Care Manual, pp 189–190. Chicago, Year Book Medical Pub, 1985
6. Wallach J: Interpretation of Pediatric Tests. Boston, Little, Brown & Co, 1983
7. Widmann FK (ed): AABB Technical Manual, 9th ed, p 303. Washington, D. C., American Association of Blood Banks, 1985
8. Widmann FK (ed): AABB Technical Manual, 9th ed, p 304. Washington, D. C., American Association of Blood Banks, 1985
9. Bowman JM, Chown B, Lewis M et al: Rh isoimmunization during pregnancy: Antenatal prophylaxis. Can Med Assoc J 118: 623–627, 1978
10. Schmidt PJ (ed): Standards for Blood Banks and Transfusion Services, 11th ed, p 32. Arlington, Virginia, American Association of Blood Banks, 1984
11. Schmidt PJ (ed): Standards for Blood Banks and Transfusion Services, 11th ed, p 32. Arlington, Virginia, American Association of Blood Banks, 1984
12. Polesky HF, Sebring ES: Detection of fetal–maternal hemorrhage: An evaluation of serological tests related to Rho(D) immune globulin. Transfusion 11: 162, 1971
13. Polesky HF, Sebring ES: Evaluation of methods for detection and quantitation of fetal cells and their effect on RhIg usage. Am J Clin Pathol 76: 525–529, 1981
14. Sebring ES, Polesky HF: Detection of fetal–maternal hemorrhage in Rh immune globulin candidates. Transfusion 22: 468–471, 1982
15. Taswell HF, Reisner RK: Laboratory medicine: Prevention of Rho hemolytic disease of the newborn: The rosette method—a rapid, sensitive screening test. Mayo Clin Proc 58: 342–343, 1983
16. Walker RH: Relevancy in the selection of serologic tests for the obstetric patient. In Garraty G (ed): Hemolytic Disease of the Newborn. p 194. Arlington, Virginia, American Association of Blood Banks, 1984

Chapter 77

Failure to Thrive

Michael W. Sullivan

Failure to thrive is a symptom, rather than a specific disease or disorder. Failure to thrive is suspected when an infant or child falls below the third percentile in size and/or weight according to the normal growth curve, or when an infant or child deviates from the growth pattern exhibited previously.[1] There is no single diagnostic category into which failure to thrive fits. Instead, it encompasses multiple etiologies such as organic diseases and psychological and/or environmental disorders.[2] Because failure to thrive can be the result of numerous pediatric disorders, the identification of an underlying cause may be very difficult.

ETIOLOGY

The definition of failure to thrive is broad. It includes those infants who are not of the appropriate size, weight, and height according to the growth curves, although they may be energetic, happy, and content, as well as those infants who appear listless, lethargic, and discontented. Because not all pediatric patients who are of small size, weight, and height have some organic or psychological disorder, a number of factors must be taken into account when failure to thrive is being considered. For example, if the parents are unusually small in height, weight, or physical stature, the child may be exhibiting a familial trait. Also, the child may have been small for his or her gestational age as a term infant, or may have been born prematurely. In any of these cases, the child may be in the low range of the normal growth curve, and may not have any organic disease.[3] Also, growth *in utero* may have some effect on postnatal growth. Maternal drug use during pregnancy and placental insufficiency cause decreased growth patterns *in utero.*[4]

Inadequate Caloric Intake

Diseases/disorders in which failure to thrive is a symptom can be categorized in a number of different ways. One is according to the amount of caloric intake.[5] Failure to thrive due to inadequate caloric intake can have the following causes:[6–11]

1. Insufficient amount of formula or breast milk given
2. Disorders of maternal bonding
3. Chronic vomiting or diarrhea
4. Congenital heart disease
5. Chronic renal disease
6. Psychosocial deprivation
7. Certain endocrine disorders.

Other Disorders

Examples of disorders in which failure to thrive is a symptom even with sufficient caloric intake follow:[12–14]

1. Malabsorption
2. Disorders in swallowing
3. Central nervous system damage
4. Trisomy 21
5. Chronic inflammatory bowel disease

Indications for Hospitalization of Children Who Fail to Thrive

Strong suspicion of organic etiology, *e.g.*, congenital heart disease
Signs of physical or emotional abuse
Suspected neglect
  Poor infant hygiene (*e.g.*, severe diaper rash, long dirty fingernails)
  No previous medical attention
History of frequent vomiting or diarrhea
Infant over 2 months of age and still near birthweight
Infant between 3 and 6 months of age with minimal weight gain over previous 2 months
Potentially life-threatening malnutrition
Mother overtly depressed or rejecting baby
Insignificant weight gain after 1 month of outpatient management

LABORATORY ANALYSES AND DIAGNOSIS

The etiology of failure to thrive is best determined through a complete, thorough, and accurate history and physical examination. The information obtained may indicate that the child should be hospitalized for observation. Indications for hospitalization that may be ascertained via a history and physical examination are listed at the top of the right-hand column.[2] During hospitalization, observations by the physician should be made of mother–child interaction during and between feedings. Observations should also be made of the child's interactions with others without the mother present. In this way, the child can be observed in a controlled environment and the physician can be assured that the infant (or child) is receiving an adequate diet.

An in-depth history of feeding practices is very useful, including how feeding is performed and by whom, stool patterns, the presence and nature of sucking or swallowing problems, and the presence of symptoms of the respiratory tract, central nervous system, or urinary tract. The emotional responsiveness of the infant in different situations should also be ascertained.[15]

Laboratory testing is used primarily to confirm diagnoses or to monitor treatment. It may be useful to perform screening tests such as a complete blood count (CBC), measurements of blood urea nitrogen (BUN), creatinine, electrolytes, and glucose, and a complete urinalysis. Abnormal results that are obtained upon admission may reflect the patient's state of malnutrition and not the underlying disease state;[16] therefore, abnormal results should be evaluated with caution. If, after a complete history, physical, and period of observation, the physician suspects a metabolic congenital disorder, specific laboratory tests should be ordered to confirm that diagnosis.

REFERENCES

1. Fulginiti VA: Pediatric Clinical Problem Solving, p 159. Baltimore, Williams & Wilkins, 1981

2. Accardo PJ: Growth and Development: An Interactional Context for Failure to Thrive. In Accardo PJ (ed): Failure to Thrive in Infancy and Early Childhood, pp 11–14. Baltimore, University Park Press, 1982
3. Illingworth RS: Common Symptoms of Disease in Children, 7th ed, p 5. Boston, Blackwell Scientific Publications, 1982
4. Rosenberg A, Jones MD: Growth Patterns of Small Infants. In Accardo PJ (ed): Failure to Thrive in Infancy and Early Childhood, p 110. Baltimore, University Park Press, 1982
5. Fulginiti VA: Pediatric Clinical Problem Solving, p 160. Baltimore, Williams & Wilkins, 1981
6. Krieger I: Growth Abnormalities in Organic Disease. In Krieger I: Pediatric Disorders of Feeding, Nutrition, and Metabolism, pp 138–144. New York City, John Wiley & Sons, 1982
7. Krieger I: Growth failure and congenital heart disease. Am J Dis Child 120:497, 1970
8. Betts PR, Magrath G: Growth pattern and dietary intake of children with chronic renal insufficiency. Br Med J 2:189, 1974
9. Illingworth RS: Common Symptoms of Disease in Children, 7th ed, p 6. Boston, Blackwell Scientific Publications, 1982
10. Abrams CA: Endocrinologic aspects of failure to thrive. Pediatr Ann 7:760–766, 1978
11. Derivan AT: Disorder of Bonding. In Accardo PJ (ed): Failure to Thrive in Infancy and Early Childhood, pp 91–103. Baltimore, University Park Press, 1982
12. Ament ME: Malabsorption syndromes in infancy and childhood. J Pediatr 81:685–697, 867–884, 1972
13. Illingworth RS: Common Symptoms of Disease in Children, 7th ed, pp 7–14. Boston, Blackwell Scientific Publications, 1982
14. Krieger I: Growth Failure Without Organic Disease. In Krieger I: Pediatric Disorders of Feeding, Nutrition, and Metabolism, pp 101–129. New York City, John Wiley & Sons, 1982
15. Fulginiti VA: Pediatric Clinical Problem Solving, p 163. Baltimore, Williams & Wilkins, 1981
16. Accardo PJ: Growth and Development: An Interactional Context for Failure to Thrive. In Accardo PJ (ed): Failure to Thrive in Infancy and Early Childhood, p 11. Baltimore, University Park Press, 1982

Part XVII

HEALTH PROMOTION/ DISEASE PREVENTION

Glenda D. Price, Associate Editor

Chapter 78

The Clinical Laboratory and Health Promotion/ Disease Prevention

Glenda D. Price

Traditionally, the health care delivery system in the United States, including the clinical laboratory and its practitioners, has been focused on disease and curative mechanisms. Little attention had been paid to preventive strategies and life-style changes designed to promote health and prevent disease. Recently, however, more and more health professionals are incorporating health promotion and disease prevention (HP/DP) methods into their practice.

The U.S. Department of Health and Human Services (formerly Health, Education, and Welfare) has actively sought to influence the nation's health through HP/DP strategies. The Surgeon General issued a report in 1979, entitled *Healthy People,* in which he stated "Further improvements in the health of the American people can and will be achieved—not alone through increased medical care and greater health expenditures—but through a renewed national commitment to efforts designed to prevent disease and to promote health."[1] This document served to focus the attention of the nation on the principles of HP/DP as well as on the establishment of five major health goals for the American people.

Health Goals for the American People. The government's initiative in health promotion and disease prevention has taken the form of goals to be accomplished by 1990 (See Table 78-1).[2] The goals are to be achieved through a combination of private- and public-sector programs focused on target populations. Economic constraints, personal attitudes, social/cultural mores, the traditional interactions between health care providers and their patients/clients, and an inadequate knowledge base are all barriers to the accomplishment of the goals. However, many believe that these barriers can be overcome and the goals achieved through the implementation of multiple projects involving large numbers of people.

A national strategy developed to meet these goals must recognize that the individual plays a central role in the process; that community and individual projects designed to develop life-styles consistent with wellbeing are essential; that risks must be identified and individuals protected against those risks; and that medical care must minimize disability and death when illness does occur. All four components must be in place and intereact or complement one another. Without attention to these basic concepts, the focus would likely be on curative approaches to disease rather than on HP/DP. Only through HP/DP can the goals be fulfilled.[3]

Promoting Health. Among the more significant advances of the past two decades is the growth in knowledge of the importance of health promotion to further reduce unnecessary death in the United States. This knowledge, unlike prior information about health, has not been restricted to health care professionals but rather has become a social phenomenon. The public is concerned about and involved in activities designed to promote their own health.

Examples of the health-promoting activities common to the general public are (1) increased awareness of the nutritional benefits of food, with a concomitant reduction in the amount of cholesterol, saturated fat, and salt intake, (2) increased exercise such as jogging, aerobic dancing, and attendance at fitness centers, (3) increased natural childbirth, and (4) concern for the environment, with greater awareness of water and air pollution and involvement in "cleanup" activities.

The health professional has a responsibility to become involved in each of these activities as an individual and as a role model for the public, as well as for professional colleagues. Additionally, health practitioners, because of their increased knowledge, have a responsibility to be educators. Every opportunity should be seized to provide necessary information to patients/clients, family members, neighbors, and the public at large.

Health professionals must also be advocates for health in the workplace, in the legislative arena, and in their professional societies. This advocacy must focus on systematically changing the health care delivery system so that the individual becomes an integral part of the system. People must individually accept the responsibility for ensuring their own health, and the practitioner must be willing to allow this to happen.

Preventing Disease. At any given point in time, each person is somewhere along a continuum of health to illness, with that place on the continuum shifting as the environment changes or as threats to health are increased or decreased. Multiple risks face us constantly, and the degree to which those risks are reduced is the degree to which we are able to maintain our health.

Earlier in this century the major cause of death in the United States was infectious disease. We have witnessed a tremendous reduction in life-threatening communicable diseases with the introduction of a large array of antibiotics and improvements in hygiene and sanitation. Worldwide programs to eradicate diseases such as smallpox have also contributed to the reduction in premature mortality and morbidity from infectious agents. Today 75% of all deaths in this country are

Table 78-1 ***Health Goals for the American People***

	Goal 1	Subgoal	Subgoal
Healthy Infants	To continue to improve infant health, and, by 1990, to reduce infant mortality by at least 35%, to fewer than nine deaths per 1000 live births	Reduce the number of low-birth-weight infants	Reduce the number of birth defects
	Goal 2		
Healthy Children	To improve child health, foster optimal childhood development, and, by 1990, reduce deaths among children ages 1 to 14 years by at least 20%, to fewer than 34 per 100,000	Enhance childhood growth and development	Reduce childhood accidents and injuries
	Goal 3		
Healthy Adolescents and Young Adults	To improve the health and health habits of adolescents and young adults, and, by 1990, to reduce deaths among people ages 15 to 24 by at least 20%, to fewer than 93 per 100,000	Reduce fatal motor vehicle accidents	Reduce alcohol and drug abuse
	Goal 4		
Healthy Adults	To improve the health of adults, and, by 1990, to reduce deaths among people 25 to 64 by at least 25%, to fewer than 400 per 100,000	Reduce heart attacks and strokes	Reduce death from cancer
	Goal 5		
Healthy Older Adults	To improve the health and quality of life for older adults, and, by 1990, to reduce the average annual number of days of restricted activity due to acute and chronic conditions by 20%, to fewer than 30 days per year for people aged 65 and older	Increase the number of older adults who can function independently	Reduce premature death from influenza and pneumonia

due to chronic and degenerative disorders such as cancer, stroke, and heart disease. Accidents are the leading cause of death in the age range between 1 and 40 years.

Specific risk factors have been associated with increased incidence of the nation's leading causes of death. Reducing these risks will clearly serve to prevent and/or delay the onset of chronic cardiovascular disease, accidents, and degenerative disorders. Risk reduction means, in many cases, life-style change that is not within the ability of health professionals to accomplish, but rather is totally controlled by the individual. It is the role of the health care provider to identify the risks, to assist the individual in developing a plan for life-style change, and to monitor the effectiveness of the change.

Smoking cessation, reduction in the misuse of drugs and alcohol, dietary control, adherence to speed laws and the use of seat belts, and the proper use and disposal of household and workplace toxic agents are all within the ability of the average U.S. citizen to control. Cigarette smoking is the leading cause of death due to lung cancer. Alcohol-related factors are identified in more than 10% of U.S. deaths. The intake of excessive calories, fat, sugar, and salt are implicated in low birthweight in infancy, premature births, and coronary artery disease as well as problems secondary to obesity. In 1983, highway accidents killed 44,600 people.[4] Evidence suggests that more than 100 chemicals are known carcinogens for humans and are associated with birth defects, and more than 1000 are toxic if ingested.

Disease prevention is imperative. Prevention saves lives, improves the quality of life, and saves health care dollars. Mechanisms of prevention should be taught at an early age in the schools and introduced to the community at large. Public-sector dollars should be employed to adopt processes designed to prevent accidents and to provide clean air and water and a safe environment. All risks cannot be eliminated. Genetic risk factors are beyond the control of the individual; however, behavioral and environmental risks are significant elements of the shift along the health-to-illness continuum.

OBJECTIVES FOR THE NATION

In 1980 the Surgeon General took the second major step in the process of improving the nation's health. Specific quantifiable objectives for attaining the five broad health goals were outlined in a report entitled *Promoting Health/Preventing Disease: Objectives for the Nation.* Fifteen priority objectives were defined within three general categories: Health Promotion, Preventive Health Services, and Health Protection[2] (see below). For each priority area, an assessment was provided of the nature and extent of the problem, appropriate prevention/promotion measures, specific objectives to be met by 1990 or earlier, principal assumptions that influence the evaluation of the outcomes, and current data sources.

Objectives for the Nation: Priority Areas

Health Promotion

Smoking and health
Misuse of alcohol and drugs
Nutrition
Physical fitness and exercise
Control of stress and violent behavior

Preventive Health Services

High blood pressure control
Family planning
Pregnancy and infant health
Immunization
Sexually transmitted diseases

Health Protection

Toxic agent control
Occupational safety and health
Accident prevention and injury control
Fluoridation and dental health
Surveillance and control of infectious diseases

Role of the Clinical Laboratory Scientist

The clinical laboratory scientist has the ability to become a fulcrum around which many programs/activities can revolve. A proactive stance is required to ensure that the public and other health care practitioners understand the significant contributions that the laboratory can make in satisfying these objectives.

Laboratory scientists can implement and/or participate in educational programs directed toward adolescents to prevent their starting to smoke and in other programs directed toward smokers to encourage them to stop. High-risk groups such as pregnant women should be specifically targeted for information on the effects of cigarette smoking on the blood vessels and circulation and its impact on the development of the fetus. Participation in research projects on the effects of smoking on various laboratory tests and working to establish a smoke-free laboratory/hospital environment are also important.

The misuse of prescription medications as well as illicit drugs is a major threat to health in the United States. Drug and alcohol misuse are implicated in many accidents, account for significant absences from work and increased birth defects, are related to increased instances of crime, and lead to premature death. Clinical laboratory scientists can provide drug information, assist in enforcing the laws related to drunk driving, assist in review and revision of medication labeling, and help to develop additional therapeutic drug monitoring procedures.

Nutritional counseling, research on the relationship of foods, vitamins, and minerals within various parameters, establishment of weight control support groups, legislative processes oriented toward package labeling, and general awareness programs are all activities for the laboratory scientist. Assessment techniques to evaluate the nutritional status of individuals as identified by laboratory tests can also be developed. Establishing cholesterol screening programs is another important activity related to laboratory practice.

Physiological measures are greatly influenced by the degree of fitness an individual exhibits. Exercise generally improves fitness and therefore enhances performance on physiological scales. In addition to designing and implementing screening programs within physiological parameters, laboratory professionals can be good role models for others. A laboratory exercise program, competitive sports teams, and monitoring programs can be developed. Advocating for the incorporation of an "exercise history" in the medical record is a worthwhile activity.

Studies have shown that the clinical laboratory is one of the most stressful worksites within the health care delivery system. Clinical laboratory scientists can develop stress management programs for the workplace, initiate stress assessment appraisals, develop support systems for colleagues, and participate in educational experiences designed to recognize stress and individuals who are at risk for suicide. Legislative action intended to control firearms and other instruments of violent behavior is likewise an appropriate approach for laboratory scientists to assist in meeting the objective of reducing violent behavior.

Providing information on the relationship of diet to blood pressure, and the effects of exercise on blood pressure, as well as blood pressure checks and the performance of tests that are altered in hypertensives are all activities for the laboratory scientist. Encouraging the monitoring of the children of hypertensives is also an important effort, as well as developing a mechanism for the periodic assessment of blood pressure for all persons associated with the worksite and/or clients of the facility.

Family planning is the process of conscious decision-making about having a child. Methods to avoid unwanted pregnancy must be communicated, especially to adolescents. Instruction on over-the-counter contraceptives that are available and their proper use is critical. Products to determine ovulation are also important for individuals who are infertile as well as for those wishing to avoid pregnancy. Working with the pharmacist, the laboratory scientist can supply much needed information.

The United States has one of the highest infant mortality rates among all of the westernized developed nations. This rate can be lowered through cooperative programs designed to touch all socioeconomic, cultural, and ethnic levels of our society. The laboratory scientist working with the March of Dimes, the Red Cross, and other organizations with programs for pregnant women can contribute to reducing the problem. Further, sharing information on the physiological and laboratory parameters that change during pregnancy should prevent unnecessary and dangerous false diagnoses during pregnancy.

Research in the production of new vaccines, providing information on the importance of vaccinating children, participating in immunization programs, and working with schools and day-care centers to ensure that all children are immunized are just a few of the activities appropriate to the priority area of immunization. Working on institutional committees to develop policies for immunization of employees is another opportunity to be involved.

Designing screening programs and providing information on methods to reduce the transmission of infectious agents during sexual contact is an obvious arena for the laboratory. Instruction to other health care professionals on the nature of the infections, the effectiveness of various antibiotics as therapeutic measures, and complications associated with sexually transmitted diseases is also warranted.

Measures to assess the toxicity of various agents, screening programs to evaluate individuals who have been exposed to potentially toxic agents, and legislative measures to control environmental hazards and to ensure accurate labeling of chemicals are the major arenas for laboratory involvement. Further ensuring that the laboratory itself properly disposes of toxic agents is a critical arena for action by the clinical laboratory scientist.

The clinical laboratory itself is potentially an unsafe workplace. Laboratory personnel must become more aware of and concerned with the dangers inherent in the environment and take steps to improve its safety. Participation in the design of facilities is as important as are day-to-day work activities to ensure safety. Advocating for and participating in an institutional occupational health program can also have positive effects.

In all aspects of our lives we are at risk of injury from accidents—at home, in the workplace, in our cars, during leisure-time activities, and in other ways. Periodic review to assess situations or objects that might cause accidents and taking action to remove the potential hazard is one approach. Wearing seat belts and requiring all others in your vehicle to do likewise is another. Learning and teaching first aid to those around you is essential to minimizing injury that might occur following an accident.

Advocating for fluoridation of the water supply in communities in which fluoridation has not yet been instituted is the most significant contribution that the laboratory professional can make to the priority area of dental health.

The clinical laboratory scientist is clearly capable of designing programs of surveillance, analyzing the data generated by these programs, and making recommendations to reduce the spread of infectious diseases. Surveillance programs can be implemented in hospitals, nursing homes, day-care centers, and other public facilities. The challenge to laboratory scientists is not to their appropriateness to design and implement the program but rather to their ability to command funding support for such activities.

HP/DP PROGRAM DEVELOPMENT

Program development in any arena follows five basic steps: (1) assess the need, (2) design the program to fulfill the need, (3) implement the program, (4) evaluate the effectiveness of the program, and (5) modify it as appropriate, based on a review of the needs assessment and program design. In health promotion/disease prevention activities, these same basic steps apply.

The major programmatic areas for laboratory involvement in HP/DP can be organized into four categories: screening activities, surveillance programs, education aimed at life-style change, and legislative activities.[5] The category used and/or the experiences planned will depend on the interest and expertise of the clinical laboratory scientist, the needs of the population to be addressed, the resources available, and the perceived effectiveness of the planned approach.

An example of a surveillance program that was designed by a laboratory scientist follows the classic program development model. The program took place in a day-care center in which the individual enrolled her young child.

Needs Assessment

In this instance, the need to develop a program of surveillance and control of infectious agents was identified by the mother, not by the day-care center staff. Shortly after enrolling her child in the center, the mother noticed an increase in the number of infections her child experienced with the routine cuts, scrapes, and bruises normal at that age. The number of upper respiratory infections also increased. Because these increases occurred following enrollment at the center, it seemed logical to consider that the infections were acquired at that site.

To determine the extent of the infectious phenomenon, a questionnaire was developed and given to other parents to ascertain their perceptions about an increase in infections among their children. When the questionnaire results were analyzed, it was clear that a problem existed at the center.

Program Design

The purpose of the program was to reduce the number of infections contracted by the children in the day-care center. The first step in the process was the identification of the source(s) of the infections. A program of environmental culturing was designed to locate the contaminated objects, as well as a parent survey form to ascertain which children might be carrying infectious agents into the center. A followup form was also developed to monitor the number of infections occurring over the next 3-month period.

Implementation

Parents and day-care center staff participated in the project implementation. A clinical laboratory microbiologist assumed responsibility for the environmental culturing and data evaluation. Weekly cultures were obtained from tables, chairs, bathroom fixtures, eating utensils, toys, and other furniture used by the children. Parents were asked to complete the two survey instruments on a weekly basis, providing information on any infections their children had that might have been brought to the center and any newly-acquired infections. The planned 3-month period was determined to be appropriate for assessment.

Evaluation

At the end of the 3-month period pilot phase, the data revealed no change in the number of infections; however, it was now evident that the infections were being transmitted primarily via the tables, chairs, and toys that were frequently handled by the children. Identifying the source was important, but no intervention had been built into the pilot program and thus no reduction in the transmission of infections had occurred.

Program Modification

Two educational activities were developed to be incorporated into the project. The first educational program was developed for the maintenance/janitorial staff of the center. They were instructed in proper methods of disinfecting, the importance of thorough cleaning, and the need for different types of disinfectants. The second program was developed for the children themselves. They were instructed in proper hand-washing techniques, the need to cover scrapes and bruises, and proper use and disposal of tissues.

The day-care center staff were also instructed to use paper covering for the tables that could be discarded daily. The staff were provided with masks for any child with an upper respiratory tract infection.

One month after the educational programs were initiated, a decrease was noted in the number of infections acquired by the children in the center. This project is a clear example of how laboratory scientists can use their expertise outside of the hospital for health promotion/disease prevention. Educational programs aimed at life-style changes, legislative activity to enact law, and screening programs to monitor segments of the population can all follow this model.

CLINICAL LABORATORY SCIENTIST AS HEALTH EDUCATOR

All health care practitioners, irrespective of their disciplines, have encountered situations in which friends, relatives, neighbors, or even casual acquaintances have asked questions of them about a health problem or health-related issue. These are moments of opportunity for practitioners to become health educators. These are "teachable moments" when the questioner is ready to listen, and ready to be affected by the response.[6] The clinical laboratory scientist should seize these opportunities.

Involvement in HP/DP will extend the practice of clinical laboratory science outside the laboratory itself. Laboratory scientists will need to integrate into their practice the necessary skills to be an educator, a counselor, or a consultant. Laboratory scientists must accept responsibility for the interpretation of laboratory data and the sharing of their knowledge about biological systems with other health professionals and the public at large. The time is past when clinical laboratory scientists can say that their role ends with the performance of clinical tests and the generation of test data.

Currently a number of barriers to functioning as health educators exist for many laboratory practitioners. The first barrier undoubtedly lies in the personal perception of the laboratorian. Many practitioners have not observed faculty and colleagues serving as role models in this arena and, therefore, do not perceive themselves in this role. Second, the personality of many laboratory practitioners is fundamentally introverted, thus making it difficult for them to initiate communications beyond the traditional scope of providing information on test values. Poor communications skills also contribute to their inability to see themselves as educators.

Historically, the medical profession, personnel practices, increasing specialization, and an undervaluing of the principles of health promotion/disease prevention have caused laboratory personnel to focus their attention only on activities within the laboratory. Their role as health educators had not been defined, nor had their abilities in this arena been tested. Today, however, with the trends in health care away from a centralized to a decentralized approach, with consumers of health care demanding more information about and involvement in their care, and with the growing number of options available for health care, all providers must reexamine their traditional stance and contribute in a new way.[7]

Laboratory scientists must begin to build coalitions with consumers and other health care professionals to move out of the laboratory and into alternative sites for practice. Working with the American Cancer Society, the American Red Cross, and other such organizations, laboratory scientists can become involved in educational programs of health promotion and screening programs of disease prevention. Independent research projects to validate the effectiveness of HP/DP educational strategies are also an important point of contribution for the laboratory health educator.

CLINICAL LABORATORY SCIENTIST AS CONSULTANT IN HEALTH PROMOTION AND DISEASE PREVENTION

Considerable need exists for clinical laboratory scientists to be involved in health promotion activities beyond the laboratory arena. Individuals will find opportunities for consultation in industry, in health care facilities, with community organizations, in academic settings, and in leisure-time facilities. They will also find opportunities for consultation with individuals, for program design and implementation, for situational assessments, and for educational programming.

As consultants, clinical laboratory scientists should

1. Be selective about those areas in which consultation will be provided
2. Start small—working in those areas in which they are known, and then moving into new areas
3. Be realistic about the time required
4. Look to colleagues for help and advice
5. Become involved with nonlaboratory agencies and organizations to extend their contacts and network

Two major areas of consultation in arenas of particular need are at-home testing and occupational disorders. The clinical laboratory scientist is especially suited to providing expertise in these areas.

At-Home Testing

The diagnostic component of over-the-counter products available in pharmacies is growing at an annual rate of approximately 25%. It is estimated that by the year 2000 every U.S. home will have at least one home testing product. Currently most at-home testing is recommended by a physician; however, it will not be long before self-initiated testing will surpass physician recommendations.[8]

At-home testing is not a new concept. Temperature, pulse, weight, vision screening, and blood pressure measurements are available to individuals interested in monitoring their own health.[9] Breast self-examination is being encouraged by the American Cancer Society as an important measure for preventing advanced cancers in women. The first laboratory products designed for lay-public use were methods for the measurement of glucose in urine. These products first appeared in the latter half of the 1920s, but were not popular until the development of dry chemical test tablets and strips in the 1950s.[10] The truly public interest in this arena came in the 1970s with the marketing of the home pregnancy test kit.

Products are now available for evaluating acetone, albumin, amebiasis, bilirubin, urea nitrogen, glucose, *p*H, occult blood, urobilinogen, leukocytes in urine, ascorbic acid, PKU, pregnancy, ovulation, gonorrhea, asthma, urinary tract infections, streptococcal antibodies, sickle cell, calcium, and sodium.[11] In addition, consumers may purchase an array of products to collect blood samples.

The development of home testing products has been encouraged by the trend toward consumers demanding more control over their own medical care. Manufacturers have taken advantage of this trend and have developed and marketed test kits that are convenient and easy to use. The trend toward attempts to reduce health care costs is also credited for the increse in these products.[12] However, home testing may actually increase an individual's personal health care costs rather than decrease them. An individual who uses a home test kit will generally consult a physician if the results are inconclusive or abnormal. The physician will then order additional tests that must be paid for by the patient. This dual testing serves to increase rather than decrease the cost.

An aging population and the cost containment measures that cause release of patients from hospitals at an earlier point enhance the need for and use of self-testing kits. Individuals have a need to monitor their own therapy through these test procedures.

Without question, advances in chemistry and

technology are also responsible for the growth of home testing products. Miniaturized circuitry, operator-independent instruments, monoclonal antibodies, and immunologic methodology have all contributed to the opportunities for lay persons to perform laboratory tests that, in the past, required sophisticated instruments and specific knowledge. These same factors will ensure the development of new tests for the at-home market.

Tests now available for the physician's office will soon be available for home use. Tests to monitor drugs, cholesterol, respiratory function, and sexually transmitted diseases, along with cancer detection techniques, are in various stages of development for home use. Instruments for laboratory procedures and a wide range of medical devices are being manufactured with the general public in mind.

Many of the objections that have been expressed about the increase in home testing products have focused on the fear that individuals may be misled by these products and thus not seek needed medical attention. This fear is based on an underlying assumption that the client cannot perform these tests with the same degree of accuracy and specificity as does the clinical laboratory. This assumption is not necessarily valid, but several factors need to be considered:

1. The Food and Drug Administration has stringent regulations affecting these products. The degree of specificity is increasing constantly, and appropriate instructions written in terms that lay persons can understand are required. The regulatory process supposedly prevents a product from coming to the marketplace before it can be used safely.
2. Individuals who do not follow the directions properly may obtain inaccurate results; however, it could be argued that persons motivated to purchase and perform their own tests are sufficiently concerned to follow directions.
3. Performing the test under proper physiological conditions, such as fasting, is also important; however, the same logic applies. With proper instructions and clear motivation these specific test conditions will be adhered to.
4. The clinical laboratory always uses controls, both positive and negative, for its procedures. Many over-the-counter tests do not include these controls, thereby providing an area for legitimate concern. The individual has no assurance that the test system is working properly.
5. Test interpretation is, of course, another problematic factor in the overall quality of these tests. The individual who is not a health professional may not understand the interferences that arise from diet, contaminated containers, and the like that might cause false-positive or false-negative results. Inconclusive results are also subject to good judgment on the part of the individual performing the test. The willingness to spend additional monies to purchase another test kit to repeat the inconclusive test will also vary from one individual to another.

In general, the motivated individual who follows the directions enclosed with the test will be able to perform and interpret certain straightforward procedures. In those cases in which there is doubt or there is a need for clarifying the instructions, the laboratory scientist should be available for assistance and should be an educator and a consultant to the pharmacist and the client. Further, the clinical laboratory scientist should be involved in the development of home test kits, the writing of package insert instructions, and the design of marketing programs.

Educational programs should be structured to define clearly the indications for performing various tests, the conditions that will result in positive values, and those that will produce negative values. The technique for performing the test, the problems that may arise in performance, and the interpretation of the results should be covered. Assisting the client in determining the appropriate health care practitioner to visit following the test is a needed consultative role that the laboratory scientist should assume. These activities can be coordinated through pharmacies, home health agencies, health maintenance organizations, community centers, fitness centers, and other facilities.

Occupational Disorders

In 1983, 11,300 deaths occurred in the United States as a result of some accident of the workplace.[4] The deaths were caused by a wide range of problems, ranging from traumas to infections to toxicity. With increased attention to prevention and early recognition of workplace hazards, a significant reduction in death could be realized.

The first task of the individual concerned with preventing occupational disorders is the identification of the potential hazards of the environment. Ergonomic, biologic, chemical, physical, and psychosocial factors may each contribute risks to health in the workplace.[13]

Ergonomics is the study of the laws of work and the interactions of various factors that either enhance or impede efficient and effective functioning. Machine design, organization of equipment, physical arrangement of furniture, and sequence of activities are issues for the ergonomist. Physiological, anatomic, and cultural factors must also be considered in the determination of the appropriateness of a worksite for the tasks to be accomplished and the people involved. Should any segment of the environment be inconsistent with the individual or with any other segment, the situation becomes a potential risk.

Biologic agents tend to cause few problems in the workplace because the laws governing infectious materials have heightened the public's awareness of proper methods for handling these materials. Nonetheless, work-acquired infectious disorders still occur on occasion. Brucella, psittacosis, Weil's disease, and contact infections of various types are still known to be problematic in certain occupations. Knowledge about the manner in which the infection is transmitted, signs and symptoms of early infections, and methods to prevent infections are essential to the individual worker.

Dust, silica, toxic gases and fumes, asbestos, and chemical liquids are hazardous environmental contributors to disease in some worksites. Physical barriers between the worker and the chemical agent are needed to reduce the risks associated with these materials.

Physical agents such as temperature, noise, radiation, and light are significant contributors to job-related injuries and illnesses. An understanding about the potential hazards of these agents and the type of injuries they cause must be communicated to workers in environments where risk exists.

Until recently, psychosocial factors associated with workplace illnesses were not recognized. It is now known that stress, job satisfaction, nutrition, fitness, compensation, and level of responsibility are important determinants of health. Health promotion programs at the workplace to reduce tobacco and alcohol dependency, increase fitness, reduce stress, and improve nutrition are successful in reducing the number of days of absenteeism.

The incidence of work days lost from injuries and illness is a measure of the severity of the problem of work-related illness. In 1984, 3.7 days per 100 workers were lost and 5.4 million persons were reported as having experienced a work-related injury or illness, along with 3,740 work-related deaths. Each of these figures is higher than those reported for 1983. Skin diseases and disorders associated with repeated trauma such as hearing loss due to continuing pressure of vibration accounted for three of every five illnesses in 1984.[14]

Involvement in the establishment of programs to reduce the probability of workplace injuries is needed. The clinical laboratory scientist has significant expertise that can be brought to this arena.

REFERENCES

1. Healthy People: The Surgeon General's Report on Health Promotion and Disease Prevention. U.S.

Department of Health, Education, and Welfare, Publication No. 79-55071, 1979

2. Promoting Health/Preventing Disease: Objectives for the Nation. U.S. Department of Health and Human Services, 1980
3. Public Health Service Implementation Plans for Attaining the Objectives for the Nation. In Public Health Reports. U.S. Department of Health and Human Services, 1983
4. World Almanac. New York City, Random House, 1985
5. Danish S: What is an effective health promotion program? Health Promotion 2:3, 1985
6. Jacobson L, Pellegrino E: Editor's Forum: The role of allied health professionals in prevention. Prev Med 6:379–385, 1977
7. Longe M, Ardell D: Wellness programs attract new markets for hospitals. Hospitals Nov:115, 1981
8. Koffer K, Gerbino P: Home laboratory testing: Part 1. Am Druggist Mar:63–72, 1986
9. Hooper J. Seven medical tests you can do yourself. Good Housekeeping March:243, 1980
10. Free A, Free H: Self-testing, an emerging component of clinical chemistry. Clin Chem 30:829, 1984
11. Gossel T: Diagnostic products. U.S. Pharmacist Feb:746–750, 1986
12. Koffer K, Gerbino P: Home laboratory testing: Part 2. Am Druggist Apr:103–111, 1986
13. Levy B, Wegman D: Occupational Health: Recognizing and Preventing Work-Related Disease. Boston, Little, Brown and Co, 1982
14. Noble K: Job-linked injuries and illness rose in 1984. The New York Times, Nov 14, 1985, p A21

Part XVIII

PHYSICIANS' OFFICE LABORATORIES

Diana Mass, Associate Editor

Chapter 79

The Physician Office Laboratory (POL)

Julia R. Crowley/Jane Sidney Oliver

Today's clinical laboratory scientist confronts an array of practice settings. Due both to new technologies and to sweeping changes in federal and third-party payment policies for health services, diagnostic tests increasingly are being performed in decentralized ambulatory care settings of all kinds. There, according to the conventional wisdom, some elements of patient care can be delivered at a cost substantially lower than that incurred in the inpatient, hospital context, and both patients and physicians can enjoy speedier test turnaround and enhanced convenience. One such decentralized laboratory test setting is that of the physician office laboratory (POL).

THE GROWTH OF TESTING IN POLs

Estimates are that currently 50% of all diagnostic tests are performed in the POL.[1] If this trend continues the POL will feel increased pressure to assure patients, insurors, and hospitals as recipients of preadmission test results that its laboratory services meet acceptable standards of quality.

As test volume has increased, concern about the quality of tests provided in POLs has escalated, especially in the last several years. Manufacturers are aggressively marketing relatively inexpensive new laboratory technologies to POLs, alleging an enhanced operating ease, convenience, and profit potential.[2, 3] At the same time, fundamental changes in Medicare and other third-party payment policies have created incentives that favor more testing in the ambulatory sector.[4, 5] Federal and state laboratory regulations, however, have not kept pace with either of these developments. Except in certain limited circumstances, federal regulation has exempted POLs from mandatory personnel, quality control, and proficiency testing standards, and in most instances state laboratory regulations ignore physician practices involving fewer than five or six physicians.[6, 7]

These twin forces, technology and the absence of potentially costly regulatory requirements, have enhanced the POL's testing capability, at the same time creating special quality challenges in the small POL.

For the physician-owner, whose education typically has omitted training in the fundamentals of laboratory management (from either a technical or a business perspective),[8] there are several challenges. From a business perspective, the first is to determine whether the POL can, in fact, deliver its promised clinical rewards and profitability. Other more serious challenges require physicians to provide adequately for their professional, medical, and legal responsibility for the POL. For the POL staff, who also typically lack formal training in clinical laboratory science,[8–11] the challenge is to deliver high-quality, cost-effective, reliable test results while at the same time providing nursing, bookkeeping, receptionist, and other services that a small private practice usually requires.

Assisting the POL in meeting these challenges is the province of the clinical laboratory scientist, as consultant, laboratory director, or bench practitioner. While the particular needs of individual POLs may vary, in general, all POLs have certain common requirements: demonstrable quality assurance, clinical relevance, and cost-effectiveness.

THE POL SETTING

Office laboratories range from highly sophisticated, computerized facilities serving a group practice of hundreds of physicians, to kitchen countertops in single-physician offices. The technology available can rival that in the largest teaching hospital, or it can consist of an outdated monocular microscope, a microhematocrit centrifuge, and a handful of urinalysis dipsticks.[9, 12] Although the term "POL" spans both extremes and all points in between, it means *any* setting in which physicians provide tests solely for the benefit of *their own* patients.

It is estimated that more than 90% of primary care physicians have access to an office laboratory.[13] Overall, however, general and family practitioners, internists, pediatricians, and ob–gyn specialists currently account for the bulk of in-office testing.[14] As a rule of thumb, the larger the practice, the more likely it is to provide the bulk of its testing in-house.[15]

Practice contexts and employment demands on the POL practitioner *differ radically* from those for the clinical laboratory scientist who functions in a hospital or independent laboratory. These differences tend to result in distinctions that, if recognized, will better equip traditionally-educated clinical laboratory scientists for POL consulting or technical direction roles.

The small office primary care laboratory demands a balance of scientific, technical, business managerial, and interpersonal competencies. That is, practitioners in a small primary care setting must be multicompetent: they are usually responsible not only for laboratory service, but also for performing chest and extremity x-rays, electrocardiograms, and nursing duties, as well as for "front office" business management and administrative services.

Apart from imposing sharp limitations on the POL practitioner's time and energy, these demands for direct involvement in several dimensions of patient care have another important and often overlooked implication: *at its best, this setting could require of the laboratory scientist clinical correlation, test interpretation, and problem-solving skills of the highest order. In fulfilling this role, the clinical laboratory scientist functions as a true colleague of the primary care physician and other members of the health care team.* This point deserves elaboration. Regardless of education or training, POL personnel work in a primary care setting and, therefore, view and provide its laboratory services from deep within a comprehensive, immediate, and direct patient care context. The POL setting thus not only requires but also *emphasizes* the POL practitioner's responsibility for patient interaction, clinical correlation, and even test interpretation, in collaboration with the primary care physician.

This important characteristic holds great promise for the POL as a practice setting. It also accounts for one crucial difference between the POL and its hospital or independent counterpart that the consultant must fully appreciate. Because primary care settings encourage the laboratory practitioner's direct involvement in patient care, the singular emphasis on purely technical and scientific procedure and quality assurance protocols that characterizes the regulated hospital and independent laboratory is not appropriate in the POL setting.

Clinical laboratory scientists in hospital and independent settings, on the other hand, typically practice in relative isolation from the patient, often removed from direct patient care involvement. Thus, hospital and independent laboratory professionals' skills generally reflect or emphasize an educational and regulatory focus on scientific and technical laboratory principles, and their practice settings may de-emphasize or even actively discourage patient interaction, clinical relevancy, and diagnostic test interpretation skills.

At present, given the lack of understanding of these fundamental differences, and given widespread deficiencies in basic training for anyone considering practice in the primary care setting, such differences can frustrate both collaborative and consultant interactions. Yet, if they are recognized and anticipated, these distinctions also point the way to a synthesis of skills through which the office laboratory practitioner, the professional clinical laboratory scientist, and the primary care physician could ultimately offer laboratory services of the highest quality available.

POL PERSONNEL

The larger the practice, the more likely that trained laboratory personnel are hired. One study of group practices averaging 18 physicians found that approximately five laboratory scientists were employed in each.[15] By contrast, about two-thirds of laboratory personnel in small office settings have received little or no formal training in clinical laboratory science.[8–11] Most often, they are licensed practical nurses, medical assistants, registered nurses or nurse practitioners, or lay persons whose laboratory techniques have been learned solely on the job (OJT).[16, 17]

Although medical assistants, nurse practitioners, and physician assistants may have received training that prepared them to perform some basic laboratory tasks, such training often does *not* address competency in quality assurance procedures, complex laboratory testing, or complex test interpretation. One study found that, while only 15% of nurses and 56% of on-the-job trainees performing tests in these settings employed quality control procedures, 78% of the certified laboratory scientists followed standard quality assurance practice.[8]

As noted above, POL practitioners have responsibilities outside the laboratory. These additional duties could result in constraints that a clinical laboratory scientist might not anticipate. For example, in a typical small office setting, the physician sees from 20 to 30 patients daily, and spends about eleven minutes with each. This caseload, in turn, imposes automatic patient interaction and administrative demands on POL practitioners, creating real limits on the amount of time they can devote to testing. One potential consequence is that time-sensitive test procedures may be interrupted to meet more urgent needs. Such contingencies must be accounted for if the professional consultant is to be of genuine service to the POL.

Moreover, the laboratory may simply be inadequate. Necessary equipment may be outdated or missing entirely; the laboratory may lack storage or counter space; pipettes, reagents, and specimens may share shelf space with office lunch bags. Whatever the case, it is important to recognize that many of the most troubling constraints facing the POL practitioner may have little to do with training deficiencies. Rather, they may arise from environmental, motivational, or practice priorities far beyond the POL practitioner's control. Sensitivity to these factors can greatly enhance the professional consultant's success in this setting.

THE INSTRUMENTS

Tests offered in the POL vary with the size and type of practice, as well as with available instrumentation and staff expertise, but tests actually offered in the POL setting do not always conform to professional recommendations for tests that are suited to its staff. Here, it is important to recognize that test selection is predominantly (if not exclusively) the province of the physician-owner, and the selection of tests may be based on any number of considerations. These include clinical relevance, habit and custom, local competition and supporting reference facilities, patient convenience, accessible instrumentation and laboratory lay-out, and considerations of pricing and profit.

Typically, however, the physician's chief source of guidance in test selection is the diagnostic equipment manufacturer's sales representative. In that case, the chief decision criterion may too often be the reported capabilities of the instrument being sold rather than the relevance, necessity, and feasibility of the procedure for a small practice laboratory.

Instrumentation, of course, is an important consideration. While a typical POL utilizes centrifuges, incubators, microscopes, glucose analyzers, and dry chemistry analyzers,[8] one study found that in 1984 40% of POLs possessed dedicated single chemistry analyzers, semi-automated hematology systems, and/or multi-chemistry semi-automated analyzers; 15% were computerized; and 5% utilized mainframe computers networked to the entire laboratory.[12] A second study predicted that annual expenditures for POL diagnostic equipment and reagents will exceed $1 billion by 1990, providing the small POL with capability for chemistry, hematology/coagulation, microbiology, immunoassay, urinalysis, and pregnancy testing.[18] Another study projected that 60% of chemistry products will be marketed to "decentralized" laboratories by 1990—up from 20% in 1984.[19] It should be noted that all of these predictions assume no change in the current federal regulatory climate for POLs, which may indeed change in the early 1990s to a more regulated market.

THE TESTS

Tests commonly performed in POLs include hemoglobin and hematocrit, rapid streptococcal slide tests, urine dipsticks and sediment examinations, glucose and other chemistries, vaginal wet preparations, and pregnancy tests.[8, 9, 12, 16] Table 79-1 illustrates tests recommended for performance by personnel according to training or competency levels.[20–22]

Clearly, there is no such thing as a master list of tests and practitioner competency levels that can provide foolproof guidance for POL test selection. First, no list can keep pace with today's rapid technological advances. Second, any test performed poorly can have serious consequences. Third, no practitioner, and no instrument, is error-proof.

NEEDS OF THE POL

POLs vary widely. The needs of large group practices differ from each other according to numerous

Table 79-1 ***Recommendations for Levels of Testing***

Personnel	Responsibilities	Testing Tasks
Nontechnical personnel	Use laboratory procedure manual as a performance guide. Follow quality assurance procedures. Maintain equipment. Observe safety precautions.	Urinalysis, hematocrit, occult blood, pregnancy test, streptococcal throat screen (rapid), preparing Gram stain, serology for mononucleosis and rheumatoid factor, any self-diagnostic test
Personnel with some formal training or demonstrated competence	As above, and—maintain and update procedure manual. Troubleshoot problems as indicated by quality assurance data, performance inconsistencies, equipment malfunction.	As above, and—white blood cell counts, modified differentials, platelet estimates, sedimentation rate, prothrombin time, simple chemistry (blood glucose, potassium, uric acid), throat, urine, and gonorrhea cultures, vaginal wet preparations, and reading Gram stains
Personnel with experience, training, and certification	As above, and—develop procedure manual. Have total responsibility for quality assurance, troubleshooting, problem-solving. Correlate test results with patient data, evaluate discrepancies, discuss with physician. Evaluate tests and equipment.	As above, and—advanced hematology, microbial culture, identification, biochemical panels. If the laboratory is large and complex, tasks may extend to coagulation, microbial sensitivity, enzyme assay, electrophoresis, and others.

factors, and large POLs as a class differ still more radically from small POLs. Moreover, practice settings and employment demands intensify differences in staff education and practice orientation. These differences may initially complicate successful interactions between the typical POL practitioner and the clinical laboratory scientist consultant who practices routinely in hospital and independent settings.

Geography also makes a difference. Reference, consultation, educational, and other external resources available to POLs in urban and suburban settings may be wholly or partly absent for POLs in isolated rural areas. Location alone may thus impose special, potentially serious constraints and considerations. Regulation that requires demonstrated competency and continuing education is lacking; therefore, the need for these two important aspects of laboratory quality is not reinforced, as it is in regulated settings. Also, the level of laboratory-specific education and training possessed by both the physician and the POL staff is very low, creating a special need for basic laboratory education.

As a class, however, all POLs present challenges and rewards unique to the direct patient care environment, and all should give adequate assurance of the quality, clinical relevancy, and cost-effectiveness of their services. These issues translate into goals and objectives for which the clinical laboratory scientist, in consultation or collaboration with the primary care physician, is ideally suited. The following discussion explores some of these special needs in greater detail.

Laboratory Direction

Although most primary care physicians have access to an office laboratory,[13] few have had the training necessary for competency in that role.[23]

For most physicians, residency training in laboratory science is usually limited to ordering tests and interpreting results.[23] Important competencies in such areas as staff and equipment selection, quality assurance procedures, and knowledge of testing complexities are all but ignored. Ironically, however, current standards for medical practice appear to hold the physician personally accountable for the adequacy of services rendered in the office laboratory.[13, 24–28] The obvious consequence currently is that, often, the paramount function of the office laboratory physician-owner is one for which he or she is ill-equipped.

Primary care physicians have several choices in order to resolve this dilemma. They can opt to acquire technical laboratory direction competencies themselves, in addition to their competencies in primary care and medical direction. Or, they can seek to provide for an appropriate level of technical direction through methods including contracting with local laboratories; retaining consultants; or hiring a full-time clinical laboratory scientist for the laboratory director function.

Although this is almost certain to change, at present the physician-owner might reject the last option almost reflexively. Focusing on short-term cost considerations, and largely unaware of the clinical, legal, and ethical requirement for professional competency in this arena, the primary care physician may overlook the fundamental advantages that a qualified clinical laboratory scientist can bring to the small office setting. The primary care physician often lacks first-hand experience of the pitfalls inherent in relying on new, complex technologies operated by staff unprepared for the myriad medical, legal, technical, and economic problems that can arise in a small POL. Thus, the primary care physician first considering a POL will have to be convinced of the cost-effectiveness of this option.

A quick review of the clinical laboratory scientist's professional training and education will help to make that case. The chart on page 981 correlates the typical needs of the small POL with the professional competencies of the clinical laboratory scientist. *It should immediately be apparent that it is easier, more cost-effective, and ultimately far more prudent to acquaint this professional with the multiple skills required for practice in the small office setting, than to attempt—unfairly—to burden individuals proficient in nursing, medical assisting, or office administration with the enormous responsibility entailed in operating a highly technical, increasingly complex office laboratory.*

Quality Assurance

Experience repeatedly has confirmed that it is extremely difficult for individuals untrained in clinical laboratory science to understand, much less implement, effective quality assurance. Yet quality assurance is the linch-pin on which the medical, legal, and clinical reliability of modern laboratory testing depends.[30]

Effective, reliable, and relevant quality assurance is, in fact, the most pressing need in the small POL. Moreover, as its share of the nation's test volume increases, pressures will mount from federal and private-sector purchasers and consumers alike for evidence that POL services meet national standards of care for laboratory practice. As hospitals increasingly rely on results of tests performed in settings beyond their direct control, it is also likely that effective quality assurance will become a fundamental consideration on which successful private practice/hospital interactions will depend.

In traditional laboratory settings, state and federal regulation both impose and enforce specific quality assurance requirements, including, generally, internal quality control procedures, external proficiency testing, periodic inspection, and personnel qualification standards. Over time, regulatory imperatives, supplemented by technological advances and increased professional sophistication, have meant that these hospital and independent laboratories have evolved a reputation for supporting high quality assurance standards.

With perhaps a few exceptions, small POLs are subject to none of these regulations, and even where standards do exist enforcement varies

The Needs of the Small Office Laboratory That Can be Addressed by the Clinical Laboratory Scientist[29]

Set-up and Purchasing

Evaluate laboratory facility.
- Space and design
- Logistics
- Equipment
- Staff

Monitor product availability.
- Instruments
- Reagents
- Specimen handling

Evaluate products.

Perform cost analyses.

Implement cost-effective purchasing.

Implement cost-effective leasing.

Evaluate/implement computer services.

Test Selection and Performance

Advise on in-house test menu

Determine referral menu.

Analyze test results.

Document test results.

Correlate results with clinical data.

Evaluate discrepancies.

Advise on test interpretation.

Quality Assurance

Develop/implement procedure manual.

Design/implement laboratory record system.

Calibrate, maintain, trouble-shoot, and repair instruments.

Validate systems.

Provide controls.

Investigate and resolve quality control problems.

Coordinate proficiency testing.

Advise on procedure/system changes.

Personnel Management

Evaluate and hire personnel.

Write job descriptions.

Supervise personnel.

Design and deliver in-service tutorials.

Regulation and Reimbursement

Advise on state/federal regulatory requirements.

Monitor and report on reimbursement policies.

Coordinate inspection/licensing compliance.

widely. In the effort to resolve this problem, there has been a protracted debate over the need for and nature of appropriate regulations for POLs, during which a dual standard has evolved.[31] Even as tests provided in POLs increase in number and complexity, small POLs in practices of fewer than six physicians are unregulated—regardless of their scope or volume.

This dual standard has had an important consequence. It has helped to inspire and fuel a growing skepticism, perhaps even a certain hostility, in POLs to traditional quality assurance practices. The problem has been exacerbated by standard training practices in small POLs, through which marginally-trained staff advise their peers and successors of technical quality assurance procedures, and impart their views on the need for and meaning of these practices. These factors, and others discussed earlier, may partially explain findings in comparative studies of regulated and unregulated laboratories, which indicate that test quality is problematic in POLs.[10, 32, 33]

It can be argued that historical and environmental forces have joined with technological, economic, regulatory, and other factors to encourage testing in decentralized settings. Simultaneously, these same forces have created a current situation in which quality assurance is both the POL's most pressing need *and* one of the greatest challenges facing the consulting or staff-based clinical laboratory scientist.

The professional literature has begun to document the quality assurance problems of the small POL:[31] out-of-date reagents; improper specimen collection, handling, documentation, and storage; instrument malfunction; and inadequate recordkeeping. Although such problems are by no means the sole province of the POL, historical factors, as well as limitations of space and practitioner education and time, can cause them to occur more frequently in the small office laboratory.

Significantly, there appears to be an emerging trend that POL practitioners, recognizing from experience the limitations of their skills for handling increased volumes and new types of testing, *want* relevant training and education.[9–12] Thus, whether as a consultant or on staff, the clinical laboratory scientist considering interacting with a small POL must be thoroughly equipped to devise, "sell," and implement basic quality assurance protocols and continuing education practices designed to keep pace with changing technologies and changing practice patterns, and yet be responsive to the needs of the POL environment described above.

Education and Information

Currently, the primary source of education and information on laboratory matters may be the manufacturer's sales representative. Industry, therefore, must responsibly ensure that optimal quality assurance safeguards are engineered into diagnostic laboratory equipment, and that its sales staff are communicating appropriate usage protocols and quality assurance instructions.

Other sources for education and training can include local hospital and reference laboratories. Even so, on balance, available resources are seldom geared to help the small POL practitioner solve the practical, patient-oriented technical problems that arise daily, or cope with the avalanche of equipment, instruments, kits, and reagents now being marketed to that setting. There is simply no substitute for adequately trained personnel.

Consequently, the typical small POL has three primary educational needs.[34] First, because few residency programs provide it, there is an immediate need for residency-level procedures designed to enable new physicians to assume responsibility for practices involving laboratory services.[23] At the very least, physicians must learn enough about contemporary laboratory management and practice to assess the importance of relying on qualified clinical laboratory scientists for POL direction. Residency programs, therefore, offer clinical laboratory science educators a prime opportunity to work collaboratively with physician faculty to develop model laboratory curricula addressing test selection, performance, and interpretation; fundamentals of quality assurance theory and practice; and laboratory management from a technical–medical–legal perspective.

A second pressing educational need is that of the staff who perform laboratory services in direct patient care settings. Because test results are often applied immediately for on-site diagnosis and treatment, a basic knowledge of the clinical context—the clinical conditions affecting reliable testing and interpretation—is at least as critical for that practitioner as knowledge of the fundamentals of test performance and quality assurance. Because physician, patient, patient support, and equipment manufacturer interactions are daily requirements for these individuals, skills and knowledge for competently managing these distinct relationships are also essential.

CONSULTING IN THE SMALL POL

A third vital need is for adequate training and education for clinical laboratory scientists who increasingly will be retained to meet the myriad challenges of the small office laboratory. An understanding of the needs of the POL that includes its distinguishing historical, environmental, and philosophical characteristics can yield both a framework for designing approaches to consultation and a starting point for consultant education curricula. Consulting to POLs and other decentralized settings is in an early developmental phase for clinical laboratory scientists. Whether it will prove to be a viable alternative career pathway will be determined by future developments in regulation, technology, and primary care physician education and training. Initially, however, consultants to small POLs will probably operate best from a base within a hospital or reference laboratory. In that model, credibility, visibility, and other marketing essentials will have been established for the consultant by the base laboratory. Moreover, education, trouble-shooting, and staff training can be offered in exchange for physician referrals. In larger POLs, however, consultants may find considerable opportunity for rewarding and profitable consulting services. Whether they function in the academic setting as instructors, or in the health care delivery setting as consultants, laboratory directors, or bench practitioners, clinical laboratory scientists must be aware of and sensitive to the unique requirements of the small POL setting, and implement adequate procedures for addressing them.

REFERENCES

1. Cooperative Agreements for Improving Performance and Utilization of Physician Office Laboratories Through Training: Availability of Funds for FY85. Federal Register 50(107):23518–23520, June 4, 1985
2. Ratafia M: The diagnosis revolution. Med Marketing Media 8:13–25, 1985
3. Ratafia M: Diagnostics in physicians' offices. Am Clin Prod Rev 11:12–22, 1985
4. Title VI, Section 1886(d), Prospective Payment or Inpatient Hospital Services, Social Security Amendments of 1983 (P.L. 98-369), enacted April 20, 1983
5. Title III, Division B, Deficit Reduction Act of 1984, The Medicare and Medicaid Budget Reconciliation Amendments of 1984 (P.L. 98-369), enacted July 18, 1984
6. Clinical Laboratories Improvement Act of 1967 (P.L. 90-174). 42 USC 263
7. Conditions for Coverage of Services of Independent Laboratories. 42 Code of Federal Regulations (CFR), Subchapter B, §405.1310 *et seq,* 1972
8. Gwyther RE, Kirkman-Liff BL: Laboratory testing in the offices of family physicians. Am J Med Technol 48:697–702, 1982
9. McKenzie SB, Kazen CM, Smith LA et al: Physician's office laboratorians: What do they do? How should they be educated? J Med Technol 2:577–597, 1985
10. Grayson RT: Effects of regulatory controls on the accuracy of clinical laboratory tests. J Med Technol 1:632–637, 1984
11. Stevens CR, LaVallee RB, Croneberger H et al: Training and educational needs in small office laboratories. J Med Technol 2:570–574, 1985
12. Center for Research in Ambulatory Health Care Administration: The present and future of in-house labs. J Med Group Management Assoc 32:24–32, 1985
13. Fischer P, Addison LA: The office laboratory director's guide. JAMA 254:2941–2945, 1985
14. Physicians' Office Laboratories Market. Report No. 303. Wethersfield, Connecticut, Theta Technology Corporation, 1983
15. Benezra N: Group practice labs: How and why they're growing. Med Lab Observer 15(12):33–38, 1983
16. Georgia Department of Human Resources: A Statewide Survey of Office Laboratory Practices Among Members of the American Medical Association of Georgia, p 3, 1982
17. Frost and Sullivan, Inc: Group practice laboratories benefiting from new federal regulations. News of International Research Reports for Business (Summer): 2, 1985
18. Duey M: Physician Office Testing: Market Trends and Implications. Robert S. First, Inc. presented at *A Blueprint for Economic Survival.* Washington G-2 Reports, Arlington, Virginia, September, 1985
19. DRGs could cut ranks of lab suppliers. Clin Chem News 11(9):13, 1985
20. Levine RZ, Wardlow SC: Cost justification for in-office laboratory testing. Diagn Dynamics 2:1–2, 4–5, 1984

21. Mass D: House adopts position papers. Am J Med Technol 46:810–812, 1980
22. Crowley JR, Tillman M: Performance audit in the selection and management of personnel in the physician office laboratory. Prim Care 13:617–632, 1986
23. Fischer P, Curtis P, Kirkmann-Liff BL: The office laboratory in family practice residency programs. J Fam Pract 13:407–410, 1981
24. Greene MA, Belsey RE: How to lessen the risk of liability. AACC SpotNews 1(1):18–19, 1985
25. Stewart TC: The staff with the right stuff. AACC SpotNews 1(2):14–15, 1985
26. Peterson RG: Malpractice liability of allied health professionals: Developments in an area of critical concern. J Allied Health 14(4):363–372, 1985
27. Morrison v. MacNamara 407 A 2d 555 (DC App 1979)
28. Halper AR, Foster HS: Laboratory Regulation Manual, Vols 1–111. Rockville, Maryland, Aspen Systems, 1976, as updated
29. Baer DM, Belsey R: Needed: Consultants to physicians' office labs. Med Lab Observer 17(9):45–48, 1985
30. Bakken CL: Quality performance in the physicians' office laboratory: The hiring, training, and continuing education of staff. Lab Med 17(6):346–349, 1986
31. American Society for Medical Technology: Quality Assurance in Physician Office Laboratories: The Setting, The Issues, and Federal, State, and Private Approaches, pp 29–63. A white paper with recommendations submitted by the Presidential Task Force on Physician Office Laboratories and adopted in February, 1986, by the Board of Directors, American Society for Medical Technology, 2021 L st NW, Washington, DC 20036
32. Kenney M: Laboratory Performance and Regulatory Requirements: An Empirical Assessment of the Quality Assurance Effects of Selected Regulatory Requirements on the Performance of Clinical Laboratories. Atlanta, Centers for Disease Control, 1985
33. Kenney M: Laboratory Quality and Director Qualifications: An Empirical Assessment of the Medicare Requirement That Directors of Independent Clinical Laboratories Possess Earned Doctorates: Unpublished doctoral dissertation, University of California, at Berkeley, 1984
34. Fischer P, Addison LA, Koneman EW et al: Education and the physician office laboratory. JAMA 255(11):1464–1467, 1986

Index

Page numbers in *italics* indicate illustrations; those followed by *t* indicate tables. All case studies are listed under the heading *Case study*; all algorithms are listed under the heading *Algorithm.*

ISBN 0-397-50860-3

90000

9 780397 508600